OXFORD MEDICAL PUBLICATIONS

Oxford Handbook of
# General Practice

**Published and forthcoming Oxford Handbooks**

# Oxford Handbook of
# General
# Practice

**Third Edition**

## Chantal Simon
General Practitioner and Executive Editor, InnovAiT

## Hazel Everitt
General Practitioner and Clinical Lecturer,
University of Southampton

## Françoise van Dorp
General Practitioner

## Guest author

**Knut Schroeder**
General Practitioner and Honorary Senior Clinical Lecturer,
University of Bristol

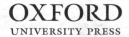

OXFORD
UNIVERSITY PRESS

# OXFORD
## UNIVERSITY PRESS

Great Clarendon Street, Oxford OX2 6DP

Oxford University Press is a department of the University of Oxford.
It furthers the University's objective of excellence in research, scholarship,
and education by publishing worldwide in

Oxford New York

Auckland Cape Town Dar es Salaam Hong Kong Karachi
Kuala Lumpur Madrid Melbourne Mexico City Nairobi
New Delhi Shanghai Taipei Toronto

With offices in

Argentina Austria Brazil Chile Czech Republic France Greece
Guatemala Hungary Italy Japan Poland Portugal Singapore
South Korea Switzerland Thailand Turkey Ukraine Vietnam

Oxford is a registered trade mark of Oxford University Press
in the UK and in certain other countries

Published in the United States
by Oxford University Press Inc., New York

First edition published 2002
Second edition published 2005
Third edition published 2010

British Library Cataloguing in Publication Data
Data available

Library of Congress Cataloging-in-Publication-Data
Data available

Typeset by Cepha Imaging Private Ltd., Bangalore, India
Printed in China
on acid-free paper by
C&C Offset Printing Co., Ltd.

ISBN 978-0-19-923610-7

10 9 8 7 6

# Contents

# Detailed contents

## 16  Neurology

# Preface

The new edition of the *Oxford Handbook of General Practice* seems to come round quicker each time, yet so much has changed in general practice in the past five years. For this edition, we welcome Françoise van Dorp as a guest editor. She has a special interest in child health within primary care.

When the second edition of the OHGP went to press, the new GP contract for British GPs was in its infancy. This contract has now become established and evolved in many ways. Furthermore, other contracting arrangements have been introduced and the idea of 'super-practices' run by private health providers is now a reality. This edition of the OHGP has been updated to include these developments. The general practice section (now edged purple) has been split so that information on different aspects of non-clinical general practice can be more easily accessed.

Since the last edition of the OHGP, medical training has changed considerably. In the UK, GPs in training now have to sit a new MRCGP examination to graduate as fully-fledged GPs. Foundation level doctors have also started placements in primary care. We now include specific reference to the requirements that both these groups face and their needs within general practice.

Within the clinical sections, as well as updating all the clinical information in line with current guidance, we have introduced several novel features. For example, the new 'Healthy living' chapter looks at preventative medicine within general practice. Throughout the book we also highlight instances where management of conditions that affect all age groups, differs for the elderly or for children.

The symptoms section of previous editions of the Oxford Handbook was liked by some and hated by others. In response to comments from our readers, we asked an excellent new guest author, Knut Schroeder, to rewrite this section. Now each clinical chapter has relevant symptoms and signs at the start of the chapter which should make them easier to find. For example, symptoms relevant to mental health are now at the start of the mental health chapter. We hope that you think that this is an improvement.

As always, we welcome any feedback from our readers. We would also like to thank the many of you who have contacted us to point out errors, omissions and ways to improve the OHGP in the past. It is thanks to you and the feedback that you provide that the OHGP continues to develop to meet your day-to-day needs.

CS

HE

# Acknowledgements

This book would not have come into being without the support of our editorial team at Oxford University Press. In particular we would like to thank our two commissioning editors—Liz Reeve and Beth Womack—who, due to their respective maternity leaves, have shared the difficult task of supporting and supervising us through the development of this edition of the OHGP.

We would also like to give special thanks to the following (in no particular order) who have all contributed either directly or indirectly to this edition of the OHGP: Gill Jenkins, Judith Harvey, Gavin Clunie, Malcolm Maclean, Meme Wijesinghe, Will Bolland, Richard Davies, Sue Connolly, Jeanette Lynch, Simon Crawford, Rick Linforth, Helen Dignum, Nick Dunn, Jonny Hobman, Ian Williamson, Anneke Lucassen, Peter Farndon, Richard Newsum, Karen O'Reilly, Robin Proctor, John Buckmaster, David Hargreaves, Jonathan Rhodes, Ben Riley, Carrie Saddler, Jo White, Helen Dunkelman, Max Watson, Anna Wilson, Lucy Yardley, Renos Ritarides, Tony Kendrick, Lasanthe Wijesinghe, Cathryn Bateman, Ruvaiz Haniffa, Rachel Hazeldene, Karen Brackley, Alexandra Pickering, Sarah Darden, Farid Bhatti, Jonathan Barratt, Audrey Fenton, Caroline McLoughlin, Danielle Peet, and Ann Drake.

If there are any omissions from this list, we apologize—please tell us and we will add your name to the list at the first opportunity.

As working GPs, much of the information that goes into this book is gleaned during the course of our everyday practice. Therefore, we would like to thank the doctors, staff, and perhaps most importantly the patients of The Banks and Bearwood Medical Centres in Bournemouth, Totton Health Centre in Hampshire and Whiteparish Surgery in Wiltshire.

Lastly we would like to thank the many unnamed reviewers asked for feedback by OUP for their criticisms and helpful hints—many of which were very constructive. You will see some of your ideas incorporated into this edition.

# Abbreviations and symbols

## Evidence-based superscripts

| | |
|---|---|
| N | NICE guideline |
| G | guideline from a major guideline producing body |
| C | Cochrane review |
| CE | Clinical evidence |
| S | systematic review or meta-analysis published in a major peer-reviewed journal |
| R | randomized controlled trial published in a major peer-reviewed journal |

## Referral times

| | |
|---|---|
| E | emergency admission |
| U | urgent referral |
| S | soon referral |
| R | routine referral |

## Handbook symbols

| | |
|---|---|
| ❶ | note |
| ⚠ | warning |
| 📖 | cross reference |
| 🖫 | web link |
| ☎ | telephone number |
| ♀ | female |
| ♂ | male |
| ●※ | controversy |
| 1° | primary |
| 2° | secondary |
| ↑ | increased/increasing |
| ↓ | decreased/decreasing |
| → | leading to/resulting in |
| ~ | approximately |
| ≈ | approximately equal to |
| ± | with or without |

## Standard abbreviations

| | |
|---|---|
| AA | Attendance Allowance |
| AAA | abdominal aortic aneurysm |
| A&E | accident and emergency |
| ABI, ABPI | ankle–brachial pressure index |

| AC | acromioclavicular |
| ACTH | adrenocorticotrophic hormone |
| ADH | antidiuretic hormone |
| ADHD | attention deficit–hyperactivity disorder |
| ADL | activities of daily living |
| AED | automated external defibrillator |
| AF | atrial fibrillation |
| AFP/αFP | alpha fetoprotein |
| AIDS | acquired immune deficiency syndrome |
| AKI | acute kidney injury |
| Alk phos | alkaline phosphatase |
| ALL | acute lymphoblastic leukaemia |
| ALO | Actinomyces-like organism |
| ALT | alanine aminotransferase |
| AMD | age-related macular degeneration |
| AML | acute myeloid leukaemia |
| ANA | antinuclear antibody |
| ANF | antinuclear factor |
| APH | ante-partum haemorrhage |
| APMS | Alternative Provider Medical Services |
| ARB | angiotensin-receptor blocker |
| ARF | acute renal failure |
| AS | ankylosing spondylitis |
| ASD | atrial septal defect |
| ASO | antistreptolysin o |
| AST | aspartate aminotransferase |
| AV | arterio-venous |
| AXR | abdominal X-ray |
| BCC | basal cell carcinoma |
| bd | twice daily |
| BJGP | *British Journal of General Practice* |
| BM | basal metabolism |
| BMA | British Medical Association |
| BMD | bone mineral density |
| BMI | body mass index |
| BMJ | *British Medical Journal* |
| BNF | *British National Formulary* |
| BP | blood pressure |
| BPH | benign prostate hypertrophy |
| bpm | beats per minute |
| | bilateral salpingo-oophorectomy |

| | |
|---|---|
| bv | bacterial vaginosis |
| Ca, $Ca^{2+}$ | calcium |
| CABG | coronary artery bypass graft |
| CAM | complementary or alternative medicine |
| CAPD | continuous ambulatory peritoneal dialysis |
| CBT | cognitive behavioural therapy |
| CCF | congestive cardiac failure |
| CD | controlled drug |
| CDH | congenital dislocation of the hip |
| CF | cystic fibrosis |
| CHD | coronary heart disease |
| CIN | cervical intra-epithelial neoplasia |
| CK | creatine kinase |
| CKD | chronic kidney disease |
| CLL | chronic lymphocytic leukaemia |
| CMV | cytomegalovirus |
| CNS | central nervous system |
| COC | combined oral contraceptive |
| COPD | chronic obstructive airways disease |
| COX2 | cyclo-oxygenase-2 |
| CPAP | continuous positive airways pressure |
| CPD | continuing personal development |
| CPR | cardiopulmonary resuscitation |
| Cr | creatinine |
| CRF | chronic renal failure |
| CRP | C-reactive protein |
| CSM | Committee on Safety of Medicines |
| CSSD | central sterile supplies department |
| CT | computed tomography |
| CTS | carpal tunnel syndrome |
| CVA | cerebrovascular accident |
| CVD | cardiovascular disease |
| CVS | cardiovascular system |
| CXR | chest X-ray |
| d | days |
| D&C | dilatation and curettage |
| DDH | developmental dysplasia of the hip |
| DES | directed enhanced services |
| DEXA | dual-energy X-ray absorptiometry |
| DH | Department of Health |

| DHEA | dehydroepiandrosterone |
|---|---|
| DI | diabetes insipidus |
| DIP | distal interphalangeal |
| DLA | Disability Living Allowance |
| DM | diabetes mellitus |
| DN | district nurse |
| DRE | digital rectal examination |
| DUB | dysfunctional uterine bleeding |
| DVLA | Driving and Vehicle Licensing Authority |
| DVT | deep vein thrombosis |
| EBM | evidence-based medicine |
| EBV | Epstein–Barr virus |
| ECG | electrocardiogram |
| Echo | echocardiogram |
| ECV | external cephalic version |
| EDD | estimated date of delivery |
| EEG | electroencephalogram |
| eGFR | estimated glomerular filtration rate |
| ENT | ear, nose and throat |
| EOC | epithelial ovarian cancer |
| EPAU | early pregnancy assessment unit |
| ERCP | endoscopic retrograde cholangiopancreatography |
| ERPC | evacuation of retained products of conception |
| ESR | erythrocyte sedimentation rate |
| ESRD | end-stage renal disease |
| FBC | full blood count |
| $FEV_1$ | forced expiratory volume in 1sec |
| FH | family history |
| FMH | feto-maternal haemorrhage |
| FOB | faecal occult blood |
| FSH | follicle stimulating hormone |
| FVC | forced vital capacity |
| g | gram |
| GA | general anaesthetic |
| GCA | giant cell arteritis, temporal arteritis |
| GGT/γGT | gamma glutamyl transferase |
| GI | gastrointestinal |
| GMC | General Medical Council |
| GMS | General Medical Services |
| | glomerulonephritis |

| GnRH | gonadotrophin-releasing hormone |
| GORD | gastro-oesophageal reflux disease |
| GP | general practitioner |
| GPC | General Practitioner Committee |
| GPwSI | GP with special interest |
| GTN | glyceryl trinitrate |
| GTT | glucose tolerance test |
| GU | genito-urinary |
| GUM | genito-urinary medicine |
| h | hour |
| Hb | haemoglobin |
| HbF | fetal haemoglobin |
| HBsAg | hepatitis B surface antigen |
| hCG | human chorionic gonadotrophin |
| HDL | high density lipoprotein |
| HIV | human immunodeficiency virus |
| HOCM | hypertrophic obstructive cardiomyopathy |
| HPV | human papillomavirus |
| HRT | hormone replacement therapy |
| HSV | herpes simplex virus |
| HV | health visitor |
| HVS | high vaginal swab |
| IBS | irritable bowel syndrome |
| ICAS | Independent Complaints Advocacy Service |
| ICP | intracranial pressure |
| IDDM | insulin-dependent diabetes mellitus |
| Ig | immunoglobulins |
| IHD | ischaemic heart disease |
| IM | intramuscular |
| INR | international normalized ratio |
| IOP | intraocular pressure |
| IPSS | International Prostate Symptom Score |
| iu | international unit |
| IUCD | intrauterine contraceptive device |
| IUGR | intrauterine growth retardation |
| IUS | intrauterine system |
| IV | intravenous |
| IVP | intravenous pyelogram |
| IVU | intravenous urography |
| JME | juvenile myoclonic epilepsy |

| | |
|---|---|
| JVP | jugular venous pressure |
| K⁺ | potassium |
| kg | kilograms |
| KUB | X-ray of kidneys, ureters, and bladder |
| L | litre |
| LA | local anaesthetic |
| LBBB | left bundle branch block |
| LDL | low density lipoprotein |
| LE | lupus erythematosus |
| LFT | liver function test |
| LH | luteinizing hormone |
| LIF | left iliac fossa |
| LMC | Local Medical Committee |
| LMN | lower motor neuron |
| LMP | last menstrual period |
| LMWH | low molecular weight heparin |
| LN | lymph node |
| LOC | loss of consciousness |
| LQTS | long QT syndrome |
| LRTI | lower respiratory tract infection |
| LSCS | lower-segment Caesarian section |
| LTOT | long-term oxygen therapy |
| LUQ | left upper quadrant |
| LVF | left ventricular failure |
| LVH | left ventricular hypertrophy |
| m | metre |
| M,C&S | microscopy, culture, and sensitivity |
| mane | in the morning |
| MAOI | monoamine oxidase inhibitor |
| MCP | metacarpophalangeal |
| MCUG | micturating cysto-urethrogram |
| MCV | mean cell volume |
| MDI | metred dose inhaler |
| Mg²⁺ | magnesium |
| mg | milligram |
| MI | myocardial infarct |
| min | minute |
| mL | millilitre |
| mmHg | millimetres of mercury |
| MMR | measles, mumps, and rubella |

| MND | motor neuron disease |
|---|---|
| mo | month |
| MRI | magnetic resonance imaging |
| MS | multiple sclerosis |
| MSU | midstream urine |
| MTP | metatarso-phalangeal |
| Na$^+$ | sodium |
| NAI | non-accidental injury |
| NASGP | National Association of Sessional GPs |
| NF | neurofibromatosis |
| NG | nasogastric |
| NHL | non-Hodgkin's lymphoma |
| NHS | National Health Service |
| NICE | National Institute of Health and Clinical Excellence |
| NNT | number needed to treat |
| nocte | at night |
| NRT | nicotine replacement therapy |
| NSAID | non-steroidal anti-inflammatory drug |
| NSF | National Service Framework |
| NT | nuchal translucency |
| NUD | non-ulcer dyspepsia |
| OA | osteoarthritis |
| od | once daily |
| OGD | oesophagogastroduodenoscopy |
| OM | otitis media |
| OOH | out of hours |
| OR | odds ratio |
| OT | occupational therapy |
| PALS | Patient Advice and Liaison Service |
| PAN | polyarteritis nodosa |
| PCO | primary care organization |
| PCOS | polycystic ovary syndrome |
| PCT | primary care trust |
| PCTMS | Primary Care Led Medical Services |
| PD | Parkinson's disease |
| PDA | patent ductus arteriosus |
| PDP | personal development plan |
| PE | pulmonary embolus |
| PEFR | peak expiratory flow rate |
| PEG | percutaneous endoscopic gastrostomy |

| PET | pre-eclamptic toxaemia |
| PH | pulmonary hypertension |
| PHCT | primary health care team |
| PHQ | Patient Health Questionnaire |
| PID | pelvic inflammatory disease |
| PIH | pregnancy-induced hypertension |
| PIP | proximal interphalangeal |
| PKU | phenylketonurea |
| PMB | post-menopausal bleeding |
| PMDD | premenstrual dysphoric disorder |
| PMH | past medical history |
| PML | progressive multifocal leucoencephalopathy |
| PMR | polymyalgia rheumatica |
| PMS | Personal Medical Services, premenstrual syndrome |
| PMT | premenstrual tension |
| PN | practice nurse |
| po | oral |
| POP | progesterone only pill |
| PPH | postpartum haemorrhage |
| PPI | proton pump inhibitor |
| PPP | primary proliferative polycythaemia |
| PR | per rectum |
| prn | as needed |
| PROM | premature rupture of membranes |
| PSA | prostate-specific antigen |
| PTH | parathyroid hormone |
| PTSD | post-traumatic stress disorder |
| PU | peptic ulcer |
| PUVA | psoralen–ultraviolet A |
| PV | per vagina |
| PVD | peripheral vascular disease, pulmonary vascular disease |
| qds | four times daily |
| QOF | Quality and Outcomes Framework |
| RA | rheumatoid arthritis |
| RAST | radio-allergosorbent test |
| RBBB | right bundle branch block |
| RCGP | Royal College of General Practitioners |
| RCT | randomized controlled trial |
| RhD | rhesus factor |
| RhF | rheumatoid factor |

| RIF | right iliac fossa |
|---|---|
| RR | relative risk, respiratory rate |
| RSI | repetitive strain injury |
| RSV | respiratory syncytial virus |
| RTA | road traffic accident |
| RTOG | Radiotherapy and Oncology Group |
| RUQ | right upper quadrant |
| RVT | renal vein thrombosis |
| s | second |
| SAH | subarachnoid haemorrhage |
| SBE | sub-acute bacterial endocarditis |
| sc | subcutaneous |
| SCC | squamous cell carcinoma |
| SD | standard deviation |
| SHBG | sex hormone binding globulin |
| SIADH | syndrome of inappropriate ADH |
| s/ling | sublingual |
| SLE | systemic lupus erythematosus |
| SLR | straight leg raise |
| SOL | space-occupying lesion |
| SSRI | selective serotonin-reuptake inhibitor |
| stat | immediately |
| STD | sexually transmitted disease |
| STI | sexually transmitted infection |
| SVT | supraventricular tachycardia |
| $T_3$ | tri-iodothyronine |
| $T_4$ | thyroxine |
| TAH | total abdominal hysterectomy |
| TB | tuberculosis |
| $^{99m}Tc$ | technetium-99m |
| TCC | transitional cell carcinoma |
| TCPR | total protein:creatinine ratio |
| tds | three times daily |
| TENS | transcutaneous electrical nerve stimulation |
| TFT | thyroid function test |
| TGs | triglycerides |
| TIA | transient ischaemic attack |
| TLC | tender loving care |
| TMJ | temporomandibular joint |
| TOF | trans-oesophageal fistula |

| TOP | termination of pregnancy |
| TPCR | total protein creatinine ratio |
| TPHA | *Treponema pallidum* haemagglutination antibody |
| TRUS | trans-rectal ultrasound |
| TSH | thyroid-stimulating hormone |
| TURP | transurethral resection of prostate |
| TV | *Trichomonas vaginalis* |
| u | unit |
| U&E | urea and electrolytes |
| UC | ulcerative colitis |
| UMN | upper motor neuron |
| URTI | upper respiratory tract infection |
| USS | ultrasound scan |
| UTI | urinary tract infection |
| VDRL | Venereal Disease Research Laboratory |
| VF | ventricular fibrillation |
| VIP | vasointestinal peptide |
| VSD | ventriculoseptal defect |
| VT | ventricular tachycardia |
| VUR | vesico-ureteric reflux |
| VZ | varicella zoster |
| VZ-Ig | zoster immunoglobulin |
| WCC | white cell count |
| wk | weeks |
| y | year |

❶ *All other abbreviations are defined in the text on the page in which they appear.*

**Elderly care and child health flags:** conditions peculiar to children or elderly people, or in which management varies for these groups, are flagged as follows:

Child health

Elderly care

## Chapter 1

# What is general practice?

# What is general practice?

In the early 19th century, when apothecaries, physicians, and surgeons provided medical care, the term 'general practitioner' became applied to apothecaries taking the Membership Examination of the Royal College of Surgeons of England.

Over the past 50y general practice has established itself as the cornerstone of most national healthcare systems. In so doing, general practitioners (GPs or family physicians) have shown that the intellectual framework within which they operate is different from, complementary to, but no less demanding than that of specialists.

GPs diagnose illness, treat minor illness within the community, promote better health, prevent disease, certify disease, monitor chronic disease, and refer patients requiring specialist services. General practice is the primary point of access to healthcare services.

Although 80% of patients have seen their GP within the past year, only 13% are referred for hospital care. Everything else is dealt with in the primary care general practice setting. In order to do this GPs must:
- Have a working knowledge of the whole breadth of medicine.
- Maintain ongoing relationships with their patients—they are the only doctors to remain with their patients through sickness and health.
- Focus on patients' response to illness rather than the illness itself taking into account personality, family patterns, and the effect of these on the presentation of symptoms.
- Be interested in the ecology of health and illness within communities and in the cultural determinants of health beliefs.
- Be able to draw on a far wider range of resources than are taught in medical school, including intuition, knowledge of medicine, communication skills, business skills, and humanity.

**Is general practice a specialty?** In English, 'generalist' and 'specialist' are opposites. GPs do not have in-depth knowledge about a specific biomedical topic unique to general practice. However, general practice is an academic discipline with its own curriculum, research base, and peer-reviewed journals. Therefore, is it a specialty?

In many countries GPs have needed to claim specialist status to achieve recognition for their level of training and to be deemed a separate discipline. In the UK this recognition has been accomplished by showing that the expertise of the generalist is complementary to that of the specialist. To achieve the same standing and status as their hospital-based colleagues, GPs must claim to be specialists—but specialists in general and holistic care of their patients.

**Defining general practice** The aim of a definition of general practice is to state the core content and function of the discipline. The breadth and comprehensiveness of general practice makes that difficult—so why define it? *Potential reasons include*:
- To allow doctors performing broadly similar roles to communicate and work together across healthcare systems and national boundaries
- To set clinical and administrative boundaries if needed, and
- To provide a framework for teaching, training, and research.

The definition should be universal and independent of country-specific systems, settings or working methods but there is no ideal definition as yet.

## Commonly used definitions

**Leeuwenhorst 1974** 'The GP is a licensed medical graduate who gives personal, primary and continuing care to individuals, families and a practice population irrespective of age, sex and illness. It is the synthesis of those functions which is unique.'

**McWhinney 1997** 9 principles of family medicine. *Family physicians:*
1 Are committed to the person rather than to a particular body of knowledge, group of diseases, or special technique.
2 Seek to understand the context of the illness.
3 See every contact with their patient as an opportunity for prevention or health education.
4 View the patients in their practice as a population at risk.
5 See themselves as part of a community-wide network of supportive and healthcare agencies.
6 Should ideally share the same habitat as their patients.
7 See patients in their homes.
8 Attach importance to the subjective aspects of medicine.
9 Manage resources.

**Olesen 2000** 'The GP is a specialist trained to work in the front line of a healthcare system and to take the initial steps to provide care for any health problem(s) that patients may have. The GP takes care of individuals in a society, irrespective of the patient's type of disease or other personal and social characteristics, and organizes the resources available in the healthcare system to the best advantage of the patients. The GP engages with autonomous individuals across the fields of prevention, diagnosis, cure, care, and palliation, using and integrating the sciences of biomedicine, medical psychology, and medical sociology.'

## Further information
**Heath I et al.** (2000) *BMJ* **320**: 326–7
**Olesen F et al.** (2000) *BMJ* **320**: 354–7
**McWhinney IR** *A textbook of family medicine* (1997) Oxford University Press ISBN: 019511518

# General practice in the UK

Today, along with opticians, dentists, and pharmacists, GPs form the 'front line' of the NHS providing primary medical care and acting as 'gatekeepers' to the secondary care system.

**Workload** ~97% of the British population are registered with a GP. Patients register with a practice of their choice in their area—whole families are often registered with the same practice. Once registered, patients stay with that practice for an average 12y GPs carry out ~300 million consultations/y—80% at the surgery and 10% at the patient's home. 70% of the GP's total workload is spent with a patient, while >20% is currently spent on administration.

**Working hours** Standard working hours are 8 a.m.–6.30 p.m. on normal working weekdays for GMS and most PMS practices. In addition, practices may provide 'extended hours' as a DES (📖 p.21). To qualify, the practice must provide 30 min of additional opening time per 1000 registered patients at times agreed with the PCO according to local need. Some practices also provide OOH care (📖 p.20). How workload is distributed between individual doctors and other PHCT staff is a matter for each practice to decide.

**Independent contractor status** 2 in every 3 GPs work as independent contractors providing core primary healthcare services and additional services as negotiated within their contract. As such, these GPs are self-employed, running small businesses or practices. They have management responsibilities for staff, premises, and equipment. Since most GPs receive a profit share, the amount that each GP is paid depends not only on income to the practice, but also on expenditure:

## Income
- *Private work* Includes private appointments (e.g. clinical assistant, industrial appointments), insurance examinations/reports, private medical examinations, and certificates (e.g. HGV licence applications).
- *Income from the NHS* GMS, PMS, or APMS contract work.

## Expenditure
- *Running costs of the practice* Staff salaries, cost of the premises (rent, rates, repairs, maintenance, and insurance), service costs (heating, water, electricity, gas and telephone bills, stationery, and postage), training costs, etc.
- *Capital expenses* Purchase of new medical and office equipment.

**Primary care contracts** The provider contract with the local PCO defines services primary care providers will provide, standards to achieve, and payment they will receive. Currently there are 4 contract types:
- General Medical Services (GMS) (📖 p.20)
- Personal Medical Services (PMS) (📖 p.28)
- Alternative Provider Medical Services (APMS) (📖 p.29)
- Primary Care Led Medical Services (PCTMS) (📖 p.29).

**Primary care provider** Term used to designate any organization providing NHS primary care services.

**Partnership** Group of self-employed contractors working together for mutual benefit. A partnership can become a primary care provider as long as ≥1 partner is a GP. Although traditionally partnerships are made up of GPs only, practice managers, nurses, allied health professionals, and pharmacists can be included within partnerships.

**Polyclinics** Also referred to as 'Darzi centres' are a new concept in the UK. Initially only intended for London, the concept has now extended throughout the UK. They may be owned and run by the NHS, large GP practices, private companies, or Foundation Trusts. Key features:
• Large premises housing up to 25 GPs and serving a population of up to 50 000 patients.
• GP services alongside other health services, e.g. dentists, pharmacists.
• Extended services—consultant out-patient appointments, physiotherapy, routine diagnostic services, e.g. ECG, X-ray.
• Extended opening—urgent care 18–24h/d and routine GP appointments in the evenings and at weekends.

**Primary care performer list** List of all doctors deemed competent to provide primary medical care.

**Salaried GP** A GP employed by a PCO, practice, or alternative provider of medical services. PCOs and GMS practices are bound by a nationally agreed model contract, with a salary within a range set by the Review Body. PMS practices can make their own arrangements.

Salaried posts have advantages for those who do not want to commit themselves to long-term working within 1 practice or to become involved with managerial tasks. Pay tends to be less than that of independent contractors.

**GP with special interest (GPwSI)** 📖 p.70

**GP retainer** Provides an opportunity for doctors with other commitments to maintain medical skills before returning to full- or part-time employment at a later date (usually within 5y). Practices approved for the retainer scheme must provide adequate education, supervision, and support. Members of the scheme must:
• Have 'right to practice' and maintain their GMC registration.
• Work ≥ 12 but ≤ 208 paid service sessions a year (1 session = 3.5h). Most work 2–4 sessions/wk.
• Undertake ≥ 28h of educational sessions/y and take a professional journal.

**Freelance GP or locum** Works for practices or PCOs by a regular or intermittent arrangement or by providing medical cover on a one-off basis. Tends to be self-employed and charge on a sessional basis. Long-term locums should make their own pension provision or apply to join the NHS scheme.

**GP registrar** 📖 p.64

# Good medical practice for GPs

*All patients are entitled to good standards of practice and care from their doctors.*

GMC: Good Medical Practice for GPs

## GMC duties of a doctor*

- Make the care of your patient your first concern.
- Treat every patient politely and considerately.
- Respect patients' dignity and privacy.
- Listen to patients and respect their views.
- Give patients information in a way they can understand.
- Respect the right of patients to be fully involved in decisions about their care.
- Keep your professional knowledge and skills up to date.
- Recognize the limits of your professional competence.
- Be honest and trustworthy.
- Respect and protect confidential information.
- Make sure your personal beliefs do not prejudice your patient's care.
- Act quickly to protect patients from risk if you have good reason to believe you or a colleague may not be fit to practise.
- Avoid abusing your position as a doctor.

In all these matters you must never discriminate unfairly against your patients or colleagues and you must always be prepared to justify your actions to them.

## Good medical practice for GPs**

- *Good clinical care* Provide the best possible clinical care for patients.
- *Maintaining good medical practice* Monitor, review, and continuously strive to improve the performance of yourself and your practice.
- *Relationships with patients* Communicate with and listen to the views and opinions of your patients; use terms/information they can understand; respect their privacy and dignity at all times.
- *Working with colleagues* Ensure effective communication channels within and outside the practice; ensure environment for personal and professional development for everyone working within the practice.
- *Teaching and training, appraising and assessing* (📖 p.60)
- *Probity* Behave in a proper fashion ensuring honesty and openness in all matters. Avoid conflicts between personal and professional roles. Research (📖 p.82).
- *Health and performance of other doctors* (📖 p.68).

---

\* Reproduced with permission of the General Medical Council. Based on information from *Good Medical Practice for General Practitioners*.
\*\* Summarized from *Good medical practice for GPs* 🖥 www.rcgp.org.uk

**Continuity of care** A patient seeing the same healthcare worker over time. In the UK this has been the norm but continuity of care is becoming less available.

*Reasons for continuity of care* A practitioner's sense of responsibility toward his/her patients ↑ with duration of relationship and number of contacts. Continuity builds trust, creates a context for healing, and ↑ practitioner's and patient's knowledge of each other.

*Evidence* ↑ patient and doctor satisfaction, ↑ compliance, ↑ uptake of preventive care, and better use of resources (time spent in the consultation, discriminatory use of laboratory tests, and admission to hospitals).

Patients' desire for personal care depends on the reason for the encounter. Most find it important to see their own GP for serious medical conditions and emotional problems.

*Reasons why continuity of care is becoming less available* Problems balancing accessibility, flexibility, and continuity of care:
• *Doctor factors* Flexible careers, special interests, and managerial responsibilities all limit the availability of GPs to their patients.
• *Patient factors* 24-h society in which patients want to be seen at their convenience rather than when their GP is available makes it impossible to maintain continuous care. For minor problems and emergencies patients do not mind who they see, as long as they see someone who can deal with their problem quickly.
• *System factors* Changing roles—nurse practitioners and other healthcare professionals commonly take on tasks which used to be done by GPs; clinical governance structures mean that patients with particular conditions are managed in clinics specifically for those conditions within the practice; other primary healthcare providers, e.g. NHS Direct, walk-in clinics, and separate OOH cover arrangements, further fragment care.

**Rationing** A full discussion of rationing healthcare is beyond the scope of this handbook, but with continued innovation, rising demand, and limited resources it will become an increasingly important factor in medicine worldwide. To some extent there is already rationing by default—medicines and certain treatments are not provided on the NHS or have very long waiting lists. Government bodies such as NICE are trying to evaluate services and develop guidelines for healthcare professionals about medicines and services which are both clinically and cost effective. Inevitably this will mean that some groups will feel that they are being deprived of the treatment they require. It will remain a contentious issue.

**Further information**
Appraisal and revalidation (📖 p.68)
**GMC/RCGP** *Good medical practice for GPs* 🖥 www.rcgp.org.uk
**GMC** *Duties of a doctor* 🖥 www.gmc-uk.org
**Hjortdahl P** (2001) *BJGP* **51**: 699–700

# Stress in general practice

Increasing stress is a feature of society as a whole. GPs score 2× the national average on stress test scores. Similar figures are seen if anxiety scores are used and 1 in 4 GPs is classed as suffering from depression if depression screening tools are used. Burnout describes the syndrome of emotional exhaustion, depersonalization, low productivity, and feelings of low achievement. A study of British GPs found that significant numbers in all age groups are affected.

**Causes of stress in general practice** Insecurity about work (particularly complaints), isolation, poor relationships with other doctors, disillusion with the role of GPs, changing demands, work–home interface, demands of the job—particularly time pressure, problem patients, and emergencies during surgery hours—patients' expectations, and practice administration.

**Roots of stress** Many of the main stressors for GPs appear to be created or perpetuated by doctors' own policies: overbooking patients, starting surgeries late, accepting commitments too soon after surgeries are due to finish, making insufficient allowances for extra emergency patients, and allowing inappropriate telephone or other interruptions. Higher than average pressure scores occur in doctors with fast consultation rates than in those with slower rates.

**General characteristics of a stressed person at work are** lack of concentration, poor timekeeping, poor productivity, difficulty in comprehending new procedures, lack of cooperation, irritability, aggressiveness, withdrawal behaviour, resentment, ↑ tendency to make mistakes, and resistance to change.

**Effects of stress** are poorly documented.
- *Effects on clinical work* One study showed that frustrated doctors are more willing to take undesirable short cuts in treating patients; another showed that those doctors with negative feelings of tension, lack of time and frustration have poor clinical performance (measured by prescription rate and lack of explanation to patients).
- *Effects on practice* Stress also has effects on the practice, resulting in mistakes, arguments or angry outbursts, poor relationships with patients and staff, increased staff sickness and turnover, and accidents.
- *Effects at home:* Stressed GPs may develop problems in their relationships with their partners and family at home, becoming uncommunicative at home or work, and more withdrawn and isolated.

Experience of stress does not necessarily result in damage. Extent of stress necessary to ↓ performance or satisfaction levels will depend on the doctor's personality, biographical factors and coping methods but a concurrent illness or co-existing life event may have additive effects, and can ↑ vulnerability to stress or ↓ ability to cope.

**Alcohol** Doctors commonly use alcohol as a coping method for stress. The BMA estimates that 7% of doctors are addicted to alcohol and/or other chemical substances, with half of those addicted to alcohol alone.

### Interventions and solutions

- *Improve your working conditions,* e.g. longer booking intervals for patient consultations; develop a specialist clinical or academic interest within or outside the practice; learn to decline extra commitments. GPs with high stress levels do not necessarily have low morale, but there is a close correlation between levels of job satisfaction and morale—job satisfaction seems to protect against stress.
- *Look at your own behaviour and attitudes* Stop being a perfectionist; resist the desire to control everything; don't judge your mistakes too harshly.
- *Look after your own health and fitness* Set aside time for rest and relaxation; make time for regular meals and exercise.
- *Allow time for yourself and your family* Do not allow work to invade family time. Consider changes in working arrangements to allow more time for leisure and family.
- *Don't be too proud to ask for help* As well as formal channels for seeking help, there are several informal doctor self-help organizations and counselling services (📖 see 'Useful contacts').

**Chronic stress** 📖 p.996

### Useful contacts

**BMA Stress Counselling Service** Service provided by the BMA to members and their families. 24-h confidential telephone counselling service for all personal, emotional, and work- or study-related problems. Also runs the 'Doctors-for-Doctors' service; ☎ 0845 9 200 169.

**British Doctors and Dentists Group** Support group of recovering medical and dental drug and alcohol users. Students are also welcomed. Gives confidential help and advice through a local recovering doctor or dentist. National contact (via the Medical Council on Alcohol): ☎ 0777 164 22682.

**Sick Doctors Trust** A confidential intervention and advisory service for alcohol- and drug-addicted doctors, run by doctors for doctors. 24 Hour Helpline: ☎ 0870 444 5163 🖥 www.sick-doctors-trust.co.uk

# General practice within the wider NHS

In 1948 the National Health Service (NHS) was formed giving free health-care for the entire population of the UK paid for by the taxpayer. The NHS is now the largest organization in Europe. Structure of the NHS varies from country to country within the UK.

**England** (Figure 1.1)
- *Secretary of State for Health* Head of the NHS. Accountable to Parliament.
- *Department of Health (DH)* Sets overall health policy in England, is headquarters for the NHS, and is responsible for developing and putting policy into practice. It also sets targets and monitors performance.
- *Strategic Health Authorities (StHA)* Key link between DH and NHS. Responsible for developing strategies for local health services, ensuring high-quality performance, and ensuring national priorities are integrated into local plans.
- *Special Health Authorities* Provide health services to the whole population of England and not just to a local community, e.g. National Blood Authority, NICE.
- *NHS Trusts* Provide hospital and specialist community services. Services are commissioned by PCTs.
- *Primary Care Trusts (PCTs)* Cornerstone of the NHS—responsible for planning, providing, and commissioning health services from service providers, and improving the health of the local population. In addition, PCTs are responsible for integrating health and social care. They control 75% of the NHS budget.

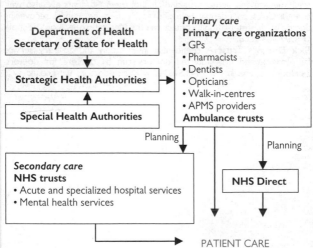

**Fig. 1.1** Structure of the NHS in England

**Northern Ireland** The *Department of Health, Social Services and Public Safety* (DHSSPS) is responsible for:
- *Health and Personal Social Services* An integrated service which includes policy and legislation for hospitals, family practitioner services, community health, and personal social services.
- *Public Health* Covers responsibility for policy and legislation to promote and protect the health and well-being of the population of Northern Ireland.
- *Public Safety* Encompasses responsibility for the policy and legislation for the Fire Authority, food safety, and emergency planning.

Four Health and Social Service Boards cover the whole of Northern Ireland (Eastern, Northern, Southern, and Western). They are agents of the DHSSPS in planning, commissioning, and purchasing services, including primary care services, for the residents in their areas.

*Further information* 🖳 www.n-i.nhs.uk

### Scotland

- *Scottish Government Health Directorate* Responsible for both NHS Scotland and the development and implementation of health and community care policy.
- *NHS Boards* Health services are delivered through 14 regional NHS Boards. These Boards provide strategic leadership and performance management for the entire local NHS system in their areas and ensure that services are delivered effectively and efficiently. NHS Boards are responsible for the provision and management of the whole range of health services in an area, including hospitals and general practice.
- *Special Boards* Scotland has 8 Special Boards delivering services across the whole of Scotland, e.g. Scottish Ambulance Service; NHS24.

*Further information* 🖳 www.show.scot.nhs.uk

**Wales** The NHS is Wales's largest employer (7% workforce).
- *Welsh Assembly Government* Responsible for policy direction and for allocating funds to the NHS in Wales.
- *Local Health Boards (LHBs)* 22 boards together receive ~¾ of the Welsh NHS Budget. Each board covers a local authority area, and LHBs and local authorities have a statutory duty to work together to produce strategies for improving health and social care for the people living in their area. LHBs are also responsible for commissioning GP services from practices, and community and secondary care services from NHS Trusts.
- *NHS Trusts* 13 Trusts manage hospitals and community health services across Wales; 1 Trust manages an all-Wales ambulance service.
- *The Health Commission Wales (Specialized services)* provides specialist services operating across the whole of Wales (e.g. blood transfusion).
- *The National Public Health Service* provides advice and guidance to Local Health Boards on a range of issues, e.g. disease protection and control, child protection.

*Further information* 🖳 www.wales.nhs.uk

# Organizations important to general practice

**British Medical Association (BMA)** Voluntary professional association and independent trade union of doctors. >80% of practising UK doctors are members. Also runs a publishing house producing books and journals (including the BMJ), negotiates doctors' pay and terms of service, provides advice about matters related to work practice, and provides educational and research facilities, accommodation, dining facilities, and financial services. The General Practitioners Committee (GPC) is a sub-group of the BMA.

*Further information* ☎ 020 7387 4499 🖳 www.bma.org.uk

**Care Quality Commission (CQC)** The CQC is an independent public body. Its functions are to:
- Assess management, provision, and quality of health and social care in England.
- Review the performance of each NHS trust and award an annual performance rating.
- Regulate the independent healthcare sector through registration, annual inspection, monitoring complaints, and enforcement.
- Publish information about the state of health and social care.
- Consider complaints about NHS organizations that the organizations themselves have not resolved.
- Coordinate reviews and assessments of health and social care.
- Carry out investigations of serious failures in the provision of health and social care.

*Further information* 🖳 www.cqc.org.uk

**General Medical Council (GMC)** Licenses doctors to practice medicine in the UK. The Council investigates complaints against doctors, and has the authority to revoke a doctor's licence if appropriate. It also monitors standards of undergraduate, postgraduate, and continuing medical education and provides information about good medical practice.

*Further information* 🖳 www.gmc-uk.org

**General Practitioners Committee (GPC)** BMA committee with authority to deal with all matters affecting NHS GPs, representing all doctors in general practice whether or not they are members of the BMA. The committee is recognized as the sole negotiating body for general practice by the DH.

*Further information* 🖳 www.bma.org.uk

**Independent Complaints Advocacy Service (ICAS)** Supports patients and their carers wishing to pursue a complaint about their NHS treatment or care.

**Local Medical Committee (LMC)** Committee of GPs representative of GPs in their area. All GPs (including locums and salaried doctors) are represented by LMCs. Functions:
- *Statutory* Consultation regarding administration of the GMS and PMS contracts, involvement with disciplinary and professional conduct committees, representation of GPs as a whole.
- *Non-statutory* Advice on all matters concerning GPs, communication between GPs; links with other bodies; helping individual GPs.

**National Association of Sessional GPs (NASGP)** Acts as a voice and resource for all NHS GPs who work independently of the traditional 'GP principal' model. This includes GP locums, retainers, salaried GPs, and GP assistants.

*Further information* 🖳 www.nasgp.org.uk

**National Institute for Health and Clinical Excellence (NICE)** Special Health Authority which aims to provide the NHS (patients, health professionals, and the public) in England and Wales with authoritative guidance on 'best practice' and thus improve the quality and consistency of health services across the country. It evaluates health technologies and reviews management of specific conditions.

*Further information* 🖳 www.nice.org.uk

**NHS Business Services Authority (NHSBSA)** 💷 p.143

**Patient Advice and Liaison Service (PALS)** Provided by all trusts running hospitals, GP services, or community health services. Aims to:
- Advise and support patients, their families and carers.
- Provide information on NHS services.
- Listen to and record concerns, suggestions, or queries. PALS can liaise directly with NHS staff and managers regarding patients' concerns.
- Help sort out problems quickly.
- Direct NHS users to sources of independent advice and support, e.g. ICAS.

**Royal College of General Practitioners (RCGP)** Founded to 'encourage, foster and maintain high standards within general practice and to act as the voice of GPs on issues concerned with education, training, research and standards'. Services include: library and educational publications (including *British Journal of General Practice and InnovAiT*); representation on committees, and research support. *Statutory responsibilities*: setting the GP training curriculum, setting and managing the UK licensing examination for general practice, and managing certification and re-certification. 3 grades of membership:
- *Members* are entitled to speak and vote at meetings, and to use the designation MRCGP (💷 p.66).
- *Fellows*: Highest grade of membership (💷 p.66).
- *Associates*: Doctors still in training. Associates can participate in RCGP activities but cannot vote or use the designation MRCGP.

*Further information* 🖳 www.rcgp.org.uk

# Practice in other countries

It is beyond the scope of this book to discuss different systems of health-care and practice regulations outside the UK. However, in most countries there is a registration body (usually termed the 'Medical Council') which ensures that doctors are qualified and fit to practice, an organization representing the interests of the medical profession generally (often termed the 'Medical Association'), and separate specialist bodies representing the interests of family practitioners. Details can be obtained from the following websites.

**International Directory of Medical Regulatory Authorities** lists worldwide medical regulatory bodies and contact details.

🖳 www.iamra.com

**World Organization of Family Doctors (WONCA)** includes a list of member organizations and contact details.

🖳 www.globalfamilydoctor.com

**Medical Association of South East Asian Nations (MASEAN)** contains contact details for medical associations in Brunei, Cambodia, Indonesia, Laos, Malaysia, Myanmar (Burma), Philippines, Singapore, Thailand, and Vietnam.

🖳 www.masean.org

## Country-specific information

### Australia
- Australian Medical Council 🖳 www.amc.org.au
- Australian Medical Association 🖳 www.ama.com.au
- Royal Australian College of General Practitioners 🖳 www.racgp.org.au

### Canada
- Medical Council of Canada 🖳 www.mcc.ca
- Canadian Medical Association 🖳 www.cma.ca
- College of Family Physicians of Canada 🖳 www.cfpc.ca

### Hong Kong
- Medical Council of Hong Kong 🖳 www.mchk.org.hk
- Hong Kong Medical Association 🖳 www.hkma.org
- Hong Kong College of Family Physicians 🖳 www.hkcfp.org.hk

### India
- Medical Council of India 🖳 www.mciindia.org
- Indian Medical Association (and IMA College of GPs)
  🖳 www.ma-india.org

### Ireland (Eire)
- Irish Medical Council ▣ www.medicalcouncil.ie
- Irish Medical Organization ▣ www.imo.ie
- Irish College of General Practitioners ▣ www.icgp.ie

### New Zealand
- Medical Council of New Zealand ▣ www.mcnz.org.nz
- New Zealand Medical Association ▣ www.nzma.org.nz
- Royal New Zealand College of General Practitioners
  ▣ www.rnzcgp.org.nz

### Pakistan
- Pakistan Medical and Dental Council ▣ www.pmdc.org.pk
- Pakistan Medical Association ▣ www.pma.org.pk

### Singapore
- Singapore Medical Council ▣ www.smc.gov.sg
- Singapore Medical Association ▣ www.sma.org.sg
- College of Family Physicians Singapore ▣ www.cfps.org.sg

### South Africa
- Health Professions Council of South Africa ▣ www.hpcsa.co.za
- South African Medical Association ▣ www.samedical.org
- South African College of Family Physicians ▣ www.collegemedsa.ac.za

### USA
- Educational Commission for Foreign Medical Graduates (ECFMG)
  ▣ www.ecfmg.org
- American Medical Association (AMA) ▣ www.ama-assn.org
- Federation of State Medical Boards ▣ www.fsmb.org
- American Board of Family Practice ▣ www.abfp.org
- American Academy of Family Physicians ▣ www.aafp.org

# Chapter 2

# Contracts

# Partnership agreements

Partnership disputes are common. A properly drafted partnership agreement may prevent disputes and, if they do occur, may lessen their impact.

**Partnership at will** A partnership without an up-to-date written agreement is a 'partnership at will', governed by the 1890 Partnership Act. A 'partnership at will' is a very unstable situation as:

- All partners are deemed to have equal profit shares unless there is clear evidence to the contrary.
- Decisions are made by simple majority.
- Notice may be served by any partner on the others without their prior knowledge or consent.
- Dissolution of the partnership may take immediate effect and no reason need be given to justify it.
- Dissolution may result in the forced sale of all partnership assets (including the surgery premises) and redundancy of all staff.
- There is nothing to prevent any partner, or group of partners, from immediately forming a new practice/partnership to the exclusion of the other partner(s) once the practice is dissolved.

**Partnership agreements** should be drawn up every time a new partner joins a practice. Employed doctors and retainers also require contracts of employment. An agreement checklist is shown in Box 2.1. Detailed guidance is produced by the BMA and further guidance can be obtained from local BMA offices and LMCs.

**Partnership disputes** However good a partnership agreement, disputes still occur. Advice on partnership and employment matters is available from the BMA and LMC, and the BMA also provides conciliation services (contact local office). Legal battles are expensive and the BMA will not fund partnership disputes. Try to resolve matters amicably.

**Discrimination** It is unlawful for any partnership to discriminate on grounds of age, gender, marital status, colour, race, nationality (including citizenship), or ethnic or national origins when appointing a new partner or in the way they treat an existing partner. The BMA will consider backing GPs to take such matters to industrial tribunals—contact the local office. Applications should be made on forms available via local Job Centres and must be made within 3mo of the last act of discrimination.

**Contracts of employment for salaried GPs** Model terms and conditions of service for a salaried GP and a model offer letter of employment are available from the BMA or DH websites. Nationally agreed salary scales apply and are compulsory for GMS but not PMS practices.

*Responsibilities towards employed GPs* 📖 p.36

## Box 2.1 Partnership agreement checklist

- *Business detail* Purpose of the business; premises and basis of occupation. If premises are owned by the partners, state procedure for valuation, payment of the retiring partner, and investment of the incoming partner.
- *Assets* Specify assets, their ownership, arrangements for valuation and interest payments. It is illegal to sell goodwill in NHS practices.
- *Income and allowances* Definition of practice income; allowable expenses.
- *Profit sharing* Distribution of practice NHS income and other NHS allowances; distribution of income from non-NHS work.
- *Accounting* Accounting and banking arrangements; cheque signing; access to accounts and bank statements.
- *Taxation* Arrangements for paying tax; obligations of each partner.
- *Pension arrangements*.
- *Retirement/suspension/expulsion* Reasons for suspension or expulsion; process of suspension/expulsion; mechanisms of voluntary leaving / retirement; division of assets in the event of retirement. May include a restrictive covenant preventing the outgoing doctor working in the practice area for a period of time after leaving—seek legal advice.
- *Leave* Holiday entitlement; basis of deciding who has holiday when; study leave; sabbatical leave; sick leave; maternity, paternity and adoption leave; compassionate leave.
- *Obligation* NHS obligations; non-NHS work within the practice; other work outside the practice; educational activities; obligations to each other; hours of work.
- *Decisions and disputes* Decision-making process; process to manage disputes; process to dissolve partnership. Ensure that it includes who pays legal fees for whom in the event of a dispute.
- *Correct procedure* Ensure that each partner has signed and dated the agreement and that their signature has been witnessed. It is recommended that each partner should take independent legal advice and not rely on the 'practice solicitor' for sole advice.

### Further information

**DH** 🖳 www.dh.gov.uk
**BMA** 🖳 www.bma.org.uk
**Equality and Human Rights Commission** ☎ 0845 604 6610 (England); 0845 604 8810 (Wales); 0845 604 5510 (Scotland)
🖳 www.equalityhumanrights.com

# The General Medical Services Contract

Although there may be some differences in process in each of the four countries of the UK, the principles of the General Medical Services (GMS) Contract apply to all.

**The Contract** The GMS Contract is a contract made between an individual practice and a PCO. All the partners of the practice, at least one of whom must be a GP, have to sign the contract. It includes:
- National terms applicable to all practices (the 'Practice Contract').
- A description of which services will be provided by that practice, i.e.
  - Essential services
  - Additional services if not opted out
  - Out-of-hours cover if not opted out
  - Enhanced services, if opted in.
- A level of quality of essential and additional services that the practice 'aspires to'.
- Support arrangements, e.g. for IT and premises.
- A summary of the total financial resources.

**Essential services** Services that all practices *must* undertake. These services include:
- *Day-to-day medical care of the practice population* Health promotion, management of minor and self-limiting illness, and referral to secondary care services and other agencies as appropriate.
- *The general management of patients who are terminally ill*, and
- *Chronic disease management*.

**Additional services** Services that the practice will *usually* undertake but may 'opt out' of. If the practice opts out, the PCO takes responsibility for providing the service instead. The practice then receives a ↓ global sum payment. The services included are:
- *Cervical screening*—opting out results in a 1.1% ↓ in global sum.
- *Contraceptive services*—opting out results in a 2.4% ↓ in global sum.
- *Vaccinations and immunizations*—opting out of vaccinations and immunizations results in a 2% ↓ in global sum; opting out of childhood immunizations leads to a 1% ↓ in global sum.
- *Child health surveillance* (excluding the neonatal check)—opting out leads to a 0.7% ↓ in global sum.
- *Maternity services excluding intrapartum care* (which is an enhanced service)—opting out results in a 2.1% ↓ in global sum.
- *Certain minor surgery procedures* Curettage, cautery, cryocautery of warts/verrucae, and other skin lesions—opting out results in a 0.6% ↓ in global sum.

**Out of hours (OOH) care** Practices can 'opt out' of providing an OOH service. The decision must be made for the whole practice—individual doctors within a practice cannot 'opt out' alone. The cost of opting out for a practice is 7% of the global sum. Practices that have opted out of OOH can offer surgeries or consultations within the OOH period as an extended opening hours directed enhanced service by agreement with their local PCO.

**Enhanced services** Enhanced services are commissioned by the PCO and paid for in addition to the global sum payment. There are 3 types:

- *Directed enhanced services (DES)* Services under national direction with national specifications and benchmark pricing that all PCOs *must* commission to cover their population. These services change from year to year and include payment targets for childhood immunizations, influenza vaccinations, and more complex minor surgery, e.g. joint injections, incisions/excisions.
- *National enhanced services (NES)* These services have national minimum standards and benchmark pricing but are not directed (i.e. PCOs do *not* have to provide these services). Examples include: anticoagulation monitoring, treatment of drug/alcohol abuse, and minor injury services.
- *Local enhanced services (LES)* Services developed locally to meet local needs, e.g. special services for refugees

**Further details** Other parts of the GMS contract covered in greater detail in this book include:

- Carr-Hill formula 📖 p.24
- Dispensing 📖 p.23
- GP pay 📖 p.22
- Minimum practice income guarantee 📖 p.23
- IT 📖 p.40
- Premises 📖 p.38
- Quality framework 📖 p.26
- Seniority 📖 p.23.

**Further information**

**DH** The GMS contract. 🖥 www.dh.gov.uk
**BMA** The GMS contract and supporting documents 🖥 www.bma.org.uk
**NHS Employers** 🖥 www.nhsemployers.org

# GP pay under the GMS Contract

A total sum for GMS services is given to each primary care trust (PCO) as part of a bigger unified budget allocation. PCOs are responsible for managing the GMS budget locally.

## Payment to practices comprises the following components:

- The Global Sum +
- Quality payments +
- Enhanced services payments +
- Payment for premises +
- IT payments +
- Dispensing payments (if applicable).

**The Global Sum** Major part of the money paid to practices. It is paid monthly and intended to cover practice running costs. It includes provision for delivery of essential services and additional/OOH services (if not opted out); staff costs; career development; and locum reimbursement (e.g. for appraisal, career development, and protected time).

**Quality payments** Payment for quality is made in two ways:
- *Aspiration payments* Advance payments to allow practices to develop services to achieve higher-quality standards. Practices agree their aspirations for quality points the following year with their PCO. Aspiration payments are made monthly alongside Global Sum payments and amount to roughly 70% of the points achieved the previous year (for 2009/10 this was equivalent to 2008/9 points achieved × £124.60/ point × 70% × adjustment for list size and composition).
- *Achievement payments* Payments made for the practice's actual achieved number of points in the Quality and Outcomes Framework (📖 p.26) as measured at the start of the following year. Aspiration payments that have already been received are deducted from the total (i.e. actual payment = achievement payment – aspiration pay already received).

**Payment for extra 'enhanced' services** Paid to practices that provide directed enhanced services, national enhanced services, and/or local enhanced services.

**Payment for premises and information technology** GP premises are funded in many different ways. The GP contract has provision to reimburse practices that rent their premises the cost of the rent, or to pay practices that own their premises for the use of those premises. The PCO also reimburses all the IT costs of the practice.

**Carr-Hill allocation formula** GMS resource allocation formula for allocating funds for the Global Sum and quality payments. The formula takes the practice population and then makes a series of adjustments based on the profile of the local community, taking account of determinants of relative practice workload and costs. The resulting 'allocation factor' is then applied to the Global Sum, and quality payments made to the practice (📖 p.24).

**Minimum practice income guarantee (MPIG)** Protects those practices that lost out under the redistribution effect of the change from the old GP contract to the new GP contract in 2004. It is calculated from the difference between the Global Sum allocation (GSA) under the new GMS contract and the Global Sum equivalent (GSE)—the amount the practice would have earned providing the same service under the old GMS contract. If GSA < GSE a correction factor (CF) will be applied as long as necessary so that GSA + CF = GSE.

**Seniority payments** Payment system based on years of NHS service. Superannuable income is used as a measure of that service. Salaried GPs will have seniority reflected in their salary scales.

**Dispensing GPs** Any GP in an area classified as rural may apply to dispense to any of his/her patients living >1 mile from the local pharmacist, as long as this would not render the pharmacist's business unviable. A series of fees are paid for providing this service in a similar way to that in which community pharmacists are funded and in addition to the GMS Global Sum.

# The Carr-Hill allocation formula

Geographical and social factors result in differing workload for GPs (see Table 2.2). The Carr-Hill formula allocates payment to practices on the basis of the practice population, weighted for factors that influence relative needs and costs in order to reflect the differences in workload that these factors generate.

**Age–sex adjustments** Older people and children <5y require the most GP care. The Carr-Hill formula uses an age–sex curve to adjust payments to practices based on the age and gender of their registered populations (Table 2.1).

**Table 2.1** Age–sex workload index (males aged 5–14 = 1)

| Age | 0–4 | 5–14 | 15–44 | 45–64 | 65–74 | 75–84 | 85+ |
|---|---|---|---|---|---|---|---|
| Male | 3.97 | 1 | 1.02 | 2.15 | 4.19 | 5.18 | 6.27 |
| Female | 3.64 | 1.04 | 2.19 | 3.36 | 4.9 | 6.56 | 6.72 |

❶ A different age–sex curve is used for Scotland.

**Nursing and residential homes** Patients in nursing and residential homes generate more workload through ↑ travelling time. The workload factor applied is 1.43.

**List turnover** Areas with high list turnovers often have higher workload, as patients tend to have more consultations in their first year of registration in a practice. A factor of 1.46 is applied to all new registrations.

**Additional needs** In the UK (apart from Scotland) Standardized Limited Long-Standing Illness (SLLI) and the Standardized Mortality Ratio for those <65y (SMR<65) are best at explaining variations in workload over and above age and sex. They are related to workload by a complex formula used to make the payment adjustment.

**Scotland** SMR <65 together with unemployment rate, elderly people (>65y) on income support, and households with ≥2 indicators of deprivation are used in the adjustment formula.

**Staff market forces factor (MFF)** Reflects geographical variation in staff costs incurred by practices.

**Rurality** Rural practices have ↑ practice costs. Adjustment is made to payments based on a complex formula using average distance patients live from the practice and population density. An additional adjustment is made for a few small practices in Scotland to allow for economies of scale (small practices incur disproportionately high costs as many expenses, particularly relating to premises, must be met regardless of practice size).

**Table 2.2** Comparison of inner city and rural practice

|  | Inner city practice | Rural practice |
|---|---|---|
| **Deprivation** | Above average unemployment; workers on low pay; ↑ single parents; ↑ sick and disabled | 1:4 rural households live in poverty; deprivation is more covert |
| **Access to care** | Highly mobile populations → fragmented care<br>Non-English speakers (e.g. refugees) have limited access to care<br>Cultural issues can restrict care | Public transport is often poor Costs of private transport are increasing making it impossible for some patients to attend the surgery or hospital. Home visiting rates are ↑ and visiting is arranged by geography rather than urgency |
| **Patterns of illness** | Social class gradients are found for many different causes of morbidity and mortality | Certain conditions are rarely seen in the town, e.g. poisoning with organophosphate insecticides |
| **Workload** | Social deprivation ↑ ↑ consultation rates, ↓ consultation times, multiple problems and heavy workload ↑ Land costs, elderly buildings and ↑ crime rates → poor premises and ↓ patient, GP, and staff morale | GPs in rural areas take longer to do home visits etc. and may need to travel further to attend meetings or educational events |
| **Recruitment** | Potential recruits are dissuaded from applying due to heavy workload, environment and high property costs | Difficulty recruiting due to ↑ working hours, ↓ income, lack of OOH cover (still the case in some rural Scottish practices), and difficulties covering time off for educational activities |

## Further information

**DH** The GMS contract—Annex D 🖥 www.dh.gov.uk

# The Quality and Outcomes Framework

The Quality and Outcomes Framework (QOF) was developed for the GMS contract, but there are similar arrangements for those working with other contracts. Financial incentives encourage high-quality care.

**The domains** The QOF is divided into 4 domains:

- Clinical
- Organizational
- Additional services
- Patient experience.

See Table 2.3

**Indicators** Every domain has a set of 'indicators' relating to quality standards that can be achieved within that domain. The indicators are developed by expert groups based on best available evidence and are updated regularly. All data should be available from practice clinical systems. Indicators are split into 3 different types:

- *Structure*, e.g. is a disease register in place?
- *Process*, e.g. is a particular measure being recorded? Is action being taken where appropriate?
- *Outcome*, e.g. how well is the condition being controlled?

**Quality points** All achievement against quality indicators converts to points. Each point has a monetary value.

- *Yes/no indicators* Points are awarded only if the result is +ve
- *Range of attainment* For most clinical indicators it is not possible to attain 100% results, so a range of satisfactory attainment is specified. Minimum standard is usually 40%. Points are allocated in linear fashion by comparison of attainment against the maximum standard, e.g. if the maximum is 90%, the minimum 40%, and the practice achieves 65%, the practice receives 25/50 (i.e. ½) of the available points
- *Minimum standard* All points are awarded if the criterion is met in more than a certain % of cases.

**Exception reporting** Prevents practices being penalized when unable to meet targets due to factors beyond their control, e.g. patients fail to attend for review, or medication is contraindicated. It applies to indicators where level of achievement is determined by % of patients reaching the designated level. Practices report number of exceptions for each indicator set and individual indicator. Ensure the reason why a patient has been 'excepted' from the QOF is identifiable in the clinical record.

**Reporting on quality** Annually each practice completes a standard return form recording achievement in the past year. Most practices use the Quality and Outcomes Framework Management and Analysis System (QMAS) to do this. There is also an annual quality review visit by the PCO. Based on achievement, the PCO confirms level of achievement funding attained and discusses points the practice will 'aspire' to in the following year. The process is confirmed in writing and signed off by both parties. PCO-wide quality is checked against other PCOs countrywide.

**QMAS** Software developed for the GMS contract in England to allow practices to continually assess their achievement under the contract and contribute to the calculation of national disease prevalence. Similar software is available for use in Scotland, Wales, and Northern Ireland.

**Table 2.3** Calculation of points for quality framework payments (2009/10)

| Components of total points score | Points | Way in which points are calculated |
|---|---|---|
| Clinical indicators | 697 | Achieving preset standards in management of:<br>• Asthma • Hypertension<br>• Atrial fibrillation • Hypothyroidism<br>• Cancer • Learning disability<br>• Chronic kidney disease • Mental health<br>• COPD • Obesity<br>• Coronary heart disease • Stroke and TIA<br>• Dementia • Palliative care<br>• Depression • Primary prevention of CVD<br>• DM<br>• Epilepsy • Smoking<br>• Heart failure |
| Organizational | 167.5 | Achieving preset standards in:<br>• Records and information about patients<br>• Information for patients<br>• Education and training<br>• Medicines management<br>• Practice management |
| Additional services | 44 | Achieving preset standards in:<br>• Cervical screening<br>• Child health surveillance<br>• Maternity services<br>• Sexual health contraception |
| Patient experience | 91.5 | Achieving preset standards in:<br>• Patient survey*<br>• Consultation length |
| Total possible | **1000** | |

In 2008/9 the average value of 1 point = £124.60

**Further information**
**DH** The GMS contract ⊟ www.dh.gov.uk
**BMA** The Quality and Outcomes Framework and supporting documents ⊟ www.bma.org.uk
**NHS Employers** ⊟ www.nhsemployers.org
**QMAS** ⊟ www.qmas.nhs.uk

* Improving Patient Questionnaire (IPQ – charge payable) – ⊟ www.cfep.co.uk or General Practice Assessment Questionnaire (GPAQ) – ⊟ www.gpaq.info

# Other provider contracts

**The Personal Medical Services (PMS) contract** The option to become or stay a PMS practice remains an alternative contracting arrangement in the UK. At present ~ 40% of GP practices in England work under PMS contracts. *Features*:

- The GMS contract is a nationally agreed, locally managed contract. The PMS contract is a locally agreed, locally managed contract.
- The PMS contract alters the way the primary care provider, not individual doctors, are paid.
- As decision-making is closer to the patient, theoretically PMS contracts give better flexibility to meet local needs and solve problems.
- Practices are paid to provide a package of services but PMS contracts do not necessarily contain all the elements of the GMS contract, and may contain others in addition by local negotiation. How the practice provides those services is up to the practice.
- As for GMS practices, payments to PMS practices are adjusted for practice factors that ↑ workload using the Carr-Hill formula.
- Practices can opt out of additional and OOH services.

**Budget** Most PMS budgets consist of:
- **Practice costs** Staffing, equipment, IT and premises costs.
- **Core services** Services patients would expect to receive from any GP. This is equivalent to the GMS contract 'essential' services.
- **Additional services** Both those usually expected from a GP (maternity, minor surgery, contraception) and those usually provided by other community/secondary care services, e.g. community nursing, or community-based specialist services (endoscopy, ultrasound, etc.). Extra services not usually provided by the GP are known as 'PMS plus'. These services are roughly equivalent to both the additional and enhanced services under the GMS contract.
- **Prescribing budget** (optional).
- **Dispensing budget** (for dispensing practices only).

**Quality payments** PMS practices can apply for aspiration and achievement payments in the same way as GMS practices. In order to reflect the local nature of the contract, quality standards do not have to be the same as those contained in the QOF. Nevertheless, all standards must be rigorous, evidence based, monitored fairly, assessed against criteria agreed between PCOs/provider, and paid at appropriate rates.

**Specialist PMS** Provide medical services to meet the needs of special groups. Patients do not need to be registered for all 'core' primary care services. This enables practices to develop innovative bespoke models of service delivery tailored to specific needs of groups poorly served in the established primary care system. Some examples are:

- Primary care services for vulnerable groups, e.g. homeless, refugees.
- Specialist services, e.g. out-patient elderly care, home-based palliative care, dermatology, ultrasound, community rehabilitation for stroke.
- Specific service provision, e.g. services for violent patients, OOH care, teenage contraceptive services, sexual health clinics.

**Alternative Provider Medical Services (APMS)** PCOs may commission APMS to provide:
• Essential services
• Additional services (including where GMS/PMS practices opt out)
• Enhanced services
• OOH services.

APMS contracts for the provision of primary medical services can be made with anyone, for example:
• Existing GMS/PMS practices—through a separate contract
• Groups of other healthcare professionals e.g. community nurses
• Individuals
• Private companies—including those from overseas
• Secondary care trusts
• Voluntary sector organizations.

APMS may be used where specific needs arise e.g. through practice vacancies, or in areas with rapidly expanding populations where extra capacity is needed.

**Primary Care Led Medical Services (PCTMS)** Under PCTMS, primary medical services are delivered directly by employees of the PCO.

**Further information**
DH ⌨ www.dh.gov.uk

# Practice based commissioning

PCOs have been responsible for deciding which health services the local population needs and ensuring the provision of these services. They do this by providing some services themselves, and commissioning others from other service providers.

**Scope of PBC** Practice based commissioning (PBC) is a voluntary scheme by which practices, rather than PCOs, either alone or in combination with other practices in commissioning groups, can use allocated funds to directly commission care and services for their patients. It is open to all practices. PCOs currently give practices financial incentives to engage in PBC.

There is no centrally directed 'menu' for PBC. Practices/PCOs are free to determine the range of services which fall within the indicative budget and which practices can commission on behalf for their patients.

**Aims of PBC** The aims of PBC are to:
• Design improved patient pathways
• Enable more efficient use of funds so that savings can be used to provide better patient services
• Enable improved community and hospital services that better meet the needs of patients.

**PBC plan** Each year a PBC plan is agreed between the practice and PCO including:
• Practice name and lead clinician
• Scope of the indicative budget
• Work to be done by each party and timescale of proposed actions
• Use of savings accrued the previous year
• Arbitration procedures.

**Indicative budget** Each practice is set an 'indicative budget'. This is a notional sum based on their patients':
• Secondary or hospital-based care costs, including laboratory costs
• Prescribing costs
• Community care costs
• Mental health care costs.

The actual funds are held by the PCO and not the practice, but the practice can decide how to use those funds to best meet the needs of their practice population.

**The commissioning cycle** (Figure 2.1)
• *Planning* An assessment is made of the needs of the practice population and resources available. Information is provided by the PCO to enable practices to do this. Where identified needs do not have matching resources, the practice should identify, attract or develop the necessary resource or capacity to meet that need.
• *Contracting* Once resource and need are matched, practices direct the PCO to commission services for their patients. Contracts should cover quality standards, access targets, volumes, prices, and other issues identified.

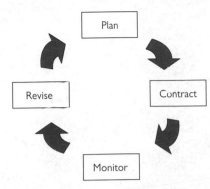

**Fig. 2.1** The commissioning cycle

- *Monitoring* Once a contract is made, it is important to monitor delivery, and ensure that it is kept on track. Funding passes from the PCO to the provider under the terms of the contract.
- *Revision* If delivery is not on track or the needs of the practice change with time, agreements should be reviewed and revised.

**Use of freed resources** 70% of profits from PBC can be used to improve or develop new services. Problems include:
- Variations in profits from year to year—this makes provision of long-term services funded through profits problematic.
- Losses—commissioning may result in losses as well as profits. Practices are expected to balance overspends with savings in <3y.

**PBC commissioning groups** Although some practices are large enough to hold their own budgets and are commissioning as single practices, smaller practices have formed groups to allow them sufficient economies of scale to be effective commissioners and also to share resources and risks with other practices.

**PBC provider companies** Recently, groups of GPs have started forming provider companies to enable them to set up new services themselves, or provide services traditionally provided by other providers through the PBC mechanism. Forming a business enables the GPs involved to pool financial resources, premises, and skills to produce sound business plans with which they can compete against other service providers. However, there are potential conflicts of interest when GPs are acting as both commissioners and providers of the same services.

### Further information
**DH** Practice based commissioning ☐ www.dh.gov.uk
**BMA** Practice based commissioning ☐ www.bma.org.uk

# Chapter 3

# Practice management

# GPs as managers

*If you have time to do something wrong; you have time to do it right.*

W. Edwards Deming

GP partners in a practice have dual roles as both clinicians and managers of small businesses. As such they must cooperate with their partners and practice manager to run the business side of the practice and with primary healthcare team members to cover all aspects of the clinical work.

**Definition** Management is the process of designing and maintaining an environment in which individuals, working together, efficiently accomplish selected aims. The manager coordinates individual effort towards the group goal. To do this he/she needs technical skill (knowledge specific to the business of the organization), human skill (ability to work with people), conceptual skill (ability to see the 'big picture'), and design skill (ability to solve problems). There are 5 managerial functions:
- *Planning* Involves selecting missions and objectives and the actions to achieve them—requires decision-making.
- *Organizing* Defining roles—ensuring all tasks necessary to accomplish goals are assigned to those people who can do them best.
- *Staffing* Ensuring all positions in the organizational structure are filled by people able to carry out those roles.
- *Leading* Influencing people so that they will contribute to organization and group goals.
- *Controlling* Measuring and correcting individual and organizational performance to ensure that events conform to plans.

**Management and teamwork** Key features contributing to successful teamwork are:
- *Communication* Information sharing, feedback, and grievance airing.
- *Clear team rules* especially with regard to responsibility and accountability. Make sure these are understood by everyone.
- *Sympathetic leadership* Any team needs a co-coordinator to direct its efforts. A weak leader may allow the team to drift, but an autocratic leader may be too directive and diminish the status of other team members and thus ↓ the effectiveness of the team.
- *Clear decision-making process* especially if differences of opinion.
- *Pooling* knowledge, experience, skills, resources, and responsibility for outcome.
- *Specialization of function* Team members must understand and respect the role and importance of other team members.
- *Delegation* Work of the team is split between its members. Each member leaves the others to carry out functions delegated to them.
- *Group support* Team members share and are committed to a common agreed purpose or goal which directs their actions.

**Practice meetings** Essential to ensure necessary decisions are made, review policies and agree standards of care, review the financial position of the practice, educate and inform practice members, aid communication, and improve morale of practice members.

**Risk management** Primary care is about risk and uncertainty, but sometimes we take unnecessary risks and cause ourselves and our patients unnecessary harm. Defence organization records suggest that ~½ of all successful negligence claims reflect poor clinical judgement on the doctor's part. The other ½ represent avoidable mishaps which would be susceptible to risk management approaches—often failures in simple administrative systems, communication failures, inadequate records, or lack of training. Risk management is the process of taking steps to minimize risk and keep ourselves and others as safe as possible. All the major defence organizations run risk management programmes for their members. There are 4 stages:

1  Identify the risk—through analysis of complaints and comments from GPs, other practice staff or patients, through significant event audit (📖 p.81), or by using material provided by the defence organizations to identify common pitfalls.
2  Assess frequency and severity of the risk.
3  Take steps to reduce or eliminate the risk.
4  Check the risk has been eliminated.

## Categories of risk relevant to general practice
- Clinical care, e.g. prescribing errors.
- Non-clinical risks to patient safety, e.g. security and fire hazards.
- Risks to the health of the workforce, e.g. hepatitis B
- Organizational risks, e.g. failure to safeguard confidential information and unlicensed use of computer software.
- Financial risks e.g. employment of new staff member.

## Key safety issues for primary care
- *Diagnosis* 28% reported errors.
- *Prescribing problems* occur at a rate of 3–5% of all prescriptions. 9% of hospital admissions are due to potentially avoidable problems with prescribed drugs. 4% of drugs are incorrectly dispensed each year.
- *Communication* Poor communication is a major cause of complaints. 40% of patients have been found to have discrepancies between the drugs prescribed at hospital discharge and those they receive in the community.
- *Organizational change* In industry, better teamwork, communication, and leadership ↓ adverse incidents.

## In each case consider
- *Organizational and management factors* Financial resources/constraints; practice policies; and organization.
- *Work environment factors* Staffing levels, skill mix, workload, equipment.
- *Team factors* Team structure, communication, supervision.
- *Individual (staff) factors* Knowledge and skills, competence, physical and mental health.
- *Task factors* Availability and use of protocols/guidelines, availability and accuracy of test results.
- *Patient factors* Condition (complexity and seriousness), language and communication, personality and social factors.

# Practice staff

Practices employ an array of staff. Staff costs are included in the Global Sum (📖 p.22) paid to a practice.

## Recruiting staff

- Review the post—does the post need to be filled or the duties changed?
- Prepare a job description stipulating duties and hours of work.
- Prepare a profile of the person required.
- Decide on a salary range. BMA can give advice.
- Advertise the post.
- Set a closing date for applications.
- Short-list candidates.
- Interview—decide who will interview, what points must be covered, and who will ask questions. Ask all candidates similar questions and score the responses at the time.
- Make a decision on the preferred candidate—if in doubt, defer the appointment or re-interview preferred candidates.
- Confirm the job offer by letter asking for a formal letter of acceptance in return.
- Plan an induction course for the new employee. A probationary period can be helpful for both employer and employee.
- Produce a contract of employment.

**Employment law** Very complex field which changes rapidly. If in doubt contact your local BMA office for advice. *Major points:*

**Contract of employment** Sample contracts are available from the BMA. All employees must have a written statement of main particulars of employment <2mo after their start date. Includes pay, hours, holidays, notice period, and disciplinary and grievance procedures.

**Pay** Workers must be paid ≥ the national minimum wage for every hour worked. Deductions can only be made if authorized by legislation, contract of employment, or in advance in writing by the employee. All employees must receive an itemized pay statement at or before the time they are paid, including all deductions.

**Notice** After 1mo employment, an employee must give ≥ 1wk notice. An employer must give an employee ≥ 1wk notice after 1 mo, 2wk after 2y, 3wk after 3y, and so on up to 12wk after ≥12y unless other notice periods are specified in the contract of employment.

**Redundancy pay** After 2y continuous employment, employers must make 'redundancy payments' related to employee's age, length of continuous service with the employer (up to a maximum of 20y), and weekly pay.

**Pensions** All employees must belong to a pension scheme. The NHS pension scheme is available to practice employees.

**Working time** Parents of children <6y old or disabled children <18y old may request flexible working patterns, and employers have a duty to consider their requests. Working Time Regulations 1998 apply to agency workers and freelancers as well as employees and include:

- Average working week ≤ 48h (though individuals can opt to work longer)
- 1d off each week
- A minimum of 4wk paid annual leave
- In-work rest break if the working day is ≥6h
- 11 consecutive hours' rest in any 24h period (night workers must work ≤ 8h/d).

**Time off** Employees are entitled to time off for illness, antenatal care, emergencies involving a dependant, certain public duties (e.g. jury service), to look for another job, and approved trade union activities.

**Maternity leave** All pregnant employees are entitled to 52wk. ordinary maternity leave, regardless of length of service. Women are entitled to return to their own or an equivalent job after their leave. Similar arrangements exist for adoptive mothers.

**Paternity leave** Employees who have worked for their employer for ≥26wk by the 15th wk before the baby is due and up to the birth of the child are entitled to 1–2wk paternity leave which must be completed within 56d of the birth

**Parental leave** After 1y employment, employees are entitled to 13 wk unpaid parental leave for each child born or adopted up to the child's 5th birthday (or 5y after adoption). Parents of disabled children can take 18wk up to the child's 18th birthday.

### Health and safety of staff 📖 p.38

**Discrimination** Employers must not either directly or indirectly discriminate against their staff on the basis of age, race, gender, or disability.

**Unfair dismissal** Employees of >1y standing (or on maternity or adoption leave) are entitled to a written statement of reasons for dismissal. Employers must not dismiss an employee unfairly.

### Further information
**ACAS** Provides advice for employers and employees ☎ 0845 747 4747 🖥 www.acas.org.uk
**Business Link** Provide advice on all aspects of running a business ☎ 0845 600 9006 🖥 www.businesslink.gov.uk
**Equality and Human Rights Commission** ☎ 0845 604 6610 (England); 0845 604 8810 (Wales); 0845 604 5510 (Scotland) 🖥 www.equalityhumanrights.com

# GP premises

**Funding of premises** GPs may either own or rent the property in which they practice.

- *GPs who own surgeries* GPs may own surgeries by themselves or in partnership. They receive a payment ('notional rent') for allowing their private buildings to be used for NHS purposes. Payment is based on the current market rental (CMR) value of the property as assessed by the district valuer. When a new GP partner joins a practice he/she will be expected to buy into the practice to contribute a share of previous investment in the practice premises and equipment.
- *GPs who rent surgeries* can claim reimbursement from their PCO for the rent they pay as long as it is 'reasonable' as assessed by the district valuer.
- *The cost rent scheme* This scheme is no longer available but many surgeries remain on it. Finance for building, refurbishment, or modification of GP premises was originally raised by the partners. The PCO reimburses the interest payments on the loans taken out to do this.
- *Improvement grants* Available via the PCO in some circumstances.

**❶** New premises/refurbishments must meet national minimum standards.

**Disabled access** The Disability Discrimination Act 1995 gives disabled people rights of access to goods, facilities, and services. A disabled person is defined as 'someone who has a physical or mental impairment that has a substantial and long-term adverse effect on his or her ability to carry out normal day-to-day activities'. Practices must:

- Not refuse to take disabled people onto a practice list, or provide a lower standard of service, due to their disability
- Make reasonable adjustments to their premises and the way they deliver their services so that disabled people can use them.

*Building regulations and access for disabled patients* The Building Regulations exist to ensure the health and safety of people in and around all types of buildings. Part M deals with access/facilities for disabled people. All new buildings and alterations to existing buildings must be accessible to and usable by anyone, including those with disabilities.

**Health and safety** The basis of British health and safety law is the Health and Safety at Work Act 1974. The Act sets out the general duties employers have towards employees and members of the public, and employees have to themselves and to each other.

*Responsibilities of GPs as employers* The Management of Health and Safety at Work Regulations 1992 (the Management Regulations) give clear guidance about employers' duties towards their staff. Employers with ≥5 employees must:

1 Carry out a risk assessment and record the significant findings. HSE leaflet *5 Steps to Risk Assessment* gives more information.
2 Make arrangements for implementing the health and safety measures identified as necessary by the risk assessment.
3 Appoint competent people (usually the practice manager) to help implement the arrangements.

4  Set up emergency procedures (e.g. fire drills).
5  Provide clear information and training to employees.
6  Work together with other employers sharing the same workplace.

## Other important pieces of health and safety legislation

- *Employers' Liability (Compulsory Insurance) Regulations 1969* require employers to take out insurance against accidents and ill health to their employees and display the insurance certificate.
- *Health and Safety Information for Employees Regulations 1989* require employers to display a poster telling employees what they need to know about health and safety.
- *Workplace (Health, Safety and Welfare) Regulations 1992* cover a wide range of basic health, safety and welfare issues such as ventilation, heating, lighting, and seating.
- *Reporting of Injuries, Diseases and Dangerous Occurrences Regulations 1985 (RIDDOR)* require employers to notify certain occupational injuries, diseases and dangerous events.
- *Health and Safety (Display Screen Equipment) Regulations 1992* set out requirements for work with visual display units (VDUs).
- *Personal Protective Equipment (PPE) Regulations 1992* require employers to provide appropriate protective clothing and equipment.
- *Provision and Use of Work Equipment Regulations (PUWER) 1992* require that equipment provided, including machinery, is safe.
- *Manual Handling Operations Regulations 1992* cover moving of objects by hand or bodily force.
- *Health and Safety (First Aid) Regulations 1981* cover requirements for first aid.
- *Control of Substances Hazardous to Health Regulations 1994 (COSHH)* require employers to assess the risks from hazardous substances and take appropriate precautions.
- *Gas Safety (Installation and Use) Regulations 1994* cover safe installation, maintenance, and use of gas systems and appliances in domestic and commercial premises.

## Further information

**Health and Safety Executive** ☎ 0845 345 0055 🖳 www.hse.gov.uk
**Business Link** Provides advice on all aspects of running a business including issues of health, safety, and premises. ☎ 0845 600 9006 🖳 www.businesslink.gov.uk

# Computers and classification

**Information for Health Strategy (1998)** Aims to provide:
- A lifelong electronic health record for every person in the country.
- Online 24h access to records and information about best clinical practice for all NHS clinicians.
- Electronic communication between general practices and hospitals.
- ↑ public access to information and services through online or telephone services.
- New ways of delivering services and care through telemedicine.

**Computers in practices** Under the GMS contract, PCOs directly fund 100% of IT costs. Almost all practices now use computers on a daily basis. All specialist GP systems must be approved by the DH (termed Systems of Choice—Table 3.1). The software covers all aspects of practice from appointment systems, through clinical care, to audit and reporting.

**Electronic GP records** Many GPs maintain all records on computer, i.e. are 'paperless'. DH/BMA good practice guidelines are regularly updated.

**Read codes** Code all aspects of patient care in general practice in the UK. They code in a hierarchical way, e.g. all operations are quantified by 7…., all appendix operations as 770.., and all emergency excisions of abnormal appendix as 77001. Characters in the code can be numerical or alphabetical. The huge number ($58^5$) of possible combinations ensures there are enough unused Read codes to accommodate changes.

**SNOMED clinical terms (CT)** New coding system that will eventually replace Read coding. The aim is that all healthcare systems in the UK will use the same coding system, allowing a single unified patient record.

**NHSnet** Intranet connecting NHS organizations which is protected from the Internet by a firewall. This enables NHS users to access the Internet but outside users cannot access protected NHSWeb sites. All GP practices in the UK are connected to the NHSnet, enabling email, Internet access, electronic exchange of information, shared learning resources, computer-based training packages, discussion forums, and many other benefits. For example, many practices now receive all laboratory and X-ray results electronically.

**Choose and book (C&B)** National service which combines electronic booking and choice of place, date and time for first outpatient appointments. Features:
- A list of available services and indicative waiting list times for the first out-patient appointment is displayed to the GP.
- Appointments can be booked by the GP in the surgery (if the secondary care provider is linked to the C&B system), or patients may take booking forms home to book appointments themselves later via the Internet or by telephone. This ensures that appointments are made at dates and times convenient for the patient.
- Patients can opt to be referred to any hospital offering services paid for by the NHS.
- Patients may cancel or alter their appointments at a later date by the same mechanism without going back to the GP.

**Table 3.1** GP Systems of Choice (GPSoC) suppliers

| System | Web address for more information |
| --- | --- |
| EMIS (*LV/PCS*) | www.emis-online.com |
| Healthy Software (*Crosscare*) | www.healthysoftware.co.uk |
| INPS (*Vision*) | www.inps.co.uk |
| Microtest (*Evolution/Practice Manager*) | www.microtest.co.uk |
| iSOFT (*Premiere/Synergy*) | www.isoftplc.com |
| CSC Computer Sciences Ltd (*SystmOne*) | www.csc.com/mms/primarycare/en |
| **Scotland** | |
| GPASS (*General Practice Administration System for Scotland*) | www.gpass.scot.nhs.uk |

- Each referral is allocated a unique number (UBRN), enabling referral letters to be submitted and retrieved electronically.
- The 'advice and guidance' facility enables GPs to contact consultants for advice via C&B.

**Use of email in the surgery** 📖 p.95

**Electronic transmission of prescriptions** The Electronic Prescription Service (EPS) allows prescribers working in primary care settings to generate and transmit electronic prescriptions from their clinical software. The electronic prescription is transmitted to the EPS where it can be downloaded by a dispenser with appropriate computer software. Patients 'nominate' a dispenser to receive their prescriptions. No paper prescription is required.

**Further information**
**NHS Connecting for Health** 📖 www.connectingforhealth.nhs.uk
- GP Systems of Choice
- Electronic prescribing
- Choose and book
- SNOMED CT

**DH** 📖 www.dh.gov.uk
- Good practice guidelines for general practice electronic patient records (v.3.1 – 2005).
- Information for Health: an information strategy for the modern NHS 1998–2005.

**British Computer Society Primary Health Care Specialist Group** 📖 www.phcsg.org.uk

# Useful websites for GPs

| Website | Description |
| --- | --- |
| **Organizations** | |
| www.nhs.uk | NHS |
| www.dh.gov.uk | Department of Health |
| www.gmc-uk.org | GMC |
| www.bma.org.uk | BMA |
| www.rcgp.org.uk | Royal College of GPs |
| www.the-mdu.com www.mps.org.uk www.mddus.com | UK medical defence organizations |
| **Guidelines/books/journals/evidence based medicine** | |
| www.library.nhs.uk | National Library for Health |
| www.nice.org.uk | NICE |
| www.sign.ac.uk | SIGN |
| www.gpnotebook.co.uk | GP Notebook—online textbook |
| www.bnf.org | BNF |
| www.bnfc.org | BNF for children |
| www.merck.com/mmpe/index.html | Merck manual textbook of medicine |
| www.cks.library.nhs.uk | NHS Clinical Knowledge Summaries |
| www.medicine.ox.ac.uk/bandolier | Bandolier |
| www.pubmed.gov | PubMed Central |
| www.npc.co.uk/ebt/merec.htm | MeReC Bulletin |
| www.bmj.com www.bmjjournals.com | BMJ and other BMJ Group journals |
| www.rcgp-innovait.oxfordjournals.org | InnovAiT—journal for GPs in training |
| www.freemedicaljournals.com | Portal to free medical journals online |
| www.freebooks4doctors.com | Portal to free medical books online |
| **Other useful medical sites** | |
| www.patient.co.uk | Patient information leaflets |
| www.rcgp-curriculum.org.uk | GP curriculum |
| www.doctors.net.uk | Doctors net |
| www.adviceguide.org.uk | Citizens Advice Bureau |
| www.direct.gov.uk | Government guide to services |
| www.nhsdirect.nhs.uk | NHS Direct |
| www.firstpracticemanagement.co.uk | First Practice Management |

**Useful non-medical sites**

| | |
|---|---|
| www.google.co.uk | Search tool |
| www.bt.com | Telephone directories |
| www.yell.com | |
| www.royalmail.com | Postcode finder |
| www.hmrc.gov.uk | Online self-assessment tax form |
| www.rac.co.uk | Online travel information—roads |
| www.nationalrail.co.uk | Train tickets and timetables |
| www.streetmap.co.uk | Maps |
| www.amazon.co.uk | Online bookshop |
| www.bbc.co.uk | General information, news |
| www.lastminute.com | Travel, gifts, and leisure |

# Eligibility for free healthcare

**Eligibility to receive free primary medical care in the UK** is determined by whether a person is resident in the UK and is not related to nationality or payment of National Insurance/taxes.

## Patients from abroad

- Anyone coming to the UK intending to stay for <6mo does not fulfill the qualifying criteria for free non-emergency NHS care.
- For patients coming to the UK intending to stay ≥6mo, entitlement to free treatment begins on arrival in the UK—there is *no* qualifying period of residency before free treatment starts.

## British nationals returning to the UK

- A British resident on extended holiday or a business trip still counts as ordinarily resident and is entitled to free healthcare on return.
- Someone who has emigrated and ordinarily lives abroad, but returns from time to time to take advantage of free NHS care, does not qualify. Treat UK Nationals resident abroad like any other overseas visitor (unless embassy staff, merchant seamen, or in the armed forces).
- Persons leaving the UK for >6mo should *not* continue to be registered with a GP. The onus is on the patients to inform the relevant authorities and surrender their medical cards.

## UK residents going abroad

- Doctors should *not* provide NHS scripts for conditions that might arise whilst the patient is away e.g. traveller's diarrhoea.
- Prescribing interval for any repeat medication should be related to the next time that medication would normally be reviewed. Generally this should not be >13wk.
- The prescribing doctor retains medico-legal responsibility for the duration of the prescription.
- If the doctor does decide to prescribe for the patient's stay abroad (e.g. if repeat supplies cannot be obtained at the destination or the drug prescribed has a narrow therapeutic index), it is essential to inform the patient of the need to consult a doctor for any regular monitoring, as well as the need to consult a doctor in the event of any unforeseen complications or symptoms.

## General rules for treatment of overseas visitors to the UK

- *Emergency or immediately necessary treatment* must be offered to overseas visitors free of charge for a period of ≤14d. There is no obligation to provide non-emergency treatment. It is the decision of the GP whether care is deemed necessary. It includes pre-existing conditions that have become worse, oxygen, and renal dialysis.
- *Non-emergency care* Provide only on a private paying basis.
- *Reciprocal healthcare arrangements* Treat in the same way as nationals from other countries. The exception is patients from European Economic Area (EEA) member states, who may also request ongoing prescriptions and routine monitoring for existing conditions free of change.
- *Refugees* (whether or not awarded leave to stay) are regarded as ordinarily resident.

- *Hospital admission* A&E services are free, as is compulsory psychiatric treatment and treatment for certain communicable diseases. Testing for the HIV virus and counselling following a test are both free of charge, but any necessary subsequent treatment and medicines may have to be paid for.
- *NHS prescriptions* can be issued, but quantities supplied should be no more than necessary for immediate purposes. Overseas visitors are charged normal NHS fees.

**General rules for British patients travelling abroad** <60 countries worldwide have any sort of healthcare agreements with the UK. When travelling abroad, always have comprehensive medical insurance.

***The European Health Insurance Card (EHIC)*** The EHIC entitles holders to reduced cost, sometimes free, medical treatment which becomes necessary whilst in another EEA country or Switzerland. The EHIC can be obtained online from 🖳 www.ehic.org.uk or at any Post Office. Countries this applies to are listed in Table 3.2. Each country has its own rules—details for individual countries are available on the DH travel advice website. British citizens moving to another EEA country are not entitled to use an EHIC to obtain medical treatment.

**Table 3.2** Countries in which an EHIC can be used

| | | |
|---|---|---|
| • Austria | • Greece | • Norway |
| • Belgium | • Hungary | • Poland |
| • Bulgaria | • Iceland | • Portugal |
| • Cyprus (but not Northern Cyprus) | • Ireland | • Romania |
| | • Italy | • Slovakia |
| • Czech Republic | • Latvia | • Slovenia |
| • Denmark | • Liechtenstein | • Spain |
| • Estonia | • Lithuania | • Sweden |
| • Finland | • Luxembourg | • Switzerland |
| • France | • Malta | |
| • Germany | • Netherlands | |

***Other reciprocal agreements*** The UK has reciprocal agreements with certain other countries for the provision of urgently needed medical treatment at ↓ cost or free. Countries and the services available are listed on the DH travel advice website. Only urgently needed treatment is provided on the same terms as for residents of that country. Proof of British nationality or UK residence is required.

**Further information**
**DH** Access to healthcare abroad
🖳 www.nhs.uk/nhsengland/healthcareabroad

# Registration and practice leaflets

**The registration process** Patients can apply to join a practice list by handing in their medical card at the practice or completing an application form. A parent or a guardian can make the application for children.

- *Open lists* Practices with open lists must consider all applications to join their list They can only refuse if they have reasonable grounds for doing so which do not relate to the applicant's race, gender, social class, age, religion, sexual orientation, appearance, disability, or medical condition. When an application is refused the practice must inform the applicant in writing of the reasons for refusal.
- *Closed lists* Practices with closed lists can only consider applications from immediate family members of patients already registered.

Once the practice has accepted the application it must then inform the PCO. The PCO confirms that the application has been accepted in writing to practice and patient.

**List closure** Practices wishing to close their lists to new registrations must inform the PCO in writing. The PCO must then enter into discussion with the practice to provide support to keep the list open. If that is not possible, the list will be closed for a specified period of time. Often closure is requested because of high list size. In that instance, a list size can be set so that the list reopens when it falls below that limit.

**Newly registered patients** When a patient has been accepted onto a practice list, or assigned to a practice list by a PCO, the practice must offer the patient a consultation for a routine health check (the 'new patient check') within 6mo of registration.

**Routine health checks for other groups** Practices must offer a consultation for a routine health check to all:
- Patients aged 16–75y who have not been seen by a healthcare professional within the practice in the past 3y.
- Patients aged >75y who have not been seen by a healthcare professional within the past year.

❶ Patients aged 40–74y will be invited every 5y for free health checks and personalized assessment of risk under a new scheme launched in 2009.

**Temporary residents** Patients may register with a practice on a short-term basis for treatment or advice if they are living temporarily (for >24h but <3mo) in the practice area.

**Emergency and immediately necessary treatment** A practice must provide services required in core hours for the immediately necessary treatment of:
- Anyone injured or acutely unwell as a result of an accident or medical emergency at any place in its practice area.
- Anyone whose application for inclusion in the practice list (as a permanent or temporary resident) has been refused and who is not registered with another provider in the area.
- Anyone who is in the practice area for <24h.

**Removing patients from the practice list** 📖 p.56

**Assignments** PCOs may assign patients to any open practice list if the patient has problems registering with a practice. PCOs can only assign patients to closed lists if all other local practice lists are also closed and an assessment panel has approved the placement.

**Practice leaflets** Each practice is required to produce a practice leaflet to distribute to patients. In Wales, the practice leaflet must be in Welsh and English. The practice leaflet aims to inform patients about the practice, the services provided, and how to access them. In addition, it informs patients of their rights and responsibilities. Most practices also take the opportunity to include general health information and information about self-management of minor illness.

***Content of the practice leaflet*** Practice leaflets *must* be updated annually *and* include details of:
- The name of the practice (and if the contract is with a partnership, names of partners and status within the partnership; if the contract is with a company, names of directors, company secretary, shareholders, and the address of the company's registered office)
- Names and professional qualifications of those providing medical care.
- Whether the practice teaches or trains healthcare professionals.
- Practice area including reference to a map, plan, or postcode
- Addresses of all practice premises, telephone and fax numbers, and website address (if any)
- Services available including details of routine health checks for patients aged >75y not seen in the past year or aged 16–75y not seen in the previous 3y.
- Access for disabled patients and, if not, alternative arrangements for providing them with services.
- Registration process.
- Opening hours and methods of accessing services (including home visits) within those hours.
- Out-of-hours arrangements (including who is responsible for their provision) and how to access them.
- Arrangements for dispensing drugs (if applicable) and repeat prescriptions.
- Name and address of any local walk-in centre, telephone number of NHS Direct, and details of NHS Direct online.
- Complaints procedure.
- Rights and responsibilities—including the right of patients to express a preference of practitioner (and the way that they can express that) and responsibility to keep appointments.
- Action that will be taken if a patient is aggressive or abusive.
- Access to patient information and the patient's rights of confidentiality.
- Name, address, and telephone number of the responsible PCO.

# The primary healthcare team

The GP does not function alone. Doctors within general practice are an integral part of a team of professionals who care for patients in the community—the primary healthcare team (PHCT). Precise composition of the PHCT depends on the overall aims of the team, needs of the practice population and practice characteristics. Team members include the GPs and:

**Practice manager** General manager of the practice in liaison with the partners. Roles include staff appointments, supervision, training, and dismissals; duty rotas; liaison with outside organizations (e.g. PCO) and other primary healthcare team members (e.g. community nurses and health visitors); maintenance of premises and equipment and financial planning. Most practice managers have management qualifications.

**Practice nurse** Duties can vary, but include 'traditional' nursing tasks, health promotion, immunizations, new registration checks, specialist clinics (e.g. asthma, DM etc.), administration, and audit.

**Nurse practitioner** Specially trained nurse who takes on clinical responsibility for specific aspects of care he/she has been trained for, e.g. filtering out-of-hours calls. Seen as a way to alleviate pressure on GPs. Nurse practitioners are at least as effective as GPs in the roles they perform.

**District nurse** Qualified nurse who has a community nursing qualification recognized by the Nursing and Midwifery Council. Most work is conducted in patients' homes, particularly in looking after the chronically ill or those recently discharged from hospital. District nurses are usually employed by local community trusts or PCOs and coordinate their own team of community nurses.

**Health visitor** works with individuals, families, and groups in preventive medicine, health promotion, and education. Health visitors visit all babies after the midwife ceases to attend, carry out developmental assessment checks, and advise on general care and immunization. Some health visitors have a role exclusively for the elderly. Health visitors must be trained nurses and registered as health visitors with the Nursing and Midwifery Council.

**Midwife** Important link between hospitals, GPs, and other members of the primary healthcare team in obstetric care. May practice independently when dealing with uncomplicated pregnancies, but are obliged to refer to a doctor in the event of complications. Midwives must be registered with the Nursing and Midwifery Council.

**Administrative and clerical staff** perform all the non-clinical tasks necessary to keep the practice running. Training varies.

**Receptionists** perform an essential role as the interface between the general public and the GPs and nursing staff. Good interpersonal skills are essential. Training varies.

**Community pharmacist** Increasing role within practices—managing repeat prescribing, monitoring prescribing practices, and advising on prescribing policy.

**Social worker** Helps people live more successfully within the local community by helping them find solutions to their problems. Social workers tend to specialize in either adult or children's services.
- *Adult services* Roles include working with people with mental health problems or learning difficulties in residential care; working with offenders by supervising them in the community and supporting them to find work; and working with older people or disabled people at home, helping to sort out problems with their health, housing, or benefits.
- *Children/young people services* Roles include providing assistance and advice to keep families together, working in children's homes, managing adoption and foster care processes, providing support to younger people leaving care or who are at risk or in trouble with the law, and helping children who have problems at school or are facing difficulties brought on by illness in the family.

**Other team members** might include dieticians, occupational therapists, physiotherapists, and/or complementary therapists (such as counsellors).

**Further information**
**Association of Medical Secretaries, Practice Administrators & Receptionists (AMSPAR)** ☎ 020 7387 6005 🖳 www.amspar.co.uk
**Nursing and Midwifery Council (NMC)** ☎ 020 7637 7181 (registrations: ☎ 020 7333 9333) 🖳 www.nmc.uk.org
**Royal College of Nursing** 🖳 www.rcn.org.uk
**Royal College of Midwives** 🖳 www.rcm.org.uk
**Community Practitioners' and Health Visitors' Association** 🖳 www.unite-cphva.org
**British Association of Social Workers** 🖳 www.basw.co.uk

# Confidentiality

The Human Rights Act 1998 establishes a right to 'respect for private and family life' and creates a general requirement to protect the privacy of individuals and preserve confidentiality of their health records. Respect for confidentiality is also an essential requirement for the preservation of trust between patient and doctor. Failure to comply with standards can lead to disciplinary proceedings and even restriction/cessation of practice.

## Caldicott principles for disclosure of patient information

- *Justify the purpose* Patients may voluntarily agree to identifiable information about themselves being released to specific individuals for known purposes. Implied consent occurs when a patient who is aware their personal information may be shared and of their right to refuse, but makes no objection. Patients must have had a realistic opportunity to refuse. If patients refuse, it should be clearly documented and respected.
- *Don't use patient identifiable information unless it is absolutely necessary* It is not necessary to seek consent to use anonymous information. If in doubt seek advice from the BMA or your defence organization. Health information used for 2° purposes (e.g. planning, teaching, audit) should—wherever possible—be anonymous.
- *Use the minimum necessary patient identifiable information.*
- *Access to patient identifiable information should be on a strict 'need to know' basis'.*
- *Everyone should be aware of their responsibilities.*
- *Understand and comply with the law.*

## Special circumstances

- *Children* Disclosure can be authorized by a person with parental responsibility. Young people mature enough to understand the implications can make their own decisions and have a right to refuse parental access to their health record.
- *Mentally incapacitated adults* Capacity must be judged in relation to the decision to be made. People with a mental incapacity can authorize or prohibit sharing of information if they broadly understand its implications. If a patient lacks the ability to understand, decisions must be based on an evaluation of the person's best interests and reflect the individual's expressed wishes and values.
- *The deceased* Legislation covering records made since 1st November 1991 permits limited disclosure in order to satisfy a claim arising from death. Where there is *no* claim, there is *no* legal right of access to information.

**Breaching confidentiality** Only breach confidentiality in exceptional cases and with appropriate justification. This includes discussing a patient with another health professional not involved currently with that patient's care. Wider disclosure to people loosely associated with care (e.g. support staff in residential care settings) requires patient consent.

### Situations where breach of confidentiality may be justified

- *Emergencies* Where necessary to prevent or lessen a serious and imminent threat to the life or health of the individual concerned or another person (unless previously forbidden by the patient).
- *Statutory requirement* Ask under which legislation it is sought—check the legislation before disclosing if unsure.
- *The public interest* What is in the public interest is not defined. The BMA has produced guidance.
- *Public health* Reporting notifiable diseases (statutory duty 📖 p.645).
- *Required by court or tribunal.*
- *Adverse drug reactions* Routine reporting to the Medicines and Healthcare Products Regulatory Agency (📖 p.148).
- *Complaints* As part of GMC performance procedures involving doctors.

### Legal considerations

- *Human Rights Act* Compliance with the Data Protection Act and common law of confidentiality should satisfy requirements.
- *Common law of confidentiality* Built up from case law where practice has been established by individual judgements. The key principle is that information confided should not be used or disclosed further, except as originally understood by the confider, or with their subsequent permission, except in exceptional circumstances (see breaching confidentiality).
- *Data Protection Act 1998* Imposes constraints on processing of personal information. Also requires personal data to be protected against unauthorized/ unlawful processing and accidental loss, destruction or damage. Also applies to personnel records.
- *Administrative law* The extent to which the NHS can access confidential information to perform its functions is set down in statutes.
- *Health and Social Care Act 2001* Allows for certain exceptions to confidentiality laws to be made, e.g. for use in cancer registries.
- *Freedom of information Act 2000* Applies to all NHS bodies including GP practices. Practices are required to produce a publication scheme detailing all information routinely published by the practice. In addition, members of the public can make written requests to see any information recorded by the practice in any format. These rights are restricted by certain exemptions, e.g. personal data.

### Further information

**GMC** Guidance on good practice—confidentiality 🖥 www.gmc-uk.org
**DH** Patient confidentiality and access to health records
🖥 www.dh.gov.uk
**BMA** Confidentiality and people under 16 🖥 www.bma.org.uk
**Information Commissioner's Office** Data Protection 🖥 www.ico.gov.uk

# Consent

**Consent** Implies willingness of a patient to undergo examination, investigation, or treatment (collectively termed 'procedure' here). It may be expressed (i.e. specifically says yes or no/signs a consent form) or implied (i.e. complies with the procedure without ever specifically agreeing to it—use with care). For consent to be valid patients:
• must be competent to make the decision
• have received sufficient information to take it, and
• not be acting under duress.

⚠ Under 'common law' touching a patient without valid consent may constitute the civil or criminal offence of battery, and if the patient suffers harm as a result of treatment, lack of consent may be a factor in any negligence claim. Never exceed the scope of the authority given by a patient, except in an emergency.

If you are the doctor carrying out a procedure, it is *your responsibility* to discuss it with the patient and seek consent. The task may be delegated but the responsibility *remains* yours.

## Information to include
• Reasons why you want to perform the procedure.
• Nature, purpose, and side effects (common and serious) of proposed procedure.
• Name of the doctor with overall responsibility.
• Whether students or other 'trainees' will be involved.
• Whether part of a research programme or outside usual procedure.
• Reminder that patients have a right to seek a second opinion and/or can change their minds about a decision at any time.

*And for therapeutic procedures/treatments:*
• Details of diagnosis and prognosis (including uncertainties).
• Management options—including the option not to treat and other options that you cannot offer—and for each option an estimation of likely risks, benefits, and probability of success.
• Details of follow-up in order to monitor progress or side effects.

❶ Document if a patient does not want to be fully informed before consenting.

**Written consent** It is good practice to seek written consent if:
• The procedure is complex, or involves significant risks ('risk' means any adverse outcome including complications and side effects).
• The procedure involves general/regional anaesthesia or sedation.
• Providing clinical care is not the primary purpose of the procedure.
• It has consequences for the employment, social life, or personal life of the patient.
• The procedure is part of a project or programme of approved research.

**Establishing capacity to make decisions** 📖 p.124

**Mentally incapacitated adults** The Mental Capacity Act 2005, and equivalents in Scotland and Northern Ireland, enables patients' advocates (usually friends, relatives, or carers) or suitable professionals (e.g. doctors, social workers) to act in patients' best interests on their behalf. This includes provision of medical care. Before acting:

- Take all factors affecting the decision into consideration.
- Involve the patient with the decision-making as far as possible.
- Take the patient's previous known wishes into consideration.
- Consult everyone else involved with the patient's care/welfare.

In situations in which there is disagreement about the patient's best interests, the decision can be referred to the Court of Protection.

**Advance statements** 📖 p.125

**Children (<16y)** A competent child is able to understand the nature, purpose, and possible consequences of a proposed procedure, as well as the consequences of not undergoing that procedure. This is termed *Gillick competence* after the court case in which the principle was established (Gillick v West Norfolk and Wisbech AHA [1986] AC 122).

A competent child may consent to treatment . However, if treatment is refused, a parent or court may authorize procedures in the child's best interests*. Where a child is not judged competent, only a person with parental responsibility may authorize/refuse investigations or treatment. If in doubt, seek legal advice.

**Emergencies** When consent cannot be obtained, you may provide medical treatment, provided that it is limited to what is immediately necessary to save life or avoid significant deterioration in the patient's health. Respect the terms of any advance statement/living will you are aware of.

**Further information**

**GMC** 🖳 www.gmc-uk.org
- Consent: patients and doctors making decisions together (2008)
- 0–18 years: guidance for all doctors (2007).

**Office of the Public Guardian** Making decisions: a guide for people who work in health and social care (2007) 🖳 www.publicguardian.gov.uk

---

* In Scotland, parents do not have this power to overrule a competent child's decision.

# Complaints

Sadly, complaints are a fact of life for most GPs. The most constructive and least stressful approach is to view them as a learning experience and a chance to improve practice risk management strategy. Always contact your local LMC ± defence organization if you are directly implicated in a complaint. Patients who complain generally want:
• Their complaint to be heard and investigated promptly
• Their complaint to be handled efficiently and sympathetically
• To receive a genuine apology if mistakes have occurred
• To be assured that steps will be taken to prevent a recurrence.

**Time limits for complaints** NHS complaints can be accepted <1y after the incident which is the subject of the complaint, or <1y after the date at which the complainant became aware of the matter. After that time complaints can only be accepted if there is good reason for delay and it is possible to investigate effectively. A 3y time limit after the incident (or after the date upon which the claimant became aware that the incident might have caused harm) is placed on civil clinical negligence cases, except for children who may claim until their 21st birthday.

**Conciliation** is a way of dealing with complaints that helps to avoid adversarial situations. Either party can ask the local PCO for conciliation, but both parties must agree to it taking place. By bringing the 2 sides together with a neutral conciliator, it aims to:
• Explain and clarify matters for both parties
• Ensure both parties are really listening to each other
• Ensure the process is unthreatening and helpful.

**Records of complaints** A file on the complaint, including a copy of all correspondence, should be kept separate from clinical records of the patient and, if the patient leaves the practice, should not be sent on with the clinical notes.

**Private sector** Most private sector healthcare providers have their own complaints resolution procedures. Patients should contact the organization concerned for details.

**Disciplinary procedures** There is no direct connection between complaints procedures and disciplinary action. If a complaints procedure reveals information indicating the need for disciplinary action, it is the responsibility of the PCO to act. If they decide that there has been a breach of the terms of service the PCO can fix a penalty, if appropriate.

**Further information**
**Risk management** 📖 p.35
**BMA** 🖥 www.bma.org.uk
**Medical defence organizations**

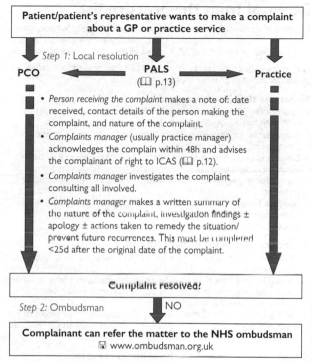

Patient/patient's representative wants to make a complaint about a GP or practice service

*Step 1*: Local resolution

PCO ← PALS (□ p.13) → Practice

- *Person receiving the complaint* makes a note of: date received, contact details of the person making the complaint, and nature of the complaint.
- *Complaints manager* (usually practice manager) acknowledges the complain within 48h and advises the complainant of right to ICAS (□ p.12).
- *Complaints manager* investigates the complaint consulting all involved.
- *Complaints manager* makes a written summary of the nature of the complaint, investigation findings ± apology ± actions taken to remedy the situation/prevent future recurrences. This must be completed <25d after the original date of the complaint.

Complaint resolved?

*Step 2*: Ombudsman ↓ NO

Complainant can refer the matter to the NHS ombudsman
🖳 www.ombudsman.org.uk

**Fig. 3.1** The NHS complaints procedure for general practice

# Removal from the practice list

Removal of a patient from a practice list can be distressing for both patient and GP. In England and Wales ~53 000 patients/y are transferred by PCOs at the request of the GP, ~1000/y because of an act or threat of violence.

**❶** Practice policies for removing patients and dealing with threats/violence should be stated in practice leaflets.

## Situations that justify removal

- *Violence* Physical violence or verbal abuse towards doctor, practice staff, premises, or other patients. Includes violence or threatening behaviour by other household members not registered with the practice and/or pets (e.g. dogs).
- *Crime and deception* Deliberate deceit to obtain a service or benefit; obtaining drugs under false pretences for non-medical reasons; use of the doctor to conceal or aid criminal activity; stealing from practice premises.
- *Distance* New residence outside the designated practice area with failure to register with another GP until such times as geographic practice areas are abolished.

## Situations that never justify removal

- *Costly treatment* GPs can apply for an ↑ in their prescribing budget to allow for this.
- *Particular conditions* If a particular condition demands costly treatment, out of area referrals, or expensive equipment, accommodation can be made at PCO level.
- *Age* General practice is about looking after patients from cradle to grave. Although patients >75y do result in higher costs this is reflected in allocation of funds to the practice.

## Situations that do not normally justify removal

- *Disagreement with the patient's views* Patients must have freedom to choose whether to accept a GP's advice. The GP can try to influence the view but should not remove a patient if he/she fails to concur.
- *Critical questioning and/or complaints* Complaints to the practice via normal in-house channels can be constructive and help improve services and do not usually justify removal of the patient from the practice list. However, personal attacks on a doctor or allegations that are clearly unfounded indicate a serious breakdown in doctor–patient relationship and could justify removal.

**Patients' rights to change doctor** Patients also have a right to change their doctor. They are not required to give reasons or any period of notice and there is no requirement for the GP to be notified.

**Other family members** Removal of other family members should not automatically follow removal of a patient from a practice list unless removal of that patient makes ongoing care of the rest of the household impossible.

**Irretrievable breakdown of the doctor–patient relationship**
The most contentious reason for removal from a practice list. Causes the most problems. As a good doctor–patient relationship is fundamental to successful care, it is in the interest of both patient and GP that the patient moves to another practice list if that relationship breaks down. Difficulty arises when the patient sees matters differently.

- *Inform appropriate members of the practice* Discuss reasons for breakdown in relationship (e.g. chronic stress, mental illness, cultural differences) and factors that contribute to the situation; consider solutions/alterations in procedures that might help.
- *Inform the patient* Consider arranging a meeting to discuss matters (can be done through the in-house complaints framework). Explain the nature of the problem and elicit the patient's perspective; be prepared to give ground and compromise.
- *If discussion fails to resolve the problem* Suggest that the patient sees another GP within the practice (though discuss the patient's feelings about the possibility of being treated by the ex-GP in an emergency). Consider giving advice about alternative practices in the area. If the situation continues, then consider removal from the practice list.

## Removing patients from the practice list
- Warn the patient—a practice can only request removal of a patient from a practice list if, within 12mo prior to the date of its request to the PCO for removal, it has warned the patient that he/she is at risk of removal and explained the reasons for that. Exceptions to this are violent patients, patients who have moved outside the practice area, and those for whom it would unsafe or impractical to issue a warning.
- Inform the PCO in writing of your decision. Give full patient details. Except in the case of violent patients, removal will not take effect until the 8th day after the request is received by the PCO unless the patient is accepted by, allocated to, or assigned to another GP sooner than this. The patient is always notified by the PCO.
- Write to the patient about the decision and reason for removal (take advice from your medical defence organization). Include information on how to register with another practice and reassurance that the patient will not be left without a GP. Take care to ensure that reasons given are factual and the tone of the letter is polite and informative.

**Immediate removal of any patient who has committed an act of violence** Includes actual or threatened physical violence or verbal abuse leading to fear for a person's safety.
- Notify the police (or in Scotland, either the police or the procurator fiscal) about the violent behaviour.
- Notify both the PCO and the patient of the removal in writing. The PCO has a duty to provide alternative primary medical care services by commissioning specialized directed enhanced services, e.g. GPs with secure facilities for consulting.

## Further information
**RCGP** 🖳 www.rcgp.org.uk
**BMA** 🖳 www.bma.org.uk

# Chapter 4

# Education, monitoring, and research

# Education in primary care

Teaching and training in primary care at every level should:
- Be based on evidence.
- Train the doctor to be part of an integrated and comprehensive healthcare system.
- Have a balanced agenda across clinical topics (prevention, diagnosis, cure, care, and palliation), practice organization and management, team working, audit, and research.

**Teaching in general practice** Most GPs are involved in teaching to some extent. This may involve:
- Teaching medical students, foundation doctors or GP registrars within the practice.
- Helping to train new practice staff.
- Arranging your own and/or your colleagues' continuing education programme.

Teaching can be very rewarding but also brings stresses (e.g. preparation of material). Payments are available to GPs who take medical students, foundation doctors, and/or GPs in training into their surgeries for teaching, and there are a few teaching posts for GPs within UK universities.

As a teacher it is your responsibility to ensure that you are competent to fulfill the task. Take steps to acquire proficiency in teaching skills. Local medical schools often run courses for prospective teachers.

**Learning styles** Different people have different learning styles. Depending on a person's preferred learning style, the starting point for an educational initiative will be different.
- *'Why'* (concrete, reflective) learners learn best when they know why something is relevant and how it will apply to their work.
- *'What'* (abstract, reflective) learners learn best when given plenty of time to think about things and link different concepts in their mind.
- *'How'* (abstract, active) learners like to work actively on well-defined tasks and learn by trial and error.
- *'What if'* (concrete, active) learners learn best by applying course material in new situations and solving problems they create for themselves.
- *Serialist* learners like to see the 'big picture' first.
- *Holist learners* like to take learning bit by bit in small chunks.
- *Individual learners* prefer to learn on their own.
- *Group learners* prefer to learn with others.

**Principles of self-directed and adult learning** The learner takes responsibility for defining learning needs, setting goals, identifying resources, implementing appropriate activities, and evaluating outcomes. Adults are motivated by education that:
- Is based on mutual trust and respect.
- Allows them to take responsibility for their own learning.
- Actively involves them.
- Is perceived as relevant.
- Is based on, and builds on, previous experience.
- Is focused on problems.

- Can be immediately applied in practice.
- Involves cycles of action and reflection.

**Personal development plans (PDPs)** Outline areas of knowledge in need of update and ways in which these needs can be met. PDPs are an integral part of junior doctor training, GP training and the appraisal process. Ask:
- *What* you need to learn—specific, measurable objectives.
- *Why* you need to learn it.
- *How* you plan to learn it.
- How you will know *whether* you have learnt it.
- How your intentions link to *past* and *future* learning.
- The *timescale* for your learning.

**'SMART' criteria**—learning objectives should be:
**S**pecific
**M**easurable
**A**chievable
**R**ealistic
**T**imed (i.e. there should be a deadline for achieving them).

**Methods of Identifying learning needs** Numerous—include:
- Gap analysis
- Significant event audit (📖 p.81)
- Objective tests of knowledge and skill
- Self-assessment through diary, log book, or weekly review
- Video assessment of performance
- Criterion-based audit (📖 p.80)
- Patient satisfaction surveys (📖 p.84)
- Risk assessment (📖 p.35)
- Peer assessment and multi-source feedback.

**Medical students** are taught in general practice as:
- *Early patient contact* is helpful to enable students to relate theoretical concepts to the reality of medical practice. General practice settings are especially good for teaching concepts of health and illness behaviour and the effect of family and social settings on illness.
- *Clinical skills* can be taught successfully in general practice, and the one-to-one teaching that can be undertaken within GP surgeries is an excellent teaching resource.

**Foundation doctors** 📖 p.62

**GP training** 📖 p.64

**Continuing professional development (CPD)** The aim of CPD is to sustain professional development of doctors and help them to provide high-quality patient care throughout their careers. Doctors need to demonstrate that they have up-to-date knowledge across the spectrum of general practice to become a registered GP, and then need to show that they are continuing to update and expand their knowledge to meet requirements of appraisal and revalidation (📖 p.68).

# Foundation doctors in primary care

Newly qualified doctors spend their first working year (F1) doing 3 hospital placements before obtaining full registration. In the second year (F2), most have a 4mo attachment to primary care, whether or not they wish to become GPs.

**Who employs foundation doctors?** Foundation programmes are hosted by acute hospital trusts. The trust recruits the doctors, arranges their placements, employs them throughout their 2y programme, provides their indemnity, appoints an educational supervisor, and is responsible for their assessment.

## F2 placements in general practice

- Placements in primary care are made by the employing trust and practices have no say over who they take.
- Educational deaneries are responsible for appointing practices for F2 placements and interested practices should contact their local deanery.
- Practices must be of adequate standard and have an approved supervisor for their F2s. The standard required of the practice is similar to that required of training practices (📖 p.64). Practices will be inspected by their deanery to check that they meet the criteria.
- GP F2 supervisors need not be trainers. To attain approval, potential supervisors undergo a short training course organized by the deanery. They are paid by the deanery at a rate related to the trainer rate.

## Expectations of F2 doctors

- Expected to do 7 clinical sessions/wk, 1 session of supervised study, 1 session of project work, and attend a ½ day group session at their host trust. No OOH work is expected. Part-time working is allowed but training must be undertaken on a ≥½ time basis.
- Entitled to study leave (up to 1 wk) and annual leave.
- Can sign prescriptions. Practical procedures must be supervised.
- Need an initial induction period working with practice staff and the wider primary health care team, and sitting in with a trained GP.
- Likely to need longer consultation times than standard 10min slots.
- Need to have a fully trained GP available whenever they are seeing patients to provide advice and support, monitor their performance, and debrief at the end of the session.

**Assessment** Workplace-based assessment and feedback are central to foundation training. 3 types of assessment are commonly used:

- *Multi-source feedback (MSF)* The F2 nominates colleagues to provide feedback—tools available: Mini Peer Assessment Tool (mini-PAT), Team Assessment of Behaviours (TAB), multi-source feedback tool (Scotland).
- *Direct observation of doctor–patient encounters* An experienced colleague watches the F2. Tools available: Direct Observation of Procedural Skills (DOPS) for practice procedures; Mini Clinical Evaluation Exercise (Mini-CEX) for clinical consultations.
- *Case-Based Discussion (CBD)* Structured case review with a senior clinician.

**Foundation learning portfolio** Compulsory record of training. The doctor must prove that he/she has attained all the competences required

(Box 4.1) before progression to specialist training. May be paper-based or electronic. Includes:

- Completed assessments
- Educational agreements
- Reflective practice
- Personal development plan
- Records of meetings with educational supervisor.

---

### Box 4.1 Foundation level competences and core skills

#### Good clinical care
- Take a history/examine patients, prescribe safely, and keep an accurate and relevant medical record.
- Manage time and organizational decision-making appropriately.
- Maintain good quality care and ensure/promote patient safety.
- ↓ risk of cross-infection.
- Understand clinical governance.
- Ensure basic nutritional care.
- Educate patients effectively
- Cope with ethical and legal issues.

#### Maintaining good medical practice
- Start self-directed lifelong learning.
- Use evidence and guidelines that will benefit patient care.
- Use audit to improve patient care.

#### Teaching and training
- Undertake a teaching role.

#### Relationship with patients/communication skills
- Communicate effectively with patients, relatives, and colleagues.

#### Working with colleagues
- Demonstrate effective teamwork skills within the clinical team and in the larger medical context.

#### Professional behaviour/probity
- Always act in a professional manner.

#### Acute care
- Recognize critically ill patients, take part in advanced life support, feel confident to initiate resuscitation, lead the team where necessary, and use the local protocol for deciding when not to resuscitate patients.
- Function safely in an acute 'take' team.
- Plan discharge for patients.
- Select, appropriately request, and accurately interpret reports of frequently used investigations, and recognize abnormalities which need immediate action.

#### Practical procedures
- Competent/confident to do routine procedures/teach them to undergraduates.

---

**Further information**
**The Foundation Programme** 🖳 www.foundationprogramme.nhs.uk

# Becoming a GP in the UK

**Vocational training for GPs** currently involves 3y full-time (or the equivalent part time) specialty training after the foundation years. Trainees must:
- Complete speciality training in posts/programmes approved by the Postgraduate Medical Education and Training Board (PMETB).
- Complete all 3y training within the 7y period immediately preceding the date of formal application for a certificate.
- Pass the nMRCGP (📖 p.66).

## Recruitment and selection
- Applications for GP training must be made online to the National Recruitment Office for General Practice Training (NRO).
- All applicants meeting GP training entry criteria are invited to attend a national short-listing assessment consisting of a machine-markable test.
- Candidates are sorted in rank order. Highest scoring applicants are invited to attend a selection centre at their highest preferred location. Selection centres in England are the regional deaneries. Scotland, Wales, and Northern Ireland each have a single selection centre.
- The selection centre assessment comprises 3 workplace-based assessments, which include a patient simulation exercise. Following assessment, highest ranked applicants are offered training places in that area.
- Appointable candidates without training places are placed on a reserve list for the deanery. Any reserve candidates not offered local places are entered into national clearing.

**Criteria for training practices** Each region sets its own criteria for selection of practices to train prospective GPs. These relate to: the trainer as a doctor, the trainer as a teacher, and the training practice. Practices must demonstrate high-quality clinical care and administration, and a commitment and capability to educate a GP registrar. Details of local requirements can be obtained from regional deanery offices.

**Training** The 3y GP training programme (see Table 4.1) must include:
- ≥12mo (and preferably 18mo) full-time employment as a GP Registrar under the supervision of an approved trainer.
- 24mo full-time employment in hospital training posts approved for GP training in relevant hospital specialties.

The mix of specialities is important. GPs in training must have completed:
- ≥6mo in each of 2 List A specialities or
- ≥4mo in each of 3 List A specialities or
- ≥3mo in each of 4 List A specialties.

In addition, training for ≤6mo in any of the list B specialties is acceptable.

**RCGP Curriculum** describes the core knowledge, skills, and attitudes required to be a competent GP. It comprises 15 sections that cover the whole breadth of general practice. Access at 🖳 www.rcgp-curriculum.org.uk

**InnovAiT** RCGP Journal for GPs in training. Provided free to all GPs in training. Acts like a rolling textbook covering the breadth of the GP curriculum every 3y.

**Table 4.1** Specialties approved for GP training

| List A specialties | List B specialties |
| --- | --- |
| • A&E medicine<br>• Paediatrics or community paediatrics<br>• General medicine or geriatrics or dermatology or GU medicine or rehabilitation medicine<br>• Gynaecology or obstetrics/gynaecology<br>• Psychiatry or old age psychiatry<br>• Palliative medicine | • Cardiology or medical oncology or clinical oncology or gastroenterology or endocrinology and DM or haematology or nephrology or respiratory medicine or rheumatology or neurology or infectious diseases<br>• Child and adolescent psychiatry or psychiatry of learning disability<br>• Ophthalmology or ENT or general surgery or paediatric surgery or urology or trauma/orthopaedics<br>• Intensive therapy<br>• Public health medicine |

**The RCGP Certification Unit** Evaluates general practice training and makes recommendations for Certificates of Completion of Training (CCT) to the PMETB. Anyone undertaking a training programme for leading to a CCT should register with the Certification Unit.

**Certification under Article 10**
• During training, on completion of each placement, the clinical supervisor completes an assessment of the trainee's performance.
• The GP educational supervisor signs this assessment off as confirmation that there has been satisfactory progress in acquiring the relevant curriculum competencies.
• The portfolio of assessments is reviewed and endorsed by the deanery at least annually.
• Submission of this portfolio together with successful completion of the nMRCGP enables a GP registrar to apply for the CCT via the RCGP certification unit.

**Certification under Article 11** Equivalency route. For those having:
• Completed some or all of their training overseas
• Completed training in >7y, or
• Worked in a post prior to its approval as an educational post.

Successful application under Article 11 results in the award of a Statement of Eligibility for Registration (SER). More information on application under Article 11 is available on the certification section of the RCGP website (🖳 www.rcgp.org.uk).

**Postgraduate Medical Education & Training Board** Non-governmental independent regulatory body responsible for approving all GP training posts, the GP training curriculum, and the nMRCGP assessments. On receipt of the CCT/SER from a doctor, the PMETB informs the GMC and the doctor is entered onto the GMC's GP register in <7d.

**Further information**
RCGP ☎ 0207 581 3232 🖳 www.rcgp.org.uk
**National Recruitment Office for General Practice Training (NRO)**
🖳 www.gprecruitment.org.uk

# Membership of the Royal College of General Practitioners

**Membership of the Royal College of General Practitioners (nMRCGP)** The 'new' MRCGP is an assessment of professional competency based on modern educational theory and an evidence-based approach to assessment. It is the compulsory assessment for all doctors wishing to become GPs in the UK. It is made up of 3 assessments.

*Applied Knowledge Test (AKT)* 200 multiple-choice questions test whether the candidate can apply knowledge in the context of general practice. Computer-based assessment held at Pearson VUE computer centres across the country. Questions are distributed as follows: clinical medicine (80%); administration and informatics (10%); research, appraisal, evidence-based medicine and statistics (10%).

*Clinical Skills Assessment (CSA)* The CSA assesses behaviour in a mock surgery. The candidate performs 13 consultations each of 10 min duration (although only 12 count towards the final mark). The candidate remains in a consulting room and the patients, played by trained actors, come in one by one. The CSA is currently only available at one centre, in Croydon, and takes place 3 times a year in February, May, and October.

*Workplace Based Assessment (WPBA)* Continuous assessment based on the e-portfolio and trainer's report.

**nMRCGP competencies** The nMRCGP assessments are designed to assess GPs in training against 12 nMRCGP competency areas (Box 4.2).

**Fellowship of the RCGP** Candidates for Fellowship of the RCGP can self-nominate. The process of becoming a Fellow involves submitting a portfolio of evidence in one, any or all of 6 'achievement categories', reflecting the range of the GP's past and current roles and activities, together with a detailed personal statement of the GP's past and current roles and activities. The achievement categories are:

- Clinical practice
- Patient-centred practice
- Leadership
- Teaching & education
- Innovation & creativity
- Academic & research.

**❶** Candidates in active clinical practice must submit in the 'clinical practice' category.

For each submitted category, candidates must give the name of a referee able to vouch for the reliability of the evidence. When applying under >1 category, candidates should identify ≥2 different referees. The portfolio of evidence will be adjudicated in the first instance by an Adjudication Group and evaluated against published criteria. The Adjudication Group may either approve the application or refer it to the National Fellowship Committee for a final decision.

**Further information**
RCGP ☎ 0207 581 3232 ⌨ www.rcgp.org.uk

## Box 4.2 The 12 nMRCGP competency areas

**1.** *Communication and consultation skills* How a GP communicates with patients and uses recognized consultation models and communication techniques.

**2.** *Practising holistically* The ability of the doctor to operate in physical, psychological, socio-economic, and cultural dimensions, taking into account feelings as well as thoughts.

**3.** *Data gathering and interpretation* Gathering and use of data for making clinical judgements, choice of physical examinations and investigations, and how they are interpreted.

**4.** *Making a diagnosis/making decisions* How a GP adopts a structured conscious approach to decision-making.

**5.** *Clinical management* How a doctor recognizes and manages common medical conditions in primary care.

**6.** *Managing medical complexity and promoting health* Aspects of care that go beyond managing straightforward problems, including the management of comorbidity, uncertainty, risk, and approaches to health rather than just illness.

**7.** *Primary care administration and information technology* The appropriate use of primary care administration systems, effective record keeping, and information technology for the benefit of patient care.

**8.** *Working with colleagues and in teams* GPs must be able to work effectively with other health professionals to ensure good patient care, including the sharing of information with colleagues.

**9.** *Community orientation* Managing the health and social care of the practice population and local community.

**10.** *Maintaining performance, learning, and teaching* This looks at how doctors maintain their performance and ensure effective continuing professional development of themselves and others.

**11.** *Maintaining an ethical approach to practice* How GPs ensure that they practice ethically, with integrity and a respect for diversity.

**12.** *Fitness to practice* The GP's awareness of when his/her own performance, conduct, or health, or that of others, might put patients at risk, and the actions taken to protect patients.

Reproduced from Riley B, Haynes J, Field S (2007) *The Condensed Curriculum Guide*, RCGP, with permission of the Royal College of General Practitioners.

# Appraisal and revalidation

**Appraisal** Requires all doctors wishing to practice medicine in the UK to undergo a formal review on a yearly basis. It aims to:
- Set out personal and professional development needs, career paths and goals, and agree plans for them to be met.
- Review the doctor's performance and consider the doctor's contribution to quality and improvement of local healthcare services.
- Optimize the use of skills and resources in achieving the delivery of high quality care.
- Offer an opportunity for doctors to discuss and seek support for their participation in activities.
- Identify the need for adequate resources to enable service objectives to be met.

Based on the GMC's document *Good Medical Practice*, the appraisal is divided into the following sections:
- Good clinical care
- Maintaining good medical practice
- Teaching and training
- Relationships with patients
- Working with colleagues
- Probity
- Health.

**The appraiser** Chief executives of NHS organizations are accountable for ensuring that appraisal takes place and that appraisers are properly trained to carry out this role and are in a position to undertake appraisal of a doctor's whole practice, including clinical performance, and where appropriate, specialist aspects of performance, e.g. research, service delivery, or management issues. In general appraisers for GPs will be other GPs.

## The appraisal process
- *Before the interview* Doctors must prepare an appraisal folder containing information and supporting evidence about their practise and personal needs. Folders should be submitted to the appraiser ≥ 2wk prior to appraisal interviews to allow adequate time for preparation. An electronic 'Toolkit' and further information are available at 🖳 www.appraisals.nhs.uk
- *At the interview* Doctor and appraiser agree a summary of achievement in the past year, objectives for the next year, key elements of a personal development plan, and actions expected of the organization.
- *After the interview* A summary document is produced (usually by the doctor being appraised) and a joint declaration signed that the appraisal has been carried out properly.

## Further information
🖳 www.appraisals.nhs.uk
**RCGP** Principles of GP Appraisal 🖳 www.rcgp.org.uk

⚠ **Concerns about performance** In the first instance, any GP with concerns about their own, or a colleague's, performance should discuss the matter confidentially with the secretary of their LMC, with the clinical governance lead/performance information manager of their PCO or with the GMC.

## Revalidation

*'The regular demonstration by doctors that they remain fit to practise.'*[1]

Regular revalidation will become a requirement for all doctors practising in the UK before the end of 2011.

**What is revalidation?** Revalidation is formed of 2 processes:
- **Relicensure** All doctors registered with the General Medical Council will be required to hold a licence to practise which will need to be renewed every 5y; and
- **Recertification** Those doctors working unsupervised within specialities have been issued with certificates and appear on either the GMC's Specialist or GP registers. In order to continue to be on these registers indicating specialist skills, doctors will need to renew their certificates every 5y.

**Proposed routes to revalidation** Doctors will need to be able to show the GMC that they have followed the standards within Good Medical Practice relevant to their specialty and practice. It is the doctor's responsibility, not that of anyone else.

In general practice it is proposed that evidence will be gathered with direction through the annual appraisal process and then submitted every five years. Exact details of the evidence needed are yet to be determined.

### Outcomes of revalidation
- **Revalidation** licence to practise and certificate of specialist skills will remain valid.
- **Insufficient information** The GMC cannot revalidate the doctor because he/she has not given it enough information. It will ask the doctor to send additional information, and then reconsider the case.
- **Inadequate information** The GMC is not persuaded by the information the doctor has provided, including any additional information that was asked for, that he/she should be revalidated.

**Withdrawing a licence to practise** The GMC will withdraw a licence if:
- The doctor tells them they no longer want it
- The doctor does not pay the appropriate fee
- The doctor does not take part in the revalidation process when they ask them to, or
- A Fitness to Practise panel directs that the doctor's registration should be suspended or erased.

A doctor has a right of appeal against any decision to withdraw, or refuse to restore, their licence to practise.

### Further information
**GMC** 🖥 www.gmc-uk.org
**RCGP** Guide to revalidation (2009) 🖥 www.rcgp.org.uk

---

[1] From General Medical Council. A license to practice and revalidation. London: GMC, 2003.

# Career options for GPs

Times are changing in general practice. Doctors considering a life as a GP want a more flexible and varied career than in the past.

## Career options within the NHS

**Clinical assistant or hospital practitioner** The GP works within a hospital setting on the wards or in out-patients, providing a specialist service under direct supervision of a hospital consultant. Posts are usually advertised in medical/GP post ± locally. Generally poorly paid.

**GP with special clinical interests (GpwSI)** GPs who, in addition to their normal GP duties, provide a specialist service to meet the needs of their local PCO. They might deliver a specialist clinical service beyond the scope of normal general practice, undertake advanced procedures, or develop services. The main difference between a GPwSI and clinical assistant is that the GPwSI receives referrals from other GPs and will decide on the appropriate treatment independently and not under direct supervision of a consultant, but with the support of secondary care. Apply to local PCO. In order to be classed as having a special interest, GPs must:
• Have undertaken particular training in the specialty, or have a proven track record of expertise in the specialty
• Regularly update knowledge through attendance at courses, conferences, or meetings, and through reading
• Look after a specific group of patients with the condition
• Audit practice in the specialty area, thereby demonstrating quality of care.

**Medical adviser or consultant in primary care** Medical advisers or directors in ambulance trusts, NHS Direct sites, etc. Some national NHS agencies also have GP advisers or directors, e.g. National Clinical Governance Support Team. Posts are either advertised or obtained by direct approach.

**Providing GMS/PMS ± enhanced medical services** 📖 p.20

**Providing postgraduate medical education** e.g. GP tutor, GP trainer (1:8 GPs are GP trainers), course organizer. Approach local director or dean of postgraduate medical education.

**Working for a local PCO** e.g. serving on a committee, clinical tutor, GP appraiser, etc. Contact local PCO.

## Opportunities outside the NHS

**Academic posts** A GP may be employed solely by a university or jointly by a university and the NHS. Posts include undergraduate teachers, lecturers, and research posts. Contact local university department of general practice or look for posts advertised in the medical/GP press.

**Clinical sessions for commercial companies and charities** e.g. school doctor for a private school.

**Complementary medicine** Seek specialist training. Contact representative bodies of the specialty chosen (📖 p.156).

**Forensic work** e.g. police surgeon, coroner, expert witness (🖥 www.ewi.org.uk).

**Media work/medical author** Some sort of professional journalism qualification is useful. The BMJ offers a 1y registrar post for doctors with 3–5y experience. Courses are also available through the BMA and Medical Journalists Association (🖳 www.mja-uk.org). If you have an idea for a book, contact the medical commissioning editor of a reputable publisher to discuss your ideas. If you would like to write or review an article for a journal, go onto the journal homepage and look for the author and reviewer instructions, or contact the journal's editorial office.

**Medical adviser posts within GP and other medical organizations** e.g. RCGP, MDU, GMC. Posts may be advertised or appointments made through election or direct approach. Contact the relevant organization.

**Medicals for benefits** Examining Medical Practitioners (EMPs) carrying out fitness to work and disability assessments on behalf of the Department for Work and Pensions (DWP).

**Medical politics** GPs serve on local medical committees (LMCs) on an elected basis. Contact local LMC and ask about standing for election.

**Work for government agencies** e.g. armed forces as a civilian medical practitioner or the territorial army. Usually civilian posts are advertised in the medical/GP press. For commissioned posts contact service recruitment offices.

**Occupational medicine** Contact: Faculty for Occupational Medicine (🖳 www.facoccmed.ac.uk).

**Prison doctor** Posts usually advertised in the medical/GP press.

**Sports medicine** e.g. for professional sportsmen, in private clinics. Doctors are required to have a knowledge of sports injuries and their treatment, rehabilitation, and prevention. They also need to know about other aspects of sport, e.g. drugs in sport, nutrition, travel problems. Contact British Association of Sport and Exercise Medicine (🖳 www.basem.co.uk).

**Work abroad** Contact RCGP International Department (email: international@rcgp.org.uk); RedR UK (🖳 www.redr.org.uk); Voluntary Service Overseas (🖳 www.vso.org.uk). Overseas posts are also advertised in the medical press.

# Clinical governance

Clinical governance is a far-reaching quality initiative. It is defined as *'a framework through which NHS organizations are accountable for continuously improving the quality of their services and safeguarding high standards of care by creating an environment in which excellence in clinical care will flourish'.*[1] Although the onus is on NHS organizations to make these changes, the legislation makes it clear that all health professionals, guided by their professional bodies, are expected to adhere to the concept.

**Essential elements of clinical governance** Figure 4.1

## What does clinical governance entail?

- Every PCO must appoint a health professional as clinical governance lead.
- PCOs must publish routine reports and an annual progress report on the local implementation of clinical governance.
- Within practices, individual doctors must consider their own professional development and educational needs.
- Performance and development of other health professionals engaged by practices must be assessed regularly.
- Within practices there must be continuous review and appraisal of procedures and standards (**RAID**):
    **R**eview—gather all stakeholders together to look at a topic
    **A**gree strategy to take forward
    **I**ntervene—make changes decided upon
    **D**emonstrate the effect of changes through audit (📖 p.80), patient satisfaction questionnaire, prescribing data etc.
- External peer review should be encouraged.
- Deficiencies in knowledge, skills, or experience must be acted upon through appropriate education and professional development.
- Resources should be provided to help develop clinical governance— time out for audit, PCO meetings, and to address educational needs; funding for courses and educational activities to address deficiencies and enable more effective assessment of standards and performance.

⚠ **Concerns about performance** In the first instance, any GP with concerns about their own, or a colleague's, performance should discuss the matter confidentially with the secretary of their LMC, with the clinical governance lead/performance information manager of their PCO, or with the GMC.

## Further information

**Clinical governance** *Quality in the new NHS* HSC 1999/065 (16 March 1999) 🖥 www.dh.gov.uk

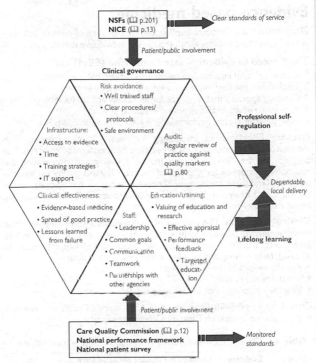

**Fig. 4.1** Model of clinical governance within the NHS quality improvement framework

1 Department of Health (1998). *A first class service: quality in the new NHS.*

# Evidence-based medicine

**Definition** Conscientious, explicit, and judicious use of current best evidence in making decisions about the care of individual patients.

### The 5 steps of evidence-based medicine (EBM) are

1 Convert clinical information needs into answerable questions.
2 Track down the best evidence with which to answer them.
3 Critically appraise that evidence for its validity and usefulness.
4 Apply the results of this appraisal in clinical practice.
5 Evaluate your clinical performance, e.g. through audit (📖 p.80).

Practising EBM involves integrating individual clinical expertise with the best available external clinical evidence from systematic research. The problem for the clinician on the ground is finding and interpreting the appropriate evidence for the clinical situation. If good quality evidence is out there (and there are many under-researched areas in medicine)—How do you access it? When do you find the time to search for it? How do you assess its quality and relevance?

**Critical appraisal** The process of assessing and interpreting evidence by systematically considering its validity, results, and relevance (Table 4.2). Essential to avoid misinterpretation and misuse of evidence in practice. In all cases, before integrating evidence into practice consider:
• Are the results of the study valid?
• What are the results?
• Will they help me in caring for my patients?

Critical Appraisal Skills Programme (CASP) appraisal tools are available from 🖥 www.phru.nhs.uk/Pages/PHD/resources.htm

**Table 4.2** Classification and grading of evidence: Most → least reliable

| Grade | Evidence level | Definition: *Evidence obtained from …* |
|-------|----------------|------------------------------------------|
| A | Ia | Meta-analysis of randomized controlled trials |
| | Ib | At least one randomized controlled trial |
| B | IIa | At least one well-designed controlled study without randomization, e.g. case-controlled study; cohort study |
| | IIb | At least one other type of well-designed quasi-experimental study |
| | III | Well-designed non-experimental descriptive studies, such as comparative studies, correlation studies, and case studies |
| C | IV | Expert committee reports or opinions and/or clinical experience of respected authorities |

**Table 4.3** Useful web resources

| | Website: http:// + suffix |
|---|---|
| General information | |
| National Electronic Library for Health | www.library.nhs.uk (has guidelines index and numerous links to EBM websites) |
| Bandolier | www.medicine.ox.ac.uk/bandolier |
| Evidence-based Medicine | ebm.bmjjournals.com |
| Guidelines | |
| NICE | www.nice.org.uk |
| Scottish Intercollegiate Guidelines Network (SIGN) | www.sign.ac.uk |
| eGuidelines | www.eguidelines.co.uk (registration needed) |
| National Guidelines Clearing House (USA) | www.guideline.gov |
| New Zealand Guidelines Group | www.nzgg.org.nz |
| Systematic reviews | |
| Cochrane library | www.cochrane.co.uk |
| Clinical Evidence (BMJ Publishing) | www.clinicalevidence.com |
| Health Technology Assessment (HTA) | www.ncchta.org |
| Drugs and Therapeutic Bulletin (DTB) | www.dtb.bmj.com (subscription required) |
| MeReC Bulletin | www.npc.co.uk/ebt/merec.htm |
| PubMed* | www.pubmed.gov |
| Knowledge summaries | |
| Clinical Knowledge Summaries (CKS) | www.cks.library.nhs.uk |

*When searching aim to retrieve all the most relevant citations with a minimum of junk. A useful tip is to use the Clinical Queries or Systematic Reviews filter to restrict the amount of information retrieved.

## Further information

**Sackett DL et al.** *Evidence-based Medicine: How to Practice and Teach EBM* (1997) Churchill Livingstone (ISBN 0443 056862)
**Crombie IK** *The Pocket Guide to Critical Appraisal* (1996) BMJ Books (ISBN 072791099X)
**Greenhalgh T** *How to Read a Paper* (2000) BMJ Books (ISBN 0727915789)

# Glossary of terms used in evidence-based medicine

**Absolute risk reduction/increase** The absolute arithmetic difference in rates of bad outcomes between experimental and control participants in a trial, calculated as the difference between experimental event rate (EER) and control event rate (CER).

**Bias** Systematic disposition of certain trial designs to produce results consistently better or worse than other trial designs. Always consider whether a study is biased before accepting its conclusions. Further information: 🖳 www.jr2.ox.ac.uk/bandolier/Extraforbando/Bias.pdf

**Case–control study** Involves identifying patients who have the outcome of interest (cases) and control patients without the same outcome, and looking back to see if they had the exposure of interest.

**Cohort study** Involves identification of two groups (cohorts) of patients: one that received the exposure of interest, and one that did not, and following these cohorts forward for the outcome of interest.

**Confidence interval (CI)** Quantifies uncertainty in measurement. Usually reported as 95% CI, which is the range of values within which we can be 95% sure that the true value for the whole population lies.

**Control event rate (CER)** The rate at which events occur in a control group. It may be represented by a percentage (e.g. 10%) or a proportion (e.g. 0.1).

**Cost–benefit analysis** Assesses whether the cost of an intervention is worth the benefit by measuring both in the same units—usually monetary units. Further information: 🖳 www.medicine.ox.ac.uk/bandolier/painres/download/whatis/Cost-effect.pdf

**Cross-sectional study** Observation of a defined population at a single point in time or time interval.

**Experimental event rate (EER)** The rate at which events occur in an experimental group. May be expressed as a percentage or proportion (see CER).

**False negative/positive** 📖 p.173

**Likelihood ratio (LR)** Likelihood that a given test result would be expected in a patient with the target disorder compared with the likelihood that the same result would be expected in a patient without the target disorder. Gives an indication of accuracy of a clinical test. The higher the likelihood ratio, the better the test at detecting the disorder.

**Meta-analysis** Systematic review that uses quantitative methods to summarise the results. Further information: 🖳 www.medicine.ox.ac.uk/bandolier/painres/download/whatis/Meta-An.pdf

**Number needed to treat (NNT)** A measure of the difference between active treatment and control treatment. An NNT of 1 describes a situation where an event occurs in every patient given the active treatment but no patient in the comparison group. There are few circumstances in which a treatment is 100% effective and placebo completely ineffective, so NNTs of 2–3 indicate an effective intervention.

*Calculating NNT:*

$A =$ number who had successful outcome with the intervention divided by total number who had the intervention

$B =$ number who had successful outcome with control divided by total number who had the control

$$NNT = \frac{1}{A - B}$$

**Number needed to harm (NNH)** Compares the number having a side effect in the intervention group with the number having that side effect in the comparison group. If no one in the control group and no one in the comparison group has an unwanted effect, the NNH will be infinity. Therefore the NNH should be as large as possible.

**Odds ratio (OR)** Odds of an event are calculated as the number of events divided by the number of non-events. The odds ratio is the ratio of the odds in the experimental group compared with the control group. For epidemiological studies looking for factors causing harm, an odds ratio >1 indicates that the factor the experimental group was exposed to caused harm. For experimental studies looking for a decrease in events through treatment, an odds ratio <1 indicates a positive result. Often expressed as a percentage.

**Positive predictive value** 📖 p.173

**Relative risk or risk ratio (RR)** Ratio of risk in the treated group (EER) to risk in the control group (CER): RR = EER/CER. It used in randomized trials and cohort studies. If RR=1 there is no difference between the two groups for that measure.

**Relative risk reduction (RRR)** Difference between the EER and CER divided by the CER: RR = (EER–CER)/CER Usually expressed as a percentage.

**Sensitivity** 📖 p.173

**Specificity** 📖 p.173

**Systematic review** Summary of the medical literature that uses explicit methods to perform a thorough literature search and critical appraisal of individual studies and uses appropriate statistical techniques to combine results of studies of acceptable quality.

# Clinical guidelines, protocols, and integrated care pathways

**Clinical guidelines** Defined as '*user-friendly statements that bring together the best external evidence and other knowledge necessary for decision-making about a specific health problem*'.[1] Over recent years there has been a dramatic ↑ in publication of guidelines and protocols. They aim to ↓ harmful or expensive variations in clinical practice, improve healthcare outcomes, and encourage rapid dissemination of useful innovations. Good clinical guidelines have 3 properties.

- They define practice questions and identify all their decision options and outcomes.
- They identify, appraise, and summarize best evidence about prevention, diagnosis, prognosis, therapy, harm, and cost-effectiveness.
- They identify the decision points at which the evidence needs to be integrated with individual clinical experience and clinical circumstances in deciding a course of action.

***Before starting to use a guideline*** Always ask:

'Is this guideline valid, important and applicable in my practice?'

*If the answer is yes then consider:*
- What barriers exist to implementation?
- Can they be overcome?
- Can you enlist collaboration of key colleagues?
- Can you meet the educational and administrative conditions that are likely to determine the success or failure of implementing the strategy?

**Protocol** is the term reserved for guidelines at the more rigid end of the spectrum. These are very specific guidelines which are expected to be followed in detail, with little scope for variation e.g. resuscitation protocols.

**Integrated care pathway (ICP)** ICPs amalgamate all the anticipated elements of care and treatment of the multidisciplinary team, for a particular patient group in order to achieve agreed outcomes. Any deviation from the plan is documented as variance—the analysis of which provides information for the review of current practice. ICPs aim to:
- Facilitate introduction of guidelines and systemic audit into clinical practice
- Improve multidisciplinary communication and care planning
- Reach or exceed existing standards
- Decrease unwanted practice variation
- Improve clinician—patient communication and patient satisfaction
- Identify research and development questions
- Cross the interface between primary, secondary, and social care.

**Grading/classification of evidence** 📖 p.74

## Box 4.3 Advantages and disadvantages of guidelines

### Advantages
- Provide guidance for busy clinicians—a consistent basis for decision-making.
- Practical framework for common problems and chronic disease.
- Summarize the available research evidence.
- Can be used as a basis for continuing medical education.
- Justification for expenditure—can aid cost-effective use of limited resources.
- Facilitate the audit cycle.

### Disadvantages
- Poor-quality guidelines can reinforce poor practice.
- Lack of relevance of the guidelines to the clinical setting—much of the 'evidence' used to develop guidelines comes from secondary care and may not reflect the situation in primary care.
- Tendency to uniformity—can stifle innovation.
- Resistance to change—new methods may not be considered until a new guideline is produced.
- Increased risk of litigation.
- Cost—they are time consuming to develop and update.
- Lack of ownership—guidelines developed by others may not feel relevant.
- Difficulties in implementation—guidelines that are not user-friendly and well disseminated will not be used.

## Further information

**National Electronic Library for Health** Guidelines database, integrated care pathways database, and useful information on development of guidelines. ☐ www.library.nhs.uk
**NICE** ☐ www.nice.nhs.uk
**Scottish Intercollegiate Guidelines Network** ☐ www.sign.ac.uk
**eGuidelines:** ☐ www.eguidelines.co.uk (free registration required)
**National Guidelines Clearing House (US)** ☐ www.guideline.gov
**New Zealand Guidelines Group** ☐ www.nzgg.org.nz

---

[1] Sackett DL et al. (1997) Evidence-based medicine. New York: Churchill Livingstone.

# Audit

Audit is defined as the systematic critical analysis of quality of health care. Its purpose is to appraise current practice (*What is happening?*) by measuring it against preselected standards (*What should be happening?*) to identify and implement areas for change (*What changes are needed?*) and thus improve performance.

Audit differs from research as research aims to establish what best practice is globally, whereas audit aims to discover how close practice is to best practice on a local level and identify ways of improving care. Audit is a continual process and an integral part of clinical governance (🕮 p.72). All practices in the UK are involved in audit in some way.

## Aims of audit

- Improved care of patients
- Enhanced professionalism of staff
- Efficient use of resources
- Aid to continuing education
- Aid to administration
- Accountability to those outside the profession.

**Criterion-based audit—the audit cycle** The process of identifying areas of care to be audited, implementing necessary changes, and periodically reviewing the same issues is known as the audit cycle (Figure 4.2).

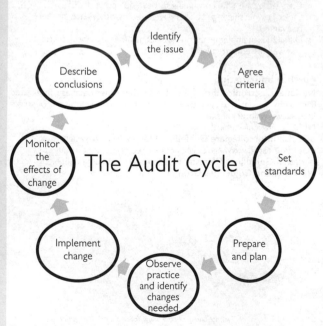

Fig. 4.2 The audit cycle

**Choosing a topic** Any practice matter—clinical or administrative. Make sure the topic is important, manageable, and clearly defined, and that data are available to assess the criteria chosen. Good starting points are significant events, QOF targets, complaints, NSF or clinical guideline topics, and personal observations.

**Choosing criteria** Criteria are specific statements of what should be happening. Criteria might be those laid down for quality payments, 'gold standard' care as defined in guidelines, or generated within the practice. Use evidence-based criteria wherever possible. All criteria have to be measurable, ideally with data already collected.

**Setting standards** Standards are minimum levels of acceptable performance for a criterion. 100% achievement of standards is unusual, so set realistic standards based on quality framework levels and standards achieved by other practices (e.g. comparative practice data, audits from other practices) or previous audits within the practice.

**Observing practice** You can collect information from computer registers, medical records, questionnaires (patients, staff, or GPs), data collection sheets (e.g. drugs in doctor's bag are all in date).

**Comparing results with standards** Consider why standards have not been met. What should be done? Who's going to do it? When? How?

**Repeating the audit cycle** to ensure action taken is effective.

**Significant event audit** Process in which individual episodes (when there has been a significant occurrence either beneficial or deleterious) are analysed in a systematic and detailed way to ascertain what can be learnt about the overall quality of care, and to indicate changes that might lead to future improvements. Methods of reporting—Table 4.4.

**Table 4.4** Methods of reporting significant event audits

| Reporting method 1 | Reporting method 2 |
| --- | --- |
| *Description of event* This should be brief and can be in note form | What happened? |
| | Why did it happen? |
| *Learning outcome* This should describe the aspects which were of high standard and those that could be improved. Where appropriate it should include why the event occurred | Was insight demonstrated? |
| | Was change implemented? |
| *Action plan* The decision(s) taken need to be contained in the report. The reasons for these decisions should be described together with any other lessons learned from the discussion | |

## Further information

**NICE** Best practice in clinical audit.
🖳 www.nice.org.uk/pdf/BestPracticeClinicalAudit.pdf
**RCGP** Occasional Paper 70: Significant event audit (1995)
🖳 www.rcgp.org.uk

# Research in general practice

Discovery of new knowledge (*research*) and spreading that knowledge (*dissemination*) is essential for provision of high-quality care. GPs may be involved in research at many levels—as part of an academic department, in a research general practice, or just taking part in a project. Drug company research—📖 p.150.

**National Institute for Health Research (NIHR)** Commissions and funds NHS and Social Care research in England, and provides infrastructure to support both studies and researchers within the NHS. 🖥 www.nihr.ac.uk

**Primary Care Research Network (PCRN)** One of a number of research networks that operate under the umbrella of the NIHR. Focuses on areas of research for which primary care has particular responsibility: disease prevention, health promotion, screening, early diagnosis, and the clinical management of long-term conditions. Studies may be accepted onto its portfolio if the topic of the research falls within the remit of the PCRN and funding has been obtained through a recognized funding body as a result of open competition and peer review. The PCRN keeps a list of all the studies in its portfolio.

Within the PCRN there are 8 local research networks. These provide support to researchers developing proposals and studies within the portfolio through network-funded staff. This can be anything from help with formulation of a study proposal, through identification of subjects and recruitment, to help with data management. 🖥 www.ukrn.org.uk

❶ A separate Primary Care Research Network operates in Scotland.

**University departments of general practice** Every UK medical school has a department of general practice, but there are very few GP academic posts. However, these departments are invaluable sources of advice and support if you contemplate doing any original research of your own.

**RCGP** Supports research by giving advice to GPs, providing research training fellowships and research funding through the Scientific Foundation Board, sponsoring research units and research practices, and administering a quality assessment scheme for research practices. 🖥 www.rcgp.org.uk.

**Ethics** An ethics committee must pass all medical research involving human participants. Information, contacts, and application forms are available from the National Research Ethics Service. 🖥 www.nres.npsa.nhs.uk.

**Funding** Numerous sources of funding for primary care research are available (including NHS, RCGP, Medical Research Council, and Wellcome Trust), but all are keenly fought for. Take time preparing your protocol. Ask for advice. It helps to have an experienced researcher as co-applicant on the application form or as project supervisor. 🖥 www.rdfunding.org.uk

**Turn your idea into a specific research question**
- What is your aim/hypothesis?
- Review the literature (□ p.74)
- Is your idea novel?
- Why does it matter?

**Design the study and develop your methods**
- Involve participants/other researchers
- Qualitative or quantitative methodology?
- Survey design/sample size
- How are you going to choose/randomize participants?
- Who is going to do the work?

**Obtain permissions, funding and PCRN acceptance**
- Ask the healthcare trust in which the research will be performed
- Ensure that you contact the research governance officer of the organization within which your research will be carried out, and comply with local and national requirements
- Obtain ethics permission
- Obtain funding to cover the costs of the study and staff required
- Gain acceptance onto the PCRN (or another research network) portfolio

**Collect and collate data** Remember the importance of data protection (□ p.74)

**Analyse and interpret data**
- Consider involving a professional statistician for quantitative data
- Think about the implications of the study findings
- Identify how findings can be put into practice

**Write up and disseminate findings**
- Journal articles
- Conference presentations
- Press releases
- Submission for higher degrees

**Fig. 4.3** The research process

# Outcomes in general practice

Within the NHS there are ↑ demands for accountability and improvements in quality of care. In general practice the outcome measures used to judge 'quality of care' are a matter of some debate. Possible measures are:

**Patient satisfaction** The definition of satisfaction is not uniform. It implies to a varying degree meeting both the wants and the needs of the patient. Questionnaires often have low validity and reliability, and satisfaction scores are closely related to the psychological health of a patient, i.e. someone who is depressed is less likely to be satisfied with services. Nevertheless, satisfaction measures are increasingly being used to judge the effectiveness of the NHS. In the surgery, patient satisfaction audits (e.g. of the appointments system) are a useful way of identifying deficiencies in the system from the user's perspective which can then be improved. Two surveys are approved for use in the 'patient experience' domain of the QOF (📖 p.26):

• *Improving Patient Questionnaire (IPQ)* ❶ charge payable. 🖳 www.cfep.co.uk
• *General Practice Assessment Questionnaire (GPAQ)* 🖳 www.gpaq.info

Surveys of satisfaction show ~80% of patients are satisfied overall with GP care. However, if questioned more specifically about different components of care (e.g. information provided, communication, etc.), <50% are completely satisfied.

**Patient recall** Many studies suggest that >50% (some estimate up to 90%) of information has been forgotten within a few minutes of leaving the surgery. Characteristics of memorable information:

• The patient perceives it as important.
• The patient understands it (avoid the use of jargon and medical terms, keep language brief and simple, support information with sketches/diagrams ± patient information sheets).
• The information is given early in the consultation.
• The information is given in ↑ small chunks (not too much at once).

**Patient concordance or compliance** Another measure of the effectiveness of a consultation is the degree to which the patient complies with advice and uses medication supplied as directed. In general practice ~1/3 follow advice closely enough to make it effective, ~1/3 follow some advice but not closely enough to make it effective, and ~1/3 follow no advice at all.

**Prescribing rates** There are wide variations in prescribing rates (e.g. variation in the rate of statin prescription cannot be accounted for by population characteristics; prescription rates for antibiotics for minor illness vary widely between GPs). Whether and how these reflect quality of care is controversial.

**Referral rates** There are wide variations in referral rates (~3–12/100 consultations) not accounted for by population characteristics. Referral rates are not related to age of the GP or GP experience, use of investigations, or postgraduate qualifications. Experience in a specialty ↑ referrals to that specialty, implying high referrers are not necessarily inadequate. Attempts have been made to judge appropriateness of referrals, but the assessor is often not aware of the full circumstances of the referral, e.g. it is appropriate to refer a child for a paediatric opinion purely to allay parental anxiety but the referral might be deemed inappropriate on clinical grounds.

**Doctors' ability to detect illness** There are wide variations between GPs in their ability to detect certain illnesses, e.g. mental illness. GPs adept at identifying mental health problems have empathy, early eye contact, use directive rather than closed questioning, and clarify the complaint at an early stage. Whether this is a marker of quality of care or just the diversity of general practice is debatable.

**Performance of procedures** Comparisons of procedure outcome (e.g. inadequate smear rates, diabetic outcome measures, immunization rates) between practices can be a way of identifying practices or GPs clearly performing less well than others. The reasons for the discrepancy must then be investigated.

# Consulting and certification

# The consultation

Good communication is an essential for all aspects of a GP's work.

**Potential barriers to effective communication** Lack of time, language problems, differing gender, age, ethnic or social background of doctor and patient, 'sensitive' issues to address, 'hidden' or differing agendas, prior difficult meetings, lack of trust between doctor and patient.

**The consultation** Cornerstone of general practice. Various models exist (📖 p.90). Focuses on successful information exchange. There is no 'correct' way to perform a consultation. Approach will vary according to situation and participants.

*Patient centredness* Patient centredness in which the patient's viewpoint is considered and integrated into the diagnosis and decision-making process, seems to improve patient satisfaction and may improve health outcomes. Consists of 6 interactive components:[1]

- Exploring the disease and illness experience
- Understanding the whole person in context
- Finding common ground regarding management
- Incorporating prevention and health promotion
- Enhancing the doctor patient relationship
- Being realistic.

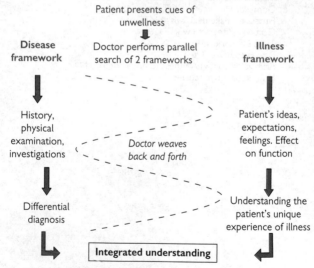

**Fig. 5.1** The patient-centred process
Reproduced from Stewart M et al. (1995) *Patient-Centred Medicine: Transforming the Clinical Method*, with permission from Sage Publications.

[1] Stewart M et al. (1995) *Patient-Centered Medicine: Transforming the Clinical Method*, Sage (ISBN 0-8039-5689-4)

**Consultation length** Average consultation length (face-to-face time) in the UK is 7min (for '10min appointments' face-to-face time is 8min). Consultation length has ↑ over the last 30y but is still shorter in the UK (~½ the length) than in Canada or New Zealand. Personality and attitudes influence consultation length—female GPs, older GPs, those with MRCGP, and those with a +ve attitude to mental health problems tend to have longer consultations.

*Beneficial effects of longer consultation times*
- ↑ patient and doctor satisfaction
- Improved doctor–patient communication
- ↑identification of psychosocial problems and health promotion
- ↓ reconsultation rates and prescriptions for minor illnesses.

However, as the length of time allocated ↑, the proportion of face-to-face time ↓.

**Consultation rate** Average number of consultations per registered patient per year is 2.5–6. Factors affecting the consultation rate:
- List size (↑ list size → ↓ rate)
- Personal lists (↓ rate)
- New and elderly patients (↑ rate)
- Not prescribing for minor ailments (↓ rate)
- Social deprivation (↑ rate)
- Time of year (↑ in winter)
- ↑ health promotion (↑ rate).

**Time-keeping** Running late is stressful and frustrating for patients. General practice does not fit conveniently into 10min (or any other size) chunks. Even the best time keepers occasionally run late. Tips:
- *Endeavour to run to time* Start on time; make appointments long enough (e.g. book double appointments for difficult problems, schedule catch-up slots in the middle of surgeries, change to longer appointments); break difficult problems or multiple problems up into chunks.
- *If you are running late* ask reception staff to apologize to patients as they check in and tell them the expected delay.

# Consultation models

The consultation process has been extensively studied—each model views it from a slightly different perspective. A brief overview of each is presented here; for more information consult the original texts:

**The medical model** Traditional model: history-taking → examination → investigation → diagnosis → treatment → follow-up. Does not recognize the complexity and diversity of the consultation in general practice.

**Balint 1957** *The Doctor, His Patient and the Illness* A philosophy rather than a consultation model.
• Psychological problems are often manifested physically
• Doctors have feelings. Those feelings have a role in the consultation
• Doctors need to be trained to be more sensitive to what is going on in the patient's mind during a consultation.
*Reference:* Churchill Livingstone (ISBN 0443064601)

**Berne 1964** *Games People Play* Describes how to recognize behaviours ('games') patients might use and roles patient and doctor might adopt— 'parent, adult, and child'.
*Reference:* Penguin Books (ISBN: 0140027688)

**RCGP 1972** 'The triaxial approach'—Physical, psychological, and social approach to consultation.
*Reference:* Working party of the RCGP, 1972

**Becker and Maiman 1975** *Health Belief Model* Involves exploration of concerns, beliefs and expectations of the patient. 5 elements:
• Health motivation
• Perceived vulnerability
• Perceived seriousness
• Perceived costs/benefits of an action
• Cues to action—stimuli/triggers for beliefs.
*Reference:* Med Care **13**,10–24

**Heron 1975** *Six Category Intervention Analysis* Six types of intervention a doctor could use with a patient:
1 Prescriptive
2 Informative
3 Confronting
4 Cathartic
5 Catalytic
6 Supportive.
*Reference:* University of Surrey

**Byrne and Long 1976** *Doctors Talking to Patients* 6 aspects:
1 Doctor establishes a relationship with the patient
2 Doctor attempts to/actually discovers the reason for attendance
3 Doctor conducts verbal ± physical examination
4 Doctor or doctor + patient or the patient consider the condition
5 Doctor (occasionally the patient) detail treatment and investigation
6 Consultation is terminated—usually by the doctor.
*Reference:* RCGP; ISBN: 0850840929

**Stott and Davis 1979** *Exceptional potential of the consultation.* 4 tasks:
1 Management of presenting problems
2 Management of continuing problems
3 Modification of help-seeking behaviour
4 Opportunistic health promotion.
*Reference:* JRCGP **29**, 201–5

**Helman's folk model 1981** *Disease vs. illness in general practice:*
- What has happened?
- Why has it happened?
- What would happen if nothing where done about it?
- What should I do and who should I consult for further help?
- Why to me?
- Why now?

*Reference:* JRCGP 1981 **31** 548–52

**Pendleton et al. 1984** *The doctor's tasks.*
- Define the reason for patient's attendance.
- Consider other problems (continuing problems and at-risk factors).
- Choose an appropriate action for each problem (involves negotiation between doctor and patient).
- Achieve a shared understanding of the problem (doctor and patient).
- Involve the patient in the management and encourage the patient to accept appropriate responsibility.
- Use time and resources appropriately.
- Establish and maintain a relationship (between doctor and patient).

*Reference:* OUPress (ISBN 01926328840)

**Neighbour 1987** *The Inner Consultation.* Checkpoints:
- Connecting (doctor establishes rapport with the patient).
- Summarizing (doctor clarifies the patient's reason for consulting).
- Handing over (doctor/patient negotiate and agree a management plan).
- Safety netting (doctor-patient plan for the unexpected—managing uncertainty).
- Housekeeping (doctor is aware of his/her own emotions).

*Reference:* Petroc Press (ISBN 1900603675)

**Fraser 1992** *Areas of competence*
1 Interviewing and history-taking
2 Physical examination
3 Diagnosis and problem-solving
4 Patient management
5 Relating to patients
6 Anticipatory care
7 Record-keeping

*Reference:* Butterworth Heinemann (ISBN 0750610057)

**Kurtz and Silverman 1996, update 2003** *Calgary–Cambridge Observation Guide.* 5 tasks:
1 Initiating the session
2 Gathering information
3 Building the relationship
4 Giving information—explaining and planning
5 Closing the session

*Reference:* Med Educ **30**, 83–9 & Acad Med **78**, 802–9

**Warren 2002** *Four avenues of analysis (BARD)*
- **B**ehaviour: non-verbal and verbal—needs of patient/personality of GP.
- **A**ims: purpose of the consultation and priorities.
- **R**oom: setting for the consultation.
- **D**ialogue: tone of voice, what is said etc.

*Reference:* Update 5.9.2002 152–4

**Launer 2002** *Narrative-based approach.* 6 key concepts:
- Conversations
- Curiosity
- Circularity
- Contexts
- Co-creation
- Caution.

*Reference:* Radcliffe Medical Press (ISBN 1857755391)

# Patient records

### General principles

- *Be factual, consistent, and accurate* Write records in an indelible fashion as soon as possible after an event/encounter has occurred. Ensure logical sequence; be clear, unambiguous, legible, and concise. Use standard coding techniques if using an electronic record. Wherever possible write notes openly whilst patients/carers are present in terms that they can understand. Date, time, and sign (or otherwise identify yourself) on all entries
- *Be relevant and useful* Record:
  - *Information you have on which to base your decisions* Problems presented to you by the patient; relevant aspects of past and family history; examination findings and test results you already have
  - *Your impression of the situation* How you see the problem—may include diagnosis, differential diagnosis, prognosis
  - *Plan of action* Negotiated between patient and doctor—may include tests requested, prescriptions given, referrals made
  - *Information shared and advice given* Relevant worries or concerns voiced by the patient; information provided to the patient; advice given—especially contingency plans if things don't go to plan and review/follow-up arrangements
  - *Include other essential information*—e.g. correspondence to and from other agencies; whether a sickness certificate was issued, and if so for how long and the reason stated on the certificate; if consent for disclosure of information (📖 p.50) or treatment/examination (📖 p.52) was given
- *Do not include* abbreviations (especially unconventional ones), jargon, or personal views about behaviour or temperament unless they have a bearing on the management of the patient.

**Electronic patient records** 📖 p.40

**Confidentiality** 📖 p.50

**Amending records** Rectify errors of fact or judgement. Any alterations or additions should be dated, timed, and signed in such a way that the original entry can still be seen. Patients may request correction of information that they believe is incorrect—you must record the patient's view. Highlight amendments and reasons for them.

**Access to records** Under the Data Protection Act 1998, patients have a right of access to health records which:
- Are about them and from which they can be identified
- Consist of information relating to their health or condition, and
- Have been made in connection with their care
- Most records doctors make are included whenever they were made.

## Who can seek access?

- Any competent person may seek access to their own health records, including competent children (📖 p.53).
- Any person with parental responsibility may apply for access to records of a child (<18y or <16y in Scotland). Where >1 person has parental responsibility, each may apply independently without consent of the other parent.
- Where the patient is incapable of managing his/her affairs, a person appointed by a court may access records necessary for the appointee to carry out his/her functions.
- A third party authorized by a competent person may seek access to that person's records (e.g. a solicitor or insurance company) but proof of permission from the patient must be provided. If there is doubt, contact the patient to verify consent has been given (📖 p.51).

## Access to dead patients' records 📖 p.50

**Requests for access** Nothing prevents doctors from giving patients access to their records on an informal basis provided that there is no reason preventing disclosure. Information must *not* be disclosed if it:

- Is likely to cause serious physical or mental harm, *or*
- Relates to a third party who has not given consent for disclosure (where that third party is not a health professional who has cared for the patient).

If unsure take advice from the BMA or your defence organization.

Formal applications for access must be in writing and accompanied by the appropriate fee. Patients are entitled to a permanent copy of information (e.g. photocopy, print-out) which must be accompanied by an explanation of any unintelligible terms. Access must be given within 40d of receipt of the fee and request. Contact BMA for current fees.

**Security of records** Do not leave records (electronic or manual) unattended in easily accessible areas. When not in use, ideally store all files and portable equipment under lock and key. Query the status of strangers. Highlight any concerns to the practice/security manager. Do not reveal how security systems operate.

- *Manual records* Store files closed and in logical order. Use a tracking system to monitor the whereabouts of files and return files taken away as soon as they are no longer required
- *Electronic records* Do not leave a terminal unattended and logged-in. Do not share log-ins or reveal your password to others. Change passwords regularly and avoid using short or obvious ones. Always clear the screen of a previous patient's information before seeing another. Use a password-protected screen-saver to prevent casual viewing of patient information by others.

## Further information

**BMA** Access to health records by patients. 🖥 www.bma.org.uk
**GMC** Guidance on good practice—confidentiality. 🖥 www.gmc-uk.org

# Telephone consulting and email

## Telephone consultations
***Emergency calls*** Nearly all requests for emergency care are made by telephone. General rules:
- *Train surgery staff* to handle distressed callers, recognize serious problems, and act appropriately when such calls are received.
- *Where possible use a single number for patients to access help.* If using an answering machine ensure that the message is easily heard and contains clear instructions. Worried patients find it difficult to cope with complicated telephone referral systems or messages.
- *Take the name and address of the patient*
- *Appear helpful* rather than defensive from the outset. Keep calm and friendly, even in the event of provocation. Worried callers often appear abrupt or demanding.
- *Record* the time of the call, date, patient's name, address and contact telephone number, brief details of the problem, and action taken (even if calls are being recorded).
- *Collect only information you need to decide whether a visit or urgent surgery appointment is necessary* If a visit is necessary, collect enough information to decide how quickly the patient should be seen and whether extra equipment or help is needed. If a visit is not necessary, decide whether other action, such as an urgent surgery appointment, would be more appropriate.
- *If giving advice* make it simple and in language the patient can understand. Repeat to make sure that it has been understood. Consider asking the patient/carer to repeat what you've told them. Always tell callers to ring back if symptoms change or they have further worries.
- *If a visit is indicated* ensure that the address is right and ask for directions if you are not sure where to go. Try to give a rough arrival time.
- *In some cases* (e.g. major trauma, large GI bleeds, MI, burns, overdoses) call for an emergency ambulance at once.
- *If a call seems inappropriate* consider the reason for it, e.g. depression might provoke recurrent calls for minor ailments.

⚠ If in doubt—see the patient.

***Routine calls*** Most GPs run telephone clinics where patients are free to ring with their problems, have telephone message books and/or bookable telephone slots in surgery time. The telephone is a useful way to answer simple queries without wasting surgery time. Examples include:
- Consultations for minor self-limiting conditions or conditions that do not require an examination
- Follow-up of surgery consultations, e.g. to give results, or to offer management advice/prescription following investigations.

The biggest draw backs of telephone consultations are:
- Inability to examine the patient
- Lack of visual cues to aid communication.

Be alert for verbal cues such as lowering of the voice, hesitation, and signs of distress. Ask about the patient's ideas and concerns, and invite the patient to ask questions. Before giving advice, always ensure that you have sufficient information upon which to base your judgement. If examination is needed, see the patient.

**Use of email in the surgery** ~ 80% of the UK population now has access to email. Cyber-savvy patients increasingly want to be able to communicate with healthcare professionals by email, but email has been used relatively little to date in healthcare settings because of concerns over quality of email content, time lag, confidentiality, and liability. Its use is likely to develop further over the next few years. Successful use of emails depends on both the doctor and patient having a clear understanding of its role, advantages, and limitations.

### Guidelines for email consultations

- Establish turnaround time for messages. Do not use email for urgent matters
- Warn users that email is not secure and that they cannot assume confidentiality just because they are communicating with a doctor
- Advise patients not to use a work or multi-user email address to correspond with the doctor
- Retain electronic and/or paper copies of email communications with patients
- Instruct patients to put the category of transaction in the subject line of the message for filtering: prescription, appointment, medical advice
- Request that patients put their name and date of birth in the message for identification purposes
- Configure automatic reply to acknowledge receipt of messages
- Send a new message to inform the patient of completion of the request. Ensure that others are not copied into the reply
- Avoid giving person-specific information or confirming information given by the patient —it may not be the patient
- Never write anything that you would not be happy to see printed on a newspaper front page
- Request that patients use reply to acknowledge reading your message
- Append a standard block of text to the end of email messages to patients, which contains the GP's full name, contact information, and reminders about security and the importance of alternative forms of communication for emergencies
- Explain to patients that their messages should be concise
- Remind patients when they do not adhere to the guidelines.

### Further information
#### Car J, Sheikh A
- Telephone consultations (2003) *BMJ* **326**, 966–9
- Email consultations in health care 1—Scope and effectiveness (2004) *BMJ* **329**, 435–8
- Email consultations in health care 2—Acceptability and safe application (2004) *BMJ* **329**, 439–42

**American Medical Association** *Guidelines for physician–patient electronic communications* (2001)

# Home visiting and referral letters

**Home visiting** Home visits may be routine checks for housebound patients or emergency visits for patients temporarily unable to get to the surgery. Home visits done in working hours are usually done by practices under their GMS/PMS contract, but in some areas home-visiting services are provided by the PCO and practices are able to 'opt out'.

**Routine visits** Conducted in much the same way as ordinary surgery consultations. Seeing patients in their own environment often gives valuable additional information.

### Emergency visits

- Try to stick to the problem you've been called about
- Take a concise history and examine as appropriate
- Make a decision on management and explain it to the patient and any carers in clear and concise terms they can understand. Repeat advice several times ± write it down
- Record history, examination, management suggested, and advice given for the patient's notes
- Always invite the patient and carers to ring you again should symptoms change, the situation deteriorate, or further worries appear
- For inappropriate calls, take time to educate the patient and/or carers about self-management and use of emergency GP visiting services
- Always consider hidden reasons for seemingly unnecessary visits.

### Being prepared

- Ensure that you have a reliable car with a full tank of fuel
- Have a good street map of the area, in-car electronic navigation system ± Ordinance Survey map
- Carry a large strong torch in the car
- Carry a mobile telephone
- Check that your drug box is fully stocked and all items are in date
- Check all equipment carried is operational and carry spare batteries
- Carry a list of emergency telephone numbers
- Know which chemists have extended opening hours and/or carry the chemist's rota.

### Safety and security

- In all cases ensure someone else knows where you are going, when to expect you back and what to do if you don't return on time.
- If going to a call you are worried about either take someone with you to sit in the car or call the police to meet you there before going in.
- If you reach a call and find you are uncomfortable, make sure you can get out. Note the layout of the property and make sure you have a clear route to the door.
- Set up your mobile phone to call the police or your base at a single touch of a button. Consider carrying an attack alarm.
- If possible have separate bags for drugs and consultation equipment.
- Leave the drug box locked out of sight in the boot of the car when doing a visit.

**Referral letters** Good communication is essential when referring patients to other doctors and agencies. Ensure that all referral letters include:
- Address of the referrer (including telephone number if possible).
- Name and address of registered GP if not the referrer.
- Date of referral.
- Name, address, and date of birth of the patient (and any other identifiers available, e.g. hospital or NHS number).
- Name of the person to whom the patient is being referred (or department if not a named individual)
- Presenting condition—history, examination, investigations already performed with results, treatments already tried with outcomes.
- Relevant past medical history and family history.
- Current medication and any intolerances/allergies known.
- Reason for referral (what you want the recipient of the letter to do), e.g. to investigate symptoms, to reassure parents.
- Any other relevant information, e.g. social circumstances.
- Signature (and name in legible format) of referrer.

❶ Consider using carbonized paper to keep copies of referral letters written in emergency situation in patients' homes.

# The doctor's bag

⚠ The GP's bag must be lockable and not left unattended during home visits. If left in the car, keep the bag locked and out of sight— preferably in the boot. Consider having a separate bag for drugs and consultation equipment and only get the drug bag out of the boot of the car if it is needed. Keep the bag away from extremes of temperature.

Consider including the following (exact contents will vary according to location and circumstances):

## Diagnostic equipment
- Stethoscope
- Sphygmomanometer
- Thermometer
- Gloves, jelly, and tissues
- Torch
- Otoscope
- Ophthalmoscope
- Tongue depressors
- Peak flow meter
- Pulse oximeter
- Fluorescein sticks
- Urine and blood dipsticks
- Tourniquet, Vacutainer (or syringe), and needles
- Patella hammer
- Swabs
- Specimen containers
- Vaginal speculum ± sponge forceps
- Fetal stethoscope/doppler.

## Administrative equipment
- Mobile telephone ± charger
- Controlled drugs record book
- Envelopes
- Headed notepaper
- Local map
- Pathology/X-ray forms
- Prescription pad
- List of useful telephone numbers
- BNF/Mimms
- Quick reference text, e.g. *Oxford Handbook of General Practice*
- Obstetric calculator
- Peak flow chart/wheel
- Book/cards/adhesive strips/ carbonized paper for keeping a record of patient encounters
- Temporary resident records
- List of local chemists and OOH opening times
- Small amount of change for public telephones, parking, etc.

## Other equipment
- Airway ± Laerdal mask
- Oxygen cylinder and mask with reservoir bag
- Automated external defibrillator
- Nebulizer
- Spacer device
- IV cannula
- IV giving set and fluids
- Needles/syringes
- Bandages
- Gauze swabs
- Adhesive plasters
- Scissors
- Steristrips
- Suturing equipment/skin glue
- Urinary catheter and bag
- Antiseptic sachets
- Dressing pack
- Sharps box.

**Drugs for the doctor's bag** *Consider:*

*Injectables*

- Adrenaline (epinephrine)
- Atropine
- Amiodarone
- Benzylpenicillin injection
- Cefotaxime injection
- Lorazepam/diazepam
- NSAID, e.g. diclofenac
- Local anaesthetic, e.g. lidocaine
- Opiate analgesic, e.g. morphine, pethidine, diamorphine
- Naloxone
- Thrombolytic therapy (if >30min from nearest acute hospital and have training)
- Antiemetic, e.g. domperidone, prochlorperazine
- Antihistamine, e.g. chlorphenamine
- Hydrocortisone injection
- Diuretic, e.g. furosemide
- Syntometrine
- Glucagon ± IV glucose
- Major tranquillizer, e.g. haloperidol, chlorpromazine.

*Oral drugs*

- Antacid
- Antibiotics (adult tablets and paediatric sachets), e.g. amoxicillin + erythromycin/clarithromycin
- Antihistamine
- Rehydration tablets/sachets
- Aspirin
- Lorazepam
- Paracetamol tablets + suspension
- Prednisolone tablets (soluble)
- NSAID, e.g. ibuprofen.

*Other drugs*

- GTN spray
- Bronchodilator for nebulizer
- Salbutamol inhaler + spacer
- Antibiotic eye drops
- GlucoGel® glucose gel
- Glycerol suppositories
- Rectal diazepam
- Diclofenac suppositories
- Domperidone suppositories.

⚠ Check drugs at least twice yearly to see they are still in date and usable. Record origin, batch number, and expiry date of *all* drugs administered to patients or dispensed to them to take themselves.

**Drugs given to patients from the doctor's bag should be**

In a suitable container and properly labelled with:

- Patient's name
- Drug name
- Drug dosage
- Quantity of tablets
- Instructions on use
- Relevant warnings
- Name and address of the doctor
- Date
- Warning: 'Keep out of reach of children'.

**Further information**

**Drugs & Therapeutics Bulletin** *Drugs for the doctor's bag 1: Adults* (Sept 2005) and *Drugs for the doctor's bag 2: Children* (Nov 2005)

# Organization of out-of-hours services

**Definition** Out of hours (OOH) is defined as 6.30pm–8.00am on weekdays, the whole weekend, Bank Holidays, and public holidays. GPs have increasingly moved away from the traditional model of personally providing care 'around the clock'. There are several reasons for this.

- *Changed attitudes of GPs* GPs find frequent on-call cover too onerous and an unacceptable intrusion into family life.
- *Daytime workload* The role of the GP has shifted and ever more work comes the GP's way.
- *Number of OOH contacts* Today society has a '24 hour' culture. Consequently the number of GP OOH contacts has risen, as has 'inappropriate' use of A&E services.

Since December 2004, PCOs have taken full responsibility for making sure that there is effective OOH provision in the UK.

**'Opting out' of OOH** Both PMS and GMS practices can 'opt out' of providing an OOH service. The decision must be made for the whole practice—individual doctors within a practice cannot 'opt out' alone. The cost of opting out for a practice is 7% of the global sum (or PMS equivalent).

**Provision of services during the OOH period by 'opted out' practices** There is nothing to stop practices that have opted out from offering surgeries or consultations within the time periods specified as OOH. These services can be paid for through the practice global sum or under the 'extended opening' DES.

**Choice of OOH provider** PCOs can consider a range of alternative OOH care providers as long as accreditation standards are met. Only where a practice is exceptionally remote will the PCO be able to require a practice to continue providing OOH care. Special arrangements for payment then exist. Several schemes operate side by side:

*In-practice rotas* Traditional model of cover. Usually organized in a rota between practice GPs. Largely based on home visiting.

*Extended rotas* GPs on-call in rotation for a small group of practices.

*GP cooperatives* GPs grouped together (often >100 in a cooperative) within a district to cover OOH care between themselves. Often several GPs are on call at any time—one doing visits; one taking calls; one seeing patients in a central clinic.

*Hospital-based OOH cover* GPs and primary care nurses in A&E departments.

*Commercial OOH services* OOH provided by a commercial profit-making organization employing GPs and specialist nurses.

*NHS Direct* 24h nurse-led telephone advice service available throughout the UK. It is designed as a first-line service and aims to have links to local primary care and OOH services. There is also an NHS Direct website and advice booths in public places.

**NHS walk-in centres** Walk-in clinics tend to offer nurse consultation and use NHS Direct algorithms. Most are sited in urban areas. They aim to provide easier access to medical care and are increasingly used to cover the OOH period.

**Enhanced paramedic services** Provide initial assessment of patients who are not able to get to OOH centres and/or patient transport to OOH centres.

**Enhanced community nursing teams** Provide care to patients who are terminally ill and initial assessment of patients who do not feel able to get to an OOH centre for other reasons.

**The future of NHS OOH care** There is a move towards an integrated model of OOH care. One suggestion is that all OOH calls are routed through NHS Direct which will act as a triage system, giving advice or directing callers to the appropriate service (e.g. A&E, ambulance call, GP OOH cover, or routine GP appointment). The use of patient-held 'smart cards' on which each patient's medical record could be stored will allow freer movement of patients between services without the danger of vital information being missed.

**Further information**

**NHS Direct.** ☎ 0845 4647 💻 www.nhsdirect.nhs.uk
Separate services for Scotland and Wales can be accessed via this website.

# Social factors in general practice

*The task of medicine is to promote health, to prevent disease and to treat the sick …these are highly social functions.*

H.E. Sigirist, *Civilization and Disease*, 1943

**Deprivation** Social deprivation is linearly associated with death from all causes with no threshold and no upper limit. The most pronounced effect is with circulatory and other smoking-related disease. A similar trend is seen with infant mortality, morbidity from chronic illness (particularly musculoskeletal, cardiovascular, and respiratory conditions), and teenage pregnancy.

This is not a new problem, nor one unique to the UK. Suggestions that it is due to smoking and eating habits may be partly correct, but this disparity was in evidence 80y ago when those of social classes I and II were more likely to smoke, eat foods high in saturated fats, and take less exercise. Disparity in health is closely related to income. In the UK an ↑ proportion of the population than 20y ago is now living on <50% of average income—the mortality gap has grown proportionately.

❶ Benefits for people with low income are summarized in Table 5.1 (📖 p.104)

**Impact on general practice** Higher incidence of illness → ↑ requirement for primary care team services and ↑ use of OOH and A&E services amongst deprived communities. This is recognized in the UK in the Carr-Hill Index which allocates funds to practices (📖 p.24).

## Homelessness

***Bed and breakfast accommodation*** Adverse effects of living in temporary bed-and-breakfast accommodation are well documented.
- Adults have an ↑ incidence of depression than people of similar social standing in their own homes.
- Homeless women are 2× as likely to have problems in pregnancy and 3× as likely to require admission in pregnancy.
- A quarter of babies born to women living in bed-and-breakfast accommodation are of low birth weight (national average <1:10).
- Children from these families are less likely to receive their immunizations, more likely to have childhood accidents, and have higher incidence of minor respiratory tract and diarrhoeal diseases.

***Sleeping rough*** Poor diet, poor accommodation, and lack of access to medical services are universal problems in this group. A study in London in 1986 found $1/3$ are psychotic, $1/4$ have severe physical problems, and $2/3$ have no contact whatsoever with medical services. Evidence shows that if services are provided, homeless people will use them.

**Divorce** Divorcees of all ages are at greater risk of premature death (2× ↑ for men aged 35–42y) than married people—mainly from cardio- and cerebrovascular disease, cancer, suicide, and accidental death. There is also a similar ↑ in morbidity. Children of divorced parents have ↑ risk of ill health from the time of separation until adult life, with children <5y old when their parents separate being particularly vulnerable. These children are also more prone to psychiatric illness later in life and are more likely to become divorced themselves.

## Employment and unemployment

*Without work all life goes rotten.*

Albert Camus

Effects of work have been compared to effects of vitamins—we need a certain amount to be healthy, then there is a plateau where extra doesn't help—and too much is harmful. There is good evidence that unemployment causes both ↑ mortality (from coronary vascular disease, cancers, suicide, violence, and accidents) and ↑ morbidity (depression, IHD). Threat of unemployment alone can cause morbidity—in one study GP consultation rates rose by 20% and referral rates by 60% after it was announced that a factory would close. Increases on service usage were also found in other family members.

**Refugees and asylum seekers** The Geneva Convention defines a refugee as any person who 'owing to well-founded fear of being persecuted for reasons of race, religion, nationality, membership of a particular social group or political opinion, is outside the country of his nationality and is unable or, owing to such fear, is unwilling to return it'. Refugees are entitled to free healthcare in the UK. *Consider:*
- *Cultural and religious issues* 📖 p.108
- *Physical needs* Health needs are diverse depending on country of origin and previous level of health care. Always consider infectious diseases, e.g. hepatitis B, HIV, TB, and malaria. Ensure that refugees claim all health-related benefits available to them (e.g. free prescriptions).
- *Psychological needs* Depression, anxiety, panic attacks, agoraphobia, and poor sleep are common. Symptoms are often reactions to past experiences and current situation. Social isolation, hostility, and racism compound them. Use medication if appropriate but also address other issues. ⚠ Although telling their story is helpful for some refugees, 'active forgetting' is the way that people cope with their difficulties in some cultures.
- *Victims of torture* may present with many non-specific health problems. Some are the result of physical trauma, but most are of mixed physical and psychological origin. Considerable time and patience are needed to manage these problems but it is worth it. Advice and support are available from the Medical Foundation for the Care of Victims of Torture (🖥 www.torturecare.org.uk).
- *Family* Many will have left other family members behind. They may not know their whereabouts, or even if they are alive or dead. The Red Cross or Red Crescent can help with tracing (🖥 www.redcross.org.uk).

## Useful contacts
**Shelter** Advice for homeless people ☎ 0808 800 4444 🖥 www.shelter.org.uk
**RELATE** Relationship counselling ☎ 0300 100 1234 (telephone counselling cost £45/h in 2009) 🖥 www.relate.org.uk
**RELATE Scotland** ☎ 0845 119 2020 🖥 www.relationships-scotland.org.uk
**Refugee Council** 🖥 www.refugeecouncil.org.uk
**Asylum Aid** ☎ 0207 354 9264 🖥 www.asylumaid.org.uk

**Table 5.1** Benefits for people with low income

| | Eligibility | How to apply | Benefits gained |
|---|---|---|---|
| *Income Support (IS)* | • ≥16y and <60y<br>• Low income, <£8000 in savings (£16 000 if in residential care) and not in receipt of JSA.<br>• <16h paid work/wk (and partner <24h/wk) | Form A1 from local Jobcentre Plus office or online at<br>🖥 www.jobcentreplus.gov.uk | *Money* Depends on circumstances<br>*Other benefits* Housing benefit, community tax benefit, health benefits, and social fund payments. Children <5y and pregnant women—free milk and vitamins. Children >5y—free school meals and, in some areas, uniform grants<br>*Christmas bonus* 📖 p.224 |
| *JobSeekers Allowance (JSA)* | • ≥19y and <60y (women) or <65y (men)<br>• Unemployed or working < 16h/wk<br>• Capable of and available for work<br>• Have a JobSeekers agreement that contracts the recipient to actively seek work | Apply by visiting local JobCentre Plus office or online at<br>🖥 www.jobcentreplus.gov.uk | *Contributions-based JSA* Can claim for up to 26wk. Age-dependent fixed weekly payment<br>*Income-based JSA* Allowance dependent on circumstances. Entitles claimants to same benefits as income support (see above)<br>*Hardship payments* Available to people disallowed JSA |
| *Child Tax Credit (CTC)* | • Age ≥ 16y and<br>• Responsible for ≥1 child (<16y or 16–19y and in full-time education)<br>• Family income <£50 000 per annum | Apply to the Tax Office<br>☎ 0845 300 3900<br>🖥 www.hmrc.gov.uk | *Tax credits*<br>• Family element: credit for any family eligible if there is a child <1y old in the family<br>• Child element: credit for each child in the family.<br>↑ if the child is disabled/severely disabled |

| | | |
|---|---|---|
| Working Tax Credit (WTC) | • Age ≥ 16y, working ≥16h/wk and responsible for a child (<16y or 16–19y in full-time education)<br>• Age ≥ 16y, working ≥16h/wk and has a disability<br>• Age ≥ 50y, working ≥16h/wk and has started work after ≥ 6mo of receiving one of certain benefits<br>• Age ≥25y and working ≥30h/wk | Apply to the Tax Office<br>☎ 0845 300 3900<br>🖥 www.hmrc.gov.uk | ***Tax credits*** Depend on adding elements together:<br>• Basic element paid to everyone entitled to WTC<br>• Second adult element<br>• Lone parent element<br>• Working >30h/wk (can combine both parents if have children)<br>• Disability (if working >16h/wk)<br>• Severe disability (if working >16h/wk)<br>• Aged ≥50y and in receipt of certain benefits before resuming work<br>• Childcare—up to 70% of childcare costs |
| Health Benefits | ***Automatic entitlement***<br>• Age >60y or <16y or 16–18 y in full-time education<br>• Patient or family receiving IS, income-based JSA, or Pension Credit Guarantee Credit<br>• Patients/families receiving WTC or Child Tax Credit who have a valid NHS Tax Credit Exemption Certificate (should be supplied automatically)<br>***By application***<br>• Low income *and*<br>• Savings <£8000 | If automatic exemption, no need to claim. If not, claim using form HC1 available from pharmacies, GP surgeries, and local Jobcentre Plus offices<br>Pregnancy 🔲 p.783<br>Free prescriptions 🔲 p.139 | ***Free***<br>• Prescriptions<br>• NHS dentistry<br>• NHS eye tests and glasses<br>• NHS wigs and fabric supports<br>• Travel to hospital<br>• Milk and vitamins for pregnant and breastfeeding women, and children <5y |
| Housing Benefit | Low income, living in rented housing<br>*Exclusions:* Full-time students without dependants, people in residential care or with savings >£16 000 | Via local authority | Pays rent for up to 60wk. Then need to reapply |

**Table 5.1** (Continued) Benefits for people with low income

| | Eligibility | How to apply | Benefits gained |
|---|---|---|---|
| Council Tax Benefit and Second adult rebate | • **Council tax benefit** Low income; exclusions as for housing benefit<br>• **Second adult rebate** Payable if someone who lives with you is aged >18y, does not pay rent or council tax, and has low income<br>• **Council tax reduction** If single occupier or disabled<br>• **Disregarded occupants** Certain people, including students, carers, and children, are not counted in calculating the number of people living at a property | Via local authority | **Council tax benefit** pays council tax.<br>**Council tax reductions:**<br>• single occupier—25% discount<br>• all disregarded occupants—50%<br>• disabled—reduction to next lowest council tax band. |
| The 6 Social Fund payments | • **Crisis loan** Anyone except students and people in residential care can apply<br>• **Budgeting loan** for large purchases. Must receive IS, pension credit or income-based JSA<br>• **Funeral payments** Must receive low-income benefit and be responsible for the funeral<br>• **Cold weather payments** Average temperature <0°C for ≥7d. Must receive IS, pension credit, or income-based JSA and live with a pensioner, child <5y, or disabled person<br>• **Maternity grant** 📖 p.783<br>• **Community care grant** 📖 p.228 | Cold weather payments should be automatic<br>All others claim via local Jobcentre Plus offices or<br>🖥 www.jobcentreplus.gov.uk | • **Crisis loan** Up to £1000 interest-free loan repayable over 78wk when crisis finished<br>• **Budgeting loan** As crisis loan<br>• **Funeral expenses** Sum towards cost of funeral—usually does not cover full expenses.<br>• **Cold weather payments** £8.50/wk |

# Multicultural medicine

Britain is a multicultural and multi-faith society. It is important that providers of care take into account cultural and spiritual needs.

⚠ Table 5.2 is a rough guide to religious differences which affect health care. Because of space limitations it is brief and cannot address all the many variations. Everyone is an individual and there is a real danger of 'pigeon-holing' patients by religion or ethnic background and making incorrect assumptions as a result. Always ask patients/family about their own preferences.

**Communication** Effective communication is essential. Do not assume English proficiency. It is important to ascertain that you understand the patient and that the patient understands you.
- Ask the patient to let you know if he/she doesn't understand. Consider using an interpreter (see below).
- Speak clearly and slowly and repeat important information. Avoid jargon, confusing phrases, double negatives, and rhetorical questions.
- Ask patients to tell you what you have said to check comprehension.
- Be wary of sounding condescending—English skills are not a reflection of a hearing disorder or level of intelligence.

**Respect beliefs and attitudes** People have different reactions towards illness, life, and death. Ask patients to provide you with information about their own ideas, e.g for newly arrived immigrants, ask: 'Could you tell me what would happen to you if you were in your country?'

**Using interpreters** Interpreters are an important resource in providing a voice for patients whose proficiency in English is poor or insufficient for the situation. In general, anyone who has been in an English-speaking country for <2y will need an interpreter. Sometimes a friend or another family member can be used, but if sensitive issues have to be discussed or it is essential that the information is translated accurately, use a professional.

## General tips
- Anticipate that an interpreter will be needed where possible and pre-book someone of the same gender who speaks the same language/dialect and will be ethnically acceptable to the patient.
- Explain that the interpreter is bound to maintain confidentiality.
- Face and speak in the first person directly to the patient, not the interpreter. Interpreters are solely there to convey information in a language both patient and doctor can understand—not to analyse information, or decide what should or should not be conveyed.

## Useful contacts
**Interpreter services (fees payable)** Language line ☎ 0800 169 2879; National Interpreting Service ☎ 0800 169 5996
**NHS Direct** Multilingual health information and advice. ☎ 0845 4647
🖳 www.nhsdirect.nhs.uk

**Table 5.2** Religious differences important in healthcare

| Religion | Dietary restrictions | Fasting | Transfusion/ transplant | Family planning | Death |
|---|---|---|---|---|---|
| Buddhist | Mainly vegetarian | N/A | No objections | No objections Abortion not allowed | Cremation preferred No objections to PM |
| Christian | None | N/A | No objections | Some approve of natural methods only | Burial or cremation No objections to PM |
| Hindu | Most do not eat beef. Some are strict vegetarians | Fasting involves limiting type of foods | No objections | No objections | Strong preference to die at home. The body should not be touched by non-Hindus. All adults are cremated No PMs unless legally required |
| Muslim | No pork. Other meat must have been killed in a special manner (Halal). Alcohol is prohibited | Fasting sunrise → sunset during Ramadan | Strict Muslims may not consent to transplant | Variable— strict Muslims do not approve | The body should not be touched by non-Muslims. All Muslims are buried No PMs unless legally required |
| Jehovah's Witness | No foods containing blood or blood products. No alcohol | N/A | No blood transfusion or organ transplant. Dialysis is usually permitted | No objections | Burial or cremation No objections to PM |
| Jewish | No pork, rabbit, or shellfish. Meat prepared in kosher fashion. Liberal Jews may not adhere to dietary restrictions | Orthodox Jews may fast for Yom Kippur | No objections | Some Orthodox Jews prohibit contraception. Most Jewish boys are circumcised 8d after birth | Burial is preferred No PMs unless legally required |
| Sikh | No beef. Most are vegetarian. Alcohol is forbidden | N/A | No objections | Allowed but not openly discussed | Children and adults are cremated |

# Breaking bad news

It is never easy to break bad news. GPs do it frequently, but police officers are rated as showing more sympathy than doctors.

## Why is breaking bad news hard?

- *Admission of failure* When we tell patients bad news it is often an admission that we have failed. When we fail we naturally question what we have done, and when looking at our practice in retrospect it is easy to find fault. Feelings of guilt are common.
- *Fear of the reaction of the patient* We all have a desire to avoid unpleasantness, but sharing information with patients may be a positive way forward. Even if news is bad it gives the patient control of the situation.

## Guidelines for sharing bad news with a patient

### DO

- Plan the consultation as far as possible. Check the facts first and ensure that you have all the information. Ensure privacy and freedom from interruption.
- Set aside enough time.
- Ask if the patient would like a relative or friend with them. Make sure that you introduce yourself and find out their name and relationship to the patient.
- Make eye contact—watch for non-verbal messages. Sit at the same level as the patient.
- Use simple and straightforward language.
- Allow silence, tears, or anger.
- Be prepared to go over facts again.
- Answer questions.
- Reflect on what the patient or relative have said to allow you to modify your understanding of their feelings.
- Take into account the patient's current health, e.g. if in pain, then sort out the pain and schedule a further discussion when the patient is more comfortable.
- Offer ongoing support.

### DON'T

- Lie or fudge the issue.
- Get your facts wrong.
- Break bad news in public.
- Give the impression of being rushed or distant.
- Give too much information. It is better to be concise— the finer points can be filled in later.
- Interrupt or argue.
- Say that 'nothing can be done'—there is always something that can be done.
- Meet anger with anger.
- Say you 'know how they feel'—you don't.
- Be frightened to admit you don't know something.
- Use medical jargon.
- Leave the patient with no follow-on contact.
- Agree to withhold information from the patient.

## Common problems

- *What if the relatives don't want you to tell the patient?* With adults of
  sound mind, information is confidential to the patient and can only be
  released, even to close relatives, with the patient's permission. Relatives
  who say that they don't want the patient to know often do so to
  protect their relative. It is important to recognize that they know your
  patient best. First, explore their worries and point out the difficulties
  of the patient not knowing. Often, once a relative realizes that the
  patient knows things are not right and needs help and support to face
  the situation, they come round to the patient being told. Stress that you
  will not lie to a patient if asked a direct question.
- *How do you know if the patient wants to know?* Most people (80–90%)
  do want to know. Assume that this is the case and then feel your way
  carefully. Give the patient ample opportunity to say that they don't
  want to know.
- *How do you respond to questions you cannot answer?* The best way
  to deal with this is to say that you don't have all the answers but will
  answer when you can, find out what you can, and say when you don't
  know.

# Confirmation and certification of death

⚠ The death certification process in England and Wales is currently under review and likely to change in the near future.

English law *does not* require a doctor:
- To confirm death has occurred or that 'life is extinct'. A doctor is only required to certify what, in their opinion, was the cause.
- To view the body of a deceased person. There is no obligation to see/examine a body before issuing a death certificate.
- To report the fact that death has occurred.

English law *does* require the doctor who attended the deceased during the last illness to issue a certificate detailing the cause of death. Certificates are provided by the local registrar of births, marriages, and deaths. A special certificate is needed for infants <28d old.

**Death in the community** A quarter occur at home.
**Expected deaths** In all cases, advise to contact the undertakers and ensure that the patient's own GP is notified.
- *Patient's home* Visit as soon as practicable.
- *Residential/nursing home* If possible, the GP who attended during the patient's last illness should visit and issue a death certificate. The 'on-call' GP is often requested to visit. There is no statutory duty to do this, but it is reassuring for the staff at the home and often necessary before staff are allowed to ask for the body to be removed.

**Unexpected and/or 'sudden' death** If called, advise the attendant to call the emergency services. Visit and take a rapid history from any attendants. Then:
- *Resuscitate if appropriate* Drowning and hypothermia can protect against hypoxic neurological damage; brains of children <5y old are more resistant to damage.
- *Report the death to the coroner* If any suspicious circumstances or circumstances of death are unknown/unclear, call the police.

*Alternatively* if police or ambulance service is already in attendance and death has been confirmed, suggest that the police surgeon is contacted.

**Cremation** The Cremation Regulations (2008) require 2 doctors to complete a certificate to establish identity and that the cause of death is not suspicious before a person can be cremated. The person arranging the funeral may see the forms and pays a fee to each doctor. There are 2 parts:
- *Cremation 4* Completed by the patient's usual medical attendant—usually his/her GP.
- *Cremation 5* Completed by another doctor who must have held full GMC registration (or equivalent) for ≥5y and is not connected with the patient in any way or directly connected with the doctor who issued cremation 4—usually a GP from another practice.

⚠ Pacemakers, certain internal fixation devices, and radioactive implants must be removed from the deceased before cremation can take place.

## Box 5.1 Deaths which must be reported to the coroner

- Sudden or unexpected deaths
- Accidents and injuries
- Industrial diseases, e.g. mesothelioma
- Service disability pensioners
- Deaths where the doctor has not attended within the past 14d
- Deaths arising from ill treatment, e.g. abuse, neglect, starvation, hypothermia
- Cause of death unknown
- Deaths <24h after hospital admission
- Poisoning (chronic alcoholism and its sequelae are no longer notifiable *per se*)
- Medical mishaps (including anaesthetic complications, short- or long-term complications of operations, drugs—whether therapeutic or addictive)
- Abortions
- Prisoners
- Stillbirths (when there is doubt about whether the baby was born alive).

**Notification of death to the coroner** The coroner can be contacted via the local police. Reporting to the coroner does not automatically entail a postmortem. Once circumstances of death are clear, the coroner may advise the GP to tick and initial box A on the back of the certificate which advises the registrar that no inquest is necessary. Deaths which *MUST* be reported to the coroner are listed in Box 5.1.

**❶** In Scotland deaths are reported to a procurator fiscal. The list of reportable deaths is the same with the addition of deaths of foster children and the newborn.

**Recording deaths at the practice** Death registers are useful. Routine communication of deaths to all members of the primary healthcare team and other agencies involved with the care of that patient (e.g. hospital consultants, social services) avoids the embarrassing and distressing situation of ongoing appointments and contacts being made. Record the death in the notes of any relatives/partner registered with the practice.

### Benefits available after a death
- For widows/widowers 📖 p.116
- Funeral payment 📖 p.106

### Patient advice and support
**Department of Work and Pensions (DWP)** 🖳 www.jobcentreplus.gov.uk
- Leaflet D49: *What to do after a death in England and Wales* (2009)
- Funeral payment: Information and on-line application form

**Scottish Executive** *What to do after a death in Scotland* (2006) Available from 🖳 www.scotland.gov.uk/Publications/2006/04/12094440/0

# Organ donation

>7200 people in the UK are waiting for an organ transplant that could save or dramatically improve their life but ~3000 transplants are carried out each year. There is a desperate need for more donors. In 2006–7, 459 people died while waiting for a transplant.

## Absolute contraindications to any organ donation

- Untreated systemic infection
- HIV
- Hepatitis B or C
- Alzheimer's disease and other diseases of unknown aetiology (e.g. MS, motor neuron disease)
- Creutzfeldt–Jakob disease
- Any high-risk factor for HIV (defined by the DH as: homosexual men, prostitutes, history of IV drug abuse, haemophiliacs, people who have had sexual relations with local people from Africa south of the Sahara since 1977, sexual partners of people in these groups).

**Donor cards and the NHS Organ Donor Register** Potential donors should always discuss their wishes with their relatives. They can register their desire to donate their organs after death by adding their names to the NHS Organ Donor Register and/or obtaining an Organ Donor Card. Contact the NHS Organ Donor Line ☎ 0300 123 23 23 or sign up online at 🖥 www.uktransplant.org.uk

**Live donation** Certain tissues can be donated whilst a donor is alive.
- *Blood* Contact the Blood Transfusion Service ☎ 0300 123 23 23 🖥 www.blood.co.uk (in South, Mid, East, and West Wales ☎ 0800 25 22 66 🖥 www.welsh-blood.org.uk).New donors age 17–59y are accepted. There is no upper age limit for established donors.
- *Bone marrow* Contact the British Bone Marrow Registry ☎ 0845 7 711 711 🖥 www.blood.co.uk (in South, Mid, East, and West Wales contact the Welsh Bone Marrow Registry ☎ 0800 25 22 66 🖥 www.welsh-blood.org.uk). A blood sample is taken on registration to allow tissue matching. Donation involves a small operation in which bone marrow is harvested—usually from iliac crests.
- *One kidney, part of lung, liver, or small intestine* Usually close relatives. Removal of the organ/part-organ involves a major operation for the donor. Risks to donor must be weighed vs. benefits to recipient.

## Donation after death

- *Heart beating donation* Donors must be maintained on a life-support machine at the time of death and until the organs are removed. The role of the GP in these situations is pre-emptive (information about organ donor register/donor cards) and to support families to make the decision whether to donate. Organs that can be donated are kidney, heart, liver, lungs, pancreas, cornea, heart valves, bone, and skin.
- *Non-heart beating donation* See Table 5.3. The most important group for GPs as donation can occur even if the patient dies in the community. The GP must initiate removal of tissues by contacting the local organ transplant coordinator or UK Transplant ☎ 0300 123 23 23.

**Table 5.3** Organs suitable for non-heart beating donation

| Organ | Criteria for donation | Specific contraindications |
|---|---|---|
| Corneas | >1y old; no upper age limit<br>May be retrieved up to 24h after death | Scarring/ulceration of cornea<br>Leukaemia/certain lymphomas<br>Malignancy otherwise is *not* a contraindication; neither is poor eyesight |
| Heart valves | 3mo—60y<br>May be retrieved up to 48h after death | Congenital valve defect<br>Rheumatic heart disease<br>Cardiac arrest/MI and malignancy are *not* contraindications |
| Skin | 16–85y<br>>1.7m tall and >70kg weight<br>May be retrieved up to 48h after death | Prolonged steroid therapy<br>Chronic skin disease, e.g. psoriasis<br>Malignancy |
| Bone | ≥16y; no upper age limit<br>May be retrieved up to 24h after death | Any history of malignancy<br>Osteomyelitis<br>Rheumatoid arthritis<br>Traumatic bone fractures |

- *Donation of whole body for medical education* Contact Human Tissue Authority 🖥 www.hta.gov.uk/donations.htm (☎ 020 7211 3137/3442). Relatives should contact the medical school with which the donor has made arrangements after their death. Medical schools arrange collection of the body and a simple funeral. Not all bodies are accepted. The donor must give authorization for donation prior to death.
- *Tissue donation after death for research purposes* Can be done in addition to donation for transplantation—organs for transplant are taken first. 🖥 www.hta.gov.uk/donations.htm

**Approach to relatives** Many families find the act of donation a source of comfort. Even with a signed donor card, the relatives of the patient must give their consent to organ donation postmortem.

**The coroner** For any patient normally referred to the coroner, coroner's permission must be gained before tissues are removed.

**Further information**
**United Kingdom Transplant** ☎ 0300 123 23 23
🖥 www.uktransplant.org.uk

# Bereavement, grief, and coping with loss

**Models of grief** In the traditional model, the bereaved person moves through phases until 'recovery'.
- *Initial shock* Sense of unreality, detachment, disbelief, or 'numbness'. Lasts from hours to days.
- *Yearning* Pangs of grief, episodes of intense pining, and a desire to search interspersed with anxiety, guilt, and self-reproach.
- *Despair* The permanence of the loss is realized. Despair and apathy, social withdrawal, poor concentration, pessimism about the future.
- *Recovery* Rebuilding an identity and purpose in life.

**Recent models** Grief represents an oscillation between loss- and restoration-focused behaviour, demonstrated by swings in mood, thoughts, and behaviour between memories of the dead person and 'getting on with life'. Avoidance or denial of the loss is common and a part of the process.

## Health consequences of bereavement
- ↑ *mortality* (↑ deaths from CHD, cirrhosis, suicide, accidents), particularly in first 6mo. Risk factors: ♂>♀, age <65y, lower social class.
- *Mental health problems* Depression, anxiety, ↑ risk of suicide, substance abuse, identification reaction (hyperchondriacal disorder—symptoms mimic those of deceased e.g. chest pain if died from MI), insomnia, self-neglect.
- *Physical problems* Fatigue, aches and pains (e.g. headaches, musculoskeletal pain), appetite change, GI symptoms, ↓ immune response (↑ minor infection).
- *Others* Interference with family life, education, and employment; social isolation/loneliness; ↓ income.

**Role of the primary care team** Develop a practice policy for dealing with bereaved patients. Flag notes. Consider staff training and active follow-up of bereaved patients. If the person who has died is registered with the practice, ensure that all medical referrals/appointments are cancelled.

**Bereaved children** Children understand what death is by 8y and even children of 2–3y have some understanding of death. Exclusion makes children isolated and often makes the death of someone they have known more, not less, painful. Prepare children for a death if possible and give them a chance to have their questions answered. If a child has problems, seek specialist help.

**Bereavement benefits** Payable to men and women whose spouses have died, including civil partnership. Cohabitation does not qualify except in Scotland. Claims can be made on forms available from benefits offices or online via 🖳 www.jobcentreplus.gov.uk. Benefits available:

*Bereavement payment* Lump sum payable if spouse has paid sufficient National Insurance contributions, or death was caused by employment, and the recipient is below state pension age at the time of the death. Claim <12mo after death.

***Widowed parent's allowance*** Paid to widows/widowers with children or if pregnant.

***Bereavement allowance*** Paid for 52wk from the date of bereavement for spouses >45y old, not bringing up children and under retirement age.

**Other benefits for widows/widowers**
- Funeral payment ◫ p.106
- War widows/widowers ☎ 0800 169 22 77 ▯ www.veterans-uk.info

**Abnormal grief reactions** Whether a grief reaction is normal or abnormal depends on individual circumstances—personality, situation surrounding death, and cultural expectations. Recognized patterns are:
- Inhibited grief—grief is absent or minimal.
- Delayed grief—late onset .
- Prolonged or chronic grief—inability to rebuild life in any way.

***If abnormal grief is suspected*** Monitor carefully. Consider referral for bereavement counselling, e.g. to CRUSE. Consider clinical depression (◫ p.998) or post-traumatic stress disorder (◫ p.996). If symptoms are persistent or worsening despite treatment, or if there is suicidal risk, refer to psychiatry for specialist advice.

---

**Risk factors for poor outcome after bereavement**

*Predisposing factors*
- Multiple prior bereavements
- History of mental illness (e.g. depression, anxiety, suicidal attempts or threats)
- Ambivalent or dependent relationship with the deceased
- Low self-esteem
- Being male
- Poor social or family support.

*Situations where the circumstances of death may cause particular problems for the bereaved*
- Sudden or unexpected death
- Death of parent when child or adolescent
- Multiple deaths (e.g. disasters)
- Miscarriage; death of baby, child, or sibling.
- Cohabiting partners, same-sex partners, extra-marital relationship
- Death due to AIDS or suicide
- Deaths where those bereaved may be responsible
- Deaths from murder, high media profile, or involving legal proceedings
- Where a postmortem and/or inquest is required.

---

**Further information**
**CRUSE** ☎ 0844 477 9400 ▯ www.crusebereavementcare.org.uk
**Royal College of Psychiatrists** information leaflet. Available at
▯ www.rcpsych.ac.uk
**National Association of Widows** ☎ 024 7663 4848
▯ www.widows.uk.net

# Occupational illness

If a patient develops an occupational disease, a doctor is obliged to notify their employer in writing with the patient's consent. The doctor does not need to make a judgement about whether the disease is, in that particular case, caused by the occupation.

Employers must then inform the Reporting of Injuries, Diseases and Dangerous Occurrences Regulations (RIDDOR) incident contact centre (☎ 0845 300 99 23 🖥 www.hse.gov.uk/riddor). Self-employed patients must contact RIDDOR themselves.

Patients who do not give consent for the doctor to notify their employer may allow the doctor to inform the employer's occupational health department or RIDDOR directly instead.

---

**Notifiable industrial diseases ❶** This is not a complete list

- Poisoning by industrial agents e.g. lead, arsenic, mercury
- Repetitive strain injury
- Vibration white finger
- Bursitis, e.g. housemaid's knee
- Occupational asthma
- Folliculitis and acne (associated with work with tar, pitch or oils)
- Occupational infection. e.g. hepatitis B in healthcare workers, anthrax in farmers
- Chrome ulceration
- Irritant dermatitis, e.g. hairdressers' dermatitis
- Tenosynovitis, e.g. as a result of repeated movements of the hand/wrist
- Pneumoconiosis
- Extrinsic allergic alveolitis
- Occupational deafness
- Occupational cancers, e.g. nasopharyngeal cancer in woodworkers, bladder cancer in plastic workers, cancers as a result of ionizing radiation, mesothelioma due to asbestos exposure.

---

**Industrial injury** Injured employees should always report details of any accident to their employer and record them in the accident book as soon as possible, however trivial the injury. Employers must inform RIDDOR of:

- Dangerous incidents even if no one was hurt
- Incidents where death or serious injury occurs
- Incidents resulting in injury requiring >3d absence from work
- Incidents involving gas.

**Industrial injuries disablement benefit** Available to employed earners for injuries resulting from accidents or certain (prescribed) illness arising as a result of employment, even if the employee was either partly or wholly to blame. 'Industrial' covers virtually all forms of work. For accidents, claims can be made at any time after the event but benefit is paid only if there are still effects of the injury after the 91st day.

**Prescribed industrial disease** Disease for which benefit is paid if the applicant worked in a job for which that disease is 'prescribed' and it is likely that the employment caused the disease. Claims may be made at any time with the exceptions of occupational deafness (claim <5y after leaving employment) and occupational asthma (claim <10y after leaving employment). The list of prescribed diseases is similar to, but *not* the same as, the list of notifiable diseases.

## Benefits that may be payable

***Disablement benefit*** If the person was a paid employee at the time of the accident or when he/she contracted the disease *and* disability is assessed at ≥14% (exceptions: occupational deafness >20%; dust-related lung disease, no level). If a patient claims benefit for >1 industrial accident or disease, assessments may be added together and benefit awarded on the total.

***Reduced earnings allowance*** Accident occurred/disease contracted prior to 1 October 1990, disablement assessment of ≥1%; *and*
• Unable to work, *or*
• Unable to work at normal job, *or*
• Working less hours at normal job.

***Retirement allowance*** Reduced earnings allowance becomes retirement allowance at age 60y (women) or 65y (men). It is paid at 25% of the rate of reduced earnings allowance when a claimant stopped work.

***Constant attendance allowance*** For people so disabled that they need constant care and attention and who are receiving disablement benefit for disability assessed at 100%. Four rates of benefit.

***Exceptionally severe disablement allowance*** For people who receive constant attendance allowance at high rate and where need for attendance is likely to be permanent.

❶ People who suffer from industrial diseases or have suffered disability as a result of an industrial accident are also eligible to apply for benefits available for any disabled individuals (📖 pp.226–230).

**Making claims** through local Jobcentre Plus or social security office. A full list of prescribed industrial diseases is also available from these places. Some claims can be made online 🖥 www.jobcentreplus.gov.uk

## Useful contacts

**RIDDOR** Incident Contact Centre ☎ 0845 300 99 23
🖥 www.hse.gov.uk/riddor
**Jobcentre Plus** 🖥 www.jobcentreplus.gov.uk
**Trade unions**

# Victims of crime

Victims of crime need treatment of injuries and emotional support.
- Note the date, time, and place of the event.
- Record injuries in detail (physical and psychological), including measuring the size of lacerations and bruises. Record all information carefully as it may be needed for legal cases.
- Arrange for photos to be taken if appropriate (police may arrange this).
- Encourage reporting of the incident to the police—the patient will not be eligible for criminal injury compensation if it is not reported.
- Give patient details of local victim support groups.
- If the patient's safety is an issue, contact the duty social worker for a place of safety.

**Rape and indecent assault** If a patient reports rape or indecent assault and is willing to report the matter to the police, do not examine her/him. The case against the assailant could be won or lost on the basis of evidence gained by examination of an alleged victim, and so it is best done by a doctor trained and experienced in such work.

### If the patient will not report the matter to the police
- Take a full history of the event. Note LMP, contraception, and sexual history.
- Suggest that the patient attends attends a Sexual Assault Referral Centre (SARC) if available locally for forensic/medical examination and specialist advice and support.

### If there is no SARC or the patient is unwilling to attend
- Make a note of any injuries and take photographs if possible and appropriate. Do not insist on examination if the patient is unwilling. Ensure a chaperone is present if any examination is attempted.
- Discuss the need for emergency contraception, prophylactic antibiotics (e.g. ciprofloxacin 250mg po stat), blood tests at 3mo to exclude transmission of syphilis and 3–6mo for exclusion of seroconversion for HIV.
- If at high risk for HIV transmission refer to A&E for consideration of prophylaxis (🕮 p.742). Discuss the need for counselling and inform the patient about the victim support scheme and rape crisis centres. Arrange follow up in 2–3wk.

**Criminal injuries compensation** For victims of violent crimes, even if the attacker is not identified. Compensation is paid for the injury, loss of earnings, and expenses. Claim by contacting the Criminal Injuries Compensation Authority, Tay House, 300 Bath Street, Glasgow G2 4LN ☎ 0800 358 3601 🖳 www.cica.gov.uk

**Post-traumatic stress disorder (PTSD)** 23% assault victims and 80% rape victims develop PTSD. ♀:♂ ≈ 2:1. Defined as significant symptoms 1mo after the event, i.e. flashbacks, nightmares, survivor guilt, mood changes, detachment, poor concentration, insomnia, anxiety, and depression. Alcohol abuse and work and relationship problems are common. Symptoms may last years. See 🕮 p.996.

**Domestic violence** 🕮 p.122

**Child abuse** 📖 p.922

**Elder abuse** 📖 p.123

## Further information

**Treating victims of crime** Guidelines for health professionals. Victim Support (National office—Cranmer House, 39 Brixton Road, London SW9 6DZ. ☎ 020 7735 9166 🖥 www.victimsupport.org)

## Patient information and support

**Victim support** ☎ 0845 3030 900 🖥 www.victimsupport.org

**Rape Crisis UK and Ireland** 🖥 www.rapecrisis.org.uk (a list of SARCs can be obtained from the website)

**Survivors UK** provides resources for men who have experienced any form of sexual violence ☎ 0845 122 1201 🖥 www.survivorsuk.org

# Domestic violence: the GP's role

Domestic violence is defined by the Home Office as 'any violence between current and former partners in an intimate relationship, wherever the violence occurs. The violence may include physical, sexual, emotional, and financial abuse'.

~80% of reported domestic violence is against women by male partners—domestic violence affects ~1:4 women and is the most common form of interpersonal crime: 60%—current partner; 21%—former partner; half suffer >1 attack; a third have been attacked repeatedly.

General practice is often the first place in which victims seek formal help but only 1:4 actually reveal they have been beaten. Without appropriate intervention, violence continues and often ↑ in frequency and severity. By the time injuries are visible, violence may be a long-established pattern. On average, victims will be assaulted 35 times before reporting it to police.

**Effects** High incidence of psychiatric disorders, particularly depression, and self-damaging behaviours including drug and alcohol abuse, suicide, and para-suicide.

## Factors preventing the victim leaving the abusive situation

• Loss of self-esteem makes victims think they are to blame.
• Fear of partner.
• Disruption of the family and children's relationship with their partner.
• Loss of intimate relationship with partner.
• Fall in income.
• Risk of homelessness.
• Fear of the unknown.

## Guidelines for care

• Consider the possibility of domestic violence—ask directly.
• Emphasize confidentiality.
• Document—accurate clear documentation over time at successive consultations may provide cumulative evidence of abuse, and is essential for use as evidence in court, should the need arise.
• Assess the present situation—gather as much information as possible.
• Provide information and offer help in making contact with other agencies.
• Devise a safety plan—e.g. give the phone number of local women's refuge; advise to keep some money and important financial and legal documents hidden in a safe place in case of emergency; help plan an escape route in case of emergency.

Do not pressurize the victim into any course of action. If the patient decides to return to the violent situation, she or he will not forget the information and support given. In time this might give her/him the confidence and back-up needed to break out of the situation.

⚠ If children are likely to be at risk you have a duty to inform social services or police, preferably with the patient's consent.

**Assault** 📖 p.120
**Child abuse** 📖 p.922

**Elder abuse** Defined as: *'A single or repeated act or lack of appropriate action, occurring within any relationship where there is an expectation of trust, which causes harm or distress to an older person'.*[1]

Older people may report the abuse but often do not. May take several forms that may coexist.

- *Physical* e.g. cuts, bruises, unexplained fractures, dehydration/ malnourishment with no medical explanation, burns.
- *Psychological* e.g. unusual behaviour, unexplained fear, appears helpless or withdrawn.
- *Financial* e.g. removal of funds by carers, new will in favour of carer.
- *Sexual* e.g. unexplained bruising, vaginal or anal bleeding, genital infections.
- *Neglect* e.g. malnourished, dehydrated, poor personal hygiene, late requests for medical attention.

**Prevalence (in own home)** Physical abuse—2%; verbal abuse—5%; financial abuse—2%.

**Signs** Inconsistent story from patient and carer, inconsistencies on examination; fear in presence of carer; frequent attendance at A&E; frequent requests for GP visits; carer avoiding GP.

**Management** Talk through the situation with the patient, carer and other services involved in care. Assess the level of risk. Consider admission to a place of safety contact social services and/or police as necessary; seek advice from Action on Elder Abuse.

### Further information

**Department of Health** *Responding to Domestic Abuse: A Handbook for Health Professionals* (2005) Available from 🖳 www.dh.gov.uk

**Home Office** 🖳 www.homeoffice.gov.uk/crime-victims/reducing-crime/ domestic-violence

**RCGP** Heath I *Domestic Violence: the GP's Role* (updated 2006). 🖳 www.rcgp.org.uk

Ramsay J *et al.* Should health professionals screen women for domestic violence? Systematic review (2002). *BMJ* **325**, 314

### Useful contacts

**Womens' aid** ☎ 0808 2000 247 🖳 www.womensaid.org.uk
**Men's advice line** ☎ 0808 801 0327 🖳 www.mensadviceline.org.uk
**Action on elder abuse** ☎ 0808 808 8141 🖳 www.elderabuse.org.uk
**Police domestic violence units** ☎ 0845 045 45 45
**Local authority social services departments**
**Local authority housing departments**

1 Action on elder abuse. What is elder abuse? London. Available at 🖳 www.elderabuse.org.uk

# Fitness to make decisions

**Definition** *Mental capacity* is the ability to take actions affecting daily life (e.g. when to get up, what to wear, what to eat) and/or make more major decisions (e.g. where to live, how to manage money).

**Mental Capacity Act 2005** came into force in 2007 in England and Wales. Similar legislation applies elsewhere in the UK. It specifies who can take decisions on behalf of other people and allows people to plan ahead for a time when they may lack capacity. 5 key principles:
- Every adult has the right to make decisions and must be assumed to have the capacity to make them unless proved otherwise.
- Every adult must be given all possible help and support to make decisions, and to communicate those decisions where necessary, before he/she can be assumed to have lost capacity.
- Making an unwise decision does not mean that a person lacks capacity to make that decision.
- Anything done or any decision made on behalf of someone who lacks capacity must be done in his/her best interests.
- Anything done or any decision made on behalf of someone who lacks capacity should be the least restrictive of his/her basic rights/freedoms.

**Assessing capacity** A GP asked to give an opinion on a patient's mental capacity should:
- Have access to the patient's records and ideally know the patient.
- Seek information from friends, relatives, carers, and/or the patient's independent mental capacity advocate, if one has been appointed.
- Examine the patient, and assess the type and degree of deficit.
- Decide if there is an impairment of, or disturbance in, the functioning of the patient's brain or mind.
- If there is a disturbance, decide if the patient is able to make the particular decision in question. In particular: Can the patient understand the information relevant to that decision, including the likely consequences of making, or not making, that decision? Can the patient retain that information? Can the patient use or weigh that information as part of the process of making the decision? Can the patient communicate that decision by any means?
- Decide if assessment should be postponed while measures are taken to improve capacity.
- Record all the above information.

**❶** Even if you think a proposed action is in the patient's best interests, you must not judge the patient capable if that is not clearly the case. If in doubt, seek a second opinion.

**Capacity to consent to medical treatment** 📖 p.52

**Lasting Power of Attorney (LPA)** Replaced Enduring Power of Attorney (EPA) in October 2007. Patients with EPAs can still use them. An LPA is a legal document which lets individuals appoint someone they trust to make decisions for them. It can be drawn up at any time whilst the

person has capacity, but has no legal standing until it is registered with the Office of the Public Guardian. 2 types:
- *Property and affairs LPA* allows the 'attorney' to make decisions about management of money, property, and affairs. Unless specified otherwise can be used even when the individual retains capacity.
- *Personal welfare LPA* allows the 'attorney' to make decisions about healthcare and welfare, including decisions to refuse or consent to treatment and decide on place of residence. Only active when the LPA is registered and the individual lacks capacity to make decisions. The attorney can make decisions about life-sustaining treatment only if the LPA specifies that.

**Court of Protection** If a person, by reason of mental disorder, becomes incapable of managing his/her affairs but has not previously signed an LPA, it may be necessary for someone, usually the nearest relative, to apply to the Court of Protection for the appointment of a 'receiver' to do so. The medical practitioner will be asked to complete form CP3. Alternatively, if the patient's affairs are simple (e.g. state pension), direct arrangements can be made with relevant authorities.

**Testamentary capacity** The capacity to make a will. Anyone can make a will provided that they understand the nature and effect of making a will, the extent of property being disposed of and claims others may have on that property, and the decision is not the result of their condition (e.g. due to a delusion).

❶ Decisions don't have to seem rational to others, especially if consistent with premorbid personality.

**Advance decision** Statement about wishes regarding medical treatment in case the individual becomes incapable of making that decision later. Advance decisions are legally binding.
- Respect any refusal of treatment as long as the decision is clearly applicable to the circumstances, there is no reason to believe the individual has altered that decision, and the decision was not made under duress.
- Advance decisions do not have to be written, except those refusing life-sustaining treatment which must be specific to a particular treatment (e.g. refusal to have CPR), written, and signed by the person making the decision (or a representative if unable to sign) and a witness.
- Advance decisions cannot include decisions about treatment the person would like, only treatment the person refuses, and cannot include directions to end the person's life prematurely.
- Doctors may not be willing to carry through an advance directive. In such cases they should refer the patient to another doctor who is.
- The BMA recommends that doctors should *not* withhold 'basic care' (e.g. symptom control) even in the face of a directive which specifies that the patient should receive no treatment.
- Where a formal advance statement is not available, take the patient's known wishes into consideration.

**Further information**
**Office of the Public Guardian** ☎ 0300 456 0300 🖥 www.publicguardian.gov.uk
**BMA local offices**
**Medical defence organizations**

# Certifying fitness to work

**Own occupation test** Applies to those claiming statutory sick pay for the first 28wk. of their illness. The doctor assesses whether the patient is fit to do their *own* job.

**Work capability assessment** Assesses a patient on a variety of different mental and physical health dimensions for ability to work. Not diagnosis dependant. Applies to:
• Everyone after 28wk incapacity
• Those who do not qualify for the own occupation test from the start of their incapacity.

The following tests are performed in the first 13 wk. of any claim for Employment and Support Allowance (ESA; 📖 p.226):

*Limited capability for work assessment* In most cases this takes the form of a medical examination assessing mental and physical ability to work. Groups who will not be considered unfit to work without medical examination include pregnant women, people with severe physical or learning disability, and those who are terminally ill.

*Limited capability for work-related activity assessment* This is usually carried out at the same time as the medical examination and is used to place the individual into one of two groups on the basis of their ability to perform any work:
• *Work related activity group* Individuals are expected to take part in work-focused interviews with their personal advisers, and a provided with a range of support to help them prepare for a return to work. Those refusing to participate will have their benefit reduced.
• *Support group* For those who have an illness/disability that has a severe effect of their ability to work. These individuals are not expected to take part in any work related activity, but can choose to do so on a voluntary basis.

*Work-focused health-related assessment* Only for those in the work-related activities group. It collects additional information about activities that individuals *can* do. It explores the individual's wishes and aspirations regarding work, and problems that the individual may face getting into work and/or staying in work. It also looks at ways to manage these difficulties and/or minimize them.

**Private certificates** Some employers request private certificates in the 1st week of sickness absence. They should request it in writing. If the GP chooses to provide the service, s/he may charge, both for a private consultation and the provision of a private certificate. The company should accept full responsibility for all fees incurred by the patient.

**Disability Discrimination Act 1995** In some circumstances requires employers to make reasonable adjustments for an employee with a long term disability. Advise patients to seek specialist advice.

## Forms for certifying incapacity to work

**SC1** Self-certification form for people not eligible to claim statutory sick pay who wish to claim incapacity benefit. Certify first 7d of illness. Available from local Jobcentre Plus offices and GP surgery.

**SC2** As SC1 but for people who can claim statutory sick pay. Available from employer, local Jobcentre Plus offices, and GP surgery.

**Med 3** Filled in by GP or hospital doctor who knows the patient for periods of incapacity to work likely to be >7d. If return within 14d is forecast give fixed date of return ('closed certificate'). If longer, specify a period of time (e.g. 2 mo) ('open certificate'). Before the patient returns to work reassess and give further certificate with fixed date of return. Only one Med 3 can be issued per patient per period of sickness. If mislaid re-issue and mark 'duplicate'.

**Med 5** Can be used if:
- A doctor has not seen the patient but on the basis of a recent (<1mo) written report from another doctor is satisfied that the patient should not work—the certificate should not cover a forward period of >1mo
- The patient returned to work without receiving a closed certificate (see Med3)
- >1d since the patient was seen (so Med3 cannot be issued) but it is clear the disability is ongoing.

**Med 6** When it is felt that putting a diagnosis on a Med 3/Med 4 would be harmful either directly to a patient or through their employer knowing their diagnosis. A vague diagnosis is put on the form and a Med 6 completed which requests the DWP to send a form to obtain more precise details.

**Mat B1** Signed by doctor or midwife. Provided to pregnant women once within 20wk of EDD. Enables her to claim statutory maternity pay and other benefits (📖 p.783).

## Further information

**Department of Work and Pensions** *Medical Evidence for Statutory Sick Pay, Statutory Maternity Pay and Social Security Incapacity Benefit Purposes: A Guide for Registered Medical Practitioners.* IB204, August 2004. 🖥 www.dwp.gov.uk/advisers/#med

**Disability Discrimination Act** 🖥 www.direct.gov.uk/disability

# Time off work

The longer a patient is off work, the lower the chances of returning—
<50% of people who have been absent for >6mo ever return to work.
- Wherever possible suggest work adjustments where appropriate
  rather than signing the patient off work. It is possible to do this through
  the 'remarks' section of the Med3 form (📖 p.127).
- Suggest work adjustments if the patient is off sick to enable early return
  to work (can be done in the 'remarks' section of the Med3 form).
- Suggest graduated work/transitional arrangements to ease the patient
  back into work.
- Involve occupational health professionals.

**Post-operative time off work** See Table 5.4.

❶These are not hard and fast rules—alter them to fit individual circumstances (e.g. laparoscopic procedures often entail less time off than open
procedures; patients performing hard manual jobs may require more time
off work).

**Time off work for emergencies** In many cases patients have the right
to take time off work to deal with an emergency involving someone who
depends on them, but they may only be absent for as long as it takes to
deal with the immediate emergency.

*Dependants* include spouse or partner, children, parents, or anyone
living with the patient as part of their family. Others who rely wholly on
the patient for help in an emergency may also qualify.

*Emergencies* include situations in which a dependant:
- Is ill and needs help
- Is involved in an accident or assaulted
- Needs the patient to arrange their longer-term care
- Needs the patient to deal with an unexpected disruption or
  breakdown in care, such as a childminder or nurse failing to turn up
- Goes into labour
- Dies and the patient needs to make funeral arrangements or attend the
  funeral.

The legal right only covers emergencies and employers do not have to pay
for time taken off.

**Certification of time off work** 📖 p.126

**Table 5.4** List of expected time off work for uncomplicated procedures

| Operation | Minimum expected (wk) | Maximum expected if no complications (wk) |
|---|---|---|
| Angiography/angioplasty | <1 | 4 |
| Appendectomy | 1 | 3 |
| Arthroscopy | <1 | <1 |
| Cataract surgery | 2 | 4 |
| Cholecystectomy | 2 | 5 |
| Colposcopy ± cautery | <1 | <1 |
| CABG or valve surgery | 4 | 8 |
| Cystoscopy | <1 | <1 |
| D&C, ERPC, or TOP | <1 | <1 |
| Femoro-popliteal grafts | 4 | 12 |
| Haemorrhoid banding | <1 | <1 |
| Haemorrhoidectomy | 3 | 6 |
| Hysterectomy | 3 | 7 |
| Inguinal or femoral hernia | 1 | 3 |
| Laparoscopy ± sterilization | <1 | <1 |
| Laparotomy | 6 | 12 |
| Mastectomy | 2 | 6 |
| Pacemaker insertion* | <1 | <1 |
| Pilonidal sinus† | <1 | <1 |
| Retinal detachment | <1 | Avoid heavy work lifelong |
| Total hip or knee replacement | 12 | 26 |
| TURP | 3 | 6 |
| Vasectomy | <1 | <1 |

* Driving—see p.130

† If time off for dressings is allowed

# Fitness to drive

⚠ Driving licence holders (or applicants) have a legal duty to inform the DVLA of any disability likely to cause danger to the public if they were to drive.

## Driving licence types

- *Group 1* Ordinary licence for driving a car/motorcycle. Minimum age 17y (16y if disabled). Old licences expire at 70th birthday and then must be renewed every 3y. Applicants are asked to confirm they have no medical disability. If so, no medical examination is necessary. New photocard licences are automatically renewed every 10y until age 70.
- *Group 2* Enables holders to drive lorries and buses. Minimum age 21y. Initially valid until 45th birthday then renewable every 5y until 65th birthday >65y renewable annually. Medical examination is needed to renew Group 2 licenses. Applicants must bring form D4 (available from post offices) with them. Examinations take ~30min. A fee may be charged by the GP.

**Determining fitness to drive** Patients with any disorder which may cause danger to others if they drove should be advised not to drive and to contact the DVLA. The DVLA gives advice on when they can restart.

**Driving after surgery** Drivers do not need to notify the DVLA unless a condition likely to affect safe driving persists >3mo (certain exceptions apply for neurological and cardiovascular disorders). It is the responsibility of the driver to ensure that he/she is in control of the vehicle at all times. It might also be advisable for the driver to check with his/her insurer before returning to drive after surgery. *Consider:*

- Recovery from the surgical procedure.
- Recovery from anaesthesia (sedation and cognitive impairment).
- Distracting effect of pain.
- Impairment due to analgesia (sedation and cognitive impairment).
- Physical restrictions due to the surgery or the underlying condition.

**Disabled drivers** who want to learn to drive or return to driving following onset of their disability should have an assessment of their driving ability and/or advice on controls and adaptations needed. Licences may be limited to adapted vehicles. A list of driving assessment centres can be obtained from the Forum of Mobility Centres ☎ 0800 559 3636 🖳 www.mobility-centres.org.uk

**Seatbelt exemption** GPs can sign a form to exempt patients (e.g. those with colostomies) from having to wear a seatbelt. Consider very carefully the reasons for exemption in view of the weight of evidence in favour of seatbelt use. A fee can be charged for this service

❶ Patients on low income can apply for a free medical examination on a form available from Department for Transport, Road Safety Division 1, Zone 2/15, Great Minster House, 76 Marsham Street, London SW1P 4DR ☎ 020 7944 2046.

**Breaking confidentiality** When a patient continues to drive despite advice by a doctor to stop, a doctor has an *obligation* to breach confidentiality and inform the DVLA.

*If the patient does not understand the advice to stop driving*—inform the DVLA immediately.

*If the patient does understand but continues to drive*
- Explain your legal duty to inform the DVLA if the patient does not stop driving.
- If he/she still refuses to stop driving, offer to refer to a colleague for a second medical opinion—on the understanding that the patient stops driving in the interim.
- If the patient still continues driving—consider action such as recruiting the next-of-kin to the cause (but beware of breach of confidentiality).
- If all else fails, inform the DVLA in confidence. Before doing this, write to the patient to inform him/her of your intended actions and consider contacting your medical defence organization for advice. Once the DVLA has been informed, you should also write to the patient, to confirm that a disclosure has been made.

**Further information**
**DVLA** *At a Glance Guide to the Current Medical Standards of Fitness to Drive for Medical Practitioners* available from 🖥 www.dvla.gov.uk
Medical advisers from the DVLA can advise on difficult issues—contact The Medical Adviser, Drivers Medical Group, DVLA, Swansea SA99 1TU or ☎ 01792 782337 or email medadviser@dvla.gsi.gov.uk (medical professionals only)
**Forum of Mobility Centres** ☎ 0800 559 3636
🖥 www.mobility-centres.org.uk
**Certificates of exemption from compulsory seatbelt wearing** can be obtained from ☎ 0300 123 1002 or online at 🖥 www.orderline.dh.gov.uk

**Patient information**
**Motoring: Medical Rules for Drivers** 🖥 www.direct.gov.uk/motoring
**DVLA** Customer enquires ☎ 0300 790 6801 🖥 www.dvla.gov.uk

# Brief guide to DVLA fitness to drive criteria

⚠ Any person driving (or attempting to drive) on the public highway, or other public place whilst unfit due to any drug, whether prescribed or illicit, is liable to prosecution.

## Neurology

- **Unexplained loss of consciousness** If >1 episode in 6mo, abnormal ECG, evidence of structural heart disease, or syncope causing injury occurring when sitting/lying, licence revoked for 6mo (1y for Group 2 licence) unless cause is found and treated. If low risk or cause is found and treated, licence revoked for 4wk (3mo for Group 2 licence).
- **First epileptic seizure/solitary fit** Licence revoked. Specified seizures with identifiable non-recurring cause (e.g. stroke or intracranial surgery) may be dealt with on a case-by-case basis by the DVLA.
  - Group 1—assessed by specialist, no abnormality found on investigation and seizure-free for 6mo to regain licence.
  - Group 2—assessed by specialist, seizure free for 5y, and good prognosis to regain licence i.e. normal brain imaging, normal EEG, no medication, seizure risk ≤2%/y.
- **Epilepsy** Licence revoked.
  - Group 1—until 1y after last attack (special rules apply if fits only occur in sleep). If withdrawing medication, stop driving during period of withdrawal and 6mo afterwards.
  - Group 2—licence revoked. Review after 1y.
- **CVA/TIA/amaurosis fugax**
  - Group 1—1mo off driving. Restart when clinically fit thereafter. If recurrent TIAs licence revoked for 3mo after last event.
  - Group 2—off medication and 10y since last fit.

## Cardiovascular disease

- **Postural hypotension/syncope** If cause is clear and not sudden or disabling continue driving.
- **Hypertension** If asymptomatic continue driving. Group 2—stop driving if systolic >180mmHg or diastolic >100mmHg until BP controlled.
- **Arrythmia** Stop driving.
  - Group 1—until attacks controlled for at least 4wk.
  - Group 2—licence revoked until arrythmia controlled >3mo and renewed only if the left ventricular ejection fraction is >0.4.
- **Pacemaker insertion** Includes box change.
  - Group 1—stop driving for 1mo.
  - Group 2—stop driving for 6wk.
  Other implantable defibrillator devices—see DVLA guidance.
- **Stable angina**
  - Group 1—stop driving if attack whilst at the wheel, at rest or with emotion until symptoms controlled.
  - Group 2—licence revoked until symptom free >6wk—renewal requires medical examination and exercise ECG or equivalent.
- **Acute coronary sydromes**
  - Group 1—if successful treatment with angioplasty—stop driving for 1wk. Otherwise stop driving 1mo.

- *Group 2*—licence revoked. Reviewed after 6wk with medical examination and exercise ECG.
- **Coronary revascularization**
  - *Group 1*—angioplasty/stenting—stop driving 1wk. Restart when clinically fit thereafter. CABG—stop driving for 1mo.
  - *Group 2*—licence revoked for 6wk after angioplasty or 3mo after CABG. Reviewed after 6wk with medical examination and exercise ECG or equivalent.

## Diabetes mellitus

- **Controlled by diet/oral hypoglycaemics** Continue driving if adequate control unless related problems (e.g. loss of vision, CHD, CVA)
- **Controlled with insulin** Stop driving if poor control, related problems that prevent driving, frequent hypoglycaemic episodes, or inability to recognize hypoglycaemia. Given a 1, 2 or 3y licence with review. *Group 2*—if issued after 1 April 1991, licence revoked. If issued before then, DVLA considers each case individually.

## Psychiatric conditions

- **Dementia** Stop if pose danger to public. *Group 2*—licence revoked on diagnosis
- **Anxiety, depression, other neuroses** Unless severe, continue driving. Stop if severe (especially if possible suicide at the wheel) or if medication inhibits ability to drive. *Group 2* licences are revoked if serious acute mental illness. Restored it symptom free and stable for ≥6mo.
- **Psychosis**
  - *Group 1*—licence revoked. Restored if well and stable for ≥3mo, compliant with treatment, and free from adverse drug effects which would impair driving. Specialist report required.
  - *Group 2*—licence revoked for 3y. Restored if stable and off anti-psychotic medication which might affect ability to drive. Specialist report required.
- **Drug or alcohol misuse or dependency** DVLA arranges assessment prior to licence restoration.
  - *Group 1*—6mo off driving (1y after alcohol- or drug-related seizure or detoxification for alcohol, opioid, cocaine, or benzodiazepine dependence).
  - *Group 2*—licence revoked 1y (3y if alcohol dependence or misuse of opiates, cocaine, or benzodiazepines; 5y if alcohol- or drug-related seizure).

## Conditions affecting vision

- **Visual acuity**
  - *Group 1*—able to read in good light (with glasses or contact lenses) a number plate containing figures 79 mm high and 57 mm wide at a distance of 20.5 m (20 m where the characters are 50 mm wide).
  - *Group 2*—corrected vision of 6/9 (best eye) and 6/12 (other eye). Stop driving if uncorrected acuity in either eye <3/60.
- **Visual field defects**—stop driving. *Group 1*—restore if able to meet DVLA criteria.
- **Diplopia**—stop driving. *Group 1*—can resume if controlled (e.g. by wearing patch).

## Miscellaneous

**Sleep apnoea**—stop driving. Restart when symptoms are adequately controlled.

# Fitness for other activities

**Fitness to fly** Passengers are required to tell the airline at the time of booking about any conditions which might compromise their fitness to fly. The airline's medical officer must then decide whether to carry them.

## Hazards of flying

- Cabin pressure—oxygen levels are lower than at ground level and gas in the body cavities expands 30% in flight.
- Inactivity and dehydration.
- Disruption of routine.
- Alcohol consumption.
- Stress and excitement.

## Contraindications to flying

- **Respiratory disease**
  - Suspected pneumothorax/pneumomediastinum—patients should not fly for 14d after complete resolution of pneumothorax.
  - Chronic lung disease—if a patient can walk >50m without getting breathless, he/she should be fit to fly. Supplementary oxygen can be provided in flight for patients unable to walk this far, but the patient must pre-book this with the airline and there is usually a charge.
- **Heart disease** Patients should not travel if they have unstable angina, poorly controlled heart failure, or an uncontrolled arrythmia. Patients should also refrain from travelling <10d post uncomplicated MI (3–4 wk if complicated recovery) and for 3–5d post angioplasty.
- **Thrombo-embolic disease** Patients should not travel with a DVT before established on anticoagulants.
- **Neurological disease** Patients should not travel for 3d post stroke or, if epileptic, within 24h of a grand mal fit.
- **Infectious disease** Patients must not travel with untreated infectious disease.
- **Psychiatric illness** Patients should not travel if they have disturbed or unpredictable behaviour whichd disrupt the flight.
- **Fractures** Flying is restricted for 24–48h (depending on the length of the flight) after the plaster cast has been fitted.
- **Haematological disease** Anaemia (<7.5g/dl) and recent sickling crisis may restrict flying.
- **Pregnancy** Most airlines will not carry women >36wk pregnant (3rd trimester if multiple pregnancy) or with history of premature delivery, cervical incompetence, bleeding, or ↑ uterine activity.
- **Ear problems** Flying with otitis media or sinusitis can result in pain ± perforation of the ear drum. Patients are advised not to fly until symptoms resolve.
- **Babies** <2d old should not fly (preferably <7d old).
- **Surgery** Patients should not travel <10d post surgery to the chest, abdomen, or middle ear. Any other procedure where gas is introduced into the body also needs careful consideration.

### Precautions

- Carry all regular medication especially relief medications (e.g. salbutamol, GTN spray) in the cabin
- For people who have to time their medication carefully keep to the times that medication was taken at home for duration of flight, e.g. diabetics (take snacks to eat and take insulin at normal times), epileptics.
- Drink plenty of liquid (non-alcoholic) to prevent dehydration.
- Do calf exercises/get up and walk up and down at intervals to prevent venous stasis in the legs—those at risk of venous thromboembolism should take prophylactic aspirin 75mg od and wear compression stockings for the flight.
- Pre-warn airlines of special needs so that they can accommodate them, e.g. extra leg room, special diet, oxygen in-flight, transport to and from plane.

### Further information
**Civil Aviation Authority (CAA)** Am I fit to fly? 🖥 www.caa.co.uk

### Fitness to perform sporting activities 📖 p.510

**Pre-employment certification** It is becoming increasingly common for GPs to be asked about the 'medical' suitability of candidates to perform a job. This is not part of the GP's terms of service and therefore a GP can refuse to give an opinion. In all cases where an opinion is given, a fee can be claimed. Common examples are:

- Forms for childminders
- Care home staff—proof of 'physical and mental fitness'
- Food handlers—certificates of fitness.

⚠ Remember—signing a form may result in legal action against you should the patient NOT be fit to undertake an activity.

Where possible include a caveat, e.g. 'based on information available in the medical notes the patient appears to be fit to …, although it is impossible to guarantee this.'

If unsure, consult your local LMC or medical defence organization for advice.

# Medicines and prescribing

# NHS prescriptions

> *A doctor is a man who writes prescriptions till the patient either dies or is cured by nature.*
>
> John Taylor (1694–1761)

At any one time, 70% of the UK population are taking medicines. $^3/_4$ of people >75y are taking prescribed medicines and 36% of older people take ≥4 different medications on a regular basis. 1.7 million prescriptions are dispensed daily within the NHS to prevent illness, cure existing illness, and give symptomatic relief costing >£6 billion/y (>10% NHS costs).

Prescribing forms a major part of any GP's workload. Bad prescribing wastes resources, deprives patients from a chance to benefit, and may cause illness. Medicines should be prescribed only when necessary, and in all cases benefits of prescribing should be weighed against risks.

❶ Currently only patients in England pay prescription charges. There are no prescription charges in Wales, Northern Ireland, or Scotland.

**Prescription pre-payment certificate (PPC)** If not entitled to free prescriptions but needing a lot of medication (>3 prescriptions/3mo or >14/y) it is cheaper for a patient to purchase a pre-payment certificate. There are 4 ways to purchase a PPC:
• Internet 🖳 www.nhsbsa.nhs.uk/HealthCosts
• Telephone ☎ 0845 850 0030.
• Post: form FP95 available from doctors' surgeries and pharmacists or 🖳 www.nhsbsa.nhs.uk/HealthCosts. Send completed form to PPC Issue Office, PO Box 854, Newcastle-upon-Tyne NE99 2DE.
• From a pharmacy registered to sell PPCs. List available at 🖳 www.nhsbsa.nhs.uk/HealthCosts

*Refunds* Send PPC a letter explaining the reason for refund to PPC Issue Office (address above).
• *Full refund* may be claimed if <1mo after purchase the holder becomes entitled to free prescriptions or dies.
• *Partial refund* may be claimed if the holder dies >1mo after issue or if the holder becomes entitled to free prescriptions 1–4mo after issue.

***Reclaiming money spent whilst awaiting an exemption certificate or PPC*** Ask for an official receipt at the pharmacy when the drug is paid for (FP57 England/EC 57 Scotland). Claim money back within 3mo.

**Drugs cheaper over-the-counter (OTC)** Many drugs commonly prescribed in primary care (e.g. paracetamol, topical steroid nasal sprays, oral antihistamines, ibuprofen) are cheaper than a prescription charge to buy OTC. Before prescribing for patients who pay prescription charges, always consider:
• Is this medication available to purchase OTC?
• Would it be cheaper to buy OTC in the quantities required?

**Table 6.1** Free prescription entitlement

| Free prescription entitlement | Action needed |
|---|---|
| • Prescription for contraception<br>• >60 or <16y of age or 16–18y of age in full-time education<br>• Patient or family receiving IS, income-based JSA, or Pension Credit Guarantee Credit<br>• Patients/families receiving Working Tax Credit or Child Tax Credit who have a valid NHS Tax Credit Exemption Certificate (should be supplied automatically) | Tick the box on reverse of prescription form |
| Pregnant women and women who have had a baby <12mo ago (MatEx) | Fill in form FW8 as soon as pregnancy confirmed. Exemption certificates last 1y from EDD. If FW8 is completed after the baby is born, the MatEx certificate lasts 12 mo after the date of birth. Includes dentists' charges |
| *Certain conditions* (MedEx):<br>• DM (unless diet controlled only)<br>• Myxoedema/requirement for thyroxine, or hypoparathyroidism<br>• Epilepsy requiring continuous anticonvulsants<br>• Permanent fistula (e.g. colostomy) needing stoma dressing/appliance<br>• Hypoadrenalism (including Addison's disease) needing replacement therapy<br>• Hypopituitarism including diabetes insipidus<br>• Myaesthenia gravis<br>• Cancer (from April 2009)<br>• Unable to go out without the help of another person because of a continuing physical disability | Fill in form FP92A (available from doctors' surgeries). Requires a doctor's signature to confirm the condition when applying for exemption. Certificate lasts 5y or until 60th birthday if sooner |
| War pensioners: prescriptions related to pensionable condition only | Apply through Veterans-UK<br>☎ 0800 169 2277 |
| Low income and <£8000 savings (higher if in residential care) or pending application for any benefit listed above | Students may be eligible. Includes opticians' and dentists' charges. Apply through the NHS Low Income Scheme (LIS) on form HC1<br>☎ 0845 850 1166 or<br>🖥 www.nhsbsa.nhs.uk/HealthCosts |

❶ Leaflet HC11 (*Help with Health Costs*) is available from Post Offices, some pharmacies, and GP surgeries or from
🖥 www.nhsbsa.nhs.uk/HealthCosts/792.aspx

# Writing prescriptions

⚠ Legal responsibility for prescribing lies with the person who signs the prescription form

**British National Formulary (BNF)** contains a list of all drugs that a registered medical practitioner can prescribe on NHS prescription. It does not include homeopathic drugs which can be prescribed on NHS prescription, or aids and appliances. There is a separate BNF concerned with prescribing for children. Dentists and nurses have their own limited formulary.

*Further information*
**BNF** 🖥 www.bnf.org
**BNF for Children** 🖥 www.bnfc.org

**Claiming for items dispensed by a non-dispensing GP** All GPs may claim payment for dispensing certain items that are supplied and personally administered by the GP, or practice staff on behalf of the GP. Claims are made on form FP10 (GP10) to the PPA and must state the name of the patient, item dispensed and manufacturer of the item. Claimable items are:

- Vaccines
- Anaesthetics
- Injections
- Sutures
- Skin closing strips
- IUCDs
- Contraceptive caps/ diaphragms
- Diagnostic reagents
- Pessaries that are appliances (e.g. ring pessary).

❶ Different arrangements apply for high-volume vaccines, e.g. influenza.

**Prescription writing** NHS prescriptions are written on form FP10 (GP10 in Scotland). They should be legible and in indelible ink. They are valid for 13wk from the date written on them. *Include*:

- Patient details—full name, address, and age/date of birth if <12y
- Date
- Full name of the drug (not abbreviated) with quantity to be supplied and dose interval (avoid the use of decimal points, e.g. quantities <1g, write in mg). If you want a description of the drug included on the label, then write it on the prescription (e.g. 'for asthma')
- Deletion of any unused space (e.g. by striking through)
- Signature of the prescriber in ink
- Name and address of the prescriber.

❶ Special rules apply for controlled drugs (📖 p.153).

**Computer issued prescriptions (form FP10(C))** should contain the same information as their hand-written equivalents. They must still be signed in ink by the responsible GP.

Guidelines are available from the Joint Computing Group of the GPC and RCGP (a summary is available in the BNF 🖥 www.bnf.org).

**Non-NHS prescriptions** The same rules apply to the writing of private prescriptions as for NHS prescriptions but private prescriptions should not be written on FP10 forms (headed notepaper is normally used). There are no restrictions upon which drugs can be prescribed.

*Private prescriptions for controlled drugs* Controlled drugs in Schedules 2 and 3 (including temazepam) presented for dispensing in the community (but not in hospitals) must be written on specially designated forms available from local PCOs. These forms must include the prescriber's unique 6-digit identification number issued specifically for their private prescribing activity.

**Nurse prescribers** (BNF—Appendix NPF). There is a list of preparations approved by the Secretary of State which may be prescribed on form FP10P (form HS21(N) in Northern Ireland, form GP10(N) in Scotland, forms FP10(CN) and FP10(PN) in Wales) by nurses for NHS patients. Nurses who have undergone additional training can prescribe from the nurse prescribers' extended formulary list.

**Dentists** (BNF—Appendix DPF). Can prescribe medication for dental conditions to their NHS patients on form FP10 (D) (GP14 in Scotland).

**Emergency supply of medicines by pharmacists** In emergency situations pharmacists can dispense prescription-only medicines (POMs). In general ≤5d supply can be dispensed.

**Patient information** Since 1994, all newly licensed/relicensed medicines dispensed in an original pack must be accompanied by a patient information leaflet (PiL). Despite the fact that most drugs are now supplied with PiLs, doctors should make patients aware of 'substantial or special risks when offering treatment'. How much information to give is unclear. Information regarded as important by patients is name of the drug, what to do if a dose is missed, purpose of treatment, precautions (e.g. effect on driving), when and how to take the medicine, problems with alcohol and other drugs, and unwanted effects and what to do about them.

**Security of prescriptions** Prescription theft and fraud is common and wastes valuable NHS resources. *Basic precautions*:
- *Prescriptions* should not be left unattended at reception desks, should not be left in a car where they might be visible; and when not in use should be kept in a locked drawer at the surgery and at home
- *Writing prescriptions* Draw a diagonal line over the blank part of the form under the prescription, write the quantity in words and figures for drugs prone to abuse (even if not controlled drugs), make alterations clear and unambiguous, and add your initials against any altered items.

If prescription fraud is suspected ☎ 0800 028 40 60

*Further information*
NHS Counter Fraud Service 🖳 www.nhsbsa.nhs.uk/CounterFraud

# Cost-effective prescribing

**Generic prescribing** Use of generic names when prescribing is one of the simplest ways to ↓ cost of drugs to the NHS, but only 63% drugs prescribed by GPs in UK are prescribed generically.

Every marketed drug has a chemical name, a generic name, and a proprietary or brand name. For as long as the drug's patent is valid, the company that developed the drug will derive income from prescription whatever the name on the prescription. Once the patent has expired, competitors can manufacture the drug and market it under its generic or an alternative brand name. If the drug is prescribed generically, the pharmacist decides which brand to supply and market forces drive price ↓.

**Advantages of generic prescribing** Cost ↓, professional convenience (there are often several brand names for one drug—by using generic names everyone knows they are talking about the same thing), ↑convenience to the patient (pharmacists do not stock each brand of a given drug and if prescribed by brand name may have to order—usually generic preparations of all commonly used drugs are available).

### Reasons not to prescribe generically
- **Drugs with a low therapeutic index,** e.g. lithium, carbamazepine, phenytoin, ciclosporin. Dosage is carefully titrated against plasma concentration or response. Small differences in plasma concentrations can be clinically significant
- **Modified release formulations,** e.g. diltiazem, nifedipine, aminophylline, or theophylline products. Composition and pharmokinetic properties are very difficult to standardize
- **Formulations containing ≥2 drugs** Some do have generic names (e.g. co-amilofruse 5/40), but others do not. Don't make up a generic name if there isn't one.

**Evidence-based prescribing** Decisions on what to prescribe when were, in the past, largely based on guesswork or faith. With the advent of information from randomized controlled trials and their evaluation using systematic reviews and other techniques, such decisions can now be based (at least in part) on scientific evidence. Failure to do this may cause patients to suffer unnecessary side effects of ineffective drugs, deprive patients the chance to benefit from effective treatments, and waste valuable resources. *Sources of information:* 📖 p.75.

**NICE** 📖 p.13

**Rationing** 📖 p.7

**Practice formularies** An agreed practice formulary is an effective way to limit prescribing and costs of prescribing. Compiling a formulary from scratch is a daunting prospect, but there are many formularies available which can be modified according to evidence that emerges and review within a practice (contact PCO prescribing lead). When compiling or reviewing a formulary consider evidence of efficacy, safety, cost effectiveness, and local policy.

**NHS Business Services Authority (NHSBSA)** Special Health Authority which provides a wide range of services to the NHS including:
- Payments to pharmacists for prescriptions dispensed in primary care
- Provision of information on costs and trends in prescribing
- Payments to dentists for work undertaken on NHS contracts and provision of information on costs of dental care
- Management of the NHS Pension Scheme
- A range of health benefits schemes (Low Income Scheme, Exemption schemes, Pre-payment Certificates)
- Administration of the European Health Insurance Card (EHIC) scheme
- Management of the NHS Injury Benefits Scheme
- Provision of the NHS Counter Fraud and Security Management service.

**Prescribing information** The NHSBSA provides practices with information on their prescribing via the ePFIP (Electronic Prescribing and Financial Information for Practices) system. This is available by registration at 🖳 www.nhsbsa.nhs.uk/963.aspx. Information can be used to improve prescribing habits, manage prescribing costs, and produce formularies and prescribing policies. 4 types of report are available:

**Practice detailed prescribing information (PDPI)** shows prescribing amounts and costs broken down according to the BNF for each prescriber in a practice. A new report is created online each time a report is requested. A data selector allows the user to choose the parameters of the report, e.g. prescribers, time periods (1–24mo), BNF groups.

**Prescribing analysis report** Analysis of practice prescribing during the reporting period. Produced at both a monthly and a quarterly level. The report shows total level of prescribing, trends in prescribing, a breakdown of prescribing in the 6 highest-cost BNF therapeutic groups, the top 20 leading cost drugs in the practice, and the top 40 BNF sections by cost in the practice. Practice prescribing is also compared with the previous year's level and with the PCO and national levels.

**Prescribing review** Each quarter the NHS Prescription Services of the NHSBSA produces an article discussing national guidance, recent clinical trial and prescribing trends for a specific area of prescribing (available from 🖳 www.nhsbsa.nhs.uk/945.aspx).

**Prescribing monitoring document (PMD)** shows the cost of prescribing to enable management of the drugs element of unified budgets. 2-page report: the first page is a practice statement (or annual return in March), and the second is an annual profile of cumulative expenditure.

**Further information**
**NHSBSA** 🖳 www.nhsbsa.nhs.uk
**UK Medicines information** 🖳 www.ukmi.nhs.uk
**Electronic medicines compendium** 🖳 www.medicines.org.uk

# Medicines management and concordance

**Medicines management** Defined as *'facilitating the maximum benefit and minimum risk for medicines for individual patients'*.[1] Encompasses the way medicines are selected, procured, delivered, prescribed, administered, and reviewed to optimize use. *Components are*:

- Optimizing a medication regime (right drug at the right time)
- Facilitating adherence to medication, addressing beliefs and fears as well as physical problems as a result of drugs
- Organizing supply and administration support, such as repeat dispensing systems
- Providing monitoring and feedback systems.

**Concordance** is a process of prescribing and medicine taking based on partnership. Patient concordance (or rather lack of it) is a major challenge in general practice. For drugs to be optimally effective they should be taken as directed by the prescriber. Concordance sufficient to attain therapeutic objectives occurs about half the time: 1:6 patients take medication exactly as directed, 1:3 take medication as directed 80–90% of the time, 1:3 take medication 40–80% of the time, and the remaining 16–17% take medication as directed <40% of the time. 20% of prescriptions are never 'cashed'.

**'White-coat concordance'** Phenomenon in which 90% of patients take regular medication as directed for a period before a check up—may mask effects of non-concordance.

**Consequences of non-concordance** Failure to attain therapeutic targets, e.g. failure to take antihypertensive medication ↓ reduction of stroke by 30-50%, wastage of precious resources (~£230 million worth of medicines are returned to pharmacies each year for disposal—the true quantity wasted is many times that).

## Causes of non-concordance

- **Patient beliefs** Strongest predictor of concordance—how natural a medicine is seen to be, the dangers of addiction and dependence, the belief that constant use may lead to ↓ efficacy have all been shown to influence concordance.
- **Lifestyle choices**
  - Unpleasant side effects (especially if not pre-warned)
  - Inconvenience (e.g. multiple daily dosage regimes, though little difference between od and bd dosage)
  - No perceived benefit.
- **Information** Instructions not understood or poor understanding of the condition/treatment.
- **Practical** Forgetfulness; inability to open containers.
- **Professional**
  - Doctor–patient relationship (there is a link between patient satisfaction with the consultation and subsequent concordance)
  - Inappropriate prescribing; mistakes in administration/dispensing.

*Improving concordance* ~70% of patients want to be more involved in decisions about treatment. Doctors underestimate the degree to which they instruct and overestimate the degree to which they consult and elicit their patients' views. The doctor's task is, by negotiation, to help patients choose the best way to manage their problem. Patients are more likely to be motivated to take medicines as prescribed when they:

- Understand and accept the diagnosis
- Agree with the treatment proposed
- Have had their concerns about the medicines specifically and seriously addressed.

### Ways to improve concordance

- Use simple language and avoid medical terms.
- Discuss reasons for treatment and consequences of not treating the condition, ensuring information is tailored, clear, accurate, accessible, and sufficiently detailed.
- Seek the patient's views on their condition.
- Agree course of action before prescribing.
- Explain what the drug is, its function, and (if known and not too complex) its mechanism of action.
- Keep the drug regime as simple as possible—od or bd dosing preferable, especially long-term.
- Seek the patient's views on how they will manage the regime within their daily schedule and try to tie in with daily routine (e.g. take one in the morning when you get up).
- Discuss possible side effects (especially common or unpleasant side effects).
- Give clear verbal instructions and reinforce with written instructions if complex regime, elderly, or understanding of patient is in doubt.
- Deal with any questions that the patient has.
- Repeat information yourself and also ask patients to repeat information back to you to reinforce information.
- If necessary, arrange review within short time of starting medicine to discuss progress or queries, or arrange follow-up by another member of the primary health care team (e.g. asthma nurse to check inhaler technique 2–3 wk after starting inhaler).
- Address further patient questions and practical difficulties at follow-up.
- Monitor repeat prescriptions.

### Further information

NICE Medicines adherence (2009) 🖳 www.nice.org.uk
Medicines Partnership 🖳 www.npc.co.uk/med_partnership/index.htm
Managing Medicines 🖳 www.managingmedicines.com

1 Hospital Pharmacist (1997) Medical management. Hospital Pharmacist, **4**: 245–259.

# Repeat prescribing

80% of NHS prescriptions are for repeat medication. Good practice is essential to ensure wastage (>10% of total prescribing costs) is kept to a minimum. *Essential elements are:*

- *Written explanation* of the repeat prescribing process for patients and carers
- *Practice personnel with dedicated responsibility* Ensure patient recall and regular medication review
- *Agreed practice policies* for repeat prescriptions, e.g. duration of supply, procedure if someone 'runs out' but isn't authorized to have more
- *Authorization check* each time a prescription is signed
- *Compliance check* for under- or over-use (prescription frequency)
- *Equivalence check* All regular prescriptions are for the same duration of treatment so that prescription requests can be synchronized
- *Regular housekeeping* Keep records of medication up to date (including dosage instructions). Particular care is needed after hospital discharge when medication could have been substantially changed
- *Training of practice staff.*

**Review process** Invite the patient ± carer. *Areas to cover:*
- *Explain* what you want to do in the review and the reasons for it
- *Compile* a list of all medicines being taken/used including prescribed medication, OTC drugs, herbal/homeopathic medicines, illicit drugs, and medicines borrowed from others. Compare the list of drugs generated with the prescription record
- *Concordance* Find out whether and how medication is taken
- *Explore* understanding of the purpose of the medication and consequences of not taking it, and how much, how often, when.
- *Discuss* misconceptions/queries
- *Ask about side effect*
- *Review relevant monitoring tests*, e.g. TFTs, INR, HbA$_{1c}$
- *Review practical aspects* Problems ordering/receiving repeat prescriptions, using medicines (e.g. problems opening containers), with formulations (e.g. difficulty swallowing tablets), reading label (can request large print), remembering to take medication (consider reminder chart, compliance aid, altering times of doses to fit in better with daily schedule)
- *Check* necessity and appropriateness of all prescriptions (Figure 6.1).

## Further information
BNF 🖳 www.bnf.org
UK Medicines Information 🖳 www.ukmi.nhs.uk
Electronic Medicines Compendium 🖳 www.medicines.org.uk

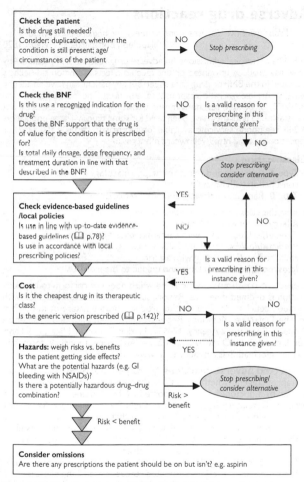

**Fig. 6.1** Deciding whether a prescribed drug is appropriate

# Adverse drug reactions

*I don't want two diseases—one nature-made and one doctor-made.*
Napoleon Bonaparte, St. Helena, 1820

In 5–17% of hospital admissions, an adverse drug reaction is implicated. Any drug may produce unwanted or unexpected effects. Common side effects are listed in the BNF or drug data sheet, but any patient can have an allergic reaction or idiosyncratic response to any drug. The possibility of rare (<1:5000) or delayed reactions means that safety of new medicines cannot be established until they have been used for some time in a large population. A 24h free-phone service is available for information (☎ 0800 100 3352) or report online at 🖳 http://yellowcard.mhra.gov.uk

## Classification
- **Type A** Common and relate to the pharmacology of the drug (eg. constipation with opioids)
- **Type B** Rare, unpredictable and often serious.

Within this classification, reactions may be:
- **Allergy** Anaphylaxis, allergic rash
- **Toxic effect,** e.g. ataxia with carbamazepine if dose is too high
- **Predictable** Well-recognized side effect, e.g. dry mouth with amitriptyline, GI bleeding with aspirin
- **Idiosyncratic** Unpredictable and unique to the individual.

**Defective medicines** A medicine which does not conform to its specification is deemed defective. Report suspected defective medicines, with as much detail as possible on the product and the nature of the defect, to The Defective Medicines Report Centre, Medicines and Healthcare Products Regulatory Agency, 17–157, Market Towers, 1 Nine Elms Lane, London SW8 5NQ ☎ 0207 084 2574. An online reporting form and further information is available at: 🖳 www.mhra.gov.uk

**Suspected adverse reactions** Any suspected adverse reaction to any therapeutic agent, whether OTC, herbal/alternative medication, or prescribed by a doctor, should be reported to the Medicines and Healthcare products Regulatory Agency (MHRA, CHM Freepost, London SW8 5BR). Forms ('Yellow Cards') are available from that address or in the back of the BNF. Alternatively, report online at 🖳 http://yellowcard.mhra.gov.uk
- **For new drugs** (marked ◆ in BNF) Doctors are asked to report all reactions whether or not causality is clear
- **For established drugs** Doctors are asked to report all reactions in children; and all serious suspected reactions even if the effect is well documented (e.g. anaphylaxis, blood disorders, renal or liver impairment, drug interactions). Well-known relatively minor side effects (e.g. constipation with opioids, insomnia with SSRIs) should *not* be reported.

## Prevention of adverse reactions

- Never use a drug unless there is a good indication
- Always ask patients if they have had reactions previously to a drug before prescribing
- Ask about other drugs patients are taking (including self-medication). Consider interactions
- Consider the effects of age and hepatic or renal impairment
- Prescribe as few drugs as possible—the more drugs, the more likelihood of interactions
- Give clear instructions about how to take the drug
- Wherever possible use drugs you are familiar with. If using a new drug be alert to side effects
- Warn patients about potentially serious side effects (e.g. risk of GI ulceration with NSAIDs).

**Consumer Protection Act 1987** If a patient is damaged by a defective product, liability falls on the producer unless outside the EC when it falls on the importer. If the importer cannot be identified, liability falls on the supplier. This is important for GPs. Those who dispense are at greatest risk, but all GPs occasionally supply drugs in an emergency or for procedures within the surgery (vaccinations, minor surgery, contraception). Always record manufacturer, batch number, and expiry date when using such drugs, and keep records of storage of drugs and maintenance of equipment.

**Poisoning** 📖 p.1112

### Poisons information

**TOXBASE poisons database** 🖥 www.toxbase.org
**UK National Poisons Information Service** 🖥 www.npis.org
Contact regional center for further information:
- Birmingham ☎ 0121 507 4123
- Cardiff ☎ 029 207 15554
- Edinburgh ☎ 0131 242 1381
- Newcastle ☎ 0191 260 6180
- Belfast ☎ 02890 632032

# Licensing

In the UK, the Medicines Act 1968 makes it essential for anyone who manufactures or markets a drug for which therapeutic claims are made to hold a licence. The Licensing Authority, working through the Medicines and Healthcare Products Regulatory Agency (MHRA), can grant both a Manufacturer's Licence and Marketing Authorization (which allows a company to market and supply a product for specified indications). Although doctors usually prescribe according to the licensed indications, they are not obliged to do so.

**Prescribing outside licence** There may be occasions when a doctor feels that it is necessary to prescribe outside a drug's licence.
- *Generic formulations* for which indications are not described. The prescriber has to assume that the indications are the same as for branded formulations
- *Use of well-established drugs for proven but not licensed indications,* e.g. amitriptyline for neuropathic pain
- *Use of drugs for conditions where there are no other treatments* (even if the evidence of their effectiveness is not well proven). This often occurs in secondary care when new treatments become accepted. GPs may become involved if a patient is discharged to the community and the GP asked to continue prescribing. ❶ The person signing the prescription is legally responsible
- *Use of drugs for individuals not covered by their licensed indications.* Frequently occurs in paediatrics.

⚠ Before prescribing any medication (whether within or outside the licence), weigh risks against benefits. The more dangerous the medicine and the flimsier the evidence-base for treatment, the more difficult it is to justify the decision to prescribe.

When prescribing licensed drugs for unlicensed indications, it is important to inform patients and carers about what you are doing and why. Explain that the patient information leaflet (PiL) will not have information about the use of the drug in these circumstances. Record in the patients notes your reasons for prescribing outside the licensed indications for the drug.

**Clinical trials** Drug discovery and development is a protracted process (>10y) costing huge sums of money (~£100 million). Clinical testing is conventionally divided into 5 stages:
- *Phase I trials:* clinical pharmacology in normal volunteers
- *Phase II trials:* preliminary small-scale studies
- *Phase III trials:* large-scale trials (often several thousand patients). Once complete application is made for a licence to sell the drug
- *Phase IV trials:* post-marketing surveillance—large-scale follow-up of patients using the drug to establish evidence of long-term efficacy and safety
- *Phase V trials:* further trials to compare efficacy and safety with other marketed compounds and explore new indications.

GPs are unlikely to be involved before phase III. Taking part in trials can benefit both patients and the practice, but consider proposals carefully before embarking on a project.

**Research in general practice** 📖 p.82

**Questions to ask before agreeing to take part in a clinical trial**

- Are the aims and objectives of the study defined?
- What is the design?
- Which drug is to be tested?
- What are the endpoints?
- Are the criteria for identifying patients clear and explicit?
- Are the numbers to be recruited specified and feasible?
- Are the observations to be made clearly and vigorously defined?
- Are the arrangements for providing information to patients and for obtaining informed consent satisfactory?
- Has ethical approval of the study been obtained?
- Are the financial arrangements clearly set out (minimum— reimbursement of patients' expenses and reimbursement of practice expenses)?
- Has adequate provision been made for compensation in the event of injury to patients in the course of the study?

# Controlled drugs

**Misuse of Drugs Act 1971** Controls manufacture, supply, and possession of controlled drugs (CDs). Penalties for offences are graded according to perceived harmfulness of the drug into 3 classes:
- *Class A* e.g. cocaine, diamorphine (heroin), methadone, LSD, ecstasy
- *Class B* e.g. oral amphetamines, barbiturates, cannabis
- *Class C* e.g. most benzodiazepines, androgenic and anabolic steroids, cannabis.

**Misuse of Drugs Regulations 2001** Defines persons authorized to supply and possess CDs while carrying out their professions and describes the way in which this is to be done. 5 schedules of drug:
- *Schedule 1* Drugs not used for medicinal purposes, e.g. LSD. Possession and supply are prohibited except with special licence
- *Schedule 2* Drugs subject to full CD controls (written dispensing record, kept in locked container, CD prescription regulations), e.g. diamorphine, cocaine, pethidine
- *Schedule 3* Partial CD controls (as Schedule 2 but no need to keep a register—some drugs subject to safe custody regulations), e.g. barbiturates, temazepam, meprobamate, buprenorphine
- *Schedules 4 and 5* Most benzodiazepines, anabolic and androgenic steroids, HCG, growth hormone, codeine. Controlled drug prescription requirements do not apply nor do safe custody requirements.

❶ Preparations in Schedules 2 and 3 are identified throughout the British National Formulary (BNF) by the symbol CD (controlled drug).

**Controlled drugs register** All healthcare professionals who hold personal stock of any Schedule 2 drugs must keep their own controlled drugs register, and they are personally responsible for keeping this accurate and up to date. Out-of-date drugs should be recorded and destroyed in the presence of an authorized witness (police, PCO official).

**Prescriber's responsibilities** If prescribing controlled drugs for medicinal purposes, you have a responsibility:
- To avoid creating dependence by unnecessarily introducing controlled drugs to patients
- For careful monitoring to ensure the patient does not gradually ↑ the dose of drug to a point where dependence becomes more likely
- To avoid being an unwitting source of supply for addicts. If you suspect an addict is going round surgeries with intent to obtain supplies, contact your PCO so that they can issue a warning to other practices.

**Writing prescriptions for CDs** Any prescription for Schedule 2 and 3 controlled drugs (with the exception of temazepam) must contain the following details, written so as to be indelible:
- The patient's full name, address, and age. If the patient is homeless, 'no fixed abode' is an acceptable address
- The patient's NHS (in Scotland, Community Health Index) number.
- Name and form of the drug, even if only one form exists
- Strength of the preparation and dose to be taken
- The total quantity of the preparation, or the number of dose units, to be supplied in both words and figures, e.g. 'Morphine sulphate 10 mg (ten milligram) tablets, one to be taken twice daily. Supply 60 (sixty) tablets, total 600 (six hundred) milligrams'
- Signature of the prescriber (must be handwritten) and date. It is good practice to include the GMC number of the prescriber as well
- The address of the prescriber.

❶ Apart from exceptional circumstances, prescriptions for CDs in Schedules 2, 3, and 4 should be limited to a supply of ≤30d treatment. The validity period of NHS and private prescriptions for Schedule 1, 2, 3, and 4 controlled drugs is restricted to 28d. Schedule 2 and 3 drugs cannot be prescribed on repeat prescriptions or under repeat dispensing schemes.

**Prescribing for drug misusers** 📖 p.191

**Notification of drug misusers** 📖 p.190

**Travelling abroad with controlled drugs** An export licence may be required for patients or doctors travelling abroad with Schedule 2 or 3 drugs. Further details are available from ☎ 020 7035 6161 or 🖳 www.drugs.gov.uk/drugs-laws/licensing/personal. Patient applications to the Home Office for an import/export licence for a CD must be accompanied by a supporting letter from the prescribing doctor stating:
- The patient's name and address
- The quantities of drugs to be carried
- The strength and form in which the drugs will be dispensed
- The country of destination
- The dates of travel to and from the UK.

For clearance to import the drug into the country of destination, it is advisable to contact the Embassy or High Commission of that country prior to departure.

**Further information**
**National Prescribing Centre (NPC)** *A Guide to Good Practice in the Management of Controlled Drugs in Primary Care (England)* (2007) 🖳 www.npc.co.uk
**Department of Health** 🖳 www.dh.gov.uk/controlleddrugs
**British National Formulary** 🖳 www.bnf.org
**Home Office** *Tackling Drugs: Changing Lives* 🖳 www.drugs.gov.uk

# Prescribing for special groups

**Borderline substances** (BNF Appendix 7)
For certain conditions, foods and toilet products can be regarded as drugs and prescribed on NHS prescription (e.g. gluten-free foods for coeliac disease, nutritional supplements for disease-related malnutrition). The Advisory Committee on Borderline Substances advises on which products are available for certain specified conditions. Products should not be prescribed for any other condition. Use form FP10 (GP10 in Scotland) and endorse with the letters ACBS.

**Renal impairment** Renal function ↓ with age but may not be reflected by raised creatinine due to ↓ muscle mass. Always assume mild–moderate renal failure if prescribing for the elderly. Renal impairment can change the effects of drugs by:
- **Inability to excrete drug** May cause toxicity. Dose reduction or increase in interval between doses may be necessary
- **Increased sensitivity to drugs** even if elimination is unimpaired
- **Poor tolerance of side effects** Nephrotoxic drugs may have more serious side effects
- **Lack of effectiveness** when renal function is reduced.

**Degree of renal impairment** Estimated glomerular filtration rate (eGFR), based on serum creatinine, age, gender, and ethnic origin, is now provided to GPs when renal function tests are done.
- **Mild renal impairment**—eGFR 60–89mL/min/1.73m$^2$
- **Moderate renal impairment**—eGFR 30–59mL/min/1.73m$^2$
- **Severe renal impairment**—eGFR <30mL/min/1.73m$^2$.

**Further information** BNF Appendix 3; patients on dialysis—consult local renal unit.

**Hepatic impairment** Problems tend not to arise until late stages of liver failure when there is jaundice, ascites, or evidence of encephalopathy. Problems are due to:
- **Impaired drug metabolism** Many drugs are metabolized by the liver. In severe liver failure dose may need to be ↓ ± dosage interval ↑. A few drugs are excreted in the bile unchanged and may accumulate in patients with obstructive jaundice (e.g. rifampicin, fusidic acid)
- **Hypoproteinaemia** Liver failure is associated with ↓ plasma protein. This affects binding of drugs. Highly protein-bound drugs (e.g. phenytoin, prednisolone) can become toxic in normal dosage
- **Hepatotoxicity** Liver toxicity will have ↑ effect if hepatic reserve is already ↓
- **Clotting** Blood clotting factors are made in the liver. In liver disease effects of oral anticoagulants are ↑
- **Encephalopathy** Drugs that depress cerebral function (e.g benzodiazepines, opioids) can precipitate encephalopathy if severe liver failure
- **Fluid retention** Drugs causing fluid retention (e.g. NSAIDs) make oedema and ascites worse.

**Further information** BNF Appendix 2

**Palliative care** 📖 pp.1026–1042

**Prescribing for the elderly** 📖 p.208

**Pregnancy** 📖 p. 782. Drugs taken by the mother can harm the fetus at any stage in pregnancy. *Mechanisms*:
- *1st trimester* Teratogenesis causing congenital malformations. Greatest risk—weeks 3–12
- *2nd and 3rd trimesters* Toxic effects, effects on growth/development
- *Around labour* May affect labour or have adverse effects on the newborn baby.

Only prescribe if essential, especially in the 1st trimester. Stick to tried and tested drugs when possible (see BNF appendix 4 for list of drugs with known effects); use smallest effective dose; avoid new drugs.

***Further information*** BNF Appendix 4; National Teratology Information Service ☎ 0191 232 1525 🖥 www.nyrdtc.nhs.uk/service/teratology.html

**Breastfeeding** Drugs taken by a mother breastfeeding can affect the child by inhibiting lactation or entering the milk and causing toxicity to the infant. Therapeutic doses in the mother can cause toxicity in the infant if the drug is concentrated in milk (e.g. iodides). Avoid prescribing wherever possible. Stick to tried and tested drugs (BNF Appendix 5).

---

### Prescribing for children

⚠ Keep all medicines out of the reach of children (and preferably in a locked box). Dispose of unwanted medicines by returning them to a supplier/GP surgery for destruction.

- Children differ from adults in their response to drugs. Consult the BNF for Children, or Paediatric Vade Mecum before prescribing unfamiliar drugs. Always check doses carefully. Many drugs are not licensed for use with children
- Paediatric suspensions often contain sugar. For long-term use or children having frequent prescriptions consider sugar-free versions.
- Do not advise adding medicines to infant feeding bottles—they may interact with milk and the dose will be ↓ if not all the contents are drunk
- Information on drugs used to treat rare paediatric conditions: Alder Hey Children's Hospital (☎ 0151 252 5381) or Great Ormond Street Hospital (☎ 020 7405 9200)
- Report *all* adverse reactions on Yellow Cards 📖 p.148

---

**Driving whilst taking drugs** 📖 p.133 or 🖥 www.dvla.gov.uk/medical/ataglance.aspx

**Drugs and sport** 📖 p.509

**Further information**
**British National Formulary** 🖥 www.bnf.org
**UK Medicines information** 🖥 www.ukmi.nhs.uk
**Electronic medicines compendium** 🖥 www.medicines.org.uk

# Complementary medicine

In the UK ~90% of the population have tried complementary or alternative medicine (CAM) at some time. But, although CAM undoubtedly helps many individuals, its use remains controversial.

## Reasons for caution

- *Lack of evidence of effectiveness* There are many anecdotal reports and small-scale observational studies of the positive effects of complementary therapies, but large-scale high-quality studies tend to be –ve
- *Lack of regulation of practitioners* At present anyone can set up as a practitioner of alternative medicine. Regulation has been proposed and is likely to come into force over the next few years. Until then, it is important to find a reputable practitioner with accredited training who is a member of a recognized professional body. It is also important to ensure any practitioner used carries professional indemnity insurance
- *Lack of regulation of products* At present, most complementary 'medicines' are sold as foods rather than medicines and do not hold a product license. No licensing authority has assessed efficacy, safety, or quality, and interactions with conventional medicines are unknown. Complementary medicines can, and do, cause adverse effects—just because they are natural does not mean they are safe.

## Legal position of GPs

***Practising complementary medicine*** Conventionally trained doctors can administer alternative treatments. The *Bolam test* applies—in other words, if a doctor has undergone additional training in a complementary discipline and practises in a way that is reasonable and would be considered acceptable by a number of other medically qualified complementary practitioners, his/her actions are defensible.

### *Referring to complementary medicine practitioners*

- *Delegation to non-medically qualified practitioner* Ask yourself:
  - *Is my decision to delegate to this complementary therapy appropriate?* Evidence-based decisions are most persuasive; commonly accepted but unproven indications are also acceptable
  - *Have I taken reasonable steps to ensure that the practitioner is qualified and insured?* Usually sufficient to ensure he/she is a member of the main professional regulatory body responsible for that discipline. Main bodies require members to be fully indemnified
  - *Has my medical follow-up been adequate?* Continue following up chronic conditions as usual. Do not issue repeat prescriptions without having sufficient information to ensure safe prescribing.
- *Referral to a medically qualified practitioner/state registered osteopath or chiropractor* Same legal situation as when referring to another conventional healthcare practitioner. As long as the decision to make the referral is appropriate, all further responsibility is taken over by the practitioner providing the service.

## Further information

Bandolier ⊠ www.medicine.ox.ac.uk/bandolier/booth/booths/altmed.html

**Table 6.2** Commonly used complementary therapies

| Therapy | Features |
|---|---|
| Acupuncture | Needles are used to alleviate symptoms or cure disease. mechanism of action remains unclear. 2 broad forms:<br>• *Traditional acupuncture* based on Chinese medicine where health is a balance between yin and yang. Illness is imbalance and treatment aims to restore balance<br>• *Modern acupuncture* uses modern anatomy and physiology<br>**Evidence** Mixed—good evidence that effective for back pain, idiopathic headache and migraine, knee pain, and post-operative nausea/vomiting<br>**Variants** Auriculotherapy, transcutaneous electrical nerve stimulation (TENS), reflexology |
| Homeopathy | From the Greek meaning 'treatment of similars'. Works on the principle that like cures like. A remedy is chosen that mimics the symptoms displayed by the patient. Most remedies are serially diluted in steps of 1:10 (decimal ×) or 1:100 (centesimal c). Manufacture is controlled by the Medicines Act<br>**Evidence** With higher dilutions (>12c) a theoretical problem arises as the solution may not contain any molecules of the mother substance. However, meta-analysis suggests it is overall effective |
| Herbal medicine | Use of plants for medicinial purposes. Although traditional medicine uses many plant extracts (e.g. digoxin, morphine), herbal medicine uses plant extracts and not isolated constituents. By 2011, all herbal medicines must be registered in order to be sold in the UK<br>**Evidence** There is evidence of effectiveness of many herbal remedies including saw palmetto (benign prostatic hyperplasia), echinacea (common cold), St John's wort (depression), feverfew (migraine)<br>**Variants** Aromatherapy is the use of concentrated aromatic plant oils. No good evidence of effectiveness. Oils commonly used include lavender oil (insomnia, burns, blisters), tea tree oil (skin infection, head lice), peppermint oil (indigestion), valerian oil (anxiety, insomnia) |
| Dietary manipulation | **Healing foods** are commonly used, e.g. cranberry juice for UTI, soya to ↓ menopausal symptoms, ginger to ↓ nausea.<br>**Nutritional medicine** involves giving supplements of vitamins, minerals, amino acids, or essential fatty acids. There is some evidence of effectiveness, e.g. glucosamine for OA, calcium and vitamin D supplements to ↓ osteoporosis, vitamin B$_6$ for premenstrual tension.<br>**Probiotics**—orally administered microbial cell preparations. Some evidence of effectiveness for treatment of GI conditions.<br>**Environmental medicine** Based on the premise that individuals develop intolerances to environmental substances, most commonly foods. Exclusion diets improve symptoms. The most common culprits are caffeine, milk, gluten, and citrus fruit |
| Osteopathy & chiropractic | Physical treatments aimed at restoring the alignment of the joints and improving functioning of the body. Already under statutory regulation. Good evidence of effectiveness, particularly for back pain |
| Hypno-therapy | Hypnotherapy consists of training the patient to relax very deeply, often with a focus (a scene, smell, touch sensation, or colour) to aid this process. May be helpful for pain relief |

# Minor surgery

*A minor operation: one performed on someone else.*
Unaccredited
Penguin Dictionary of Humorous Quotations (2001)

# Providing minor surgery

**Minor surgery in GMS practices** Under the new GMS contract, minor surgery can be provided as an additional service or directed enhanced service.

**Minor surgery as an additional service**
- Includes curettage and cautery and, in relation to warts, verrucae, and other skin lesions, cryocautery
- In all cases a record of consent of the patient to treatment and a record of the procedure itself should be kept
- Payment is included within the global sum payment. If a practice does not want to provide this service it must 'opt out' and global sum payment is ↓ by 0.6%.

**Minor surgery as a directed enhanced service** Extends the range of procedures beyond those practices are expected to do as an additional service. For the purpose of payment, procedures have been divided into three groups.
- Injections—muscles, tendons and joints
- Invasive procedures, including incisions and excisions
- Injections of varicose veins and piles.

*Payment* Treatments are priced according to the complexity of the procedure, involvement of other staff, and use of specialized equipment. Terms for this must be negotiated locally. Typical figures are £40 for a joint injection or £80 for a simple excision.

**Minor surgery in PMS practices** PMS contracts are negotiated on an individual basis with the local PCO. In most cases, however, the contract provides for similar arrangements and payments to those in place for GMS practices.

**Qualification to provide minor surgery** Practices can provide minor surgery as a directed enhanced service if they can demonstrate that they have the necessary facilities and personnel (partner, employee, or subcontractor) with the necessary skills. This includes:
- Adequate equipment
- Premises compliant with national guidelines as contained in Health Building Note 46 General Medical Practice Premises (DH)
- Nursing support
- Compliance with national infection control policies—sterile packs from the local Central Sterile Services Department (CSSD), disposable sterile instruments, using approved sterilization procedures, etc
- Ongoing training in minor surgery, related skills, and resuscitation techniques
- Regular audit and peer review to monitor clinical outcomes, rates of infection and procedure.

**Location and equipment** A suitable room, adequate lighting, the appropriate equipment, and sufficient uninterrupted time are needed for successful minor surgery. An experienced assistant is also a great help. Sterile instruments and gloves and aseptic technique are essential.

- *Basic minor surgery sets* Contain a scalpel, several sizes of blade (e.g. sizes 11 and 15), toothed forceps, needle holder, fine scissors, artery forceps, skin hook, and curette
- *Additional equipment required* Skin preparation liquid (e.g. chlorhexidine), local anaesthetic (e.g. lidocaine 1%), suitable sized needles and syringes, sterile towels, swabs, sterile specimen pots, suture materials, and dressings for the wound. For joint injection ensure you have steroid and local anaesthetic drawn up and suitable sized needles available before starting.

⚠ Always make sure you know how many blades, sutures, needles and swabs you have and ensure that you have accounted for and safely disposed of them at the end of the procedure.

**Consent** Patient consent for the procedure must be sought and recorded in the notes. This involves giving enough information about the procedure and other possible treatment options to allow the patient to make an informed decision about whether to proceed; the patient and consenting doctor should then both sign the consent form, and the form should be filed in the patient's medical records.

**Histological examination** All tissue removed by minor surgery should be sent for histological examination unless there are exceptional or acceptable reasons for not doing so.

**Documentation** Maintain full, legible, and accurate records. Include:
- History of the complaint
- Examination findings
- Diagnosis
- Full details of the procedure undertaken—include dose, batch number, expiry date and quantities of drugs, size and number of sutures
- Follow-up arrangements
- If the patient is not registered with the practice undertaking the minor surgery, a complete record of the procedure must be sent to the patient's registered practice for inclusion in the GP notes.

**Follow-up and outcome** Should be recorded in the patient's notes. Advise the patient:
- What to expect after the procedure
- Precautions to take after the procedure
- When to return for suture removal
- Signs that would indicate the need for reconsultation
- About the expected recovery/healing time.

Arrange a follow-up appointment for all but the most straightforward procedures.

# Basic techniques

⚠ Never attempt a procedure if you are unsure about it—know the boundaries of your experience and abilities.

### Local anaesthesia
- Lidocaine and procaine are the most commonly used preparations.
- Adrenaline (epinephrine) (1:200 000) added to local anaesthetic ↓ bleeding and prolongs anaesthesia but do not use epinephrine in areas supplied by end arteries (i.e. fingers, toes, penis, ear, nose).
- The safe maximum dose of local anaesthetic in adults is 20mL of 1% solution (less in elderly and children)—overdose causes fits or cardiac arrhythmias.

#### *Administering local anaesthetic*
- Pre-warn patients that local anaesthetic stings before numbing and that they will still be able to feel pressure—but not pain. If pain is felt more anaesthetic is needed
- Clean the skin, insert a small needle intradermally, and raise a small bleb before infusing more deeply
- Always pull back on the syringe plunger before injecting to check that you are not in a blood vessel
- Anaesthetic must be infused all around the excision site. This may require several needle insertions—try to do this through an area that is already numb to ↓ discomfort for the patient
- Allow time for anaesthetic to take effect (2–5min) before proceeding.

### Suturing (suture and needle types 📖 p.165)
- Various techniques for suturing and knot tying can be used (e.g. interrupted, continuous, subcuticular)
- Always make a careful record of the number of stitches and when they should be removed
- Usually stitches need removal after 3–5d on the face, 7–14d on the back and legs, and 5–7d elsewhere
- Steri-Strips™ can be used instead of or in addition to stitches in some circumstances.

**Cautery** Chemical (silver nitrate) or electrocautery are used alone, or in combination with other methods (e.g. curettage), to secure haemostasis or destroy tissue. *Suitable conditions:* nose bleeds, spider naevi, telangiectasia.

⚠ *Do not* use electrical cautery for patients with a cardiac pacemaker.

**Implants** Subcutaneous implants are prescribed for several conditions (e.g. prostate cancer). Most implants come pre-packaged with an insertion cannula and information leaflet—always read and follow the instructions if administering a new product and ensure that position of implant and timing of administration is correct.

**Joint and soft tissue injection** Steroids can have a potent local anti-inflammatory effect and dramatically improve certain musculoskeletal problems. Most joint injections are straightforward and can be undertaken within a general practice setting.

### General rules
- Always use aseptic technique
- Do not inject if there is local sepsis (e.g. cellulitis) or any possibility of joint infection
- Never inject into the substance of a tendon— this may cause rupture (in tenosynovitis steroid is injected into the tendon sheath)
- Injections should not require pressure on the syringe plunger—if so the needle is probably not correctly located (tennis elbow is an exception)
- Undertake as few injections as possible to settle the problem—often 1 is sufficient. If no improvement after 2–3, reconsider the diagnosis
- Do no more than 3–4 injections/patient/appointment and no more than 3–4 in any single joint per year—more than this ↑ risk of systemic absorption and joint damage.

### Preparation for the procedure
- Take a history, make a careful examination, and have a clear diagnosis before considering Injecting steroids.
- Gather the needles, syringes, a sterile container (for sending aspirated fluid), steroid, local anaesthetic, skin preparation fluid (e.g. chlorhexidine), cotton wool, and adhesive plaster beforehand.
- The injected joint should be rested for 2–3d afterwards if possible— certainly avoid heavy activity. Make sure that the patient is comfortable, has given informed consent, and knows what to expect.

*Steroid preparations* (↑ order of potency) hydrocortisone acetate, methylprednisolone acetate, triamcinolone hexacetonide.

*Local anaesthetic (LA),* e.g. lidocaine 1%, can be mixed with the steroid for some injections. LA effect occurs immediately and lasts 2–4h. The patient may then experience some return of symptoms (pain) before the steroid takes effect–warn the patient.

### Follow-up
- Some injections are painful at administration—this is normal for tennis elbow and plantar faciitis
- Severe or increasing pain ~48h after injection may indicate sepsis— advise the patient to return urgently if this occurs
- If steroid is injected close to the skin surface (as in tennis elbow), skin dimpling and pigment loss can occur—warn the patient.

### Further information
**Silver T** *Joint and Soft Tissue Injection Injecting with Confidence* (2007). Radcliffe Publishing Ltd (ISBN 1 846 191 909).

Most hospital rheumatology departments have a joint injection clinic and are happy to allow GPs to watch to gain experience.

# Removal of skin lesions

Ensure that you have had training in the techniques—learning by experience is much better than from a book. There are many courses available.

## Excision of skin lesions

- Gain written consent—ensure that you have warned the patient about the likely size of the scar and the possibility of keloid (especially if the lesion is on a risk area, e.g. upper back and chest)
- Work out the direction of the skin contour lines; clean and anaesthetize the area (📖 p.162)
- An elliptical incision ~3× as long as it is wide is suitable for most lesions. Place the incision in the skin contour lines if possible (marking the incision line can be helpful)
- Cut through the skin at right angles to the surface with a smooth sweep of the blade
- Use a skin hook to lift the skin from one end of the ellipse
- Use the scalpel blade to remove the skin from the subcutaneous fat.
- Save the excised specimen for histology
- Close the wound by carefully apposing the edges (slightly everted) using interrupted non-absorbable sutures. Avoid tension in the sutures and knot securely. Large wounds may benefit from the use of deep absorbable sutures to reduce skin tension.

## Curettage

- Useful for seborrhoeic warts, pyogenic granuloma, keratoacanthoma, or single viral warts. Not suitable for naevi
- Use only if the diagnosis is certain—scrapings can be sent for histology but the architecture of the lesion is lost
- Numb the area with local anaesthetic and remove the lesion with gentle scooping movements using a curette spoon
- Finally, cauterize the base of the lesion.

## Cryotherapy

- Liquid nitrogen can be used to treat viral and seborrhoeic warts and solar keratoses
- Local arrangements for delivery of liquid nitrogen differ—often a clinic session to treat all suitable lesions at the same time is helpful
- If diagnosis is uncertain, excise the lesion or take a biopsy prior to freezing
- A cotton wool bud or nitrogen spray gun can be used to apply liquid nitrogen for approximately 10s until a thin frozen halo appears at the base of the lesion
- A blister forms <24h after treatment—the lesion then falls off with the blister
- Repeat treatment may be needed after 4wk.

*Side effects* Pain, failure to remove the lesion, skin hypopigmentation, ulceration of lower leg lesions (especially in elderly patients).

## ⚠ Rules for removing skin lesions

- **Only** remove benign lesions—refer suspicious lesions to a specialist for expert management
- **Only** remove lesions that you are confident that you can cope with. Take special care with lesions on the face or lip margin—the scar may be very noticeable
- **Send all** excised lesions for histology—place in formalin and carefully label with the site and side.

---

**Suture types**
- *Absorbable,* e.g. catgut, Dexon, Vicryl—used to stitch deep layers to help ↓ tension
- *Non-absorbable,* e.g. silk, prolene, nylon—used for closure of skin wounds after minor surgery

**Needle types** Straight, curved, cutting, or round-bodied. Surgical site and personal preference dictate which to use—a cutting needle is usually used for skin.

**Suture thickness (gauge)** Indicated by a number (10/0 is fine and 2/0 is thick). For skin closure 6/0 or 5/0 is usually used for the face, 3/0 on legs and back, and 4/0 elsewhere.

# Lower and upper limb injections

**The knee** Joint effusions are common (e.g. trauma, ligament strains, OA, RA, gout). Aspirated fluid should be clear/slightly yellow and not purulent. Send any fluid aspirated for analysis. Aspiration of fluid can:

• Help make a diagnosis e.g. gout
• Be a therapeutic procedure—draining a tense effusion can relieve pain
• Precede administration of steroids e.g. RA flare.

⚠ Any sign of infection within the joint prohibits steroid use.

### Technique for aspiration and joint injection

• Lie the patient on couch with knee slightly bent—place a pillow under the knee as this relaxes the muscles
• Palpate the joint space under the lateral or medial edge of the patella and inject/aspirate just below the superior border of the patella with the needle horizontal (Figure 7.1)
• Use a green (21 gauge) needle
• If aspirating and then injecting steroids, maintain the needle in position and swap the syringe
• Normal doses of steroid are triamcinolone 20mg or methylprednisolone 40mg
• In prepatella bursitis, aspiration and injection of hydrocortisone 25mg into the bursa can help settle inflammation.

**Plantar faciitis** Painful area in the middle of the heel pad. Steroid injection (e.g. triamcinolone 10–20mg) into the most tender spot can help. Injection hurts, so advise analgesia. Mixing lidocaine 1% with the steroid can help.

### Technique Two methods are commonly used (Figure 7.2):

• Injection through the tough skin of the sole (more accurate) or
• Lateral approach (less painful).

Rest the foot for several days afterwards and use an in-shoe heel pad. Rupture of the plantar fascia is a rare complication.

**Tenosynovitis** Causes pain and stiffness in the line of the tendon, and crepitus over the affected tendon. The most common site is the base of the thumb (*de Quervain tenosynovitis*). Injecting steroid and LA (e.g. hydrocortisone 25mg + 1mL 1% lidocaine) into the space between tendon and the sheath can help.

### Technique

• Insert the needle along the line of the tendon just distal to the point of maximum tenderness.
• Advance the needle proximally into the tendon (felt as a resistance) and then slowly withdraw until the resistance disappears. The tip of the needle is now in the tendon sheath.
• It is now safe to inject—the tendon sheath may swell.
• Advise the patient to rest the affected area for several days and avoid the precipitating activity.

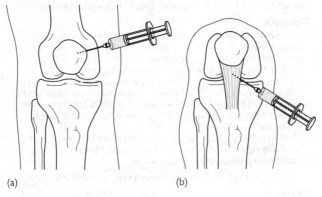

(a)                                                      (b)

**Fig. 7.1** Knee joint injection or aspiration

Adapted from Collier et al. *Oxford Handbook of Clinical Specialties* 6e (2003) with permission from Oxford University Press.

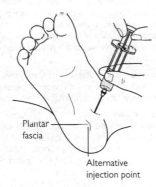

Plantar fascia

Alternative injection point

**Fig. 7.2** Injection of plantar fasciitis

## Patient information

**Arthritis Research Campaign (ARC)** Patient information leaflet: *Local Steroid Injection* ☎ 0870 850 5000 🖳 www.arc.org.uk

**Carpal tunnel syndrome** can be relieved by steroid injection.

*Technique*
- Sit the patient with hand resting on a firm surface, palm up. Palmaris longus tendon can be seen by wrist flexion against resistance.
- Insert the needle at the distal skin crease at 45° to the horizontal, pointing towards the fingers, just ulnar (little finger side) to the palmaris tendon (Figure 7.3). If palmaris longus is absent (10%), inject between flexor digitorum superficialis and flexor carpi radialis tendons.
- Use a green (21 gauge) needle. Advance it to half its length. If sudden pain in the fingers, you have hit the median nerve—withdraw the needle and reposition it.
- Inject steroid e.g. 10mg triamcinolone. If there is resistance, needle is not in the right place. Do not use LA as it causes finger numbness.
- Rest the hand for several days afterwards.

**Elbow** Tennis and golfer's elbows respond well to steroid injection.

*Technique*
- Sit the patient with the elbow flexed to 90°.
- Palpate the most tender spot and insert the needle into that spot.
- Inject 0.1–0.2mL of steroid (e.g. hydrocortisone 25mg/mL). There will be resistance. Without taking the needle out, move the needle in a fan shape injecting small amounts of steroid—try to inject all the tender area. Warn about the possibility of skin dimpling or pigment loss.
- Pain of injection may last 48h—warn the patient in advance. Advise resting the arm and analgesia.

**Shoulder** Injection may help rotator cuff problems, frozen shoulder, subacromial bursitis, and RA. Use an anterior or posterior approach for shoulder joint injection and lateral approach for the subacromial space.

*Technique* Anterior approach
- Sit patient with the arm relaxed at the side, slightly externally rotated.
- Insert the needle (green, 21 gauge) horizontally into the gap between the head of humerus and the coracoid process, ensuring that it is lateral to the coracoid process—Figure 7.4(a). Insert the needle for most of its length to reach the joint space.
- Inject 1mL steroid, e.g. triamcinolone 20mg +1mL 1% lidocaine. There should be no/little resistance to injection. If there is, the needle is wrongly positioned.

*Technique* Lateral approach to subacromial space: Sit the patient with arm hanging down to the side. Palpate the posterolateral corner of the acromion. Insert the needle horizontally into the space under the acromion—Figure 7.4(b). Inject 5mL 0.5% bupivacaine + triamcinolone 20mg.

**AC joint injection** Can help the pain of OA.

*Technique*
- Palpate the joint space. Insert the needle anteriorly or superiorly—if you go too far you may enter the shoulder joint—Figure 7.4(c).
- Only 0.2–0.5mL can be injected as joint space is small. Use a blue (23 gauge) needle and do not add LA.

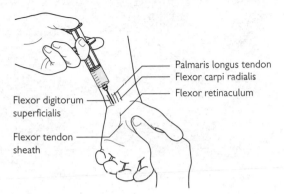

Palmaris longus tendon
Flexor carpi radialis
Flexor retinaculum
Flexor digitorum superficialis
Flexor tendon sheath

**Fig. 7.3** Injection of the carpal tunnel

⚠️Warn patients that pain may worsen for up to 48h after injection before it improves.

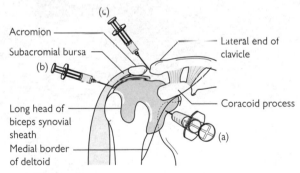

Acromion
Subacromial bursa
(b)
Long head of biceps synovial sheath
Medial border of deltoid
Lateral end of clavicle
Coracoid process
(a)

**Fig. 7.4** Shoulder joint injection

Adapted from Collier et al. Oxford Handbook of Clinical Specialties 6e (2003) with permission from Oxford University Press.

❶ A recent RCT showed that, for tennis elbow, steroid injection has significantly better effects in the short term (~6wk) but poorer outcome long term compared with physiotherapy.

# Healthy living

# Prevention and screening

In all disease, the goal is prevention.

## Definitions

- *Primary prevention* Prevention of disease occurrence
- *Secondary prevention* Controlling disease in early form
  (e.g. carcinoma *in situ*)
- *Tertiary prevention* Prevention of complications once the disease is
  present (e.g. DM).

## Barriers to prevention

- *Patient* Blinkering ('It'll never happen to me'); rebellion ('I know it's
  bad—but it's cool'); poor motivation (path of least resistance).
- *Doctor* Time; money—health promotion takes time and personnel;
  motivation—health promotion is repetitive and boring.
- *Society* Pressure from big business (e.g. cigarette advertising and
  Formula 1); other priorities; ethics (e.g. public uproar at threats not to
  offer cardiac surgery to smokers).

## Prevention of coronary heart disease 📖 p.246

**Screening** The idea of screening is attractive—the ability to diagnose and
treat a potentially serious condition at an early stage when it is still treatable.
An ideal screening test must pick up all those who have the disease (have
high sensitivity) and must exclude those who do not (high specificity).
It must detect *only* those who have the disease (high positive predictive
value) and should exclude *only* those who do not have the disease (high
negative predictive value). See Table 8.1.

*The Wilson–Jungner criteria\** All screening tests should meet the fol-
lowing criteria before they are introduced to the target population.
- The condition being screened for is an important health problem.
- Natural history of the condition is well understood.
- There is a detectable early stage.
- Treatment at early stage is of > benefit than treatment at late stage.
- There is a suitable test to detect early stage disease.
- The test is acceptable to the target population.
- Intervals for repeating the test have been determined.
- Adequate health service provision has been made made for the extra
  clinical workload resulting from screening.
- Risks, both physical and psychological, are < benefits.
- Costs are worthwhile in relation to benefits gained.

## UK screening programmes

- Cervical cancer 📖 p.726
- Breast cancer 📖 p.692
- Colon cancer 📖 p.404
- Antenatal 📖 p.794
- Neonatal bloodspot 📖 p.848
- Neonatal hearing 📖 p.855
- Child health surveillance 📖 p.844
- Diabetic retinopathy 📖 p.365
- Chlamydia 📖 p.738

---

\* Wilson JMG, Jungner G *Principles and Practice of Screening for Disease* (1968). Public Health Paper
No. 34. WHO, Geneva.

**Table 8.1** Performance of screening tests

| | | Disease | |
|---|---|---|---|
| | | *Present* | *Absent* |
| **Test** | **Positive** | True positive ($a$) | False positive ($b$) |
| | **Negative** | False negative ($c$) | True negative ($d$) |
| Sensitivity = $a/(a+c)$ | | Negative predictive value = $d/(c+d)$ | |
| Specificity = $d/(b+d)$ | | Positive predictive value = $a/(a+b)$ | |

***Performance of screening tests*** For a screening programme to be effective and ↓ morbidity and mortality there must be:
- Adequate participation of the target population
- Few false-negative or false-positive results
- Screening intervals shorter than the time taken for the disease to develop to an untreatable stage
- Adequate follow-up of all abnormal results
- Effective treatment at the stage detected by screening.

⚠ There is **no** ideal screening test. Always explain:
- Purpose of screening
- Likelihood of positive/negative findings and possibility of false-positive/negative results
- Uncertainties and risks attached to the screening process
- Significant medical, social, or financial implications of screening for the particular condition or predisposition
- Follow-up plans, including availability of counselling and support services.

**Table 8.2** Benefits and disadvantages of screening

| Benefits | Disadvantages |
|---|---|
| • Improved prognosis for some cases detected by screening | • Longer morbidity in cases where prognosis is unaltered |
| • Less radical treatment for some early cases | • Overtreatment of questionable abnormalities |
| • Reassurance for those with negative test results. | • False reassurance for those with false-negative results |
| • Increased information on natural history of disease and benefits of treatment at early stage | • Anxiety and sometimes morbidity for those with false-positive results |
| | • Unnecessary intervention for those with false-positive results |
| | • Hazards of the screening test |
| | • Diversion of resouces to the screening programme |

# Prevention of travel-related illness

**Pre-travel assessment** 8wk pre-departure where possible. *Check:*
- Age
- General health
- Where and when intending to travel (including areas within a country and stopovers elsewhere)
- Type of accommodation
- Purpose of travel
- Previous experience (including experience with antimalarials)
- Current vaccination status.

**Health risks**
- *Environmental hazards (e.g. changes in altitude/climate)* Avoid rapid changes of altitude and take time to readjust; avoid sunburn
- *Accidents* Avoid potentially dangerous tasks under the influence of alcohol, e.g. swimming, driving. Avoid motorbikes—especially without helmets and protective clothing
- *Illness abroad* MI causes 61% of deaths related to international travel. Don't travel if unwell. Ensure adequate insurance, including repatriation costs. Take enough supplies of regular medication when travelling to last the entire trip and take preventative steps to avoid infection
- *Transport related problems*
  - Fitness to fly 📖 p.134
  - Motion sickness—take OTC medication if afflicted
  - Jet lag
  - DVT—drink plenty of water on long haul flights; avoid alcohol; regularly get up and walk around; consider prophylactic aspirin ± support stockings
- *Psychological effects of travel*.

**Vaccination** 4% deaths related to travel are due to infectious disease—ensure fully vaccinated for areas intending to visit. Information is available via the Travax website (🖥 www.travax.nhs.uk) and travel information clinics.

**Prevention of travellers' diarrhoea** 50% of travellers experience some diarrhoea. Most cases last 4–5 d; 1–2% last >1mo.
- Take care to eat and drink uncontaminated food and water
- Food should be freshly cooked and hot
- Avoid salads and cold meats/fish
- Eat fruit that can be peeled
- Stick to drinks made with boiling water or bottled drinks and water with intact seal; avoid ice in drinks
- Use water purification tablets if necessary.

*Action* If diarrhoea occurs when abroad advise patients to use oral rehydration fluids. Only take anti-diarrhoeals if impossible to get to a toilet. Seek medical advice if blood in stool, fever, or not resolving in 72h (24h for elderly or infants).

⚠ Do not use anti-diarrhoeals if blood in stool, fever, or <10y old.

## Prevention of malaria[ND]

- *Awareness of risk* High-risk areas are Central and South America, South East Asia, Pacific islands, and sub-Saharan Africa—however brief the time there. Pregnant and asplenic patients are at particular risk.
- ↓ *mosquito bites* Mosquitos bite at night.
  - *Accommodation*—sleep in screened accommodation. Spray screens with insecticide each evening and use a pyrethroid vaporizer. If screens are not available, use a permethrin-impregnated bed net (kits are available)
  - *Person*—In the evenings wear long-sleeved shirts and trousers; protect limbs with repellant containing diethyltoluamide.
- *Chemoprophylactic drugs* Regimes vary with location and time of year. Information is available via the Travax website (🖥 www.travax.nhs.uk) and travel information clinics. For all anti-malarials, apart from mefloquine, start 1 wk prior to departure. Start mefloquine 3 wk before leaving to allow change to alternative if there are adverse side effects. Continue all anti-malarials for 4 wk after return.
- *Awareness of residual risk* Chemoprophylaxis is not 100% effective. Advise all travellers to malaria regions to seek medical advice if unwell for up to 6 mo after return. Malaria is a great mimic. Have a high level of suspicion.

## Prevention of HIV and hepatitis B and C

- Avoid casual sexual contacts. If these occur use barrier methods of contraception (Femidom, condoms)
- Avoid shared needles (e.g. tattooing, ear piercing, drugs)
- Medical kits—if travelling to a high-risk area, take a clearly labelled medical kit containing sutures, syringes, and needles for use in an emergency
- Avoid blood transfusion. $^2/_3$ of blood donations in the developing world are unscreened. Know your blood group. Have good travel insurance including repatriation costs. In an emergency the Blood Care Foundation can arrange screened blood to be provided anywhere in the world (☎ 01403 262652; 🖥 www.bloodcare.org.uk)
- Vaccination for hepatitis B prior to travelling.

## Useful information

**Health Protection Agency (HPA)** *Guidelines for Malaria Prevention in Travellers from the UK* (2007) 🖥 www.hpa.org.uk
**Fit for Travel** Information for people travelling abroad from the UK. Includes a list of yellow fever vaccination centres 🖥 www.fitfortravel.nhs.uk
**Travax** Information for health professionals 🖥 www.travax.nhs.uk (registration required)

# Diet

### The role of the GP and primary care team
- **Screening** Identification of obese patients and patients in need of dietary advice for other reasons
- **Assessment** Current diet, motivation, and barriers to change
- **Discussion and negotiation** Exploration of knowledge about diet; negotiation of goals
- **Goal-setting** Provide information and 2–3 food-specific goals on each occasion. Set a series of mini-targets that appear realistic and achievable; tailor them to existing diet and usual schedule
- **Monitoring progress**.

### Barriers to a good diet
- Ignorance: posters in surgeries/leaflets may help
- Cultural differences: modify information to be relevant
- Enjoyment: perception that healthy diet is not enjoyable
- Poverty: fresh fruit/vegetables and lean meat/fish are expensive—some elements are cheap (e.g. potatoes, pasta, rice)
- Lifestyle: convenience foods contain a lot of salt, sugar, and fat
- Peer pressure: children are under pressure to eat sweets, crisps, etc
- Habits of a lifetime: we like the foods we have grown up with
- Confusion about what is good: packaging may be misleading, e.g. breakfast cereals claiming health messages but containing high sugar
- Mixed messages: one minute the press says something is good for you, the next that it causes some horrible disease and should be avoided
- Fatalism/apathy.

**The ideal diet** See Figure 8.1 📖 p.178. Adjust composition/portion size of each meal to maintain a healthy weight. Include a variety of foods:
- **Use starchy foods** (e.g. bread, rice, pasta, potatoes) as the main energy source
- **Eat plenty of fruit and vegetables** (>5 portions of fruit+vegetables/d). Do not overcook vegetables; steaming is preferable to boiling. Keep the delay between cutting and eating fruit/vegetables to a minimum
- **Eat plenty of fibre** Good sources are high-fibre breakfast cereals, beans, pulses, wholemeal bread, potatoes (with skins), pasta, rice, oats, fruit/vegetables
- **Eat fish** at least 2×/wk including 1 portion (max. 2 portions if pregnant) of oily fish (e.g. mackerel, herring, pilchards, salmon). ↓ cooked red or processed meat; consider substituting meat with vegetable protein (e.g. pulses, soya)
- **Choose lean meat** Remove excess fat/poultry skin and pour off fat after cooking; avoid fatty meat products (e.g. sausages, salami, meat pies); boil, steam, or bake foods in preference to frying; when cooking with fat use unsaturated oil (e.g. olive oil, sunflower oil) and use cornflour rather than butter and flour to make sauces
- **Use skimmed milks** and low-fat yoghurts/spreads/cheese (e.g. Edam or cottage cheese)
- **Avoid adding salt** to foods. Aim for <6g salt/d. Avoid processed foods, crisps, and salted nuts.

- *Avoid adding sugar* and cut down on sweets, biscuits, and desserts
- *Drink at least 4–6 pints (2–3L) of fluid*—preferably not tea, coffee, or alcohol. Drinking a large glass of water with meals and instead of snacks can reduce the urge to overeat.
- *Avoid excessive alcohol intake* < 21u/wk for men and <14u/wk for women 📖 p.186.

## Obesity 📖 p.180

**Weight loss** Non-specific symptom. Treat the cause. *Consider*:
- *GI causes* Malabsorption, malnutrition, dieting
- *Chronic disease* Hyperthyroidism, DM, heart failure, renal disease, degenerative neurological/muscle disease, chronic infection (e.g. TB, HIV) or infestation
- *Malignancy*
- *Psychiatric causes* Depression, dementia, anorexia.

**Malnutrition** 50% of women and 25% of men aged >85y are unable to cook a meal alone. Malnutrition is common amongst the elderly.

**Poor nutritional status** slows rate of wound healing, ↑ risk of infection, ↓ muscle strength, is detrimental to mental well-being, and ↓ the ability of elderly people to remain independent.

### Risk factors
- Low income
- Living alone
- Mental health problems (e.g. depression)
- Dementia
- Recent bereavement
- Gastric surgery
- Malabsorption
- ↑ metabolism
- Difficulty eating and/or swallowing (stroke, neurological disorder, MND)
- Presence of chronic disease (e.g. Crohn's disease, UC, IBS, cancer, COPD, CCF).

### Management
- *General nutritional advice* Encourage to eat more and ↑ consumption of fruit and vegetables; consider using nutritional, vitamin (e.g. vitamin D for the housebound and institutionalized), and mineral supplements
- *Inability to prepare meals/shop* Consider referral to social services, Meals on Wheels, community dietician, community day centre, local voluntary support organization
- *Difficulty with utensils* Consider aids/equipment, e.g.special cutlery, non-slip mats—consider OT referral
- *Nausea* Consider antiemetics
- *Difficulty with swallowing* Investigate cause. If none found or unable to resolve the problem, consider pureed food and/or thickened fluids.

## Further information
**Scientific Advisory Committee on Nutrition (SACN)**
🖥 www.sacn.gov.uk
**Food Standards Agency** 🖥 www.eatwell.gov.uk
**British Nutrition Foundation** 🖥 www.nutrition.org.uk
**Malnutrition Universal Screening Tool (MUST)**
🖥 www.bapen.org.uk/must_tool.html
**NICE** Nutrition Support in Adults (2006) 🖥 www.nice.org.uk

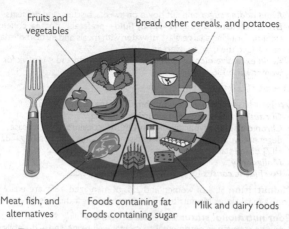

Fruits and vegetables

Bread, other cereals, and potatoes

Meat, fish, and alternatives

Foods containing fat
Foods containing sugar

Milk and dairy foods

**Fig. 8.1** The plate model. Developed nationally to communicate current recommendations for healthy eating. It shows rough proportions of the various food groups that should make up each meal.

Reproduced from the Food Standards Agency under the terms of the Click-Use Licence.

### What is a portion of vegetables or fruit?

**One** portion of vegetables or fruit is roughly equivalent to:
- 1 normal portion (2 tablespoons) of any vegetable
- 1 dessert bowl of salad
- 1 large fruit, e.g. apple, banana, orange, pear, peach, large tomato or a large slice of pineapple or melon
- 2 smaller fruits, e.g. satsumas, plums, kiwi fruits, apricots
- 1 cup of small fruits, e.g. strawberries, raspberries, blackcurrants, cherries, grapes
- 1 tablespoon of dried fruit.
- 2 large tablespoons of fruit salad, stewed or canned fruit in natural juices.
- 1 glass (150mL) of fresh fruit juice.

**Avoiding snacking** Discourage uncontrolled snacking of junk food between meals. Advise patients to ask themselves the following questions when they feel like eating between meals:
- *Am I hungry?* If unsure, wait 20min and then ask the same question again.
- *When was the last time I ate?* If <3h ago, it may not be real hunger.
- *Could a small snack tide me over until the next meal?* Have ready-to-eat fruits or vegetables on hand for this.

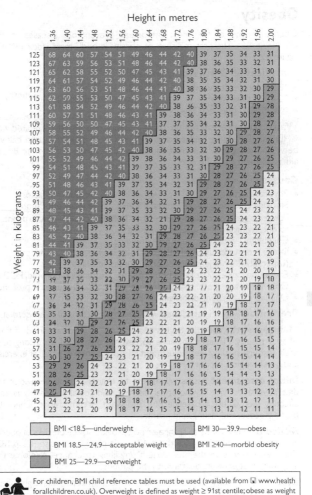

Height in metres

Weight in kilograms

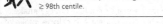

BMI <18.5—underweight

BMI 18.5—24.9—acceptable weight

BMI 25—29.9—overweight

BMI 30—39.9—obese

BMI ≥40—morbid obesity

For children, BMI child reference tables must be used (available from ⬜ www.health forallchildren.co.uk). Overweight is defined as weight ≥ 91st centile; obese as weight ≥ 98th centile.

**Fig. 8.2** Body mass index (BMI) ready reckoner for adults

# Obesity

Obesity is one of the most important preventable diseases in the UK (Table 8.3). The best measure of obesity is body mass index (BMI)—Figure 8.2.

**Classification** BMI [weight in kg/(height in $m^2$)]

- 18.5–24.9 Healthy weight
- 25—29.9 Overweight
- 30–34.9 Obesity I
- 35–39.9 Obesity II
- >40 Morbid obesity (Obesity III).

} Obesity

**Waist circumference** Alternative measure of body fat correlated with CHD risk, DM, hyperlipidaemia, and ↑ BP (Table 8.4). Measured halfway between the superior iliac crest and the rib cage. Use in addition to BMI to aid assessment of health risks.

## Causes

- Physical inactivity
- Smoking cessation - mean weight ↑ 3–4kg
- Cultural factors
- Low education
- Polygenic genetic predisposition ( ~1 in 3 obese people)—more prone to obesity again after successful dieting
- Childbirth—especially if not breastfeeding
- Drugs—steroids, antipsychotics (e.g. olanzapine), contraceptives (especially depo-injections), sulphonylureas, insulin
- Endocrine causes (rare)—hypothyroidism, Cushing's syndrome, PCOS. Only investigate if other symptoms/signs of endocrine disease present
- Ongoing binge eating disorder (📖 p.1013).

**Prevention** Begins in childhood with healthy patterns of exercise/diet.

**Management** When the body's intake > output over a period of time, obesity results. Management aims to reverse this trend on a long-term basis through healthy diet, adjustment of calorie intake, physical exercise, and psychological support.

*Initial assessment* Assess willingness to change, eating behaviour and diet, physical activity, psychological distress, and social and family factors affecting diet. Check a baseline BMI and waist circumference. Check BP, blood glucose, and fasting lipid profile.

*Advice* Whether willing to change or not, provide advice on risks of obesity, and benefits of *healthy eating* (📖 p.176) and *physical exercise* (📖 p.182). Tailor your advice to the individual. If unwilling to change, reinforce this information at each encounter with the patient.

*Diet* Advise a weight loss diet for any patient who is overweight/obese and willing to change:

- ↓ *calorie diets* All obese people lose weight on a low energy intake. Aim for weight loss of 1–2lb (0.5–1kg)/wk using a ↓ in calorie intake of ~600kcal/d with a target BMI of 25 in steps of 5–10% of original weight. There is no health benefit of weight loss below this. If simple diet sheets are not effective, refer to a dietician
- *Very low calorie diets* (<1000kcal/d) Only limited place in management—use for a maximum of 12wk for obese patients when weight loss has plateaued.

**Table 8.3** Health risks of obesity

| Greatly increased risk (RR >3) | Slightly increased risk (RR 1–2) |
|---|---|
| Mortality (BMI>30) | Cancer (breast in post-menopausal women, endometrial, oesophageal, colon)—14–20% of cancer deaths are due to obesity |
| Type 2 DM (BMI = 35 confers a 92× ↑ risk of DM) | |
| Gallbladder disease | |
| Dyslipidaemia | Reproductive hormone abnormalities |
| Insulin resistance | PCOS |
| Breathlessness | Impaired fertility |
| Sleep apnoea | Low back pain |
| **Moderately increased risk (RR 2–3)** | Stress incontinence |
| | Anaesthetic and post-operative risk |
| CHD (5–6% deaths are due to obesity) | Fetal defects associated with maternal obesity |
| ↑ BP | |
| OA (knees) | Suicide |
| Hyperuricaemia/gout | School/workplace prejudice |

**Table 8.4** Waist circumference with excess risk (RR ≥3) of CHD and DM

| Waist circumference | White Caucasians | Asians |
|---|---|---|
| Male | ≥ 102cm (40 inches) | ≥ 90cm (36 inches) |
| Female | ≥ 88cm (35 inches) | ≥ 80cm (32 inches) |

**❶** For every 1cm↑ in waist circumference, the RR of a CVD event ↑ by ~2%

**Drug therapy** (BNF 4.5) 3 drugs are licensed for treatment of obesity:
- Orlistat (120mg tds with food)—acts by ↓ fat absorption
- Sibutramine (10–15mg od—monitor BP and pulse rate closely) and rimonabant (20mg mane)—centrally acting appetite suppressants.

Consider if BMI ≥30kg/m$^2$ or >28kg/m$^2$ + comorbidity (e.g. DM, ↑BP). Do not use combination therapy with >1 anti-obesity drug. Continue treatment >3mo only if weight ↓ is ≥5% of initial body weight.

**Surgery** Consider if BMI >40kg/m$^2$ and non-surgical measures have failed. Gastroplasty is the most common procedure. Surgery ↓ cancer risk. *Complications:* dumping (20%); anastomosis complications (12%); abdominal hernias (7%); infections (6%); pneumonia (4%). *Mortality:* 0.2%.

**Group and behavioural therapy** Group activities, e.g. Weight Watchers, have higher success rates in producing/maintaining weight loss. Behavioural therapy together with low calorie diets is also effective.

**Maintenance of weight loss** Once a patient has lost weight, continue to monitor diet. *Ongoing follow-up* helps to sustain weight loss. Weight fluctuation (yo-yo dieting) may be harmful.

### Further information
**NICE** Obesity: the prevention, identification, assessment and management of overweight and obesity in adults and children (2006) ☐ www.nice.org.uk
**National Obesity Forum** ☐ www.nationalobesityforum.org.uk

# Exercise

In the UK, 60% of adults are not active enough to benefit their health.

### Recommended amounts of activity
- *Adults* ≥ 30 min/d moderate intensity exercise on ≥ 5 d/wk
- *Children* ≥ 1h/d moderate intensity exercise every day.

**Assessing levels of physical activity** Use a validated tool to assess levels of physical activity, e.g. General Practitioner Physical Activity Questionnaire (GPPAQ—Table 8.5).

**Health benefits of exercise** Regular physical activity:
### ↓ *risk of*
- DM through ↑ insulin sensitivity[S].
- Obesity[S] 📖 p.180
- Cardiovascular disease—physically inactive people have ~2× ↑ risk of CHD and ~3× ↑ risk of stroke[S].
- Osteoporosis—exercise ↓ risk of hip fractures by half[S].
- Cancer—↓ risk of colon cancer ~40%. There is also evidence of a link between exercise and ↓ risk of breast and prostate cancers[S].

### Is a useful treatment for
- ↑ BP—can result in 10mmHg drop of systolic and diastolic BP; can also delay onset of hypertension[S]
- Hypercholesterolaemia—↑ high density lipoprotein (HDL); ↓ low density lipoprotein (LDL)[C]
- MI (📖 p.266) and COPD (📖 p.324)
- DM—improves insulin sensitivity and favourably affects other risk factors for DM including obesity, HDL/LDL ratio, and ↑BP
- HIV—↑ cardiopulmonary fitness and psychological well-being[C]
- Arthritis and back pain—maintains function[C]
- Mental health problems —↓ intensity of depression; ↓ anxiety[S].

### Benefits the elderly
- Maintains functional capacity
- ↓ levels of disability
- ↓ risk of falls & hip fracture
- Improves quality of sleep[C].

**Negotiating change** Figure 8.3

### Effective interventions
- *Healthcare* Counselling is as effective as more structured exercise sessions. Specialist rehabilitation schemes are available for patients with specific conditions (e.g. post-MI, COPD); exercise schemes offering low-cost supervised exercise for patients who might otherwise find it unacceptable to visit a gym operate in some areas, and are accessed via GP 'prescription'; many sports facilities offer special sessions for pregnant women, the over-50s, and people with disability
- *Workplace* Interventions to ↑ rates of walking to work are effective
- *Schools* Appropriately designed and delivered PE curricula can enhance physical activity levels. A whole-school approach to physical activity promotion is effective
- *Transport* Well-designed interventions ↑ walking and cycling to work
- *Communities* Community-wide approaches are effective in ↑ activity.

**Table 8.5** Physical activity index (PAI) derived from the GPPAQ

| Physical exercise and/or cycling (h/wk) | Occupation | | | |
|---|---|---|---|---|
| | Sedentary | Standing | Physical | Heavy manual |
| 0 | Inactive | Moderately inactive | Moderately active | Active |
| Some but <1 | Moderately inactive | Moderately active | Active | Active |
| 1–2.9 | Moderately active | Active | Active | Active |
| ≥3 | Active | Active | Active | Active |

Reproduced from *The General Practice Physical Activity Questionnaire* with permission of the Department of Health.

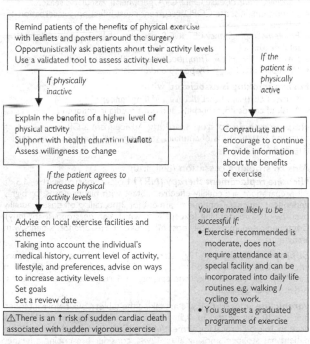

Remind patients of the benefits of physical exercise with leaflets and posters around the surgery
Opportunistically ask patients about their activity levels
Use a validated tool to assess activity level

*If physically inactive*

Explain the benefits of a higher level of physical activity
Support with health education leaflets
Assess willingness to change

*If the patient agrees to increase physical activity levels*

Advise on local exercise facilities and schemes
Taking into account the individual's medical history, current level of activity, lifestyle, and preferences, advise on ways to increase activity levels
Set goals
Set a review date

⚠ There is an ↑ risk of sudden cardiac death associated with sudden vigorous exercise

*If the patient is physically active*

Congratulate and encourage to continue
Provide information about the benefits of exercise

*You are more likely to be successful if:*
- Exercise recommended is moderate, does not require attendance at a special facility and can be incorporated into daily life routines e.g. walking / cycling to work.
- You suggest a graduated programme of exercise

**Fig. 8.3** Management plan for increasing activity levels

### Further information
**NICE** Physical activity guidance (2006) ⌨ www.nice.org.uk
**DH** The General Practice Physical Activity Questionnaire (2006)
⌨ www.dh.gov.uk

# Smoking

**Facts and figures** In the UK, 12 million adults (23% ♂, 26% ♀) smoke cigarettes and a further 3 million smoke pipes or cigars. *Prevalence:* highest aged 20–24y. Government targets aim to ↓ smoking to ≤24% by 2010; surveys of smokers show 73% want to stop and 30% intend to give up in <1y, but only ~2%/y successfully give up permanently.

1% school children are smokers when they enter secondary school; by 15y, 26% ♀ and 16% ♂ are smoking. 82% of smokers start as teenagers. Government targets aim to ↓ smoking amongst children to ≤9% by 2010.

**Risks of smoking** Smoking is the greatest single cause of illness and premature death in the UK. Half of all regular smokers will die as a result of smoking—106 000 people/y. Smoking is associated with ↑ risk of:

- *Cancers* ~30% of ALL cancer deaths. Common cancers include lung (>90% are smokers), lip, mouth, stomach, colon, bladder.
- *Cardiovascular disease* CHD, CVA, peripheral vascular disease.
- *Chronic lung disease* COPD, recurrent chest infection, exacerbation of asthma.
- *Problems in pregnancy* PET, IUGR, pre-term delivery, neonatal and late fetal death.
- DM
- Osteoporosis
- *Thrombosis* (especially if also on the COC pill)
- *Dyspepsia and/or gastric ulcers*

***Passive smoking is associated with:***
- ↑ risk of coronary heart disease and lung cancer (↑ by 25%)
- ↑ risk of cot death, bronchitis, and otitis media in children

**Helping people to stop smoking** Advice from a GP about smoking cessation results in 2% of smokers stopping—5% if advice is repeated[CE] (Figure 8.4).

### Aids to smoking cessation (BNF 4.10)

***Nicotine replacement therapy (NRT)*** ↑ chance of stopping by ~1.5×[N]. All preparations are equally effective[C]. Start with higher doses for highly dependent patients. Continue treatment for 3mo, tailing off dose gradually over 2wk before stopping (except gum which can be stopped abruptly). Contraindicated immediately post MI, stroke, or TIA, and for patients with arrhythmia.

***Bupropion*** Smokers (>18y) start taking the tablets 1–2wk before intended quit day (150mg od for 3d, then 150mg bd for 7–9wk). Cessation rate ↑ by >2×[N]. *Contraindications:* epilepsy or ↑ risk of seizures, eating disorder, bipolar disorder.

***Varenicline*** Smokers (>18y) start taking the tablets 1wk before intended quit day (0.5mg od for 3d, 0.5mg bd for 4d, then 1mg bd for 11wk). ↓ dose to 1mg od if renal impairment/elderly. Cessation rate ↑ by >2×. If the patient has stopped smoking after 12wk., consider prescribing a further 12 wk treatment to ↓ chance of relapse. *Contraindications:* caution in psychiatric illness.

***Alternative therapies*** Hypnotherapy may be helpful in some cases[C].

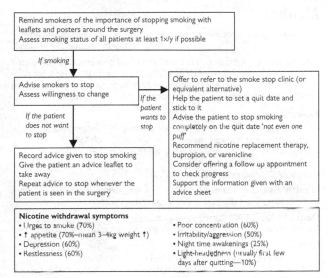

Remind smokers of the importance of stopping smoking with leaflets and posters around the surgery
Assess smoking status of all patients at least 1×/y if possible

*If smoking*

Advise smokers to stop
Assess willingness to change

*If the patient does not want to stop*

*If the patient wants to stop*

Offer to refer to the smoke stop clinic (or equivalent alternative)
Help the patient to set a quit date and stick to it
Advise the patient to stop smoking completely on the quit date *'not even one puff'*
Recommend nicotine replacement therapy, bupropion, or varenicline
Consider offering a follow up appointment to check progress
Support the information given with an advice sheet

Record advice given to stop smoking
Give the patient an advice leaflet to take away
Repeat advice to stop whenever the patient is seen in the surgery

**Nicotine withdrawal symptoms**
• Urges to smoke (70%)
• ↑ appetite (70%—mean 3–4kg weight ↑)
• Depression (60%)
• Restlessness (60%)
• Poor concentration (60%)
• Irritability/aggression (50%)
• Night time awakenings (25%)
• Light-headedness (usually first few days after quitting—10%)

**Fig. 8.4** Management plan for smokers in the surgery

⚠ **Smoking cessation medication** Prescibe *only* for smokers who commit to target stop date. Initially prescribe only enough to last 2wk after the target stop date, i.e 2wk nicotine replacement therapy, 3–4wk bupropion, or 3wk varenicline. Only offer a second prescription if the smoker demonstrates continuing commitment to stop smoking.

❶ If unsuccessful the NHS will not fund another attempt for ≥6mo.

**Support** In many areas 'stop smoking' services are provided by PCOs. These programmes vary from area to area but generally consist of a combination of group education, counselling, and support ± individual support in combination with nicotine replacement, bupropion, or varenicline.

## Further information
**NICE** 🖥 www.nice.org.uk
• Nicotine replacement therapy and bupropion for smoking cessation (2002)
• Brief interventions and referral for smoking cessation in primary care and other settings (2006)
• Varenicline for smoking cessation (2007).

## Useful contacts
**NHS Smoking Helpline** ☎ 0800 022 4332 🖥 www.gosmokefree.nhs.uk
**Action on Smoking and Health (ASH)** 🖥 www.ash.org.uk
**Quit** ☎ 0800 00 22 00 🖥 www.quit.org.uk

# Alcohol

*An alcoholic is someone you don't like who drinks as much as you do.*
Dylan Thomas (1914–1953)

Alcohol misuse is a major public health and social concern. Alcohol-related problems cost the NHS ~£1.7 billion/y. Most harm is caused by non-dependent drinkers. Screening and brief interventions in primary care can identify drinkers in this group and ↓ consumption and harm.

## Prevalence

- Hazardous/harmful drinking—excess drinking causing potential or actual harm but without dependence. Affects 32% ♂; 15% ♀
- Binge drinking—defined as drinking >8u for ♂ or >6u for ♀ in 1d. Affects 21% ♂; 9% ♀
- Alcohol dependence—affects 6% ♂, 2% ♀.

**Health risk** Continuum—individual risk also depends on other factors (e.g. smoking, heart disease). Alcohol-associated problems:

**Death** 15 000–22 000 deaths/y in the UK are associated with alcohol misuse (most related to stroke, cancer, liver disease, accidental injury/suicide).

### Social

- Marriage breakdown
- Absence from work
- Loss of work
- Social isolation
- Poverty
- Loss of shelter/home.

**Mental health** Anxiety, depression, and/or suicidal ideas; dementia and/or Korsakoff's ± Wernicke's encephalopathy (📖 p.589).

### Physical

- ↑ BP
- CVA
- Sexual dysfunction
- Brain damage
- Neuropathy
- Myopathy
- Cardiomyopathy
- Infertility
- Gastritis
- Pancreatitis
- DM
- Obesity
- Fetal damage
- Haemopoietic toxicity
- Interactions with other drugs
- Fatty liver
- Hepatitis
- Cirrhosis
- Oesophageal varices ± haemorrhage
- Liver cancer
- Cancer of the mouth, larynx, and oesophagus
- Breast cancer
- Nutritional deficiencies
- Back pain
- Poor sleep
- Tiredness
- Injuries due to alcohol-related activity (e.g. fights).

**Beneficial effects of alcohol** Moderate consumption (1–3u/d) ↓ risk of non-haemorrhagic stroke, angina pectoris, and MI.

**Table 8.6** Recommended levels of alcohol consumption

| Recommended limits (units) | Men | Women | As a rough guide: 1 unit = 8g of alcohol |
|---|---|---|---|
| Weekly | <21 | <14 | • ½ pint of beer (strong beer >1.5u) |
| Daily | <8 | <6 | • A small glass of wine/sherry or • A spirit measure of spirits (in Scotland 1.2u) |

## Box 8.1 Alcohol use disorders identification test (AUDIT)

| Questions assessing hazardous alcohol use | Questions assessing dependence symptoms | Questions assessing harmful alcohol use | | |
|---|---|---|---|---|
| **Question** | **0** | **1** | **2** | **3** | **4** |
| 1. How often do you have a drink containing alcohol? | Never | <1× /mo | 2–4× /mo | 2–3× /wk | ≥4× /wk |
| 2. How many drinks containing alcohol do you have on a typical day when you are drinking? | 1–2 | 3– | 5–6 | 7–9 | ≥10 |
| 3. How often do you have 6 or more drinks on one occasion? | Never | <1× /mo | Monthly | Weekly | Daily/ almost daily |
| 4. How often during the last year have you found that you were not able to stop drinking once you started? | Never | <1× /mo | Monthly | Weekly | Daily/ almost daily |
| 5. How often during the last year have you failed to do what was normally expected of you because of drinking? | Never | <1× /mo | Monthly | Weekly | Daily/ almost daily |
| 6. How often during the last year have you needed a first drink in the morning to get yourself going after a heavy drinking session? | Never | <1× /mo | Monthly | Weekly | Daily/ almost daily |
| 7. How often during the last year have you had a feeling of guilt or remorse after drinking? | Never | <1× /mo | Monthly | Weekly | Daily/ almost daily |
| 8. How often during the last year have you been unable to remember what happened the night before because of your drinking? | Never | <1× /mo | Monthly | Weekly | Daily/ almost daily |
| 9. Have you or someone else been injured because of your drinking? | No | | Yes—not in the last year | | Yes—in the last year |
| 10. Has a relative, friend, doctor, or other healthcare worker been concerned about your drinking or suggested that you cut it down? | No | | Yes—not in the last year | | Yes—in the last year |
| | | | Total: | | |

**Action*:**

| | |
|---|---|
| Audit score 0–7 | Alcohol education |
| Audit score 8–15 | Simple advice |
| Audit score 16–19 | Simple advice + brief counselling + continued monitoring |
| Audit score 20–40 | Referral to specialist for evaluation and treatment |

* Provide the next highest level of intervention to patients who score ≥2 on Questions 4, 5, and 6, or 4 on Questions 9 or 10.

# Management of alcohol misuse

### Assessing drinking
**Suspicious signs/symptoms** ↑ and uncontrolled BP; excess weight; recurrent injuries/accidents; non-specific GI complaints; back pain; poor sleep; tired all the time.

**Ask** Use standardized questionnaires to identify patients with harmful and hazardous patterns of alcohol consumption, e.g. AUDIT (Box 8.1, 📖 p.187).

### Risk factors
- Previous history
- Family history
- Poor social support
- Work absenteeism
- Emotional and/or family problems
- Financial and legal problems
- Drug problems
- Alcohol associated with work, e.g. publican.

**Examination** Smell of alcohol, tremor, sweating, slurring of speech, ↑ BP; signs of liver damage.

**Investigations** FBC (↑ MCV), LFTs (↑ GGT identifies ~25% of heavy drinkers in general practice, ↑ AST, ↑ bilirubin). USS—fatty liver/cirrhosis. Often incidental findings.

### Alcohol management strategies (Figure 8.5)
**Patients drinking within acceptable limits** Reaffirm limits.

**Non-dependent drinkers** Brief GP intervention → ~24% ↓ drinking. Present results of screening interventions, e.g. AUDIT (📖 p.187), and identify risks. Provide information about safe amounts of alcohol and harmful effects of exceeding these. Assess whether the patient is receptive to change. If so, agree targets to ↓ consumption, give encouragement, and negotiate follow-up.

**Alcohol-dependent drinkers** suffer withdrawal symptoms if they ↓ alcohol consumption, e.g. anxiety, fits, delirium tremens (📖 p.1066).
- If wanting to stop drinking, refer to the community alcohol team, suggest self-help organizations (e.g. Alcoholics Anonymous), involve family and friends in support
- Detoxification in the community usually uses a reducing regimen of chlordiazepoxide over a 1 wk period (20–30mg qds on days 1 and 2, 15mg qds on days 3 and 4, 10mg qds on day 5, 10mg bd on day 6, 10mg od on day 7, then stop)
- Community detoxification is contraindicated for patients with:
  - Confusion or hallucinations
  - History of previously complicated withdrawal (e.g. withdrawal seizures or delirium tremens)
  - Epilepsy or fits
  - Malnourishment
  - Severe vomiting/diarrhoea
  - ↑ risk of suicide
  - Poor cooperation
  - Failed detoxification at home
  - Uncontrollable withdrawal symptoms
  - Acute physical or psychiatric illness
  - Multiple substance misuse
  - Poor home environment

**If ambivalent/unwilling to change** provide information, reassess and re-inform on each subsequent meeting, and support the family.

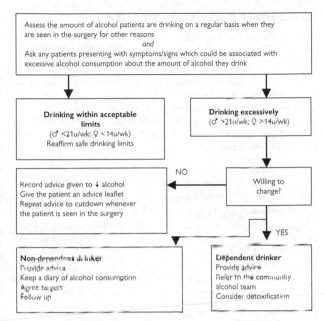

Assess the amount of alcohol patients are drinking on a regular basis when they are seen in the surgery for other reasons

*and*

Ask any patients presenting with symptoms/signs which could be associated with excessive alcohol consumption about the amount of alcohol they drink

**Drinking within acceptable limits**
(♂ <21u/wk; ♀ <14u/wk)
Reaffirm safe drinking limits

**Drinking excessively**
(♂ >21u/wk; ♀ >14u/wk)

Record advice given to ↓ alcohol
Give the patient an advice leaflet
Repeat advice to cutdown whenever the patient is seen in the surgery

NO

**Willing to change?**

YES

**Non-dependent drinker**
Provide advice
Keep a diary of alcohol consumption
Agree targets
Follow up

**Dependent drinker**
Provide advice
Refer to the community alcohol team
Consider detoxification

**Fig. 8.5** Alcohol management strategy

**Vitamin B supplements** People with chronic alcohol dependence are frequently deficient in vitamins, especially thiamine—give oral thiamine indefinitely (if severe 200—300mg/d; if mild 10—25mg/d)[G]. During detoxification in the community, give thiamine 200mg od for 5—7d

**Relapse** Common. Warn patients and encourage them to re-attend. Be supportive and maintain contact (↓ frequency and severity of relapses[G]). Consider drugs to prevent relapse, e.g. acamprosate, disulfiram (specialist initiation only).

**Delerium tremens** 📖 p.1066      **Alcohol and driving** 📖 p.133

**Further information**

**WHO** Alcohol Use Disorders Identification Test (AUDIT): guidelines for use in primary care. 🖥 www.who.int

**SIGN** Management of harmful drinking and alcohol dependence in primary care (2003 and 2004 update) 🖥 www.sign.ac.uk

**Patient advice and support**

**Drinkline** (government-sponsored helpline) ☎ 0800 917 8282
**Alcoholics Anonymous** ☎ 0845 769 7555
🖥 www.alcoholics-anonymous.org.uk
**ADFAM** Support for families ☎ 020 7553 7640 🖥 www.adfam.org.uk

# Assessment of drugs misuse

14% of men and 8% of women aged 16–59 report taking illicit drugs in the previous year. The majority of patients on treatment programmes report opioid misuse (heroin, 54%; methadone, 13%), but the most frequently abused drugs are cannabis, amphetamine, ecstasy, and cocaine. Three factors appear important: availability of drugs, vulnerable personality, and social pressures—particularly from peers.

**Detection** Warning signs suggesting drug misuse:

**Use of services** Suspicious requests for drugs of abuse (e.g. no clear medical indication; prescription requests are too frequent)

## Signs and symptoms

- Inappropriate behaviour
- Lack of self-care
- Unexplained nasal discharge
- Unusually constricted/dilated pupils
- Evidence of injecting (e.g. marked veins)
- Hepatitis or HIV infection.

**Social factors** Family disruption, criminal history.

**Assessment** Assess on >1 occasion before deciding how to proceed. Exceptions are severe withdrawal symptoms and/or evidence of an established regime requiring continuation. Points to cover:

## General information

- Check identification (ask to see an official document)
- Contact with other agencies (including last GP)—check accuracy
- Current residence; family—partner, children
- Employment/finances
- Current legal problems
- Criminal behaviour - past and present.

## History of drug use/risk taking behaviour

- Reason for consulting now and willingness to change
- Current and past usage
- Knowledge of risks
- Unsafe sexual practices.

## Medical and psychiatric history

- Complications of drug abuse, e.g. HIV, hepatitis, accidents
- General medical and psychiatric history and examination
- Alcohol abuse
- Overdose—accidental/deliberate.

## Investigations

- Consider urine toxicology to confirm drug misuse.
- Consider blood for FBC, LFTs, hepatitis B, C, and HIV serology (with consent and counselling 🕮 p.743), and other tests according to medical history/examination.

**Specific drugs** Table 8.7, 🕮 p. 192

**Notification of drug misusers** Doctors are expected to report patients who start treatment for drug abuse to the National Drug Treatment Monitoring Centres or regional equivalents (Table 8.6). All types of problem drug misuse should be reported. Databases cannot be used as a check on multiple prescribing, as data are anonymized.

**Driving and drugs misuse** 🕮 p.133

**Overdose** 🕮 p.1112

**Table 8.6** Regional and national drug misuse databases/centres

| Region | *Area code* telephone number (fax) |
| --- | --- |
| South East | *01865* 334725 (334733) |
| Eastern | *01223* 597598 (597601) |
| London | *020* 7261 8820 (7261 8883) |
| North West | *0151* 231 4533 (231 4515) |
| North East | *0191* 334 0372 (334 0391) |
| South West | *0117* 970 6474 ext. 311 (970 7021) |
| Yorkshire and the Humber | *0113* 295 3714 (295 3720) |
| West Midlands | *0121* 415 8556 (414 8197) |
| East Midlands | *0115* 971 2738 (971 2740) |
| Scotland | *0131* 275 6655 (275 7511) |
| Wales | *029* 2050 3343 (2050 2330) |
| Northern Ireland | *028* 9052 2421 (9052 0718) |

**Controlled drugs regulations** 📖 p.152

**Prescribing for drug misusers** Approach with special caution. Some controlled drugs can be dispensed to substance misusers in instalments providing they are prescribed on special NHS prescription forms (England, FP10 MDA; Wales, WP10 MDA; Scotland, GP10; NI, HS21). As a general principle, prescribe substitute opioid medicines in daily instalments. Specify number of instalments, intervals to be observed between instalments and if necessary instructions for supplies at weekends or bank holidays, total quantity of CD providing treatment for a period ≤ 14 d, and quantity to be supplied in each instalment.

❶ The prescription must be dispensed on the date on which it is due

**Other equipment for drug misusers** Doctors, pharmacists, and drug workers may provide supplies of alcohol swabs, sterile water (≤10 ampoules of ≤2mL), mixing utensils, filters, and citric acid to drug misusers for the purposes of harm reduction.

**Travelling abroad with controlled drugs** 📖 p.153

### Advice and support for patients and their families

**Talk to FRANK** (England and Wales) Government-run information, advice and referral service. ☎(24h) 0800 77 6600 🖥 www.talktofrank.com
**Know the Score** (Scotland) ☎ 0800 587 5879
🖥 www.knowthescore.info
**Drugscope** Information about drug abuse and how to get treatment.
🖥 www.drugscope.org.uk
**Drugs-info** Information about substance abuse for families of addicts.
🖥 www.drugs-info.co.uk
**ADFAM** Support for families of addicts. ☎ 020 7553 7640
🖥 www.adfam.org.uk
**Benzodiazepines** 🖥 www.benzo.org.uk
**Solvent abuse** ☎ 01785 810762 🖥 www.re-solv.org

**Table 8.7** Commonly misused substances in the UK

| Name (street/trade names include) | How usually taken | Effects sought | Harmful effects |
|---|---|---|---|
| *Heroin* (smack, horse, gear, H, junk, brown, stag, scag, jack) | Injected, snorted, or smoked | Drowsiness, sense of warmth and well-being | Physical dependence, tolerance<br>Overdose can lead to coma and death<br>Sharing injecting equipment brings risk of HIV or hepatitis infection |
| *Cocaine* (coke, charlie, snow, C) | Snorted in powder form, injected | Sense of well-being, alertness and confidence | Dependence, restlessness, paranoia<br>Damage to nasal membranes |
| *Crack* (freebase, rock, wash, stone) | Smokable form of cocaine | Similar to those of snorted cocaine but initial feelings are much more intense | As for cocaine but, because of the intensity of its effects, crack use can be extremely hard to control<br>May additionally cause lung damage ('crack lung') |
| *Ecstasy* (E, XTC, doves, disco bisuits, echoes, scooby doos) Chemical name: MDMA | Swallowed, usually in tablet form | Alert and energetic but with a calmness and a sense of well-being towards others; heightened sense of sound and colour | Possible nausea and panic<br>Overheating and dehydration if dancing, which can be fatal.<br>Use has been linked to liver and kidney problems<br>Long-term effects are not clear but may include mental illness and depression |
| *LSD* (acid, trips, tabs, dots, blotters, microdots) | Swallowed on a tiny square of paper | Hallucinations, including distorted or mixed-up sense of vision, hearing and time; an LSD trip can last as long as 8–12h | There is no way of stopping a bad trip, which may be a very frightening experience<br>Increased risk of accidents<br>Can trigger long-term mental problems |
| *Magic mushrooms* (shrooms, mushies) | Eaten raw or dried, cooked in food, or brewed in a tea | Similar effects to those of LSD but the trip is often milder and shorter | As for LSD, with the additional risk of sickness and poisoning |
| *Amphetamines* (speed, whizz, uppers, billy, sulph, amp) | In powder form, dissolved in drinks, injected, sniffed/snorted | Stimulates the nervous system, wakefulness, feeling of energy and confidence | Insomnia, mood swings, irritability, panic<br>The comedown (hangover) can be severe and last for several days |

**Table 8.7** *(Continued)*

| Name (street/trade names include) | How usually taken | Effects sought | Harmful effects |
|---|---|---|---|
| *Barbiturates* (barbs, downers) | Swallowed as tablets or capsules, injected—ampoules | Calm and relaxed state, larger doses produce a drunken effect | Dependency and tolerance<br>Overdose can lead to coma or death<br>Severe withdrawal symptoms |
| *Cannabis* (hash, dope, grass, blow, ganja, weed, shit, puff, marijuana) | Rolled with tobacco into a spliff, joint, or reefer and smoked, smoked in a pipe, or eaten | Relaxed, talkative state, heightened sense of sound and colour | Impaired coordination and increased risk of accidents<br>Poor concentration, anxiety, depression<br>Increased risk of respiratory diseases, including lung cancer |
| *Tranquillizers* (brand names include: Valium® Ativan® Mogadon® (moggies), temazepam (wobblies, mazzies, jellies) | Swallowed as tablets or capsules, injected | Prescribed for the relief of anxiety and to treat insomnia, high doses cause drowsiness | Dependency and tolerance<br>Increased risk of accidents<br>Overdose can be fatal<br>Severe withdrawal symptoms |
| *Anabolic steroids* (many trade names) | Injected or swallowed as tablets | With exercise can help to build up muscle; however, there is some debate about whether drug improves muscle power and athletic performance | *For men:* erection problems, risk of myocardial infarction or liver disease<br>*For women:* development of male characteristics<br>Injecting equipment brings risk of HIV or hepatitis infection |
| *Poppers* (alkyl nitrates, including amyl nitrate with trade names such as Ram, TNT, Thrust) | Vapours from small bottle of liquid are breathed in through mouth or nose | Brief and intense head-rush caused by a sudden surge of blood through the brain | Nausea and headaches, fainting, loss of balance, skin problems around the mouth and nose<br>Particularly dangerous for those with glaucoma, anaemia, breathing or heart problems |
| *Solvents* (including lighter gas refills, aerosols, glues) Some painter thinners and correcting fluids | Sniffed or breathed into the lungs | Short-lived effects similar to being drunk, thick-headed, dizziness, possible hallucinations | Nausea, blackouts, increased risk of accidents<br>Fatal arrythmias can cause instant death |

❶The RCGP Substance Misuse Unit provides certificate courses in management of drug abuse. 🖥 www.rcgp.org.uk

# Management of drugs misuse

**Aims to** ↓ risk of infectious diseases, ↓ drug-related deaths, and ↓ criminal activity used to finance drug habits

Avoid working in isolation. Anyone involved in substitute prescribing should wherever possible be doing so through their local shared care arrangements. The GP and primary healthcare team have a vital role in:
- Identifying drug misusers
- Assessing health/willingness to modify drug behaviour (Figure 8.6)
- Referring for specialist assessment and treatment of drug abuse
- Routine screening/prevention (e.g. cervical screening, contraception).

**General measures** If ongoing care, at each meeting consider:

### Education
- Safer routes of drug administration, e.g. smoking/rectal administration for heroin abusers. Discourage IM/subcutaneous administration
- Specific risks of drugs (e.g. psychosis with amphetamines, local risks such as contaminated street drugs)
- Safe injecting advice and overdose prevention
- Safe sexual practices/condom use
- Driving and drug misuse (🕮 p.133)
- Other local services.

### Medical care
- Treatment of/advice about complications of drug misuse
- Testing/treatment for blood-borne disease, e.g. hepatitis B or C, HIV.

**Hepatitis B immunization** for injecting drug misusers not already infected/immune and close contacts of those already infected. Use accelerated regime—immunization at 0, 7, and 21d and a booster after 12 mo.

### Treatment of dependence
- Set realistic goals—aim to help the patient remain healthy until, with appropriate care and support, he/she can achieve a drug-free life. Consider ↓ in illicit drug use, ↓ duration of periods of drug use, ↓ risk of relapse, ↓ need for criminal activity to finance drug misuse, improving personal and social functioning. These aims are often best met by maintenance substitute prescribing, e.g. with methadone/buprenorphine for heroin abuse
- Set conditions for acceptable behaviour/treatment withdrawal. Agree on the pharmacy to be used and involve the pharmacist
- Review regularly and include the whole team
- Give contact numbers for community support organizations (🕮 p.191).
- Send National Drug Treatment Monitoring Service notification (🕮 p.190) if this has not been done
- Seek advice/refer to a Community Substance Misuse Team as needed.

## Further information

**DH** Drug misuse and dependence—guidelines on clinical management (2007) 🖳 www.dh.gov.uk
**NICE** Substance misuse interventions (2007) 🖳 www.nice.org.uk
**National Treatment Agency for Substance Abuse** 🖳 www.nta.nhs.uk
**Substance Misuse Management in General Practice (SMMGP)** 🖳 www.smmgp.org.uk

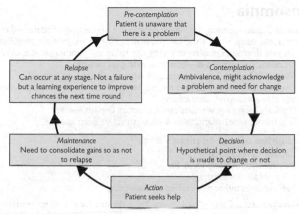

**Fig. 8.6** Stages of change in addiction

---

### Safe injecting advice

- Never inject alone
- Always inject with the blood flow and rotate sites—avoid neck, groin, penis, axilla, foot and hand veins, and any infected areas/swollen limbs—even if veins are distended
- Use sterile new injecting equipment with the smallest bore needle possible and dispose of all equipment safely after use
- Avoid unsuitable preparations, e.g. crushed tablets and/or injecting cocktails of drugs (injection of heroin and cocaine together is known as 'speedballing' or 'snowballing')
- Learn basic principles of first aid and CPR (provide information on courses available). Encourage calling for an ambulance
- Poor veins indicate poor technique—find out what the patient is doing.

**Preventing overdose** Be aware of risk factors:

- Injecting heroin
- Recent non-fatal overdose
- Longer injecting career
- High levels of use/intoxication
- High levels of alcohol use
- Lowered tolerance through detoxification/imprisonment
- Depression, suicidal thoughts
- Multiple drug use, particularly CNS depressants
- Sharing equipment/other high-risk injecting behaviour—may indicate low concern about personal risk
- Not being on a treatment programme or premature exit from a methadone programme.

# Insomnia

From the Latin meaning 'no sleep': describes a perception of disturbed or inadequate sleep. ~1:4 of the UK population (♀>♂) are thought to suffer in varying degrees. *Prevalence*: ↑ with age rising to 1:2 amongst the over-65s. Causes are numerous—common examples include:

- *Minor, self-limiting* Travel, stress, shift work, small children, arousal
- *Psychological* About half have mental health problems: depression, anxiety, mania, grief, alcoholism
- *Physical* Drugs (e.g. steroids), pain, pruritus, tinnitus, sweats (e.g. menopause), nocturia, asthma, obstructive sleep apnoea.

## Definition of 'a good night's sleep'

- <30min to fall asleep
- Maintenance of sleep for 6–8h
- < 3 brief awakenings/night
- Feels well rested and refreshed on awakening.

**Management** Careful evaluation. Many do not have a sleep problem themselves but a relative feels there is a problem, e.g. the retired milkman continuing to wake at 4a.m. Others have unrealistic expectations, e.g. they need 12 h sleep/d. Reassurance alone may be all that is required.

### For genuine problems

- **Eliminate as far as possible any physical problems preventing sleep,** e.g. treat asthma or eczema, give long-acting pain killers to last the whole night, consider HRT or fluoxetine for sweats, refer if obstructive sleep apnoea is suspected (📖 p.346)
- **Treat psychiatric problems** e.g. depression, anxiety
- **Sleep hygiene** Box 8.2
- **Relaxation techniques** Compact discs (borrow from libraries or buy from pharmacies); relaxation classes (often offered by local recreation centres/adult education centres); many physiotherapists can teach relaxation techniques
- **Consider drug treatment** Last resort. Benzodiazepines may be prescribed for insomnia 'only when it is severe, disabling, or subjecting the individual to extreme distress'.

**Drug treatment** Benzodiazepines (e.g. temazepam), zolpidem, zopiclone, and low-dose TCA (e.g. amitriptyline 10–50mg) nocte are all commonly prescribed for patients with insomnia.

- *Side effects*: amnesia and daytime somnolence. Most hypnotics affect daytime performance and may cause falls in the elderly. Warn patients about their effect on driving and operating machinery
- Only prescribe a few weeks supply at a time because of potential for dependence and abuse.

⚠ Beware the temporary resident who has 'forgotten' his/her night sedation.

**Complications of insomnia** ↓ quality of life; ↓ concentration and memory affecting performance of daytime tasks; relationship problems; risk of accidents. 10% of motor accidents are related to tiredness.

## Box 8.2 Principles of 'sleep hygiene'

- Don't go to bed until you feel sleepy
- Don't stay in bed if you're not asleep
- Avoid daytime naps
- Establish a regular bedtime routine
- Reserve a room for sleep only (if possible). Do not eat, read, work, or watch TV in it
- Make sure the bedroom and bed are comfortable, and avoid extremes of noise and temperature
- Avoid caffeine, alcohol, and nicotine
- Have a warm bath and warm milky drink at bedtime
- Take regular exercise, but avoid late night hard exercise (sex is OK)
- Monitor your sleep with a sleep diary (record both the times you sleep and its quality)
- Rise at the same time every morning regardless of how long you've slept.

## Patient information and support

**Royal College of Psychiatrists** Patient information sheets.
🖳 www.rcpsych.ac.uk
**Patient UK** 🖳 www.patient.co.uk

# Chronic disease and elderly care

> ❶ In other sections of this book, where management differs from the norm for elderly patients, the text is highlighted in a box marked with this symbol.

# Chronic disease management

The predominant disease pattern in the developed world is one of chronic or long-term illness. In the UK, 17.5 million adults are currently living with a chronic disease. Long-term conditions frequently seen and managed in general practice include:

- Arthritis of all types
- Back pain
- Cancer
- Chronic lung disease
- HIV
- Renal or liver failure
- Irritable bowel syndrome
- Inflammatory bowel disease
- Chronic neurological conditions, e.g. Parkinson's disease, MS
- Cardiovascular disease, e.g. ↑ BP, heart disease, stroke
- DM
- Dementia
- Psychiatric illness, e.g. depression, psychosis.

Although details of chronic illness management depend on the illness, people with chronic diseases of all types have much in common with each other. They all:

- Have similar concerns and problems (📖 p.202)
- Must deal not only with their disease(s) but also with the impact it has on their lives and emotions.

## Common elements of effective chronic illness management

- *Involvement of the whole family* Chronic diseases affect not only the patient but everyone in a family.
- *Collaboration between service providers and patients/carers* Negotiate and agree a definition of the problem; agree targets and goals for management; develop an individualized self-management plan.
- *Personalized written care plan* Take into account patient's/carers' views and experience and the current evidence base.
- *Tailored education in self-management* A diabetic spends ~3h/y with a health professional—the other 8757h he/she manages his/her own condition. Helping patients with chronic disease understand and take responsibility for their conditions is imperative. User-led (i.e. led by someone who suffers from the condition) self-management education programmes are most effective.
- *Planned follow-up* Proactive follow-up according to the careplan—use of disease registers and call–recall systems is important.
- *Monitoring of outcome and adherence to treatment* Use of disease and treatment markers; monitoring of concordance, e.g. checking prescription frequency; medicine management programmes (📖 p.144).
- *Tools and protocols for stepped care* Provide a framework for using limited resources to greatest effect; step professional care in intensity—start with limited professional input and systematic monitoring, and then augment care for patients not achieving an acceptable outcome; initial and subsequent treatments are selected according to evidence-based guidelines in light of a patient's progress (📖 p.78).
- *Targeted use of specialist services* for those patients who cannot be managed in primary care alone.
- *Monitoring of process* Continually monitor management through clinical governance mechanisms (📖 p.72).

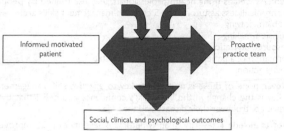

**Community**
- *Resources*: collaboration with voluntary organizations, social services, and other community agencies
- *Policies*: government policy at national and local level to support people with chronic disease and enable resource allocation; incentives for improved care

**Healthcare system**
- *Self-management support* (training, education, easy access to further information)
- *Clinical information systems* (e.g. computer-based disease templates, disease registers)
- *Delivery system design* (convenient, user-friendly)
- *Decision support* (guidelines, protocols)

Informed motivated patient

Proactive practice team

Social, clinical, and psychological outcomes

**Fig. 9.1** Model for chronic disease care

**National Service Frameworks (NSFs)** Models of how services should be provided. They were developed to improve patient care and address variations in service provision across the UK and are a key part of NHS quality initiatives. They cover all areas of service delivery, not just clinical practice. Relevant NSFs and related programmes include:
- Blood pressure
- Cancer
- Children
- COPD
- DM
- Coronary heart disease
- Long-term (neurological) conditions
- Older people
- Mental health
- Renal
- National stroke strategy
- End-of-life care programme.

**Depression screening and chronic disease[N]** Depression is common among people with chronic disease. Use the NICE depression screening questions to detect depression:
- During the last month, have you often been bothered by feeling down, depressed or hopeless?
- During the last month, have you often been bothered by having little interest or pleasure in doing things?

A positive response to either of these questions should prompt further assessment. Depending on the severity of the depression consider additional support, e.g. with counselling or through disease-specific organizations and/or drug therapy with antidepressants.

# The expert patient

Most doctors acknowledge that many of their patients with chronic conditions know their own condition best. Expert patient programmes (or patient self-management programmes) utilize this fact to improve patient care. The aim is to promote effective partnerships in management of chronic disease by combining the expertise of patient and doctor (Figure 9.2).

**Chronic disease self-management programmes** have been developed over the last 20y. They are a system of patient education and empowerment. As well as using health professionals, they use trained lay people with chronic illness as tutors. The 5 core self-management skills are:
- Problem-solving
- Decision-making
- Resource utilization
- Formation of a patient–professional partnership
- Taking action.

However, none of these is in itself the key to effective self-management. The key is the change in the individual's confidence and belief that they can take control over their disease and their life.

***Benefits*** include ↓ severity of all symptoms, ↓ severity of pain, improved life control and activity, improved resourcefulness and life satisfaction, enhanced doctor-patient relationship, and ↓ use of health services.

## Common patient concerns may include
- Finding and using health services.
- Finding and using other community resources.
- Knowing how to recognize and respond to changes in a chronic disease.
- Dealing with problems and emergencies.
- Making decisions about when to seek medical help.
- Using medicines and treatments effectively.
- Knowing how to manage the stress and depression that accompany a chronic illness.
- Coping with fatigue, pain, and sleep problems.
- Getting enough exercise.
- Maintaining good nutrition.
- Working with your doctor(s) and other care providers.
- Talking about your illness with family and friends.
- Managing work, family, and social activities.

## Further information
**DH** The expert patient: a new approach to chronic disease management for the 21st century 🖳 www.dh.gov.uk
**EPP** Expert Patients Community Interest Company
🖳 www.expertpatients.co.uk

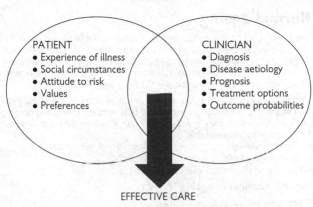

**Fig. 9.2** The patient–professional partnership

# Normal ageing

The UK is home to 60.2 million people. Average age is 38.8y and rising. By 2004, women aged 65 could expect to live to the age of 85. Projections suggest that this will ↑ by another 3y by 2021. Over the past 35y, the population aged >65y has grown by 31% from 7.4 to 9.7 million. The largest percentage growth in population is in the >85y age group.

**What is ageing?** Ageing is a gradual series of changes over time that lead to the loss of function of organs and cells, with the eventual outcome of death. Individuals vary greatly in the rate at which they age. Several factors seem to influence this:

- Genetic make-up
- Psychological health
- Lifestyle—diet, physical exercise, smoking.
- Socio-economic factors
- Environment

**Normal changes of ageing** Table 9.1.

**Difficulties assessing the elderly**

- Communication problems—hearing, cognition, speech.
- Multiplicity of cause—a single symptom may be caused by different concurrent processes, e.g. breathlessness as a result of COPD + heart failure.
- Non-specific symptoms/signs—confusion, falls or 'off legs' may be the only overt sign of underlying disease, e.g. UTI, MI, stroke.
- Symptoms may be absent despite disease, and signs harder to elicit.
- Polypharmacy (📖 p.208) may result in side effects and interactions.
- Laboratory tests may be unreliable, especially white cell counts and ESR (always check CRP).

**Disease** The ageing process is compounded by overt disease. This may affect functional capacity, quality of life, and independence, cause frailty, ↓ well-being and independence, and result in ↑ care and mobility needs.

**Effects of multiple conditions** Older people are more likely to have several ongoing chronic illnesses which can act in combination to cause disability greater than any one of those illnesses alone and/or result in:

- Direction of care at some problems, with relative neglect of others.
- Polypharmacy (📖 p.208).
- Involvement of multiple specialist teams which can cause inconvenience to the patient and family, and result in conflicting advice, and opposing opinions on cause/effect of symptoms.

**Frailty** Many elderly people are described as being 'frail'. This term is used to describe individuals who are physically weak and fragile. It can occur on a background of natural ageing or be precipitated by a disease process. It is not a disease or disability in itself, but a vulnerability or inability to withstand physical/psychological stressors. Common features of frailty include:

- Unintentional weight loss (>5kg in a year)
- Feeling of exhaustion
- Weakness (measured by grip strength)
- Slow walking speed
- Low levels of physical activity.

**Table 9.1** Normal changes of ageing

| System | Clinical/functional effects |
|---|---|
| Cardiovascular | Cardiac enlargement/left ventricular hypertrophy |
| | ↓ cardiac output →↓ exercise capacity |
| | ↓ response of heart rate to exercise |
| | Systolic hypertension |
| | Left ventricular failure |
| Respiratory | ↓ FEV$_1$/FVC and ↑ residual volume |
| | ↑ susceptibility to infection |
| | ↑ susceptibility to aspiration |
| Endocrine | ↓ insulin sensitivity → impaired glucose regulation |
| | ↓ thyroid hormone production |
| Gastrointestinal | ↑ gastric acid production |
| | Constipation |
| Genito-urinary | ↓ glomerular filtration rate not reflected by ↑ creatinine |
| | Benign enlargement of the prostate (25–50% of men >65y) → prostatism |
| | Slowing of sexual function; erectile dysfunction |
| | Dry vagina and ↑ susceptibility to urinary infections (♀) |
| Musculoskeletal | Sarcopenia—↓ muscle strength/power, ↓ lean body mass (30–40%), ↑ fat body mass |
| | ↓ mobility |
| | ↑ likelihood of falls |
| | ↑ osteoporosis/susceptibility to fractures |
| Nervous | Slower thought processes/reaction times |
| | General decline in performance |
| | ❶ Dementia is *not* a normal change of ageing |
| Vision | Presbyopia (difficulty focusing on near objects), ↓ visual acuity, cataract, impaired dark adaptation |
| Hearing | High-frequency hearing loss/presbyacusis—deafness affects 80% of 80y olds |
| | Degenerative changes in the inner ear → impairment of balance, causing falls |
| Immune | Atrophy of the thymus |
| | Reduced immune function resulting in ↑ infectious disease, reactivation of latent disease (e.g. TB, shingles), ↑ cancer, ↑ autoimmune disease |
| Skin/hair | Dry skin, wrinkles, tendency to bruise easily, and slower healing |
| | Greying of the hair |
| | ↓ sweating, heat generation, and heat conservation → heat stroke; hypothermia |
| | ↓ sensitivity to touch, pain and temperature discrimination → burns, pressure sores |

# Elderly care and rehabilitation

*Use strengthens, disuse debilitates.*

Hippocrates (460–357BCE)

13–14% of the population have some disability. This is increasing as populations age and people survive longer with disability. Many more are just elderly and frail. 35% of people aged >80y cannot live an independent life. Most patients are best managed by a multidisciplinary team in their home environment (if practicable) with a problem-oriented approach. Good interdisciplinary communication and coordination is essential and many patients benefit from specialist rehabilitation services. Psychological and sociocultural aspects are as important as medical aspects.

**Role of the GP** Maintain an open-door policy and encourage patients and carers to seek help for problems early. Try to become familiar with patients' diseases, even if rare. It is impossible to plan care without knowledge of course and prognosis, and an easy way to lose a patient's confidence is to appear ignorant of their condition.

The GP of any elderly patient or patient receiving rehabilitation in the community is a team member and is often the key worker who coordinates care. Information alone can improve outcome.

> ### Consider
> - *Can physical symptoms be improved?*
> - *Can psychological symptoms be improved?* (including self-esteem)
> - *Can functioning within the home be improved?* (aids and adaptations within the home, extra help)
> - *Can functioning in the community be improved?* (mobility outside the home, work, social activities)
> - *Can the patient's or carer's financial state be improved?*
> - *Does the carer need more support?*

If progress is slower than expected, or stalls, consider other medical problems (e.g. anaemia, hypothyroidism, dementia), a neurological event, depression, or communication problems (e.g. poor vision/hearing).

## Principles of rehabilitation and elderly care
- **Use of assessments/measures** Central to the management of frailty/disability. Use validated measures accepted by all team members (e.g. Barthel index 📖 p.592). Reassess regularly.
- **Teamwork** Good outcomes are associated with clinicians working as a team towards a common goal with patients and their families (or carers) included as team members.
- **Goal-setting** Goals must be meaningful and challenging, but achievable. Use short- and long-term goals. Involve the patient ± carer(s). Regularly renew, review, and adapt.
- **Underlying approach to therapy** All approaches focus on modification of impairment and improvement in function within everyday activities. Patients derive benefit from therapy focused on the management of frailty/disability.

- *Intensity/duration of therapy* How much therapy is needed? Is there a minimum threshold below which there is no benefit at all? Studies on well-organized services show it is rare for patients to receive >2h therapy/d. No-one knows what is ideal.

**Multidisciplinary working** A multidisciplinary approach is ideal, e.g.
- *DNs* provide nursing care and equipment, advice on all aspects of nursing care and teach carers how to do everyday tasks (e.g. emptying catheter bags, lifting). They are sources of information on local services and provide support for carers of patients on their caseload.
- *Community matrons* provide specialist nursing support on all aspects of care for patients with chronic conditions who are high users of health services.
- *Community physiotherapists* are invaluable sources of help, advice, and equipment for practical problems relating to mobility.
- *Occupational therapists* can help patients and carers cope with difficulties in everyday living caused by disability by providing aids and appliances and arranging alterations.
- *Speech therapists* can help with communication problems.

## Referral
- *Medical opinion* for clarification of diagnosis (e.g. if diagnosis is in doubt or patient has symptoms/signs incongruous with diagnosis).
- *Specialist rehabilitation services* New or deterioration in existing impairment, disability, or handicap, or advances in management that warrant referral for specialist care.
- *Social services* for assessment of the home for modification, assessment to allow application for mobility aids or services to help the disabled person and/or carer to cope.
- *Voluntary organizations and self-help groups* Useful sources of support for patients and carers.
- *Citizen's Advice Bureau* for independent advice on benefits and services.
- *Disabled Living Foundation* for independent advice on equipment and appliances.

## Common neurological rehabilitation problems 📖 p.590

## Equipment and adaptations 📖 p.230

## Driving 📖 p.130          Benefits 📖 p.224

## Employment 📖 p.126          Carers 📖 p.222

## Patient information and support

**Disabled Living Foundation** Advice about equipment and appliances ☎ 0845 130 9177 🖥 www.dlf.org.uk

**Age Concern** Wide range of information and factsheets ☎ 0800 00 99 66 🖥 www.ageconcern.org.uk

**Royal Association for Disability and Rehabilitation (RADAR)** ☎ 020 7250 3222 🖥 www.radar.org.uk

**Disablement Information and Advice Line (DIAL)** ☎ 01302 310123 🖥 www.dialuk.info

# Prescribing for the elderly

Use of medicines ↑ as people get older. 1 in 3 NHS prescriptions are issued to patients >65y. 90% of these prescriptions are for repeat medications. Adverse drug events are common reasons for hospital admission in the >75y age group. Many are avoidable. Regular review is essential.

## Problems commonly encountered

***Polypharmacy*** Elderly people often have multiple problems—it is easy to keep adding drugs for each new problem → polypharmacy. This ↑ confusion about drug regimes, and results in poor concordance and multiple interactions/side effects.

- Before prescribing a new drug, consider whether it is necessary—avoid treating normal changes of ageing; use non-pharmacological therapies wherever possible; avoid 'a pill for every ill' approach and try to treat the underlying condition, not the symptoms
- Balance the potential risks of the drug against the benefits. Drug trials of efficacy of medication often exclude older participants—the applicability of evidence to elderly patients cannot be assumed. For prophylactic medication (e.g. warfarin, statins), consider the likelihood of concordance and benefits in the context of the whole person (including other comorbidities).
- Review medication regularly. Stop ineffective/redundant drugs and consider whether the overall drug regime can be simplified.

***Form of the medicine*** Swallowing tablets can be difficult for elderly people. Consider using liquid preparations/giving explicit advice to take medication with plenty of water and sitting upright.

***Confusion post-discharge*** Up to half of all patients are inadvertently prescribed the wrong medication after hospital discharge.

***Drug hoarding/self-medication*** Especially if recent changes in medication. It is common for elderly people to have a back stock of drugs and continue taking their old drugs alongside new ones. A written list may be helpful. Many elderly people also self-medicate extensively with OTC preparations. If necessary, do a home visit to sort out the drugs.

**↑ susceptibility to side effects** Common due to altered:
- Pharmacodynamics—↑ susceptibility to GI side effects (e.g. constipation with opioids; gastric irritation with NSAIDs) and ↑ sensitivity to effects of CNS drugs (e.g. benzodiazepines, opioids—use with care).
- Pharmacokinetics—↓ renal function is particularly important. Always assume any elderly person has moderate impairment if renal function is not known.

***Social and personal factors*** Low level of home support, physical factors (e.g. poor vision, poor hearing, or poor manual dexterity), and mental state (e.g. confusion/disorientation, depression) can all affect ability of an older person to take medication.

**Specific medicines** Beer's list is a list of agents to be avoided/used with extreme caution in elderly patients. It can be accessed via:
🖥 www.dcri.duke.edu/ccge/curtis/beers.html

### Box 9.1 Guidelines for prescribing for the elderly

*Think before prescribing*
- Is the drug needed?
- Is there another non-pharmacological way of management?
- Are you treating the underlying condition or its symptoms?
- What are the pros and cons of the patient taking this drug?
- What is the evidence base for its use in this age group?
- Will the patient be able to take the drug (formulation; packaging)?
- Will the patient be concordant?
- Will the patient comply with any necessary monitoring?

*Limit the range of drugs that you use* Prescribe from a limited array of drugs that you know well.

*Repeats and disposal*
- Tell patients how to get more tablets and monitor frequency of repeat prescriptions.
- Review repeat prescriptions regularly (📖 p.146).
- Tell patients what to do with any left over if a drug is stopped.

*↓ the dose*
- Start with 50% of the adult dose.
- Avoid drugs likely to cause problems (e.g. long-acting antidiabetic agents such as glibenclamide).

*Review regularly*
- Consider on each occasion whether each drug could be stopped or the regime simplified.
- Consider lowering dosage of drugs if renal function is deteriorating.
- Involve carers, community pharmacists, and other PHCT members.

*Simplify regimes*
- Use od or bd regimes wherever possible.
- Avoid polypharmacy.

*Explain clearly*
- Put precise instructions on the drug bottle—avoid 'use as directed'.
- Give written instructions about how the drug should be taken.
- Ensure explanations are given to both carers as well as patients where appropriate.

*Consider method of administration*
- Bottles with child-proof tops are often impossible for arthritic hands to open. Suggest the patient asks for a standard screw cap.
- Drug administration boxes in which the correct tablets are stored in slots marked with the day and time of administration can be helpful. They are available from pharmacists and can be filled by the patient, carer, friend or relative, or the pharmacist.
- Medication reminder charts can also be helpful.

### Further information

**Gallagher P et al.** STOPP (Screening Tool of Older Persons Prescriptions) and START (Screening Tool to Alert doctors to Right Treatment). Consensus validation *Int J Clin Pharmacol Ther* (2008) **46**, 72–83.

# Falls amongst the elderly

Falls are a major cause of disability and the leading cause of mortality due to injury in people aged >75y. Tendency to fall ↑ with age. Assessment of a patient who has fallen is a common primary care emergency.

**Risk factors for falls** Recurrence ↑ with number of risk factors:

- ♀:♂ ≈ 2:1 in the over 75s
- ↑ age
- Multiple previous falls
- Disorders of gait or balance
- Visual impairment
- Cognitive impairment
- Low morale/depression
- High level of dependence
- ↓ mobility
- Foot problems
- Lower limb weakness or arthritis
- History of stroke or PD
- Use of psychotropic drugs, sedatives, diuretics, or β-blockers
- Alcohol
- Environmental factors, e.g. loose rugs, poor lighting, ice, high winds
- Infection, e.g. pneumonia, UTI.

**History** Deal with the injuries first—ask about pain, loss of function, headache. Ask carers about behaviour.

**Examination** Check for bruising, ↓ function, confusion, BP, pulse, neurology, and fundi. Consider hypothermia if on the floor for any duration.

**Investigate the cause of the fall** *Consider:*

- *Physical problems* Neurological problems (e.g. stroke); visual loss; cardiac abnormalities (e.g. arrhythmia, postural hypotension); muscular abnormalities (e.g. steroid-induced myopathy); skeletal problems (e.g. osteoarthritis); infection (pneumonia, UTI).
- *Environmental problems* Climbing ladders to do routine maintenance; loose/holed carpets; slippery floor or bath; chair or bed too low.

**Management**

- Treat acute injury (20%). Exclude fracture (mainly Colles'/neck of femur). ❶ Subdural haematoma may take days/weeks to reveal itself.
- Even if uninjured, older people might not be able to get up off the floor without help. The result may be a prolonged period of lying on the floor until help arrives. Apart from the indignity/helplessness this causes, 2° problems (e.g. pneumonia, pressure sores, hypothermia, UTI, and dehydration) may follow.
- Perform/refer to a specialist falls service for a falls assessment.
- Undertake measures to ↓ risk of falls or damage from falling.

**Refer to A&E if**

- Significant head injury (🕮 p.1108)
- Any suspicion of fracture
- Any other significant injury (e.g. lacerations).

**Admit to the acute medical team or elderly care team if**

- Cause of the fall was an acute medical problem (e.g. stroke).
- The patient is unable to cope at home.

**Refer to the specialist elderly care team if**

- The cause of recurrent falls remains unclear
- The patient or carer is worried about the possibility of further falls, *or*
- There is doubt about whether the patient can cope.

**Prevention of falls** Falls are one of the biggest risk factors for fracture. All elderly people should have risk of falls assessed regularly.

❶ Any fall may seriously undermine an elderly person's confidence and cause worry about the possibility of recurrence. As a result, there may be restriction of activities → ↓ fitness and ↑ dependency on others.

*Is a falls assessment needed?* Ask if patients fall—they may not volunteer the information spontaneously.

The *Get up and Go test*—People who can get up from a chair without using their arms, walk several paces, and return with no difficulty or unsteadiness are at low risk of falling. People who have difficulty with the *Get Up and Go test*, have to stop walking whilst talking, present following a fall, or have recurrent falls need a falls assessment.

**Falls assessment** If available, refer to a specialist falls service. *Record:*
- Frequency and history of circumstances around any previous falls.
- Drug therapy—polypharmacy, hypnotics, sedatives, diuretics, antihypertensives may all cause falls.
- Assessment of vision.
- Examination of gait and balance, including abnormalities due to foot problems or arthritis, and motor disorders (e.g. stroke, PD)
- Examination of basic neurological function, including mental status (impaired cognition and depression), muscle strength, lower extremity peripheral nerves, proprioception, and reflexes.
- Assessment of basic cardiovascular status including BP (exclude postural hypotension), heart rate, and rhythm.
- Assessment of environmental risk factors, e.g. poor lighting particularly on the stairs, loose carpets or rugs, badly fitting footwear or clothing, lack of safety equipment such as grab rails, steep stairs, slippery floors, or inaccessible lights or windows.

**Measures to ↓ risk of falls and damage from falling**
- Assess and correct vision, if possible.
- Correct postural hypotension—alter medication; consider compression stockings, but many elderly people cannot apply stockings tight enough to be of any use themselves.
- Treat other medical conditions, e.g. refer to cardiology if arrhythmia.
- Review medication and discontinue/alter inappropriate medication.
- Remove environmental hazards—arrange bath at a day centre, refer to OT to identify and correct hazards in the home (e.g. remove loose carpets, wheeled trolley for use indoors, commode or urine bottle for night-time use, moving the bed downstairs, etc.).
- Liaise with other members of the PHCT and social services to provide additional support if needed; refer to local council for 'carephone' or alarm system to call for help if any further falls.
- Refer to rehabilitation/physiotherapy to improve confidence after falls and for weight-bearing exercise (focusing on strength and flexibility) and balance training (↓ risk of falls). Use of hip protectors ↓ fracture risk in patients at high risk, but compliance is a problem[C].

**Osteoporosis and prevention of fracture** 📖 p.516

# Assessment of pain

Take a history to ascertain:
- what the patient means when he/she complains of pain
- the cause of the pain
- the severity of the pain.

**❶** Don't jump to conclusions or make assumptions about a patient's pain.

**Assessment questions** There are many approaches to assessing pain. The specifics of each scheme are not crucial, but it is important that the scheme used has a logical outline which works for the individual clinician. A simple mnemonic approach is detailed in Figure 9.3.

**Elderly patients and patients with difficulty communicating** High prevalence of pain in the elderly population is now well recognized. 40–80% of elderly people in institutions are in pain. The reason for this lies in the difficulty in assessing those with communication difficulties. Additionally, the elderly often minimize their pain, making it even more difficult to evaluate.

***Methods of evaluation*** Unusual behaviour and its return to normal with adequate analgesia may be the only confirmation of pain in patients with communication difficulties. Examples include:

***Verbal expression*** e.g.
- Crying when touched
- Shouting
- Becoming very quiet
- Swearing
- Grunting
- Talking without making sense.

***Facial expression*** e.g.
- Grimacing/wincing
- Closing eyes
- Worried expression
- Withdrawn/no expression.

***Behavioural expression*** e.g.
- Jumping on touch
- Hand pointing to body area
- Increasing confusion
- Rocking/shaking
- Not eating
- Staying in bed/chair
- Grumpy mood.

***Physical expression*** e.g.
- Cold
- Pale
- Clammy
- Change in colour
- Change in vital signs if acute pain (e.g. BP, pulse).

**Pain assessment tools** Sometimes it is helpful to use pain scales to assess the degree of pain that a patient is in, particularly if communication is difficult. The most commonly used tool is a simple visual analogue pain scale—this consists of a line marked in graduations from 0 to 10. Ask patients to point to the place on the line which represents how much pain they are in, where 10 is the most possible pain and 0 is no pain.

**Examine the patient** The cause of the problem may be clear to you from history alone, but examine the patient to confirm/refute your proposed diagnosis.

⚠ Beware of emergency requests for opioids from patients unknown to you or your practice.

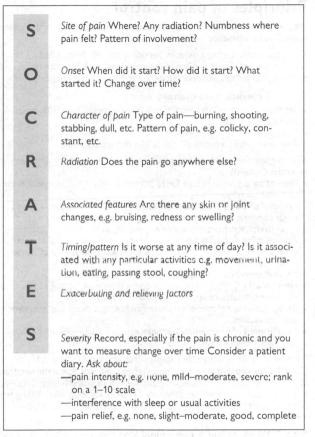

**S** — *Site of pain* Where? Any radiation? Numbness where pain felt? Pattern of involvement?

**O** — *Onset* When did it start? How did it start? What started it? Change over time?

**C** — *Character of pain* Type of pain—burning, shooting, stabbing, dull, etc. Pattern of pain, e.g. colicky, constant, etc.

**R** — *Radiation* Does the pain go anywhere else?

**A** — *Associated features* Are there any skin or joint changes, e.g. bruising, redness or swelling?

**T** — *Timing/pattern* Is it worse at any time of day? Is it associated with any particular activities e.g. movement, urination, eating, passing stool, coughing?

**E** — *Exacerbating and relieving factors*

**S** — *Severity* Record, especially if the pain is chronic and you want to measure change over time Consider a patient diary. *Ask about:*
—pain intensity, e.g. none, mild–moderate, severe; rank on a 1–10 scale
—interference with sleep or usual activities
—pain relief, e.g. none, slight–moderate, good, complete

**Fig. 9.3** Points to consider when taking a history of pain

### Further information
**British Pain Society** Assessment of pain in older people: National guidelines (2007) ⌨ www.britishpainsociety.org

### Patient support contacts
**Action on Pain** ☎ 0845 603 1593 ⌨ www.action-on-pain.co.uk
**Pain Concern** ☎ 01620 822 572 ⌨ www.painconcern.org.uk
**Pain Association of Scotland** ☎ 0800 783 6059
⌨ www.painassociation.com

# Principles of pain control

**Acute pain** Symptom of injured/diseased tissue. Subsides as the injury heals. Can be worsened by fear. Treat the underlying cause.

**Chronic pain** Defined as pain persisting for >3–6mo. Affects ~7% of adults in the UK. Cause is often multidimensional, with physical, social, and psychological factors all contributing to the overall feeling of pain.

## Goals of chronic pain management

- Set realistic targets. Abolition of pain may be impossible—70% have pain despite analgesia.
- If analgesia is not helping—stop it.
- The aim is often rehabilitation with ↓ in distress/disability.

**Strategies for pain management** A multidisciplinary approach is essential. *Consider*:

- *Prevention*, e.g. wrist splints for carpal tunnel syndrome, analgesia prior to minor surgery.
- *Removal of cause* Treat medical causes of pain, e.g. infection, ↓ blood sugar (diabetic neuropathy). Refer surgical causes for surgery if appropriate, e.g. hip osteoarthritis—joint replacement.
- *Pain-relieving drugs* Start with a single drug at low dose and step up dose or add another drug as needed. Especially in situations of acute pain, step down if pain diminishes.
- *Physical therapies* Acupuncture, physiotherapy, or TENS.
- *Nerve blocks* Consider referral for epidural (low back pain), local nerve block, or sympathectomy (e.g. vascular rest pain).
- *Modification of emotional response* Psychotropic drugs, e.g. anxiolytics, antidepressants.
- *Modification of behavioural response*, e.g. back pain—consider referral to a back rehabilitation scheme.

**The analgesic ladder** Use a step-by-step approach (Figure 9.4).

*Step 1. Non-opioid* Start treatment with paracetamol. Stress the need for REGULAR dosage. Adult dose is 1g every 4–6 h (maximum daily dose 4g). If this is not adequate in 24h, either try a NSAID, e.g. ibuprofen 400mg tds (if appropriate) alone or in combination with paracetamol, or proceed to step 2.

*Step 2. Weak opioid + non-opioid* Start treatment with a combined preparation of paracetamol + codeine/dihydrocodeine. Combining 2 analgesics with different mechanisms of action enables better pain control than using either alone. Combinations have ↓ dose-related side effects but the range of side effects is ↑ (additive effects of 2 drugs). Combinations using 30mg of codeine are more effective than paracetamol alone, but it is cheaper and more flexible if constituents are prescribed separately. Advise patients to take tablets regularly and not to assess efficacy after only a couple of doses.

❶ There is no proven additional analgesic benefit for preparations containing paracetamol + 8mg of codeine compared with paracetamol alone.

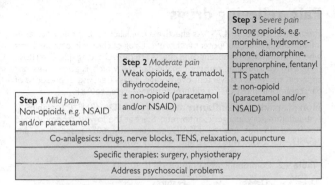

**Fig. 9.4** World Health Organization analgesics ladder
Reproduced with permission of the World Health Organization

### Step 3. Strong opioid + non-opioid

- Use immediate release morphine tablets or morphine solution.
  2 tablets of co-codamol (30/500) contain 60mg of codeine which is
  equi-analgesic to ~6mg of oral morphine. If changing to morphine,
  use a minimum dose of 5mg (6mg is hard to prescribe).
- Chronic pain may be only partially opioid sensitive. Give for a 2wk trial
  and only continue if of proven benefit. Worries of tolerance/addiction
  are unfounded for patients with true opioid-sensitive pain. If the pain
  seems responsive to opioids and there are no undue side effects, ↑ the
  dose upwards by 30–50% every 24h until pain is controlled (🔲 p.218).

⚠ Take care if the patient is elderly or in renal failure—consider starting
with a ↓ dose of morphine.

**Addition of co-analgesics and adjuvant drugs** In combination with
analgesics, can enhance pain control. Examples include:
- **Antidepressants** in low dose for nerve pain and sleep disturbance
  associated with pain; in larger doses for secondary depression.
- **Anticonvulsants** for neuropathic pain.
- **Corticosteroids** for pain due to oedema.
- **Muscle relaxants** for muscle cramp pain.
- **Antispasmodics** for bowel colic.
- **Antibiotics** for infection pain.
- **Night sedative** when lack of sleep is lowering pain threshold.
- **Anxiolytic** when anxiety is making pain worse (relaxation exercises may
  also help in these circumstances).

**Referral** If unable to remove cause and unable to achieve adequate pain
relief consider referral to a specialist pain control clinic or palliative care
(depending on the context of the pain).

⚠ Be aware of 2° gain from pain if symptoms seem out of proportion
(outstanding compensation claims are a significant negative factor in
success of pain management).

# Pain-relieving drugs

**Paracetamol** (BNF 4.7.1) As effective a painkiller as ibuprofen. No anti-inflammatory effect but potent antipyretic. Drug of choice in osteoarthritis where inflammation is absent. Side effects are rare. Dose 1g qds. Overdose (>4g/24h) can be fatal, causing hepatic damage which is sometimes not apparent for 4–6d. Inadvertent overdosage is easy because of presence of paracetamol in most OTC cold preparations—refer to A&E.

**Non-steroidal anti-inflammatories (NSAIDs)** (BNF 10.1.1; Table 9.2) Anti-inflammatory, analgesic, antipyretic. Start at the lowest recommended dose and do not use >1 NSAID concurrently. 60% respond to any NSAID—for those who don't, another may work.

**Table 9.2** Commonly used NSAIDs (BNF 10.1.1)

| Drug | Dosage | Features |
|------|--------|----------|
| Ibuprofen | 1.2–1.6g/d in 3–4 divided doses | Fewer side effects than other NSAIDs. Anti-inflammatory properties are weaker. Do not use if inflammation is prominent, e.g. gout |
| Naproxen | 0.5–1g/d in 1–2 divided doses | Good efficacy with a low incidence of side effects. |
| Diclofenac | 75–150mg/d in 2–3 divided doses | |
| Meloxicam | 7.5–15mg od | Selective COX2 inhibitors. As effective as non-selective NSAIDs and share side effects but risk of serious upper GI events is lower. Only use if at low risk of cerebro- or cardiovascular disease and high risk of GI side effects |
| Celecoxib | 200mg od or bd | |

**GI side effects** Common (50%), including GI bleeds (¼ GI bleeds in UK). ↑ with age. Risks are dose related and vary between drugs. For the elderly, and those on steroids or with past history of GI ulceration or indigestion, protect the stomach with misoprostol or a proton pump inhibitor (PPI). Selective inhibitors of cyclo-oxygenase-2 (COX2) are equally effective but should not be given to any patient with pre-existing or high risk of cardio- or cerebrovascular disease.

**Other side effects** Hypersensitivity reactions—5–10% asthmatics develop bronchospasm; fluid retention—relative contraindication in patients with ↑BP/cardiac failure; renal failure—rare, more common in patients with pre-existing renal disease; hepatic impairment—particularly diclofenac.

❶ COX2 inhibitors
• have NO effect on platelet aggregation
• have no benefit if used in patients on continuous low-dose aspirin, and
• combining a COX2 inhibitor with PPI/misoprostol does NOT give extra stomach protection.

**Topical NSAIDs** Of proven benefit for acute and chronic conditions[S] and can be as effective as oral preparations. They have lower incidence of GI and other side effects, although these still occur.

**Codeine** (BNF 4.7.2) Most commonly used weak opioid in the UK. Dose is 30–60mg every 4h to a maximum of 240mg/24h. Analgesic effect is ↑ by regular ingestion.

**Equipotence with morphine** 60mg codeine 4×/d equals 240mg codeine in 24h. 10mg of codeine is equipotent to 1mg of morphine, so the equivalent morphine dose would be 24mg/24h.

**Side effects** The most common side effects are nausea, vomiting, constipation, and drowsiness (📖 p.218). Codeine is effective for the relief of mild to moderate pain but is too constipating for long-term use. Always consider prescribing a laxative (e.g. bisacodyl 1–2 tablets nocte) with codeine to prevent constipation.

### Reasons for decreased effectiveness
- 5–10% of Caucasians have CYP2D6 genotype. They lack the hepatic enzyme necessary to convert codeine to morphine and will obtain less analgesia when taking codeine-containing analgesics.
- Effects of codeine are reduced by concurrent use of:
  - Anti-psychotics, e.g. chlorpromazine, haloperidol
  - Metoclopramide
  - Tricyclic antidepressants, e.g. amitriptyline.

**Dihydrocodeine** has analgesic efficacy and side effect profile similar to that of codeine. The dose of dihydrocodeine by mouth is 30–60mg every 4h. A 40mg tablet is now also available.

**Tramadol** is a synthetic analogue of codeine. It is not a controlled drug. Dose range 50mg bd, increasing to a maximum of 400mg/24h. Produces analgesia by two mechanisms:
- An opioid effect, and
- An enhancement of serotonergic and adrenergic pathways.

### Advantages over codeine and dihydrocodeine
- Rapid absorption of oral doses—analgesia in <1h, peaks at 1–2h.
- Metabolized in the liver—safer for the elderly/those with renal failure.
- Fewer typical opioid side effects (notably, ↓ respiratory depression, constipation, and addiction potential).
- May have a significant effect on neuropathic pain.

### Disadvantages
- Psychiatric reactions have been reported.
- Nausea and vomiting can be a problem with high doses.

**Morphine and other strong opioids** 📖 p.218

### Further information
**British Pain Society** 🖥 www.britishpainsociety.org
- Recommendations for the appropriate use of opioids for persistent non-cancer pain (2005)
- A practical guide to the provision of chronic pain services for adults in primary care (2004)

**Oxford Pain Internet Site**
🖥 www.medicine.ox.ac.uk/bandolier/booth/painpag
**Bandolier** Topical NSAIDs (2003)
🖥 www.medicine.ox.ac.uk/bandolier/band110/b110-6.html

# Morphine and other strong opioids

Morphine is the strong opioid of first choice for moderate to severe pain in both malignant and non-malignant conditions.

**Starting a patient on oral morphine** Start with 4 hourly immediate release morphine. Give clear instructions. *Initial dosage*:
- *Adults not pain controlled with regular weak opioids* (e.g. co-codamol 500/30 2 tablets qds)—5–10mg every 4h.
- *Elderly, cachectic, or not taking regular weak opioids* 2.5–5mg every 4h (2.5mg if very elderly/frail).

*Titration of dose* ↑ dose as needed by 25–50%/d until pain is controlled/ unacceptable side effects. There is no 'maximum' daily allowance, e.g. 5→ 10→15→20→30→40→60→80→100→130→160→200mg

**Maintenance** Once pain is controlled, consider a long-acting preparation of equivalent dose (e.g MST® bd, MXL® od). Calculate total daily dose of morphine by adding together the 4h doses.

*Increasing dose* If dose ↑ is necessary, use ⅓–½× dose increments. ↑ dose rather than frequency as tablets are designed for od or bd dosing.

**Breakthrough pain** Pain of rapid onset, and moderate/severe intensity despite background analgesia. *Management*:
- Prescribe immediate release morphine for breakthrough pain—give the equivalent 4 hourly dose as an additional dose.
- If pain starts to occur regularly before the next dose of analgesia is due, ↑ the regular *background dose*.

**Common side effects of opioid drugs** Warn patients:
- *Nausea and vomiting* affects >1:3 patients for the first 2wk of opioid use. Prescribe a regular antiemetic for 2wk (e.g. haloperidol 1.5mg nocte). If nausea/vomiting continues, consider an alternative opioid.
- *Constipation*. Consider prescribing prophylactic laxatives (e.g. bisacodyl 1–2 tablets nocte). Fentanyl causes less constipation than morphine.
- *Drowsiness/cognitive impairment* usually wears off in <1wk. Advise not to drive, perform other skilled tasks, or work with dangerous machinery for ≥1wk after starting morphine (longer if drowsiness persists), or after ↑ in dose. If not improving, consider an alternative opioid or refer for specialist advice.

**Conversion to injectable morphine and other opioids** Table 9.3

**Reasons to chose/switch to an alternative strong opioid** Unacceptable side effects; renal failure (fentanyl is licensed for use; oxycodone is safe in mild–moderate renal failure); patient unable to take oral medication regularly (consider fentanyl or buprenorphine patch, or syringe driver); choice (morphine is unacceptable for some patients).

**Alternative strong opioids** Diamorphine; oxycodone; fentanyl; buprenorphine; hydromorphone; pethidine (not suitable for severe continuing pain—used for acute pain relief/obstetric pain).

❶ Never attempt dose titration for unstable pain using a fentanyl patch— convert from oral morphine once a stable dose is attained.

**Table 9.3** Quick conversions of oral morphine

| From | To | Conversion | Example |
|---|---|---|---|
| Oral morphine (total dose) e.g. 10mg morphine 4 hourly = 60mg oral morphine in 24h | sc diamorphine | ÷ by 3 | 60÷3=20mg diamorphine by syringe driver over 24h |
| | sc morphine | ÷ by 2 | 60÷2=30mg morphine by syringe driver over 24h |
| | oral oxycodone | ÷ by 2 | 60÷2=30mg oral oxycodone in divided doses over 24h |
| | oral hydromorphone | ÷ by 7.5 | 60÷7.5=(60×2)÷15=8mg hydromorphone in divided doses over 24h |

❶ If total 24h dose is equivalent to 360mg morphine or more—get specialist advice

**Opioid toxicity** Intentional or unintentional overdose produces:
- Drowsiness or coma
- Hypotension
- Pinpoint pupils
- Vomiting
- Hypotension
- Confusion—including auditory and/or visual hallucinations
- Respiratory depression:
  - *If respiratory rate ≥ 8/min and the patient is easily rousable and not cyanosed* adopt a policy of 'wait and see'. Consider reducing or omitting the next regular dose of opioid. Stop syringe drivers temporarily to allow plasma levels to ↓; then restart at lower dose.
  - *If respiratory rate < 8/min and the patient is barely rousable/unconscious and/or cyanosed* dilute naloxone 400 micrograms to 10mL with sodium chloride 0.9%. Administer 0.5–1mL IV every minute until respiratory status is satisfactory. If respiratory function still does not improve, question diagnosis. Further doses may be needed later as naloxone is shorter acting than morphine.
- Muscle rigidity/myoclonus—consider renal failure (can produce myoclonus alone). Treat by rehydration, stopping other medication which may exacerbate myoclonus, switching opioid, or with clonazepam 2–4mg/24h depending on circumstances.

**Subacute overdosage** Slowly progressive somnolence and respiratory depression—common in patients with renal failure. Withhold morphine for 1–2 doses and then reintroduce at 25% lower dose.

**Opioid toxicity may be ↑ by**
- Renal failure
- Other change in disease status, e.g. hepatic function, weight loss
- Dehydration
- Other analgesics, e.g. NSAIDs
- Co-administration of amitriptyline.

**Syringe drivers** 📖 p.1027

**Further information**
**British Pain Society**. Recommendations for the appropriate use of opioids in persistent non-cancer pain (2005) 🖥 www.britishpainsociety.org
**DTB** Opioid analgesics for cancer pain in primary care (2005).
**Online converter for fentanyl patches**
🖥 www.globalrph.com/fentconv.htm

# Neuropathic pain

Neuropathic pain occurs as a result of damage to neural tissue. Examples include post-herpetic neuralgia, complex regional pain syndrome (reflex sympathetic dystrophy), peripheral neuropathy (e.g. due to DM), compression neuropathy, and phantom limb pain.

Pain typically occurs in association with altered sensation, e.g. burning, stabbing or numbness. Pain may also be provoked by non-noxious stimuli (allodynia) e.g. gentle heat or cold. Neuropathic pain is generally managed with tricyclic antidepressants or antiepileptic drugs.

## Tricyclic antidepressants

**Amitriptyline** is prescribed most frequently (unlicensed indication). Start at a dose of 25 mg nocte—10mg nocte if elderly. ↑ dose by 10–25mg nocte every 5–7d to a maximum of 75mg nocte as needed (higher doses under specialist supervision). Some patients do not derive benefit for 4–6 wk.

*Alternatives include*
- Nortriptyline—also given at an initial dose of 10–25 mg nocte. May produce fewer side effects than amitriptyline.
- Dosulepin—25–75mg nocte.
- Lofepramine—particularly suitable for the elderly/frail. Start at 70mg nocte increasing to 70mg bd as necessary after 5–7d.

## Anticonvulsants

**Gabapentin and pregabalin** Both licensed for treatment of neuropathic pain. Dose regimes:
- **Gabapentin** 300 mg on day 1; 300 mg bd on day 2; 300 mg tds on day 3; then increase dose according to response in steps of 300 mg daily (in 3 divided doses) to a maximum of 1.8 g/d.
- **Pregabalin** Initially 150 mg/d in 2–3 divided doses; increased if necessary after 3–7d to 300 mg daily in 2–3 divided doses; increased further if necessary after 7 d to a maximum of 600 mg daily in 2–3 divided doses.

**Carbamazepine** Traditionally the drug of choice for neuropathic pain but it is unlicensed and often poorly tolerated. Start with 100–200mg 1–2×/d (less if elderly or frail). Build up dose slowly to minimize adverse effects to the usual dose of 0.8–1.2g daily in divided doses. Oxcarbazepine is an alternative for trigeminal neuralgia.

**Sodium valproate, lamotrigine, and phenytoin** Also occasionally used for neuropathic pain but are reserved for use under specialist supervision.

**NSAIDs** Sometimes effective for neuropathic pain either because there is mixed nociceptive pain or because they ↓ inflammatory sensitization of nerves. There is considerable variation in individual patient tolerance and response (📖 p.216).

**Opioids** Neuropathic pain often responds only partially to opioid analgesics. Oxycodone, tramadol, and methadone are probably the most effective of the opioids—consider when other measures fail.

## Other drug treatments

*Corticosteroids* may help relieve pressure in compression neuropathy and, indirectly, pain. Start with a high initial dose to achieve rapid results (dexamethasone 8mg/d works in 1–3d); then rapidly ↓ dose to the minimum that maintains benefit.

*Capsaicin* is a topical treatment licensed for neuropathic pain. Apply a small amount 3–4×/d. Acts by counter-irritation, but intense burning during initial treatment limits use. Advise patients to wash hands after application and avoid application after a hot shower/bath (↑ burning sensation).

*Topical lidocaine* Plasters impregnated with lidocaine 5% are licensed for post-herpetic neuralgia. Apply od for up to 12h, followed by a 12h plaster-free period; discontinue if no response after 4 wk. Up to 3 plasters may be used to cover large areas; plasters may be cut.

## Non-drug treatments

- Patients with chronic neuropathic pain often require a multidisciplinary approach including physiotherapy and psychological support.
- TENS and/or acupuncture help in some cases.
- Nerve blocks and/or central electrical stimulation may help in some cases—refer for specialist advice.

**Referral** If unable to achieve adequate pain relief, consider referral to a specialist pain control clinic (or palliative care team if more appropriate).

**Trigeminal neuralgia** 📖 p.565

**Post-herpetic neuralgia** 📖 p.651

**Diabetic neuropathy** 📖 p.366

## Further information

**British Pain Society** Recommendations for the appropriate use of opioids in persistent non-cancer pain (2005) 🖳 www.britishpainsociety.org

## Information for patients

**Neuropathy Trust** 🖳 www.neurocentre.com

# Support for informal carers

In the UK there are 6 million informal carers who are vitally important to the well-being of disabled people in the community. Most are relatives or friends of the person being cared for. Many are elderly with health problems themselves. There is good evidence their health suffers as a result of caring - 52% report treatment for a stress-related illness since becoming a carer and 51% report being physically injured as a result of caring. Young carers (<18y) are at particular risk of social, educational, and mental health problems.

Record whether patients are carers in their notes. GPs and their primary care teams are often the 1st point of access for any help needed and 88% of carers have seen their GP in the past 12 mo. Carers see the GP as the professional most able to improve their lives but few GPs have had any training about their problems and 71% carers believe their GPs are unaware of their needs.

## Physical help
- *Practical advice on nursing skills* Ask DNs to review problems.
- *Advice on management* Specialist nurses (e.g. respiratory nurses, cancer care nurses, Macmillan nurses, etc.) provide special expertise.
- *Additional help* Social services can provide home care. Voluntary organisations provide sitting services e.g. Crossroads schemes.
- *Home modification* Local authorities can arrange modifications. DNs have access to equipment needed for nursing. The Red Cross loans commodes, wheelchairs, etc.
- *Respite* Hospitals, charity organizations, and local authorities provide day care (to give regular breaks each week) and respite care (for a week or more at a time).

## Emotional support
- *Carer centres* Provide practical advice, may provide counselling, and give carers an opportunity to share experiences with people in similar situations.
- *Always ask carers how they are when visiting*, even if they are not your patients themselves.
- *If the patient and/or carer have a religion, the clergy will often provide ongoing support*
- *Maintain good lines of communication* Make sure that you inform both carer and patient fully. Make appointments for review. Don't be short with a carer, patronising, or impossible to contact.

**Financial support** Many patients who have carers are entitled to Attendance Allowance or Disability Living Allowance (&#x1F4D6; p.227). If the patients are not expected to live >6mo, they are entitled to claim under Special Rules. This benefit is *not* means tested. Other benefits:
- *Low income* &#x1F4D6; p.104
- *Given up work to look after the patient* May be eligible for carers allowance (&#x1F4D6; p.228)
- *Substantial modification to home* Council tax may be payable at lower rate (consult local council).

**GP services**
- Consider appointing a carers lead to champion the needs of carers within the practice.
- Try to identify carers e.g. notice in reception, question on registration form, scanning discharge summaries for patients with long-term conditions likely to need carers, opportunistically.
- Provide appointments for carers at times when they can attend. Consider offering home visits for the carer if unable to get to the sugery as a result of caring duties.
- Offer carers an annual influenza vaccination.
- Include carers as partners in care.
- Consider asking the cared-for for written consent to share medical information about them with their carers.

The RCGP and Princess Royal Trust for Carers have developed a self-assessment checklist and action guide for GP practices to help them to support carers. *Supporting carers: an action guide for general practitioners and their teams* is available from 🖳 www.carers.org

**Social services assessment** Every carer has a right to ask for a full assessment of their needs by the social services. Emergency planning is part of the carer's assessment

**Emergency planning** Advise carers to make an emergency plan. Emergency plans are lodged on a database and the carer is provided with a card to carry with the emergency contact number printed on it
- If carers have an unexpected crisis and cannot provide care, they can ring the emergency line with the knowledge that short-term replacement care will be available.
- Carers are advised to carry the cards with them in an obvious place (e.g. wallet or purse). In the event of mishap, this will alert that the person is a carer and allow the emergency plan to be activated.

**Support organizations for carers**
**NHS Carers Direct** ☎ 0808 802 0202 🖳 www.nhs.uk/carersdirect
**Disability and carers service**
🖳 www.direct.gov.uk/carers or 🖳 www.direct.gov.uk/disability
**Carers UK** ☎ 0808 808 7777 🖳 www.carersuk.org
**Princess Royal Trust for Carers** ☎ 0844 800 4361
🖳 www.carers.org
**Benefits Enquiry Line** ☎ 0800 882200; 0800 243355 (minicom facility); 0800 441144 (for help with form completion)
**Citizens Advice Bureau** 🖳 www.adviceguide.org.uk
**Age Concern** ☎ 0800 00 99 66 🖳 www.ageconcern.org.uk
**Counsel and Care** ☎ 0845 300 7585 🖳 www.counselandcare.org.uk
**Support organizations for the patient's condition**

> ❶ **Carer skills** A carer skills course has been developed by Caring with Confidence. Further information is available at
> 🖳 www.caringwithconfidence.net

# Pensions and benefits

**Retirement pension** A state retirement pension is currently payable to women aged ≥60y and men aged ≥65y, even if still working. Entitlement age will rise to 65y for women between 2010 and 2020 (affects those born April 1950 to April 1955). Claim forms should be received automatically—if not, request one through the local Jobseeker Plus office. Pensions are taxable.

**Basic pension** Flat rate amount—different for single people and married couples. If not enough National Insurance (NI) contributions have been paid, amounts may ↓. >80y a higher rate is payable which is not dependent on NI contributions.

**Increase for dependants** Paid if:
- The claimant's spouse is <60y and earns under a set amount/does not receive certain other benefits.
- The claimant has children (if claim made before April 2003).

**Additional pension** State second pension (replaced SERPS). Based on NI contributions and earnings. Workers can opt out of the additional pension scheme, pay into a private or company scheme instead, and pay lower NI.

**Graduated pension** Some people may be entitled to a graduated pension. This is based on earnings between 1961 and 1975.

**Extra pension** For a person who defers claiming retirement pension for up to 5y. Extra pension is payable when retirement pension is claimed.

❶ If hospitalized, retirement pension is payable for 1y at full rate. After 12 mo, basic pension is ↓ but additional pension stays the same.

**Pension Credit** Apply on form PC1 ☎ 0800 991 234

**Guarantee credit** ≥60y and income below the 'appropriate amount'. Appropriate amount varies according to circumstances. Capital (excluding value of own home) >£6000 is deemed to count as income at the rate of £1/wk/£500 capital. Confers automatic eligibility for housing benefit, community tax benefit, and social fund payments.

**Savings credit** ≥65y and income > savings credit starting point—currently >£167/wk for a single person or >£245 if one of a couple. Depends on level of income and circumstances.

## Other benefits just for pensioners
- *Free colour TV licence* All pensioners >75y.
- *Winter fuel payment* Annual payment to all pensioners >60y.

**Home Responsibilities Protection (HRP)** Scheme which protects basic state pension for people who don't work or have low income and are caring for someone. 🖥 www.thepensionservice.gov.uk

**Christmas bonus** One-off payment made to people receiving a retirement pension or income support a few weeks before Christmas.

**Cold weather payment** 📖 p.106.

**Benefits for**

**Help with mobility**

**Adaptations and equipment**

**War pensions** For people injured whilst serving in the armed forces and their dependants (if injury caused or hastened death). Administered by the Veterans Agency, Ministry of Defence. No time limit for claims.

*War pensions scheme* for ex-service personnel whose injuries, wounds, and illnesses arose prior to 6 April 2005.

*War Disablement Pension*
- *Basic benefits:* based on percentage disablement:
  - if <20% disabled—lump sum
  - if >20% disabled—weekly sum (pension).
- *Other benefits* Allowances if severely disabled, e.g.
  - War Pensioners Mobility Supplement for walking difficulty. Holders can apply for the motability scheme and road tax exemption.
  - Constant Attendance Allowance for high levels of care.

*Medical treatment* Some services and appliances may be paid for by the Veterans' Agency (includes prescription charges, nursing home fees).

*War widows' and widowers' pensions* for spouses/civil partners of service/ ex-service personnel:
- where death was a result of service or
- if the deceased was in receipt of a War Pensions Constant Attendance Allowance
- if the deceased was in receipt of a War Disablement Pension at the rate of ≥80% and was getting unemployability supplement.

*War widows' and widowers' allowances* Automatic age allowance when widows/widowers reach 65y and further increase at 70y and 80y.

**Armed Forces Compensation Scheme (AFCS)** provides benefits for illness, injury, or death caused by service on or after 6 April 2005. Time limit is 5y from the event, from the time when medical advice was first sought, or after retirement, whichever is soonest. There is an exceptions list for late onset conditions. Provides:
- Lump sum for significant illnesses/injuries—15 levels of award.
- Tax-free Guaranteed Income Payment (GIP) for life for injuries at the higher tariff levels (1–11) to compensate for loss of earnings capacity.
- Guaranteed Income Payment for Survivors (SGIP) where an attributable death occurs.

**Further information**
**The Pension Service** 🖥 www.thepensionservice.gov.uk
**Pensions Advisory Service (TPA)** ☎ 0845 601 2923
🖥 www.pensionsadvisoryservice.org.uk
**Citizens Advice Bureau** 🖥 www.adviceguide.org.uk
**Veterans Agency** ☎ 0800 169 22 77 🖥 www.veterans-uk.info

**Table 9.4** Benefits for disability and illness

| | Eligibility | How to apply | Amount |
|---|---|---|---|
| **Statutory Sick Pay** | • Employee age ≥16y and <65y<br>• Incapable of work due to sickness or disability<br>• Earning ≥ NI lower earnings limit<br>• Unable to work ≥4d and <28wk (inc. days when would not normally work)<br>• Those ineligible may be eligible for incapacity benefit or maternity allowance | Notify employer of illness; self-certification first 7d (SC2); Med 3 after that time (📖 p.127) | £79.15/wk<br>Some employers have more generous arrangements. Paid through normal pay mechanisms |
| **Employment and Support Allowance (ESA)** | • Age ≥16y and <60y (woman) or <65y (man)<br>• Not entitled to statutory sick pay<br>• Unable to work due to sickness or disability—SC1 certificate for first 7d then Med3 certificate until work capability assessment (done <13wk into period of sickness/disability) 📖 p.126<br>• Not receiving income support, income based Job Seeker's Allowance or Pension Credit<br>**2 types of ESA**<br>• *Contributory ESA*—paid if sufficient NI contributions (unless unfit for work under the age of 20 (25 if in full time education)<br>• *Income related ESA*—full rate is paid if savings ≤£16,000 and income is less than a minimum income; reduced rates may be payable if income is greater than this minimum amount. | Claim from<br>🌐 www.jobcentreplus.gov.uk<br>or ☎ 0800 055 6688<br>(textphone: 0800 023 4888) | *First 3d*—no payment<br>*Assessment phase* (>3d but <14wk)<br>• <25y—up to £50.95<br>• ≥25y—up to £64.30<br>*Main phase* (≥ 14wk)<br>• Work related activity group—up to £89.80<br>• Support group —up to £95.15<br>❶ Figures are for a single person. Additional payments may be available for dependents if receiving income-related ESA |

❶ Incapacity Benefit—Since 27.10.2008, ESA has replaced Incapacity Benefit for new claims. Those people already receiving Incapacity Benefit will continue to do so at present

| | | |
|---|---|---|
| **Disability Living Allowance (DLA)**[†] | • Disability >3mo and expected to last >6mo more*. <br> • <65y at time of application <br> **Mobility component** Help needed to get about outdoors <br> • *Higher rate* —unable/virtually unable to walk (age >3y) <br> • *Lower rate* —help to find way in unfamiliar places (age >5y) <br> **Care component** Help needed with personal care <br> • *Lower rate* —attention/supervision needed for a significant proportion of the day or unable to prepare a cooked meal. <br> • *Middle rate* —attention/supervision throughout the day or repeated prolonged attention or watching over at night. <br> • *Higher rate* —24h attention/supervision or terminal 'illness'* | ☎ 0800 882200 (0800 220674 in Northern Ireland) or Leaflet DLA A5DCS available from Post Offices or Using claim packs available at Citizen's Advice Bureau and social security offices or 🖥 www.direct.gov.uk | **Mobility component** <br> *Higher rate*—£49.10/wk <br> *Lower rate*—£18.65/wk <br> **Care component** <br> *Higher rate*—£70.35/wk <br> *Middle rate*—£47.10/wk <br> *Lower rate*—£18.65/wk |
| **Attendance Allowance (AA)**[†] | • Disability > 3mo and expected to last > 6 mo more*. <br> • Aged ≥ 65y <br> • Not permanently in hospital or accommodation funded by the local authority <br> • Needs attention/supervision—higher rate if 24hour care required/terminal illness* | ☎ 0800 882200 (0800 220674 in Northern Ireland) or Leaflet AA A5DCS available from Post Offices or 🖥 www.direct.gov.uk | *Lower rate* £70.35 <br> *Higher rate* £47.10 (for people who need day and night care or are terminally ill) |

[†]No need to receive help to apply. Not means tested.

*Terminal illness (not expected to live >6mo)—claim under Special Rules. Claims are processed much faster and the highest care rate is automatically awarded. GP or hospital specialist fills in form DS1500 to provide clinical information to support application (fee can be claimed)

**Table 9.4** (continued) Benefits for disability and illness

| | Eligibility | How to apply | Amount |
|---|---|---|---|
| **Community Care Grant** | Receiving Income Support, income-related ESA, pension credit, or income-based Jobseeker's Allowance *and*:<br>• Want to re-establish or help the applicant or a family member stay in the community<br>• To ease exceptional pressure on the applicant or a family member<br>• To help with certain travel costs | Form SF300 from local social security offices or ⬚ www.direct.gov.uk | Minimum payment £30<br>No maximum amount |
| **Disabled Facilities Grant** | For work essential to help a disabled person live an independent life; means tested | Apply via local housing department | Any reasonable application for funds is considered |
| **Carer's Allowance** | • Aged ≥16y *and*<br>• Spends ≥35h/wk caring for a person with a disability who is getting AA or constant attendance allowance or middle or higher rate care component of DLA, *and*<br>• Earning ≤£95.00/wk after allowable expenses<br>• Not in full-time education | Complete form in leaflet CAA5DCS available from local social security offices or ⬚ www.direct.gov.uk | £53.10/wk<br>plus additions for dependants (❶ no new claims for dependant children have been accepted since April 2003) |

❶
• People who need someone's help to get out of the house are entitled to free prescriptions (⬚ p.139).
• Severe Disablement Allowance is still paid to those who applied prior to April 2001.

**Table 9.5** Mobility for elderly and disabled people ❶ Local public transport schemes also exist

| | Eligibility | How to apply | Benefits received |
|---|---|---|---|
| **Blue Badge Scheme** | Age >2y and ≥1 of the following: <br>• War Pensioner's Mobility Supplement <br>• Higher rate of the mobility component of DLA <br>• Motor vehicle supplied by a government health department <br>• Registered blind <br>• Severe disability in both upper limbs preventing turning of a steering wheel <br>• Permanent and substantial difficulty walking | Apply through local social services department. <br>❶ In most circumstances the disabled person does not have to be the driver. The badge should not be used if the disabled person is not in the car <br>☎ (207 944 2914 <br>🖥 www.dft.gov.uk | Entitles holder to park: <br>• in specified disabled spaces <br>• free of charge or time limit at parking meters or other places where waiting is limited <br>• or single yellow lines for up to 3h (no time limit in Scotland) |
| **Motability Scheme** | • Higher rate mobility component of DLA or <br>• War Pension Mobility Supplement. <br>❶ Driver may be someone else | Contact Motability. <br>Application guide available at <br>🖥 www.motability.co.uk | Registered Charity <br>Mobility payments can be used to lease or hire-purchase a car, powered scooter, or wheelchair <br>Grants may also be available for advance payments, adaptations, or driving lessons |
| **Road Tax Exemption** | • Higher rate mobility component of DLA or <br>• War Pension Mobility Supplement or <br>• Person nominated as someone who regularly drives for a disabled person or <br>• Certain types of powered invalid carriages | Usually received automatically if not and claiming DLA <br>☎ 0845 712 456. <br>If claiming War Pension <br>☎ 0800 169 2277 | Exemption from Road Tax |
| **Seatbelt Exemption** | Certain medical conditions, e.g. colostomy | Medical practitioner must complete exemption certificate | Exemption from wearing seatbelt |

**Table 9.6** Adaptations and equipment for elderly and disabled people ● All purchases related to disability are VAT exempt

| | Eligibility | How to apply | Benefits received |
|---|---|---|---|
| Wheelchairs | Anyone requiring a wheelchair(s) for >3mo<br><br>Short-term loan of equipment is often available via the Red Cross | Referral by GP or specialist to the wheelchair service centre<br><br>Directory of service centres is available at 🖥 www.wheelchairmanagers.nhs.uk | Provision of suitable wheelchair<br><br>Vouchers enable disabled patients to purchase their chairs privately |
| Occupational therapy (OT) assessment | All elderly or disabled people | Request a needs assessment by an occupational therapist via local social services department | Enables provision of equipment and adaptations necessary to maintain an independent lifestyle |
| Disabled Living Centres<br><br>Disability Living Foundation | All elderly or disabled people | 49 *Disabled Living Centres* in the UK—list available from 🖥 www.assist-uk.org<br><br>*Disabled Living Foundation* 🖥 www.dlf.org.uk | *Disabled Living Centres* look at and try out equipment with OTs on hand to advise<br><br>*Disabled Living Foundation* information on aids and adaptations |
| Telephone | People who have physical difficulty using the telephone or communication problems | British Telecom produce a booklet *Communication Solutions* obtainable from ☎ 0800 800150 or 🖥 www.bt.com<br><br>If difficulty using a telephone directory register to use directory enquiries free ☎0800 5870195 | Gadgets and services that make it easier for disabled or elderly people to use the telephone |
| Alarm systems | Any disabled or elderly person who is alone at times, at risk, and mentally capable of using an alarm system | Arrange via local social services or housing department. Alternatively, charities for the elderly have schemes e.g.<br>Age Concern—Aid-Call ☎ 0800 772266 | Enables a call for help when the phone cannot be reached |

# Cardiology and vascular disease

# Blood pressure measurement

### Taking blood pressure

- Regularly maintain and calibrate your sphygmomanometer.
- Use a cuff of correct width:
  - *Most adults* 12 × 26cm bladder size
  - *Large adults (arm circumference >33cm)* 12 × 40cm bladder size
  - *Thin adults and children with arm circumference ≤ 26cm* 10 × 18cm bladder size.
- Seat the patient with arm at the level of the heart.
- In patients with symptoms of postural hypotension (falls or dizziness) measure BP when standing as well as seated. If there is a drop in systolic BP of >20mmHg consider specialist referral.
- Measure BP to the nearest 2mmHg.
- Measure diastolic pressure when heart sounds completely disappear ($K_5$). Only use the pressure at which they suddenly muffle ($K_4$) when $K_5$ cannot be determined.
- BP varies throughout the day and can ↑ as a response to having BP checked ('white coat phenomenon'—prevalence 10%). Take ≥2 measurements on two occasions before classifying a patient as hypertensive.
- If BP is very variable consider ambulatory BP monitoring (gives average BP over 24h) or intermittent home BP monitoring.

**Home monitoring and ambulatory BP monitoring** Both may have advantages in eliminating variation between readings (by taking the average), in decreasing 'white coat' hypertension, and in reduced observer bias. Finger and wrist devices are not recommended. Electronic devices for patient use loaned from GP premises are popular but require regular calibration and maintenance, and not all patients adhere to instructions for use.

**Table 10.1** Threshold values for treatment for ambulatory BP monitoring

|             | Abnormal |
| ----------- | -------- |
| Daytime     | >140/90  |
| Night-time  | >125/75  |
| 24h         | >135/85  |

The threshold for treatment for home monitoring is usually taken as 135/85mmHg.

The British Hypertension Society recommend downward adjustment of clinic readings by 12/7mmHg, in order to make a valid comparison with home monitoring reading.

❶ NICE does not recommend the routine use of ambulatory or home BP monitoring methods at present because of lack of research evidence.

**Hypertension** 📖 p.252

**Hypotension** Suggests fluid loss or heart pump failure.

*Postural hypotension* BP drops on moving from supine or sitting position to standing position. Confirm diagnosis by checking BP lying and then standing. Standing usually causes a slight ↓ in the systolic BP (<20mmHg) and a slight ↑ in the diastolic BP (<10mmHg). In postural hypotension there is a marked ↓ in both systolic and diastolic BP.

- *Review medication* Stop any non-essential medication contributing to symptoms (e.g. night sedation, unnecessary diuretics).
- *Optimize treatment* of intercurrent heart disease, Parkinson's disease, or DM.
- *Advice* Patients should take care when standing, especially if getting up from their beds or out of a hot bath/shower, and after meals.

*Cardiogenic shock* Due to heart pump failure e.g. MI, arrhythmia, tamponade. *Signs:*
- Hypotension—systolic BP <80–90mmHg.
- Pulse rate may be normal, ↑, or ↓.
- Severe breathlessness ± cyanosis.
- Pallor and sweating.

⚠ **Acute management of cardiogenic shock**
- Sit the patient up if possible.
- Call for ambulance assistance.
- Treat any underlying cause found, e.g. atropine for bradycardia; diamorphine, furosemide and GTN spray for acute LVF.
- Gain IV access if possible.
- If available give 100% oxygen (unless COPD, when give 24%).

# Examining the heart

**Apex beat** Normal position is in the 5th intercostal space, in the midclavicular line. Moved sideways/inferiorly if the heart is enlarged (e.g. CCF) or displaced (e.g. pneumothorax). May not be palpable if the patient is obese, or has hyperexpanded lungs (e.g. COPD) or a pericardial effusion. In infants/children apex beat is superior/more lateral.

**Parasternal heave** Detect by placing the heel of the hand over the left parasternal region. If present, the heel of the hand is lifted off the chest wall with each heart beat. *Causes:* usually right ventricular enlargement; rarely, left atrial enlargement.

**Heart sounds** (Table 10.3) Low/medium-frequency sounds (e.g. 3rd/4th heart sounds) are more easily heard with the bell applied lightly to the skin. High-frequency sounds (e.g. 1st/2nd heart sounds and opening snaps) are more easily heard with a diaphragm.

**Heart murmurs** Due to abnormalities of flow within the heart and great vessels. Very common. Often incidental findings. Described by:
• *Location*—where heard loudest.
• *Quality*, e.g. blowing, harsh.
• *Intensity*—graded out of 6 (1, virtually undetectable; 6, heard by an observer with no stethoscope); grades 4–6 are usually palpable (*thrills*).
• *Timing*—systolic or diastolic
• *Radiation*—does the murmur spread elsewhere, e.g. to axilla, carotids?

⚠ *Red flag symptoms*

• Cyanosis    • Lethargy/tiredness    • Weight loss (or failure
• Breathlessness    • Collapse                 to thrive)

*Always* refer for echo. Differential diagnosis—Table 10.2.

**Table 10.2** Differential diagnosis of heart murmurs

| Type of murmur | Description | Causes |
|---|---|---|
| Ejection systolic murmur | ↑ to reach a peak midway between the heart sounds | Flow murmurs e.g children, pregnancy, with fever, during/after exercise<br>Aortic stenosis or sclerosis (📖 pp.288–289)<br>Pulmonary stenosis (📖 p.289)<br>HOCM (📖 p.286) |
| Pan-systolic murmur | Uniform intensity between the 2 heart sounds; merges with 2nd heart sound | Mitral valve regurgitation/prolapse (📖 p.288)<br>Tricuspid regurgitation (📖 p.289)<br>VSD (📖 p.290)<br>ASD (📖 p.290) |
| Early diastolic murmur | Occurs just after the 2nd heart sound; high pitched; easily missed | Aortic regurgitation (📖 p.289)<br>Pulmonary regurgitation (📖 p.289)<br>Tricuspid stenosis (mitral stenosis coexists) |
| Mid-diastolic murmur | Midway between 2nd heart sound of 1 beat and 1st of the next; rumbling/low pitch | Mitral stenosis (📖 p.288)<br>Aortic regurgitation (Austin Flint murmur 📖 p.289) |

**Table 10.3** Heart sounds, abnormalities, and their causes

| Heart sound | | Causes |
|---|---|---|
| 1st heart sound<br>Heard loudest<br>at the apex<br>Caused by<br>closing of the<br>mitral and<br>tricuspid valves | Soft | Mitral regurgitation, low BP, rheumatic carditis, severe heart failure, LBBB |
| | Loud | AF, tachycardia, atrial premature beat, mitral stenosis |
| | Variable intensity | Varying duration of diastole, complete AV block |
| | Split | RBBB, paced beat from the left ventricle, left ventricular ectopics, ASD, Ebstein's anomaly, tricuspid stenosis |
| 2nd heart sound<br>Caused by<br>closure of the<br>aortic (A2) and<br>pulmonary (P2)<br>valves<br>A2 and P2 split<br>on inspiration<br>so that P2 is<br>heard after A2 | Soft | —A2: calcification of the aortic valve, dilatation of the aortic root<br>—P2: pulmonary stenosis |
| | Loud | —A2: ↑BP; thin patients<br>—P2: pulmonary hypertension, ASD |
| | Wide splitting | May be the result of early A2 or delayed P2<br>—Early A2: mitral regurgitation; VSD<br>—Delayed P2: RBBB, pulmonary stenosis, ASD, right ventricular failure |
| | Reversed splitting | A2 is delayed. P2 occurs before A2 so the split between the sounds ↓ on inspiration<br>Delayed A2—LBBB, systolic hypertension, HOCM, severe aortic stenosis, PDA, left heart failure |
| | Single | Calcification of the aortic valve, pulmonary stenosis, Fallot's tetralogy, Ebstein's anomaly, pericardial effusion, large VSD, obesity, emphysema |
| Clicks and snaps | Early systolic | Caused by opening of the aortic or pulmonary valves<br>—Aortic: aortic stenosis, bicuspid valve<br>—Pulmonary: pulmonary stenosis, pulmonary hypertension |
| | Mid/late systolic | Mitral valve prolapse |
| | Diastolic | Caused by opening of the mitral or tricuspid valves; silent in the healthy heart<br>—Mitral: mitral stenosis, rapid mitral flow, e.g. PDA, VSD, severe mitral regurgitation<br>—Tricuspid (rare): rheumatic stenosis, ASD |
| 3rd heart sound<br>Heard in<br>diastole after<br>the 2nd heart<br>sound | Right ventricle | Loudest at lower left sternal edge; never normal. *Causes:* right heart failure, tricuspid regurgitation, ASD, constrictive pericarditis |
| | Left ventricle | Loudest at the apex when inclined to the left. Can be normal in children and pregnancy. *Other causes:* LVF, mitral regurgitation, anterior MI |
| 4th heart sound<br>Heard in late<br>diastole | | Maximal at the apex or lower left sternal edge; never normal. *Causes:* ventricular hypertrophy or fibrosis and HOCM |

# Examination of the arterial system

The main conditions affecting the abdominal and peripheral arteries are:
- Aneurysms (📖 p.292).
- Atherosclerosis resulting in ischaemia of the legs and intermittent claudication, atrophic chamges, and/or rest pain.
- Embolization resulting in acute ischaemia of the limbs.

## General scheme
- Look at the limbs. Are there any signs of ischaemia? Are the extremities warm or cold? What colour are they?
- Examine the abdomen looking for a pulsatile mass which might suggest abdominal aortic aneurysm (📖 p.292). Auscultation may reveal a bruit.
- Check the peripheral pulses.

⚠ Tenderness on palpation of an abdominal aortic aneurysm suggests need for urgent operative repair.

**Carotid pulse** Ask the patient to lie supine with head/neck at 45° to the horizontal. When assessing the carotid pulse, consider:

### Rate
- *Tachycardia*: >100bpm (📖 p.276)
- *Bradycardia*: <60bpm (📖 p.280).

### Rhythm
- *Irregularly irregular*: AF, multiple ectopics.
- *Regularly irregular*: 2nd degree heart block.

**Character and volume** Always assess with a central pulse, e.g. carotid or femoral.
- *Small volume*: shock, pericardial tamponade, aortic stenosis (slow-rising).
- *Large volume*: hyperdynamic circulation (e.g. pregnancy), aortic incompetence (water-hammer, collapsing pulse), PDA.
- *Pulsus paradoxus*: pulse weakens in inspiration by >10mmHg—asthma, cardiac tamponade, pericarditis.

**Carotid bruits** May signify stenosis (>30%) often near the origin of internal carotid. Heard best behind the angle of the jaw. Usual cause is atheroma.

## Peripheral pulses
**Location** Table 10.4

### Examination
- Check whether each pulse is present. If present check:
  - Rate
  - Rhythm
  - Amplitude
  - Compare pulses in the 2 legs/2 arms.
- Check for radiofemoral delay—palpate radial and femoral pulses simultaneously. Delay suggests coarctation of the aorta.

**Table 10.4** Location of the limb pulses

| Pulse | Location |
|---|---|
| Brachial | ~2cm medial to the central point of the antecubital fossa over the elbow skin crease. |
| Radial | ~0.5–1cm on the radial (lateral) side of the flexor carpi radialis tendon at the wrist |
| Femoral | Below inguinal ligament, $^1/_3$ of the way up from pubic tubercle |
| Popliteal | With knee flexed at right angles palpate deep in the midline |
| Posterior tibial | 1cm behind medial malleolus |
| Dorsalis pedis | Variable—on the dorsum of the foot just lateral to the tendons to the big toe. ❶ Many healthy people have only 1 foot pulse |

Check for bruits over the femoral and/or carotid pulses—these indicate disturbed blood flow, usually 2° to narrowing due to atherosclerosis.

⚠ Character and waveform of the pulse should *only* be assessed using the femoral or carotid pulse.

## Signs of ischaemia

**Acute ischaemia** Acutely pale, cold, and pulseless limb (📖 p.1122). Refer immediately– keep the limb cool in the interim.

### Chronic ischaemic changes
- Atrophic skin changes—pallor, cool to the touch, hairless, shiny.
- On lowering the leg turns a dusky blue-red colour; on elevation, pallor and venous guttering.
- Ulceration—check under the heel and between the toes.
- Swelling suggests the patient is sleeping in a chair to avoid rest pain or, rarely, pain from deep infection
- Absent foot pulses—if pulses are present consider alternative diagnosis
- Ankle–brachial pressure index <0.95.

### Checking the ankle–brachial pressure index (ABPI)
- Check BP in one arm (📖 p.234). The systolic measurement is the brachial pressure (B).
- Then inflate a BP cuff around the lower calf just above the ankle.
- Using a Doppler ultrasound probe, record the maximum cuff pressure at which the probe can still record a pulse (ankle pressure (A)).
- Calculate the ankle–brachial pressure index by dividing the ankle pressure by the brachial pressure, i.e. ABPI = A÷B.

### Interpretation of ABPI results
- ABPI <0.95—ischaemia
- ABPI < 0.5—critical ischaemia.

❶ Arterial calcification (e.g. due to DM) can result in falsely elevated ankle pressure readings.

# Other symptoms and signs of cardiovascular disease

**Chest pain** 📖 p.1076

**Breathlessness or dyspnoea** 📖 p.302

**Crackles in the chest** 📖 p.307

**Peripheral oedema** Swelling of the ankles/Legs (or sacrum if bed bound) occurs when the rate of capillary filtration > rate drainage.
- Increased capillary filtration occurs due to ↑ venous pressure, hypoalbuminaemia, or local inflammation.
- Decreased drainage occurs due to lymphatic obstruction.

Consider whether swelling is acute or chronic, symmetrical or asymetrical, localized or generalized. Ask about associated symptoms, e.g. breathlessness. Treat according to cause. *Causes:*

### Acute
- DVT
- Superficial thrombophlebitis
- Joint effusion/haemarthrosis
- Cellulitis
- Haematoma
- Baker's cyst
- Arthritis
- Fracture
- Acute arterial ischaemia
- Dermatitis

### Chronic
- Gravitational oedema, e.g due to immobility. Common in the elderly. Advise elevation of feet above waist level, support stockings (ideally apply stockings before getting out of bed), avoid standing still. Diuretics are not a long-term solution.
- Heart failure
- Hypoproteinaemia, e.g. nephrotic syndrome
- Idiopathic oedema
- Reflex sympathetic dystrophy
- Post-thrombotic syndrome
- Chronic venous insufficiency/ venous obstruction
- Lipodermatosclerosis
- Lymphoedema: infection, tumour, trauma
- Congenital vascular abnormalities

**Pulmonary oedema** Accumulation of fluid in the pulmonary tissues and air spaces. *Causes include:*

### Cardiac/vascular
- Left heart failure
- Mitral stenosis
- MI
- Hypertension
- Pulmonary venous obstruction
- IV fluid overload.

### Other
- High altitude
- Kidney failure
- Nephrotic syndrome
- Cirrhosis
- Lymphatic obstruction, e.g. due to tumour
- PE.

### Lung
- Pneumonia
- Pneumonitis due to inhalation of toxic substances, e.g. gases, radiation.

**Cyanosis** Dusky blue skin

**Central cyanosis** Cyanosis of mucus membranes, e.g. mouth. *Causes:*
- Lung disease resulting in inadequate oxygen transfer (e.g. COPD, PE, pleural effusion, severe chest infection).

- Shunting from pulmonary to systemic circulation (e.g. Fallot's tetralogy, PDA, transposition of the great arteries).
- Inadequate oxygen uptake (e.g. met- or sulf-haemoglobinaemia).

**Peripheral cyanosis,** e.g. cyanosis of fingers. *Causes:* as for central cyanosis plus
- Physiological (cold, hypovolaemia)
- Local arterial disease (e.g. Raynaud's syndrome).

❶ Feet can be a dusky blue colour due to venous disease. If this occurs without central cyanosis, it does not imply abnormal oxygen saturation.

**Mitral facies** Dusky bluish red flushing of the cheeks (a form of peripheral cyanosis) associated with a low cardiac output.

**Clubbing** Loss of the angle between nail fold and plate; bulbous finger tip and nail fold feels boggy (📖 p.607).

⚠ Refer any patient with unexplained nail clubbing for urgent CXR[N].

**Jugular venous pressure** Observe internal jugular vein at 45° with head turned slightly to the left. Vertical height is measured in relation to the sternal angle. Raised if >4cm. Causes of ↑ JVP:

- Fluid overload
- Right heart failure and CCF
- SVC obstruction (non-pulsatile)
- Tricuspid or pulmonary valve disease
- Pulmonary hypertension
- Arrhythmia: AF or atrial flutter, complete heart block
- ↑ intrathoracic pressure, e.g pneumothorax, PE, emphysema,

**Kussmaul's sign** The JVP usually drops on inspiration along with intrathoracic pressure. The reverse pattern is called Kussmaul's sign. Caused by raised intrathoracic pressure or constrictive pericarditis.

## Signs of infective endocarditis
- *Infective*—fever, weight ↓, clubbing, splenomegaly, anaemia.
- *Cardiac*—murmurs (particularly new murmurs) ± heart failure.
- *Embolic*—neurological deficit due to stroke
- *Vasculitic*—microscopic haematuria, splinter haemorrhages, conjunctival haemorrhages, Roth's spots (retinal vasculitis), Osler's nodes (painful lesions on finger pulps), Janeway lesions (palmar macules).

## Signs of hypercholesterolaemia

**Corneal arcus** Whitish opaque line surrounding the margin of the cornea, separated from it by an area of clear cornea. Rarely congenital—more commonly occurs bilaterally in patients >50y (*arcus senilis*). Sometimes associated with ↑ blood lipids, particularly familial hypercholesterolaemias. Check lipids. If lipids are normal, no treatment is needed.

**Xanthomata** Localized collections of lipid-laden cells. Appear as yellowish-coloured lumps. Often caused by ↑ lipids. Commonly seen on the eyelids (*xanthelasma*), on the skin, or in tendons (appear as mobile nodules in the tendon).

# Cardiac investigations

**Electrocardiogram (ECG)** Graphic recording of electric potentials generated by the heart. Most surgeries now have ECG machines which interpret themselves and print out their findings. Analysis is easier, but it is still important to be able to understand significance of abnormalities and check computer analysis in the clinical context.

*Interpreting ECGs* Many mistakes in ECG interpretation are errors of omission, so a systematic approach is best. Check:

- Standardization (calibration) and technical features (including lead placement and artefacts).
- Heart rate—usual speed (25mm/s). Each big square represents 0.2s (small square—0.04s). Rate = 300÷R–R interval (in large squares).
- Rhythm—regular/irregular.
- P–R interval—normal if <0.2s.
- QRS interval—abnormal if >0.12s.
- Q–T interval—varies with rate. At 60bpm normal if 0.35–0.43s.
- P waves—present or absent, shape.
- QRS voltages— height of complexes (see Table 10.5, 📖 p.245).
- Mean QRS electrical axis—sum of all ventricular forces during ventricular depolarization. Normal axis: −30° to +120°.
  - If more −ve = left axis deviation; if more +ve = right axis deviation.
  - *Rule of thumb 1:* if the majority of the QRS complex is above the baseline (+ve) in leads I and II the axis is normal.
  - *Rule of thumb 2:* the axis lies at 90° to a QRS complex where the height above the baseline = height below the baseline.
- Precordial R-wave progression.
- Abnormal Q waves: >25% of the succeeding R wave and/or >0.04s wide.
- ST segments—elevation/depression, shape.
- T waves—height, inversion, shape.
- U waves—small rounded deflection (≤1 mm); follows T wave and usually has the same polarity.

*Brief guide to common ECG changes* 📖 p.244

**24h/ambulatory ECG** ECG monitoring equipment is worn for 24h. Continuous monitoring may detect intermittent arrhythmias or ischaemia.

**Exercise ECG** ECG testing whilst the patient undergoes graded exercise on a treadmill/exercise bicycle. Local referral criteria vary. Mortality ~ 1:10 000. Used for:

- Diagnosis of IHD—75% have a +ve test. False +ve rate of ~5%.
- Assessment of exercise tolerance.
- Response to treatment.
- As a prognostic indicator.
- Assessment of exercise-related arrhythmias.

*Contraindications* Recent MI (<7d), unstable angina, electrolyte disturbance, aortic stenosis, severe heart failure, known left main coronary artery stenosis, LBBB (may not be possible to interpret the trace).

**Cardiac enzymes** Biochemical blood assay of molecules released when the heart is damaged. Used in diagnosis of MI.
- *Troponins T and I* Preferred markers as more sensitive/specific than CK, AST, or lactate dehydrogenase (LDH). Together with CK, earliest to ↑ after MI.
- *Creatine kinase (CK)* ↑ in MI, muscle damage, e.g. prolonged running or seizures, after IM injection, and with dermatomyositis (e.g. due to statins). CK-MB assay may help clarify whether a cardiac event has occurred <48 h previously.
- *AST* 2nd to ↑                    • *LDH* Last to ↑

**Echocardiogram (Echo)** Heart USS. Local referral procedures vary.
- *2-dimensional* Produces a fan-shaped cross-sectional moving real-time image of the heart. May be transthoracic or transoesophageal. Used to assess valvular abnormalities and prosthetic heart valves, aortic aneurysm/dissection, heart failure, pericardial effusion, masses within the heart, myocardial abnormalities (e.g. aneurysms, hypertrophy), IHD, congenital heart disease.
- *M-mode* Plotted on a scrolling screen. Stationary structures appear as straight lines across the screen; moving structures appear as undulating lines. Usually displayed with an ECG trace to enable identification of phases of the cardiac cycle. Used to investigate movement of individual structural elements, e.g. valves, chamber walls.
- *Doppler* Enables flow across valves and ASD/VSDs to be quantified.

**Cardiac catheterization** Refer via 2° care. Involves passing a catheter, usually via the femoral or brachial artery, to the heart. Used to;
- Measure pressures within the heart and great vessels. Assess oxygen saturation via blood samples.
- Perform coronary angiography—contrast is injected into the coronary arteries to assess their anatomy and/or patency.
- Perform intravascular ultrasound.
- Perform other procedures, e.g. angioplasty, valvuloplasty, cardiac biopsy.

**Complications** Arrhythmia (0.56%), MI (0.07%), stroke (0.07%), death (0.14%), haemorrhage at the site of insertion (0.56%), thromboembolism, trauma to heart and vessels, infection.

**Radionucleotide imaging** Refer via 2° care. Involves IV administration of a γ-emitting radionucleotide and gamma camera monitoring.
- *Radionucleotide angiography* Uses $^{99m}$Tc-labelled RBCs to calculate left ventricular ejection fraction and assess ventricular action.
- *Myocardial perfusion scintigraphy* Uses thallium-201 injected IV during exercise testing to demonstrate areas of poorly perfused myocardium.

**Cardiac MRI/magnetic resonance angiography** Used increasingly in 2° care to provide detailed structural information about the heart and rapid angiographic images.

### Patient information
**British Heart Foundation** ☎ 0845 708 070 🖳 www.bhf.org.uk

# Brief guide to common ECG changes

❶ For detailed analysis of ECGs refer to a specialist text, e.g. Hampton JR (2003)*The ECG Made Easy* Churchill Livingstone (ISBN 0443072523).

❶ Always compare with previous ECGs if available.

**Table 10.5** Common ECG abnormalities and their causes

| ECG abnormality | | Possible causes |
|---|---|---|
| Tachycardia | Rate >100bpm | Physiological, AF, atrial flutter, SVT, VT. |
| Bradycardia | Rate <60bpm | Physiological, drugs (e.g. β-blockers, digoxin), heart block (see ▢ p.280), sick sinus syndrome. |
| Irregular | Assess whether any pattern or not | AF (no pattern), sick sinus syndrome (no pattern), ventricular ectopics (normally no pattern), heart block (pattern). |
| P–R interval | Short P–R interval | Nodal rhythm, Wolff–Parkinson–White (WPW) syndrome (▢ p.277) |
| | Prolonged >0.2s | Heart block (▢ p.280), sick sinus syndrome, drugs (e.g. β-blockers, digoxin) |
| Left bundle branch block (LBBB)* | QRS >0.12s. wide; last peak is below the isoelectric line in V1 | IHD, ↑BP, cardiomyopathy, aortic valve disease, SVT. Artificial pacemakers may produce a similar QRS complex |
| Right bundle branch block (RBBB) | QRS >0.12s wide. Last peak is above the isoelectric line in V1 | May be normal; congenital heart disease (e.g. ASD), valvular heart disease, IHD, pulmonary hypertension, during SVT. |
| Incomplete bundle branch block | QRS <0.12s with abnormal-shaped QRS complex | As for RBBB or LBBB |
| Q–T interval abnormalities | Prolonged Q–T interval | ↓$K^+$, drugs (e.g. TCAs, phenothiazines, amiodarone), SAH, or CVA, hypothermia |
| | Shortened Q–T interval | ↑$Ca^{2+}$, digoxin |
| Abnormal P-waves | ↑P-wave amplitude (>2.5mm) | Right atrial overload—tricuspid stenosis, pulmonary hypertension, pulmonary stenosis |
| | Biphasic P-wave in V1 ± broad (>0.12s) often notched P wave in ≥ 1 limb lead | Left atrial abnormality—mitral stenosis, aortic stenosis, conduction abnormalities |

*No comment can be made about ST segment or T wave if LBBB.

**Table 10.5** *(Continued)* Common ECG abnormalities and their causes

| ECG abnormality | | Possible causes |
|---|---|---|
| Right ventricular hypertrophy (RVH) | Strain pattern—ST depression and T-wave inversion in leads V1–3. Dominant R in V1 with narrow QRS | Pulmonary stenosis, mitral stenosis, pulmonary hypertension, ASD (±RBBB). Similar changes seen with inferior MI (T-wave upright), WPW syndrome |
| Left ventricular hypertrophy (LVH) | Strain pattern—ST↓ and T-wave ↓ in leads V4–6. Large voltages of QRS complex—sum of S in V1 and R in V5 or V6 alone >35mm | ↑BP, aortic stenosis, coarctation of the aorta, HOCM |
| Right axis deviation | 📖 p.242 | RVH/strain (e.g. following PE), cor pulmonale, pulmonary stenosis. Alone with normal QRS = left posterior hemiblock |
| Left axis deviation | 📖 p.242 | LVH/strain (e.g. ↑BP, aortic stenosis, HOCM), VSD, ASD. If occurs alone with normal QRS = left anterior hemiblock |
| Poor R-wave progression | Small or absent R waves in the R Ð mid-precordial leads | L or R ventricular enlargement, LBBB, left pneumothorax, dextrocardia, COPD |
| | Reversed R wave progression— ↓ in R-wave amplitude from V1 → mid/Lateral precordial leads | Right ventricular enlargement |
| Abnormal Q-waves | >25% of succeeding R-wave and/or >0.04s wide. | Normal, left pneumothorax, dextrocardia, MI, myocarditis, hyperkalaemia, cardiomyopathy, amyloid, sarcoid, scleroderma, LVH, RVH, LRBB, WPW syndrome |
| ST elevation | ST segment raised >1mm above baseline | MI, Prinzmetal angina, pericarditis, ventricular aneurysm |
| ST depression | ST segment lowered >0.5mm below baseline | Angina, ventricular strain, drugs (digoxin, verapamil), hyperkalaemia, myocarditis, cardiomyopathy, fibrosis, Lyme disease |
| T-wave inversion | Abnormal if inverted in leads I, II, or V4–6 | MI (inverts <24h after MI), angina, ventricular strain (see above), PE (III), digoxin (V5–6) |
| U-waves | ↑ amplitude >1mm | Drugs (e.g., quinidine, procainamide, disopyramide), ischaemia or ↓K⁺ |
| Inversion in precordial leads | | Subtle sign of ischaemia |

# Prevention of coronary heart disease

Coronary heart disease (CHD) is the most common cause of death in the UK (1:6 deaths). Mortality is falling but morbidity is rising.

**Primary prevention** Aims to stop heart disease developing.

*Population strategy* Influences factors that ↑ CHD risk in an entire population, e.g. anti-smoking campaigns. GPs can do this by displaying health education posters/Literature (e.g. in waiting room, practice leaflet).

*High-risk strategy* Most cardiovascular diseases occur in individuals at medium risk as that is the largest group. However, individuals at high risk have the most to gain from risk reduction. This strategy aims to identify individuals with 10y CVD risk ≥20% and ↓ their risk through lifestyle modification ± medication.

*Selection of patients for intervention* is based on overall risk.
• All patients aged >75y or with a familial monogenic dyslipidaemia are at high risk.
• Most patients with DM are at high risk (📖 p.362).
• For patients aged 40–74y, use a systematic strategy using information already recorded on practice computers to identify those with risk factors for CVD, and invite them for formal risk assessment (recording smoking status, alcohol consumption, BMI, BP, and lipid profile).

*Estimation of risk* NICE recommends using the Framingham risk score to estimate CVD risk for individuals who are <75y and do not have a past medical history of CVD or DM (📖 p.248 or 🖥 http://cvrisk.mvm.ed.ac.uk/calculator/framingham.htm). Alternatives include QRISK2 (🖥 www.qrisk.org) or ASSIGN (🖥 www.assign-score.com).

❶ If the risk score is near the threshold for intervention, consider other factors that may predispose to CVD and are not included in the score.
• Low socio-economic group.
• BMI—risk ↑ if BMI>40.
• Is the person already taking antihypertensive/Lipid modification therapy?
• Has the person recently stopped smoking?
• Is the person taking anti-psychotic medication?
• Are other conditions present that ↑ risk (e.g. CKD, RA, SLE, HIV)?

**Secondary prevention** Aims to stop progression of symptomatic CHD. 46% people who die from MI are already known to have CHD. There is strong evidence that targeting patients with CHD for risk-factor modification is effective in ↓ risk of recurrent CHD.[S]

**The GP's role** GPs have a role in:
• Identification of patients who would benefit from 1° prevention.
• Ensuring patients who are at high risk of atherosclerotic disease (established CVD, DM, CVD risk ≥ 20% over 10y, elevated BP with systolic ≥160 and or diastolic ≥100 and target organ damage, ↑ total cholesterol:HDL ratio ≥6, familial dyslipidaemia) have ongoing follow-up through disease registers, routine recall and follow-up by the practice, PCO, and/or 2° care services, and monitoring of drug prescriptions.[G]

- Promoting lifestyle modification in at-risk patients.
- Ensuring current best care guidelines are followed and treatment regimes are updated as policies change. This is a major challenge for primary care as guidelines change frequently and often conflict.
- Checking the process through audit.

**Risk factors for heart disease** See Table 10.6. ❶ Patients aged 40–74y in the UK are entitled to free cardiovascular risk assessments every 5y.

**Table 10.6** Risk factors for heart disease

| Non-modifiable | Modifiable (proven benefit) | Modifiable (unproven benefit) |
|---|---|---|
| Age—↑ with age | Smoking* 📖 p.184 | Haemostatic factors—↑ plasma fibrinogen, and factors VII and VIIIc |
| Sex—♂ > ♀ in those <65y | Hyperlipidaemia 📖 p.258 | |
| Ethnic origin—in the UK people who originate from the Indian subcontinent have ↑ risk, Afro-Caribbeans have ↓ risk | Hypertension* 📖 p.252 | Apolipoproteins—↑ lipoprotein(a)* |
| | DM* 📖 p.362 | |
| | Diet* 📖 p.176 | Homocysteine -↑ blood homocysteine |
| Socio-economic position* | Obesity (particularly waist-hip ratio)* 📖 p.180 | |
| Personal history of CVD | Physical inactivity* 📖 p.182 | Vitamin levels—↓ blood folate, vitamins $B_{12}$ and $B_6$ |
| Family history of CVD—<55y ♂; <65y ♀ | Alcohol consumption* 📖 p.186 | Depression |
| Low birth weight (IUGR) | Left ventricular dysfunction/ heart failure (2° prevention) 📖 p.268 | |
| | Coronary-prone behaviour—competitiveness, aggression and feeling under time pressure (2° prevention)–behaviour modification is associated with ↓ risk | |

* These 9 factors account for 90% of risk for acute MI.

## Further information

**NICE** 🖥 www.nice.org.uk
- Cardiovascular risk assessment and the modification of blood lipids for the primary and secondary prevention of cardiovascular disease (2008)
- The management of type 2 diabetes (2008)
- Identifying and supporting people most at risk of dying prematurely (2008)

**SIGN** Guideline 97: Risk estimation and the prevention of cardiovascular disease (2007) 🖥 www.sign.ac.uk

**DH** National Service Framework: Coronary Heart Disease (2000, update 2005) 🖥 www.dh.gov.uk

**Joint British Societies** JBS2 Joint British Societies' guidelines on prevention of cardiovascular disease in clinical practice (2005). *Heart* **91** (Suppl. 5), v1–52

## Patient information

**British Heart Foundation** ☎ 0845 708 070 🖥 www.bhf.org.uk

# Estimating cardiovascular risk

⚠ The Framingham Score overestimates risk in UK populations.

**Total CVD risk** = 10y stroke risk +10y CHD risk.

**Stroke risk** Add the points for each row together.

## Men

| Points | 0 | 1 | 2 | 3 | 4 | 5 | 6 | 7 | 8 | 9 | 10 |
|---|---|---|---|---|---|---|---|---|---|---|---|
| Age | ≤56 | 57–59 | 60–2 | 63–5 | 66–8 | 69–72 | 73–5 | 76–8 | 79–81 | 82–4 | 85 |
| Untreated SBP | ≤105 | 106–115 | 116–125 | 126–135 | 136–145 | 146–155 | 156–165 | 166–175 | 176–185 | 186–195 | ≥196 |
| Treated SBP | ≤105 | 106–112 | 113–117 | 118–123 | 124–129 | 130–135 | 136–142 | 143–150 | 151–161 | 162–176 | 177–205 |
| DM | No | | Yes | | | | | | | | |
| Smoking | No | | | Yes | | | | | | | |
| CVD | No | | | | Yes | | | | | | |
| AF | No | | | | Yes | | | | | | |
| LVH | No | | | | | Yes | | | | | |

## Women

| Points | 0 | 1 | 2 | 3 | 4 | 5 | 6 | 7 | 8 | 9 | 10 |
|---|---|---|---|---|---|---|---|---|---|---|---|
| Age | ≤56 | 57–9 | 60–2 | 63–5 | 65–7 | 68–70 | 71–3 | 74–6 | 77–8 | 79–81 | 82–4 |
| Untreated SBP | <95 | 95–106 | 107–118 | 119–130 | 131–143 | 144–155 | 156–167 | 168–180 | 181–192 | 193–204 | ≥205 |
| Treated SBP | <95 | 95–106 | 107–113 | 114–119 | 120–125 | 126–131 | 132–139 | 140–148 | 149–160 | 161–204 | ≥205 |
| DM | No | | | Yes | | | | | | | |
| Smoking | No | | | Yes | | | | | | | |
| CVD | No | | Yes | | | | | | | | |
| AF | No | | | | | | Yes | | | | |
| LVH | No | | | | Yes | | | | | | |

### Converting points to 10y % stroke risk

| Points | 1 | 2 | 3 | 4 | 5 | 6 | 7 | 8 | 9 | 10 | 11 | 12 | 13 | 14 | 15 | 16 | ≥17 |
|---|---|---|---|---|---|---|---|---|---|---|---|---|---|---|---|---|---|
| %risk ♂ | 3 | 3 | 4 | 4 | 5 | 5 | 6 | 7 | 8 | 10 | 11 | 13 | 15 | 17 | 20 | ≥22 | |
| %risk ♀ | 1 | 1 | 2 | 2 | 2 | 3 | 4 | 4 | 5 | 6 | 8 | 9 | 11 | 13 | 16 | 19 | ≥23 |

⚠ If ♂ of South Asian background, ↑ Framingham CVD risk ×1.4; if FH of premature heart disease (<55y for ♂; <65y for ♀)—↑ risk ×1.5 if 1 relative affected; ×2 if >1 relative affected.

## CHD risk

### Step 1 Age

| Age | 30–4 | 35–9 | 40–4 | 45–9 | 50–4 | 55–9 | 60–4 | 65–9 | 70–4 |
|---|---|---|---|---|---|---|---|---|---|
| Score ♂ | –1 | 0 | 1 | 2 | 3 | 4 | 5 | 6 | 7 |
| Score ♀ | –9 | –4 | 0 | 3 | 6 | 7 | 8 | 8 | 8 |

### Step 2 LDL cholesterol—add correction factor to age score

| Total cholesterol (mmol/L) | <4.14 | 4.15–5.17 | 5.18–6.21 | 6.22–7.24 | ≥7.25 |
|---|---|---|---|---|---|
| ♂ | | –3 | 0 | +1 | +2 | +3 |
| ♀ | | –2 | 0 | +1 | +1 | +3 |

### Step 3 Adjust score for HDL cholesterol

| HDL cholesterol (mmol/L) | <0.9 | 0.91–1.16 | 1.17–1.29 | 1.3–1.55 | ≥1.56 |
|---|---|---|---|---|---|
| ♂ | +2 | +1 | 0 | 0 | –2 |
| ♀ | +5 | +2 | +1 | 0 | –3 |

### Step 4 Adjust score for BP

| BP (mmHg) | | <120 | 120–129 | 130–139 | 140–159 | ≥160 |
|---|---|---|---|---|---|---|
| | Systolic | <120 | 120–129 | 130–139 | 140–159 | ≥160 |
| | Diastolic | <80 | 80–84 | 85–89 | 90–99 | ≥100 |
| ♂ | | 0 | 0 | +1 | +2 | +3 |
| ♀ | | –3 | 0 | 0 | +2 | +3 |

❶ When systolic and diastolic pressures provide different estimates for point scores, use the higher number

### Step 5 Adjust score for diabetes and smoking

| | | Diabetes | | Smoking | |
|---|---|---|---|---|---|
| | | Yes | No | Yes | No |
| ♂ | | +2 | 0 | +2 | 0 |
| ♀ | | +4 | 0 | +2 | 0 |

### Step 6 Calculate 10y CHD risk from total score

| Score | ≤–2 | –1 | 0 | 1 | 2 | 3 | 4 | 5 | 6 | 7 | 8 | 9 | 10 | 11 | 12 | 13 | 14 | 15 | 16 | ≥17 |
|---|---|---|---|---|---|---|---|---|---|---|---|---|---|---|---|---|---|---|---|---|
| %risk –♂ | 2 | 2 | 3 | 3 | 4 | 5 | 7 | 8 | 10 | 13 | 16 | 20 | 25 | 31 | 37 | 45 | | | | ≥53 |
| %risk –♀ | 1 | 2 | 2 | 2 | 3 | 3 | 4 | 4 | 5 | 6 | 7 | 8 | 10 | 11 | 13 | 15 | 18 | 20 | 24 | ≥27 |

## Computerized risk assessment tools

- Framingham score 🖳 http://cvrisk.mvm.ed.ac.uk/calculator/framingham.htm
- QRISK2 🖳 www.qrisk.org
- ASSIGN (Scotland) 🖳 www.assign-score.com

# Aspirin for cardiovascular prevention

Antiplatelet therapy is effective in ↓ cardiovascular morbidity and mortality. Aspirin 75mg od for maintenance treatment, and 300mg for acute stroke/MI, is the agent most widely used.

⚠ Patients treated with aspirin are 2.5× more likely to have a GI bleed (NNH to cause 1 GI bleed = 100). There is no evidence that using enteric-coated aspirin ↓ risk of GI bleeding. Consider prescribing stomach protection with a PPI or H₂ receptor antagonist in high-risk individuals. Avoid concomitant use of warfarin except on specialist advice as it significantly ↑ risk of bleeding.

## Indications for aspirin

**Acute cardiovascular disease** Patients with suspected acute MI or unstable angina should receive a stat dose of 300mg aspirin.

**Established cardiovascular disease** Aspirin 75mg od ↓
- All-cause mortality by 18% (NNT to prevent 1 death = 67)
- Number of strokes by 20%
- MI by 30%
- Other vascular events by 30%.

❶ For patients in AF, warfarin may be used in preference to aspirin to prevent stroke (📖 p.572) if previous ischaemic stroke/TIA, >65y, ↑ BP, DM, cardiac failure, Echo showing LV dysfunction or mitral valve calcification.

**Primary prevention** Aspirin ↓ risk of MI by 40% but ↑ risk of haemorrhagic stroke by 40% and ↑ risk of major GI bleeding by 70%. Risk outweighs benefit when 10y CVD risk is ~15%. Current recommendations are that people with 10y CVD risk ≥20% should be considered for aspirin therapy.

**DM** Control systolic BP to <145/90mmHg before starting treatment. Give 75mg od to:
- All type 1 diabetics with ↑ risk of arterial disease (age >35y, from the Indian subcontinent; family history of premature CVD or personal history of CVD; ≥ 2 features of metabolic syndrome; abnormal lipids; ↑BP; micoalbuminuria/proteinuria).
- All type 2 diabetics aged >50y.
- Type 2 diabetics <50y with other CVD risk factors (overweight, ↑BP, micoalbuminuria, smoker, high-risk lipid profile, personal or family history of cardiovascular disease).

**Hypertension** Treat with aspirin 75mg od if 10y CVD risk ≥ 20%, target organ damage or DM *and* blood pressure is treated to <150/90mmHg.

**Use of clopidogrel** Clopidogrel 75mg od is indicated as:
- An alternative to aspirin for patients unable to tolerate aspirin
- In combination with aspirin for patients with proven troponin-positive acute coronary syndromes for 12mo following the acute event (📖 p.266) or for patients who receive drug-eluting stents (first 12mo only).

## Further information

**NICE** 🖥 www.nice.org.uk
- Cardiovascular risk assessment and the modification of blood lipids for the primary and secondary prevention of cardiovascular disease (2008)
- The management of type 2 diabetes (2008)
- MI: secondary prevention (2007)

**SIGN** Guideline 97: risk estimation and the prevention of cardiovascular disease (2007) 🖥 www.sign.ac.uk

**DH** National Service Framework: Coronary Heart Disease. (2000, update 2005) 🖥 www.dh.gov.uk

**Joint British Societies** JBS2 Joint British Societies' guidelines on prevention of cardiovascular disease in clinical practice (2005) *Heart* **91** (Suppl. 5), v1–52

## Patient information

**British Heart Foundation** ☎ 0845 708 070 🖥 www.bhf.org.uk

# Hypertension[N]

Hypertension is a major risk factor for CHD and CVA. ↑BP is normally symptomless until it causes organ damage. ~50% aged 65–74y have ↑BP. Management aims to detect and treat ↑BP before damage occurs. Hypertension is under-diagnosed and under-treated in the UK.

**Measurement of blood pressure** 📖 p.234.

**Diagnosis of hypertension** BP is a continuous variable—the higher the BP the greater the risk of CVD. There is no figure above which hypertension can be diagnosed definitively, although currently treatment is considered at BP >140/90 (see management guidelines).

**Isolated systolic hypertension**[G] Offer patients with isolated systolic hypertension (systolic BP >160mmHg) the same treatment as patients with both raised systolic and diastolic blood pressure.

## Causes
- Unknown—95% (essential hypertension). Alcohol (10%) or obesity may be contributory factors.
- Renal disease—📖 p.448
- Endocrine disease —Cushing's (both syndrome and 2° to steroids), Conn's syndrome, phaeochromocytoma, acromegaly, hyperparathyroidism, DM (📖 pp.349–379).
- Pregnancy—📖 p.824
- Coarctation of the aorta—📖 p.290

## Presentation
- Usually asymptomatic and found during routine BP screening or incidentally. Occasionally headache or visual disturbance.
- May be symptoms of end-organ damage—LVH, TIAs, previous CVA/MI, angina, renal impairment, PVD.

**Examination** Check BP, heart size, heart sounds, heart failure, examine the fundi.

## Investigation
- *Blood* FBC, U&E, creatinine, eGFR, glucose, lipid profile; consider GGT if excess alcohol is a possibility
- *Urine* RBCs, glucose, protein
- *ECG*
- *Echo* Consider referral if left ventricular hypertrophy is suspected

⚠ **Malignant hypertension** *Presents with* headache, very elevated BP (diastolic >140mmHg), renal failure, fits, coma (encephalopathy), severe retinopathy. Life-threatening condition. If malignant hypertension is suspected, admit as an acute medical emergency.

## Summary of hypertension management
(Based on updated NICE guidance 2006 and JBS 2 guidance 2005)
- *Provide lifestyle modifications* for all those with high, borderline, or high normal BP.
- *Discuss the need to formally assess cardiovascular risk with patients.*
- *Consider specialist referral* for patients with signs or symptoms of 2° hypertension.
- *Initiate antihypertensive drug therapy* in those with sustained systolic BP ≥160 and/or diastolic ≥100mmHg.
- *Systolic BP141–159mmHg and/or diastolic BP 91–99mmHg* Treat those with DM, a history of cardiovascular disease (CVD), target organ damage, or estimated risk of CVD of ≥20% over 10y.
- *Optimal BP treatment goals*
  - In non-diabetics: systolic BP <140mmHg, diastolic <85mmHg (JBS2) or <140/<90mmHg (NICE).
  - In diabetics, chronic renal disease, or established CVD: systolic <130mmHg, diastolic <80mmHg.
- *Most patients with ↑BP require ≥2 BP lowering drugs* to achieve BP targets.
- *Use low-dose aspirin 75mg/d* (unless contraindicated) for 2° prevention of ischaemic CVD and for 1° prevention in patients with 10y CVD risk ≥20% when BP is controlled at <150/<90mmHg.
- *Statin therapy* is recommended for all those with ↑BP complicated by CVD irrespective of baseline cholesterol or LDL levels, and for 1° prevention in patients with ↑BP and 10y CVD risk ≥20%.

## Further information
**NICE/BHS** Hypertension—management of hypertension in adults in primary care (2004, update 2006) 🖳 www.nice.org.uk
**NICE** Cardiovascular risk assessment and the modification of blood lipids for the primary and secondary prevention of cardiovascular disease (2008) 🖳 www.nice.org.uk
**SIGN** Guideline 97: Risk estimation and the prevention of cardiovascular disease (2007) 🖳 www.sign.ac.uk
**Joint British Societies Guidelines 2 (JBS2)** (2005) Available from 🖳 www.bhsoc.org

# Management of hypertension[N]

**Malignant hypertension** 📖 p.252

**Education** Patients will not take tablets regularly, be motivated to change lifestyle, or turn up for regular checks if they don't understand why treating their ↑ BP is important or the side effects of treatment they are likely to experience. On the other hand, some patients who were fit and well prior to their diagnosis, will assume a sick role unless it is explained that they are well and treatment is designed to stop illness developing. Reinforce management at follow up and give opportunities for discussion.

## Initial treatment

- Treat other modifiable risk factors for CHD (📖 p.247), and CVA (📖 p.572).
- Aim to ↓BP to <140/85mmHg (diabetics <130/80mmHg).
- Benefits of treatment remain in patients up to 85y of age—and probably beyond. Offer patients >80y the same treatment as young patients taking into account any comorbidity and existing drug use.

**Non-drug treatment** Offer to all hypertensives and those with family history of ↑BP. Reinforce advice with written information.

- Offer smoking cessation advice and help (📖 p.184).
- ↓ weight to optimum for height (📖 p.180).
- Encourage regular exercise—dynamic is best, e.g. walking, swimming, cycling (📖 p.182).
- ↓ alcohol to <21u/wk for ♂ and <14u/wk for ♀ (📖 p.186).
- ↓ dietary salt intake.
- ↑ dietary fruit and vegetable intake—aim for ≥5 portions/d.
- ↓ excess coffee consumption and other caffeine-rich products.
- Encourage relaxation and stress management.
- *Don't* offer $Ca^{2+}$, $Mg^{2+}$, or $K^+$ supplements as a method to ↓ BP.

**Drug treatment**

- *BP-lowering drugs* 📖 p.256
- *Aspirin* (📖 p.250) Recommend 75mg od for hypertensive patients if:
  - Aged ≥50y
  - Satisfactory control of BP (<150/90mmHg) *and*
  - Target organ damage, DM, or 10y CVD risk ≥ 20%.
- *Statin therapy* (📖 p.260) Prescribe:
  - If ↑BP complicated by CVD irrespective of baseline cholesterol or LDL levels *or*
  - For 1° prevention in patients >40y with ↑BP and 10y CVD risk ≥20%.

❶ Side effects of drug treatment for hypertension are common. 40–50% started on an antihypertensive drug discontinue regardless of which class of drug is used. 80% of side effects are seen in the 1st year of treatment.

**Follow up** Regular review of patients with ↑ BP is essential. Once ↑ BP is controlled, routine review of BP can be undertaken by properly trained practice nurses but annual review of medication should be undertaken by a GP and the GP must review if BP is not controlled.

**Review interval** Depends on stability of BP:
- *After starting treatment* Review after 1mo.
- *If BP is controlled* Review after a further 3mo and then every 3–6 mo.
- *If BP is not controlled*
  - Bring the patient back to repeat the BP reading. *Don't* alter medication on the strength of a single BP reading.
  - If ↑BP is sustained, alter medication (📖 p.256). Most patients need >1 drug.
  - If ↑ dose causes ↑ side effects without improvement in response, alter medication.
  - Review in the same way monthly until BP is controlled.

*Format of the annual review*
- Check BP.
- Look for signs of end-organ failure, including annual urine test for proteinuria.
- Discuss symptoms and medication.
- Assess and treat other modifiable risk factors for CHD/CVA.
- Reinforce non-drug treatment.

**Referral to cardiology/general medicine**
(*E*=Emergency admission; *U*=Urgent; *S*=Soon; *R*=routine)
- Malignant hypertension—*E*
- Renal impairment—*U/S/R*
- Suspected 2° hypertension—*S/R*
- Patients <35y  *R*
- Multiple risk factors—*R*
- BP difficult to treat—*R*
- Pregnancy—to obstetrician. Urgency depends on stage of pregnancy and clinical features (📖 p.824).

**Reducing or stopping treatment** ↓ BP too far (<120/80mmHg) may ↑ mortality, especially in the elderly.
- *Don't* stop medication if high CVD risk or end-organ damage.
- If diastolic BP <80mmHg and systolic BP <140mmHg consistently, consider decreasing or stopping medication. 1–2 y after withdrawal of medication 50% are normotensive and 40% stay off drug therapy permanently.
- Elderly people are prone to postural hypotension. Check for postural drop (sitting and standing BP). If present, ↓ dose of antihypertensive.
- Continue BP follow-up life-long even if off medication.

**Further information**
**NICE/BHS** Hypertension—management of hypertension in adults in primary care (2004, update 2006) ⌨ www.nice.org.uk
**Joint British Societies Guidelines 2 (JBS2)** (2005) Available from ⌨ www.bhsoc.org
**SIGN** Guideline 97: Risk estimation and the prevention of cardiovascular disease (2007) ⌨ www.sign.ac.uk

**Patient information**
**British Heart Foundation** ☎ 0845 708 070 ⌨ www.bhf.org.uk

# Drug treatment of hypertension

## Recommendations for drug treatment

### General rules
- *If a drug is not tolerated* stop and move on to next line of therapy.
- *If a drug is tolerated but the BP target isn't met* add in the next line of therapy.
- *Where possible* recommend treatment with drugs taken only once a day and prescribe non-proprietary drugs which minimize cost.

**≥55y or black-skinned (any age)** First choice initial therapy is a dihydropyridine calcium-channel blocker or thiazide-type diuretic.

*Second line* If initial treatment was with a dihydropyridine calcium-channel blocker or thiazide-type diuretic and a second drug is required, add an ACE inhibitor (or angiotensin-receptor blocker (ARB) if an ACE inhibitor is not tolerated)

**<55y** First-choice initial therapy is an ACE inhibitor (or ARB if the ACE inhibitor is not tolerated).

*Second line* If initial therapy was with an ACE inhibitor and a second drug is required, add a dihydropyridine calcium-channel blocker or a thiazide-type diuretic

**If treatment with three drugs is needed** Combine an ACE inhibitor, dihydropyridine calcium-channel blocker, and thiazide-type diuretic.

**If treatment with four drugs is needed** Consider adding an α-blocker or further diuretic therapy *or* a β-blocker

❶ If blood pressure remains uncontrolled with the addition of a fourth drug, refer for specialist advice.

**Beta-blockers** are no longer recommended as a routine initial therapy for hypertension.

*Exceptions* β-blockers may be considered as first line treatment for:
- Younger women of child-bearing potential *or*
- Patients with hypertension and evidence of ↑ sympathetic drive *or*
- Patients intolerant of/with contraindications to ACE inhibitors/ARBs.

In these circumstances, if initial therapy is with a β-blocker and a second drug is required, add a dihydropyridine calcium-channel blocker.

**Patients already on ß-blockers** If a patient's blood pressure is well controlled on a β-blocker, there is no need to change it. If not controlled, change treatment according to the recommendations above. Gradually step down dose of β-blockers when withdrawing them.

⚠ Do NOT withdraw β-blockers in patients with other good reasons to take them, e.g. angina or post-MI

## Further information
**NICE/BHS** Hypertension—management of hypertension in adults in primary care (2004, update 2006) ▣ www.nice.org.uk

**Table 10.7** Antihypertensive drugs

| Class of 1st-line drug | Reasons to choose drug | Reasons to avoid drug |
|---|---|---|
| *ACE inhibitors* (BNF 2.5.5.1) ❶ Check U&E, Cr and eGFR before starting and at first follow-up | Heart failure or left ventricular dysfunction Post MI or established CVD Diabetic nephropathy 2° stroke prevention | *Do not use* if known renovascular disease (can precipitate renal failure) or in pregnancy *Use with caution* if aortic or mitral valve stenosis and in obstructive hypertrophic cardiomyopathy |
| *Angiotensin receptor blockers (ARBs)* (BNF 2.5.5.2) ❶ Check U&E, Cr and eGFR before starting and monitor $K^+$ at follow-up | ACE inhibitor intolerance Diabetic nephropathy ↑BP + LVH Heart failure if ACE intolerant Post MI | |
| *Thiazide diuretics* (BNF 2.2.1) ❶ Use the lowest dose. Higher doses don't have additional effect on BP | More effective than β-blockers in the elderly | Avoid in patients with gout. May adversely affect lipid profile |
| *Calcium-channel blockers* (BNF 2.6.2) ❶ Different agents have different therapeutic effects | *Dihydropyridine agents* of proven efficacy in the elderly and those with isolated systolic hypertension *Rate-limiting agents:* useful in those with angina or post-MI | *Rate-limiting agents:* avoid in patients with heart block or heart failure. Do not combine with β-blockers |
| *α-blockers* (BNF 2.5.4) | Prostatism Dyslipidaemia | Urinary incontinence worsens Postural hypotension is common |
| *β-blockers* (BNF 2.4) ❶ May accumulate in patients with renal failure—↓ dose | No longer recommended as a first-line drug | *Avoid in patients with* asthma, COPD, heart block, heart failure, peripheral vascular disease, hyperlipidaemia *In patients with DM may* → small deterioration in glucose tolerance and ↓ awareness of hypoglycaemia |

❶ Most patients require >1 drug to control their BP

⚠ Avoid combination of β-blockers and rate-limiting calcium antagonists (verapamil, diltiazem) because of risk of bradycardia/asystole.

# Hyperlipidaemia

Average cholesterol level in a population is a predictor of CVD risk and dependent on diet but, on an individual level, it is a much poorer predictor—only 42% who develop CVD have ↑ cholesterol. However, lowering cholesterol is of proven benefit in 1° and 2° prevention of CVD. Concern that low cholesterol is associated with ↑ risk of death from other causes (e.g. suicide, cancer) is unfounded.

**Cholesterol** Fatty substance manufactured by the body (mainly liver) which plays a vital role in functioning of cell membranes. Total plasma cholesterol consists of:

- *LDL (low-density lipoprotein) cholesterol*—high levels associated with ↑ risk CVD.
- *HDL (high-density lipoprotein) cholesterol*—low levels associated with ↑ risk CVD.
- *Triglycerides (TGs)*—independent risk factor for CVD. If >10 mmol/L refer for specialist opinion.
- *Ratio of total cholesterol: HDL*—used to predict risk. No threshold—the higher the ratio the greater the risk. High risk if ≥6.

**Testing for hyperlipidaemia** Blood cholesterol concentration is not steady over time. 1:4 ↑ cholesterols are normal on repeat testing. Check ≥2 samples at different times:

- *Before initiating treatment or if screening for familial dyslipidaemia* take fasting samples checking total cholesterol, LDL-cholesterol, HDL-cholesterol, and triglycerides.
- *Screening and routine follow-up*—take non-fasting samples testing total blood cholesterol and total cholesterol:HDL ratio.

## Screening

- *1° prevention* Whole-population screening + dietary advice has little effect on cholesterol levels. It may ↓ impact of population strategies (less inclination to alter diet if cholesterol levels are known to be normal) and allow sufferers to assume a sick role. The alternative is systematic targeting of those age 40–75y with other risk factors, or signs of ↑ cholesterol (corneal arcus <50y, xanthelasma, xanthomata).
- *2° prevention* All those who have proven CVD—check cholesterol levels annually.
- *Familial hyperlipidaemia* Screen first-degree blood relatives (even children) with fasting lipids if:
  - FH of familial hyperlipidaemia
  - FH of premature CVD (men <55y, women <65y) or other atherosclerotic disease.
  Screening interval has not been determined—5y seems reasonable.

**Familial hyperlipidaemia** There are many types of familial dyslipidaemia. If suspected, refer. Common forms include:

* *Polygenic hypercholesterolaemia*—most common form of familial dyslipidaemia. Presents with FH of premature CHD + ↑ total cholesterol >6.5 mmol/L.
* *Familial combined hyperlipidaemia*—Polygenic hyperlipidaemia affecting 0.5–1% of the population and ~15% of those suffering MI <60y. Associated with obesity, insulin resistance/DM, ↑BP, xanthelasma, corneal arcus, and premature IHD. ↑ total cholesterol (6.5–10 mmol/L); ↑ TGs (2.3–12 mmol/L).
* *Familial hypercholesterolaemia* (type IIa)—autosomal dominant. Heterozygous form present in 1:500. Associated with tendon xanthomata and FH of premature IHD. ↑ LDL (>4.9 mmol/L); ↑ total cholesterol (>7.5 mmol/L); normal TGs.
* *Familial hypertriglyceridaemia* (type IV/V)—autosomal dominant. Affects ~1% of the general population and ~5% having MI<60y. Associated with DM, obesity, gout, eruptive xanthomas and pancreatitis. Normal (or slightly ↑) total cholesterol; ↑ TGs (2.3->10 mmol/L).

**Secondary hyperlipidaemia** Conditions associated with 2° hyperlipidaemia include:

* Drugs:
  * Steroids
  * β-blockers
  * Thiazides
  * COC pill
  * Isotretinoin
  * Antipsychotics
  * Tamoxifen
  * Antiretrovirals
* Obesity
* DM (📖 pp.354–371)*
* Excess alcohol
* Smoking (lowers HDL)
* Pregnancy
* ↓T₄**
* Renal failure
* Nephrotic syndrome
* RA/SLE
* HIV
* Cholestasis
* Cushing's syndrome
* Porphyria
* Myeloma
* Lipodystrophies
* Glycogen storage disease.

*Treatment of hyperglycaemia in DM ↓ 2° hyperlipidaemia.

**Patients with hypothyroidism should receive adequate thyroid replacement before assessing need for lipid-lowering treatment. Correction of hypothyroidism may resolve the lipid abnormality and untreated hypothyroidism ↑ risk of myositis with statins.

**Management of hypercholesterolaemia** 📖 p.260.

### Further information

**NICE** 🖥 www.nice.org.uk
* Cardiovascular risk assessment and the modification of blood lipids for the primary and secondary prevention of cardiovascular disease (2008)
* Familial hypercholesterolaemia (2008).

**SIGN** Guideline 97: Risk estimation and the prevention of cardiovascular disease (2007) 🖥 www.sign.ac.uk

**Joint British Societies Guidelines 2 (JBS2)** (2005) Available from 🖥 www.bhsoc.org

### Patient information

**British Heart Foundation** ☎ 0845 708 070 🖥 www.bhf.org.uk

# Management of hypercholesterolaemia

Lowering LDL and raising HDL ↓ progression of coronary atherosclerosis—whatever the age of the patient.

**Calculating cardiovascular disease (CVD) risk** Always consider ↑ cholesterol in the context of other risk factors for CVD—🕮 p.247.

**Non-drug therapy** Offer to all patients with ↑ cholesterol, ↑ CVD risk, and those with DM or FH of CHD/CVD. Reinforce advice with written information.

• ↓ intake of fats to <30% of total energy intake (saturated fats <10%) and ↓ cholesterol intake to <300 mg/d. Replace saturated fats with mono-unsaturated/poly-unsaturated fats. If cholesterol level >5mmol/L, low cholesterol diets result in average ↓ in cholesterol of 8.5% at 3mo.
• Eat ≥5 portions of fruit or vegetables/d and ≥2 portions of fish/wk including 1 of oily fish (max. 2 portions of oily fish/wk if pregnant).
• ↓ alcohol intake to <3–4u/d (♂) or <2–3u/d (♀).
• Weight ↓—in patients with BMI ≥30kg/m², weight ↓ of 10kg → 7% ↓ in LDL and 13% ↑ in HDL.
• ↑ physical activity enhances cholesterol-lowering effects of diet and weight ↓ Advise 30min moderate exercise ≥ 5×/wk.
• Stop smoking (🕮 p.184).

❶ Foods enriched with plant sterol/stanol esters inhibit cholesterol absorption from the GI tract and can ↓ serum cholesterol in those on an average diet by 10%. Effect on individuals already on a low fat diet is less and effect on CVD risk is unknown.

**Drug therapy with statins** Consider statin therapy for:
• *Primary prevention* if ≥20% 10y CVD risk (including adjustments for high-risk ethnic groups and FH), aged >75y, or DM (unless at particularly low CVD risk—🕮 p.362)—start treatment after optimizing lifestyle intervention and treatment of other modifiable risk factors/secondary causes of dyslipidaemia.
• *Secondary prevention* if history of CVD—start treatment immediately irrespective of initial cholesterol levels.

***Before starting treatment*** assess:
• Fasting total cholesterol, LDL cholesterol, HDL cholesterol, and TGs (if fasting levels not already available)

• Fasting blood glucose
• Renal function

• Liver function (transaminases)
• TSH if dyslipidaemia is present.

***Factors to consider before starting a statin***
• Statins are contraindicated in pregnancy, breastfeeding, and for those with active liver disease. Transaminases that are ↑ but <3× upper limit of normal are not a contraindication.
• Important drug interactions—↑ effect warfarin; ↑ risk myositis when taken with other lipid-lowering drugs, macrolide antibiotics (e.g. erythromycin), or ciclosporin.
• Statins are most effective taken in the evening.

### Primary prevention (except DM)
- Start simvastatin 40mg od.
- There is no target level for total or LDL cholesterol for 1° prevention.
- Check liver function 3mo and 1y after initiating statin. Do not recheck again unless clinically indicated. Do not recheck lipid levels.
- Review drug therapy at least annually. If statin is not tolerated, consider fibrate, anion exchange resin, or ezitimibe

### Secondary prevention and DM
- Start simvastatin 40mg od. If acute coronary syndrome higher intensity statin therapy may be used.
- Aim to ↓ total cholesterol by 25% or to <4mmol/L—whichever is the lower value *and* to ↓ LDL cholesterol by 30% or to < 2.0 mmol/L—whichever is the lower value.
- Measure total cholesterol (non-fasting) 3mo after starting treatment or after any dose change. If stable measure 6–12 monthly.
- Consider ↑ simvastatin to 80mg od if target lipid levels are not met.
- Check liver function 3mo and 1y after initiating statin therapy. Do not recheck again unless clinically indicated.
- If statins are not tolerated, consider fibrate, anion exchange resin, nicotinic acid (not for DM) or ezetimibe.

❶ <50% will achieve total cholesterol <4 mmol/L or LDL cholesterol <2 mmol/L. Use an 'audit' standard of total cholesterol <5 mmol/L.

### Adverse effects of statins
- NNH for any adverse event with statin treatment is 197
- The most important adverse effect is myositis (11/100 000 person-year). Ask to report any unexplained muscle pain/weakness. If this occurs check CK—If >5× upper limit of normal withdraw therapy.
- Stop statins and seek specialist advice if unexplained peripheral neuropathy develops (12/100 000 person-year).
- Discontinue if serum transaminase ↑ (and stays at) >3× normal.

### Benefits of statins[M] NNT to prevent 1 adverse event is 34.5 for 1° prevention, 13.8 for 2° prevention. For each mmol/L ↓ in LDL:
- Major coronary events ↓ 23%
- First stroke ↓ 17%
- CHD death ↓19% (14/1000 fewer deaths if pre-existing CHD; 4/1000 if no history of CHD)
- Overall death rate ↓ 12%.

### Referral to cardiology/general medicine (R=routine)
- Familial hypercholesterolaemia (± referral to genetics)—R
- High triglycerides—R
- Hypercholesterolaemia resistant to treatment or difficult to treat—R

### Further information
**NICE** ⌨ www.nice.org.uk
- Statins for the prevention of cardiovascular disease (2006)
- Cardiovascular risk assessment and the modification of blood lipids for the primary and secondary prevention of cardiovascular disease (2008)

**Joint British Societies Guidelines 2 (JBS2)** (2005) Available from ⌨ www.bhsoc.org

# Angina

Affects ~2% population in UK. Incidence ↑ with age. ♂ > ♀. Coronary artery disease is the most common cause. Rarer causes include HOCM, valve disease, hypoperfusion during arrhythmia, arteritis, anaemia, or thyrotoxicosis. Mortality (usually sudden death or after MI or acute LVF) is ~0.5–4%/y—doubled if coexistent left ventricular dysfunction.

**Presentation of stable angina** Diagnosis is usually made on history:
- *Pain* Episodic central-crushing or band-like chest pain that may radiate → jaw/neck and/or one or both arms. Pain in the arms/neck may be the only symptom. Ask about frequency, severity, duration, and timing.
- *Precipitating/relieving factors* Precipitated by exertion, cold, emotion, and/or heavy meals. Pain stops with rest or GTN spray.
- *Associated symptoms* May be associated with palpitations, sweating, nausea, and/or breathlessness during attacks.
- *Presence of risk factors* Smoking history, family history, history of other vascular disease (e.g. CVA/TIA, peripheral vascular disease).

**Examination** There are usually no physical signs although anaemia may exacerbate symptoms. Check BMI and BP. Look for murmurs (especially ejection systolic murmur of aortic stenosis) and evidence of peripheral vascular disease and carotid bruits (especially in diabetics).

**First-line investigations**
- *Blood* FBC, fasting lipid profile, fasting blood glucose. Consider checking ESR (to exclude arteritis) and TFTs if clinical suspicion of thyrotoxicosis.
- *12-lead resting ECG* Provides information on rhythm, presence of heart block, previous MI, myocardial hypertrophy, and/or ischaemia.

❶ A normal ECG does not exclude coronary artery disease, but an abnormal ECG identifies those at higher risk of cardiac events in the next year—consider referral for further investigation.

**Differential diagnosis** Chest pain—📖 p.1076

**Referral of patients with suspected stable angina** For patients with new onset intermittent chest pains, refer to a rapid access chest pain clinic for prompt specialist assessment to:
- confirm/refute angina
- perform an exercise ECG (📖 p.242) and/or other investigations as appropriate, and
- provide information on treatment options available including the merits of revascularization for the individual.

❶ Patients with pre-existing cardiac disease (e.g. previous MI, valve disease, cardiomyopathy) are often excluded from rapid access chest pain clinic referral. Refer to cardiology direct.

## Management of patients with stable angina
### General advice
- *Driving* Patients who drive should inform the DVLA and their insurance company of the diagnosis. Vocational drivers—📖 p.132.

- *Occupation* Patients may not be able to undertake heavy work—give advice and support. Special rules apply to some occupations (e.g. merchant seamen, airline pilots)—advise patients to consult their occupational health department.

**Non-drug treatment** Aimed at 2° prevention of CHD
- *Smoking cessation* 📖 p.184
- *Hypertension* Check BP and treat if >140/90mmHg (📖 p. 254).
- *Diet* Advise healthy diet (oily fish, low cholesterol, ↑ fruit and vegetables, ↓ salt) and, if obese, aim to ↓ weight until BMI <25.
- *Alcohol* ↓ excess consumption. Targets: <3u/d ♂, <2u/d ♀.
- *Exercise* ↑ aerobic exercise within the limits set by the disease state.
- *Diabetes* Treat any underlying DM (📖 p.352–369).
- *Cardiac rehabilitation* May be helpful for patients with severe angina and/or after surgery.

**Drug treatment** 📖 p.264

**Referral to cardiology** (*E*=Admit; *U*=Urgent; *S*=Soon; *R*=Routine)
- Unstable angina/rapidly progressive symptoms—*E*
- Aortic stenosis with angina—*U*
- Angina following MI—*U/S*
- Abnormal ECG at diagnosis—*U/S*
- Angina not controlled by medication—*U/S/R*
- If diagnosis is in doubt—*S/R*
- Strong family history—*R*
- Other factors e.g. occupation affected—*R*

**Unstable angina** Pain on minimal or no exertion, pain at rest (may occur at night), or angina which is rapidly worsening in intensity, frequency, or duration. *Incidence:* 6/10,000/y; 15% suffer MI in <1mo.

**Management** Urgent referral to cardiology. Admit if attacks are severe, occur at rest, or last >20min even with GTN spray.

**Bypass surgery (CABG) and coronary angioplasty** CABG ↓ mortality over 5y, 7y, and 10y and ↓ symptoms in 80–90%. Angioplasty → improves symptoms in 70% although evidence of ↓ in mortality is lacking; coronary artery stenting improves symptom control and relapse rate.

**Prinzmetal (variant) angina** Angina at rest due to coronary artery spasm. ECG shows ST elevation. *Management:* refer to cardiology to exclude MI and atherosclerotic angina. GTN alleviates immediate episodes. Calcium-channel blockers are used to prevent angina. *M. Prinzmetal (1908–1987) US cardiologist.*

**Further information**
**NICE** Management of stable angina (due for publication in 2011) 🖥 www.nice.org.uk
**SIGN** Management of stable angina (2007) 🖥 www.sign.ac.uk
**Cardiac rehabilitation** 🖥 www.cardiacrehabilitation.org.uk

**Patient information**
**British Heart Foundation** ☎ 0845 708 070 🖥 www.bhf.org.uk

# Drug treatment of angina

**Symptom control** (BNF 2.6)

### As required medication

- Glyceryl trinitrate (GTN) spray is used for 'as required' symptom relief for angina.
- Advise 1–2 puffs as needed in response to pain and before engaging in activities that bring on pain.
- If response to GTN spray is poor, consider a buccal preparation.

❶ Sublingual GTN tablets are an alternative to GTN spray but deteriorate after 8wk.

⚠ Warn patients to call for help (dial for an emergency ambulance or ring emergency GP) if chest pain lasts >20min despite GTN spray.

### Regular treatment

Drugs for regular symptomatic treatment—see Table 10.8. Within any drug class use the cheapest preparation that the patient can tolerate, will comply with, and which controls symptoms.

All patients with angina should be taking a β-blocker (e.g. atenolol 50–100mg od) unless contraindicated/intolerant. Consider a highly-selective agent if asthma, COPD, or LV dysfunction. Thereafter, introduce medication in a stepwise manner according to response:

- **Step 2** If symptoms are not controlled with a β-blocker, or a β-blocker is contraindicated/not tolerated, add a long-acting dihydropyridine calcium-channel blocker (e.g. amlodipine 5mg od).
- **Step 3** There is little evidence to support combination therapy with 3 agents. If treatment with a β-blocker and calcium channel blocker is ineffective, consider adding a long-acting nitrate or nicorandil, and/or referral for specialist assessment.

⚠ Avoid combination of a β-blocker and a rate-limiting calcium-channel blocker (verapamil, diltiazem) because of risk of bradycardia/asystole.

### 2° prevention

**Aspirin** ↓ mortality by 34%. Unless contraindicated, give 75mg od to *all* patients with angina. Consider clopidogrel 75mg od if aspirin intolerant.

**Statins** ↓ in total cholesterol and LDL by 25–35% using statin therapy → ↓ CHD mortality by 25–35%.[S] Trial data suggest *all* patients with proven CHD benefit from ↓ in total cholesterol and LDL irrespective of initial cholesterol concentration[S] (📖 p.261).

**ACE inhibitors** Significantly ↓ cardiovascular deaths (RR 0.83) and all-cause mortality (RR 0.87), even in the absence of left ventricular dysfunction.

**Table 10.8** Drug treatment of angina

| Drug | Treatment notes |
|------|-----------------|
| β-blockers (BNF 2.4) ❶ May accumulate in patients with renal failure—↓ dose. | Effective for symptom control and to prevent vascular events |
| | Check fully β-blocked by monitoring heart rate—resting heart rate ≤65bpm; post-exercise (e.g. walking up 2 flights of stairs) heart rate ≤90bpm. Further increases in dose once adequately β-blocked are usually unhelpful |
| | Warn patients not to stop drug suddenly or run out |
| | If the patient needs to stop the drug, tail off over 4wk |
| | In patients with asthma/COPD in whom β-blockade is essential, use cardioselective β-blockers (e.g. bisoprolol, nebivolol) with care |
| Dihydropyridine calcium-channel blockers (BNF 2.6.2) | Amlodipine, felodipine, isradipine, lacidipine, lercanidipine, nicardipine, nifedipine, nimodipine |
| | All equally effective in symptom control. No evidence of cardioprotective effect |
| | *Contraindications* vary. Don't use if aortic stenosis, <1mo post-MI, or uncontrolled heart failure except with specialist advice |
| Rate limiting calcium-channel blockers (BNF 2.6.2) | Diltiazem and verapamil |
| | *Contraindications:* avoid in patients with heart block or heart failure. Do not combine with β-blockers |
| Long acting nitrates (BNF 2.6.1) e.g. isosorbide mononitrate (ISMN) | Oral and patch preparations (dosages > 10mg/24h) are available |
| | Start with a low dose and ↑ as tolerated. Side effects are common |
| | *Side effects:* headache, postural hypotension and dizziness—wear off with use. Reflex tachycardia may ↓ coronary blood flow and worsen angina |
| | *Tolerance:* many patients rapidly develop tolerance with ↓ therapeutic effect. To avoid this allow a nitrate-free period of ↑ 8h/d overnight by removing patches at night or giving the 2nd dose of ISMN at 4pm |
| | *Contraindications:* HOCM, aortic stenosis, constrictive pericarditis, mitral stenosis, severe anaemia, closed-angle glaucoma |
| Potassium-channel activator (BNF 2.6.3) | Nicorandil |
| | Similar efficacy to other anti-anginal drugs in controlling symptoms |
| | May produce additional symptomatic benefit in combination with other anti-anginal drugs (unlicensed) |
| | Headache is common—usually transitory |
| | *Contraindications:* left ventricular failure; hypotension |

# After myocardial infarction

**Acute myocardial infarct** 📖 p.1078

## Management post MI

### Modification of risk factors 2° prevention

- *Cholesterol* All patients with proven CHD benefit from ↓ in total cholesterol and LDL irrespective of initial cholesterol concentrations. ↓ in total cholesterol and LDL by 25–35% using statin therapy → ↓ CHD mortality by 25–35%. Serum cholesterol levels ↓ after MI and remain ↓ for several weeks.
- *ß-blockers* Unless contraindicated, start all patients on an oral β-blocker (e.g. atenolol) soon after MI and continue indefinitely. Estimated to prevent 12 deaths/1000 treated/y.

**ACE inhibitors** ↓ myocardial work and deaths <1mo post MI by 5/1000 treated. Survival advantage is sustained >1y even if treatment is not continued long-term. Effects are greater for patients with heart failure at presentation. *Long-term ACE inhibitors*: trials show ↓ mortality for all patients.

### Anti-platelet medication

- Starting aspirin 75mg od <24h after MI prevents 80 vascular events over the next 2y/1000 patients treated. Unless contraindicated, continue life long.
- For non-ST-segment-elevation acute coronary syndrome treat with a combination of low-dose aspirin and clopidogrel (75mg od) for 12mo Then continue aspirin alone long term.
- For ST-segment-elevation MI treated with dual therapy (aspirin + clopidogrel); continue for 4 wk. Continue aspirin alone long term.
- Occasionally (e.g. left ventricular aneurysm, AF) anticoagulation is indicated.

**Heart failure/left ventricular dysfunction** For patients who have had an acute MI and have symptoms/signs of heart failure and left ventricular systolic dysfunction, treatment with an aldosterone antagonist licensed for post-MI treatment (e.g.eplerenone 25mg od increasing in <1mo to 50mg od) should be initiated within 3–14 d of the MI, preferably after ACE inhibitor therapy.

**Exercise testing** Routine exercise testing identifies those likely to have angina post MI who might benefit from early angiography ± angioplasty/ stenting or CABG.

**Cardiac rehabilitation** ↓ risk of death by 20–25%. Provided by specialist multidisciplinary teams. *Components include*: psychological support, information about CHD, modification of risk factors.

## The role of the GP

### Support after discharge

*Return to work—guide*

- Sedentary workers: 4–6wk after uncomplicated MI.
- Light manual workers: 6–8 wk after uncomplicated MI.
- Heavy manual workers: 3mo after uncomplicated MI.

*Physical activity* Advise gradual ↑ in activity. Ensure goals given match those given by local cardiac rehabilitation. Guide to exercise post-MI:
• Up to 2wk—stroll in garden or street.
• From 2–6wk—walk 0.5 mile/d aiming to ↑ to 2 miles/d by 6wk.
• From 6wk—↑ speed of walking (aim 2 miles in <30min).

*Sexual activity* Resume after 6wk. A leaflet is available from the British Heart Foundation.

*Psychological effects* ~½ are depressed 1wk after MI and 25% after 1y. Educate about CHD. Check for depression (📖 p.998), counsel, and treat as needed.

*Driving* No driving for 1mo after MI. Inform car insurance company but no need to inform DVLA. HGV and PSV licence holders must notify the DVLA. Driving may be allowed after assessment.

*Flying* Most airlines will not carry passengers for 2 wk post MI and then only if able to climb 1 flight of stairs without difficulty.

### Ongoing follow-up

*Monitoring health* Continue regular reviews at least annually lifelong. Check for symptoms and signs of cardiac dysfunction (breathlessness, palpitations, angina); depression, carer stress.

*Monitoring drug therapy* Ongoing prescription of drugs, monitoring of compliance and side effects, changing medication if clinical circumstances or best practice alter.

### 2° prevention

• *Smoking cessation* 📖 p.184. ↓ risk of death by 50% over 15y.
• *Hypertension* Check BP and treat if >140/90 (📖 p.254).
• *Diet* Advise healthy diet (low cholesterol, ↑ fruit and vegetables, ↓ salt) and, if obese, aim to ↓ weight until BMI <25. Diets rich in omega-6 and omega-3 fatty acids (found in oily fish, vegetables, and nuts) ↓ CHD in 2° prevention but effect is through ↓ in risk of thrombosis and not associated with ↓ cholesterol.
• *Alcohol* ↓ excess consumption. Targets: <3u/d ♂; <2u/d ♀.
• *Exercise* ↑ aerobic exercise within the limits set by the disease state.
• *Diabetes*—Treat any underlying DM—📖 pp.352–369.
• Reinforce information given during cardiac rehabilitation.

**Dressler syndrome (Post-MI syndrome)** Develops 2–10 wk after MI or heart surgery. Thought to be due to autoantibodies to heart muscle. Presents with recurrent fever and chest pain ± pleural and/or pericardial effusion. *Management:* Refer urgently for cardiology/general medical advice. Treatment is with steroids and NSAIDs. *W. Dressler (1890–1969) US physician.*

### Further information

**NICE** Myocardial infarction: secondary prevention (2007) 🖳 www.nice.org.uk
**Cardiac rehabilitation** 🖳 www.cardiacrehabilitation.org.uk

### Patient information

**British Heart Foundation** ☎ 0845 708 070 🖳 www.bhf.org.uk

# Chronic heart failure

Chronic heart failure occurs when output of the heart is inadequate to meet the needs of the body. It is the end-stage of all diseases of the heart. *Prevalence*: 3–20/1000 population (1-1.6%). *Incidence* ↑ with age.

## Causes of chronic heart failure

**High output** The heart is working at normal or ↑ rate but the needs of the body are ↑ beyond that which the heart can supply, e.g. hyperthyroidism, anaemia, Paget's disease, AV malformation.

**Low output** ↓ heart function. Causes:
- ↑ *pre-load* e.g. mitral regurgitation, fluid overload.
- *Pump failure*
  - Cardiac muscle disease—IHD (46%), cardiomyopathy.
  - ↓ expansion of heart and restricted filling—restrictive cardiomyopathy, constrictive pericarditis, tamponade.
  - Inadequate heart rate—β-blockers, heart block, post MI.
  - Arrhythmia—AF commonest, ~30% patients with heart failure.
  - ↓ power—negatively inotropic drugs e.g. verapamil, diltiazem.
- *Chronic excessive afterload* ↑ BP (70%—, may be in combination with IHD), aortic stenosis.

**Primary right heart failure** e.g. pulmonary hypertension (📖 p.274), tricuspid incompetence.

## Risk factors

- Smoking
- DM
- Obesity
- Alcohol—toxic effect on the heart; cause of heart failure in 2–3%
- High total cholesterol to HDL ratio
- LVH on Echo.

**Presentation** Clinical diagnosis is difficult. 20–30% patients diagnosed by their GP as having heart failure do not have any demonstrable abnormality of cardiac function on Echo testing. Take a detailed history and do a clinical examination to exclude other disorders.

**Algorithm for diagnosing heart failure** Figure 10.1 (📖 p.270)

## Classification and symptoms

**Left ventricular failure (LVF)** Failure of the left ventricle causing back pressure into pulmonary system and giving symptoms and signs within the respiratory system. Symptoms include:
- Shortness of breath (on exertion, orthopnoea, PND)
- ↓ exercise tolerance
- Lethargy/fatigue
- Nocturnal cough (may bring up pink froth or have haemoptysis)
- Wheeze.

**Right ventricular failure (RVF)** Failure of the right ventricle causing back pressure into peripheral circulation resulting in symptoms/signs in the abdomen or limbs. Symptoms include:
- Swelling of ankles
- Abdominal discomfort due to liver distention
- Nausea and anorexia
- Fatigue and wasting
- Often ↑ weight.

**Congestive cardiac failure (CCF)** Failure of both ventricles.

### Signs
- Cachexia and muscle wasting
- ↑ RR ± cyanosis
- ↑ pulse rate
- Cardiomegaly and displaced apex beat
- Right ventricular heave
- ↑ JVP
- Pulsus alternans
- 3rd heart sound
- Basal crepitations ± pleural effusions and/or wheeze
- Pitting oedema of the ankles
- Hepatomegaly
- Ascites.

## Other conditions that may present with similar symptoms
- Obesity
- Respiratory disease
- Venous insufficiency in lower limbs
- Drug-induced ankle swelling (e.g. calcium-channel blockers) or fluid retention (e.g. NSAIDs)
- Hypoalbuminaemia
- Depression and/or anxiety
- Severe anaemia
- Thyroid disease
- Bilateral renal artery stenosis.
- Intrinsic renal or hepatic disease
- Pulmonary embolic disease

### Complications
- Arrhythmias, especially AF & VT
- Stroke or peripheral embolus
- DVT/PE
- Malabsorption
- Hepatic congestion/dysfunction
- Muscle wasting.

**Management** 📖 p.272

**Screening for depression** 📖 p.998

**Prognosis** Progressive deterioration to death. • ½ die suddenly, probably due to arrhythmias. Mortality:
- Mild/moderate heart failure —20–30% 1y mortality
- Severe heart failure —>50% 1y mortality.

**Acute heart failure** 📖 p.1084

### Further reading
**NICE** Chronic heart failure (2003) 🖥 www.nice.org.uk

### Patient information
**British Heart Foundation** ☎ 0845 708 070 🖥 www.bhf.org.uk

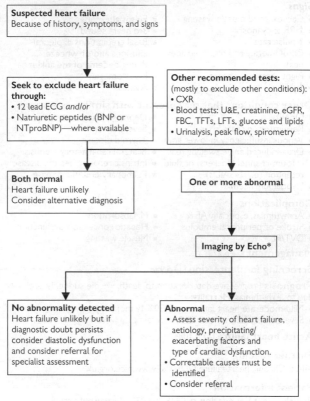

*Consider alternative methods of imaging if a poor image
is produced, e.g. trans-oesophageal Echo, radionuclide imaging,
or cardiac MRI.

**Fig. 10.1** NICE algorithm for diagnosing heart failure

Figures 10.1 and 10.2 are both reproduced from National Collaborating Centre for Chronic
Conditions. *Chronic heart failure: management of chronic heart failure in adults in primary and secondary care* (2003), London: Royal College of Physicians with permission of NICE. Full document
available at ⌨ www.nice.org.uk

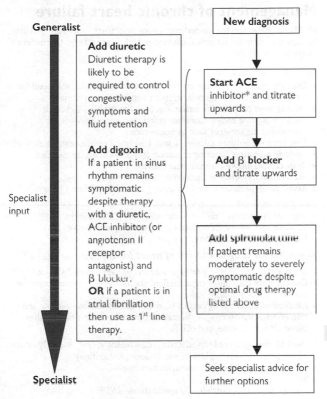

**Fig. 10.2** NICE algorithm for pharmacological treatment of symptomatic heart failure due to left ventricular systolic dysfunction

# Management of chronic heart failure

❶ Always look for the underlying cause and treat wherever possible. Review the basis for historical diagnoses and arrange Echo to confirm if diagnosis is in doubt.

## Non-drug measures

- *Educate* about the disease, current/expected symptoms, and need for treatment. Discuss prognosis. Support with written information.
- *Discuss ways to make life easier*, e.g. benefits, mobility aids, blue disability parking badge. Consider referral to social services for assessment for services such as home care.
- *Diet* Ensure adequate calories, ↓ salt, ↓ weight if obese, restrict alcohol.
- *Lifestyle measures* Smoking cessation (📖 p.184); regular exercise.
- *Restrict fluid intake* if severe heart failure.
- *Vaccination* Influenza and pneumococcal vaccination.
- *Assess for depression* Common among patients with heart failure.

## Drug treatment Table 10.9. *Aims to:*

- Improve symptoms—diuretics, digoxin, and ACE inhibitors, *and*
- Improve survival—ACE inhibitors, β-blockers, oral nitrates plus hydralazine, spironolactone.

## *Algorithm for drug treatment of heart failure* Figure 10.2 (📖 p.271).

## Monitoring Review every 6mo or more often as required. Check:

- *Clinical state* Functional capacity, fluid status, cardiac rhythm, cognitive and nutritional status, mood.
- *Medication* Ensure drug record is up to date, review compliance and side effects, change drugs if clinical circumstances/best practice alter.
- *Blood* U&E, creatinine, and eGFR.

## Referral to general medicine, cardiology, or elderly care
(*E*=Emergency admission; *U*=Urgent; *S*=Soon; *R*=Routine)

- Heart failure unable to be managed at home—*E*
- Severe heart failure—*U/S*
- Heart failure not controlled by medication—*U/S/R*
- Angina, AF, or other symptomatic arrhythmias—*U/S/R*
- If diagnosis is in doubt—*S/R*
- To initiate an ACE inhibitor or β-blocker—*S/R*
- Heart failure due to valve disease or diastolic dysfunction—*R*
- Comorbidity that may impact on heart failure (COPD, renal dysfunction, anaemia, thyroid disease, peripheral vascular disease, urinary frequency, gout)—*R*
- Women with heart failure planning pregnancy—*R*.

## Further reading
**NICE** Chronic heart failure (2003) 🖥 www.nice.org.uk

## Patient information
**British Heart Foundation** ☎ 0845 708 070 🖥 www.bhf.org.uk

**Table 10.9** Drugs used in the treatment of chronic heart failure

| Drug class | Treatment notes |
|---|---|
| Diuretics (BNF 2.2) | **Loop diuretics** e.g. furosemide or **thiazides** e.g. bendroflumethiazide. Use the minimum effective dose to control congestive symptoms and fluid retention (e.g. furosemide 20mg od). Monitor for ↓ $K^+$—co-treat with amiloride, ACE inhibitor, or $K^+$ supplement as necessary |
| ACE inhibitors (BNF 2.5.5.1) ❶ Check U&E and Cr before starting, at first follow-up, and after each ↑ dose ⚠ Do not use if renovascular disease, in pregnancy, if the patient has HOCM or if significant valve disease | Improve symptoms,↑exercise capacity, ↓ progression of disease , ↓ hospital admissions, and ↑survival in symptomatic and asymptomatic patients. Start at low dose (e.g.ramipril 1.25mg od) and titrate upwards Refer for specialist initiation if: • Age ≥70y • Severe or unstable heart failure • ↓ hypovolaemia • ↓ hypotension—systolic BP <90mmHg • Hyponatraemia ($Na^+$ <130mmol/L) • Renal impairment (creatinine >150µmol/L) • Receiving multiple or high dose diuretic therapy (e.g. >80mg furosemide/d) or high-dose vasodilator therapy If ACE inhibitors are not tolerated consider an angiotensin receptor blocker (ARB). |
| β-blockers (BNF 2.4) ❶ Refer for specialist initiation if any contraindication, elderly or severe heart failure | Start a β-blocker licensed for heart failure (e.g. bisoprolol 1.25mg mane) after diuretic and ACE inhibitor in all those with left ventricular dysfunction regardless of whether symptoms persist Use in a 'start low, go slow' manner with assessment of pulse, BP, and clinical status after each titration |
| Digoxin (BNF 2.1.1) | Use when symptoms persist despite ACE inhibitor, β-blocker, and diuretics, and for patients with AF + heart failure. 2 effects—antiarrhythmic and +ve inotrope. Improves symptoms, exercise tolerance and → ↓ admissions to hospital. No improvement in overall survival |
| Other drugs to consider depending on coexistent conditions | **Anticoagulation**—Patients with heart failure and AF, PH, thromboembolism, left ventricular aneurysm, or intra-thoracic thrombus (📖 p.670) **Aspirin**—75–150mg od if heart failure + atherosclerotic arterial disease (including CHD) **Statins**—Only if other indications (📖 p.260) **Amlodipine**—Can be used for treatment of angina and ↑ BP in patients with heart failure. ❶ Avoid verapamil, diltiazem or short-acting dihydropyridine agents |
| Drugs initiated under specialist supervision only | **Amiodarone**— All patients require clinical review, LFTs, and TFTs every 6mo **Spironolactone**—↑ survival if severe heart failure. Refer if moderate or severe symptoms despite optimal therapy. Dose 12.5-50mg od —monitor for ↑$K^+$ and ↓ renal function. If ↑ $K^+$, ½ the dose and recheck **Isosorbide/hydralazine combination** **Inotropic agents** |

# Pulmonary hypertension and cor pulmonale

Normal pulmonary arterial pressure is $<1/5$ of that in the systemic circulation. Pulmonary hypertension occurs by one of three mechanisms:
- High pulmonary blood flow (e.g. L→ R shunt)
- ↑ pulmonary vascular resistance
- Chronic pulmonary venous hypertension.

## Causes of pulmonary hypertension

*Lung disease*
- Asthma
- Bronchiectasis
- Pulmonary fibrosis.

*Hypoventilation*
- Sleep apnoea
- Enlarged adenoids in children
- CVA.

*Neuromuscular disease*
- MND
- Polio
- Myasthenia gravis.

*Cardiac disease*
- Mitral stenosis
- Congenital heart disease
- Severe LVF.

*Pulmonary vascular disease*
- PE
- Sickle cell disease.

*Thoracic cage abnormalities*
- Kyphosis
- Scoliosis.

**Consequences of pulmonary hypertension** With time ↑ pressure in the pulmonary vascular tree → permanent damage to smaller pulmonary vessels and pulmonary hypertension becomes irreversible—even if the cause is removed. If a shunt is present, when pulmonary pressure > systemic pressure the shunt reverses and the patient becomes cyanotic.

**Diagnosis** Under-diagnosed—delay between onset of symptoms and diagnosis ~2y.

**Presentation** CCF ± infective bronchitis, chest pain, breathlessness, lethargy and fatigue, haemoptysis, syncope, nausea.

**Examination** Check for cyanosis, peripheral oedema, ↑ JVP, 4th heart sound, diastolic murmur from pulmonary regurgitation, hepatomegaly ± ascites, crepitations at lung bases ± pleural effusion.

## Investigations
- **CXR**—cardiomegaly + enlargement of proximal pulmonary arteries.
- **ECG**—right axis deviation, tall peaked P waves, and dominant R wave in right precordial leads *or* RBBB.

**Management** Refer to cardiologist or chest physician. Doppler Echo is used to assess ventricular function and pulmonary arterial pressure. In the UK, ongoing care is now organized into designated multidisciplinary pulmonary hypertension units.

### Treatment
- Remove the underlying cause if possible.
- Oxygen therapy for symptomatic relief.
- Epoprostenol analogues have now become the mainstay of treatment and ↑ exercise tolerance and survival. Bosentan is also used.
- Vasodilation with calcium-channel blockers (in the 10–15% of patients who are responsive) can dramatically improve prognosis.
- Treat left ventricular failure with ACE inhibitors, β-blockers, and diuretics.
- Anticoagulation.

**Prognosis** If the cause is irreversible, a steady decline towards cor pulmonale and death is the likely outcome and heart–lung transplantation the only option. However, newer drugs are improving prognosis.

**Cor pulmonale** Right heart failure as a result of chronic hypoxia causing chronic pulmonary hypertension. Due to diseases of the lung, its vessels or the thoracic cage.

### Further reading
**British Heart Foundation Factfile** Pulmonary hypertension (1/2003)
▣ www.bhf.org.uk

### Patient information
**Pulmonary Hypertension Association (PHA) UK** ☎ 01709 761450
▣ www.phassociation-uk.com

# Tachycardia

Tachycardia is a heart rate >100bpm. It is often felt as palpitations. Tachycardia is common and may be an incidental finding. History and examination can exclude significant problems in most patients.

**History** Ask about:
- *Palpitations* Duration, frequency and pattern, rhythm (ask the patient to tap it out if not present when seen).
- *Precipitating/relieving factors*.
- *Associated symptoms* Chest pain, collapse or 'funny turns', sweating, breathlessness, or hyperventilation.
- *Past history*, e.g. previous episodes, heart disease, thyroid disease.
- *Lifestyle* Drug history, caffeine/alcohol intake, smoking.
- *Occupation* Arrhythmias may affect to driving (📖 p.132) and/or work.

> ⚠ **Red flag symptoms**
> - Pre-existing cardiovascular disease.
> - Family history of syncope, arrhythmia, or sudden death.
> - Arrhythmia associated with falls and/or syncope.

## Examination
- *General examination* for anaemia, thyrotoxicosis, anxiety, other systemic disease.
- *Cardiovascular examination* Heart size, pulse rate and rhythm, JVP, BP, heart sounds and murmurs, evidence of left ventricular failure.

## Investigations
*First-line* Resting ECG is all that is needed for many patients.

*Further investigations* Consider if ECG is abnormal or other concerning features: ambulatory ECG or cardiac memo; Echo if <50y or murmur/left ventricular failure detected; exercise tolerance test if exercise related. *Blood:* TFTs, FBC, ESR, U&E, eGFR fasting blood glucose, $Ca^{2+}$, albumin.

> **Ventricular tachycardia (VT)** Broad (>3 small squares) QRS complexes at a rate of >100bpm on ECG. Admit as a 'blue-light' emergency. Meanwhile give $O_2$ if available ± 100mg IV lidocaine. If no pulse treat as VF cardiac arrest (📖 p.1054).
>
> **Recurrent VT** may require surgery, insertion of a pacemaker or implantable cardioverter defibrillator.

**Ventricular ectopic beats** Additional broad QRS complexes, without P waves, superimposed on regular sinus rhythm. Common and usually of no clinical significance. Rarely may be the presenting feature of viral myocarditis. *Management:*
- *Frequent ectopics (>100/h) on ECG* Refer urgently to cardiology
- *R on T phenomenon on ECG* Rarely ectopics can → VF particularly if they coincide with the T wave of a preceding beat ('R on T phenomenon'). If this occurs >10×/min on ECG, admit.
- *After MI* Ventricular extrasystoles after MI are associated with ↑ mortality. Refer to cardiology.

- *No sinister features on ECG* Explain benign nature of the condition. Advise avoidance of caffeine, alcohol, smoking and fatigue. β-blockers can be helpful if unable to tolerate ectopics despite reassurance.

**Long Q–T syndrome (LQTS)** Heart condition associated with syncope/sudden death due to ventricular arrhythmias, often associated with exercise/excitement. ECG—prolonged Q–T interval. Genetic form is autosomal dominant or recessive, and may be associated with syndactyly or neural deafness. Refer any patient with a family history of sudden cardiac death for specialist assessment. Antenatal screening is possible.

**Paroxysmal supraventricular tachycardia (SVT)** Narrow QRS complex tachycardia with a regular rate > 100bpm on ECG.

### Management

*If seen during an attack* Get an ECG if possible. Try carotid sinus massage (unless elderly, IHD, digoxin toxic, carotid bruit, history of TIAs), the Valsalva manoeuvre, and/or ice on the face (especially effective for children). Admit as an emergency if the attack continues. If the attack terminates, refer to cardiology for advice on further management. Include a copy of the ECG trace during an attack if available.

*If diagnosed from history or ambulatory ECG trace, or if attack terminates rapidly* Refer to cardiology for confirmation of diagnosis and initiation of treatment—urgent referral if chest pain, dizziness, or breathlessness during attacks. Include ECG trace during an attack if available.

*Ongoing care* Advise patients to avoid caffeine, alcohol, and smoking. Treatment options are sotalol, verapamil, or amiodarone.

**Sinus tachycardia** Consider infection, pain, MI, shock, exercise, emotion (including anxiety), heart failure, thyrotoxicosis, drugs.

**Atrial fibrillation/flutter** 📖 p.278

**No tachycardia and no ECG abnormalities** Reassure. Explore the possibility of anxiety disorder (📖 p.988–991).

**Wolff–Parkinson–White (WPW) syndrome** A congenital accessory conduction pathway is present between atrium and ventricle (bundle of Kent). Clinical features:
- Predisposes to SVT and AF.
- *ECG* Short P–R interval followed by slurred upstroke ('delta wave') into the QRS complex.
- *Management* Refer to cardiology. Treatment is with anti-arrhythmics (SVT—verapamil; AF—amiodarone or DC shock) ± ablation of the accessory pathway.

*L. Wolff (1898–1972), P.D. White (1886–1973) US physicians; J. Parkinson (1885–1976) English physician.*

### Further information

**Morris F et al.** *ABC of electrocardiology* (2002) BMJ Books.
**British Heart Foundation Factfile** Palpitations: their significance and investigation (04/2004) 🖥 www.bhf.org.uk

# Atrial fibrillation (AF)

Common disturbance of cardiac rhythm which may be episodic (*paroxysmal*) or chronic. Characterized by rapid irregularly irregular narrow QRS complex tachycardia with absence of P waves. Affects <1% <60y, but >8% aged >80y. Associated with 5× ↑ risk of stroke. *Causes:*

- No cause (isolated AF) ~12%
- Coronary heart disease
- Valvular heart disease (especially mitral valve disease).
- ↑ BP (especially if LVH)
- Cardiomyopathy

**Acute AF** May be precipitated by acute infection, high alcohol intake, surgery, electrocution, MI, pericarditis, PE, or hyperthyroidism.

**Symptoms** Often asymptomatic, but may cause palpitations, chest pain, stroke/TIA, dyspnoea, fatigue, lightheadedness, and/or syncope.

## Examination

- *General examination* Check for anaemia, thyrotoxicosis, anxiety, and other systemic disease
- *Cardiovascular examination* Heart size, pulse rate and rhythm (apex rate > radial pulse rate if in AF), JVP, BP, heart sounds/murmurs, LVF.

## Investigations

- *Routine investigations* Resting ECG, CXR. *Blood*: TFTs, FBC, U&E, eGFR.
- *Further investigations* Ambulatory ECG or cardiac memo if paroxysmal AF; Echo if <50y or murmur/left ventricular failure detected; consider exercise tolerance test if exercise related.

**Management** (Figure 10.3). Aims to: relieve symptoms, e.g. palpitations, fatigue, dyspnoea; prevent thromboembolism and ↓ risk of stroke; maintain cardiac function.

**'Pill-in-the-pocket' approach to paroxysmal AF** Consider self-medication with a β-blocker prn (e.g. atenolol 50–100mg od) if infrequent symptomatic paroxysms *and* no history of LV dysfunction or valvular/ischaemic heart disease; systolic BP >100mmHg and resting heart rate >70bpm; able to understand when and how to take the medication.

### *Referral to cardiology, general medicine, or elderly care*

- Fast rate and compromised by arrhythmia (chest pain, ↓ BP or more than mild heart failure)—*E.*
- Candidate for DC or chemical cardioversion—*E/U.*
- Uncertainty about diagnosis or treatment—*S/R.*
- Symptoms are uncontrolled by standard treatment—*S/R.*
- Paroxysmal AF for consideration of sotalol or other anti-arrhythmic drugs when standard β-blockers have failed—*S/R.*

E=Emergency admission; U=Urgent; S=Soon; R=Routine.

**Atrial flutter** ECG shows regular sawtooth baseline at a rate of 300bpm with a narrow QRS complex tachycardia superimposed at a rate of 150 or 100bpm. Manage in the same way as AF (specialist drug treatment may differ).

## Further information

**NICE** The management of atrial fibrillation (2006) ⌨ www.nice.org.uk

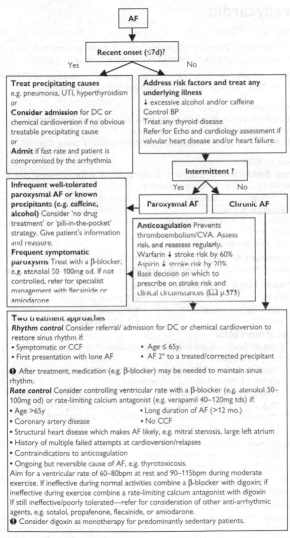

**AF**

↓

**Recent onset (≤7d)?**

Yes → / No →

**Treat precipitating causes**
e.g. pneumonia, UTI, hyperthyroidism
*or*
**Consider admission** for DC or chemical cardioversion if no obvious treatable precipitating cause
*or*
**Admit** if fast rate and patient is compromised by the arrhythmia

**Address risk factors and treat any underlying illness**
↓ excessive alcohol and/or caffeine
Control BP
Treat any thyroid disease
Refer for Echo and cardiology assessment if valvular heart disease and/or heart failure.

↓

**Intermittent ?**

Yes → **Paroxysmal AF** / No → **Chronic AF**

**Infrequent well-tolerated paroxysmal AF or known precipitants (e.g. caffeine, alcohol)** Consider 'no drug treatment' or 'pill-in-the-pocket' strategy. Give patient's information and reassure.
**Frequent symptomatic paroxysms** Treat with a β-blocker, e.g. atenolol 50–100mg od. If not controlled, refer for specialist management with flecainide or amiodarone

**Anticoagulation** Prevents thromboembolism/CVA. Assess risk, and reassess regularly.
Warfarin ↓ stroke risk by 60%
Aspirin ↓ stroke risk by 20%
Base decision on which to prescribe on stroke risk and clinical circumstances (☐ p.573)

**Two treatment approaches**
*Rhythm control* Consider referral/ admission for DC or chemical cardioversion to restore sinus rhythm if:
- Symptomatic or CCF
- First presentation with lone AF
- Age ≤ 65y.
- AF 2° to a treated/corrected precipitant

❶ After treatment, medication (e.g. β-blocker) may be needed to maintain sinus rhythm.
*Rate control* Consider controlling ventricular rate with a β-blocker (e.g. atenolol 50–100mg od) or rate-limiting calcium antagonist (e.g. verapamil 40–120mg tds) if:
- Age >65y
- Coronary artery disease
- Long duration of AF (>12 mo.)
- No CCF
- Structural heart disease which makes AF likely, e.g. mitral stenosis, large left atrium
- History of multiple failed attempts at cardioversion/relapses
- Contraindications to anticoagulation
- Ongoing but reversible cause of AF, e.g. thyrotoxicosis.
Aim for a ventricular rate of 60–80bpm at rest and 90–115bpm during moderate exercise. If ineffective during normal activities combine a β-blocker with digoxin; if ineffective during exercise combine a rate-limiting calcium antagonist with digoxin If still ineffective/poorly tolerated—refer for consideration of other anti-arrhythmic agents, e.g. sotalol, propafenone, flecainide, or amiodarone.
❶ Consider digoxin as monotherapy for predominantly sedentary patients.

**Fig. 10.3** Management of AF in primary care[N]

# Bradycardia

Heart rate < 60bpm.

**Presentation** Often an incidental finding but may present with faints or blackouts, drop attacks, dizziness, breathlessness, or lack of energy.

**Examination** Slow pulse rate; normal or low BP ± evidence of 2° heart failure. There may also be symptoms/signs of associated disease.

## Investigations
- *ECG* Ambulatory ECG may help with diagnosis of intermittent bradycardia (e.g. sick sinus syndrome).
- *Blood* TFTs, FBC, ESR, U&E, LFTs, digoxin levels (if taking digoxin).

## ECG changes
**Sinus bradycardia** Constant bradycardia. P waves present and P–R interval <0.2s (1 large square). *Causes:*

- Physiological, e.g. athletes
- Vasovagal attack
- Drugs, e.g. β-blockers, digoxin
- Inferior MI
- Sick sinus syndrome
- Hypothyroidism
- Hypothermia
- ↑ ICP
- Jaundice.

**Management** Admit acutely if symptomatic. Refer for cardiology opinion if asymptomatic but HR <40bpm despite treatment of reversible causes.

*AV node block (heart block)* *Causes:*

- IHD
- Drugs (digoxin, verapamil)
- Myocarditis
- Cardiomyopathy
- Fibrosis
- Lyme disease (rare).

*Types of heart block*
- *1st degree block*—fixed P–R interval >200ms (1 large square)
- *2nd degree block*
  - Mobitz type I (Wenckebach)—progressively lengthening P–R interval followed by a dropped beat.
  - Mobitz type II—constant P–R interval with regular dropped beats (e.g. 2:1—every 2nd beat is dropped; consider drug toxicity).
- *3rd degree block* (complete heart block)—P–P intervals are constant and R–R intervals are constant but not related to each other.

**Management** Untreated 2nd and 3rd degree heart block have a mortality of ~35%. Refer all patients to cardiology even if asymptomatic. If symptomatic (↓BP <90mmHg systolic, left ventricular failure, heart rate <40bpm) admit as an emergency—give IV atropine and O$_2$ (if available) whilst awaiting admission.

**Stokes–Adams attacks** Cardiac arrest due to AV block. Results in sudden loss of consciousness ± some limb twitching due to cerebral anoxia. The patient becomes pale and pulseless but respiration continues. Attacks usually lasts ~30s though occasionally are fatal. On recovery the patient becomes flushed. Refer to cardiology if suspected. *W. Stokes (1804–1878) Irish physician; R. Adams (1791–1875) Irish surgeon.*

**Sick sinus syndrome** Due to sinus node dysfunction causing brady-cardia ± asystole, sino-atrial block (complete heart block), AF or SVT alternating with bradycardia (tachy/brady syndrome). Common amongst elderly patients. If symptomatic, heart rate <40bpm or pauses >3s on ECG. Refer to cardiology for pacemaker insertion.

**Pacemakers** Electrically stimulate the heart to beat. Indications:
• Symptomatic bradycardia.
• 2nd or 3rd degree heart block.
• Suppression of resistant tachycardia.

*Insertion* Pacemaker box is usually attached under LA to the left, upper, antero-lateral chest wall, under the skin of the chest.

*Types* Classified according to:
• Chamber paced—atrium, ventricle or both ('dual').
• Chamber sensed—atrium, ventricle or both ('dual').
• Mode of response to sensing—inhibited output, triggered, inhibited and triggered ('dual').

Thus a V V I pacemaker both paces and senses the ventricle in inhibited mode, i.e. if the ventricle beats spontaneously the pacemaker will not fire.

*ECG changes with a pacemaker* If the pacemaker is in operation a pacing 'spike' (vertical line) is seen on ECG.

❶ In devices pacing on demand a spike will not be seen if the natural rate is in excess of the rate set on the pacemaker.

*Lifespan* Pacemakers last 7–15y. Regular checks are made by pacemaker clinics to ensure that the pacemaker remains operational. Reprogramming through the skin is possible. Batteries can be changed via a small surgical procedure under local anaesthetic.

*Driving with a pacemaker* Inform DVLA and insurance company (📖 p.132). Stop driving for 1mo after insertion.

⚠ Pacemakers must be removed after death before cremation can occur. A fee is payable.

**Further information**
**Morris F et al.** *ABC of electrocardiology* (2002) BMJ Books (ISBN: 0727915363)
**NICE** Bradyarrhythmias: dual chamber pacing (2005) 🖳 www.nice.org.uk

# Infective endocarditis

⚠ New murmur + fever = endocarditis until proven otherwise.

Infective endocarditis occurs when there is infection of a heart valve. The valve may be normal (50%—may be associated with IV drug abuse), rheumatic, degenerative, congenitally abnormal or prosthetic. Uncommon but consequences may be disastrous and often detected late.

## Causes
- *Common organisms* Strep. viridans (35–50%), Staph. aureus (20%).
- *Non-bacterial causes* SLE, malignancy.

**Presentation** May be acute (acute heart failure) or subacute (course worsening over days/weeks). *Symptoms/signs:*
- *Infective* Fever, weight ↓, night sweats, malaise, lethargy, clubbing, splenomegaly, anaemia, mycotic aneurysms.
- *Heart murmurs* ▸◂ heart failure.
- *Embolic* Stroke, lung abscesses (right heart endocarditis).
- *Vasculitic* Microscopic haematuria, splinter haemorrhages, Osler's nodes (painful lesions on finger pulps), Janeway lesions (palmar macules), Roth's spots (retinal vasculitis), renal failure.

**Management** Have a high index of suspicion for patients at ↑ risk, i.e. with valve lesions or prosthetic valves. Admit as an emergency if suspected. Avoid starting antibiotics prior to admission as this might cause delay in diagnosis by rendering the blood cultures sterile. Hospital treatment is with prolonged IV broad spectrum antibiotics (≥2wk).

**Prognosis** 20–25% of those admitted with a diagnosis of infective endocarditis die; 80% have major complications during admission, e.g. heart failure. Valve replacement may be required, especially if endocarditis is on a prosthetic valve.

## High-risk patients Those with:
- Acquired valvular heart disease with stenosis or regurgitation.
- Valve replacement.
- Structural congenital heart disease, including surgically corrected or palliated structural conditions, but excluding: isolated atrial septal defect, fully repaired ventricular septal defect or fully repaired patent ductus arteriosus, and closure devices that are endothelialized.
- Hypertrophic cardiomyopathy.
- Previous infective endocarditis.

**Prevention of infective endocarditis** New guidance advises against routine antibiotic prophylaxis because:
- There is no consistent association between having an interventional procedure and development of infective endocarditis.
- Regular toothbrushing presents a greater risk of infective endocarditis than a single dental procedure because of repetitive exposure to bacteraemia with oral flora.
- Clinical effectiveness of antibiotic prophylaxis is not proven.
- Antibiotic prophylaxis against infective endocarditis may lead to a greater number of deaths through fatal anaphylaxis than a strategy of no antibiotic prophylaxis, and is not cost effective.

***Advise instead*** about:
- The importance of maintaining good oral health.
- Symptoms that may indicate infective endocarditis and when to seek expert advice.
- The risks of undergoing invasive procedures, including non-medical procedures such as body piercing or tattooing.

❶ Do not offer chlorhexidine mouthwash as prophylaxis against infective endocarditis to people at risk undergoing dental procedures.

**Further information**
**NICE** Prophylaxis against infective endocarditis (2008) 🖳 www.nice.org.uk

# Rheumatic fever, myocarditis, and pericarditis

**Rheumatic fever** There has been a dramatic ↓ in incidence of rheumatic fever in industrialized countries since 1950s, but recently numbers of cases have ↑. Rheumatic fever is still an endemic disease in developing countries. *Peak incidence*: age 5–15y.

*Cause* Rheumatic fever is due to an abnormal immunological response to β-haemolytic streptococcal infection (e.g. 2–4wk after sore throat). Its importance lies in the permanent damage caused to heart valves in some of those affected and subsequent risk of endocarditis.

*Diagnosis* Can be made if revised Jones criteria are met (Table 10.10)

*Management* If suspected refer for specialist care. Specialist management includes evaluation of heart lesions with Echo, bed rest; penicillin, and symptom control (e.g. analgesia, sedatives for chorea). Anti-inflammatory agents such as corticosteroids and aspirin may be used to try to ↓ complications of carditis but their use is controversial.

*Prognosis*
- 60% develop chronic rheumatic heart disease (70% mitral valve; 40% aortic; 10% tricuspid; 2% pulmonary). Likelihood correlates with severity of initial disease.
- Recurrence may occur after further streptococcal infection or be precipitated by pregnancy or the COC pill.

**Table 10.10** Revised Jones criteria for diagnosis of rheumatic fever

**Requirements for diagnosis of rheumatic fever:**

Evidence of previous streptococcal infection (scarlet fever, +ve throat swab and/or ↑ ASO titre >200u/mL)

*and*

2 major criteria

*or*

1 major + 2 minor criteria

| Major criteria: | Minor criteria: |
|---|---|
| *Carditis* (45–70%)—arrhythmia, new murmur, pericardial rub, heart failure, conduction defects | Prolonged P–R interval on ECG (but not if carditis is one of the major criteria) |
| *Migratory polyarthritis* ('flitting'—75%), red tender joints | Arthralgia (but not if arthritis is one of the major criteria) |
| *Sydenham's chorea* (St. Vitus' dance—10%) | Fever |
| *Subcutaneous nodules* (2–20%) | ↑ESR or ↑CRP |
| *Erythema marginatum* (2–10%) | History of rheumatic heart disease or rheumatic fever |

**2° prevention** Penicillin 250mg bd po or sulfadiazine 1g od (500mg od for patients <30kg) for ≥5y to prevent recurrence. Duration of prophylaxis is dependent on whether there was carditis in the initial attack (no carditis—continued for 5y; if cardiac involvement—continued until age 25y or longer).

**Acute myocarditis** Inflammation of the myocardium. May present in a similar way to MI or with palpitations. Causes: viral infection, e.g. Coxsackie virus; diptheria; rheumatic fever; drugs.

*Management* Admit for specialist cardiologist care. Treatment is supportive. Some recover spontaneously—others progress to intractable heart failure requiring transplantation.

**Pericarditis** Sharp constant sternal pain relieved by sitting forwards. May radiate to left shoulder ± arm or into the abdomen. Worse lying on the left side and on inspiration, swallowing, and coughing. A pericardial rub may be present at the left sternal edge on auscultation. *Causes:*

- Infection, e.g. Coxsackie virus, TB
- Malignancy
- Uraemia
- MI (Dressler syndrome 📖 p.267)
- Trauma
- Radiotherapy
- Connective tissue disease
- Hypothyroidism.

*Investigations* ECG—concave (saddle-shaped) ST elevation in all leads.

*Management* Refer to cardiology; treat the cause (if possible); symptomatic treatment with NSAID for pain, steroids in resistant cases.

### Complications

- *Pericardial effusion* Fluid in the pericardial sac. *Presentation:* left or right heart failure, cardiac tamponade (inability of the heart to dilate in diastole resulting in tachycardia, ↓ BP, ↑ JVP). CXR—large, globular heart. Echo is diagnostic. *Management:* admit for urgent cardiology assessment.
- *Constrictive pericarditis* Pericardium becomes fibrosed and non-expansile. Most common cause is TB. *Presentation:* right heart failure, hepatosplenomegaly, ascites, ↓ BP, ↑ JVP. *Management:* refer to cardiologist for confirmation of diagnosis. Treatment involves surgical release of the pericardium.

# Cardiomyopathy and heart transplant

**Cardiomyopathy** Primary disease of the heart muscle.

**Dilated (congestive) cardiomyopathy** Prevalence ~35/100 000 population. ♂>♀. Dilation of left ± right ventricle and ↓ contractility. Presents with heart failure. ECG shows non-specific ST abnormalities. CXR shows cardiac enlargement and pulmonary venous hypertension. Echo is diagnostic. *Causes:*

- Idiopathic
- Familial (20%)
- Cardiovascular—IHD, ↑ BP, congenital heart disease, rheumatic heart disease
- Alcohol
- Infection (Coxsackie virus)
- Endocrine disease—myxoedema, thyrotoxicosis, acromegaly
- Cardiotoxic drugs
- Pregnancy
- Connective tissue disease (SLE, PAN, systemic sclerosis)
- Sarcoidosis
- Amyloidosis
- Haemachromatosis
- Malignancy
- Muscular dystrophy.

**Management and prognosis** Advise patients to stop drinking alcohol as alcohol may make the cardiomyopathy worse. Specialist management is needed in all cases and involves treatment of heart failure and arrhythmias. Most patients require long-term anticoagulation. Surgical options include cardiomyoplasty and/or heart transplantation. *Mortality:* 40% in 2y (sudden death, cardiogenic shock).

**Hypertrophic cardiomyopathy** Familial inheritance (autosomal dominant) though 1:2 cases are sporadic—in its most common form causes asymetrical septal hypertrophy ± aortic outflow obstruction (obstructive hypertrophic cardiomyopathy or HOCM).

**Presentation** Most cases are diagnosed in childhood (<14y) through screening of asymptomatic patients with FH using echocardiography. *Symptoms/signs:*

- Palpitations—associated with arrhythmias—5% have AF.
- Breathlessness on exertion.
- Chest pain—may be angina or atypical pain.
- Murmur—due to outflow obstruction and/or mitral valve dysfunction.
- Faints/collapses.

**Investigations**

- *ECG*—LVH and ischaemic changes, e.g. T wave inversion.
- *CXR*—normal until disease is in its late stages.
- *Echo*—diagnostic. Refer if suspicious symptoms or family history.

**Management and prognosis** Ongoing specialist care is essential to provide symptomatic treatment, e.g. β-blockers for chest pain, amiodarone for arrhythmia (digoxin is contraindicated). Surgical options include myotomy and myectomy. *Mortality:* major cause of mortality is sudden death unrelated to severity of symptoms. Though ultimately fatal in the majority, interval between diagnosis and death is often decades.

**Restrictive cardiomyopathy** Stiff ventricle which limits filling. Presents with heart failure. Echo is diagnostic. *Causes:* amyloid, sarcoidosis, haemachromatosis. *Management:* Specialist management is required. Treatment is symptomatic.

***Obliterative cardiomyopathy*** Rare in Western countries—idiopathic fibrosis of inflow tract prevents filling. Leads to cavity obliteration.

**Family history of sudden death** Refer 1st degree relatives of victims of sudden cardiac death who died aged <40y to cardiology. Antenatal screening for familial cardiomyopathy and LQTS syndrome is possible if familial mutation is known. If FH HOCM and no genetic test:
- Children under <10 y—screen with ECG and Echo every 3–5y.
- Children aged 10–16y—screen every 6–12mo if there is FH of HOCM. Disease is likely to become apparent at this age.
- Young people aged 16–20y—screen annually.
- >20y—screen every 5y if FH late-onset hypertrophic cardiomyopathy.

❶ Screening intervals are not established for other cardiomyopathies but should be adapted to the pattern of disease within that particular family.

**Heart transplantation** Considered in patients with estimated 1y survival <50%. *Indications/contraindications*—Table 10.11.

***Assessment*** Each eligible patient is assessed for psychosocial factors and physical factors (e.g. renal failure, obesity, age, peripheral vascular disease) which affect prognosis before a decision whether to place the patient on the transplant list is made.

***Post-operatively*** Patients require lifelong immunosuppression—usually with ciclosporin A. Follow-up is undertaken in specialist clinics.

***Prognosis*** 1:4 patients die on the transplant list; 60% receive transplant in <2y. Perioperative mortality: <10%. 1y survival 92%, 5y survival 75%; 10y survival 60%. Patients have accelerated graft atherosclerosis. Complications of immunosuppression include ↑ risks of infection and cancer.

**Table 10.11** Indications and contraindications for heart transplant

| Indications | Contraindications |
|---|---|
| All patients must have end-stage heart disease. *Causes:* <br> • IHD (50%) <br> • Cardiomyopathy (40%) <br> • Valvular and congenital heart defects (5%) | Systemic disease likely to affect life expectancy (e.g. malignancy) <br> Active infection (HIV, hepatitis B or C) <br> Significant pulmonary vascular disease <br> Continued excess alcohol consumption <br> Significant cerebral/systemic vascular disease <br> Upper age limit generally taken at ~60y |

**Further reading**
**DH** National Service Framework for CHD (2005) ▣ www.dh.gov.uk

**Patient information and support**
**Cardiomyopathy Association**. ☎ 01923 249 977
▣ www.cardiomyopathy.org
**Transplant Support Network** ☎ 0800 027 4490/1
▣ www.transplantsupportnetwork.org.uk
**Heart Transplant Families Together** ▣ www.htft.org.uk

# Valve disease

**Heart murmurs** 📖 p.236

⚠ All patients with newly detected valve disease, except those with mitral valve prolapse or aortic sclerosis, require cardiology referral.
- Admit if suspected endocarditis.
- Refer urgently/admit if symptomatic valve disease or if valve disease underlies the presenting condition, e.g. heart failure caused by aortic stenosis, AF caused by mitral valve disease.

**Mitral stenosis** Usually due to rheumatic fever.

### Presentation
- *Symptoms* Breathlessness, palpitations, fatigue. May result in pulmonary hypertension which presents with right heart failure, haemoptysis and/or recurrent bronchitis.
- *Signs* Peripheral cyanosis ('malar flush' on cheeks), left parasternal heave, tapping apex beat, AF, rumbling mid-diastolic murmur at apex.

***Management*** Confirm with Echo. Refer to cardiology. Treatment is medical (digoxin, diuretics, anticoagulation) ± surgical (valvotomy, balloon valvoplasty, valve replacement).

**Mitral regurgitation (incompetence)** *Causes:*

- Congenital
- Rheumatic fever
- Mitral valve prolapse
- Ventricular dilatation
- Endocarditis
- Cardiomyopathy
- Ruptured papillary muscle/chordae tendinae following MI
- RA.

### Presentation
- *Symptoms* Dyspnoea, fatigue.
- *Signs* Displaced apex (→ left axilla), pansystolic murmur at the apex radiating to axilla, AF, left ventricular failure.

***Management*** Confirm with Echo. Refer to cardiology. Treatment is medical (digoxin and anticoagulation for AF, diuretics) ± surgical (valve replacement).

**Mitral valve prolapse** Prevalence ~1:20.

### Presentation
- *Symptoms* Usually none. Rarely, atypical chest pain, palpitations, syncope, postural hypotension, emboli.
- *Signs* late systolic murmur over apex.

***Management*** Confirm with Echo. If syncope or palpitations refer to cardiology—a rare complication is ventricular arrhythmia.

**Aortic sclerosis** Senile thickening and stiffening of the aortic valve not associated with outflow obstruction. Clinically an ejection systolic murmur is present but no other symptoms or signs. CXR may show a calcified valve. No treatment required.

**Aortic stenosis** *Causes:*

- Congenital
- Rheumatic fever
- Bicuspid valve
- Degenerative calcification
- Hypertrophic cardiomyopathy.

### Presentation

- *Symptoms* Angina, breathlessness, syncope or 'funny turns', dizziness, sudden death.
- *Signs* Small volume pulse, low pulse pressure (difference between systolic and diastolic BP), ejection systolic murmur loudest in the aortic area which radiates to carotids and apex.

**Management** Echo is diagnostic and gives an estimate of the gradient across the valve and thus severity of the condition. Refer to cardiology. Surgery (valve replacement or transcutaneous valvuloplasty) is considered for those with syncope or if systolic gradient across the valve is >50mmHg. Avoid treatment with ACE inhibitors.

**Aortic regurgitation** *Causes:*

- Congenital, e.g. VSD
- Bicuspid aortic valve
- Rheumatic fever
- Aortic dissection
- Endocarditis
- Cardiomyopathy
- Syphilis
- Marfan's or Ehlers–Danlos syndrome.

### Presentation

- *Symptoms* Dyspnoea, palipitations (extrasystoles).
- *Signs* Prominent pulse ('water-hammer'), wide pulse pressure, visible neck pulsation (Corrigan's sign), head nodding in time with pulse (de Musset's sign), visible capillary pulsations (e.g. in nail bed—Quincke's sign), displaced apex beat, high-pitched early diastolic murmur (easily missed).

**Management** Confirm with Echo. Refer to cardiology for consideration of surgery.

**Right heart valve disease** Echo is diagnostic. Always requires specialist management.

- **Tricuspid stenosis** Mitral valve disease always coexists. *Cause:* rheumatic fever. *Murmur:* early diastolic (left sternal edge in inspiration). Treatment is with diuretics ± surgery (valvotomy or replacement).
- **Tricuspid regurgitation** *Causes:* RV enlargement, endocarditis (IV drug abusers), carcinoid, rheumatic fever, congenital. Presents with oedema, breathlessness, pulsatile hepatomegaly (± jaundice), ascites, pansystolic murmur loudest at left sternal edge. Treatment is with diuretics, vasodilators ± surgery (valve replacement or annuloplasty).
- **Pulmonary stenosis** *Causes:* congenital (Fallot's tetralogy), rheumatic, carcinoid. *Murmur:* ejection systolic murmur (loudest to left of upper sternum, radiating to left shoulder). *ECG:* RVH. *CXR:* dilated pulmonary artery. Treatment (if required) is with pulmonary valvotomy.
- **Pulmonary regurgitation** Caused by pulmonary hypertension (📖 p.274). *Murmur:* decrescendo early diastolic murmur at left sternal edge.

⚠ Women planning pregnancy who have known valve disease require review for specialist advice.

# Other structural abnormalities of the heart

**Coarctation of the aorta** Localized narrowing of the descending aorta, usually distal to the origin of the left subclavian artery.

*Presentation* Heart failure, ↑ BP, murmur heard incidentally (ejection systolic murmur over the left side of the chest radiating to the back), lack of femoral pulses or radio-femoral delay. Rarely, presentation is with a complication, e.g. subarachnoid haemorrhage or endocarditis. *CXR*: prominent left ventricle. *ECG*: left ventricular hypertrophy.

*Management* Refer to cardiology—surgery to remove the narrowed portion of the aorta is usually indicated.

**Atrial septal defect (ASD)** A hole connects the 2 atria. Holes high in the septum (ostium secundum) are most common (2/1000 live births); holes lower in the septum (ostium primum) are associated with AV valve abnormalities. Blood flows L → R through the shunt and the right heart takes the burden.

*Presentation*
- *Ostium secundum defects* Symptoms are rare in infancy and uncommon in childhood. If detected in these groups presents as a murmur (systolic—loudest in the 2nd left interspace) found incidentally, with breathlessness or tiredness on exertion or recurrent chest infections. Presentation is usually in the 3rd or 4th decade with heart failure, pulmonary hypertension, and/or atrial arrhythmias.
- *Ostium primum defects* Heart failure commonly develops in infancy/childhood ± severe pulmonary hypertension. In addition to the ASD murmur, there may be a pansystolic murmur signifying mitral or tricuspid valve regurgitation.

*Investigation*
- *CXR* Cardiomegaly with a prominent right atrium ± pulmonary artery ± pulmonary plethora.
- *ECG* Right axis deviation (ostium secundum defect) or left axis deviation (ostium primum defect), RVH ± RBBB.
- *Echo* Diagnostic.

*Management* Refer to cardiology. Cardiac surgery to close the defect is usually indicated.

**Ventricular septal defect (VSD)** A hole connects the 2 ventricles. Blood flows initially L → R through the hole. May be congenital (2/1000 live births) or acquired (usually septal rupture post MI).

*Congenital VSD*
*Small VSD (maladie de Roger)* Normally asymptomatic.
- *Examination* Thrill palpable at lower left sternal border; harsh pansystolic murmur—small holes give loud murmurs.
- *Investigations* CXR and ECG are normal. Diagnosis is confirmed on Echo.
- *Management* Refer to cardiology.

*Moderate VSD* Symptoms usually appear in infancy—breathlessness on feeding/crying, failure to thrive, recurrent chest infections. As the child gets older symptoms improve (relative size of the defect ↓).
- *Examination* Cardiomegaly, thrill palpable at left sternal edge, pansystolic murmur.
- *Investigations* Cardiomegaly ± prominent pulmonary arteries ± pulmonary plethora. Diagnosis is confirmed on Echo.
- *Management* Refer to cardiology.

*Large VSD* Presents with heart failure at ~3mo of age though there may be symptoms of breathlessness on feeding/crying prior to this.
- *Examination* Baby is obviously unwell—underweight, breathless, pulmonary oedema ± cyanosis, large heart, thrill over left sternal edge ± parasternal heave, murmur—often not pansystolic due to high right ventricular pressures.
- *Management* Admit to paediatrics—medical treatment ± surgery is always needed.

**Acquired VSD** Suspect if new pansystolic murmur ± heart failure develops after MI. Investigate as for congenital VSD. Refer to cardiology (speed of referral will depend on state of the patient) for advice on further management.

**Marfan's syndrome** Autosomal dominant connective tissue disease causing abnormalities of fibrillin (a glycoprotein in elastic fibres). *Features include*:
- Arachnodactyly (long spidery fingers).
- High-arched palate.
- Arm span > height.
- Lens dislocation ± unstable iris.
- Aortic dilatation (β-blockers appear to slow this).
- Aortic incompetence may occur, e.g. in pregnancy.
- Aortic dissection may cause sudden death—Echo screening may be helpful for affected individuals.

If suspected refer to cardiology ± genetics. There is currently no antenatal screening test available. *E.J.A. Marfan (1858–1942) French paediatrician.*

**Other congenital heart disease** 📖 p.878

# Aneurysms

An arterial aneurysm forms when there is a 50% ↑ in normal diameter of the vessel. Aneurysms may affect any medium/large artery—aorta/iliac arteries > popliteal > femoral > carotid. FH of aneurysm is a risk factor.

**Causes** Atheroma (most common); injury; infection (e.g. endocarditis, syphilis—mycotic aneurysms).

**Abdominal aortic aneurysm (AAA)** Prevalence is ~5% and increasing. The typical patient with an AAA is a ♂ smoker >65y. Risk ↑ ×4-10 if there is an affected 1st degree relative.

### Screening
- Acute rupture of AAA in the community has ~90% mortality.
- Elective surgical repair has ~5–7 % mortality.
- Single abdominal USS in men age 65y would exclude 90% of the population from future AAA rupture. A large RCT of population screening in the UK showed 44% ↓ in death due to AAA in the screened group.
- An NHS AAA Screening Programme will be operating in England from 2009 and Scotland from 2011. Men are screened with USS at 65y.
- If aortic diameter <3cm, discharged; 3–4.4cm, yearly follow up with USS; 4.5–5.4cm, 3 monthly follow up with USS; ≥5.5cm referred for specialist vascular assessment.

*Problems with screening* Identifies small aneurysms not requiring repair but surveillance. This may cause morbidity in low-risk healthy individuals.

*Presentation* Often discovered as an incidental finding on abdominal examination, X-ray (calcification of aneurysm wall in 50% cases), or USS (¾ asymptomatic at diagnosis). Otherwise presents with:
- *Local symptoms*—vague abdominal or back pain
- *Distant symptoms*—embolization /acute ischaemia of a limb. Multiple small infarcts (e.g. of toes) with good peripheral pulses suggests an aneurysm proximally.
- *Collapse due to rupture*—hypovolaemic shock ± pulsatile abdominal mass ± abdominal or back pain (🕮 p.1070).

---

### Factors predisposing to rupture of AAA

- Diameter (risk ↑ with diameter)
- COPD
- Smoking
- ↑ diastolic BP
- FH

- Fast rate of expansion
- Inflammation within the aneurysm wall
- Thrombus-free surface area of aneurysm sac.

---

*Investigation* USS confirms diagnosis, diameter, site and extent.

### Management of abdominal aortic aneurysm
- *Acute rupture* 🕮 p.1070
- *Referral for elective surgery*
  - Refer if risk of rupture > risk of elective repair.

- The greater the diameter, the more the risk (5.5cm diameter ≈ 10% 1y rupture rate; 10cm diameter >75% 1y rupture rate).
- AAAs >5.5cm are routinely repaired unless other factors ↑ risk of surgery. There is no survival benefit in treating smaller aneurysms.
- Refer urgently if symptomatic. May indicate rapid expansion, or inflammation—both risk factors for rupture.
- *USS surveillance* Patients with AAAs <5.5cm diameter. Annual screening. Routine repair takes place when and if the aneurysm expands to >5.5cm. 3:5 eventually warrant surgery.

**Inflammatory aneurysms** Characterized by inflammatory infiltrate in the aneurysm wall. May be adherent to surrounding structures. *Presentation:* fever, malaise, and abdominal pain. Associated with ↑ mortality at operation.

**Thoracoabdominal aneurysm** Involves thoracic and abdominal aorta, including the origins of the visceral and renal arteries. Surgery is more complex and carries higher mortality.

**Dissecting thoracic aortic aneurysm** 📖 p.1070

**Popliteal aneurysms** 80% peripheral aneurysms. Most are >2cm diameter; 50% are bilateral. Associated with AAA (40%).

*Presentation* Acute below-knee ischaemia 2° aneurysm thrombosis or embolization. Popliteal pulses are pronounced. Diagnosis is confirmed on USS.

### Management
- Acute ischaemia—📖 p.1122
- Elective surgery (popliteal bypass) when aneurysm >2.5cm diameter.

**Femoral artery aneurysms** *Presentation:* local pressure symptoms, thrombosis, or distal embolization. *Surgical treatment:* bypass surgery.

**Carotid artery aneurysm** Rare. Presents with pulsatile lateral neck swelling ± carotid territory TIAs. Rarely can rupture. Treatment is surgical. Refer to vascular surgery.

**Carotid body tumour** Slow-growing tumour arising in the carotid body at the carotid bifurcation. Presents with slowly enlarging mass which transmits carotid pulsation. Refer to vascular surgery for angiographic confirmation of diagnosis. Treatment is with surgical excision. If untreated, becomes locally invasive and may eventually metastasize.

**Cerebral artery aneurysms** 📖 p.570

### Further information
**British Heart Foundation Factfiles** Abdominal aortic aneurysms (3/2003) 🖳 www.bhf.org.uk

### Patient information and support
**British Vascular Foundation** 🖳 www.bvf.org.uk
**Vascular Society of GB & Ireland** 🖳 www.vascularsociety.org.uk

# Chronic peripheral ischaemia

Peripheral vascular disease (normally atherosclerotic) commonly affects arteries supplying the legs. *Incidence*: 10% patients age 60–70y; 20% >70y.

**Natural history** Most remain stable. A few (2% over 10y) progress from intermittent claudication to critical limb ischaemia. Management of cardiovascular risk factors is essential.

**Intermittent claudication** Restriction of blood flow causes pain on walking. *Risk factors*:

- ♂>♀
- Smoking
- Obesity
- ↑BP
- Hyperlipidaemia
- DM
- Physical inactivity
- Hypercoagulable states
- Post-menopausal.

*Presentation* Presents with muscular cramp-like pain in calf, thigh, or buttock on walking that is rapidly relieved on resting. The leg is cool and white with atrophic skin changes and absent pulses (Table 10.12).
- *Disease in the superficial femoral artery* Absent popliteal and foot pulses. Causes calf claudication.
- *Disease of the aorta or iliac artery* Weak or absent femoral pulse ± femoral bruit. Causes calf, thigh, or buttock claudication.

*Differential diagnosis* Nerve root compression, e.g. sciatica; spinal stenosis. Usually bilateral pain which may occur after prolonged standing as well as exercise—not rapidly relieved by rest.

### Investigation
- *Blood* FBC, U&E, Cr, eGFR (peripheral vascular disease is associated with renal artery stenosis—🕮 p.451), glucose, lipids.
- *Ankle–brachial systolic pressure index (ABPI)*
  - Good history + ABPI <0.95 confirms diagnosis.
  - If good history but normal ABPI (=1), consider exercise testing.*
- *Duplex USS* Used to determine site of disease.*

### Management
- ↓ *risk factors* Patients with claudication have a 3× ↑ risk of death from MI/stroke. Advise to stop smoking and lose weight. Ensure optimum treatment of ↑ BP, lipids, and DM.
- *Foot care* Regular chiropody.
- *Drugs*
  - Aspirin (75–300mg od) ↓ risk of cardiovascular events. Alternatives are dipyridamole (200mg bd) or clopidogrel (75mg od).
  - Naftidrofuryl may ↑ walking distance—unclear whether influences outcome. Reassess after 3–6mo Discontinue if no improvement.
  - Cilostazol ↑ walking distance in those with ongoing symptoms despite risk factor management.
- *Exercise* Training for ≥6mo by regularly walking as far as possible before being stopped by pain ↑ pain-free and maximum walking distances. Effect is greater than the effect of angioplasty.

* May only be available via 2° care referral

**Table 10.12** Location of the pulses of the lower limbs

| Pulse | Location |
|---|---|
| Femoral | Below inguinal ligament; 1/3 of the way up from pubic tubercle |
| Popliteal | With knee flexed at right angles palpate deep in the midline |
| Posterior tibial | 1cm behind medial malleolus |
| Dorsalis pedis | Variable—on the dorsum of the foot just lateral to the tendons to the big toe. ❶ Many healthy people have only one foot pulse |

### Referral to vascular surgery

(*E*=Emergency admission; *U*=Urgent; *S*=Soon; *R*=Routine)

- Critical limb ischaemia—*E/U*
- Severe symptoms—*S*
- Job affected—*S/R*
- Uncertainty about diagnosis—*R*
- No better after exercise training—*R*

### The diabetic foot ☐ p.368

### Critical limb ischaemia

**Presentation** Deteriorating claudication and nocturnal rest pain (usually just after fallen asleep—hanging the foot out of bed improves the pain) Ulceration or gangrene results from minor trauma.

**Examination** Look for:

- Atrophic skin changes—pallor, cool to the touch, hairless, shiny.
- On lowering, the leg turns a dusky blue-red colour; on elevation, there is pallor and venous guttering.
- Ulceration—check under the heel and between the toes.
- Swelling suggests that the patient is sleeping in a chair to avoid rest pain or, rarely, pain from deep infection.
- Absent foot pulses—if present, consider alternative diagnosis.
- ABPI<0.5—❶ arterial calcification can result in falsely high readings.

**Management** Analgesia (often requires opiate); refer for urgent vascular surgical assessment.

### Specialist management

- **Angiography** to assess extent and position of disease.
- **Percutaneous transluminal angioplasty ± stenting** Most suitable for short occlusions/stenoses of the iliac and superficial femoral vessels. 1y patency rate 80–90%.
- **Surgery** Most suitable for longer occlusions/multiple stenoses— aortobifemoral bypass grafts have 5y patency rates >90%; femoropopliteal bypass grafting gives 5y patency rates of <70%. Aspirin ↓ risk of re-occlusion. Amputation is a last option.

### Acute limb ischaemia ☐ p.1122

### Further information

**British Heart Foundation Factfiles** Peripheral vascular disease (9/2001) ☐ www.bhf.org.uk

### Patient information and support

British Vascular Foundation ☐ www.bvf.org.uk

# Varicose veins

Tortuous, twisted, or lengthened veins. Prevalence: 17-31%. ♂ > ♀ (~5:4).
The vein wall is inherently weak → dilatation and separation of valve cusps
so they become incompetent. Blood flows backwards from the deep to
superficial venous system, causing back pressure and further dilatation.

Most varicose veins are primary. Risk factors: age, parity, occupations
requiring a lot of standing, obesity (women only). 2°causes: DVT, pelvic
tumour, pregnancy, or AV fistula.

## Types
- *Trunk* Varicosities of the long or short saphenous vein or their
  branches. May be symptomatic.
- *Reticular* Usually asymptomatic. Dilated tortuous subcutaneous veins
  not belonging to the main branches of the long or short saphenous
  vein.
- *Telangectasia* Spider veins, star bursts, thread veins, or matted veins.
  Intradermal venules <1 mm. Unsightly, but otherwise asymptomatic.

## Presentation *Consider*:
- *Why is the patient consulting now?* Patients are often worried about
  appearance of varicose veins or prognosis if left untreated but have no
  other symptoms attributable to the veins (1:3 consultations).
- *Symptoms* Heaviness, tension, aching (worse on standing and in the
  evening; improved by elevating the leg and support stockings), itching.
- *PMH* Previous surgery or injection for varicose veins; pregnancy; past
  history of DVT or thrombophlebitis; COC pill or HRT.
- *FH* Varicose veins or DVT.

## Examination
- *Abdominal examination* to exclude 2° causes.
- *Veins* With the patient standing, inspect distribution of the veins and
  any 2° skin changes. Patterns of distribution:
  - *Long saphenous distribution*—thigh and medial aspect of the calf.
  - *Short saphenous distribution*—below the knee on the posterior and
    lateral aspects of the calf.

**Management** Reassurance is often all that is needed.
- *If symptoms are troublesome* Advise support stockings; avoid standing
  for prolonged periods and if standing do not stand still; walk regularly;
  ↓ weight (if obese).
- *If any complications or severe symptoms* Refer for surgical assessment.
  In general, patients with purely cosmetic problems are not treated
  under the NHS.

**Bleeding varicose veins** Bleeding can be stemmed by raising the foot
above the level of the heart and applying compression. If the patient is fit
for surgery, refer for surgical assessment. Once recovered from the bleed,
advise compression hosiery.

## Complications
- Haemorrhage
- Varicose eczema
- Skin pigmentation
- Thrombophlebitis
- Oedema
- Venous ulceration—40% do not have visible varicose veins.
- *Atrophie blanche*—white lacy scars
- Lipodermatosclerosis—fibrosis of the dermis and subcutis around the ankle → firm induration.

**COC pill and HRT** Women with varicose veins taking the COC pill or HRT are not at ↑ risk of DVT but are at ↑ risk of thrombophlebitis.

**Saphena varix** Dilatation of the saphenous vein at its confluence with the femoral vein which transmits a cough impulse. May have bluish tinge and disappear on lying down. A cause of a lump in the groin. Action only needed if symptomatic.

**Thrombophlebitis** Presents as severe pain, erythema, pigmentation over and hardening of the vein. Thrombophlebitis in varicose veins results from stasis. Consider underlying malignancy or thrombophilia if thrombophlebitis occurs in normal veins; there is recurrent thrombophlebitis in varicose veins.

*Management* There is no indication for antibiotics.
- Crepe bandaging to compress vein and minimize propogation of thrombus.
- Analgesia—preferably NSAID.
- Ice packs and elevation.
- Low dose aspirin 75 150mg od.

⚠ If phlebitis extends up the long saphenous vein towards the saphenofemoral junction, refer for urgent duplex scanning—saphenofemoral ligation may be indicated if thrombus extends into the femoral vein.

*Follow-up* If the patient is fit for surgery, refer for surgical assessment as thrombophlebitis tends to recur if the underlying venous abnormality is not corrected.

❶ History of thrombophlebitis is a contraindication to the COC pill and a reason to stop for current users. Evidence regarding HRT is less clear.

**Thrombophlebitis migranes** Recurrent tender nodules affecting veins throughout the body. Associated with carcinoma of the pancreas.

## Patient information
**British Vascular Foundation** 🖳 www.bvf.org.uk

# Deep vein thrombosis (DVT)

Deep vein thrombosis may be proximal—involving veins above the knee—or isolated to the calf veins. May also occur in the cerebral sinus, and veins of the arms, retina, and mesentery. *Incidence:* 1 in 1000 people/y in developed countries.

## Risk factors
- Age >40y
- Smoking
- Obesity
- Immobility
- Recent long-distance travel
- Pregnancy
- Puerperium
- COC pill/HRT use
- Surgery
- Recent trauma
- Malignancy
- Heart failure
- Nephrotic syndrome
- Inflammatory bowel disease
- PMH of venous thromboembolism
- Inherited thrombophilic clotting disorders
- Other chronic illness.

**Presentation** Unilateral leg pain, swelling, and/or tenderness ± mild fever, pitting oedema, warmth, and distended collateral superficial veins.

## Differential diagnosis
- Cellulitis
- Haematoma
- Ruptured Baker's cyst
- Superficial thrombophlebitis
- Chronic venous insufficiency
- Venous obstruction
- Post-thrombotic syndrome
- Acute arterial ischaemia
- Lymphoedema
- Fracture
- Hypoproteinaemia.

**Immediate action** Clinical diagnosis is unreliable. <50% with clinically suspected DVT have diagnosis confirmed on diagnostic imaging. Refer all suspected DVTs for further assessment. Specialist assessment: Clinical probability scores are used to decide whether patients fall into high or low probability groups for DVT.
- *If low probability* a blood D-dimer test is done (detects a degradation product of fresh venous thrombus). If the D-dimer test is –ve DVT is excluded. If +ve, the patient is assessed as if medium/high probability.
- *If medium/high probability* USS assessment is undertaken. If USS is negative and low probability or –ve D-dimer, DVT is excluded. If USS is +ve, diagnosis of DVT is confirmed. If USS is –ve and medium/high probability or +ve D-dimer, USS is repeated after 1wk or the patient is assessed with venography, CT, or MRI.

## Management of patients with confirmed DVT
- Initial anticoagulation is with low molecular weight heparin (LMWH) followed by oral anticoagulation (warfarin), usually as an out-patient.
- LMWH should be continued for at least 4d and until INR is in therapeutic range for ≥2d. Target INR 2.5 (range 2–3).
- Oral anticoagulants ↓ risk of further thromboembolism and should be continued for 3–6mo after a single DVT (📖 p.670).
- Graduated elastic compression stockings should be worn for >2y as they ↓ risk post-thrombotic leg syndrome by 12–50%.

**Management during pregnancy** 📖 p.823

**Isolated calf DVT** There is some debate as to whether anticoagulation is necessary. Untreated 40–50% extend to proximal DVT and anticoagulation ↓ risk extension. Some specialists prefer to treat with compression stockings and follow with serial USS.

## Complications of DVT

- *Pulmonary embolus* Without treatment 20% with proximal DVT develop PE (📖 p.1086).
- *Post-thrombotic syndrome* Occurs after DVT. Results in chronic venous hypertension causing limb pain, swelling, hyperpigmentation, dermatitis, ulcers, venous gangrene, and lipodermatosclerosis.
- *Recurrent venous thromboembolism* Patients with history of DVT or PE have ↑ risk of recurrence in high-risk situations (trauma, surgery, immobility, pregnancy) and should receive prophylaxis with heparin/oral anticoagulants in such situations.

# Respiratory medicine

# Breathlessness

**Dyspnoea** Sensation of shortness of breath. Speed of onset helps diagnosis (Table 11.1). Try to quantify exercise tolerance (e.g. dressing, distance walked, climbing stairs).

**Acute breathlessness** 📖 p.1084

**Exertional dyspnoea** Breathlessness with exercise. Causes are the same as dyspnoea generally. The New York Heart Association classifies 4 grades of severity.

- *Normal*
- *Moderate* Walking on the level causes breathlessness.
- *Severe* Has to stop due to breathlessness when walking on the flat. All but the lightest housework is impossible.
- *Gross* Slightest effort → severe breathlessness. The patient is almost bed/chair bound.

**Orthopnoea** Dyspnoea on lying flat and relieved by sitting up. Associated with left heart dysfunction, e.g. LVF.

**Paroxysmal nocturnal dyspnoea** Acute form of dyspnoea that causes the patient to awake from sleep. The patient is forced to sit upright or stand out of bed for relief. Associated with pulmonary oedema.

**Combined chest pain and dyspnoea** *Consider*:

- MI
- Pericarditis
- Dissecting aneurysm
- PE
- Oesophageal pain
- Musculoskeletal pain
- Chest infection
- Pulmonary malignancy.

⚠ Refer any patient with symptoms/signs of superior vena cava obstruction (acute breathlessness, headache worse on stooping, swelling of the face and/or neck with fixed elevation of jugular venous pressure) for immediate medical or oncology assessment.[N] Refer any patient with unexplained dyspnoea of >3wk duration for urgent CXR.[N]

**Respiratory rate** Normal rate for an adult is 14 breaths/min at rest. Higher in children:

- Neonate: 30–60 breaths/min
- Infant: 20–40 breaths/min
- 1–3y: 20–30 breaths/min
- 4–10y: 15–25 breaths/min
- >10y: 15–20 breaths/min

↑ **respiratory rate** *Consider*:

- Lung disease, e.g. pneumonia, asthma
- Heart disease, e.g. LVF
- Metabolic disease, e.g. ketoacidosis
- Drugs, e.g. salicylate overdose
- Psychiatric causes, e.g. hyperventilation

↓ **respiratory rate** *Consider*:

- CNS disease, e.g. CVA
- Drugs, e.g. opioids

**Cheyne–Stokes respiration** Breathing becomes progressively deeper and then shallower (± episodic apnoea) in cycles. Causes: brainstem lesions/compression (stroke, ↑ ICP), chronic pulmonary oedema, poor cardiac output. It is enhanced by narcotics.

**Table 11.1** Causes of dyspnoea

| Cause | Acute | Subacute | Chronic |
|---|---|---|---|
| Cardiac disease | Acute LVF<br>Arrhythmia<br>Air hunger due to shock, e.g. 2° to MI, dissecting thoracic aneurysm<br>Pericarditis | Arrhythmia<br>Subacute bacterial endocarditis | CCF<br>Mitral stenosis<br>Aortic stenosis<br>Congenital heart disease |
| Lung disease | Pneumothorax<br>Acute asthma attack<br>PE<br>Acute pneumonitis, e.g. due to inhaling toxic gas | Asthma<br>Infection<br>Exacerbation of COPD<br>Pleural effusion<br>Pneumonia | COPD<br>Cystic fibrosis<br>Fibrosing alveolitis<br>Occupational lung diseases<br>Mesothelioma<br>Lung cancer |
| Other | Hyperventilation<br>Foreign body inhalation<br>Guillain–Barré syndrome<br>Altitude sickness<br>Ketoacidosis<br>Polio<br>Musculoskeletal chest pain<br>Oesophageal pain | Aspirin poisoning<br>Myaesthenia gravis<br>Thyrotoxicosis | Kyphoscoliosis<br>Anaemia<br>MND<br>MS |

**Hyperventilation** May be fast (>20 breaths/min) or deep (tidal volume ↑). If inappropriate results in palpitations, dizziness, faintness, tinnitus, chest pains, perioral and peripheral tingling (due to plasma $Ca^{2+}$ ↓). *Causes include:*
- Anxiety (most common cause)
- Early pulmonary oedema
- PE
- Hyperthyroidism
- Fever
- Lymphangitis
- Weakness of the respiratory muscles.

**Kussmaul respiration** Deep sighing breathing that is principally seen in metabolic acidosis e.g. diabetic ketoacidosis and uraemia.

**Neurogenic hyperventilation** Due to stroke, tumour, or CNS infection.

**Hypoventilation** Abnormally decreased pulmonary ventilation. Respiration may be too slow or tidal volume ↓. *Causes include:*
- Respiratory depression, e.g. opioid analgesia, anoxia, trauma.
- Neurological disease, e.g. Guillain–Barré syndrome, polio, motor neuron disease, syringobulbia.
- Lung disease, e.g. pneumonia, collapse, pneumothorax, pleural effusion.
- Respiratory muscle disease, e.g. myasthenia gravis, dermatomyositis.
- Limited chest movement, e.g. kyphoscoliosis.

**Pneumothorax** 📖 p.1086

**Further information**
**NICE** Referral guidelines for suspected cancer (2005) 🖳 www.nice.org.uk

# Cough

A cough is a reaction to irritation anywhere from pharynx to lungs.

**Acute cough (<3wk)** *Causes:*

- URTI
- Croup
- Tracheitis
- Acute bronchitis
- Pneumonia—productive, loose cough
- Acute exacerbation of asthma normally well controlled
- Inhaled foreign body—especially in well children.

Reserve CXR for patients with marked focal chest signs or where inhalation of foreign body or lung cancer is suspected.

**Management** Treat the cause where possible; advise OTC cough mixture as needed, e.g. simple linctus; steam inhalation often eases symptoms temporarily; review if not clearing.

**Reasons to prescribe antibiotics immediately[N]** Investigate further and/or give antibiotics (e.g. amoxicillin 250mg tds/erythromycin 250mg qds) immediately if the patient:

- Is systemically very unwell or has symptoms/signs suggestive of serious illness and/or complications e.g. pneumonia.
- Is at high risk of serious complications because of pre-existing comorbidity, e.g. significant heart, lung, renal, liver or neuromuscular disease, immunosuppression, CF, and young children born prematurely.
- Is aged >65y with acute cough and ≥2 or more of the following, or aged >80y with acute cough and ≥1 of the following:
  - Hospitalization in the previous year
  - Type 1 or type 2 DM
  - History of congestive heart failure
  - Current use of oral glucocorticoids.

**Chronic cough (>3wk)** *Causes:*

- Post-nasal drip
- Post viral
- COPD/asthma
- Lung cancer
- Pertussis
- TB
- Bronchiectasis
- Pulmonary oedema
- Foreign body
- Vocal cord palsy
- GORD
- LVF
- Drug-induced (e.g. ACE inhibitors)
- Smoker's cough
- Idiopathic
- Ear wax
- Psychogenic.

⚠ **Red flags** Weight ↓, night sweats.

**Management** Refer any patient with a persistent cough for >3wk for urgent CXR.[N] Treat the cause. If no cause is found, refer.

## Sputum

- Absolutely clear sputum is probably saliva.
- Smoking is the leading cause of excess sputum production—look for black specks of inhaled carbon.
- Yellow-green sputum is due to cell debris (bronchial epithelium, neutrophils, eosinophils) and is not always infected.
- Bronchiectasis causes copious greenish sputum.
- Blood-stained sputum (haemoptysis) always needs full investigation.
- Pink froth suggests pulmonary oedema.

**Haemoptysis** Expectoration of blood/blood-stained sputum. *Causes:*

- Infection—bronchitis, pneumonia, lung abscess, TB
- Violent coughing
- Bronchiectasis
- Lung cancer
- PE (blood is not mixed with sputum)
- Inhaled foreign body
- Iatrogenic: anticoagulation, endotracheal tube
- Trauma
- Cardiac: acute LVF, mitral stenosis
- Blood dyscrasia/bleeding diathesis
- Idiopathic pulmonary haemosiderosis
- Bronchial adenoma
- Mycosis, e.g. aspergilloma
- Goodpastures syndrome
- Collagen vascular disease, e.g. PAN, Wegener's granulomatosis
- Unknown.

❶ Differentiate from haematemesis or local bleeding from the nasopharynx or sinuses. Melaena may occur if enough blood is swallowed.

*Management* *Always* requires investigation to find the cause.

- Admit as an acute medical emergency if the patient is compromised by the bleeding (i.e. tachycardia, low BP, postural drop) or has symptoms/signs of a cause requiring acute admission (e.g. PE, acute LVF).
- If not compromised by the bleeding, refer for urgent CXR.[N]
- Refer for urgent chest physician assessment if abnormal CXR, persistent haemoptysis with normal CXR, aged >40y and smoker/ex-smoker, or normal CXR but high suspicion of lung cancer.[N]

❶ In patients with lung cancer who have a massive haemoptysis, consider whether it is a terminal event. If so, consider treating with IV morphine/diamorphine and a sedative (e.g. midazolam or rectal diazepam) rather than admitting.

**Bronchiectasis** Consider in any patient with persistent or recurrent chest infections. Permanently dilated bronchi act as sumps for infected mucus. *Causes:*

- *Congenital* CF, Kartagener syndrome.
- *Post-infection* TB, pertussis, measles, pneumonia.
- *Other* Bronchial obstruction, aspergillosis (🕮 p.336), hypogammaglobulinaemia (🕮 p.681), gastric aspiration.

*Presentation*

- *Mild cases* Asymptomatic with winter exacerbations consisting of fever, cough, purulent sputum, pleuritic chest pain, dyspnoea.
- *More severe cases* Persistent cough and sputum, haemoptysis, clubbing, low-pitched inspiratory and expiratory crackles and wheeze.

*Investigations* CXR; sputum—M,C&S; spirometry—reversible airways obstruction is common; high-resolution CT detects disease in 97% cases.

*Management* Refer to a respiratory physician. Treatment includes physiotherapy, antibiotics, bronchodilators, vaccination (influenza and pneumococcal), and (rarely) surgery.

**Further information**

NICE 🖳 www.nice.org.uk

- Referral guidelines for suspected cancer (2005)
- Respiratory tract infections—antibiotic prescribing (2008).

# Chest signs

### Chest deformity

- *Barrel chest* The antero-posterior diameter of the chest is high compared with the lateral diameter, and expansion is ↓. Ribs move in a pump-handle up-and-down motion. Associated with chronic hyperinflation (e.g. asthma or COPD).
- *Pigeon chest (pectus carinatum)* Prominent sternum and flat chest associated with history of chronic childhood asthma or rickets.
- *Funnel chest (pectus excavatum)* The lower end of sternum is depressed. Often inherited or idiopathic and usually harmless.
- *Kyphosis* ↑ forward spinal convexity usually affecting thoracic spine.
  - *Postural* ('drooping shoulders' or 'roundback'): is common and voluntarily correctable.
  - *Structural:* cannot correct voluntarily. Causes: osteoporosis, Paget's disease, ankylosing spondylitis, Scheuermann's disease. May cause a restrictive ventilatory defect and eventually respiratory failure.
- *Scoliosis* 📖 p.486
- *Harrison's sulcus* Groove deformity of the lower ribs at the diaphragm attachment site. Suggests chronic childhood asthma or rickets.
- *Scars* Are there any scars indicative of previous chest surgery?

**Chest expansion** Expansion should be symmetrical and equal. If not, suspect chest pathology (e.g. consolidation, collapse, pneumothorax, effusion) on the side with ↓ movement.

### Vocal fremitus or resonance

- ↑ *transmission* implies consolidation. Even whispered sounds are heard clearly with a stethoscope (**whispering pectoriloquy**).
- ↓ *transmission* implies something in the way blocking the transmission of sound. Consider air (e.g. pneumothorax), fluid (e.g. effusion), pleural thickening (e.g. mesothelioma).

**Percussion** Define any areas of dullness to percussion by percussing from a resonant to dull area. *Interpretation:*

- ↑ resonance—emphysema or pneumothorax (📖 p.1086).
- ↓ resonance—consolidation, collapse, abscess, tumour, fibrosis.
- Stony dullness—pleural effusion.

**Breath sounds** Assess character of breath sounds and added sounds:

- *Bronchial breathing* Breath sounds are harsher than normal and there is an audible gap between inspiration and expiration—often caused by lung consolidation, e.g. due to pneumonia.
- ↓ *breath sounds* Consider pleural effusion, pneumothorax, emphysema, lung collapse.
- *Added sounds* Pleural rub, wheeze, crepitations/crackles.

**Wheeze** Musical sound heard during expiration.

- *Polyphonic wheeze* indicates narrowing of many small airways—typical of asthma or COPD.
- *Monophonic wheeze* indicates single large airway obstruction, e.g. due to foreign body or tumour.

**Crackles in the chest** Produced by air flow moving secretions.
- *Fine crackles* Consider pulmonary oedema (early inspiratory—usually best heard at the lung bases at the back); early pneumonia; fibrosing alveolitis (late inspiratory).
- *Coarse crackles* Consider TB; resolving pneumonia; bronchiectasis; lung abscess.

**Pleural rub** Creaking sound produced by movement of visceral over parietal pleura when both are inflamed (e.g. pneumonia, infarction).

**Pleural effusion** Fluid in the pleural cavity. Simple effusions may be transudates (<30g/L protein) or exudates (>30g/L protein). Effusions may also be blood, lymph, or pus (empyema). *Causes of simple effusion:*
- Malignancy e.g. lung cancer, mesothelioma, Meig's syndrome
- Infection (e.g pneumonia, TB)
- Infarction (PE)
- Heart failure
- Constrictive pericarditis
- Inflammation (SLE, RA, pancreatitis, asbestos exposure)
- Hypoproteinaemia
- Hypothyroidism.

**Presentation** May be incidental finding on CXR. *Symptoms:* dyspnoea, pleuritic pain, symptoms of underlying cause. *Signs:* absent breath sounds, dullness to percussion, ↓ tactile vocal fremitus, ↓ vocal resonance. Above the effusion there is usually a zone of bronchial breathing. Early on there may be a pleural rub. Large effusions shift the mediastinum away from the affected side and there may be ↓ chest wall movement. Confirm with CXR. If cause is not immediately apparent refer for diagnostic tap.

**Management** Treat the underlying cause. Refer for drainage if symptomatic. Repeated drainage ± pleurodesis may be necessary.

**Surgical emphysema** Air in the subcutaneous tissue. Can be caused by spontaneous pneumothorax or trauma to the chest wall. Tissues appear swollen and crackle on palpation.

**Table 11.2** Chest signs associated with common chest pathology

|  | Consolidation e.g. pneumonia | Pleural effusion | Collapsed lung | Pneumothorax |
|---|---|---|---|---|
| Mediastinum | Not displaced | Normal or displaced away from the effusion | Displaced towards the side of collapse | Displaced away from the side of pneumothorax |
| Expansion | ↓ | ↓ | ↓ | ↓ |
| Percussion | Dull | Stony dull | Dull | Hyper-resonant |
| Breath sounds | Bronchial breathing | ↓ | ↓ | ↓ |
| Added sounds | Crackles ± rub | Bronchial breathing above effusion | None | None |
| Other | ↑ vocal resonance, whispering pectoriloquy | ↓ vocal resonance | | ↓ vocal resonance |

⚠ Refer all patients with unexplained chest signs lasting > 3wk for urgent CXR[N]

# Other signs of respiratory disease

**Weight loss** Non-specific symptom or sign. *Consider:*
- *GI causes* Malabsorption, malnutrition, dieting.
- *Chronic disease* Hyperthyroidism, DM, COPD, heart failure, renal disease, degenerative neurological/muscle disease, chronic infection (e.g. TB, HIV).
- *Malignancy.*
- *Psychiatric causes* Depression, dementia, anorexia.

⚠ Refer any patient with unexplained weight loss for urgent CXR.[N]

**Cachexia** Severe generalized muscle wasting. *Causes:* neoplasia, malnutrition, chronic infection (e.g. TB), prolonged inactivity, dementia.

**Night sweats** *Consider:* TB, lymphoma, leukaemia, solid tumour (e.g. renal carcinoma), menopause, anxiety states.

**Erythema nodosum** 📖 p.601.

**Peripheral oedema** 📖 p.240.

**Horner's syndrome** Sympathetic nerve disruption to the iris causes
- Small (meiotic) pupil with lack of pupil dilation in the dark
- Partial lid ptosis
- Anhydrosis of the forehead *and*
- Enophthalmos.

*Causes*
- Pancoast, cervical cord, or mediastinal tumour
- Aortic aneurysm
- Posterior inferior cerebellar artery or basilar artery occlusion
- Hypothalamic lesion
- Syringomyelia.

*J.F. Horner (1831–1886)—Swiss ophthalmologist.*

**Pallor** Check eyes/mucous membranes for pallor suggesting anaemia.

**Cyanosis** 📖 p.240.

**Flapping tremor/asterixis** Bilateral motor disturbance. Ask the patient to hold his hands straight out in front of him and dorsiflex them—this provokes a flapping, asynchronous tremor which is absent at rest. Due to $CO_2$ retention in severe COPD.

**Lymphadenopathy** 📖 p.936.

⚠ Refer any patient with supraclavicular or cervical lymphadenopathy persisting >3wk for urgent CXR.[N]

⚠ Refer any unexplained lump in the neck of recent onset or any previously undiagnosed neck lump that has changed over a period of 3–6wk for urgent further investigation.[N]

**Clubbing** 📖 p.607.

⚠ Refer any patient with unexplained nail clubbing for urgent CXR.[N]

**Yellow nails** 📖 p.606.
**Hoarseness** 📖 p.934.

⚠ *Refer urgently for chest X-ray (CXR)*[N] ALL patients with hoarseness for >3wk—particularly smokers aged >50y and heavy drinkers.
- *If there is a POSITIVE finding on CXR* refer urgently to a team specializing in the management of lung cancer.
- *If there is a NEGATIVE finding on CXR* refer urgently to a team specializing in the management of head and neck cancer.

**Stridor** 📖 p.935.
**Jugular venous pressure** 📖 p.241.

**Trachea**
- Palpate the trachea in the supraclavicular notch in the midline.
- Deviation to the left or right suggests a shift of the upper mediastinum to that side.
- The distance between the suprasternal notch and cricoid cartilage in an adult is 2–3 finger-breadths. If it is less than this, the lungs are probably hyperinflated.

**Further information**
**NICE** Referral guidelines for suspected cancer (2005) 🖥 www.nice.org.uk

# Respiratory investigations

## Indications for urgent CXR[N]

- Haemoptysis
- Any of the following if unexplained or present for more >3wk:
  - cough
  - chest/shoulder pain
  - dyspnoea
  - weight loss
  - chest signs
  - hoarseness
  - finger clubbing
  - cervical/supraclavicular lymphadenopathy
  - signs suggesting metastases (brain, bone, liver, skin).

**Peak flow** A simple and cheap test. Peak flow is not a good measure of airflow limitation as it tends to overestimate lung function. It is best used to monitor progress of disease and effects of treatment for patients with asthma. Link with self-management plan (📖 p.318). Peak flow meters are available on NHS prescription. Since 2004, EN 13826/EU standard peak flow meters are supplied. Peak flow charts are available from NHS supplies (form FP1010) and drug companies.

## Measuring peak expiratory flow rate (PEFR)

- Ask the patient to stand up (if possible) and hold the peak flow meter horizontally. Check the indicator is at zero and the track clear.
- Ask the patient to take a deep breath and blow out forcefully into the peak flow meter ensuring lips are sealed firmly around the mouthpiece.
- Read the PEFR off the meter. The best of three attempts is recorded.
- Consider using a low-range meter if predicted or best PEFR is <250L/min.
- Normal values—see Table 11.4 (📖 p.312).

**Spirometry** Measures the volume of air the patient is able to expel from the lungs after a maximal inspiration.

- $FEV_1$ Volume of air the patient is able to exhale in the first second of forced expiration.
- **FVC** Total volume of air the patient can forcibly exhale in 1 breath.
- $FEV_1/FVC$ Ratio of $FEV_1$ to FVC expressed as a percentage.

## Measuring $FEV_1$ and FVC

- Sit the patient comfortably.
- Ask the patient to take a deep breath in.
- Ask the patient to blow the whole breath out as hard as possible until there is no breath left to expel, ensuring lips are sealed firmly around the mouthpiece.
- Encourage the patient to keep breathing out.
- Repeat the procedure twice (i.e. three attempts in all).
- At least two readings should be within 100mL or 5% of each other.
- Normal values—see Table 11.5 (📖 p.313).

**Flow–volume measurement** Available with some spirometers (Figure 11.1).

**RCP three questions** Useful tool to identify patients with poor asthma control in general practice and monitor effect of changes of treatment. Morbidity categories correlate with lung function.

### In the last month
- Have you had any difficulty sleeping because of your asthma symptoms (including cough)?
- Have you had your usual asthma symptoms during the day (cough, wheeze, chest tightness, or breathlessness)?
- Has your asthma interfered with your usual activities, e.g. housework, work/school etc?

NO to all questions = low morbidity
1 × YES = medium morbidity
2× or 3× YES = high morbidity

❶ Alternatives include the Asthma Control Questionnaire (ACQ) and Asthma Control Test (ACT). These questionnaires are not designed for use during an acute attack.

**Table 11.3** Interpretation of spirometry results

|  | **Restrictive lung disease** e.g. fibrosing alveolitis | **Obstructive lung disease** e.g. COPD |
|---|---|---|
| FEV$_1$ (% of predicted normal) | ↓(<80%) | ↓(<80%) |
| FVC (% of predicted normal) | ↓(<80%) | Normal or ↓ |
| FEV$_1$/FVC | Normal (>70%) | ↓(<70%) |

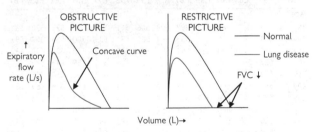

**Fig. 11.1** Flow–volume curves for patients with restrictive and obstructive lung disease

Reproduced from the British Thoracic Society Guidelines. Spirometry in practice: a practical guide to using spirometry in primary care. 🖳 www.brit-thoracic.org.uk

### Further information
**NICE** Referral guidelines for suspected cancer (2005) 🖳 www.nice.org.uk
**British Thoracic Society** Spirometry in practice: a practical guide to using spirometry in primary care. Available from 🖳 www.brit-thoracic.org.uk
**ARTP/BTS Certificate in Spirometry** Further details and list of approved training centres is available from ☎ 0121 354 8200

# Normal spirometry and peak flow values

**Table 11.4** Predicted PEFR measurements in L/min (EU scale)

**Children** Height is the only determinant of PEFR in children. With ↑ age the pattern of adult values takes over.

| Height (ft) | 3' | 3'4" | 3'8" | 4' | 4'4" | 4'8" | 5' | 5'4" | 5'8" | 6' |
|---|---|---|---|---|---|---|---|---|---|---|
| m | 0.9 | 1 | 1.1 | 1.2 | 1.3 | 1.4 | 1.5 | 1.6 | 1.7 | 1.8 |
| PEFR (L/min) | 88 | 105 | 136 | 172 | 220 | 265 | 313 | 371 | 427 | 487 |

## Women

| Ht (ft) | 4'10" | 4'11" | 5' | 5'1" | 5'2" | 5'3" | 5'4" | 5'5" | 5'6" | 5'7" | 5'8" | 5'9" | 5'10" |
|---|---|---|---|---|---|---|---|---|---|---|---|---|---|
| m | 1.47 | 1.5 | 1.52 | 1.55 | 1.57 | 1.6 | 1.62 | 1.65 | 1.67 | 1.7 | 1.72 | 1.75 | 1.77 |
| **Age** | | | | | | | | | | | | | |
| 15y | 379 | 382 | 385 | 389 | 391 | 394 | 397 | 400 | 402 | 405 | 407 | 411 | 413 |
| 20y | 402 | 406 | 409 | 413 | 416 | 419 | 422 | 425 | 428 | 431 | 434 | 437 | 439 |
| 25y | 415 | 419 | 422 | 426 | 429 | 433 | 435 | 439 | 441 | 445 | 447 | 451 | 453 |
| 30y | 419 | 424 | 427 | 431 | 433 | 437 | 440 | 444 | 446 | 450 | 452 | 456 | 458 |
| 35y | 418 | 423 | 425 | 430 | 432 | 436 | 439 | 443 | 445 | 449 | 451 | 454 | 457 |
| 40y | 413 | 417 | 420 | 424 | 427 | 431 | 433 | 437 | 439 | 443 | 445 | 449 | 451 |
| 45y | 405 | 409 | 412 | 416 | 418 | 422 | 425 | 428 | 431 | 434 | 436 | 440 | 442 |
| 50y | 394 | 399 | 401 | 405 | 407 | 411 | 414 | 417 | 419 | 423 | 425 | 428 | 430 |
| 55y | 383 | 387 | 389 | 393 | 395 | 399 | 401 | 404 | 407 | 410 | 412 | 415 | 417 |
| 60y | 370 | 373 | 376 | 379 | 382 | 385 | 387 | 391 | 393 | 396 | 398 | 401 | 403 |
| 65y | 356 | 360 | 362 | 366 | 368 | 371 | 373 | 376 | 378 | 381 | 383 | 386 | 388 |
| 70y | 343 | 346 | 348 | 351 | 353 | 356 | 358 | 361 | 363 | 366 | 368 | 371 | 372 |

## Men

| Ht (ft) | 5'2" | 5'3" | 5'4" | 5'5" | 5'6" | 5'7" | 5'8" | 5'9" | 5'10" | 5'11" | 6' | 6'1" | 6'2" |
|---|---|---|---|---|---|---|---|---|---|---|---|---|---|
| m | 1.57 | 1.6 | 1.62 | 1.65 | 1.67 | 1.7 | 1.72 | 1.75 | 1.77 | 1.8 | 1.82 | 1.85 | 1.87 |
| **Age** | | | | | | | | | | | | | |
| 15y | 479 | 485 | 489 | 494 | 498 | 503 | 506 | 511 | 515 | 520 | 523 | 528 | 531 |
| 20y | 534 | 540 | 545 | 551 | 555 | 561 | 565 | 571 | 575 | 580 | 584 | 589 | 593 |
| 25y | 568 | 575 | 580 | 587 | 591 | 598 | 602 | 608 | 612 | 618 | 622 | 628 | 632 |
| 30y | 587 | 594 | 599 | 606 | 611 | 617 | 622 | 628 | 633 | 639 | 643 | 649 | 653 |
| 35y | 594 | 601 | 606 | 613 | 618 | 625 | 629 | 636 | 640 | 646 | 650 | 657 | 661 |
| 40y | 592 | 599 | 604 | 611 | 615 | 622 | 627 | 633 | 637 | 644 | 648 | 654 | 658 |
| 45y | 582 | 590 | 594 | 601 | 606 | 612 | 617 | 623 | 627 | 634 | 638 | 644 | 647 |
| 50y | 568 | 575 | 580 | 586 | 591 | 597 | 601 | 608 | 612 | 618 | 622 | 627 | 631 |
| 55y | 550 | 557 | 561 | 568 | 572 | 578 | 582 | 588 | 592 | 598 | 602 | 607 | 611 |
| 60y | 529 | 536 | 540 | 546 | 550 | 556 | 560 | 566 | 570 | 575 | 579 | 584 | 588 |
| 65y | 507 | 513 | 517 | 523 | 527 | 533 | 536 | 542 | 545 | 551 | 554 | 559 | 562 |
| 70y | 484 | 490 | 493 | 499 | 503 | 508 | 511 | 517 | 520 | 525 | 528 | 533 | 536 |

❶ For normal values in age groups/heights not represented on these charts or for conversion from the old Wright scale peak flow meters see 🖥 www.peakflow.com

Table 11.4 adapted from Gregg I, Nunn AJ (1989) *BMJ* **298**, with permission of the BMJ Publishing Group.

**Table 11.5** Predicted $FEV_1$ and FVC measurements (in L)

❶ These values apply for Caucasians. ↓ values by 7% for Asians and 13% for people of African Caribbean origin.

## Women

| Height | ft | 4'11" | 5'1" | 5'3" | 5'5" | 5'7" | 5'9" | 5'11" |
|---|---|---|---|---|---|---|---|---|
|  | m | 1.5 | 1.55 | 1.6 | 1.65 | 1.7 | 1.75 | 1.8 |
| **Age** | | | | | | | | |
| 38–41y | $FEV_1$ | 2.3 | 2.5 | 2.7 | 2.89 | 3.09 | 3.29 | 3.49 |
|  | FVC | 2.69 | 2.91 | 3.13 | 3.35 | 3.58 | 3.80 | 4.02 |
| 42–45y | $FEV_1$ | 2.2 | 2.4 | 2.6 | 2.79 | 2.99 | 3.19 | 3.39 |
|  | FVC | 2.59 | 2.81 | 3.03 | 3.25 | 3.47 | 3.69 | 3.91 |
| 46–49y | $FEV_1$ | 2.1 | 2.3 | 2.5 | 2.69 | 2.89 | 3.09 | 3.29 |
|  | FVC | 2.48 | 2.7 | 2.92 | 3.15 | 3.37 | 3.59 | 3.81 |
| 50–53y | $FEV_1$ | 2 | 2.2 | 2.4 | 2.59 | 2.79 | 2.99 | 3.19 |
|  | FVC | 2.38 | 2.6 | 2.82 | 3.04 | 3.26 | 3.48 | 3.71 |
| 54–57y | $FEV_1$ | 1.9 | 2.1 | 2.3 | 2.49 | 2.69 | 2.89 | 3.09 |
|  | FVC | 2.27 | 2.49 | 2.72 | 2.94 | 3.16 | 3.38 | 3.6 |
| 58–61y | $FEV_1$ | 1.8 | 2 | 2.2 | 2.39 | 2.59 | 2.79 | 2.99 |
|  | FVC | 2.17 | 2.39 | 2.61 | 2.83 | 3.06 | 3.28 | 3.5 |
| 62–65y | $FEV_1$ | 1.7 | 1.9 | 2.1 | 2.29 | 2.49 | 2.69 | 2.89 |
|  | FVC | 2.07 | 2.29 | 2.51 | 2.73 | 2.95 | 3.17 | 3.39 |
| 66–69y | $FEV_1$ | 1.6 | 1.8 | 2 | 2.19 | 2.39 | 2.59 | 2.79 |
|  | FVC | 1.96 | 2.18 | 2.4 | 2.63 | 2.85 | 3.07 | 3.29 |

For women ≥ 70y use the formulae:
- $FEV_1 = (0.0395 \times \text{height in m} \times 100) - (0.025 \times \text{age in y}) - 2.6$
- $FVC = (0.0443 \times \text{height in m} \times 100) - (0.026 \times \text{age in y}) - 2.89$.

## Men

| Height | ft | 5'3" | 5'5" | 5'7" | 5'9" | 5'11" | 6'1" | 6'3" |
|---|---|---|---|---|---|---|---|---|
|  | m | 1.6 | 1.65 | 1.7 | 1.75 | 1.8 | 1.85 | 1.9 |
| **Age** | | | | | | | | |
| 38–41y | $FEV_1$ | 3.2 | 3.42 | 3.63 | 3.85 | 4.06 | 4.28 | 4.49 |
|  | FVC | 3.81 | 4.1 | 4.39 | 4.67 | 4.96 | 5.25 | 5.54 |
| 42–45y | $FEV_1$ | 3.09 | 3.3 | 3.52 | 3.73 | 3.95 | 4.16 | 4.38 |
|  | FVC | 3.71 | 3.99 | 4.28 | 4.57 | 4.86 | 5.15 | 5.43 |
| 46–49y | $FEV_1$ | 2.97 | 3.18 | 3.4 | 3.61 | 3.83 | 4.04 | 4.26 |
|  | FVC | 3.6 | 3.89 | 4.18 | 4.47 | 4.75 | 5.04 | 5.33 |
| 50–53y | $FEV_1$ | 2.85 | 3.07 | 3.28 | 3.5 | 3.71 | 3.93 | 4.14 |
|  | FVC | 3.5 | 3.79 | 4.07 | 4.36 | 4.65 | 4.94 | 5.23 |
| 54–57y | $FEV_1$ | 2.74 | 2.95 | 3.17 | 3.38 | 3.6 | 3.81 | 4.03 |
|  | FVC | 3.39 | 3.68 | 3.97 | 4.26 | 4.55 | 4.83 | 5.12 |
| 58–61y | $FEV_1$ | 2.62 | 2.84 | 3.05 | 3.27 | 3.48 | 3.7 | 3.91 |
|  | FVC | 3.29 | 3.58 | 3.87 | 4.15 | 4.44 | 4.73 | 5.02 |
| 62–65y | $FEV_1$ | 2.51 | 2.72 | 2.94 | 3.15 | 3.37 | 3.58 | 3.8 |
|  | FVC | 3.19 | 3.47 | 3.76 | 4.05 | 4.34 | 4.63 | 4.91 |
| 66–69y | $FEV_1$ | 2.39 | 2.6 | 2.82 | 3.03 | 3.25 | 3.46 | 3.68 |
|  | FVC | 3.08 | 3.37 | 3.66 | 3.95 | 4.23 | 4.52 | 4.81 |

For men ≥ 70y use the formulae:
- $FEV_1 = (0.043 \times \text{height in m} \times 100) - (0.029 \times \text{age in y}) - 2.49$
- $FVC = (0.0576 \times \text{height in m} \times 100) - (0.026 \times \text{age in y}) - 4.34$.

# Bronchodilators and steroids

**Bronchodilators** Cause relaxation of bronchial smooth muscle.

*Short-acting ß₂ agonists* (e.g. salbutamol, terbutaline) Safest and most effective $\beta_2$ agonists for use as quick relievers in asthma and COPD.
- Duration of action: ~3–5h. Oral preparations are less effective than inhaled preparations. Prescribe as 1–2 puffs prn.
- Warn patients to seek medical advice if usual dose does not relieve symptoms or relieves symptoms for <3h.
- Regular treatment with bronchodilators alone may be linked with worsening of asthma and asthma deaths. If asthmatic and using >1×/d, consider starting prophylaxis (🕮 p.321).

*Longer-acting ß₂ agonists* (e.g. salmeterol, formoterol)
- *Asthma*, e.g. salmeterol 50–100 micrograms bd as an adjunct to existing corticosteroid treatment (🕮 p.321). Particularly useful for night-time asthma. Usual duration of action is ~12h. Not for relief of acute attacks.
- *COPD* 🕮 p.324.

**Steroids** Short- and long-term treatment of inflammatory conditions.
- *Oral steroids* Prescribe as a single dose in the morning. Often started at high dose (e.g. 40–50mg od) to suppress disease process and then stopped after improvement. If used as maintenance therapy, use the minimum dose that controls disease. Supply with a 'steroid card'.
- *Inhaled steroids* Use regularly to obtain maximum benefit. Alleviation of symptoms occurs 3–7d after initiation. If causes coughing, try a short-acting $\beta_2$ agonist before use. Common unwanted effects are oral candidiasis (5%) and hoarseness—↓ by use of a large volume spacer or mouth washing after use.

**❶** CFC-free beclometasone inhalers should be prescribed by brand name

### Side effects
- ↑BP
- Osteoporosis ± fracture
- Proximal muscle wasting
- Euphoria
- Paranoid states/depression, especially if PMH of psychiatric disorder
- Peptic ulceration—soluble or EC versions may ↓ risk
- Suppression of clinical signs—may allow diseases, e.g. septicaemia, to reach advanced stage before being recognized
- Spread of infection, e.g. chickenpox
- DM/worsening of diabetic control in diabetic patients
- Cushing's syndrome—moon face, striae, and acne
- Adrenal atrophy—can persist years after stopping long-term steroids. Illness/surgical emergencies may need steroid supplements
- Growth suppression in children
- $Na^+$ and water retention; $K^+$ loss.

**Steroid cards** Should be carried by patients on oral/high doses of inhaled steroids. The card informs other practitioners that the patient is on steroids and gives the patient advice on use of steroids and risk of infection.

### Obtaining steroid cards
- England and Wales: R.R. Donnelley ☎ 0161 6832390
- Scotland: Banner Business Supplies: ☎ 01506 448 440.

***Withdrawal of steroids*** Stop abruptly if disease is unlikely to relapse, the patient has received treatment for ≤3wk and is not included in the patient groups described below. Withdraw gradually if disease is unlikely to relapse and the patient has:

• Recently had repeated steroid courses (particularly if taken for >3wk)
• Taken a short course <1y after stopping long-term therapy
• Other possible causes of adrenal suppression
• Received >40mg od of prednisolone (or equivalent)
• Been given repeat doses in the evening
• Received treatment with steroids for >3wk.

During corticosteroid withdrawal, ↓ dose rapidly to physiological levels (~prednisolone 7.5mg od)—thereafter ↓ more slowly. Assess the disease during withdrawal to ensure that relapse does not occur.

## Use of spacers with metred dose inhalers (MDIs)

***Advantages of using a spacer*** Allows more time for evaporation of propellant so a larger proportion of active drug is deposited in the lungs; there is no need to coordinate actuation with inhalation; results in fewer oropharyngeal side effects (e.g. thrush, hoarseness with inhaled steroids).

***Use of spacers*** Both large volumatic spacers and medium-volume devices (e.g. AeroChamber®) are widely available, acceptable, and portable. Inhale the drug from the spacer immediately after actuation as effect of the drugs is short-lived. Spacers should be washed and air-dried weekly to prevent build up of electrostatic charge affecting drug delivery, and replaced every 6–12mo.

***Home nebulizer therapy*** In England and Wales nebulizers are not available via the NHS (but are free of VAT). Some nebulizers are available in Scotland on form GP10A. Nebulizers convert a solution of drug into an aerosol for inhalation. They are used to deliver a higher dosage of drug than is usual with inhalers over a short period of time (5–10min). List of available devices—BNF 3.1.5. *Indications:*

• Acute exacerbations ± regular treatment of asthma/COPD.
• Antibiotic treatment—for patients with chronic purulent infection, e.g. CF, bronchiectasis; prophylaxis and treatment of pneumocystis pneumonia with pentamidine in patients with AIDS.
• Palliative care—palliation of breathlessness and cough, e.g. bronchodilators, lidocaine, or bupivacaine for dry persistent cough.

***Use in asthma/COPD*** Before suggesting long-term use:

• Review diagnosis, technique using hand-held device ± spacer, and compliance.
• Try ↑ dose of bronchodilator via a hand-held device for at least 2wk.
• Perform a 2wk trial of nebulizer therapy and monitor therapeutic effect (e.g. with PEFR in asthma, or dyspnoea score with COPD).
• Provide clear instructions on the use of the nebulizer, monitoring, and when to seek help. Follow up regularly

## Further information

**British Thoracic Society** Current best practice for nebulizer treatment (1997). *Thorax* **52** (Suppl 2), S4–24 ▣ www.brit-thoracic.org.uk

# Asthma in adults

### Symptoms/signs of a severe asthma attack

- Unable to talk in sentences
- Intercostal recession
- PEFR <50% best
- Tachypnoea (respiratory rate > 25 breaths/min)
- Tachycardia (heart rate >110bpm).

### Life threatening signs

- Central cyanosis
- Silent chest (inaudible wheeze)
- Confusion or exhaustion
- PEFR < 33% predicted or best
- Hypotension
- Bradycardia.

### Management of an acute asthma attack 📖 pp.1088–1090

Asthma is a condition of paroxysmal reversible airways obstruction and has three characteristic features:
- Airflow limitation—usually reversible spontaneously or with treatment
- Airway hyper-responsiveness to a wide range of stimuli
- Inflammation of the bronchi.

**Prevalence** European Respiratory Health Survey figures:
- 25% adults aged 20–44y suffer from wheeze
- 15% suffer from wheeze with breathlessness
- 7% have doctor-diagnosed asthma
- Occupational asthma accounts for 1–2% of adult asthma (📖 p.344).

### Asthma in special groups

- *Children* 📖 pp.880–885
- *Occupational asthma* 📖 p.344
- *Pregnancy* 📖 p.820

**Diagnosis of asthma** is based on recognition of a characteristic pattern of symptoms/signs in the absence of an alternative explanation.

### Clinical features that ↑ probability of asthma >1 of the following:

- Wheeze
- Breathlessness
- Chest tightness
- Cough

Particularly if:
- Symptoms are worse:
  - At night/early morning
  - With exercise, allergen and/ or cold air exposure
  - After aspirin/β-blockers
- PH of atopy
- FH asthma and/or atopy
- Widespread wheeze
- Unexplained low $FEV_1$ or PEFR
- Unexplained eosinophilia

### Clinical features that ↓ probability of asthma

- Prominent dizziness, light-headed-ness, peripheral tingling
- Chronic productive cough without wheeze/breathlessness
- Normal examination of chest when symptomatic
- Voice disturbance
- Symptoms with colds only
- Smoking history (>20 pack y)
- Cardiac disease
- Normal PEFR/spirometry when symptomatic

❶ Normal spirometry when asymptomatic does not exclude asthma.

**Tests** Spirometry is the preferred initial test. Interpret PEFR records with caution. They are more useful for monitoring established asthma.

**Differential diagnosis** Airflow obstruction = $FEV_1/FVC < 0.7$

### Airflow obstruction
- COPD
- Bronchiectasis*
- Inhaled foreign body*
- Obliterative bronchiolitis
- Large airway stenosis
- Lung cancer*
- Sarcoidosis*.

### No airflow obstruction
- Chronic cough syndromes
- Hyperventilation syndrome
- Vocal cord dysfunction
- Rhinitis
- Gastro-oesophageal reflux
- Heart failure
- Pulmonary fibrosis.

\* May also be associated with non-obstructive spirometry

## Action

**High probability of asthma** Give trial of treatment with inhaled beclometasone 200 micrograms bd (or equivalent) for 6–8wk. If response is poor despite adequate inhaler technique/concordance, investigate further.

❶ If significant airflow obstruction, there may be inhaled steroid resistance. Treat with oral prednisolone 30mg od for 2wk instead.

### Intermediate probability of asthma
- If $FEV_1/FVC$ <0.7 (i.e. significant airways obstruction) offer reversibility testing and/or trial of treatment. If significant reversibility and/or trial of treatment is beneficial, treat as asthma. If insignificant reversibility and treatment trial is not beneficial, consider tests for alternative diagnoses
- If $FEV_1/FVC$ >0.7 (i.e. no evidence of airways obstruction), arrange further investigations before commencing treatment ± refer.

**Low probability of asthma** Consider alternative diagnoses and investigate/manage accordingly. Reconsider asthma if no response.

**Reversibility testing** for patients with diagnostic uncertainty:
- If airflow obstruction is present at the time of assessment—assess $FEV_1$ (or PEFR) and/or symptoms before and after 400 micrograms inhaled salbutamol via MDI and spacer.
- If no airflow obstruction is present, or response to inhaled salbutamol is uncertain—assess $FEV_1$ (or PEFR) and/or symptoms after trial of treatment with inhaled (beclometasone 200 micrograms bd or equivalent) or oral steroids (prednisolone 30mg od for 14d).

>400 mL ↑ in $FEV_1$ suggests asthma. If smaller improvement, decide whether to continue treatment based on assessment of symptoms. Trial of treatment withdrawal may be helpful if there is doubt.

**Other investigations to consider in primary care** CXR—consider atypical/additional symptoms; eosinophil count

**Reasons for referral** (E=Emergency; U=Urgent; S=Soon; R=Routine)
- Severe asthma exacerbation E
- Monophonic wheeze/stridor E/U
- CXR shadowing U
- Prominent systemic features (myalgia, fever, weight loss) U/S
- Diagnosis unclear S/R
- Unexpected clinical findings (e.g. crackles, clubbing, cyanosis) S/R
- Constant breathlessness S/R
- Poor response to treatment S/R
- Unexplained restrictive spirometry R
- Suspected occupational asthma R
- Chronic sputum production R
- Eosinophilia (>1 × $10^9$/L) R

# Asthma management in practice

**Aims of treatment** to:
- ↓ symptoms and impact on lifestyle (e.g. absence from work/school).
- Minimize the need for reliever medication.
- Prevent severe attacks/exacerbations.

**GP services** Routine asthma care should be carried out in a specialized clinic. Doctors/nurses involved need appropriate training and regular updates. Practices should keep an asthma register to ensure adequate follow up and allow audit. ❶ Not all patients want to attend a pre-arranged appointment. Telephone reviews may be as effective as face-to-face consultations.

**Reviews and monitoring** Frequency depends on needs. Aim to review all patients with asthma at least annually (Figure 11.2).
- Check symptoms since last seen. Use objective measures, e.g. RCP three questions (🕮 p.311)
- Record smoking status and advise smokers to stop.
- Record any exacerbations/acute attacks since last seen.
- Check medication—use, concordance (prescription count—🕮 p.144), inhaler technique, problems, side effects.
- Check influenza/pneumococcal vaccination received.
- Review objective measures of lung function, e.g. home PEFR chart, PEFR/spirometry at review.
- Address any problems or queries and educate about asthma.
- Agree management goals and date for further review.

**Self-management** All patients should receive:
- *Self-management education* Brief simple education linked to patient goals is most likely to be successful. Include information about: nature of disease, nature of the treatment and how to use it, self-monitoring/self-assessment, recognition of acute exacerbations, allergen/trigger avoidance, patients' own goals of treatment.
- *Written action plan* Focus on individual needs. Include information about symptom triggers and peak flow levels which indicate when asthma is worsening, and guidance about what to do under those circumstances. Action plans ↓ morbidity and health costs from asthma.[S]
- *PEFR monitoring* Record PEFR at asthma review and if acute exacerbation. Home monitoring + action plan can be useful, especially for patients with severe asthma, brittle asthma (i.e. rapid development of acute asthma attacks), and/or if poor perceivers of symptoms.

⚠ Be aware that those from ethnic minorities, socially disadvantaged groups, those with communication problems, adolescents, and the elderly have complex needs.

**Management of acute asthma** 🕮 pp.1088–1093.

**Non-pharmacological measures**
- *Smoking* Smoking may ↑ symptoms of asthma—advise to stop.[G]
- *Weight* There is some evidence that weight ↓ in obese patients with asthma results in ↑ asthma control.[R]

- *Allergen avoidance*
  - *House dust mite* There is little evidence that ↓ house dust mite results in clinical improvement.[C] In committed families advise complete barrier bed coverings, removal of carpets, removal of soft toys from bed, high-temperature washing of bed linen, acaricides to soft furnishings, dehumidification. There is no evidence that air ionizers have any beneficial effect.
  - *Pets* There is no evidence that removing pets from a home results in improved symptoms but many experts still advise removal of the pet for patients with asthma who also have an allergy to the pet.

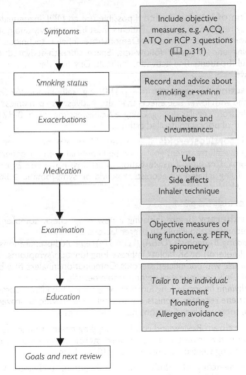

**Fig. 11.2** Summary of the annual asthma review

Reproduced from Lynch J and Simon C. *Respiratory Problems* (2007), with permission of Oxford University Press.

**Drug therapy** 📖 p.320.

**Patient information and support**

**Asthma UK** ☎ 0800 121 6244 🖥 www.asthma.org.uk

# Drug treatment of asthma

**Management of acute asthma** 🕮 pp.1088–1093.

**Use a stepwise approach** (Figure 11.3) Start at the step most appropriate to the initial severity of symptoms. The aim is to achieve early control of the condition and then to ↓ treatment by stepping down.

**Exacerbations** Treat exacerbations early. In adult patients on 200 micrograms inhaled steroids, a 5× ↑ in dose → ↓ severity. Alternatively, and in all other cases, use prednisolone 30-40mg od for 1–2wk.

**Selection of inhaler device** If possible use an MDI. Inadequate technique may result in drug failure. Patients must inhale slowly and hold their breath for 10s after inhalation. Demonstrate inhaler technique before prescribing and check at follow-ups. Spacers/breath-activated devices are useful if patients find activation difficult. Dry powder inhalers are an alternative.

**Short-acting ß₂ agonists** (🕮 p.314), e.g. salbutamol. Work more quickly and with fewer side effects than alternatives. Use prn unless shown to benefit from regular dosing. Using ≥2 canisters/mo. or >10–12 puffs/d is a marker of poorly controlled asthma.

**Inhaled corticosteroids** (🕮 p.314). Most effective preventer for achieving overall treatment goals. May be beneficial even for patients with mild asthma. Consider if exacerbation of asthma in the last 2y requiring steroids, using inhaled ß₂ agonists >3×/wk, or symptomatic ≥3×/wk or ≥1 night/wk.

**Oral steroids** 🕮 p.314

**Add-on therapy** Before initiating a new drug, check compliance and inhaler technique and eliminate trigger factors.
• *Long-acting ß₂ agonists (LABA)* (🕮 p.314)—inhaled preparations (e.g. salmeterol) or SR tablets improve lung function/symptoms. Do not use without inhaled steroids. Combination inhalers may be helpful. Only continue if of demonstrable benefit.
• *Theophylline* Improves lung function/symptoms. Side effects common.
• *Leukotriene receptor agonists*, e.g. montelukast. Provide improvement in symptoms and lung function and ↓ exacerbations.

**Stepping down** Review and consider stepping down at intervals ≥3mo. Maintain on the lowest dose of inhaled steroid-controlling symptoms. When reducing steroids, cut dose by 25–50% each time.

**Complementary therapies** Buteyko breathing technique ↓ symptoms/bronchodilator use. Immunotherapy in specialist clinics is effective for patients with specific allergies. Other complimentary therapies—no convincing evidence of effectiveness.

**Difficult asthma** Persistent symptoms and/or frequent exacerbations despite treatment at step 4/5. Check diagnosis and exacerbating factors. Assess adherence to medication. Find out about family, psychological, or social problems that may be interfering with effective management.

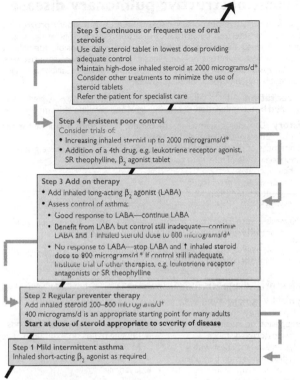

*All doses given refer to hydrofluoroalkane-beclomethasone dipropionate (BDP-HFA) equivalent inhalers. For other drugs/formulations adjust dose accordingly (see BNF Section 3).

**Fig. 11.3** Summary of stepwise management in adults

Reproduced from the 2008 British Guideline on the Management of Asthma with permission from the British Thoracic Society and SIGN.

## Further information
**British Thoracic Society/SIGN** British guideline on the management of asthma (2009) 🖥 www.sign.ac.uk
**BNF** Section 3 🖥 www.bnf.org

# Chronic obstructive pulmonary disease

Chronic obstructive pulmonary disease (COPD) is a slowly progressive disorder characterized by airflow obstruction. Affects 16% of the population in the 40–68y age group ($\male > \female$) and is responsible for ~5% of deaths. Causes: cigarette smoking; genetic (bronchial hyperresponsiveness; $\alpha_1$-antitrypsin deficiency); race (Chinese and African Caribbeans have ↓ susceptibility); diet (poor diet and low birthweight).

**Presentation** Affects different patients in different ways. Diagnosis is suggested by a combination of history, signs, and baseline spirometry.

*History* Consider diagnosis in any patient >35y with a risk factor for COPD (generally smoking) and ≥ 1 of:
- Shortness of breath on exertion—use an objective measure, e.g. MRC dyspnoea scale (Table 11.6) to grade breathlessness.
- Chronic cough.
- Regular sputum production.
- Frequent winter 'bronchitis'.
- Wheeze.

*If diagnosis is suspected also ask about* weight ↓, effort intolerance, waking at night, ankle swelling, fatigue, and occupational hazards.

⚠ Chest pain or haemoptysis are uncommon in COPD—if present consider an alternative diagnosis

**Differential diagnosis** Asthma, bronchiectasis, CCF, lung cancer

**Signs** May be none. *Possible signs:*
- Hyperinflated chest ± poor chest expansion on inspiration
- ↓ cricosternal distance
- Hyperresonant chest with ↓ cardiac dullness on percussion
- Use of accessory muscles
- Paradoxical movement of lower ribs
- Tachypnoea
- Wheeze or quiet breath sounds
- Pursing of lips on expiration (purse lip breathing)
- Peripheral oedema
- Cyanosis
- ↑ JVP
- Cachexia.

**Tests**

*Spirometry* (📖 p.310) Predicts prognosis but not disability/quality of life. A diagnosis of airflow obstruction can be made if:
- $FEV_1/FVC$ <0.7 (<70%) and
- $FEV_1$<70% predicted (QOF criterion) and
- <15% response to a reversibility test.

Reversibility testing may be confusing but is currently required for the quality and outcome framework targets:
- >400mL ↑ in $FEV_1$ following trial of bronchodilator or prednisolone (30mg od for 2wk) suggests asthma.
- Clinically significant COPD is *not* present if $FEV_1$ and $FEV_1/FVC$ return to normal after drug therapy.

*PEFR* (📖 p.310) Patients with COPD have little variability in PEFR. Serial home PEFR measurements can help distinguish between asthma and COPD. PEFR may underestimate severity of airflow limitation, and a normal PEFR does not exclude airflow obstruction.

### Other investigations
- *CXR* indicated to exclude other diagnoses, e.g. lung cancer.
- *FBC* to identify polycythaemia or anaemia.
- *BMI*
- $\alpha_1$-*antitrypsin* if early onset COPD or family history 📖 p.433.
- *ECG/Echo* if cor pulmonale is suspected.
- *Sputum culture* if purulent sputum persistent.

**Table 11.6** MRC Dyspnoea Scale

| Grade | Degree of breathlessness related to physical activity |
|-------|-------------------------------------------------------|
| 1 | Not troubled by breathlessness except on strenuous exercise |
| 2 | Short of breath when hurrying or walking up a slight hill |
| 3 | Walks slower than contemporaries on level ground because of breathlessness or has to stop for breath when walking at own pace |
| 4 | Stops for breath after walking about 100m or after a few minutes on level ground |
| 5 | Too breathless to leave the house or breathless on dressing/undressing. |

Reproduced from Fletcher CM, Elmes PC, Fairbairn MB et al. The significance of respiratory symptoms and the diagnosis of chronic bronchitis in a working population. (1959) BMJ **2**, 257–26, with permission from the BMJ Publishing Group.

**Table 11.7** Comparison of COPD and asthma

| | COPD | Asthma |
|---|------|--------|
| *Symptoms <35y* | Rare | Common |
| *Smoking history* | Nearly all | Maybe |
| *Breathlessness* | Persistent and progressive. Poor response to inhaled therapy—if good reconsider diagnosis | Variable throughout the day and from day to day. Good response to inhaled therapy is typical |
| *Chronic productive cough* | Common | Uncommon |
| *Waking at night with cough/wheeze* | Uncommon | Common |

**Table 11.8** Severity of COPD and expected clinical picture

| Severity | Clinical state | Spirometry |
|----------|----------------|------------|
| *Mild* | Cough but little or no breathlessness. No abnormal signs. No ↑ use of services | FEV$_1$ 50–80% predicted |
| *Moderate* | Breathlessness, wheeze on exertion, cough ± sputum and some abnormal signs. Usually known to GP-intermittent complaints | FEV$_1$ 30–49% predicted |
| *Severe* | SOBOE. Marked wheeze and cough. Usually other signs too. Likely to be known to GP and hospital consultant with frequent problems/admissions | FEV$_1$ <30% predicted |

# Management of COPD

Record values of spirometric tests performed at diagnosis and review. At each review record current symptoms, problems since last seen, exercise tolerance, and smoking status. Educate the patient and family about the disease, medication, and self-help strategies.

## Non-drug therapy

- *Smoking cessation* Most important to improve outcome (Figure 11.4).
- *Vaccination* All patients with COPD should have influenza and pneumococcal vaccination.
- *Exercise* Lack of exercise ↓ FEV₁. Pulmonary rehabilitation is of proven benefit—refer via respiratory physicians if available locally.
- *Nutrition* Weight ↓ in obese patients improves exercise tolerance.

## Screening for depression 📖 p.998.

**Drug therapy** Document effects of each drug treatment on symptoms, quality of life, and lung function as tried (Figure 11.5).

## Management of acute exacerbations 📖 p.326.

## Referral for specialist care

- Uncertain diagnosis
- Age <40y
- Severe COPD
- Rapid decline in FEV₁
- Cor pulmonale
- Frequent infections
- Haemoptysis
- α₁ antitrypsin deficiency

- Assessment for:
  - LTOT
  - Long-term oral steroids
  - Withdrawal of long-term steroids
  - Long-term nebulizer therapy
  - Pulmonary rehabilitation
  - Surgery, e.g. lung transplant.

**Long-term oxygen therapy (LTOT)** *Only* prescribe after evaluation by a respiratory physician. Refer patients with:

- Severe airflow obstruction (FEV₁<30%: consider if 30–49%)
- Cyanosis
- Polycythaemia

- Peripheral oedema
- ↑JVP
- Hypoxaemia (oxygen saturation ≤ 92% breathing air).

Treatment for >15h/d ↑ survival and quality of life. Ambulatory oxygen therapy can ↑ exercise tolerance in some patients. ❶Always warn patients about the fire risks of having pure oxygen in their home.

*O₂ cylinders and associated equipment* Arrangements for supply of oxygen are different in England and Wales, Scotland, and Northern Ireland—see BNF section 3.6. Specify amount of O₂ required (h/d) and flow rate. O₂ concentrators are more economical for LTOT. Supply back-up cylinders in case of breakdown or power cut.

## Further information

**RCP/NICE** Management of chronic obstructive pulmonary disease in adults in primary and secondary care (2004) *Thorax* **59** (Suppl.1), 1–232. 🖳 www.nice.org.uk

## Patient support

**British Lung Foundation** ☎ 0845 850 50 20 🖳 www.lunguk.org

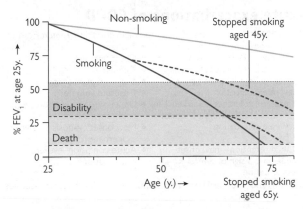

**Fig. 11.4** Effect of smoking on progression of COPD

Reproduced in modified format from: Fletcher CM, Peto R (1977) The natural history of chronic airflow obstruction *BMJ* **1**, 1645–8, with permission from the *BMJ* Publishing Group.

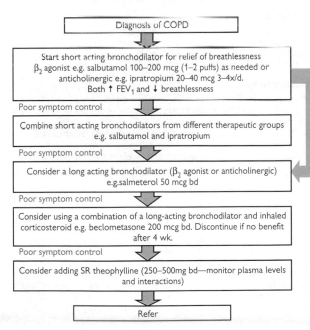

**Fig. 11.5** Drug management of COPD

# Acute exacerbations of COPD

**Presentation** Worsening of previous stable condition. *Features:* ≥ 1 of

- ↑ dyspnoea—marked dyspnoea, tachypnoea (>25breaths/min), use of accessory muscles at rest and purse lip breathing are signs of severe exacerbation
- ↓ exercise tolerance—marked ↓ in activities of daily living is a sign of severe exacerbation
- ↑ fatigue
- ↑ fluid retention—new onset oedema is a sign of severe exacerbation
- ↑ wheeze
- Chest tightness
- ↑ cough
- ↑ sputum purulence
- ↑ sputum volume
- Upper airways symptoms e.g. colds, sore throats,
- New onset cyanosis—severe exacerbation
- Acute confusion—severe exacerbation.

❶ Fever and chest pain are uncommon presenting features—consider alternative diagnosis.

**Causes of exacerbations** 30% have no identifiable cause

- *Infections* Viral upper and lower respiratory tract infections, e.g. common cold, influenza; bacterial lower respiratory tract infections.
- *Pollutants* e.g. nitrous oxide, sulphur dioxide, ozone.

## Differential diagnosis

- Pneumonia
- LVF/pulmonary oedema
- Lung cancer
- Pleural effusion
- Recurrent aspiration.
- Pneumothorax
- PE
- Upper airway obstruction.

## Investigations

- *Pulse oximetry* If available can be used as a measure of severity (saturation ≤92% breathing air suggests hypoxaemia—consider admission) and to monitor progress.
- *CXR* Consider if diagnostic doubt and/or to exclude other causes of symptoms.
- *Sputum culture* Not recommended routinely in the community.[G]

**Management** Decide whether to treat at home or admit to hospital (Table 11.9).

## Home treatment of acute exacerbations

- *Add or ↑ bronchodilators* Consider if inhaler device and technique are appropriate.
- *Start antibiotics* Use broad-spectrum antibiotic, e.g. erythromycin 250–500mg qds if sputum becomes more purulent *or* clinical signs of pneumonia *or* consolidation on CXR.
- *Oral corticosteroids* Start early in the course of the exacerbation if ↑ breathlessness which interferes with daily activities. Dosage—30mg/d prednisolone for 1–2 wk. Consider osteoporosis prophylaxis with a bisphosphonate if frequent courses are required (📖 p.516).

**Table 11.9** Deciding whether to treat acute exacerbations at home or in hospital

*The more features in the 'Treat in hospital column', the more likely the need for admission.*

|  | Treat at home | Treat in hospital* |
|---|---|---|
| Ability to cope at home | Yes | No |
| Breathlessness | Mild | Severe |
| General condition | Good | Poor—deteriorating |
| Level of activity | Good | Poor/confined to bed |
| Cyanosis | No | Yes |
| Worsening peripheral oedema | No | Yes |
| Level of consciousness | Normal | Impaired |
| Already receiving LTOT | No | Yes |
| Social circumstances | Good | Living alone/not coping |
| Acute confusion | No | Yes |
| Rapid rate of onset | No | Yes |
| Significant comorbidity (e.g. cardiac disease, IDDM) | No | Yes |
| Changes on CXR (if available) | No | Present |

* Hospital-at-home schemes and assisted discharge schemes are a suitable alternative

Adapted from Gravil JH, Al Rawas OA, Cotton MM *et al.* Home treatment of exacerbations of chronic obstructive pulmonary disease by an acute respiratory assessment service (1998), *Lancet* **351**: 1853–5, with permission from Elsevier.

## Follow-up

- Reassess as necessary. If the patient deteriorates reconsider the need for hospital admission. If not fully improved in within 2wk consider CXR and hospital referral.
- Reassess patients who have been admitted 4–6wk after discharge. Assess their ability to cope at home. ~1:3 are readmitted within 3mo.
- Reassess inhaler technique and understanding of treatment regime.
- In severe cases, reassess the need for LTOT and/or home nebulizer.
- Check FEV$_1$.
- Emphasize the potential benefit of lifestyle modification—smoking cessation, exercise, weight loss if obese.
- Arrange ongoing regular follow-up.

## Further information

**NICE** Management of chronic obstructive pulmonary disease in adults in primary and secondary care (2004). *Thorax* **59** (Suppl. 1), 1–232
www.nice.org.uk

# Lung cancer

## Referral for suspected lung cancer
### Immediate referral/acute admission
- Stridor
- Superior vena cava obstruction (swelling of face/neck with fixed ↑ JVP).

*Urgent referral* to a team specializing in manage ment of lung cancer
- Persistent haemoptysis (in smokers/ex-smokers aged ≥40y)
- CXR suggestive of lung cancer (including pleural effusion and slowly resolving consolidation)
- Normal CXR where there is high suspicion of lung cancer
- History of asbestos exposure and recent onset of chest pain, shortness of breaath, or unexplained systemic symptoms where a CXR indicates pleural effusion, pleural mass, or any suspicious lung pathology.

### Urgent referral for CXR
- Haemoptysis
- Any of the following if unexplained or present for >3 wk*
  - Cough
  - Chest/shoulder pain
  - Dyspnoea
  - Weight loss
  - Chest signs
  - Hoarseness (refer urgently ENT if CXR is normal)
  - Finger clubbing
  - Cervical or supraclavicular lymphadenopathy
  - Features suggestive of metastases from a lung cancer, e.g. secondaries in the brain, bone, liver, or skin.

* Do not delay for 3wk if high risk of lung cancer, i.e. smoker/ex-smoker, COPD, history of asbestos exposure, previous history of cancer (especially head/neck cancer).

Lung cancer is the most common cancer and 3rd most common cause of death in the UK. Incidence ↑ with age—85% are aged >65y and 1% <40y at presentation. ♂:♀ ≈ 2:1, but incidence is increasing in women.

## Types
- *Small cell lung cancer* Accounts for ~¼ all cases. Often disseminated by the time of diagnosis. Spreads to liver, bones, brain, and adrenals.
- *Non-small cell lung cancer* Mainly adenocarcinoma or squamous cell carcinoma. Not always smoking related.

**Screening** A 2003 Cochrane review concluded that current evidence does not support screening for lung cancer with chest radiography or sputum cytology. Frequent CXR screening might be harmful. results of trials of screening with CT scanning are awaited from the USA but preliminary results do not suggest this will be an effective screening strategy.

## Prevention
- *Smoking cessation* 90% of lung cancer patients are smokers or ex-smokers. The younger a person is when he/she starts smoking, the greater the risk of developing lung cancer. Risk also ↑ with amount smoked (duration of smoking and number of cigarettes smoked/d).

- *Diet* ↑ consumption of fruit, carrots, and green vegetables may ↓ incidence but there is no evidence that vitamin supplements are beneficial and they might be harmful.[C]

**Presentation** >90% have symptoms at the time of diagnosis. Common presenting features:

- Cough (56%)
- Chest/shoulder pain (37%)
- Haemoptysis (7%)
- Dyspnoea
- Hoarseness
- Weight ↓
- Finger clubbing
- General malaise
- Distant metastases
- Incidental finding on CXR.

**Pancoast syndrome** Apical lung cancer + ipsilateral Horner's syndrome. *Cause:* invasion of the cervical sympathetic plexus. *Other features:* shoulder and arm pain (brachial plexus invasion C8-T2) ± hoarse voice/ bovine cough (unilateral recurrent laryngeal nerve palsy and vocal cord paralysis). *H.K. Pancoast (1875–1939)—US radiologist.*

**Paraneoplastic syndromes**, e.g. ectopic ACTH production, SIADH, hypercalcaemia, hypercoagulability. Affect 10–20% of patients with lung cancer particularly small cell. Have a high index of suspicion and refer for specialist management if suspected.

**Management** Once the diagnosis has been confirmed, liaise with the chest physician, specialist lung cancer team, primary health care team, and specialist palliative care services (e.g. Macmillan Nurses). Active treatment options depend on type and extent of tumour, and include surgery, radiotherapy, and/or chemotherapy. Follow up regularly. 80% die in <1y.

*Palliative radiotherapy* Radiotherapy is a key component of symptomatic treatment for:

- Haemoptysis
- Chest pain
- Breathlessness due to bronchial occlusion
- Pain from bone metastasis
- Symptoms from brain metastasis.

Radiotherapy may be combined with palliative chemotherapy, particularly for patients with non-small cell lung cancer.

**Mesothelioma** 📖 p.345.

**Palliative care** 📖 p.1026–1043.

**Further information**
**NICE** 🖥 www.nice.org.uk
- Referral guidelines for suspected cancer (2005)
- The diagnosis and treatment of lung cancer (2005)
**SIGN** Management of lung cancer (2005) 🖥 www.sign.ac.uk

**Information and support for patients**
**Lung Cancer Resources Directory** 🖥 www.cancerindex.org
**Roy Castle Lung Cancer Foundation** ☎ 0800 358 7200
🖥 www.roycastle.org
**Macmillan Cancer Support** ☎ 0808 808 0000 🖥 www.macmillan.org.uk
**British Lung Foundation** ☎ 0845 850 50 20 🖥 www.lunguk.org

# Colds and influenza

**The common cold** Acute, usually afebrile, respiratory tract infection.
- *Causes* Rhino (30–50%), picorna, echo, and Coxsackie viruses. At any one time only a few viruses are prevalent.
- *Spread* Contaminated secretions on fingers and droplet infection. Most people are infected 2–3×/y.
- *Management* Advise patients to take plenty of fluids and paracetamol for symptom relief. Usually symptoms resolve in <1½ wk.
- *Complications* Exacerbation of asthma/COPD; 2° infection (bronchitis, pneumonia, conjunctivitis, OM, sinusitis, tonsillitis). Similar symptoms are caused by the adeno and parainfluenza viruses.

**Acute bronchitis** Inflammation of major bronchi. Often follows viral URTI especially in winter months. Symptoms include cough ± sputum, breathlessness, and wheeze. If signs are present, they include wheeze and scattered coarse crepitations.

*Management* Self-limiting illness (settles in <3wk) in normally healthy people. *Consider:* bronchodilators if wheeze is heard; antibiotics—may shorten symptoms but weigh benefits against possible side effects from antibiotics, ↑ in community antibiotic resistance, and 'medicalizing' a self-limiting condition. If recurrent bronchitis, consider a diagnosis of COPD.

*Reasons to prescribe antibiotics immediately*[N] Investigate further and/or give antibiotics (e.g. amoxicillin 250mg tds/erythromycin 250mg qds) immediately if systemically very unwell; symptoms/signs of serious illness, or complications (e.g. pneumonia); at high risk of serious complications because of pre-existing comorbidity (e.g. significant heart, lung, renal, liver or neuromuscular disease, immunosuppression, CF, or young children born prematurely); aged >65y with acute cough and ≥2 or more of the following, or aged >80y with acute cough and ≥1 of the following:
- Hospitalization in the previous year
- Type 1 or type 2 DM
- History of CCF
- Current use of oral steroids.

**Influenza** Sporadic respiratory illness during autumn and winter causing ~600 deaths/y with epidemics every 2–3y → 10× ↑ in deaths. *Causes:* influenza viruses A, B, or C. *Spread:* droplet infection, person-to-person contact, or contact with contaminated items. *Incubation:* 1–7d.

*Presentation* In mild cases symptoms are like those of a common cold. In more severe cases fever begins suddenly accompanied by prostration and generalized aches/pains. Other symptoms may follow: headache, sore throat, respiratory tract symptoms (usually cough ±coryza). Acute symptoms resolve in <5d, but weakness, sweating, and fatigue may persist longer. 2° chest infection with *Staph. aureus* or *Strep. pneumoniae* is common. Rarely, patients with influenza A (Asian flu) may develop severe viral pneumonia.

*Management* Rest, fluids, and paracetamol for fever/symptom control. Treat complications, e.g. antibiotics for chest infection, treatment of exacerbations of COPD or asthma.

*Antivirals* Zanamivir (10mg bd for 5d by inhalation) and oseltamivir (75mg bd for 5d) are not a 'cure' for influenza but may shorten duration of symptoms and ↓ incidence of complications if started <72h after onset of symptoms. Zanamivir should only be used for adults; oseltamivir can be used for adults or children. Only use:
- For treatment of high-risk groups (Box 11.1—except pregnancy), *and*
- When influenza is prevalent in the community[N]—determined by community-based virological surveillance schemes.

⚠ Zanamivir may cause bronchospasm—avoid in severe asthma and ensure a short-acting bronchodilator is available if the patient has asthma.

### Prevention
- Influenza vaccine is prepared each year from viruses of the 3 strains thought most likely to cause flu that winter. It is ~70% effective (range 30–90%). Protection lasts 1y. Give to high-risk groups (Box 11.1).
- Oseltamivir is recommended for prophylaxis in high-risk patients >13y who are not effectively vaccinated or who live in residential care where a staff member has influenza-like symptoms only when influenza is prevalent in the community. Use at a dose of 75mg od for 7–10d from diagnosis of the latest case in the establishment.[N]

**Pandemic flu** In 2009, pandemic 'swine flu' affected the UK. Emergency arrangements for antiviral provision were put in place and a swine flu vaccination was developed and offered to high risk groups. A severe form of 'bird flu' has affected poultry flocks and other birds in Asian countries. Concern remains that the virus might develop the ability to pass from person to person, sparking a further flu pandemic.

### Box 11.1 Risk factors for severe disease with influenza
- Aged ≥65y *or*
- With ≥ 1 of the following conditions:
  - Chronic respiratory disease including COPD and asthma, or weak respiratory muscles (e.g. MS, MND, CVA)
  - Significant cardiovascular disease excluding hypertension
  - Chronic renal disease
  - Immunosuppression (including hyposplenism)
  - DM.

#### Indications for influenza vaccination
- ≥ 65y
- Chronic renal disease
- DM
- Chronic liver disease
- Chronic lung disease, e.g, asthma, COPD
- Cardiovascular disease (except ↑BP alone)
- Immunocompromised or asplenic patients
- Carers of patients with disabilities
- Patients living in long-stay residential care establishments
- Health professionals expected to be in contact with influenza.

### Further information
NICE ⊡ www.nice.org.uk
- Guidance on the use of zanamivir, oseltamivir and amantadine for the treatment of influenza (2003)
- Respiratory tract infections—antibiotic prescribing (2008).

# Pneumonia in adults

Common condition with annual incidence of ~8 cases/1000 adult population. Incidence ↑ with age and peaks in the winter. Mortality for those managed in the community is <1% but 1 in 4 patients with pneumonia are admitted to hospital and mortality for those admitted is ~9%.

**Presentation** Acute illness is characterized by:
- Symptoms of an acute lower respiratory tract illness (cough + ≥1 other lower respiratory tract symptoms, e.g. purulent sputum, pleurisy)
- New focal chest signs on examination (consolidation or ↓ air entry, coarse crackles, and/or pleural rub).
- ≥1 systemic feature:
  - Sweating, fevers, shivers, aches, and pains *and/or*
  - Temperature ≥38°C.
- No other explanation for the illness.
- ❶ The elderly may present atypically, e.g. 'off legs' or acute confusion.

## Common causative organisms
- *Strep. pneumoniae* (36%) 📖 p.652
- *H. influenzae* (10%)—more common amongst the elderly (📖 p.654).
- Influenza A&B (8%)—annual epidemics during the winter months, ~3% develop pneumonia (📖 p.330).
- *Mycoplasma pneumoniae* (1.3%)—less common in the elderly. Epidemics occur every 4y in the UK (📖 p.336).
- Gram –ve enteric bacteria (1.3%).
- *C. psittaci* (1.3%)—~20% have history of bird contact (📖 p.336).
- *Staph. aureus* (0.8%)—more common in the winter months. May be associated with viral infection, e.g. flu (📖 p.653).
- *Legionella* spp. (0.4%)—most common in September/October; >50% related to travel.

**TB** 📖 p.334          **Immunocompromised patients** 📖 p.648

## Prevention
- Influenza vaccination 📖 p.331
- Pneumococcal vaccination 📖 p.652.

**Differential diagnosis** Pneumonitis, e.g. 2° to radiotherapy, chemical inhalation; pulmonary oedema (may coexist in the elderly); PE

**Investigations** Often unnecessary in general practice. *Consider:*
- *Pulse oximetry* (if available). Use to assess severity. If oxygen saturation is ≤ 92% in air, the patient is hypoxic and requires admission.
- *CXR* If diagnostic uncertainty or symptoms not resolving. CXR changes may lag behind clinical signs but should return to normal <6wk after recovery. Persistent changes on CXR >6wk after recovery require further investigation.
- *Sputum culture* If not responding to treatment. If weight ↓, malaise, night sweats, or risk factors for TB (ethnic origin, history of TB exposure, social deprivation, or elderly), request mycobacterium culture.
- *Blood FBC* ↑ WCC; ESR ↑; acute and convalescent titres to confirm 'atypical' pneumonia (*Legionella, C. psittaci, M. pneumoniae*).

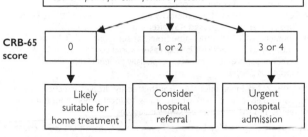

Any of:
- **C**onfusion*
- **R**espiratory rate ≥ 30 breaths/min
- **B**lood pressure (systolic <90mmHg; diastolic ≤ 60mmHg
- Age ≥ **65**y.
*Score 1 point for each feature present*

**CRB-65 score**

| 0 | 1 or 2 | 3 or 4 |

| Likely suitable for home treatment | Consider hospital referral | Urgent hospital admission |

* Defined as new disorientation in person, place, or time

**Fig. 11.6** Assessment of severity and management of pneumonia

Reproduced from the British Thoracic Society Guidelines for the management of community acquired pneumonia in adults (2009)  www.brit-thoracic.org.uk

## Management
- *Consider the need for admission* (Figure 11.6). Have a low threshold for admission if ill but apyrexial, concomitant illness (e.g.CCF, chronic lung, renal or liver disease, DM, cancer), or poor social situation. If life-threatening infection or considerable delay (>2h), consider administering antibiotics before admission.
- *If a decision is made to treat at home*
  - Advise not to smoke, to rest, and to drink plenty of fluids.
  - Start antibiotics, e.g. amoxicillin 500mg–1g tds, erythromycin 500mg tds, or clarithromycin 500mg bd.
  - Treat pleuritic pain with simple analgesia, e.g. paracetamol 1g qds
  - Review within 48h. Reassess clinical state. If deteriorating or not improving consider CXR or admission.

**Complications** Require specialist management—refer.
- Pleural effusion (may be reactive or empyema—pus in the lung cavity).
- Lung abscess (presents with swinging fever and worsening pneumonia).
- Septicaemia.
- Respiratory failure.
- Metastatic infections.
- Jaundice.

## Further information
**British Thoracic Society** Guidelines for the management of community acquired pneumonia in adults (2009)  www.britthoracic.org.uk
**Chapman S** et al. *Oxford Handbook of Respiratory Medicine* (2005) Oxford University Press (ISBN 0198529775).

# Tuberculosis<sup>ND</sup>

Caused by *Mycobacterium tuberculosis*. Worldwide 1.5 billion people have tuberculosis (TB). In the UK 7000 cases of TB are reported each year and 350 patients die. Incidence is increasing and 10% of cases are antibiotic resistant.

**Risk factors** In the UK:
- 40% cases of TB occur in London. TB is an urban disease.
- 70% cases occur in ethnic minority populations—60% in those born abroad (half are diagnosed <5y after entering the country).
- Contacts—if living in the same house as someone with TB, risk is 1:3; if school/work contact risk is 1:50; casual social contact risk is 1:100 000.
- Immunnosuppressed patients—especially patients with HIV.
- Homeless people.

**Primary TB** Initial infection. Transmitted by droplet infection. A lesion forms (usually pulmonary) which drains to local lymph nodes. Immunity develops and the infection becomes quiescent.

*Symptoms/signs* May be none. Fever, night sweats, persistent cough ± sputum/haemoptysis, pneumonia and/or pleural effusion, anorexia and weight loss, erythema nodosum.

*Investigations and management* CXR, sputum samples for culture (state on the form that you are looking for acid-fast bacilli), Tuberculin test +ve (may be −ve if immunocompromised). If diagnosis is confirmed, refer for treatment and contact tracing.

**Post-primary TB** Reactivation of a primary infection. Initial lesions, usually in the upper lobes of the lung, progress and fibrose. Other sites may develop disease. Multiple small lesions throughout the body result in miliary TB which is common in immunocompromised patients. Symptoms and signs relate to the organs infected. In all cases refer for specialist treatment. *Extrapulmonary disease sites:*
- CNS
- Lymph nodes
- Pericardia
- Spine (rarely, other bones/joints)
- Peripheral cold abscess
- Miliary.

**Screening** TB is a notifiable disease. Every time a case of TB is notified, contact tracing is initiated, usually through chest clinics. All contacts are screened for TB with a tuberculin test (Table 11.10).

**Tuberculin skin test** Useful in diagnosis of TB and must be carried out before BCG immunization except for infants <3mo old who have not had any recent contact with TB. Interpretation—Table 11.10. The tuberculin test can be suppressed by: glandular fever infection, viral infections, live viral vaccines (do not do a tuberculin test within 3wk of vaccination), Hodgkin's disease, sarcoidosis, corticosteroid therapy, and immunosuppressant treatment or diseases, including HIV.

⚠ If a patient has a +ve tuberculin test—DO NOT give BCG vaccination.

**Table 11.10** Tuberculin testing and interpretation of results

| Heaf test | Mantoux test | Grade |
|---|---|---|
| No induration at puncture sites | 0mm induration | 0—Negative |
| Discrete induration at ≥4 sites | 1–4mm induration | 1—Negative |
| Ring of induration with clear centre | 5–14mm induration | 2—Positive* |
| Disc of induration 5–10mm wide | ≥15mm induration | 3—Refer to chest clinic |
| Solid induration>10mm wide ± vesiculation or ulceration | | 4—Refer to chest clinic |

*In school children, a grade 2 response requires no further action. In other circumstances, refer to a chest clinic.

**Treatment**<sup>G</sup> ❶ Always refer to the chest clinic.

*Asymptomatic patients* If +ve tuberculin skin test (Mantoux >10mm) but normal CXR, treatment is with isoniazid for 6mo or isoniazid + rifampicin for 3mo to prevent development of the clinical disease.

*Symptomatic patients* Combination of 3–4 antibiotics for first 2mo, then 2 antibiotics for a further 4mo. Antibiotics used are rifampicin, isoniazid, pyrazinamide, and ethambutol. All have potentially serious side effects and require blood monitoring. Compliance is imperative to prevent antibiotic resistance. Those found to be non-compliant are treated with directly observed therapy (DOT)—drugs are dispensed by and taken in the presence of a health professional.

**Prevention** BCG vaccination is vaccination with a live attenuated strain of bacteria derived from *M.bovis*. BCG vaccination provides immunity lasting ≥15y to 70–80% of recipients. It is given by intradermal injection into the left upper arm. Target groups:

- All infants living in areas where incidence of TB is ≥40:100 000 and infants whose parents or grandparents were born in a country with TB incidence of ≥40:100 000.
- Previously unvaccinated new immigrants from countries where there is a high prevalence of TB.
- Those at risk because of their occupation, e.g. healthcare workers, vetinary staff, prison staff.
- Contacts of known cases or those living or working in high prevalence countries for extended periods (generally ≥1mo).

⚠ Do not give other immunizations in to the same arm for 3mo.

### Further information
**Health Protection Agency (HPA)** Topics A–Z: Tuberculosis.
🖳 www.hpa.org.uk
**DH** Stopping tuberculosis in England: an action plan from the Chief Medical Officer (2004) 🖳 www.dh.gov.uk

### Information for patients
**Immunization** NHS website for patients 🖳 www.immunization.org.uk
**Health Protection Agency (HPA)** TB and BCG 🖳 www.hpa.org.uk
**British Lung Foundation** ☎ 0845 850 50 20 🖳 www.lunguk.org

# Other respiratory infections

**Mycoplasma** *Mycoplasma pneumoniae* causes epidemics of lower respiratory tract infection every 3–4y. Spread by droplet infection.
- *Incubation* 12–14d.
- *Presentation* Dry persistent cough ± arthralgia. CXR shows bilateral patchy consolidation. Infection is confirmed with serology.
- *Management* Erythromycin 500mg qds for 2wk (alternative is tetracycline). Relapse is common. Severe infections may require hospital admission.

## Respiratory chlamydial infection
- *C.pneumoniae*—responsible for 6–19% of community-acquired pneumonia, especially in children and young adults. May be clinically indistinguishable from pneumonia caused by Mycoplasma. Treat with tetracycline or erythromycin po for 2wk or azithromycin 500mg od for 3d.
- *C.psittaci*—infects many animals, but human infection is closely related to contact with birds. Treat as for *C.pneumoniae*.

## Pertussis (whooping cough)[ND] *Caused by Bordetella pertussis.*
- *Incubation* 7d.
- *Symptoms*
  - Catarrhal stage—symptoms and signs of URTI. Lasts 1–2wk.
  - Coughing stage—increasingly severe and paroxysmal cough with spasms of coughing followed by a 'whoop'. Associated with vomiting, cyanosis during coughing spasms, and exhaustion. Lasts 4–6wk and then cough improves over 2–3wk.
- *Examination* Chest is clear between coughing bouts.
- *Investigation* Microscopy and culture of pernasal swabs (special swab and culture medium available from the lab); FBC—lymphocytosis.
- *Management* Erythromycin in the catarrhal stage. Once coughing stage has started, treatment is symptomatic.
- *Complications:* Pneumonia, bronchiectasis, convulsions, subconjunctival haemorrhages, and facial petechiae.

### Prevention
- *Proven contacts* Treat with erythromycin.
- *Vaccination* Routinely given in childhood ([book] p.643). Children with a personal or family history of febrile convulsion, FH of epilepsy, and children with well-controlled epilepsy can be vaccinated—give advice on fever prevention. Defer vaccination for children with any undiagnosed or evolving neurological condition or poorly controlled epilepsy until the condition is stable—if in doubt refer to paediatrics.

**Aspergillosis** A spectrum of diseases. *Cause:* Aspergillus fungus present in the soil and decaying vegetation. Its spores can be inhaled at any time of the year but reach peak levels in autumn and winter. Inhaled fungal spores colonize bronchial mucosa and nasal sinuses. If suspected refer to a chest physician.

*Presentations*
- *Extrinsic asthma* 📖 p.316
- *Allergic bronchopulmonary aspergillosis* Grows in the walls of the bronchi. Presents with episodes of eosinophilic pneumonia (characterised by wheeze, cough, fever, and malaise) throughout the year but worse in late autumn. CXR shows fleeting lung shadows (cleared by expectorating firm brown plugs of mucus). Untreated → upper lobe fibrosis and 'proximal' bronchiectasis.
- *Invasive aspergillosis* Only occurs in the immunocompromised. Aspergillus disseminates from lung → brain, kidneys and other organs. Carries very poor prognosis.
- *Aspergillus sinusitis* Nasal congestion, headache, and facial discomfort.
- *Aspergilloma* Growth within existing lung cavities (e.g. from previous TB or sarcoidosis). A ball of fungus forms. CXR shows a round lesion with air halo above it. Occasionally results in haemoptysis.

*Management* Refer for specialist management.

**Pneumocystis jiroveci** (formerly known as PCP) May be classified as a protozoan or fungus. Causes pneumonia in immunocompromised patients.
- *Presentation* Fever, breathlessness, tachypnoea, dry cough, respiratory failure (± cyanosis).
- *Investigation* CXR normal or 'ground-glass' appearance; sputum culture may be diagnostic.
- *Management* If suspected refer for specialist care. Treatment is with co-trimoxazole or dapsone.
- *Prevention* Prophylactic antibiotics (usually co-trimoxazole) are given to AIDS patients with CD4 counts <200 cells/mm$^3$.

**SARS (severe acute respiratory syndrome)** SARS was first reported in China in 2002. Since then there have been several further clusters in Far East Asia and one in Canada. SARS is caused by a coronavirus (SARS-CoV) and spread by direct contact with an infected individual or rarely aerosol transmission. Incubation is 2–10d.

*Two stages*
- *Prodrome*—fever (>38°C), malaise, headache, myalgia.
- *Respiratory phase*—develops after 3–7 d—dry cough and breathlessness. A high proportion progress to respiratory failure. 70% also develop diffuse watery diarrhoea.

❶ Cases in the UK are most likely to occur within 10 d of return from an affected area—especially one where transmission is thought to be continuing. Admit to a specialist infectious diseases unit. Symptomatic suspected cases should wear a surgical mask during transit.

**Further information**
**Health Protection Agency (HPA)** Topics A–Z: Aspergillus; Pertussis, Pneumocystis, SARS 🖳 www.hpa.org.uk
**Aspergillus Website** 🖳 www.aspergillus.man.ac.uk

# Cystic fibrosis and Kartagener syndrome

**Cystic fibrosis (CF)** is the most common inherited disorder in the UK (prevalence: 1:2500). Median survival has ↑ dramatically and is now >40y but, of the 7500 CF patients in the UK, 6000 are <25y old.

**Genetics** Results from mutation of a single gene on chromosome 7 (cystic fibrosis transmembrane conductance regulator) essential for salt and water movement across cell membranes → thickened secretions. >1200 different mutations have been described. Autosomal recessive inheritance—1:4 chance of having a child with CF if both parents are car-riers. ~1:25 adults in the UK carries the CF gene (~2.3 million adults). Most common in Caucasians—rare in people of African Caribbean origin.

**Screening** Several possibilities:
- **Preconceptual screening** Buccal smears to karyotype prospective parents.
- **Antenatal screening** Chorionic villous sampling at ~10wk for parents with an affected child already or where both parents are +ve on karyotyping.
- **Neonatal screening** 📖 p.848.

**Common problems associated with CF** Figure 11.7.

**Diagnosis**
- Screening
- If clinical suspicion of CF, refer to paediatrics. A +ve sweat test ($Na^+$ > 70mmol/L; $Cl^-$ >60mmol/L on 2 occasions) is diagnostic as is ↑ potential difference across the nasal respiratory epithelium.

**Management** CF is a multisystem disease requiring a holistic approach to care which aims to maintain patients' independence, improve quality of life, *and* extend life expectancy. A multidisciplinary team in a specialist CF centre is best placed to achieve this. Patients usually have direct access. Management involves:
- Treatment of lung disease e.g. with exercise, physiotherapy, antibiotics, and mucolytics.
- Maintaining good nutritional state, e.g pre-meal oral pancreatic enzymes, high-calorie diet, and fat-soluble vitamin supplements (A, D, & E).
- Treatment of complications, e.g. DM, osteoporosis.

**Further information for patients and professionals**
CF Trust 🖥 www.cftrust.org.uk

**Kartagener syndrome (immotile cilia syndrome)** Combination of bronchiectasis, chronic sinusitis, and male infertility plus situs inversus (transposed heart and abdominal organs). Caused by a defect in cilia function. Otitis media and salpingitis are frequent. *M. Kartagener (1897–1975)— Swiss physician.*

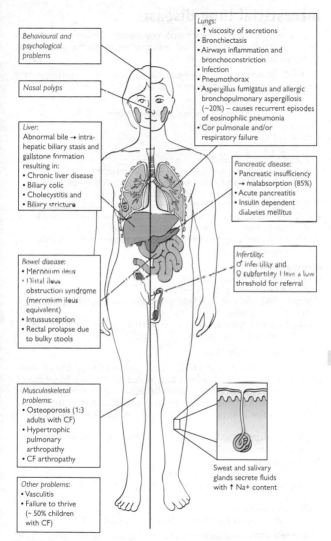

**Fig. 11.7** Features of cystic fibrosis

Figure 11.7 without annotations is reproduced from Porter RS (ed) *The Merck Manual of Medical Information*, Second Home Edition, copyright 2003 by Merck & Co. Inc., Whitehouse Station, NJ. Available at 🖳 www.merck.com/mmhe

# Interstitial lung disease

Also known as diffuse parenchymal lung disease. Comprises >200 different diseases (many rare) in which inflammation affects the alveolar wall, leading to fluid in the alveolar air spaces.

**Presentation** Increasing dyspnoea ± cough. More rarely wheeze, pleurisy, and/or haemoptysis. May present incidentally with changes on CXR.

**Further assessment**
- History of the condition—acute, episodic, chronic?
- Severity—exercise tolerance
- Possible causes
  - Smoking
  - Hobbies and occupation
  - Usual environment (e.g. lives on a farm) and travel
  - Past medical history (particularly rheumatological symptoms and immunosuppression e.g. HIV) and family history
  - Drugs
- Examine looking for fine inspiratory crackles in the chest, and evidence of systemic disease e.g. fever, rashes or other skin changes, eye signs (particularly red eye), hepatomegaly and/or splenomegaly, arthritis
- Pulse oximetry—decreased saturations.

*Investigations*
- *Chest X-ray*—diffuse shadowing
- *Urine dipstick*—for protein and blood
- *Blood*—FBC, ESR, liver and kidney function tests, thyroid function tests, autoimmune profile
- *Lung function tests*—usually show restrictive picture—rarely no abnormalities or obstructive picture.

**Classification** Table 11.11

**Hypersensitivity pneumonitis** Also known as extrinsic allergic alveolitis, farmer's lung, and bird fancier's lung. Inhaled particles (e.g. fungal spores, avian proteins) cause an allergic reaction in lungs of hypersensitive individuals. May present as an acute or chronic reaction, or both may occur together.
- *Acute reaction* 2–4h post exposure. Fever, malaise, dry cough, shortness of breath.
- *Chronic reaction* Malaise, weight ↓, exertional dyspnoea, fine crepitations in both lung fields.

*Investigations*
- *Blood* FBC: ↑ neutrophils (acute reaction); ESR ↑ (acute reaction).
- *CXR* may be normal or show typical changes (shadowing, widespread small nodules or ground glass appearance).
- Diagnosis is based on history and high-resolution CT scan findings. Serum precipitins to the provoking factor are found in ≥90%.

*Management* If possible prevent further exposure to the allergen. In all cases refer for specialist advice. Treatment is usually with corticosteroids. If occupational exposure, may qualify as industrial disease and be eligible for compensation (📖 p.118).

**Table 11.11** Classification of interstitial lung disease

| Classification | Causes |
|---|---|
| Acute | Infective:<br>• Bacterial (TB)<br>• Viral (chickenpox, measles)<br>• Fungal.<br>Allergy—drugs, fungi, helminths<br>Toxins—drugs, gases<br>Haemodynamic—LVF, fluid overload, renal failure<br>Vasculitis<br>Adult respiratory distress syndrome |
| Episodic | Eosinophilic pneumonia, e.g. allergic bronchopulmonary aspergillosis<br>Vasculitis, e.g. Churg–Strauss syndrome<br>Hypersensitivity pneumonitis<br>Cryptogenic organizing pneumonia |
| Chronic due to occupational or environmental exposure | Dust induced (🕮 p.344): asbestosis, silicosis, coal worker's pneumoconiosis, siderosis (iron)<br>Farmer's lung<br>Bird fancier's lung<br>Radiation<br>Drugs e.g. nitrofurantoin, sulfasalazine, gold, penicillamine, aspirin, amiodarone, bleomycin, methotrexate, hydralazine, heroin, methadone, oxygen |
| Chronic with evidence of systemic disease | Connective tissue disease, e.g. RA, Sjögren's syndrome, SLE<br>Neoplastic, e.g. lymphoma<br>Vasculitis, e.g. Wegener's granulomatosis, Goodpasture's syndrome<br>Sarcoidosis<br>Inherited disorders, e.g. tuberose sclerosis, neurofibromatosis<br>Miscellaneous, e.g. HIV, inflammatory bowel disease, post bone marrow transplant, amyloidosis |
| Chronic without evidence of systemic disease | Idiopathic pulmonary fibrosis<br>Chronic aspiration |

⚠ Advise all patients with interstitial lung disease to stop smoking. This results in better prognosis for their interstitial lung disease. Furthermore, patients with chronic interstitial lung disease are at substantially increased risk of lung cancer.

**Idiopathic pulmonary fibrosis (IPF)** Incidence ↑ with age. Most patients are >50y. Progressive condition of unknown cause with insidious onset. Can only be diagnosed if other causes of interstitial lung disease have been excluded and symptoms present >3mo.

### Presentation
- Progressive exertional dyspnoea
- Dry cough
- Clubbing (>50%)
- Fine 'velcro-like' crepitations
- Malaise
- Weight ↓
- Central cyanosis and right heart failure (advanced cases).

### Investigations
- **CXR** Diffuse shadowing (although may be normal).
- **Lung function tests** Restrictive picture.

### Differential diagnosis
- LVF
- COPD
- Drugs
- Inhalant exposure ($O_2$, $NO_2$)
- Radiation.
- Other causes of lung fibrosis—dust exposure (coal, asbestos, silica, farmer's lung, bird fancier's lung)

**Management** Refer to a respiratory physician for diagnosis and advice on management. Treatment, where appropriate, is with oral steroids + azathioprine. Pulmonary rehabilitation may be helpful. Lung transplant is a last option. Most patients have poor prognosis with media survival 3y (5y survival 10-15%), but the sub-group with fibrotic non-specific interstitial pneumonia (NSIP) have substantially better prognosis with >50% surviving 5y.

❶ Patients with IPF have a 10×↑ risk of lung cancer. This risk is multiplicative with that from a smoking. Patients with IPF who smoke 20 cigarettes a day may have a 200 × ↑ risk of lung cancer compared with non-smokers without IPF.

**Sarcoidosis** Multisystem inflammatory disease of unknown cause characterized by non-caseating granuloma. Incidence in the UK is 3/100 000/y. Typically presents with lung granuloma in a young adult. ♀>♂.

### Non-respiratory manifestations of sarcoidosis
- Fever and malaise
- Erythema nodosum
- Lupus pernio (blue red nodules on the nose, face and/or hands)
- Scar infiltration
- Enlarged lacrimal glands
- Hypopyon
- Uveitis
- Arthralgia
- Arrhythmias
- Heart failure
- Pericardial effusion
- Cranial and/or peripheral nerve palsies
- Seizures
- Hypercalcaemia
- Renal stones
- Lymphadenopathy
- Hepatosplenomegaly.

### Acute sarcoidosis (Löfgren syndrome)
- Polyarthralgia
- Swinging fever
- Erythema nodosum
- Bilateral hilar lymphadenopathy on CXR.

***Insidious onset*** CXR shows hilar lymphadenopathy—incidental finding in 30–50%. If symptomatic, usually presents with tiredness, malaise, weight ↓ and/or arthralgia. 15% have lung symptoms with gradual onset of progressive exertional dyspnoea and dry cough.

**Management** Refer any patient with bilateral hilar lymphadenopathy for further investigation. For patients with confirmed sarcoidosis, specialist management is needed. Steroids are the first-line treatment but should only be used if:
- Progressive disease (on imaging or lung function testing)
- Significant symptoms, or
- Extrapulmonary disease requiring treatment.

Rarely, if steroids are not controlling disease progression or symptoms, methotrexate will be added. Inhaled steroids may be helpful to control cough but do not influence disease progression. For patients with severe symptoms, pulmonary rehabilitation may be helpful. Lung-transplant may be considered for patients with end-stage pulmonary sarcoidosis.

**Prognosis** Remits without treatment in 2:3 cases. Acute sarcoidosis has good prognosis with most resolving in <2y. ~30% have chronic progressive disease. Mortality is <3%—usually death is due to CCF and/or cor pulmonale.

**Occupational lung disease** 📖 p.344.

**Further information**
**British Thoracic Society** Interstitial lung disease (2008) *Thorax* **63:** v1–v58 🖥 www.brit-thoracic.org.uk

**Patient support**
**British Lung Foundation** ☎ 0845 850 50 20 🖥 www.lunguk.org

# Occupational lung disease

Exposure to gases, vapours, and dusts at work can lead to lung disease.

**Coal-worker's pneumoconiosis** 90% of all compensated industrial lung disease in the UK. 'Pneumoconiosis' means accumulation of dust in the lungs and tissue reaction to its presence. Incidence is related to total dust exposure. Divides into:

- *Simple pneumoconiosis* Deposition of coal dust in the lung. Graded on CXR appearance. Grading determines whether disability benefit is payable in the UK. Effect on lung function is debated. Predisposes to progressive massive fibrosis.
- *Progressive massive fibrosis* Round fibrotic masses several cm in diameter form in the upper lobes. Presents with exertional dyspnoea, cough, black sputum, and eventually respiratory failure. Symptoms progress (or may even start) after exposure to coal dust has ceased. Lung function tests show a mixed restrictive and obstructive picture with loss of lung volume, irreversible airflow limitation, and ↓ gas transfer.

**Asbestosis** Before legislation banning its use, exposure was widespread and occurred particularly in naval shipyards and power stations. Effects of asbestos exposure—Table 11.12. Also consider diagnosis in relatives who came into contact with asbestos whilst washing clothes etc.—they can claim compensation if affected.

**Silicosis** Uncommon. Affects stonemasons, pottery workers, workers exposed to sand-blasting, and fettlers (remove sand from metal casts). Caused by inhalation of silica. CXR appearance is distinctive. Presents with exertional dyspnoea ± cough. *Lung function tests*: as for progressive massive fibrosis. Associated with ↑ risk of lung cancer and TB.

**Byssinosis** Affects cotton mill workers. Symptoms (tightness in the chest, cough and breathlessness) start on first day back at work after a break (Monday sickness) with improvement as the week progresses. CXR is normal.

**Berylliosis** Rare. Long latent period. Affects workers in the aerospace, nuclear power, and electrical industries and their close relatives. Presents similarly to sarcoidosis (📖 p.342).

**Iron (siderosis), barium (baritosis), and tin (stannosis) dust inhalation** Result in dramatic dense nodular shadowing on the CXR but effects on lung function and symptoms are often minimal.

**Occupational asthma** >200 industrial materials cause occupational asthma. Important causes are recognized occupational diseases in the UK—patients may be eligible for statutory compensation if they apply <10y after leaving the occupation in which asthma developed. Suspect if a patient has symptoms which improve on days away from work/holiday.

**Hypersensitivity pneumonitis (farmer's lung)** 📖 p.340.

**Management** In all cases refer to a respiratory physician for confirmation of diagnosis (essential if seeking compensation) and advice on management.

**Table 11.12** Conditions caused by asbestos exposure

| Condition | Asbestos exposure | Features/management |
|---|---|---|
| Benign pleural effusion | Usually occurs <20y after exposure | Increasing dyspnoea ± pleuritic pain |
| | | Refer for drainage of effusion |
| | | May be recurrent and require pleurodesis |
| Bilateral diffuse pleural thickening* | Follows light or moderate exposure to asbestos | Defined as pleural thickening >5mm thick covering >¼ of the chest wall |
| | May progress even in absence of further exposure | *Symptoms:* exertional dyspnoea. |
| | | *Lung function tests:* restrictive picture |
| | | Treatment is symptomatic |
| Asbestosis* | Follows heavy exposure after a 5–10y interval | Presents with progressive dyspnoea, finger clubbing, and basal end-expiratory crackles. |
| | | *CXR:* 'honeycomb lung' diffuse streaky shadowing |
| | | *Lung function tests:* severe restrictive defect and ↓ gas transfer |
| | | Treatment is symptomatic |
| Mesothelioma* | Can follow even light exposure to asbestos. | Presents with increasing shortness of breath ± pleuritic pain |
| | 20–40y time lag between exposure and appearance of disease | Examination and CXR reveal unilateral (rarely bilateral) effusion |
| | | No effective active treatment—palliative care (p.1026–1043) |
| | | Median survival is 2y from diagnosis |
| Asbestosis-related lung cancer* | Patients exposed to asbestos who have evidence of that exposure (pleural plaques, bilateral pleural thickening or asbestosis) have an ↑ risk of bronchial carcinoma—usually adenocarcinoma. Smokers exposed to asbestos have a 5× ↑ risk compared with non-smokers exposed to asbestos ||
| | Manage as for lung cancer (p.328) ||

* Eligible for industrial injuries benefit in the UK

**Benefits** p.224.

**Notification and compensation** p.118.

**Patient support**
**British Lung Foundation** ☎ 0845 850 50 20 🖥 www.lunguk.org

# Snoring and obstructive sleep apnoea

**Snoring** During sleep, the pharyngeal airway narrows due to ↓ dilator muscle tone. Snoring is vibratory noise generated from the pharynx and soft palate as the air passes through this narrowed space. Further narrowing produces louder snoring, laboured inspiration, and eventually apnoeic episodes. Social consequences are the usual reason for the patient to seek help. They can be distressing: banishment from the bedroom, marital disharmony, no holidays, fear of travelling or falling asleep in a public place, etc.

❶ Snoring may be used by the spouse as an excuse to leave the marital bed and may actually be trivial/absent. If suspected, ask the patient to bring a cassette recording of the offending noise.

**Obstructive sleep apnoea** Occurs when the pharyngeal airway completely closes during sleep, resulting in apnoeic episodes. ↑ inspiratory effort is sensed by the brain and a transient arousal provoked. A few of these arousals don't matter, but many (sometimes hundreds) per night → fragmented sleep and consequent daytime sleepiness.

## Clinical features
- **Dominant features** Excessive daytime sleepiness (not tiredness—Epworth Sleepiness Scale is a useful assessment tool), impaired concentration, snoring.
- **Other features** Unrefreshing sleep, choking episodes during sleep, witnessed apnoeic episodes, restless sleep, irritability/personality change, nocturia, ↓ libido.

## Causes of snoring and sleep apnoea
Overweight (neck circumference >16 inch), nasal congestion, evening alcohol/sedatives, large tonsils, receding lower jaw, smoking, hypothyroidism, menopause.

## Management
### Snoring without sleep apnoea
- **Initial approaches** Suggest changing sleeping position (discourage from sleeping on back); elevate head of bed (e.g. prop up on bricks—can ↓ nasal congestion); limit number of pillows to 1 thick/2 thin pillows to maximize pharyngeal size; ↓ weight if obese; ↓ or stop evening alcohol/sleeping tablets; suggest partner tries ear plugs (purchase from chemist—takes several nights to get used to wearing them).
- **If clinically indicated**
  - Nasal congestion—start beclometasone nasal spray (applied head downwards) 2 puffs bd ± ipratropium bromide nasal spray 2 puffs nocte.
  - Check TFTs to exclude hypothyroidism.
  - Discuss the use of HRT in menopausal women (📖 p.710).
- **If simple measures fail** refer to
  - Dentist or ENT for a mandibular advancement device.
  - ENT for surgery—septal straightening, polypectomy, turbinate reduction, tonsillectomy, or uvulopalatopharyngoplasty.

### Sleep apnoea

- Advise patients to ↓ weight if obese, ↓ or stop evening alcohol/sleeping tablets, *and*
- Refer to a sleep unit or physician with a special interest in sleep problems. If diagnosis is proven and causing significant daytime sleepiness, usual treatment is with CPAP therapy at night. Mandibular advancement devices are alternatives for patients who cannot tolerate CPAP or have very mild symptoms with no daytime sleepiness. Occasionally, if large tonsils, referral to ENT for surgery is warranted.

⚠ **Driving** Warn patients NOT to drive if sleepy. Once diagnosis is confirmed they must inform the DVLA and their insurance company (📖 p.133).

 **Sleep apnoea in children** Common in children aged 2–7y in association with tonsil enlargement during URTI. Sleep disruption can cause daytime sleepiness, hyperactivity, poor attention span, and bad behaviour. If tonsils are big enough to produce sleep apnoea in the absence of current infection, refer to ENT for consideration of tonsillectomy.

**The Epworth Sleepiness Scale** How likely are you to doze off or fall asleep in the following situations, in contrast to feeling just tired?

This refers to your usual way of life in recent times. Even if you have not done some of these things recently try to work out how they would have affected you.

| Situation | Chance of dozing |
|---|---|
| Sitting and reading | ☐ |
| Watching TV | ☐ |
| Sitting inactive in a public place (e.g. a theatre or a meeting) | ☐ |
| As a passenger in a car for an hour without a break | ☐ |
| Lying down to rest in the afternoon when circumstances permit | ☐ |
| Sitting and talking to someone | ☐ |
| Sitting quietly after a lunch without alcohol | ☐ |
| In a car, while stopped for a few minutes in traffic | ☐ |
| *0 = no chance of dozing*     *2 = moderate chance of dozing* | |
| *1 = slight chance of dozing*     *3 = high chance of dozing* | |

*If score > 10—consider sleep apnoea.*

### Further information

**SIGN/British Thoracic Society** Management of obstructive sleep apnoea/hypopnoea syndrome in adults (2003) 🖥 www.sign.ac.uk

### Patient support

**Sleep Apnoea Trust (SATA)** 🖥 www.sleep-apnoea-trust.org

# Endocrinology

# Symptoms of endocrine disease

Because of the wide range of functions of hormones secreted by the endocrine system, clinical presentation of different endocrine disorders varies widely from non-specific symptoms such as tiredness to very specific signs such as delayed puberty. Specific features depend on the gland and hormones involved.

**Polydipsia** Over-frequent drinking of fluid—often associated for logical reasons with polyuria. Ask if it is associated with thirst. Take a history of fluid intake. If no history of excess fluid intake and BM/fasting blood glucose is normal, investigate further with U&E, Cr, and $Ca^{2+}$.

### Common causes
- Change in lifestyle: diet/activity/exercise level—may be associated with polyuria but no other symptoms. No history of thirst.
- DM—usually accompanied by a history of thirst.

**Other causes** Diarrhoea, diabetes insipidus, ↑ $Ca^{2+}$, compulsive water drinking (may be a feature of psychotic illness), phosphorus poisoning.

**Polyuria** Passage of excessive urine. Check that the patient does not mean frequency of urination. It can be difficult to distinguish the two. Causes are similar to those of polydipsia and the 2 symptoms are related. Take a history of fluid intake. If no history of excess fluid intake and BM/fasting blood glucose is normal, investigate further with MSU (for M,C&S), U&E, Cr, and $Ca^{2+}$.

### Consider
- DM—always check a BM and/or fasting blood glucose if a patient complains of polyuria.
- Diabetes insipidus.
- Hypercalcaemia.
- Excessive intake due to change in lifestyle or psychiatric conditions, e.g. schizophrenia.
- Chronic renal failure.
- Drugs—diuretics, caffeine, alcohol.

**Tiredness and lethargy** 📖 p.536.

**Hirsutism** Affects 10% ♀s. Excess hair in androgenic distribution. *Causes:*
- Most cases are idiopathic. There may be a family history.
- Drugs—phenytoin, corticosteroids, ciclosporin, androgenic oral contraception, anabolic steroids, minoxidil, diazoxide.
- Polycystic ovarian syndrome (PCOS).
- Late-onset congenital adrenal hyperplasia (rare).
- Cushing's syndrome.
- Ovarian tumours (rare).

### Assessment
- *History* Long-standing or recent onset, family history, ethnic origin (more common in Mediterranean countries), menstrual history.
- *Examination* Distribution of excess hair.

*Investigation* Women with long-standing hirsutism (since puberty) and regular periods need no further investigation unless abnormal signs. *Otherwise: blood*—testosterone (↑ in PCOS, androgen-secreting tumour, late-onset congenital adrenal hyperplasia); LH/FSH ratio (>3:1 suggests PCOS).

**Refer to gynaecologist or endocrinologist if** recent onset, abnormal blood tests, virilism, galactorrhoea, menstrual disturbance, infertility, and/ or pelvic mass.

### Treatment of idiopathic hirsutism
- Cosmetic—bleaching, shaving, waxing, depilatory creams, electrolysis.
- Weight ↓ in obese individuals.
- Psychological support.
- Topical eflornithine—↓ growth of unwanted facial hair. Continuous use for 8wk is required before benefit is seen. Must be used indefinitely to prevent regrowth. Discontinue if no improvement in 4mo.
- Oral medication—all take ≥6 mo to take effect and none abolish the problem. In all cases continue treatment until acceptable level of hair growth and then stop. Relapse usually follows withdrawal and repeat courses are then required. Drugs used: COC pill containing desogestrel, co-cyprindiol, or spironolactone.

**Obesity** 📖 p.180.

**Sweating and facial flushing** 📖 p.604–605.

**Delayed or precocious puberty** 📖 p.891.

# Diabetes

Diabetes mellitus (DM) is a common syndrome affecting 3% of the population of the UK. It is caused by lack or ↓ effectiveness of endogenous insulin. It is characterized by ↑ blood sugars and abnormalities of carbohydrate and lipid metabolism.

**Glycosuria** Often detected incidentally on urine dipstick. *Causes:*
- DM
- Pregnancy
- Sepsis
- Renal tubular damage
- Low renal threshold.

In all cases check fasting blood glucose (+ glucose tolerance test if pregnant). Check immediate BM if other symptoms suggestive of DM.

## Presentation

- *Acute* Ketoacidosis or hyperosmolar non-ketotic coma (📖 p.1096).
- *Sub-acute* Weight ↓, polydipsia, polyuria, lethargy, irritability, infections (candidiasis, skin infection, recurrent infections slow to clear), genital itching, blurred vision, tingling in hands/feet.
- *With complications* Presentation with skin changes, neuropathy, nephropathy, arterial or eye disease (📖 pp.362–369).
- *Asymptomatic* DM may be detected on routine screening during well man/woman checks or opportunistic urine screening for glucose. A national screening programme is under consideration.

## Diagnosis of diabetes

*If symptomatic* ↑ venous plasma glucose—random ≥ 11.1 mmol/L; fasting ≥7.0 mmol/L. For *all* children, and adults with suspected ketoacidosis or who are unwell, do not delay to get a laboratory sample, but admit or refer for same-day specialist assessment on BM alone. Otherwise only make a diagnosis on laboratory sample.

*If asymptomatic* ↑ venous plasma glucose on two separate measurements on different days—random ≥ 11.1mmol/L; fasting ≥7.0mmol/L.

*Impaired fasting glycaemia* Fasting plasma glucose ≥6.1 and <7mmol/L. Do a glucose tolerance test to clarify diagnosis.

*Glucose tolerance test* Performed if impaired fasting glycaemia, borderline random plasma glucose, or inconsistent results on repeat testing of fasting blood glucose. Ask the patient to fast overnight. Give 75g of glucose (350mL Lucozade). Check plasma glucose after 2h.
- If ≥11.1mmol/L the patient is diabetic.
- If ≥7.8 and <11.1mmol/L the patient has impaired glucose tolerance.
- If <7.8 mmol/L the patient is not diabetic.

❶ Both impaired glucose tolerance and impaired fasting glucose are risk factors for DM and cardiovascular disease. Follow-up with annual fasting blood glucose—4%/y develop DM. Treat CVD risk factors aggressively.

⚠ Blood glucose may be temporarily ↑ during acute illness, after trauma or surgery, or during short courses of blood-glucose-raising drugs (see 2° causes). If HbA_{1c} >7%, DM is likely.

**Diabetes and pregnancy** 📖 p.826.

## Classification of primary diabetes

**Type 1 (insulin-dependent (IDDM), juvenile onset)** May occur at any age but more common in patients <30y. Autoimmune disease. Islet cell antibodies may initially be present. Associated with other autoimmune disease and certain genotypes (HLA DR3/4, although identical twin concordance ~30%.). Patients are prone to profound weight ↓ and ketoacidosis. Insulin is needed from diagnosis.

**Type 2 (non-insulin-dependent (NIDDM), maturity onset)** 80–90% patients with DM. ♂:♀ ≈ 3:2. Prevalence is rising. Lifetime risk of developing type 2 DM is >10% and ~½ remain undiagnosed. *Risk factors*:

- Age >65
- Obesity
- FH of DM (identical twin concordance ~100%)
- Impaired glucose tolerance
- Ethnic group (South Asians/African Caribbeans/Hispanics have 5–10× ↑ risk)
- PMH of gestational diabetes or baby >4kg at birth.

Type 2 DM is due to impaired insulin secretion and insulin resistance. It is a 'silent killing disease' in which life expectancy is ↓ by 30–40% in the age range 40–70y—a loss of 8–10y of life. Onset tends to be insidious. Treatment is usually with diet ± tablets. Type 2 DM is progressive and many patients eventually require insulin treatment (although the patient is still a type 2 diabetic). Half have complications at diagnosis.

## 2°causes of DM

- **Drugs** Steroids, thiazides
- **Pancreatic disease** Pancreatitis, surgery, cancer, haemachromatosis, cystic fibrosis
- **Endocrine disease** Cushing's disease, acromegaly, thyrotoxicosis, phaeochromocytoma
- **Others** Glycogen storage diseases, insulin receptor antibodies.

**Metabolic syndrome** Insulin resistance syndrome or syndrome X. Consists of impaired glucose tolerance or DM, insulin resistance (in patients on insulin, insulin resistance is suggested by insulin doses >1 unit/kg/d) + other metabolic disorders of ↑ cardiovascular risk including:

- Truncal obesity—waist circumference >0.9m (♀), >1.0m (♂). Use 0.1m lower figures for people of South Asian extraction.
- ↑BP—>135/80mmHg.
- Dyslipidaemia—serum HDL <1.2mmol/L (♀) or <1.0mmol/L (♂); fasting serum triglycerides >1.8mmol/L.

Associated with high risk of CVD. Treat risk factors aggressively.

## Further information

**WHO** Definition, diagnosis and classification of diabetes mellitus and its complications (2000) ⌨ www.diabetes.org.uk
**NICE** ⌨ www.nice.org.uk
- Type 1 diabetes: diagnosis and management (2004)
- Type 2 diabetes (2009).

## Patient advice and support

**Diabetes UK** ☎ 0845 120 2960 ⌨ www.diabetes.org.uk

# Organization and monitoring of care

## Aims of diabetic care
- Alleviation of symptoms
- Minimization of complications
- Reduction of early mortality
- Quality of life enhancement
- Education of the patient and family.

GP diabetic clinics can be as effective as hospital clinics in achieving diabetic control. High-quality diabetic care is rewarded within the quality and outcomes framework.

## Features of well-organized care
- Use of a register and structured records (usually available as part of in-house computer software).
- Regular review, follow-up of defaulters, following a protocol for care.
- Thorough annual review with recall system.
- Provision of protected time for the clinic.
- Availability of good-quality written information for patients.
- Open access for patients to receive advice.
- Multidisciplinary team covering all aspects of diabetes care—GPs, diabetes nurse specialists/assistants, and educators.
- Access to dieticians and podiatrists.
- Quality monitoring through audit and patient feedback.
- Continuing education for professional staff.

**Routine diabetic review** Each diabetic patient requires 6 monthly review (or more frequent as necessary). This should include a thorough annual review of all aspects of disease and care. Reviews should cover:
- *Problems* Recent life events; new symptoms; difficulties with management since last visit.
- *Review of*
  - Indices of control, e.g. $HbA_{1c}$
  - Self-monitored results and discussion of their meaning
  - Dietary behaviours
  - Physical activity
  - Smoking
  - Diabetes education
  - Skills, e.g. injection technique
  - Foot care
  - Blood glucose, lipid, and BP therapy and results
  - Other medical conditions and therapy affecting DM.
  - Immunizations—influenza ± pneumococcal vaccination
  - Depression screening (📖 p.998).
- *Review of complications* Annual review—more frequent if established complications. Cardiovascular disease, nephropathy, neuropathy, eye disease, foot problems, erectile dysfunction (📖 pp.362–369).
- *Review of services* Annual review—more frequent if problems.
- *Analysis and planning* Agreement on the main points covered, targets for coming months, changes in therapy, interval to next consultation.
- *Recording* Completion of computer record ± patient-held record.

❶ 7–10% of patients in long-term residential care have DM. Patients in residential care with DM tend to be neglected. Agree a diabetes care plan for each affected resident and ensure at least annual diabetic review.

**Monitoring blood glucose** All patients can achieve good levels of control (Table 12.1). Poorer control is acceptable in the elderly or others with limited life expectancy as long as they are symptom free.

• *Urine monitoring* Adequate for those who do not require tight control or those who cannot cope with more complex techniques.
• *Blood monitoring* Essential for all patients using insulin. Use for patients on oral medication is controversial and usually not indicated.
  • Explain the range of suitable monitoring devices available (BNF 6.1.6) and train in the use of the selected method.
  • Frequency of self-monitoring varies according to need.
  • Set targets for pre-prandial glucose levels.
  • Assess skills (and meters) yearly or if problems self-monitoring.
  • Evaluate reliability of results by comparison with HbA$_{1c}$ results and results obtained at review.
• *Glycosylated haemoglobin (HbA$_{1c}$)* Measure at least 2×/y. Represents an average of blood sugar control over the previous 6–8 wk.

**Table 12.1** Indices of control

| Measure | Target |
|---|---|
| Fasting blood glucose (mmol/L) | 4–7 (postprandial <9) mmol/L—adults<br>4–8 (postprandial <10) mmol/L—children |
| Urine | –ve (postprandial sugars <0.5%) |
| HbA$_{1c}$ (normal 4.0–6.0% or 20–42 mmol/mol)—measure every 2–6mo depending on control | 6.5% or 48 mmol/mol (but set realistic targets for each individual) |
| Serum cholesterol (mmol/L)—2° prevention, type 2 DM or type 1 DM with risk factors for CVD, metabolic syndrome or microalbuminuria | ↓ total cholesterol by 25% or to <4mmol/L, whichever is the lower value<br>*or* ↓ LDL cholesterol by 30% or to <2.0 mmol/L, whichever is the lower value |
| BMI | 25–30 kg/m$^2$ |
| BP—without macrovascular disease | <135/85mmHg |
| BP—with macrovascular disease | <130/80mmHg |

❶ From 2009 onwards, HbA$_{1c}$ levels have been reported in both 'DCCT aligned' % units, and 'IFCC' units of mmol glucose/mol haemoglobin.

**Further information**

**DH** National service framework for diabetes (2001) ⌨ www.dh.gov.uk

# Management of diabetes: education

Education is an essential aspect of diabetic care. Diabetes is a chronic condition, and however well it is managed in the clinic, the patient has to manage his/her own disease the rest of the time. Education enables patients and their carers to become equal partners in the management of their disease. *Topics to cover:*

**General knowledge** Information about:
- DM, its progressive nature and complications.
- Aims of management.
- Structure of diabetic services and ways to access them.
- Equipment required and usage instructions—syringes, needles, blood testing equipment, etc.
- Free prescriptions for patients requiring drugs or insulin to control their diabetes.
- Problems of pregnancy (women of childbearing age only).
- Alert bracelets—Medic-Alert (☎ 0800 581 420) provides stainless steel bracelets or necklets, and identity tags are also available from Medi-Tag (☎ 0121 200 1616).

**Diet** Patients do *not* need a separate diet from the rest of the family or expensive 'diabetes' food products. A diabetic diet is a healthy diet.
- ≥ 50% of calorie intake should be from fibre-rich carbohydrate, with a minimum of fat (especially saturated fat), refined carbohydrate and alcohol.
- Adjust total calorie intake according to desired BMI.
- Recommend at least 5 portions of fresh fruit or vegetables /d.
- Spread food intake evenly across the day for patients controlled with tablets or diet.
- Diet sheets are available from Diabetes UK and should be provided.
- Ready-made meals, processed foods, and alcohol are often sources of hidden sugar.

**Immunizations** Offer influenza and pneumococcal vaccine to all diabetics.

**Psychological problems** Discuss concerns underlying the diagnosis of DM or development of complications. Arrange counselling/refer to self-help resources as needed. Teenagers with diabetes can be a particularly difficult group to manage. Often control is poor because of a combination of rapid bodily changes and rebellion against the diagnosis of DM. Support information and advice given in specialist clinics.

**Exercise** Encourage regular exercise.
- Review activity at work and in getting to and from the workplace, hobbies and physical activity in the home.
- Advise physical activity can ↑ insulin sensitivity, ↓ BP, and improve blood lipid control.
- If appropriate, suggest regular physical activity tailored to individual ability (e.g. brisk walking for 30min/d, exercise prescription).

**Smoking** Advice on and assistance with smoking cessation.

**Driving** Advise all drivers that they must notify their car insurance company and the DVLA, unless their diabetes is controlled by diet alone. Be aware of insurers who cater for diabetic drivers.

**Foot care** 📖 p.368.

**Employment** Advise those on insulin that certain jobs are no longer possible:
• Working on scaffolding or with dangerous machinery.
• Joining the police or the armed services.
• Driving a heavy goods or public service vehicle.

Jobs without these hazards should pose no problems although the patient might wish to tell his/her employer. Special advice may be needed for shift work.

**Travel** Give advice on:
• Management of change in time zones (📖 p.135).
• Transport of insulin.
• Keeping monitoring and injection equipment in hand-luggage.
• Differences in insulin types and concentrations between countries.
• Travel related illness (especially gastroenteritis).
• Need for immunization and travel insurance.

Be aware of insurers who cater for diabetic travellers.

**Further information**
**DH** Structured patient education in diabetes: report from the Patient Education Working Group (2005) 🖥 www.dh.gov.uk
**NICE** Type 2 diabetes (2009) 🖥 www.nice.org.uk

**Patient advice and support**
**Diabetes UK** ☎ 0845 120 2960 🖥 www.diabetes.org.uk

# Treatment of type 2 diabetes

Tight control of type 2 DM ↓ complications. Optimal results are obtained if $HbA_{1c}$ is maintained <7%. Benefits are only evident after a decade of good control.[R]

⚠ *Always* combine treatment of hyperglycaemia with modification of other risk factors for vascular complications (📖 p.362).

**Healthy eating and exercise** Diet is the cornerstone of treatment. Diet sheets are available from Diabetes UK. ↑ physical activity is beneficial (↓ weight, ↓ lipids, and ↑ insulin sensitivity) but not always possible.

**First-line oral hypoglycaemic agents** (Figure 12.1 and BNF 6.1.2)

**Biguanides** Metformin 500mg od-qds. ↓ gluconeogenesis and ↑ peripheral utilization of glucose. Only effective if some endogenous insulin production. Initiate metformin (except if contraindicated) for all patients if $HbA_{1c}$ remains ≥6.5 after a trial of diet and lifestyle interventions. Avoid in very elderly patients and those with serious heart disease, liver/ renal failure, or high alcohol intake, as ↑ risk of lactic acidosis. Hypoglycaemia is not a problem. Start with the minimum dose and ↑ monthly until control is achieved/maximum dose reached.

**Sulphonylureas** e.g. gliclazide 40–80mg od. Act by augmenting insulin secretion—effective only if there is some residual endogenous insulin production. All are equally effective. If one sulphonylurea does not work, another is not likely to either. Advise patients to take before meals—warn about possible hypoglycaemia if meals are omitted. Start at the minimum dose and ↑ until blood sugar is controlled/maximum dose is reached. Wait ≥1mo between adjustments. Main side effect is weight ↑.

**Other oral hypoglycaemic agents** BNF 6.1.2

**Glitazones** e.g. rosiglitazone 4mg od, pioglitazone 15mg od. ↑ insulin secretion, ↑ insulin sensitivity, and slightly ↓ BP. Pioglitazone also ↓ total cholesterol. Use:
- Alone for patients who are obese and intolerant to metformin
- In combination with metformin and/or sulphonylurea for patients with poor glycaemic control on metformin and/or sulphonylurea.

❶ Glitazones cause fluid retention and ↑ risk of heart failure. Do not use if known/suspected heart failure. Rosiglitazone may ↑ risk of coronary ischaemia. Do not use if history of CHD or peripheral vascular disease.

**Acarbose** Delays digestion/absorption of starch and sucrose. Lowers blood glucose alone or in combination with metformin/sulphonylurea. Often unacceptable as it causes flatulence—but this ↓ with time.

### Add-on treatments
- *Exenatide (bd injection) and liraglutide (od injection)*—may be an alternative to insulin in obese patients. Stimulate insulin production and ↓ rate of glucose absorption from the gut. Licensed for use in addition to metformin and/or a sulphonylurea.
- *Sitagliptin and vildagliptin*—↑ incretin levels. Licensed to treat type 2 DM in combination with metformin or glitazone tablets.

- *Nateglinide and repaglinide* Stimulate insulin release. Rapid onset of action and short duration of activity. Both can be given in combination with metformin. Repaglinide is also licensed as monotherapy.

**Indications to start insulin\*** (📖 p.360)
- Continuing weight loss and/or persistent symptoms.
- Non-obese patients on maximum oral therapy with poor diabetic control.
- Patients planning pregnancy.

\*Continue metformin and sulphonylurea except if planning pregnancy.

**Drug treatment of obesity** Only prescribe for patients with type 2 DM if BMI ≥27kg/m² (sibutramine) or ≥28kg/m² (orlistat), and if they have made attempts to ↓ weight by diet and exercise.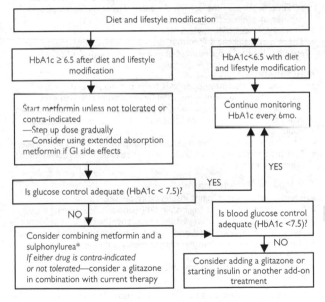

Fig. 12.1 Using oral hypoglycaemic agents in type 2 DM

**Further information**
**NICE** 🖥 www.nice.org.uk
- Type 2 diabetes (2009)
- Obesity: the prevention, identification, assessment and management of overweight and obesity in adults and children (2006).

# Treatment with insulin

First-line treatment for type 1 DM. Also used when diet ± oral therapy have failed for type 2 DM. Local guidelines agreed between 1° and 2° care govern 'who does what' and targets of care. Starting a patient on insulin is usually done by a specialist clinic with ongoing care involving the primary care team.

⚠ All drivers must notify the DVLA and their insurance company.

## Monitoring

- Ask patients to keep a written diary of blood sugar values and time and date they are taken.
- Advise patients to measure their blood sugar pre-prandially ≥1×/d at different times of the day—more often if using multiple injection regimes, after dose changes, or during intercurrent illness.
- Record episodes of hypoglycaemia.
- *Target:* blood glucose 4–7mmol/L pre-meals with hypoglycaemic episodes kept to a minimum (4–8 mmol/L pre-meals if <18y old).

## Administration

- Deep SC injection into upper arm, thigh, buttock, or abdomen.
- Fat hypertrophy/scarring minimized by rotation of injection sites.
- 'Pen' devices and conventional syringe and needle are equally effective. In all cases prime the needle using an 'air shot' (an empty needle ↓ insulin dose by ~2u).
- Rock 'pens' containing pre-mixed insulins to mix contents before use.
- ↑ absorption can occur if a limb is used in strenuous exercise following injection into it.

## Common injection regimes*

- Intermediate ± short-acting insulin od (type 2 only).
- Short + intermediate-acting insulin bd (mane and pre-evening meal).
- Short + intermediate-acting insulin mane, short-acting or rapid-acting* insulin before evening meal, and intermediate-acting insulin before bed.
- Short- or rapid-acting* insulin tds pre-meals and intermediate-acting insulin before bed.
- Combinations of oral therapy and od or bd long or intermediate acting insulin.

*Rapid-acting insulin should be used as an alternative to meal-time soluble insulin where nocturnal or late inter-prandial hypoglycaemia is a problem or to eliminate the need for snacks between meals. Rarely, continuous SC infusion is needed to achieve control[N]—needs specialist supervision.

**Inhaled insulin (Exubera®)[N]** Used for type 1 and type 2 DM if other treatment options, e.g. diet, oral hypoglycaemic agents, injected insulin have been unsuccessful, or needle phobia confirmed by an endocrine or mental health specialist. ❶ Contraindicated if smoker/stopped smoking <6mo ago. Regular lung function checks are needed.

**Exercise** ↓ insulin dose acting at the time of exercise *or* take 1–2 glucose tablets before exercise; then check blood glucose afterwards. Adjust alterations/glucose dose with experience of effects of exercise.

**Intercurrent illness** Continue insulin in usual dose and keep a regular check (≥qds) of blood sugar. Maintain glucose intake even if not eating (with e.g. Lucozade or milk):

- If glucose >13 mmol/L, ↑ insulin by 2u/d until control is achieved or use top-up injections of short-acting insulin qds prn.
- Admit to hospital if: condition warrants admission; unable to take glucose; persistent vomiting and/or dehydration; ketotic (check urine if blood sugar >13mmol/L).

## Poor control

- Exclude intercurrent illness.
- Consider diet and/or gastroparesis
- Check insulin is being used as directed and injection sites are not scarred or hypertrophic.
- Consider psychosocial factors which might be upsetting control.
- Consider changing insulin dose—ask the patient to record a glucose profile (blood sugar pre-meals and before bed).
- If using >1 insulin adjust one at a time.
- Alter by ≤10% each time; allow ≥48h between dose adjustments; alter dose of insulin acting at the time blood sugar is most out of control.
- If blood sugar is too high, ↑ insulin dose and vice versa.

## Hypoglycaemia
**Emergency management** 📖 p.1096.

### Advice for patients

- Check blood sugar before driving and every 2h during a long journey.
- Carry glucose everywhere and sandwiches on long journeys.
- If hypoglycaemia occurs stop hazardous activities and take action.
- Wait until fully recovered before resuming activities.

**In case of severe hypoglycaemia** Supply a responsible member of the family with glucose gel (e.g. GlucoGel®) and glucagon injection—teach him/her to use it. Response is short-lived—give oral glucose (e.g. Lucozade, glucose tablets, milk) as soon as the patient is conscious.

### Recurrent hypoglycaemia

- If hypoglycaemia occurs in a regular pattern, check pattern of meals and activity and alter insulin to match needs.
- If erratic consider: erratic lifestyle, alcohol, problems with absorption, errors in administration, gastroparesis.
- If no obvious cause, consider change in underlying insulin sensitivity (e.g. age, renal impairment).

**Hypoglycaemia unawareness** Associated with human insulins (but can occur with any). To restore warning signs adjust insulin and food intake to stop glucose levels dropping to <4 mmol/L. Consider undetected night-time hypoglycaemia ($HbA_{1c}$ < expected from blood sugar diary). Driving is not permitted if hypoglycaemic awareness has been lost.

## Further information

**NICE** 🖥 www.nice.org.uk

- Type 1 diabetes: diagnosis and management (2004)
- Type 2 diabetes (2009).

# Diabetic complications: cardiovascular

Diabetics are at ↑ risk of MI (2–5×), stroke (2–3×) and peripheral vascular disease. Protective effect of female sex is lost. Atherosclerotic disease accounts for most of the excess mortality due to DM. Check arterial risk factors annually:

- Age
- Family history of arterial disease
- Abdominal adiposity
- BP
- Lipid profile (LDL, HDL cholesterol and triglycerides)
- Albumin excretion rate
- Blood glucose control
- Smoking—give smoking cessation advice at every opportunity. Help patients who want to give up with advice, medication, and support.

## ⚠ High-risk groups

**Type 1 diabetics** Consider at increased risk if:
- >35y
- Originate in the Indian subcontinent
- Family history of premature heart disease
- Pre-existing CVD
- ≥ 2 features of the metabolic syndrome (📖 p.353)
- Abnormal lipids
- ↑ BP
- Microalbuminuria/proteinuria.

**Type 2 diabetics** Consider to be at high CVD risk *unless all* the following apply:
- Not overweight for ethnic group
- Normotensive (BP<140/80 mmHg without antihypertensive therapy)
- No microalbuminuria
- Non-smoker
- No high-risk lipid profile
- No history of cardiovascular disease
- No family history of cardiovascular disease.

**Aspirin** Control systolic BP to <145/90mmHg before starting treatment. Give 75mg od to:
- All type 1 diabetics with ↑ risk of arterial disease
- All type 2 diabetics aged >50y
- Type 2 diabetics <50y with other CVD risk factors.

**Statin** Give simvastatin 40mg od to:
- All type 1 diabetics with ↑ risk of arterial disease
- All type 2 diabetics aged >75y
- Type 2 diabetics of any age with any high risk factors
- Type 2 diabetics >40y with no high risk factors, but who have 10y CVD risk >20% calculated using special diabetic risk tables e.g. UKPDS risk engine (🖥 www.dtu.ox.ac.uk/riskengine).

Start with simvastatin 40mg od. Re-check lipid profile 1–3mo after starting treatment. Aim to ↓ total cholesterol to <4mmol/L or ↓ LDL cholesterol to <2.0 mmol/L. If treatment does not bring lipids within target levels increase simvastatin to 80mg od if needed. If pre-existing or new CVD, or albuminuria, consider addition of ezetimibe or changing to higher-intensity statin, e.g. atorvastatin.

### Triglycerides
- If triglycerides are >4.5 mmol/L despite optimal glycaemic control, start a fibrate. If this is ineffective, consider a trial of high-concentration omega-3 fish oils.
- If high CVD risk and triglycerides are 2.3–4.5 mmol/L despite statin treatment, consider adding a fibrate.

**Blood glucose** Target $HbA_{1c}$ = 6.5% (or 48 mmol/mol).

**BP** Any ↓ in average BP ↓ risk of cardiovascular complications. Measure BP annually if not hypertensive and no renal disease. If BP is higher than target, repeat in 1mo if >150/90mmHg, 2 mo if >140/80mmHg, and 2mo if >130/80mmHg and type 1 DM, or type 2 DM with kidney, eye, or cerebrovascular damage.
- *Type 1 DM[N]* Treat if systolic BP >135 or diastolic BP >85mmHg *unless* microalbuminuria/proteinuria or ≥2 features of the metabolic syndrome (📖 p.353) when treat if systolic BP >130 or diastolic BP >80 mmHg.
- *Type 2 DM[N]* Treat if systolic BP ≥140 or diastolic BP ≥80mmHg regardless of absolute risk of CVD. Aim to ↓ BP to <140/80mmHg (or <130/80mmHg if kidney, eye, or cerebrovascular damage).

### Choice of antihypertensive
- In all cases, discuss lifestyle modifications (📖 p.254).
- If already on antihypertensives at the time of diagnosis of DM, review BP and medication use. Change only if BP is poorly controlled or current medication is inappropriate.
- For those with new hypertension, start with an ACE inhibitor (unless possibility of becoming pregnant, when start with $Ca^{2+}$ channel blocker). Titrate dose to the maximum tolerated. If side effects with ACE inhibitor, ARB is an alternative. For people of African Caribbean descent offer ACE inhibitor + diuretic/calcium-channel blocker. Monitor BP every 1–2mo until stable within target.
- If BP remains above target add a diuretic (e.g. bendroflumethiazide 2.5mg od) and/or calcium-channel blocker (e.g. amlodipine 5mg od)—in whichever order is most appropriate for the patient.
- Fourth-line agents include α-blockers, β-blockers, or further diuretic therapy.

**Monitoring** Monitor BP every 4–6mo once stable on treatment. Check for possible adverse side effects of medication (including postural drop).

### Further information
**NICE** 🖥 www.nice.org.uk
- Type 1 diabetes: diagnosis and management (2004)
- Type 2 diabetes (2009).

**Lancet** MRC/BHF Heart Protection Study of simvastatin in diabetic patients (2003) *Lancet* **362**, 2005–16.

# Diabetic complications: renal and eye

### Renal disease
**Urinary tract infections** More common in patients with poorly controlled DM. May exacerbate renal failure and → renal scarring. Consider papillary necrosis if recurrent (more common in DM).

### Nephropathy
- Most common cause of end-stage renal failure in adults starting dialysis in the UK. 25% diabetics have renal damage—more common if of Asian or African ethnic origin.
- Nephropathy is characterized by proteinuria, ↑BP, and progressive ↓ in renal function.
- Before overt nephropathy occurs there is a phase (microalbuminuria or incipient nephropathy) in which the urine contains traces of protein not detected by standard protein dipstick. Presence of ↑ urine albumin levels and/or ↑ serum creatinine is associated with ↑ risk of premature cardiovascular events and renal failure.
- Check renal function annually (first-pass urine specimen for albumin: creatinine ratio; dipstick for protein and haematuria; serum creatinine and eGFR).

### Interpretation of albumin: creatinine ratio
- Microalbuminuria is defined as albumin:creatinine ratio ≥2.5mg/mmol (♂) or ≥3.5mg/mmol (♀) or albumin concentration ≥20mg/L in the absence of overt proteinuria or urinary tract infection.
- If albumin:creatinine ratio is abnormal, repeat the test 2× over the next 3–4mo. Microalbuminuria is confirmed if ≥1 of the repeat results is also abnormal.

### Suspect other renal disease if
- Albumin:creatinine ratio is ↑ *without* retinopathy.
- BP is particularly high or resistant to treatment.
- Heavy proteinuria (albumin:creatinine ratio>100mg/mmol) but previously documented as normal.
- Significant haematuria.
- eGFR has worsened rapidly.
- The person is systemically unwell.

### Management of nephropathy
- Optimize blood glucose control.
- Monitor and treat ↑BP (target BP <130/80mmHg) and treat other arterial risk factors aggressively.
- Modify diet (↓ salt intake, ↓ protein intake with target of 0.8g/kg).
- Treat all patients with DM and microalbuminuria or CKD with ACE inhibitor (or ARB) titrating dose to the maximum tolerated. Protects renal function and ↓ proteinuria even if the patient is not hypertensive.
- Refer to a nephrologist if proteinuria (albumin: creatinine ratio >70mg/mmol, or total protein: creatinine ratio >100mg/mmol and UTI excluded), eGFR <30, or ↓ eGFR >15% between tests (CKD 📖 p.448).

**Eye disease** ~1:3 diabetics have eye problems at the time of diagnosis.

***Blurred vision*** May occur if control is poor—caused by osmotic changes in the lens; corrects with normalization of blood sugar. Wait before changing glasses.

***Cataract*** Juvenile 'snowflake' cataracts are more common and can develop rapidly (over days). Senile cataracts occur ~10y earlier in DM.

***Glaucoma*** DM is a risk factor for developing glaucoma.

***Retinopathy*** Most common cause of blindness in people of working age in industrialized countries (risk ↑ ×20 compared with non-diabetics). 20–40% type 2 diabetics have retinopathy at diagnosis. 20y after diagnosis, 95% type 1 diabetics and 60% type 2 diabetics have retinopathy—sight-threatening in 5–10%.

***Pathogenesis*** Small retinal blood vessels become blocked, swollen (aneurysms), or leaky causing exudate formation, oedema, or new vessels. Laser treatment (photocoagulation) halts progression but does not restore vision.
- Good diabetic control slows development of retinopathy. Aim for $HbA_{1c}$ of 6.5% (or 48 mmol/mol).
- Monitor and treat risk factors—BP, lipids (hard exudates), smoking.
- Measure visual acuity (with glasses or pinhole) annually. Digital retinal photography is available throughout the UK. Screen at least annually to detect retinopathy before visual loss occurs.

### Refer to ophthalmologist if
(*E*=Emergency; *U*–urgent; *R*=routine)
- Sudden loss of vision—*E*
- Rubeosis iridis—*E*
- Pre-retinal or vitreous haemorrhage—*E*
- Retinal detachment—*E*
- New vessel formation—*U*
- Maculopathy—*R*
- Pre-proliferative retinopathy—*R*
- Cataract affecting visual acuity—*R*
- Unexplained drop in visual acuity—*R*.

### Further information
**NICE** ⊟ www.nice.org.uk
- Type 1 diabetes: diagnosis and management (2004)
- Type 2 diabetes (2009).

# Diabetic complications: nerve and skin

**Neuropathy** Enquire annually about painful and other symptomatic neuropathy, impotence in men, and manifestations of autonomic neuropathy especially if renal complications or erratic blood glucose control. Optimize blood sugar control.

**Symmetrical sensory progressive polyneuropathy** 40–50% patients with DM. Starts distally feet>hands. Glove and stocking distribution. May be asymptomatic or cause numbness, tingling, or neuropathic pain. Pain can be depressing and disabling. Be supportive. If simple analgesia with paracetamol or NSAID is ineffective, try neuropathic painkillers (Figure 12.2). When pain is controlled, review regularly and consider reducing dose/stopping.

**Mononeuropathies/mononeuritis multiplex** especially cranial nerves III and VI (📖 p.546).

**Amyotrophy** Painful wasting of quadriceps muscles—reversible with improved blood sugar control.

## Autonomic neuropathy
- **Postural ↓ BP** Common especially in the elderly. Increasing dietary salt intake may help. Other treatments are all unlicensed. They include fludrocortisone 100–400 micrograms od (uncomfortable oedema is a common side effect) ± flurbiprofen or ephedrine hydrochloride (30–60mg tds to relieve oedema), and midodrine (α-agonist).
- **Urinary retention** 📖 p.462
- **Diabetic diarrhoea** Exclude other causes of change in bowel habit (📖 p.414). Diabetic diarrhoea can be treated with 2 or 3 doses of tetracycline (250mg—unlicensed). Otherwise treat with codeine phosphate 30mg tds/qds prn.
- **Erectile dysfunction** 📖 p.774
- **Gastric paresis** Treat with an antiemetic which promotes gastric transit e.g. domperidone 30mg tds. When this fails, erythromycin may be used but evidence of effectiveness is lacking.
- **Gustatory sweating** Can be treated with an antimuscarinic such as propantheline bromide, but side effects are common. Hyperhidrosis (📖 p.604).

**Depression** Some physical illnesses, including DM, predispose patients to depression. Screen for depression as part of the annual diabetic check (📖 p.998).

**Skin changes associated with DM** Numerous skin problems are associated with DM. These include:
- Predisposition to infection e.g. candidiasis, staphylococcal infection e.g. folliculitis, boils.
- Pruritus.
- Xanthomas.
- Vitiligo (type 1 DM).
- Neuropathic and/or ischaemic ulcers—see the diabetic foot (📖 p.368).

- Fat atrophy/hypertrophy at insulin injection sites.
- Necrobiosis lipoidica—50% associated with DM. Small dusky red, nodules with well-circumscribed borders—can be single or multiple. Usually on outside of shin. Enlarge slowly, becoming brownish yellow, irregular, and flattened/depressed. Long-standing lesions may ulcerate. No effective treatment.
- Diabetic dermopathy—pigmented scars over shins.
- Granuloma annulare ⬤—asymptomatic dermal nodules. Association with DM is controversial.
- Diabetic cheiroarthropathy—waxy skin-thickening over the dorsum of the hand with restricted mobility.

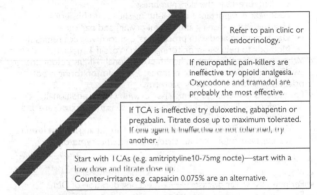

Refer to pain clinic or endocrinology.

If neuropathic pain-killers are ineffective try opioid analgesia. Oxycodone and tramadol are probably the most effective.

If TCA is ineffective try duloxetine, gabapentin or pregabalin. Titrate dose up to maximum tolerated. If one agent is ineffective or not tolerated, try another.

Start with TCAs (e.g. amitriptyline10-75mg nocte)—start with a low dose and titrate dose up.
Counter-irritants e.g. capsaicin 0.075% are an alternative.

Fig. 12.2 Diabetic neuropathy—steps to pain control

## Further information
**NICE** ▢ www.nice.org.uk
- Type 1 diabetes: diagnosis and management (2004)
- Type 2 diabetes (2009)
- Depression: management of depression in primary and secondary care (2007).

# The diabetic foot

Foot problems are common amongst diabetics. 5% develop a foot ulcer in any year and amputation rates are 0.5%/y. Foot problems are due to:
- Peripheral neuropathy (affects 20–40% diabetic patients) → ↓ foot sensation (Table 12.2) *and*
- Peripheral vascular disease (affects 20–40% diabetic patients) → pain and predisposition to ulceration (Table 12.2).

## Information about foot care
- Self-care and self-monitoring:
  - Daily examination of the feet for problems—colour change, swelling, breaks in the skin, numbness
  - Footwear—importance of well-fitting shoes and hosiery
  - Hygiene (daily washing and careful drying) and nail care
  - Dangers associated with procedures, e.g. corn/verruca removal
  - Methods to help self-monitoring, e.g. mirrors if ↓ mobility.
- When to seek advice from a health professional—if any colour change, swelling, breaks in the skin or numbness, or self-monitoring is not possible (e.g. due to mobility problems).
- For patients at increased or high risk or with ulcers, additionally advise no barefoot walking and that, because of ↓ sensation, extra care and attention are needed.
- If skin lesions, advise patients to seek help if any change in the lesion, ↑ swelling, pain, odour, colour change, or systemic symptoms.

## Risk factors
- Neuropathy
- Peripheral vascular disease
- Previous ulceration or amputation
- Age >70y
- Plantar callus
- Foot deformities
- Poor footwear
- Long duration of DM
- Social deprivation and isolation
- Poor vision
- Smoking.

**The foot check** Check the feet as part of the annual review.
### History
- Foot problems since last review.
- Visual or mobility problems affecting self-care of feet.
- Self-care behaviours and knowledge of foot care.
- History of numbness, tingling or burning—may be worse at night.

### Examination
- Foot shape, deformity, joint rigidity, and shoes.
- Foot skin condition—fragility, cracking, oedema, callus, ulceration, sweating, presence of hair.
- Foot and ankle pulses.
- Sensitivity to 10g monofilament or vibration.

## Management
### General points
- Optimize diabetic control and risk factors for vascular disease (including smoking cessation).

- Review drug therapy—stop β-blockers if peripheral vascular disease.
- Educate about foot care.

**Specific management** Classification—Table 12.3
- *Low risk* Foot care education.
- *Increased risk* Foot care education. Refer to the foot protection team. Check feet every 3–6mo. Consider referral for vascular assessment. Consider regular podiatry if poor vision, immobility or, poor social conditions/foot hygiene. If previous foot ulcer, deformity or skin changes manage as high risk.
- *High risk* Stress importance of foot care. Refer to the foot protection team for specialist podiatry. Inspect feet every 3–6mo. Review need for vascular assessment. Treat fungal infection.
- *Foot ulcer* Refer to the multidisciplinary specialist foot care team urgently. Assess ischaemia using Doppler. Consider referral for angiography. Treat infection. If new ulceration, cellulitis, or discoloration refer to a specialized podiatry/foot care team within 24h.

❶ Diabetics may have coexisting peripheral neuropathy and peripheral vascular disease. ABPI may be artificially ↑ due to calcification of vessels.

**Charcot osteoarthropathy (Charcot's joint)** Neuropathic foot damaged because of trauma 2° to loss of pain sensation. If suspected, refer immediately to the multidisciplinary footcare team for immobilization and long term management.

**Table 12.2** Clinical features of neuropathic and vascular foot ulcers

| Neuropathic | Vascular |
|---|---|
| Warm foot | Cool foot |
| Bounding pulses, normal ABPI | Absent pulses, ↓ ABPI |
| Located at pressure points | Located at extremities (e.g. between toes) |
| Painless | Painful |
| Clearly defined or 'punched out'. Surrounded by callus. | Less clearly delineated |

**Table 12.3** Classification of foot risk

| Foot risk | Features |
|---|---|
| Low current risk | Normal sensation, palpable pulses |
| Increased risk | Neuropathy, absent pulses or other risk factors |
| High risk | Neuropathy or absent pulses + deformity or skin changes or previous ulcer |
| Ulcerated foot | Foot ulcer on examination |

**Further information**

NICE 🖳 www.nice.org.uk
- Type 1 diabetes: diagnosis and management (2004)
- Type 2 diabetes: Prevention and management of foot problems (2004).

# Lumps in the thyroid gland and goitres

Faced with a lump in the pre-tracheal region of the neck, ask:
- Is it in the thyroid (moves up and down on swallowing)?
- Is it a solitary lump or more generalized (a goitre)?
- Is the patient thyrotoxic, euthyroid, or hypothyroid?
- Is the trachea being compressed (patient is breathless)?

## Management of thyroid lumps[N]

**Refer immediately to a thyroid surgeon** If symptoms of tracheal compression including stridor due to thyroid swelling.

**Refer urgently to a thyroid surgeon** If thyroid swelling + any of:
- Patient aged ≥65y
- Solitary nodule increasing in size
- History of neck irradiation
- FH of an endocrine tumour
- Unexplained hoarseness/voice changes
- Cervical lymphadenopathy
- Very young (pre-pubertal) patient.

**Investigation of patients who do not require urgent referral**
Request TFTs if thyroid swelling without stridor or any of the features listed above. ❶ Do not request USS or isotope scanning.
- **Refer non-urgently to endocrinology** Patients with hyper- or hypothyroidism and an associated goitre.
- **Refer non-urgently to a thyroid surgeon** Patients with goitre and normal thyroid function tests without any of the features listed above.

**Solitary thyroid nodules** Investigate *all* solitary nodules. Check TFTs and refer as above. Differential diagnosis:
- **Benign** (~90%): cyst, adenoma, discrete nodule in a nodular goitre.
- **Malignant** (~10%): *primary*—thyroid adenocarcinoma, lymphoma, medullary carcinoma; *secondary*—direct spread from local tumour, metastatic spread from breast, colon/rectum, kidney, lung, lymphoma.

**Carcinoma of the thyroid** Primary tumours:
- **Papillary adenocarcinoma** (60%). Typical age range: 10–40y. ♀ > ♂. Low-grade malignancy. Rarely fatal. Spreads to local LNs and/or lung. Sensitive to TSH. Treated with thyroidectomy, then lifelong thyroxine.
- **Follicular carcinoma** (25%) Typical age range: 40–60y. ♀ > ♂. May arise in a pre-existing multinodular goitre. Spreads via bloodstream. Bony secondaries are common. Treatment is with surgery and thyroxine suppression therapy and/or radioactive iodine.
- **Lymphoma** (5%) Occurs at any age. May be 1° or 2°. Associated with Hashimoto's thyroiditis. Staged/treated as for lymphomas elsewhere (📖 p.678). Prognosis is good.
- **Anaplastic carcinoma** (rare) Typical age range: 50–60y. ♀ > ♂. Aggressive tumour. Grows rapidly and infiltrates tissues of the neck. Tracheal compression is common. Metastasizes locally to LNs and via lymphatics. Poor response to treatment.
- **Medullary carcinoma** (rare) Occurs at any age. ♀ = ♂. Familial incidence; associated with adenomas elsewhere. Often secretes calcitonin (used as tumour marker). Spreads to local LNs. Treated by excision then chemotherapy ± radiotherapy.

**Goitre** There are 5 main types of goitre (Table 12.4).

**Thyroid cyst** Usually degenerative part of a nodular goitre, though true cysts do occur. Rapid enlargement/pain may be caused by haemorrhage into a cyst. Refer for confirmation of diagnosis.

**Thyroid adenoma** Four types classified according to histological appearance—papillary, follicular, embryonal, hurtle cell. A few produce thyroxine → thyrotoxicosis. Haemorrhage is rare and results in rapid ↑ in size. Refer for confirmation of diagnosis ± surgery.

**Table 12.4** Types of goitre—presentation and management

| Type | Features | Management |
|---|---|---|
| Congenital | Enlarged thyroid gland present at birth ± hypo- or hyperthyroidism | Hypothyroid babies are treated with thyroxine; if there is tracheal compression or hyperthyroidism treatment is surgical |
| Physiological | Occurs at puberty, during pregnancy, and in conditions of iodine deficiency | Usually requires no treatment. If iodine deficient, treat with iodine supplements |
| Nodular | Benign enlargement of the thyroid gland with areas of hyperplasia and involution | No treatment is necessary unless:<br>• Thyrotoxic<br>• Compression of the neck structures → dyspnoea or dysphagia<br>• Worried by cosmetic appearance<br>• Focal ↑ in size or recurrent laryngeal nerve palsy (hoarseness)—suggest malignant change<br><br>If treatment is needed, refer to surgery or endocrinology depending on symptoms |
| Toxic | *Graves' disease*: Smooth thyroid enlargement + thyrotoxicosis | See management of hyperthyroidism 📖 p.372 |
| Inflammatory | *Hashimoto's thyroiditis*: ♀>♂ Antibodies to thyroid tissue are produced. Initially goitre and thyrotoxicosis. Later myxoedema<br><br>*De Quervain's thyroiditis*: Inflammation due to viral infection—usually Coxsackie virus. Acutely swollen and tender thyroid gland and transient thyrotoxicosis often preceded by sore throat/malaise. Settles spontaneously<br><br>*Riedel's thyroiditis*: Rare. Thyroid becomes infiltrated by scar tissue → hypothyroidism ± recurrent laryngeal nerve palsy ± stridor | In all cases refer to endocrinology for confirmation of diagnosis and management guidance |

**Further information**
**NICE** Referral guidelines for suspected cancer (2005) 🖥 www.nice.org.uk

# Thyroid disease

**Hyperthyroidism** Affects 2% ♀ and 0.2% ♂. *Peak age: 20–49y. Causes:*
- Graves' disease
- Toxic nodular goitre—older women with past history of goitre
- Thyroiditis
- Amiodarone
- Kelp ingestion.

### Presentation
- Weight loss
- Tremor
- Palpitations
- Hyperactivity
- AF
- Hyperhidrosis
- Eye changes
- Infertility
- Alopecia.

❶ In elderly patients symptoms may be less obvious and include confusion, dementia, apathy and depression.

**Management** Refer to endocrinology at presentation. Treatment:
- *ß-blockers* (e.g. propranolol, atenolol) Useful for symptom control until anti-thyroid drug therapy takes effect.
- *Carbimazole* Inhibits synthesis of thyroid hormones. Ineffective for treatment of thyroiditis. May be given short term to render a patient euthyroid prior to surgery/treatment with radioactive iodine or long term (12–18 mo) in an attempt to induce remission (but >50% relapse). 3:1000 patients have serious adverse effects—agranulocytosis, hepatitis, aplastic anaemia, or lupus-like syndromes.
- *Radioactive iodine ($^{131}$I)* Effects take 3–4mo to become apparent. Withdraw carbimazole >4d prior to treatment and do not restart until >3d after. Advise women of child-bearing age to avoid pregnancy for 4mo. Most become hypothyroid at some point (sometimes years) after treatment. Continue monitoring TFTs long-term (Table 12.5). Associated with small ↑ risk of thyroid malignancy.
- *Surgery* Partial or total thyroidectomy—reserved for patients with large goitres or who decline radioactive iodine. Carries risk of damage to recurrent laryngeal nerve or parathyroids.

⚠ Warn *all* patients starting carbimazole to stop the drug and seek urgent medical attention if they develop sore throat or other infection.

**Thyrotoxic crisis/storm** 📖 p.1097

**Graves' disease** Most common cause of hyperthyroidism. ♀:♂≈5:1. *Peak age: 30–50y.* Associated with smoking and stressful life events. Auto-immune disease in which antibodies to the TSH receptor are produced. *R.J. Graves (1797–1853)—Irish physician.*

### Clinical features
- Hyperthyroidism.
- Diffuse goitre ± thyroid bruit due to ↑ vascularity.
- Extrathyroid features: eye disease 25–50% (bilateral in >90%); pretibial myxoedema 5%; thyroid acropachy (rare); clubbing, finger swelling; onycholysis (rare).

**Management** As for hyperthyroidism.

**Table 12.5** Interpretation of thyroid function test results

| Results of TFTs | Interpretation | Notes |
|---|---|---|
| TSH↓, T₄↑ | Thyrotoxic | Occasionally T₄ is normal but T₃ ↑ |
| TSH↑, T₄↓ | Hypothyroid | TSH ↓ if hypothyroidism is secondary to pituitary failure (rare) |
| TSH↑, T₄↔ | Subclinical hypothyroidism | If any symptoms (including depression and non-specific symptoms or hypercholesterolaemia) consider a trial of treatment. If no symptoms monitor annually |

**Thyroid eye disease** Presents with:
- Double vision
- Eye discomfort ± protrusion (exopthalmos and proptosis)
- Lid lag
- Ophthalmoplegia (especially of upward gaze)
- TFTs can be ↑ or normal.

**Management** Refer to ophthalmologist. If ↓ acuity or loss of colour vision—refer urgently as there may be optic nerve compression.

**Hypothyroidism (myxoedema)** Common—10% ♀ >60y, ♀:♂≈8:1.

**Causes** Chronic autoimmune thyroiditis, post ¹³¹I administration, thyroidectomy.

**Presentation** Onset tends to be insidious and may go undiagnosed for years. Always consider hypothyroidism when a patient has non-specific symptoms, depression, fatigue, lethargy, or general malaise. Other symptoms—weight ↑, constipation, hoarse voice, or dry skin/hair. Signs are often absent—there may be a goitre, slow-relaxing reflexes, or non-pitting oedema of the hands, feet, or eyelids.

**Screening** Check TFTs in patients:
- With persistent symptoms of tiredness/lethargy without clear cause
- On amiodarone or with a history of ¹³¹I administration
- With hypercholesterolaemia, infertility, depression, dementia, obesity, DM, other autoimmune disease, Turner's syndrome, or congenital hypothyroidism.

**Management** Patients taking thyroxine replacement are entitled to apply for free prescriptions (📖 p.139).
- **<65y and healthy** 150 micrograms od levothyroxine. Re-check TFTs after 12wk. Adjust dose to keep TSH in normal range. Once dose is stable and TSH is within normal range monitor annually and if symptomatic or worries about compliance.
- **If elderly or pre-existing heart disease** Start 25 micrograms od levothyroxine and ↑ dose every 4wk according to TFTs. Consider adding propranolol if history of IHD as levothyroxine can provoke angina.

**Withdrawal of levothyroxine** Usually needed lifelong. If diagnosis is in doubt, stop and re-measure TFTs after 4–6wk.

**Hypothyroid coma** 📖 p.1097

**Information for patients**
**British Thyroid Foundation** 🖥 www.btf-thyroid.org

# Hyper- and hypocalcaemia

**Checking Ca²⁺** Check serum calcium level on an *uncuffed* sample (to avoid falsely high readings) and correct for serum albumin—for every mmol/L less than 40, a correction of 0.02 mmol/L should be added to the serum calcium concentration measured. For example :

Calcium 2.40              Corrected calcium    $= (40 - 24) \times 0.02 + 2.4$
Albumin 24                                              $= 0.32 + 2.4 = \mathbf{2.72}$

**Hypocalcaemia** ↓ serum calcium (<2.15 mmol/L). *Causes:*
- *If phosphate* ↑ CRF, hypoparathyroidism (may be congenital or 2° to thyroid or parathyroid surgery, or malignant infiltration), pseudohypoparathyroidism (insensitivity to parathyroid hormone).
- *If phosphate normal or* ↓ Vitamin D deficiency (osteomalacia, rickets), malabsorption, overhydration, pancreatitis.

*Presentation* May be subtle. Includes:
- Tetany
- Irritability, depression or psychosis
- Perioral paraesthesia
- Carpopedal spasm (wrist flexion and fingers drawn together)
- Neuromuscular excitability (tapping over parotid causes facial muscles to contract—Chvostek's sign).

❶ Apparent hypocalcaemia may be an artefact of hypoalbuminaemia.

*Management* Supplement with calcium. Secondary care referral is usually needed to investigate and treat the underlying cause.

**Hypercalcaemia** Presence of ↑ level of serum calcium (>2.55 mmol/L). Prevalence ≈ 1/1000; ♂:♀ ≈ 1:3. Rare <age 50y.

**Common causes**
- Primary hyperparathyroidism
- Malignancy (10% tumours—usually myeloma, breast, lung, kidney, thyroid, prostate, ovary or colon)
- Chronic renal failure.

**Uncommon causes**
- Familial benign hypercalcaemia
- Sarcoidosis
- Thyrotoxicosis
- Milk alkali syndrome
- Vitamin D treatment.

*Presentation* Often very non-specific but if increasing serum Ca²⁺ is left untreated, it can be fatal. May be an incidental finding. Other symptoms: *'bones, stones, groans and abdominal moans'*
- Tiredness
- Lethargy
- Weakness
- Mild aches and pains
- Anorexia
- Weight loss
- Low mood
- Stone formation
- Nausea/vomiting (often intractable)
- Polyuria and polydipsia
- Abdominal pain
- Constipation
- Confusion
- Corneal calcification.

*Management*
- Treat according to cause (Figure 12.3)—malignancy (📖 p.1028); hyperparathyroidism (📖 p.375).
- If diagnosis is unclear refer to endocrinology. Urgency depends on serum Ca²⁺ and severity of symptoms.

⚠ If $Ca^{2+}$ > 3.5 mmol/L or severe symptoms, admit for lowering of $Ca^{2+}$ with forced diuresis and IV bisphosphonate.

**Hyperparathyroidism** ↑ secretion of parathyroid hormone (PTH).
• *1° hyperparathyroidism* Incidence 0.5/1000. Peak age 40–60y ♀:♂≈2:1. Circulating level of PTH is inappropriately high. Most patients are hypercalcaemic (but may be normocalcaemic if coexistent vitamin D deficiency). Due to ↑ secretion of PTH from one or both parathyroid glands. Refer. Treatment is usually surgical.
• *2° hyperparathyroidism* ↑ PTH in response to chronic hypocalcaemia or hyperphosphataemia. Treat cause.
• *3° hyperparathyroidism* Inappropriately ↑ PTH → ↑$Ca^{2+}$. Follows prolonged 2° hyperparathyroidism. Most common in patients with chronic renal failure (especially if on dialysis) or chronic malabsorption. Treatment is usually surgical.

**Familial benign hypercalcaemia** Asymptomatic. Inherited condition in which serum calcium concentrations are mildly ↑ throughout life. Confirm (if possible) by demonstrating ↑ $Ca^{2+}$ in other family members. No adverse consequences and no treatment needed.

**Milk alkali syndrome** Usually due to ingestion of OTC indigestion remedies. $Ca^{2+}$ levels revert to normal on stopping. Investigate the reason why the patient is taking these remedies (? peptic ulcer).

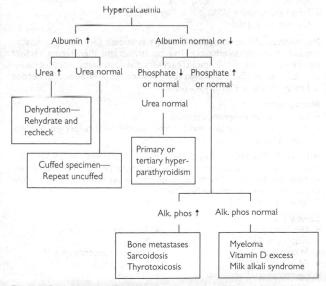

**Fig. 12.3** Guide to the diagnosis of cause of hypercalcaemia (must be taken in clinical context)

# Adrenal disorders

**Disorders of the adrenal cortex** The adrenal cortex produces three classes of steroids:
- Glucocorticoids, e.g. cortisol
- Mineralocorticoids, e.g. aldosterone
- Sex hormones, e.g. androstenedione, testosterone, oestrogen.

Disorders result from disturbance in production of these steroids:

**Cushing's syndrome** In the majority of cases, Cushing's syndrome is iatrogenic—caused by exogenous administration of prednisolone or other corticosteroids. Non-iatrogenic Cushing's syndrome is much rarer with annual incidence of 1–2/million ($♀:♂≈3:1$):
- 80% have a pituitary adenoma which secretes adrenocorticotrophic hormone (ACTH) causing hypersecretion of glucocorticoids and sex hormones (Cushing's disease).
- 20% are due to ectopic ACTH secretion by other tumours (e.g. small cell lung cancer) or hypersecreting tumours of the adrenal cortex.

*H.W. Cushing (1869–1939)—US neurosurgeon.*

**Presentation** Cushing's syndrome has high morbidity and mortality. Clinical features include:

- Moon face (90%)
- Truncal obesity (85%)
- Hypertension (80%)
- Menstrual disturbance (80%)
- Striae and bruising (60%)
- Osteoporosis (60%)
- Lethargy/depression (60%)
- Hirsutism
- Acne
- Pigmentation
- Feminization in men
- Polyuria and polydipsia
- Psychosis.

**Investigation of non-iatrogenic Cushing's syndrome** Dexamethasone suppression test—dexamethasone 1mg po at midnight then serum cortisol measured at 9a.m. If <50mmol/L excludes diagnosis unless cortisol secretion is episodic. False positives are common. Expert advice is needed before proceeding with further tests.

**Management**
- Stop/minimize exogenous steroids.
- If no exogenous steroids and Cushing's syndrome is suspected, refer to endocrinology. Usually treated surgically.

**Addison's disease** Primary adrenocortical insufficiency. In the UK most cases are due to autoimmune disease, surgery, or cessation of therapeutic steroids (or failure to ↑ dose to cover stress)—worldwide TB is a major cause. Prevalence 50/million ($♀:♂≈3:1$).

*T. Addison (1795–1860)—English physician.*

**Clinical features**
- Tiredness (95%)
- Weakness (95%)
- Anorexia (95%)
- Weight loss (90%)
- Pigmentation (buccal, palmar creases, new scars (90%))
- Abdominal pain (30%)
- Myalgia (20%)
- Postural hypotension and fainting (15%)
- Nausea
- Arthralgia.

*Presentation*
- Can be dramatic with coma and severe hypoglycaemia or insidious with vague symptoms of malaise and lassitude.
- 50% of patients with autoimmune Addison's disease have or will develop another autoimmune disease (e.g. Graves' disease, pernicious anaemia) and 5% of women develop premature ovarian failure, so review regularly with these possibilities in mind.

*Investigation*
- Biochemical abnormalities—↑$K^+$, ↓$Na^+$, ↓ glucose (may not be symptomatic), uraemia, ↑$Ca^{2+}$, abnormal LFTs.
- FBC—neutropoenia, lymphocytosis.

*Management*
- Refer to endocrinology. Patients have a normal lifespan if treated.
- Treatment usually involves replacing deficient steroids with hydrocortisone and fludrocortisone. Adjust doses carefully.
- Warn patients not to stop steroids abruptly and to tell any doctor treating them about their condition (and wear warning bracelet in case of emergency).
- Double dose of hydrocortisone prior to dental treatment or if intercurrent illness (e.g. URTI). If vomiting, replace hydrocortisone po with IM hydrocortisone.

**Hyperaldosteronism (Conn's syndrome)** Suggested by presence of ↑BP with ↓$K^+$, but normokalaemic cases are also described. Two-thirds have an aldosterone-secreting adenoma. Referral for endocrine assesment is important as adenomas can be removed surgically. Spironolactone is an effective alternative treatment.
*J.W. Conn (1907–1994)—US endocrinologist.*

**Congenital adrenal hyperplasia** 📖 p.892.

## Disorders of the adrenal medulla

**Phaechromocytoma** Rare but serious disorder affecting 0.1% of hypertensive patients. Usually caused by catecholamine-secreting tumours: 10% are bilateral; 10% extra-adrenal; 10% occur in children; 10% are malignant.

*Presentation* May present with a huge array of symptoms and signs. ↑BP may be sporadic or sustained. Suspect in young patients with ↑BP, patients with very labile BP or if associated headaches, sweating, and/or palpitations. May be associated with other conditions (e.g. neurofibromatosis).

*Investigation* Urine catecholamine/metabolite levels.

*Management* Consult local guidelines. Refer for specialist opinion if suspected. Treatment is usually surgical.

## Patient advice and support
**Pituitary Foundation** ☎ 0845 450 0375 🖳 www.pituitary.org.uk (booklet on Cushing's disease and GP Factfile)
**Addison's Disease Self Help Group** 🖳 www.addisons.org.uk

# Pituitary problems

**Hypopituitarism** ↓ production of all pituitary hormones (ACTH, growth hormone, FSH, LH, TSH, and prolactin). *Causes:*

- Surgery.
- Irradiation.
- Tumour (may be non-secreting or secrete one pituitary hormone with ↓ secretion of the others).
- Infection—TB.
- Sheehan's syndrome—pituitary necrosis after postpartum haemorrhage. *H.L. Sheehan (b. 1900)—English pathologist.*

*Presentation*

- Hypothyroidism
- Hypogonadism
- Anorexia
- Headache
- Depression
- Hair loss
- Hypotension
- Visual field defect.

*Management* If suspected refer to neurology or endocrinology for further investigation and advice on treatment.

**Pituitary tumours** 10% intracranial tumours. Almost all are benign. Classified by histological type (chromophobic, acidophilic, or basophilic) or by the hormone secreted:

- No hormone (30%).
- Prolactin (35%).
- Growth hormone (20%).
- ACTH (7%).
- Prolactin and growth hormone (7%).
- LH, FSH and TSH (1%).

*Presentation* Present with symptoms caused by:

- Local pressure (bilateral hemianopia, cranial nerve palsies, headache)
- Hormone secretion *and/or*
- Hypopituitarism.

*Management* Refer for further investigation and treatment if suspected.

**Pituitary apoplexy** Rapid expansion of a pituitary tumour due to infarction or haemorrhage. Suspect if sudden onset of headache in a patient with a known pituitary tumour. Admit as a medical/neurosurgical emergency.

**Craniopharyngioma** Tumour originating from Rathke's pouch. 50% present with local pressure effects in children (see 'pituitary tumours'). Refer as for pituitary tumours.

**Hyperprolactinaemia** The most common pituitary disorder. Due to pituitary adenoma.

*Presentation* Tends to present earlier in women than men. Symptoms are due to pressure effects or ↑ prolactin. Symptoms of ↑ prolactin.

- ♀: Loss of libido, weight gain, apathy, vaginal dryness, menstrual disturbance, infertility, galactorrhoea.
- ♂: Impotence, ↓ facial hair.

***Investigation*** Check basal plasma prolactin (ask the lab for conditions under which they would like the sample taken).

***Management*** If suspected refer for specialist opinion.

### Other causes of ↑ prolactin
- Pregnancy
- Breast-feeding
- Stress
- Sleep
- Hypothyroidism
- Drugs—phenothiazines, metoclopramide, α-methyldopa, oestrogens
- Chronic renal failure
- Sarcoidosis.

**Acromegaly** Rare condition due to a growth hormone secreting pituitary tumour. *Typical age at presentation:* 30-50y.

### Presentation
- Local pressure symptoms.
- Changes in appearance—coarse oily skin; change in facial appearance with coarsening of features; ↑ foot size; ↑ teeth spacing.
- Other effects—deepening of voice, sweating, paraesthesiae, proximal muscle weakness, progressive heart failure, goitre.
- Complications  DM, ↑BP, cardiomyopathy, large bowel tumours.

***Investigation and management*** Refer to endocrinology

**Diabetes insipidus (DI)** Caused by impaired water resorption by the kidney. Two mechanisms:
- **Cranial DI** ↓ADH secretion from the posterior pituitary. 50% idiopathic. *Other causes:* head injury, tumour, infection, sarcoidosis, vascular, inherited.
- **Nephrogenic DI** Impaired response of the kidney to ADH. *Causes:* drugs (e.g. lithium), hypercalcaemia, pyelonephritis, hydronephrosis, pregnancy (rare).

***Presentation*** Polydipsia, polyuria, dilute urine, dehydration.

***Investigations*** U&E (↑Na⁺), Ca²⁺, plasma and urine osmolality (↑ plasma, ↓ urine). Specialist investigations (e.g. water deprivation test) confirm diagnosis.

***Management*** Treat the cause.
- Cranial DI may be treated with intranasal desmopressin or surgery.
- Nephrogenic DI may be treated with dietary restriction of protein and salt and/or bendroflumethiazide.

**Syndrome of inappropriate ADH (SIADH)** Important cause of hyponatraemia. Diagnosis is made by finding a concentrated urine (sodium >20mmol/L) in the presence of hyponatraemia (<125mmol/L) or low plasma osmolality (<260mmol/kg), and absence of hypovolaemia, oedema, or diuretics. Always requires specialist management. *Causes:*
- **Malignancy** e.g. small-cell lung cancer, pancreas, lymphoma.
- **CNS disorders** e.g. stroke, subdural haemorrhage, vasculitis (SLE).

### Patient advice and support
**Pituitary Foundation** ☎ 0845 450 0375 🖳 www.pituitary.org.uk (also GP Factfile)

# Gastrointestinal medicine

# Assessment of abdominal pain

❶ Signs may be unclear in elderly patients, children or those on steroids.

**History** Consider:
- Site of pain—Figure 13.1.
- Onset: How long? How did it start? Change over time?
- Character of pain: Colicky pain comes and goes in waves—results from GI obstruction, renal/biliary colic, gastroenteritis, or IBS.
- Radiation.
- Associated symptoms, e.g nausea, vomiting, diarrhoea.
- Timing/pattern, e.g constant, colicky, relationship to food.
- Exacerbating/relieving factors—including previous treatments tried.
- Severity.

## Examination
- Temperature, pulse, BP.
- Anaemia or jaundice?
- Abdomen—site of pain (Figure 13.1); guarding/rebound tenderness?
- Rectal/vaginal examination as needed.

**Management** Treat the cause (Table 13.1).

⚠ If acute or sub-acute onset severe pain, admit as a surgical emergency to hospital. Do not give analgesia prior to surgical assessment as it may mask vital diagnostic signs.

**Table 13.1** Differential diagnosis of abdominal pain

| Renal/urological | Gastrointestinal | Other intra-abdominal |
|---|---|---|
| Renal colic | *Surgical* | Sickle cell crisis |
| UTI | Perforated bowel | Ruptured spleen |
| Pyelonephritis | Bowel obstruction | Leaking/ruptured AAA |
| Hydronephrosis | Intussusception | Mesenteric ischaemia |
| Henoch–Schönlein purpura | Strangulated hernia | Mesenteric adenitis |
| Torsion of the testis | Volvulus | Subphrenic abscess |
| | Appendicitis | |
| **Gynaecological** | Meckel's diverticulum | **Metabolic** |
| Ectopic pregnancy | Gall bladder disease | DM—ketoacidosis |
| Dysmenorrhoea | Pancreatitis | Porphyria |
| Endometriosis | GI malignancy | Addison's disease |
| Pelvic inflammatory disease | | Lead poisoning |
| Ovarian torsion | *Medical* | |
| Ovarian cyst—bleed/ rupture | Gastritis | **Other extra-abdominal** |
| Gynaecological malignancy | Peptic ulcer | Shingles/post-herpetic neuralgia |
| | Gastroenteritis | Spinal arthritis |
| | Crohn's/UC | Muscular pain |
| | IBS | MI |
| | Constipation | CCF |
| | Diverticular disease | Pneumonia |
| | Liver disease | |

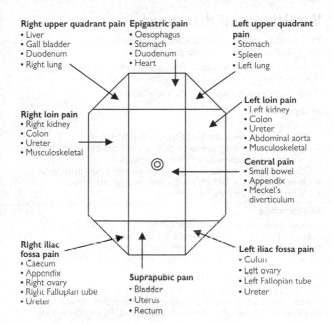

**Right upper quadrant pain**
• Liver
• Gall bladder
• Duodenum
• Right lung

**Epigastric pain**
• Oesophagus
• Stomach
• Duodenum
• Heart

**Left upper quadrant pain**
• Stomach
• Spleen
• Left lung

**Right loin pain**
• Right kidney
• Colon
• Ureter
• Musculoskeletal

**Left loin pain**
• Left kidney
• Colon
• Ureter
• Abdominal aorta
• Musculoskeletal

**Central pain**
• Small bowel
• Appendix
• Meckel's diverticulum

**Right iliac fossa pain**
• Caecum
• Appendix
• Right ovary
• Right Fallopian tube
• Ureter

**Suprapubic pain**
• Bladder
• Uterus
• Rectum

**Left iliac fossa pain**
• Colon
• Left ovary
• Left Fallopian tube
• Ureter

**Fig.13.1** Location of pain and organs likely to be involved

**Pelvic pain** 📖 p.712.

**Anal/perianal pain** Treat the cause. *Consider:*

• Anal fissure
• Haemorrhoids/perianal haematoma (thrombosed pile)
• Perianal abscess
• Anal/perianal fistula
• Pilonidal sinus
• Skin infection (e.g. hidradenitis suppurativa)
• Functional pain (proctalgia fugax)
• Rectal/anal carcinoma.

**Tenesmus** Sensation of incomplete rectal emptying following defecation—as if something has been left behind which cannot be passed. Common in irritable bowel syndrome. Can be caused by tumour.

> **Abdominal migraine or periodic syndrome**
> Seen in children. Presents as stereotyped attacks in which nausea, vomiting, and headache accompany abdominal pain. Treat as for migraine. Some of these children develop classical migraine later.

# Vomiting and diarrhoea

Most episodes of acute vomiting and diarrhoea are due to viral infection, short-lived (2–5d) and self-limiting.

**Nausea** Unpleasant symptom. The patient feels as if he/she might vomit. Most conditions which cause vomiting can also cause nausea.

**Vomiting** Common symptom. *Causes*—Table 13.2.

### History
- Duration.
- Ability to retain food and fluids/relationship to eating.
- Nature of vomitus, e.g. presence of blood or 'coffee grounds', bilious.
- Contact with anyone else with similar symptoms?
- Other associated symptoms, e.g. fever, abdominal pain, diarrhoea.
- Other illnesses, e.g. DM, Ménière's disease, migraine, cancer.
- Medication, e.g. opioids, chemotherapy.

### Examination
- Assess hydration status—BP, pulse rate, dry mouth, ↓ skin turgor, sunken eyes, or sunken fontanelle (babies) are all late signs.
- Abdomen—masses, distention, tenderness, bowel sounds.
- For children—look for other sources of infection, e.g. ENT, chest, UTI.

**Haematemesis** 📖 p.1072.

**Slimy stool** Caused by overproduction of mucus in the large bowel. Almost always associated with colonic disease/irritable bowel syndrome. Investigate unless all other features are typical of IBS and age is <40y.

**Diarrhoea** Establish what the patient means by diarrhoea. Diarrhoea is the abnormal passage of loose or liquid stools. Causes—Table 13.2.

### History
- Duration—termed 'chronic' if persists >4wk.
- Nature of the diarrhoea—colour, consistency, blood/mucus.
- Contact with anyone else with similar symptoms?
- Travel history.
- Associated symptoms, e.g. fever, abdominal pain, vomiting, weight ↓.
- Past medical history—surgery (especially ileal resection or cholecystectomy); pancreatic disease; systemic disease (e.g. DM, thyrotoxicosis).
- Family history—inflammatory bowel or coeliac disease; bowel cancer.
- Alcohol consumption—high intake is associated with diarrhoea.
- Medication, e.g. antibiotics, NSAIDs, regular medications (cause of 4% chronic diarrhoea).

### Examination
- Assess hydration status—BP, pulse rate, dry mouth, ↓ skin turgor, sunken eyes, or sunken fontanelle (babies) are all late signs.
- Abdomen—masses, distention, tenderness, bowel sounds, stool.

**Investigation** send a stool sample for M,C&S if any of the following:

| | | |
|---|---|---|
| • Fever | • Recent return from a | • Resident in an institution |
| • Blood in stool | tropical climate | • Persists >7d. |
| • Food worker | • Immunocompromise | |

**Table 13.2** Causes of vomiting and diarrhoea

| Vomiting | Diarrhoea |
| --- | --- |
| Physiological—e.g. posseting in babies | *Acute diarrhoea* |
| Travel/motion sickness | Dietary indiscretion |
| GI infection—e.g. viral gastroenteritis, food poisoning | Infection e.g. food poisoning, traveller's diarrhoea |
| Other infection (particularly children)—tonsillitis, otitis media | Constipation with overflow |
| | Pseudomembranous colitis—recent history of oral antibiotics |
| Other GI causes—GI obstruction; pyloric stenosis; 'acute abdomen' | Onset of inflammatory bowel disease or other chronic diarrhoea |
| CNS causes—raised intracranial pressure, head injury, migraine, vertigo | |
| | *Chronic diarrhoea* |
| Metabolic causes—pregnancy; uraemia; ketoacidosis | Table 13.11 (📖 p.415) |
| Psychiatric causes—anorexia; bulimia | |
| Malignancy | |
| Drugs and toxins—e.g. alcohol, opioids, cytotoxic agents | |

## Management of acute diarrhoea and/or vomiting

- Treat any identified cause
- Rehydration—encourage clear fluid intake (small amounts frequently) ± rehydration salts (use a commercial preparation, e.g. Dioralyte®)
- Food—stick to a bland diet, avoiding dairy products until symptoms have settled. Babies who are breastfed or have not been weaned should continue their normal milk.
- If dehydrated and unable to replace fluids, e.g. diarrhoea with concomitant vomiting or child/elderly person refusing to drink—admit.

⚠ Never give children antidiarrhoeal agents.

❶ *If no cause is found and diarrhoea lasts >4wk, or any atypical features* consider referral for urgent investigation (📖 p.414).

**Gastroenteritis** 📖 p.418

**Chronic diarrhoea and malabsorption** 📖 p.414

**Faecal incontinence** 📖 p.416

**Melaena or rectal bleeding** 📖 p.1072

**Factitious diarrhoea** 📖 p.415

- Some children may become cow's milk intolerant after a bout of gastroenteritis (📖 p.887).
- Think of haemolytic uraemic syndrome in any child with diarrhoea who passes blood in the stool.

## Further information

**NICE** Diarrhoea and vomiting in children under 5 (2009) 🖥 www.nice.org.uk

# Constipation

3 million GP consultations/y in the UK are because of constipation. Differentiate normal stools a few days apart (normal, needs no treatment) and infrequent hard stools (suggests constipation).

**Definition** Two or more of the following for ≥3 mo:
• Straining at defecation ≥¼ of the time.
• A sensation of incomplete evacuation ≥ ¼ of the time.
• ≤2 bowel movements/wk. Lumpy and/or hard stools ≥¼ of the time.

❶ Most patients consulting in general practice do not meet these criteria.

**Children with constipation** 📖 p.886

**Young patients <40y with lone constipation** ♀:♂ ≈ 9:1. Establish symptoms—constipation is usually long-standing in this group. Include drug history. Ask about health beliefs—80% believe that their bowels should open daily. Explore concerns about underlying disease. If long-standing ask why the patient is consulting now. Examine the abdomen. Investigate if symptoms/signs suggestive of organic disease (Table 13.3).

*Management* Treat organic causes. Otherwise:
• Give lifestyle advice—↑ fluid intake to ≥ 2L/d (8–10 cups); avoid alcohol; ↑ exercise if possible; add fibre to diet (↑ fruit/vegetables, eat whole-grain foods, and coarse bran to food); open bowel when needed.
• If lifestyle advice alone fails and symptoms are causing distress, start an osmotic laxative, e.g. magnesium hydroxide 15mL bd.
• If an osmotic laxative fails, try a short course of a stimulant laxative, e.g. senna 1–2 tablets at 5p.m., either alone or in combination with an osmotic laxative. Long-term use of some stimulant laxatives is reported to cause cathartic atonic colon. Although there is no evidence that senna causes this, in young fit patients only use short courses or use intermittently, e.g twice weekly.
• If still constipated specialist referral is warranted.

**Irritable bowel syndrome with constipation** 20% develop symptoms of irritable bowel syndrome (IBS) in their lifetime (📖 p.426). Constipation is the predominant symptom in 30%. Other symptoms are usually present. Establish symptoms. Examine the abdomen. Investigation is usually unnecessary unless atypical features

*Management* If <40y, examination is normal, and constipation is associated with abdominal pain that is relieved by opening bowels, IBS can be diagnosed. Manage as for young patients with lone constipation but avoid osmotic laxatives as they make bloating worse.

**Constipation in the over-40s** Any sustained change in bowel habit for >6wk should be taken seriously and investigated if appropriate. Establish symptoms and onset. Specifically ask about tenesmus, blood in stool, abdominal pain, and diarrhoea. Check current medication. Examine the abdomen for masses and hepatomegaly. Rectal examination is essential to exclude low rectal or anal carcinoma and detect faecal impaction.

**Table 13.3** Organic causes of constipation

| Colonic disease | Carcinoma | Stricture |
|---|---|---|
| | Diverticular disease | Intussusception |
| | Crohn's disease | Volvulus |
| Anorectal disease | Anterior mucosal prolapse | Anal fissure |
| | Distal proctitis | Perianal abscess |
| Pelvic disease | Ovarian tumour | Endometriosis |
| | Uterine tumour | |
| Endocrine/metabolic disorders | Hypercalcaemia | DM with autonomic |
| | Hypothyroidism | neuropathy |
| Drugs | Opioids | Antiparkinsonian drugs |
| | Antacids containing calcium or | Anticholinergics |
| | aluminium | Anticonvulsants |
| | Antidepressants | Antihistamines |
| | Iron | Calcium antagonists |
| Other | Pregnancy | Poor fluid intake |
| | Immobility | |

## Management

- Check FBC, ESR, renal function tests, LFTs, TFTs, and serum glucose.
- Image the lower bowel by colonoscopy or barium enema if new symptoms that persist >6wk.
- Treat any reversible underlying organic cause (Table 13.3).
- Give lifestyle advice (see management of young people with lone constipation).
- Treat symptomatically if no cause is found/cause is untreatable
- Laxatives—consider an osmotic laxative (e.g. lactulose, magnesium hydroxide) or bulk-forming laxative (e.g. ispaghula, sterculia) ± a stimulant laxative (e.g. senna). Titrate dose to response.
- Long-term use of stimulant laxatives including co-danthrusate is acceptable in the very elderly. Otherwise use prn or intermittently.
- If oral laxatives are ineffective consider adding rectal measures. If soft stool, try bisacodyl suppositories (❶ must come into direct contact with rectum); if hard stools try glycerol suppositories (act in 1–6h)
- If still not cleared/faecal impaction—refer to the district nurse for lubricant ± high phosphate (stimulant) enema (acts in ~20min).
- Once constipation has been cleared, leave the patient with clear instructions about what to do if symptoms recur.

⚠ **High-risk patients**, e.g. patients on opioids; those who are immobile or have medical conditions which predispose them to constipation. Pre-empt constipation by putting high-risk patients on regular aperients.

 **Occult presentations of constipation** are common in the elderly and include:
- Confusion
- Urinary retention
- Abdominal pain
- Overflow diarrhoea
- Loss of appetite and nausea.

# Other abdominal symptoms and signs

**Dyspepsia** 🕮 p.390.

**Abdominal distention** Consider abdominal/pelvic masses and:

- Fluid—ascites or full bladder
- Fat
- Faeces
- Flatus—intestinal obstruction, air swallowing
- Fetus
- Food, e.g. malabsorption.

**Abdominal masses** Distinguished from pelvic masses by the ability to get beneath them. *Causes:* malignancy—any intra-abdominal organ or kidney, stool, abdominal aortic aneurysm, heptato- and/or splenomegaly, appendix mass/abscess, Crohn's mass, lymph nodes, or TB mass. ❶ Hernia may present as mass in abdominal wall/groin lump (🕮 p.400).

**Pelvic masses** *Causes:* fetus, full bladder, fibroids, gynaecological malignancy, bladder cancer.

**Splenomegaly** *Causes:*
- *Haematological* Lymphoma, leukaemia, myeloproliferative disorders, sickle cell disease (children usually), thalassaemia.
- *Inflammatory* RA or Sjögren's syndrome, sarcoid, amyloid.
- *Infection* Glandular fever, malaria, SBE, TB, leishmaniasis.

**Hepatomegaly** *Causes:*
- *Apparent* Reidel's lobe, low-lying diaphragm.
- *Tumours* Secondary (most common), primary.
- *Venous congestion* Heart failure, hepatic vein occlusion.
- *Haematological* Leukaemia, lymphoma, myeloproliferative disorders, sickle cell disease.
- *Biliary obstruction* Particularly extra-hepatic.
- *Inflammation* Hepatitis, abscess, schistosomiasis.
- *Metabolic* Fatty liver, early cirrhosis, amyloid, glycogen storage disease.
- *Cysts* Polycystic liver, hydatid.

**Ascites** Free fluid in the peritoneal cavity. *Signs:* abdominal distention, shifting dullness to percussion, fluid thrill. *Causes:* malignancy—any intra-abdominal organ, ovary, or kidney; hypoproteinaemia, e.g. nephrotic syndrome; right heart failure; portal hypertension.

**Fistula** Abnormal communication between one organ and another usually due to cancer or complication of surgery (Table 13.4). Refer urgently if suspected.

**Table 13.4** Presentation of fistula

| Connection | Presentation |
|---|---|
| Bowel → skin | Faecal discharge through surgical wound |
| Bladder/ureters → skin | Clear watery discharge which smells of urine |
| Bowel → vagina | Faeculent material in vagina |
| Bladder → vagina | Leakage of urine per vaginum |
| Bowel → bladder | Air or faeculent material in urine, recurrent UTI |

**Urgent referral for upper GI symptoms[N]** Consider checking FBC when referring, depending on local protocols.

*Urgent referral to a team specializing in upper GI malignancy* Patients presenting with:
- Dysphagia.
- Unexplained upper abdominal pain and weight ↓ ± back pain.
- Upper abdominal mass without dyspepsia.
- Obstructive jaundice (depending on clinical state)—consider urgent USS if available.

*Consider urgent referral to a specialist in upper GI malignancy* Patients presenting with:
- Persistent vomiting and weight ↓ in the absence of dyspepsia.
- Unexplained weight ↓ or iron deficiency in the absence of dyspepsia.
- Unexplained worsening of dyspepsia in a patient who had peptic ulcer surgery > 20y previously, with Barrentt's oesophagus, dysplasia, atrophic gastritis or intestinal metaplasia.

*Consider urgent specialist referral or referral for urgent endoscopy* Patients of any age with dyspepsia and:

- Chronic GI bleeding
- Dysphagia
- Progressive unintentional weight ↓
- Persistent vomiting
- Iron deficiency anaemia
- Epigastric mass
- Suspicious barium meal result.

**Urgent referral for endoscopy** Any patient ≥55y with unexplained (no obvious cause (e.g NSAIDs)) and persistent recent-onset dyspepsia alone, GPs should not allow symptoms to persist >4–6wk before referral.

❶ *Helicobacter pylori* status should not affect the decision to refer for suspected cancer. Consider checking a FBC to exclude iron deficiency anaemia in all patients presenting with new-onset dyspepsia.

**Urgent referral for lower GI symptoms[N]** Refer urgently to a team specializing in lower GI malignancy if:

*Any age* with:
- Right lower abdominal mass consistent with involvement of large bowel.
- Palpable rectal mass (intraluminal, not pelvic; a pelvic mass outside the bowel would warrant an urgent referral to a urologist).
- Unexplained iron deficiency anaemia (Hb ≤110g/dL for ♂, ≤100g/dL for a non-menstruating ♀).

*Aged ≥40y* Reporting rectal bleeding with a change of bowel habit towards looser stools and/or increased stool frequency persisting ≥6wk.

*Aged ≥60y* with:
- Rectal bleeding persisting for ≥6wk without a change in bowel habit and without anal symptoms.
- Change in bowel habit to looser stools and/or more frequent stools persisting for ≥6 wk without rectal bleeding.

❶ In a patient with equivocal symptoms who is not unduly anxious, it is reasonable to 'treat, watch and wait'.

# Dyspepsia and *H. pylori*

In any year, up to 40% of the adult population suffer from dyspepsia—1:10 seek their GP's advice and ~10% of these are referred.

## Causes
- Gastro-oesophageal reflux disease (GORD): 15–25% (📖 p.394)
- Peptic ulcer (PU): 15–25% (📖 p.396)
- Stomach cancer: 2% (📖 p.398)
- The remaining 60% are classified as *non-ulcer dyspepsia* (NUD) ('functional' dyspepsia)—manage as for uninvestigated dyspepsia.
- Rare causes: oesophagitis from swallowed corrosives, oesophageal infection (especially in the immunocompromised).

**Differential diagnosis** Cardiac pain (difficult to distinguish); gallstone pain; pancreatitis; bile reflux.

**Presentation** Common symptoms include retrosternal or epigastric pain, fullness, bloating, wind, heartburn, nausea and vomiting. Examination is usually normal though there may be epigastric tenderness. Check for clinical anaemia, epigastric mass/hepatomegaly and LNs in the neck.

**Management** Figure 13.2.

**Helicobacter pylori** Infection is associated with:
- *GI disease*—peptic ulcer disease; gastric cancer; non-ulcer dyspepsia; oesophagitis
- *Non-GI disease*—ranging from cardiovascular disease and haematological malignancy to cot death.

***Testing for H. pylori***[N] 'Test and treat' all patients with dyspepsia who do not meet referral criteria (Figure 13.2). In practice choice of test is limited by availability, ease of access, and cost. Options in the community are serology, urea breath test, and faecal antigen test. A 2 wk washout period following proton pump inhibitor (PPI) use is necessary before testing for *H. pylori* with a breath test or a stool antigen test.

***Eradication***[N] Clears 80–85% *H. pylori* infections. Options:
- *PAC$_{500}$ regimen* Full-dose PPI (e.g. omeprazole 20mg bd) + amoxicillin 1g bd + clarithromycin 500mg bd for 1 wk *or*
- *PMC$_{250}$ regimen* Full-dose PPI (e.g. omeprazole 20mg bd) + metronidazole 400mg bd + clarithromycin 250mg bd for 1 wk.

❶ Do not re-test even if dyspepsia remains unless there is a strong clinical need. Re-test if needed using a urea breath test.

**Lifestyle advice** Give advice on healthy eating, weight ↓, and smoking cessation. Advise patients to avoid precipitating factors e.g. coffee, chocolate, fatty foods. Raising the head of the bed and having a main meal well before going to bed may help some people. Promote continued use of antacids/alginates.

## Further information
**NICE** Management of dyspepsia in adults in primary care (2004) 🖳 www.nice.org.uk

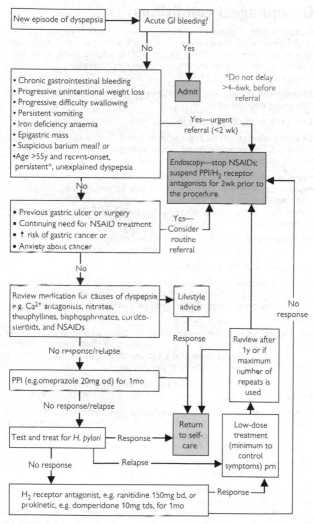

**Fig.13.2** Algorithm for management of uninvestigated dyspepsia in general practice

# Oesophageal conditions

**Oesophagitis** Common condition. Reflux of acid from the stomach to the oesophagus causes mucosal damage resulting in inflammation and ulceration. *Other causes:* drugs (e.g. NSAIDs); infection (e.g. CMV, HSV, Candida, especially in the immuno-compromised); ingestion of caustic substances.

**Management** Treat reflux induced oesophagitis as for GORD (🕮 p.394). Otherwise treat the cause.

**Barrett's oesophagus** 🕮 p.395.

**Chronic benign stricture** Recurrent oesophagitis (e.g. 2° to GORD, NSAIDs, $K^+$ preparations) scars the oesophagus resulting in stricture formation. Most common among elderly women.

**Presentation** Long history of reflux with more recent dysphagia. If obstruction is severe, undigested food may be regurgitated immediately after swallowing. May be associated with night-time coughing paroxysms due to aspiration of gastric contents into the chest. Examination is usually normal.

**Management** Refer for urgent endoscopy to confirm diagnosis and exclude carcinoma. Treatment is by endoscopic dilatation of the stricture.

**Carcinoma of the oesophagus** 🕮 p.398.

**Presbyoesophagus** Common among the elderly. Intermittent sensation that food is getting stuck—usually at the back of the throat. Examination is normal, as is endoscopy. Barium swallow may reveal oesophageal spasm. Reassure.

**Globus pharyngis (or hystericus)** Sensation of a lump in the throat without difficulty in swallowing is common. It may indicate anxiety. Reassure if no organic signs and treat any dyspepsia. If not responding refer to ENT for exclusion of an organic cause.

**Oesophageal achalasia** Failure of relaxation of the circular muscles at the distal oesophagus. *Peak incidence:* 30–40y. ♀ slightly >♂.

**Presentation** Gradual onset of dysphagia over years accompanied by regurgitation of stagnant food and foul belching. Night-time coughing fits are due to aspiration which can result in recurrent chest infections. Examination is usually normal though may be signs of aspiration pneumonia.

**Management** CXR to exclude aspiration pneumonia; endoscopy confirms diagnosis. Refer for surgery.

**Plummer–Vinson syndrome** Iron deficiency anaemia + dysphagia due to a post-cricoid web in the oesophagus. ♀ > ♂. Peak incidence: 40–50y. Presents with high dysphagia with food sticking in the back of the throat ± retching/choking sensation. This is a pre-malignant condition so refer for biopsy and dilatation of pharyngeal web; replace iron.
*H.S. Plummer (1874–1936), P.P. Vinson (1890–1959)— US physicians.*

**Pharyngeal pouch** Pulsion diverticulum of the pharyngeal mucosa through Killian's dehiscence (area of weakness between the two parts of the inferior pharyngeal constrictor). ♂>♀; ↑ with age. Usually develops posteriorly and then protrudes to one side—L>R. As the pouch becomes larger the oesophagus is displaced laterally.

**Presentation** Dysphagia—the first mouthful is swallowed easily and then fills the pouch which makes further swallowing difficult. Accompanied by regurgitation of food from the pouch ± symptoms of aspiration (nighttime coughing, recurrent chest infection). A swelling is palpable in the neck in two-thirds of cases.

**Management** Refer for further investigation. Diagnosis is confirmed with barium swallow. Treatment is surgical if bleeding.

**Oesophageal varices** Result from portal hypertension (📖 p.433) and can bleed massively—admit as a 'blue-light' emergency if bleeding.

**Impacted oesophageal foreign body** Usually the patient notices something has stuck resulting in pain, difficulty swallowing ± retching. If suspected refer immediately to A&E for further investigation ± removal of the foreign body.

**Oesophageal perforation** Rare—usually a complication of endoscopy. Less commonly due to violent vomiting. The patient becomes very distressed with pain relating to the site of perforation which is worse on swallowing. Examination reveals tachycardia, shock ± pyrexia ± breathlessness ± surgical emphysema in neck. Admit as a surgical emergency.

---

 **Oesophageal atresia and/or tracheo-oesophageal fistula** 1:2500 live births. 5% have oesophageal atresia alone; 5% tracheo-oesophageal fistula (TOF) alone; the remainder have both. Risk factors for sudden infant death syndrome.

**Presentation**
- **Antenatal** At routine USS or following investigation of polyhydramnios
- **Postnatal** Cough or breathing difficulties in a newborn infant; choking on the first feed; inability to swallow saliva → bubbling of fluid from the mouth developing soon after birth.
- **Later in childhood** 'H-type' fistulas where there is no atresia but just a fistula. May present late with recurrent chest infections.

**Management** Diagnosis is confirmed with X-ray. Treatment is surgical. Post-operatively children may have a barking cough (*TOF cough*) and/or dysphagia—both settle before 2y.

# Gastro-oesophageal reflux and gastritis

**Gastro-oesophageal reflux disease (GORD)** Caused by retrograde flow of gastric contents through an incompetent gastro-oesophageal junction. Affects ~5% of the adult population.

## Risk factors

- Smoking
- Alcohol
- Coffee
- Fatty food
- Big meals

- Obesity
- Hiatus hernia
- Tight clothes
- Pregnancy

- Drugs (TCAs, anticholinergics, nitrates, alendronate)
- Systemic sclerosis
- Surgery for achalasia.

## Conditions caused by GORD

- Oesophagitis (defined by mucosal breaks) ± oesophageal ulcer
- Benign oesophageal stricture (📖 p.392)
- Intestinal metaplasia: Barrett's oesophagus
- Oesophageal haemorrhage
- Anaemia.

## Presentation

- **Heartburn** Most common symptom. Burning retrosternal or epigastric pain which worsens on bending, stooping, or lying, and with hot drinks. Relieved by antacids.
- **Other symptoms**
  - Waterbrash—mouth fills with saliva
  - Reflux of acid into the mouth, especially on lying flat
  - Nausea and vomiting
  - Nocturnal cough/wheeze due to aspiration of refluxed stomach contents.
- **Examination** Usually normal. Check for clinical anaemia, epigastric mass/hepatomegaly, and LNs in the neck.

**Investigation** Endoscopy if indicated (Figure 13.2, 📖 p.391).

❶ Symptoms are poorly correlated with endoscopic findings. Reflux may remain silent in patients with Barrett's oesophagus but heartburn can severely affect quality of life of patients with –ve endoscopy results.

## Initial management[N]

- In all cases give lifestyle advice (📖 p.390).
- If diagnosis is clinical (i.e. patient presents with 'reflux-like' symptoms), treat as for uninvestigated dyspepsia (Figure 13.2, 📖 p.391).
- For patients with reflux confirmed on endoscopy or barium swallow, offer treatment with a PPI (e.g. omeprazole 20mg od) for 1–2 mo. If oesophagitis at endoscopy and the patient remains symptomatic double the dose of PPI for a further 1 mo.
- If inadequate response to PPI, try an H₂ receptor antagonist (e.g. ranitidine 150mg bd) or prokinetic (e.g.domperidone 10mg tds) for 1mo.

**Long-term management** of endoscopically/barium-confirmed GORD[N]:
- Patients who have had dilatation of an oesophageal stricture should remain on long-term full-dose PPI therapy.
- For all other patients, if symptoms recur following initial treatment, offer a PPI at the lowest dose possible to control symptoms, with a limited number of repeat prescriptions. Discuss using the treatment on an as-required basis with patients to manage their own symptoms.
- Refer for consideration of surgery if quality of life remains significantly impaired despite optimal treatment. Surgery of any type is >90% successful though results may deteriorate with time.

**Hiatus hernia** Common (30% of over-50s). 50% have GORD. Obesity is a risk factor. The proximal stomach herniates through the diaphragmatic hiatus into the thorax.
- 80% have a 'sliding' hiatus hernia where the gastro-oesophageal junction slides into the chest.
- 20% have 'rolling' hernias where a bulge of stomach herniates into the chest alongside the oesophagus. The gastro-oesophageal junction remains in the abdomen.

**Management** Treat as for GORD

**Barrett's oesophagus** Usually found incidentally at endoscopy for symptoms of GORD and caused by chronic GORD. The squamous mucosa of the oesophagus undergoes metaplastic change and the squamo-columnar junction appears to migrate away from the stomach. The length affected varies. It carries a 40x ↑ risk of adenocarcinoma of the oesophagus so regular endoscopy is essential. Treatment is with long-term PPIs (e.g omeprazole 20–40mg od) ± laser therapy ± resection.
*N.R. Barrett (1903–1979)—British surgeon.*

**Acute gastritis** Mucosal inflammation of the stomach with no ulcer.
- **Type A** Affects the entire stomach; associated with pernicious anaemia; pre-malignant.
- **Type B** Affects antrum ± duodenum; associated with *H. pylori*.
- **Type C** Due to irritants, e.g. NSAIDs, alcohol, bile reflux.

**Presentation and investigation** Dyspepsia—see 📖 p.390.

**Management**
- Treat the cause where possible (e.g. vitamin $B_{12}$ injections, *H. pylori* eradication, avoidance of alcohol).
- Acid suppression—$H_2$ receptor antagonist (e.g. ranitidine, nizatidine) or PPI for 4–8wk.
- Re-endoscope to confirm healing.

**Complications** Haemorrhage; gastric atrophy ± gastric cancer (type A only).

# Peptic ulceration

Peptic ulceration (PU) is a term which includes both gastric and duodenal ulceration. Most patients present with dyspepsia ($\square$ p.390). Specific features of gastric and duodenal ulcers are listed in Table 13.5.

## Management

### For patients not taking NSAIDs

- *Eradicate H. pylori if present* ($\square$ p.390)—speeds ulcer healing and $\downarrow$ relapse; confirm eradication with a urea breath test (duodenal ulcer) or repeat endoscopy (gastric ulcer), and re-treat if still present.
- *If H. pylori negative* Treat with full-dose PPI (e.g omeprazole 20mg od) for 1–2mo. If gastric ulcer, re-endoscope to check ulcer is healed.

### For patients taking NSAIDs

- Stop NSAIDs where possible. If not possible, consider changing to a safer alternative (e.g.paracetamol, $\downarrow$ dose of NSAID, COX2 selective NSAID), and/or adding gastric protection with a PPI or misoprostol.
- Offer full-dose PPI or $H_2$ receptor antagonist ($H_2$RA) therapy for 2mo and if *H. pylori* is present, subsequently offer eradication therapy.
- Check eradication with repeat endoscopy (gastric ulcer) or urea breath test (duodenal ulcer).

### For all patients

- *Lifestyle measures* Avoid foods (or alcohol) which exacerbate symptoms; eat little and often, and avoid eating for 3h before bed. Stop smoking.
- *If symptoms recur following initial treatment,* offer a PPI at lowest dose to control symptoms, with a limited number of repeat prescriptions. Discuss using the treatment on a prn basis.
- *Offer $H_2$RA therapy* if there is an inadequate response to PPI.
- *In patients with unhealed ulcer or continuing symptoms* despite adequate treatment, exclude non-adherence, malignancy, failure to detect *H. pylori*, inadvertent NSAID use, other ulcer-inducing medication, and rare causes such as Zollinger–Ellison syndrome or Crohn's disease.
- *Once symptoms are controlled,* review at least annually to discuss symptom control, lifestyle advice, and medication.
- *Refer* if gastric ulcer fails to heal or if symptoms do not respond to medical treatment. Possible surgical procedures include: gastrectomy, vagotomy, and drainage procedure; highly selective vagotomy.

**Zollinger–Ellison syndrome** Association of peptic ulcer with a gastrin-secreting pancreatic (rarely duodenal) adenoma—50–60% are malignant, 10% are multiple, and 30% are associated with multiple endocrine neoplasia (MEN I). *Incidence:* 0.1% of patients with duodenal ulcer disease. Suspect in those with multiple peptic ulcers resistant to drugs, particularly if associated with diarrhoea ± steatorrhoea or a family history of peptic ulcers (or islet cell, pituitary, or parathyroid adenomas). Refer for further investigation. Treatment is with PPI (e.g omeprazole 10–60mg bd) ± surgery.
*R.M. Zollinger (1903–1992), E.H. Ellison (1918–1970)—US surgeons.*

**Table 13.5** Features of gastric and duodenal ulcers

| | Gastric ulcer (GU) | Duodenal ulcer (DU) |
|---|---|---|
| **Population** | Typically affects middle aged/elderly ♂'s | Typically affects young–middle-aged ♂'s though can affect any adult ♂>♀ |
| **Risk factors** | H. pylori (70-90% of gastric ulcer patients)<br>NSAID use (↑ risk ×3-4)<br>Delayed gastric emptying<br>Reflux from the duodenum (↑ by smoking) | H. pylori (>90%)<br>NSAID use<br>Gastric hyperacidity<br>Rapid gastric emptying<br>Smoking<br>Stress (controversial) |
| **Presentation** | May be asymptomatic<br>Epigastric pain worsened by food and helped by antacids or lying flat ± weight loss<br>With complications (see below) | May be asymptomatic or spontaneously relapse and remit<br>Epigastric pain typically relieved by food and worse at night ± weight ↑ ± waterbrash (saliva fills the mouth).<br>With complications (see below) |
| **Examination** | In uncomplicated gastric ulceration, examination is usually normal though there may be epigastric/left upper quadrant tenderness | In uncomplicated duodenal ulceration, examination is usually normal though there may be epigastric tenderness |
| **Investigation** | As for dyspepsia (🕮 p.390) | |
| **Complications** | **Bleeding** Acute GI bleeding—🕮 p.1072; Iron deficiency anaemia—🕮 p.662<br>**Perforated peptic ulcer** DU>GU; GUs may perforate posteriorly into the lesser sac; DUs usually perforate anteriorly into the peritoneal cavity. There may not be a past history of indigestion. Presents with sudden onset severe epigastric pain which rapidly becomes generalized. When a GU perforates into the lesser sac symptoms may remain localized or be confined to the right side of the abdomen. *Examination*: generalized peritonism with 'board-like rigidity'. *Management*: acute surgical admission<br>**Pyloric stenosis in adults** Duodenal stenosis 2° to scarring from a chronic DU. Characterized by copious vomiting of food 1–2 days old. There may not be a past history of indigestion. *Examination*: if prolonged vomiting may be evidence of dehydration ± weight ↓. Succussion splash may be audible. *Management*: surgical referral for confirmation of diagnosis and surgical relief | |

**Further information**
**NICE** Management of dyspepsia in adults in primary care (2004)
🖥 www.nice.org.uk

# Gastro-oesophageal malignancy

**Carcinoma of the oesophagus** Common cancer accounting for 7,000 deaths/y in the UK. Most common in patients >60y Overall ♂:♀ ≈ 5:1. Usually presents late when prognosis is poor. Two types:
- *Squamous cell carcinoma* (50%)—predominant form in upper two-thirds of the oesophagus.
- *Adenocarcinoma* (50%)—predominant in lower third of the oesophagus. Incidence is increasing. ♂:♀ ≈ 5:1.

## Common risk factors

*Squamous cell carcinoma*—accounts for 89% of cases

- Smoking*
- Alcohol
- Low fruit/vegetable intake

*risk ↓ to that of a non-smoker 10y after giving up.

*Adenocarcinoma*—accounts for 79% of cases

- Smoking*
- Obesity
- Low fruit/vegetable intake
- GORD, particularly Barrett's oesophagus (risk ↑ >30×—the longer the affected segment, the higher the risk).

## Other risk factors
- Previous mediastinal radiotherapy (↑ 2× for patients treated for breast cancer; ↑ 20× for patients treated for Hodgkin's lymphoma)
- Plummer–Vinson (or Patterson–Kelly) syndrome—oesophageal web and iron deficiency anaemia
- Tylosis—rare inherited disorder with hyperkeratosis of the palms. 40% develop oesophageal cancer.

**Presentation** Short history of rapidly progressive dysphagia affecting solids initially then solids and liquids ± weight loss ± regurgitation of food and fluids (may be bloodstained). Retrosternal pain is a late feature. Other symptoms include hoarseness and/or cough (due to aspiration or fistula formation). Examination may be normal. Look for evidence of recent weight loss, hepatomegaly, and cervical lymphadenopathy.

**Management** Refer for urgent endoscopy if suspected. Rapid access dysphagia clinics run in many areas. Specialist management involves resection (treatment of choice but only 1:3 patients are suitable), chemotherapy, radiotherapy, and/or palliation with a stenting tube. Tubes commonly become blocked. Good palliative care is essential—refer early. Overall 7% 5y survival.

**Stomach cancer** Stomach cancer causes ~5,500 deaths/y in the UK. 95% are adenocarcinomas. Disease affecting older people with 90% diagnosed >55y. ♂ > ♀ (5:3). Incidence has halved over the past 30y in the UK probably due to improved diet.

## Other risk factors include:
- Geography—common in Japan
- Blood group A
- *H. pylori* infection (not clear if eradication ↓ risk)
- Atrophic gastritis
- Pernicious anaemia
- Smoking
- Adenomatous polyps
- Social class
- Previous partial gastrectomy.

**Presentation** Often non-specific. Presents with dyspepsia, weight ↓, anorexia or early satiety, vomiting, dysphagia, anaemia and/or GI bleeding. Suspect in any patient >55y with recent onset dyspepsia (within 1y) and/or other risk factors. Examination is usually normal until incurable. Look for epigastric mass, hepatomegaly, jaundice, ascites, enlarged supraclavicular LN (Virchow's node), acanthosis nigricans.

**Management** If suspected refer for urgent endoscopy. In early stages total/partial gastrectomy may be curative. Most present at later stage. Overall 5y survival is 12%.

## Post-gastrectomy syndromes

**Abdominal fullness** Feeling of early satiety ± weight loss. Advise to take small frequent meals.

**Bilious vomiting** Affects ~10% patients post-gastrectomy. Intermittent sudden attacks of bilious vomiting 15–30min after eating ± epigastric cramping pain relieved by vomiting. Usually settles spontaneously. Metoclopramide or domperidone may be helpful in the interim. If symptoms are severe or fail to settle request surgical review. Surgical bile diversion or stomach reconstruction may alleviate symptoms.

**Dumping** Abdominal distension, colic, and vasomotor disturbance (e.g. sweating, fainting) after meals. Affects 1–2% of gastrectomy patients (more common early after surgery—most settle within 6mo). Two types:
- **Early dumping** Due to rapid gastric emptying. Starts immediately after a meal. Consists of: sweating, flushing, tachycardia, palpitations, epigastric fullness, nausea. Occasionally there may be vomiting, diarrhoea ± colicky abdominal pain. Advise small dry meals with restricted carbohydrate. Take drinks between meals. If severe, re-refer for surgery.
- **Late dumping** Due to rapid gastric emptying → hyperglycaemia. The resultant hyperinsulinaemia causes a rebound hypoglycaemia. Starts 1–2h after meals. Consists of faintness, sweating, tremor, and nausea. Advise patients to ↓ sugar content of meals, rest for 1h after each meal, and take glucose if symptoms occur. If severe, re-refer.

**Diarrhoea post-gastrectomy** 50% of patients who have had a truncal vagotomy or gastrectomy suffer some frequency of defecation; 5% require treatment. The diarrhoea is typically episodic and unpredicatable. The exact mechanism is not clear. Treatment is with codeine phosphate or loperamide prn. Antibiotic treatment is occasionally successful—seek expert advice. Surgical measures are rarely necessary.

**Anaemia** Gastrectomy can result in both vitamin $B_{12}$ deficiency and iron deficiency anaemia. Prophylactic $B_{12}$ injections may be advised by the operating surgeon. Many advise iron supplements for life. An annual FBC to monitor for anaemia is advisable. Treat with iron/$B_{12}$ supplements.

**Stomach cancer** Risk of stomach cancer is ↑ after partial gastrectomy (2× after 20y and 7× after 45y).

## Advice and support for patients
**Cancer Research UK** ☎ 0800 226 237 ▯ www.cancerhelp.org.uk
**Macmillan Cancer Support** ☎ 0808 808 0000 ▯ www.macmillan.org.uk

# Hernias

### Irreducible hernia
- Most types of hernia may become irreducible.
- It may be the first presentation of a hernia or a complication of a longstanding hernia.
- If obstructed (incarcerated) or strangluated (blood supply to bowel contained within the hernia sac is compromised), the hernia is tender and there are symptoms/signs of small bowel obstruction.

⚠ In all cases, if you are unable to reduce a hernia, admit urgently for surgical assessment.

**Inguinal hernia** Protuberance of peritoneal contents through the abdominal wall where it is weakened by the presence of the inguinal canal. Common condition (♂>♀) which can occur at any age.

***Presentation*** Lump in the groin ± discomfort on straining/standing for any length of time. There may be a distinct precipitating event (e.g. heavy lifting). *Risk factors:* chronic cough (e.g. COPD); constipation; urinary obstruction; heavy lifting; ascites; previous abdominal surgery. *2 types:*
- *Indirect (80%)* Follow the course of the spermatic cord or round ligament down the inguinal canal through the internal inguinal ring (located at the mid-point of the inguinal ligament, 1.5cm above the femoral pulse) and sometimes out through the external inguinal ring into the scrotum/vulva.
- *Direct (20%)* Pass through a defect in the abdominal wall into the inguinal canal. Rare in children and more common in the elderly.

***Differential diagnosis of groin lumps*** Table 13.6.

***Examination*** Examine the patient standing up. Look for a bulge in the groin above the line of the inguinal ligament. Unless incarcerated, the lump should have a cough impulse. Check that you are able to reduce he hernia—sometimes it is easier if the patient lies down. Ask the patient to reduce the hernia if you cannot.

***Management*** Small hernias often require no treatment. For larger hernias/those that are symptomatic, consider referral for surgical repair. Various methods are used—all have a high level of success (<2% recurrence). Trusses can be useful for symptomatic hernias in elderly patients, or those unfit for or awaiting surgery (prescribe on FP10).

***Inguinal hernias in children*** 📖 p. 888.

**Femoral hernia** Less common than inguinal hernias. ♀>♂. The patient is usually elderly, though can occur at any age. The peritoneal contents protrude down the femoral canal. Risk of strangulation is high. Presents as a painful lump in the groin and/or small bowel obstruction.

***Examination*** Rounded swelling medially in the groin and lateral to the pubic tubercle; if reducible, a soft palpable lump remains after reduction.

***Management*** Always refer for urgent surgical repair. Admit as surgical emergency if obstructed or irreducible.

**Incisional hernia** Breakdown of the muscle closure in an abdominal wound some time after surgery. There may be a history of wound sepsis, haematoma or breakdown. Presents with a bulge at the site of the operation scar ± discomfort.

***Examination*** The hernia is usually visible when the patient stands—it can be made more obvious by asking the patient to cough or straight leg raise whilst lying flat. The margins of the muscular defect are palpable under the skin. Note whether fully reducible or not.

***Management*** Often reassurance suffices. If obstructed/strangulated or causing discomfort, refer for surgical assessment.

**Umbilical hernia** Most common in infants (📖 p.888). In adults paraumbilical hernias, presenting as a bulge adjacent to the umbilicus, may occur due to weakness in the linea alba. ♀ > ♂. Refer adults for surgical assessment—usually repaired as risk of strangulation is high. Admit as a surgical emergency if obstructed/irreducible.

**Epigastric hernia** Midline hernia through a defect in the linea alba above the umbilicus. Never contains bowel. Usually symptomless, though occasionally causes epigastric pain ± vomiting. *Examination:* epigastric mass with cough impulse. Refer for surgical repair.

**Spigelian hernia** A hernial sac protrudes lateral to the rectus sheath midway between umbilicus and pubic bone. Presents with discomfort ± vomiting. Refer for surgical repair.

**Obturator hernia** Hernia protrudes out from the pelvis through the obturator canal. Usually presents with strangulation ± pain referred to the knee. Admit for surgery.

**Richter hernia** A knuckle of the side wall of the gut is caught in a hernia sac and becomes strangulated but the bowel is not obstructed. Presents with abdominal pain which rapidly becomes worse ± shock. Admit as for acute abdomen, diagnosis is usually made at surgery.

**Table 13.6** Differential diagnosis of groin lumps

| Position relative to the skin | Groin lump | Position relative to the inguinal ligament | |
|---|---|---|---|
| | | Above | Below |
| *In the skin* | Lipoma, fibroma, haemangioma and other skin lumps | ✓ | ✓ |
| *Deep to the skin* | Femoral or inguinal lymph nodes | ✓ | ✓ |
| | Saphena varix of the femoral vein | ✗ | ✓ |
| | Femoral artery aneurysm | ✗ | ✓ |
| | Femoral hernia | ✗ | ✓ |
| | Inguinal hernia | ✓ | ✗ |

❶ The inguinal ligament runs from the pubic tubercle medially to the anterior superior iliac spine laterally.

# Appendicitis and small bowel disease

**Acute appendicitis** Most common surgical emergency in the UK—lifetime incidence ~6%. *Peak age:* 10-30y. Presents with central abdominal colic that progresses and localizes in the right iliac fossa, becoming worse on movement (especially coughing, laughing); anorexia; nausea ± vomiting; dysuria; constipation or rarely diarrhoea.

*Further assessment* Watch for discomfort on walking (tend to walk stooped) and coughing. May be flushed and unwell—pyrexial (~37.5°C); furred tongue and/or foetor oris; tenderness and guarding in the right iliac fossa (especially over McBurney's point—two-thirds of the distance between the umbilicus and anterior superior iliac spine); pain in the right iliac fossa on palpation of the left iliac fossa (Rovsing's sign). Urinalysis is normal or +ve for protein and/or leucocyte esterase but −ve for nitrites.

### Differential diagnosis
- Mesenteric adenitis
- UTI
- Gastroenteritis
- Meckel's diverticulum
- Intussusception
- Crohn's disease
- Gynaecological cause (pelvic inflammatory disease; ectopic pregnancy)
- Non-abdominal cause, e.g. otitis media, diabetic ketoacidosis, pneumonia.

**Management** Admit as a surgical emergency—expect to be wrong ~½ the time. *Complications:* generalized peritonitis 2° to perforation; appendix abscess; appendix mass; subphrenic abscess; female infertility.

*Subphrenic abscess* Rarely follows 7–21d after generalized peritonitis, particularly after acute appendicitis. Presents with general malaise, swinging fever, nausea and weight ↓ ± pain in the upper abdomen radiating to the shoulder tip. Breathlessness can be associated due to reactive pleural effusion or lower lobe collapse. *Examination:* subcostal tenderness ± liver enlargement. FBC—↑ WCC. If suspected admit for surgical assessment.

⚠ **Appendicitis in pregnancy** Appendicitis affects 1:1000 pregnancies. Mortality is ↑ and perforation more common (15-20%). Fetal mortality is 5-10% for simple appendicitis; 30% when there is perforation. Due to the pregnancy, the appendix is displaced—pain is often felt in the paraumbilical region or subcostally. Admit immediately if suspected.

 **Children with appendicitis** Symptoms/signs of appendicitis may be atypical—especially in very young children—as children localize pain poorly and signs of peritonitis can be difficult to elicit.
- If unsure of diagnosis, and the child is unwell, admit.
- If unsure of diagnosis, and the child is well, either arrange to review a few hours later or ask the carer to contact you if there is any deterioration or change in symptoms.

**Mesenteric adenitis** Inflammation of the mesenteric LNs causing abdominal pain in children. May follow URTI. Can mimic appendicitis. Check MSU to exclude UTI. If guarding/rebound tenderness, refer for acute surgical assessment. Settles spontaneously with simple analgesia and fluids. If not settling in 1–2wk refer for paediatric assessment.

**Meckel's diverticulum** Remnant of the attachment of the small bowel to the embryological yolk sac. It is 2 inches (~5cm) long, ~2ft (100cm) proximal to the appendix, and presents in 2% of the population. Meckel's diverticulum may not cause any problems or may cause an appendicitis-like picture; acute intestinal obstruction, or GI bleeding. Symptoms can occur at any age but are most common in children.
*J.F. Meckel (1781–1833)—German anatomist*

**Intussusception** 📖 p.889  **Coeliac disease** 📖 p.420

**Crohn's disease** 📖 p.422  **Obstruction and ischaemia** 📖 p.408

**Adhesions** arise as a result of intra-abdominal inflammation. Bowel loops become adherent to each other, omentum, mesentery, and abdominal wall. Fibrous bands may form, connecting adjacent structures. Presents with abdominal pain ± obstruction. *Causes:* surgery; intra-abdominal sepsis (e.g. appendicitis, cholecystitis; salpingitis); inflammatory bowel disease; endometriosis Refer to a surgeon. Treatment is difficult as any surgery may result in new adhesions; conservative management with analgesia and stool softeners is preferred. Open or laparoscopic division of adhesions is occasionally necessary.

**Intestinal non-Hodgkin's lymphoma** The majority of intestinal NHLs are B-cell type lymphomas, but coeliac disease is associated with T-cell intestinal lymphoma. *Abdominal symptoms:* non specific abdominal pain (70–80%); perforation (up to 25%); bowel obstruction; abdominal mass; intussusception; malabsorption (usually lymphoma associated with coeliac disease) or alteration in bowel habit (small intestine NHL may present like Crohn's disease). *Systemic symptoms:* weight loss (30%), fatigue, sweats, unexplained fevers. ❶ Lymphadenopathy and hepatosplenomegaly are usually absent.

**Management** (📖 p.678) Gastric lymphoma may remit with treatment of *H. pylori* infection.

**Carcinoid tumours** Slow-growing tumours of low malignancy which arise from neuroendocrine cells or their precursors. *Incidence:* 3–4/100 000. *Peak age:* 61y. ♀ > ♂. 60% are in the mid-gut (especially appendix and terminal ileum)—examination may reveal an abdominal mass and/or enlarged liver. Rarely, presents with bowel obstruction. Ileal carcinoids are multiple in 30%. *Non-intestinal sites:* lung, testes, and ovary.

**Carcinoid syndrome** Affects <10% of patients with a carcinoid tumour. Develops when serotonin (5HT) is released by the tumour and not degraded by the liver because of hepatic metastases. *Features:*
• Paroxysmal flushing, e.g. following alcohol or certain foods
• Watery explosive diarrhoea  • Bronchoconstriction (like asthma)
• Abdominal pain  • Right heart failure
• Rash—symmetrical pruritic erythematous rash which blisters/crusts.

**Management** Refer for urgent assessment if suspected. Therapeutic options include somatostatin analogues such as octreotide or radiofrequency ablation of liver metastases. Prognosis—if no metastases, median survival is 5–8y; with metastases median survival is 38mo.

# Colorectal cancer screening

Screening for colorectal cancer is available throughout the UK. Patients presenting with tumour confined to the bowel wall have >90% long-term survival. Without screening, most tumours are detected at advanced stages and overall 5y survival is ~40%. Screening aims to detect colorectal cancer at an early stage to ↑ survival chances.

**Screening test** Faecal occult blood (FOB) test kits are sent every 2y to all patients aged 60–69y with instructions for completion/return. Patients >70y may also request test kits. The test kit has 3 flaps, each with 2 windows underneath. 2 samples are taken from a bowel motion and spread onto the 2 windows under the first flap using the cardboard sticks provided. The flap is then sealed and the process repeated using the remaining 2 flaps for the subsequent 2 bowel motions. Once all 6 windows have been used, the kit is returned. Kits must be returned <14d after the first sample is taken. Results are sent to the patients in <2wk.

**Screening outcomes** (Tables 13.7 and 13.8). If 60% of those aged 60–69y do the FOB test, 1,200 deaths will be prevented each year.

**Family history** If a patient has one first degree relative (mother, father, sister, brother, daughter, or son) with colorectal cancer, risk of developing colorectal cancer is ↑ 2–3×.

*Refer for colonoscopy* at presentation or aged 35–40y (whichever is later) and repeat colonoscopy aged 55y if:
- 2× first-degree relatives with a history of colorectal cancer or
- 1× first-degree relative with a history of colorectal cancer aged <45y.

*Refer for specialist follow-up and genetic counselling if*
- >2× first-degree relatives with a history of colorectal cancer or
- Family history of:
  - *Familial adenomatous polyposis (FAP)*—usually develop cancer aged <40y. Lifetime risk of colorectal cancer is 1:2.5.
  - *Juvenile polyposis*—lifetime risk of colorectal cancer is 1:3.
  - *Peutz–Jehger syndrome*—autosomal dominant disorder. Benign intestinal (usually small intestine) polyps in association with dark freckles on lips, oral mucosa, face, palm, and soles. May cause GI obstruction or GI bleeding. Malignant change occurs in ~3%.
  - *Hereditary non-polyposis colorectal cancer*—≥3 family members with colorectal cancer where ≥2 generations have been affected and ≥1 affected family member developed the disease <50y of age; 40% lifetime risk of colorectal cancer
  - MMR (mismatch repair) oncogene.

**Ulcerative colitis** ↑ risk of colorectal cancer. Offer all patients a follow-up plan agreed with their specialist. In some cases, prophylactic colectomy is appropriate.

**Previous colorectal cancer** ↑ risk of developing a second colorectal primary. After successful treatment, younger patients are routinely followed up with colonoscopy every 5y until 70y. Remain vigilant for recurrences and re-refer urgently if suspected.

**Table 13.7** FOB test outcomes

| FOB result | Explanation | Action |
|---|---|---|
| Normal | 0 +ve spots | Screening offered again in 2y if <70y |
| Unclear ~4% tested | 1–4 +ve spots | Test repeated |
| | | If the second test is abnormal colonoscopy is offered |
| | | If the second test is normal, a third test is requested |
| | | If the third test is normal repeat screening in 2y is offered if <70y |
| | | If the third test is abnormal, colonoscopy is offered |
| Abnormal | 5–6 +ve spots | Colonoscopy is offered |
| Technical failure or spoilt kit | Laboratory or patient error | Repeat testing is offered |

**Table 13.8** Colonoscopy outcomes

- ~2% of those FOB tested are referred on for colonoscopy—uptake of colonoscopy is ~80%.
- Sensitivity of colonoscopy to detect significant abnormalities is ~90%.
- Polyps found during colonoscopy are usually removed.
- Complications of colonoscopy include heavy bleeding (1:150), bowel perforation (1:1500), death (1:10 000).

| Colonoscopy result | | Explanation | Action |
|---|---|---|---|
| Normal (50%) | | No abnormalities detected | FOB screening offered again in 2y if <70y |
| Polyp (40%) | Low risk | 1–2 small (<1cm) adenomas | FOB screening offered again in 2y if <70y |
| | Intermediate risk | 3–4 small (<1cm) adenomas or ≥1 adenoma ≥ 1cm | 3 yearly colonoscopy until 2× negative examinations |
| | High risk | ≥5 adenomas or ≥3 adenomas of which at least 1 is ≥1cm | Colonoscopy at 12mo then 3 yearly colonoscopy until 2× negative examinations |
| Cancer (10%) | | Colorectal cancer detected at colonoscopy | Refer urgently for further treatment |
| Other pathology | | Other pathology (e.g. UC) detected at colonoscopy | Refer/treat/advise as necessary |
| Technical difficulty (5%) | | Unable to negotiate the colonoscope around the bowel | Repeat colonoscopy or alternative imaging |

**Further information**

**NICE** Referral guidelines for suspected cancer (2005) 🖳 www.nice.org.uk
**NHS Bowel Cancer Screening Programme**
🖳 www.cancerscreening.nhs.uk

**Information for patients**

*Bowel Cancer Screening—The Facts* 🖳 www.cancerscreening.org.uk

# Colorectal cancer

Lifetime risk of developing colorectal cancer is 1/18–20. Colorectal cancer accounts for 13% of all cancers and 16 000 deaths/y in the UK. Two-thirds arise in the colon and one-third in the rectum. 83% of tumours occur in patients >60y. >95% are adenocarcinomas.

**Adenomatous polyps** Bowel cancers arise from polyps over many years. Polyps may be removed because of risk of malignant change. Follow-up surveillance with repeated colonoscopy may be necessary depending on the number of polyps and their size (📖 p.405).

## Protective and risk factors

*Geography* More common in the developed world—dietary factors are thought to be responsible for variations.

### Lifestyle factors
- *Obesity*—↑ risk by 15% if overweight and 30% if obese. Effect is most marked in pre-menopausal women.
- *Dietary factors*—diets with less red and processed meat, and more vegetables, fibre, fish, and milk are associated with ↓ risk.
- *Alcohol*—↑ risk for heavy drinkers, especially if also low folate.

### Medication history
- *HRT*—risk ↓ by 20% if ever taken; ↓ by 30% if taking HRT currently.
- *COC pill*—risk ↓ by 18% if ever taken.
- *Statins*—risk ↓ after 5y use.

### Other medical history
- *History of gall bladder disease and/or cholecystectomy*—50% ↑ in risk.
- *Type II (non-insulin-dependent) diabetes*—30% ↑ risk.
- *UC or Crohn's disease*—↑ risk.

### Family history 📖 p.404.

### Bowel cancer screening 📖 p.404.

**Presentation** May be found at bowel cancer screening. Clinical presentations depends on site involved:
- **Change in bowel habit** Diarrhoea ± mucus, constipation or alternating diarrhoea and constipation, tenesmus.
- **Intestinal obstruction** Pain, distension, absolute constipation ± vomiting. May be an acute sudden event (20% of patients not detected by screening present with an acute obstruction) or gradually evolve.
- **Rectal bleeding** Bright red rectal bleeding or +ve faecal occult blood test—60% rectal tumours. Rarely, melaena if high tumour.
- **Perforation** causing generalized peritonitis, or into an adjacent viscus (e.g. bladder) resulting in a fistula.
- **Spread** Abdominal distension 2° to ascites, jaundice, rectal/pelvic pain.
- **General effects** Weight ↓, anorexia, anaemia, malaise.

## Examination and investigation
- General examination—cachexia, jaundice, anaemia.
- Abdominal mass—palpable mass is present in 70% of right-sided tumours and 40% of left-sided tumours.

- Hepatomegaly.
- Ascites.
- Rectal examination detects >75% of rectal tumours.
- Check FBC for anaemia.

**Suspicious lower GI symptoms and signs** that should prompt urgent referral (to be seen in <2wk) to a team specializing in lower GI malignancy

*Any age* with:
- Right lower abdominal mass consistent with involvement of large bowel.
- Palpable rectal mass (intraluminal, not pelvic; a pelvic mass outside the bowel would warrant an urgent referral to a urologist).
- Unexplained iron deficiency anaemia (Hb ≤11g/dL for ♂; ≤10g/dL for non-menstruating ♀).

*Aged ≥40y* reporting rectal bleeding with a change of bowel habit towards looser stools and/or increased stool frequency persisting ≥6wk.

*Aged ≥60y* with:
- Rectal bleeding persisting for ≥6wk without a change in bowel habit and without anal symptoms.
- Change in bowel habit to looser stools and/or more frequent stools persisting for ≥6wk without rectal bleeding.

**❶** In a patient with equivocal symptoms who is not unduly anxious, it is reasonable to 'treat, watch, and wait'.

**Specialist management** Confirmation of the diagnosis is with sigmoidoscopy/colonoscopy and/or barium enema. If diagnosis is confirmed, further investigations include LFTs, tumour markers (carcinoembryonic antigen (CEA)—produced in >80% advanced tumours), CXR, CT/MRI, and USS to evaluate spread.

**Treatment** Surgical resection is undertaken whenever possible. Staging based on findings at surgery dictates further management with chemotherapy. For patients with more advanced disease, resection of or radioablation of hepatic metastases may be an option.

*Adverse pathological features*
- Presence/number of involved LNs
- Lymphovascular, perineural or venous invasion
- Depth of penetration through the bowel wall
- Positive resection margin
- Mucinous histology.

*Adverse clinical features*
- Emergency presentation with bowel obstruction or perforation
- Incomplete resection
- Metastatic disease
- Presentation aged <50y.

**Further information**
**NICE** Referral guidelines for suspected cancer (2005) 🖳 www.nice.org.uk
**SIGN** Management of colorectal cancer (2003) 🖳 www.sign.ac.uk

**Patient advice and support**
**Macmillan Cancer Support** ☎ 0808 808 0000 🖳 www.macmillan.org.uk
**Colostomy Association** ☎ 0800 328 4257 🖳 www.colostomyassociation.org.uk

# Other large bowel conditions

**Intestinal obstruction** Blockage of the bowel due to either mechanical obstruction or failure of peristalsis (ileus). *Causes:*

- *Obstruction from outside the bowel* Adhesions or bands; volvulus; obstructed hernia (📖 p.400); neighbouring malignancy (e.g. bladder).
- *Obstruction from within the bowel wall* Tumour; infarction; congenital atresia; Hirschprung's disease; inflammatory bowel disease (📖 p.422); diverticulitis.
- *Obstruction in the lumen* Impacted faeces/constipation (📖 p.386); bolus obstruction (e.g. swallowed foreign body); gallstone ileus; intussusception (📖 p.889); large polyps.
- *Ileus/functional obstruction* Post-op; electrolyte disturbance; uraemia; DM; back pain; anticholinergic drugs.

**Presentation** Anorexia; nausea; vomiting (may be faeculent) gives relief; colicky central abdominal pain and distension; absolute constipation for stool and gas (although if high obstruction, constipation may not be absolute). *Examination:* uncomfortable and restless; abdominal distention ± tenderness (though no guarding/rebound); active tinkling bowel sounds or quiet/absent bowel sounds (later).

**Management** Admit as surgical emergency.

**Diverticulosis** Common condition of the colon associated with muscle hypertrophy and ↑ intraluminal pressure. Mucosa-lined pouches are pushed out through the colonic wall, usually at the entry points of vessels. These pouches are the diverticula. 95% are in the sigmoid colon, though they may occur anywhere in the bowel. They are present in >⅓ of people >60y in the UK. Risk factors include low-roughage diet and age. Diverticular disease implies the diverticula are symptomatic (Table 13.9).

**Ischaemic bowel** Interruption of the blood supply of the bowel.

- *1° ischaemia* Usually due to either mesenteric thrombosis comes from the left heart or venous thrombosis. Typically occurs in elderly patients who might have pre-existing heart or vascular disease.
- *2° ischaemia* Usually due to intestinal obstruction (e.g. strangulated hernia, volvulus, intussusception).

**Presentation** Sudden onset of abdominal pain which rapidly becomes severe. There may be a history of pain worse after meals prior to this event (mesenteric angina). *Examination:* very unwell; shocked; may be in AF; generalized tenderness but normally no guarding/rebound. Often signs are out of proportion to symptoms.

**Management** Give opioid analgesia. Admit as surgical emergency.

**Sigmoid volvulus** Occurs in people who have redundant colon on a long mesentery with a narrow base. The sigmoid loop twists causing intestinal obstruction. The loop may become ischaemic. *Risk factors:* constipation, laxatives, tranquillizers. Presents with acute onset of abdominal distention and colicky abdominal pain with complete constipation and absence of flatus. There may be a history of repeated attacks.

**Management** Admit acutely to hospital. Treatment is release by passing a flatus tube and/or surgery. Once treated, ↓ recurrences by preventing constipation and stopping tranquillizers if possible.

**Hirschprung's disease** Caused by absence of the ganglion cells of the myenteric plexus in the distal bowel. Presents with delay in passing meconium, abdominal distension, vomiting and poor feeding in a neonate. If only a short segment is affected, presentation may be much later with chronic constipation. Diagnosis is confirmed with rectal biopsy. Refer to surgery. Treatment is surgical removal of the affected area of bowel.

H. Hirschprung (1830–1916)—Danish paediatrician

**Table 13.9** Presentation and management of diverticular disease

| | Presentation | Management |
|---|---|---|
| *Chronic diverticulitis* (painful diverticular disease) | Presents with altered bowel habit, abdominal pain (often colicky and left sided), nausea and flatulence.<br>Symptoms are often improved by defaecation | Investigate for change in bowel habit (☐ p.389)<br>Once diverticular disease is confirmed, treat with high-fibre diet ± antispasmodics (e.g. mebeverine 135mg tds)<br>Refer if severe symptoms |
| *Acute diverticulitis* | Presents with:<br>• Altered bowel habit<br>• Colicky left sided abdominal pain—may become continuous and cause guarding/peritonism in the left iliac fossa<br>• Fever<br>• Malaise ± nausea<br>• Flatulence<br>❶ There may be few abdominal signs in the elderly | Treat with oral antibiotics (e.g. co-amoxiclav 250mg tds or cefaclor 250–500mg tds and metronidazole 400mg bd or ciprofloxacin 500–750mg bd)<br>There may also be some benefit from a low residue diet<br>If severe symptoms, uncertain diagnosis, or not settling, admit as an acute surgical emergency |
| *Diverticular abscess* | Presents with swinging fever, general malaise ± other localizing symptoms, e.g. pelvic pain | Refer for urgent surgical assessment/admit as a surgical emergency |
| *Perforated diverticulum* | Presents with ileus, peritonitis, and shock. | Admit as an acute surgical emergency |
| *Fistula formation* | A fistula may form if a diverticulum perforates into bladder, vagina or small bowel (☐ p.388) | Refer for surgical assessment<br>Treatment is usually surgical |
| *Haemorrhage from a diverticulum* | Common cause of rectal bleeding—usually sudden and painless | Gain IV access<br>Admit as an acute surgical emergency (☐ p.1072) |
| *Post-infective stricture* | Fibrous tissue formation following infection can cause narrowing of the colon → obstruction | Keep stool soft<br>If recurrent problems refer for surgery |

**Carcinoma of the colon** ☐ p.406.

**Anal conditions** ☐ p.410.

**Inflammatory bowel disease** ☐ p.422.

# Anal and perianal problems

**Haemorrhoids ('piles')** Common in all age groups from mid-teens onwards. Represent distention of the submuscosal plexus of veins in the anus. Three main groups situated at 3, 7, and 11 o'clock positions (relative to the patient viewed in lithotomy position). *Risk factors:* constipation; FH; varicose veins; pregnancy; ↑ anal tone (cause not understood); pelvic tumour; portal hypertension. *Classification:*

- **1st degree** Piles remain within the anal canal.
- **2nd degree** Prolapse out of anal verge but spontaneously reduce.
- **3rd degree** Prolapse out of anus and require digital reduction.
- **4th degree** Permanently prolapsed.

**Presentation** Discomfort or discharge ± fresh red rectal bleeding (blood on toilet paper, coating stool, or dripping into pan after defecation); feeling of incomplete emptying of the rectum; mucus discharge; pruritus ani. *Rectal examination:* prolapsing piles are obvious, 1st degree piles are not visible or palpable.

**Management** If piles are not obvious on examination, arrange proctoscopy ± sigmoidoscopy for all patients >40y. *Treatment:* soften stool (bran, ispaghula) and recommend topical analgesia (e.g. lidocaine 5% ointment or OTC preparation). If not responding to treatment, uncertainty over diagnosis, or severe symptoms (e.g. soiling of underwear), refer for surgical assessment. *Complications:*

- **Strangulation** Circulation to the pile is obstructed by the anal sphincter. Results in intense pain and anal sphincter spasm. Treat with analgesia. If severe pain or symptoms are not settling, may require admission.
- **Thrombosis** Pain/anal sphincter spasm—analgesia, ice packs and bed rest. Consider referral for surgery to prevent recurrence.

**Perianal haematoma (thrombosed external pile)** Due to a ruptured superficial perianal vein causing a subcutaneous haematoma. Presents with sudden onset of severe perianal pain. A tender 2–4mm 'dark blueberry' under the skin adjacent to the anus is visible. Give analgesia. Settles spontaneously over ~1wk. If <1d old can be evacuated via a small incision under LA.

**Rectal prolapse** Occurs in two age groups—the very young, and those >60y. Presents with mass coming down through the anus ± anal discharge. In adults there are two types:

- **Mucosal** Bowel musculature remains in position but redundant mucosa prolapses out of the anal canal. Occurs in adults with 3rd degree piles
- **Complete** Descent of the upper rectum into the lower anal canal. Usually due to weak pelvic floor from childbirth. Bowel wall is inverted and passed out through the anus. May be associated uterine prolapse.

Refer for surgery. A supporting ring may be used if unfit for surgery.

**Anal fissure** The anal mucosa is torn, usually on the posterior aspect of the anal canal. May occur at any age. Presents with pain on defecation ± constipation ± fresh rectal bleeding ('blood on toilet paper'). The fissure is often visible as is a 'sentinel pile' (bunched up mucosa at the base of the tear). Rectal examination is very tender due to muscle spasm.

**Management** Soften stool (e.g. ispaghula); try analgesic suppositories (e.g. 5% lidocaine ointment; OTC haemorrhoid preparations). If unsuccessful add glyceryl trinitrate ointment (0.2–0.3%) which relieves pain and spasm, but may cause headache. If interventions fail refer to surgeon.

**Perianal abscess** Usually caused by infection arising in a perianal gland. Tends to lie between the internal and external sphincters and points towards the skin at the anal margin. May affect patients of any age and presents with gradual onset of perianal pain which becomes throbbing and severe. Defecation and sitting are painful—characteristically patients sit with one buttock raised off the chair. Examination may reveal the abscess in the skin next to the anus. Refer as an acute surgical emergency for drainage.

**Perianal fistula** Abnormal connection between the lumen of the anus (or rectum) and skin. Usually develops from a perianal abscess. Fistulas are either 'high' (open into the bowel above the deep external anal sphincter) or 'low' (open into the bowel below this point). High fistulas are rare and usually due to UC, Crohn's disease, or tumour—they are more complex to repair. Presents with persistent perianal discharge and/or recurrent abscesses. The external opening is usually visible lateral to the anus; the internal opening may be palpable on rectal examination. Refer for surgical repair.

**Pilonidal sinus** Obstruction of a hair follicle in the natal cleft. The ingrowing hair triggers a foreign body reaction → pain, swelling, abscess and/or fistula formation ± foul smelling discharge. *Management*: refer for surgery.

**Pruritus ani** Itching around the anus. Occurs if the anus is moist or soiled, e.g. poor personal hygiene; anal leakage or faecal incontinence; fissures; nylon/tight underwear. *Other causes*: dermatological conditions (e.g. contact dermatitis, lichen sclerosus); threadworm infection; anxiety; other causes of generalized pruritus ( p.598). Treat cause if possible; avoid spicy food; moist wipe post-defecation.

---

 **Threadworm** Common in the UK, especially in children. *Enterobius vermicularis* causes anal itch as it leaves the bowel to lay eggs on the perineum. Often seen as silvery thread-like worms at the anus of children. *Treatment*: mebendazole (available OTC). Treat household contacts as well as the index case.

---

**Anal ulcers** Rare. Consider Crohn's disease, syphilis, tumour.

**Anal cancer** usually squamous cell cancer (>50%). *Risk factors*: anal sex; syphilis; anal warts (HPV). Presents with bleeding, pain, anal mass or ulcer, pruritus, stricture, change in bowel habit. A mass may be palpable on rectal examination. Check for inguinal LNs.

**Management** Refer for urgent surgical review and confirmation of diagnosis. Treatment is usually with a combination of radiotherapy ± chemotherapy. AP resection is reserved for salvage therapy post-chemoradiotherapy failure.

# Patients with ostomies

The first iatrogenic stoma was constructed in France in 1776 for an obstructing rectal cancer. Stomas (from the Greek meaning 'mouth') may be temporary or permanent (Table 13.10).

**Stoma retraction** Can → leakage and severe skin problems. Most common reason for re-operation. Refer for specialist advice.

**Prolapse** Seen most frequently with loop colostomy. If persists and disrupts pouching, refer for consideration of revision.

**Peristomal hernia** Common complication. Symptomatic cases require referral for repair.

**Stenosis** Narrowing of the stoma may result in difficulty or pain passing stool and/or obstruction. If problematic refer for revision.

**Skin complications** Skin irritation can be due to:
• Leakage onto the skin
• Allergic reactions to the adhesive material in a skin barrier
• Fungal infection or
• Inadequate hygiene.

## Prevention of skin complications
• Advise patients to clean, rinse, and pat the skin dry between pouch changes.
• Avoid using an oily soap, which can leave a film that interferes with proper adhesion of the skin barrier.
• Ensure that the pouch system fits.
• Treat any infection with oral antibiotics and/or oral or topical antifungals.
• Apply skin barrier cream.
• If the skin is uneven (e.g. due to scarring), fill irregularities with stoma paste to give a better fit.
• Consider the use of convex discs or stoma belts (refer to specialist stoma nurse for advice).

**Drugs** Enteric-coated and modified release preparations are unsuitable for people with bowel stomas, particularly for patients with ileostomy.

## Diet
• Avoid foods that cause intestinal upset or diarrhoea.
• In the case of descending/sigmoid colostomy, avoid foods that cause constipation. If constipation does occur, ↑ fluid intake and/or dietary fibre.
• Certain foods (e.g. beans, cucumbers, and carbonated drinks) can cause gas, along with certain habits such as talking or swallowing air while eating, using a straw, breathing through the mouth, and even chewing gum.
• A daily portion of apple sauce, cranberry juice, yogurt, or buttermilk can help control odour. If odour is strong and persistent, consider use of charcoal filters.

**Table 13.10** The 3 main types of stoma

| Colostomy | Ileostomy | Urostomy |
|---|---|---|
| Age Most >50y | Peak age range 10–50y | Age Most >50y |
| *Output* Depends on site<br>• Transverse colostomy soft stool<br>• Descending/sigmoid colostomy—formed stool | *Output* Soft/fluid stool | *Output* Urine—continent procedures using bowel to fashion a bladder which is then drained with a catheter through the stoma are becoming common |
| *Reasons for colostomy*<br>Carcinoma<br>Diverticular disease<br>Trauma<br>Radiation enteritis<br>Bowel ischaemia<br>Hischprung's disease<br>Congenital abnormalities<br>Obstruction<br>Crohn's disease<br>Faecal incontinence | *Reasons for ileostomy*<br>Ulcerative colitis<br>Crohn's disease<br>Familial polyposis coli<br>Obstruction<br>Radiation enteritis<br>Trauma<br>Bowel ischaemia<br>Meconium ileus<br>Carcinoma | *Reasons for urostomy*<br>Carcinoma<br>Urinary incontinence<br>Fistulas<br>Spinal column disorders |

**Psychosocial problems** Self-help groups provide information and tips on lifestyle and stoma care; specialist stoma nurses can provide support and counselling.

**Activities** Advise patients to avoid rough contact sports and heavy lifting as these might → herniation around the stoma. Patients with stomas may swim. Because of peristalsis water will not enter a stoma, so stomas do not need to be covered when bathing.

**Travel** Advise patients to pack sufficient supplies of their stoma products and carry supplies with them in case baggage is misplaced. Avoid storing supplies in a very hot environment as heat may damage pouches.

❶ In all cases liaise with a specialist stoma nurse if possible.

**Patient advice and support**
**Colostomy Association** ☎ 0800 328 4257
🖥 www.colostomyassociation.org.uk

# Chronic diarrhoea and malabsorption

**Chronic diarrhoea** Diarrhoea persisting >4wk. Patients' perceptions of diarrhoea vary widely. Clarify what is meant. Chronic diarrhoea affects ~4–5% of adults in the UK. There are many causes (Table 13.11) and all patients require investigation. Careful history is vital.

### Symptoms suggestive of organic disease
- History of <3mo duration.
- Mainly nocturnal or continuous (as opposed to intermittent) diarrhoea.
- Significant weight ↓
- Liquid stools with blood and/or mucus.

### Symptoms suggestive of malabsorption
- Pale and/or offensive stools.
- Steatorrhoea—excess fat in faeces. The stool is pale coloured, foul smelling, and floats ('difficult to flush').

**Examination and investigation** Full examination. Look for signs of systemic disease and examine abdomen thoroughly. Check:
- *Blood* FBC, ESR, $Ca^{2+}$, LFTs, haematinics, TFTs, coeliac serology.
- *Stool* M,C&S.

### Management
- If obvious identifiable cause, e.g. GI infection, constipation, drug side effect, then treat and review. Refer to gastroenterology if treatment does not relieve symptoms.
- If symptoms suggestive of functional bowel disease and <45y with normal investigations, irritable bowel syndrome is likely. Reassure, offer advice, and review as necessary. Refer to gastroenterology if atypical symptoms appear or the patient is unhappy with the diagnosis.
- Otherwise refer to gastroenterology for assessment. Speed of referral depends on age and severity of symptoms.

⚠ **Refer urgently** to a team specializing in lower GI malignancy if:

*Any age* with
- Right lower abdominal mass consistent with involvement of large bowel
- Palpable rectal mass (intraluminal, not pelvic; a pelvic mass outside the bowel would warrant an urgent referral to a urologist)
- Unexplained iron deficiency anaemia (Hb ≤11g/dL for ♂; ≤10g/dL for a non-menstruating ♀).

*Aged ≥40y* reporting rectal bleeding with a change of bowel habit towards looser stools and/or increased stool frequency persisting ≥6wk.

*Aged ≥60y* with
- Rectal bleeding persisting for ≥6wk without a change in bowel habit and without anal symptoms
- Change in bowel habit to looser stools and/or more frequent stools persisting for ≥6wk without rectal bleeding.

❶ In a patient with equivocal symptoms who is not unduly anxious, it is reasonable to 'treat, watch, and wait'.

**Table 13.11** Causes of chronic diarrhoea

| Colon | Small bowel | Pancreas |
|---|---|---|
| Colonic cancer | Crohn's disease | Pancreatic cancer |
| Ulcerative colitis | Coeliac disease | Chronic pancreatitis |
| Crohn's disease | Other enteropathies, e.g. | CF |
| Constipation with | Whipple's disease | |
| overflow diarrhoea | Bile acid malabsorption | **Other** |
| | Ischaemia | Bowel resection |
| **Endocrine** | Enzyme deficiencies, e.g. | Intestinal fistula |
| DM (autonomic | lactase deficiency | Drugs |
| neuropathy) | Radiation damage | Alcohol |
| Hyperthyroidism | Bacterial overgrowth | Autonomic neuropathy |
| Hypoparathyroidism | Lymphoma | 'Factitious' diarrhoea |
| Addison's disease | Infection, e.g. giardiasis, | |
| Hormone-secreting | *Cryptosporidium* | |
| tumours, e.g. carcinoid | Irritable bowel syndrome | |

**Malabsorption** Presents with chronic diarrhoea, weight ↓, steatorrhoea, vitamin/iron deficiencies, and/or oedema due to protein deficiency. Refer to gastroenterology for investigation/treatment of the cause.

*Usual causes*
- Coeliac disease (📖 p.420)
- Chronic pancreatitis (📖 p.438)
- Crohn's disease (📖 p.122).

*Rarer causes*
- CF
- Pancreatic cancer (📖 p.440)
- Whipple's disease
- Biliary insufficiency
- Bacterial overgrowth
- Chronic infection (e.g. giardiasis, tropical sprue)
- Following gastric surgery.

**Whipple's disease** A cause of malabsorption which usually occurs in ♂ >50y. *Other features:* arthralgia, pigmentation, weight ↓, lymphadenopathy, ± cerebellar or cardiac signs. *Cause: Tropheryma whippelii.* Refer for gastroenterology assessment. Jejunal biopsy is characteristic. *Treatment:* long-term broad-spectrum antibiotics.

**Malabsorption in children** 📖 p.886.

**Factitious diarrhoea** Responsible for 4% of referrals to gastroenterology departments and 20% of tertiary referrals. Due to laxative abuse or adding of water or urine to stool samples. Difficult to spot—have a high index of suspicion, especially in patients with history of eating disorder or somatization.

## Further information

**British Society of Gastroenterology** Guidelines for the investigation of chronic diarrhoea (2nd edn) (2002) 🖥 www.bsg.org.uk
**NICE** 🖥 www.nice.org.uk
- Referral guidelines for suspected cancer (2005)
- Diarrhoea and vomiting in children under 5 (2009).

# Faecal incontinence

Affects ~2% of all ages, causing great personal disability. It is a common reason for carers to request placement in a nursing home.

## Causes
- Age and frailty
- Constipation (overflow incontinence)
- Childbirth
- Colonic resection/anal surgery
- Rectal prolapse/haemorrhoids
- Loose stools or diarrhoea from any cause, e.g. inflammatory bowel disease
- After radiotherapy
- Systemic sclerosis
- Neurological disorders
- Cognitive deficit
- Congenital disorders (e.g. anal atresia, Hirschprung's disease)
- Emotional problems, e.g. encoparesis in children.

**History** Aimed at establishing the underlying causes of the incontinence (may be >1) and other factors that might be contributing to it. *Ask about:*
- Onset and nature of symptoms ❶ Always consider faecal incontinence when patients present with anal soreness and/or itching.
- Bowel habit including timing and frequency of incontinence.
- Difficulties with toileting and help available.
- Other medical conditions.
- Medication.
- Diet.
- Social circumstances.

⚠ Persistent change in bowel habit to looser stools may be a sign of GI malignancy (📖 p.389).

**Examination** General and rectal examination (to detect abnormalities of anal tone, local anal pathology (e.g. rectal prolapse), and constipation causing overflow incontinence). Further examination depends on age group and history, e.g. cognitive assessment if suspected cognitive deficit; neurological examination if ↓ anal tone.

## Primary care management
### Treatment of cause
- Clear any constipation/faecal loading (📖 p.386). Use rectal preparations initially to clear faecal load. If unsuccessful/rectal preparations are inappropriate, switch to oral laxatives. Take steps to prevent recurrence, e.g. add fibre to diet, ↑ fluid intake, consider regular laxatives.
- Treat other reversible causes, e.g. infective diarrhoea, UC.
- Consider alternatives to any contributing medications, e.g. tranquillizers.

### General measures where cause cannot be treated
- Advise fluid intake of at least 1.5L/d.
- Encourage bowel emptying after a meal—advise patients to assume a seated/squatting position and not to strain.
- Ensure that toilet facilities are private, accessible, and safe—refer for OT assessment if needed.
- Manipulate diet to promote optimal stool consistency and predictable bowel emptying. A food/fluid diary may be helpful. Only change one food at a time. Consider referral to a dietician.
- If stool must be in the rectum at a set time (e.g. when a carer is there), manipulate bowel action with PR/PO laxatives and/or loperamide.

- If loose stools, consider treatment with loperamide, co-phenotrope, or codeine phosphate prn or continuously. When using loperamide, introduce at a very low dose (consider syrup for doses<2mg) and ↑ dose until desired stool consistency is reached. Dose and/or frequency can be adjusted ↑ or ↓ in response to stool consistency and lifestyle.
  ❶ Do not use if hard stools, undiagnosed diarrhoea, or flare-up of UC.
- Review regularly. If no improvement with simple strategies, consider referral for specialist care.

***Patients with faecal incontinence as a result of enteral feeding***
Discuss with the patient's dietician. Modifying type/timing of feeds may help.

***Patients with spinal injury or disease*** Bowel function is a reflex action which we learn to override as children. If the lesion is above the level of this reflex pathway ($T_{12}$ for bowel function), then automatic emptying will still occur when the bladder or bowel is full although there is no control. If the lesion is below this level, there is no emptying reflex. Bowel care programmes reflect this. Useful leaflets are available from the Spinal Injuries Association (☎ 0800 980 0501 🖳 www.spinal.co.uk).

**Referral** Consider if symptoms are not controlled:
- To continence adviser—for advice on skin care/hygiene and supplies of incontinence pads. Pelvic floor muscle training, bowel retraining, biofeedback, electrical stimulation, and/or rectal irrigation may be useful. Devices, e.g. anal plugs or faecal collectors, can help in some situations.
- To surgeon—for sphincter repair if significant sphincter defect; for consideration of implanted sacral nerve stimulation device; for appendicostomy/continent colonic conduit for anterograde irrigation in patients with colonic motility disorders; for stoma formation (last resort).
- To old age psychiatry if cognitive deficit and incontinence.
- To paediatrics if encoparesis due to chronic constipation, or child psychiatry if encoparesis due to emotional distress.

**Encoparesis in children** 📖 p.913.

**Further information**
**NICE** Faecal incontinence (2007) 🖳 www.nice.org.uk

**Patient information**
**Bladder and Bowel Foundation** Provides information and support as well as 'Just can't wait' or JCW cards. This card allows patients with bowel problems access to staff toilet facilities in many high street stores on production of their access card. ☎ 0845 345 0165
🖳 www.bladderandbowelfoundation.org.uk

**RADAR keys** The National Key Scheme (NKS) offers independent access to disabled people to around 7,000 locked public toilets around the country. Keys are available to purchase from 🖳 www.radar.org.uk If the patient has an ongoing disability, purchase can be made VAT free.

# Gastroenteritis and food poisoning

Ingestion of viruses, bacteria, or their toxins commonly causes diarrhoea and/or vomiting. Rotavirus is the most common cause in children and accounts for ~1:5 GP consultations with the under 5s.

**Prevention** Handwashing after using the toilet; longer cooking and rewarming times; prompt consumption of food.

**Presentation**
- *History* Severity and duration of symptoms; food eaten and water drunk; time relationship between ingestion and symptoms; other affected contacts; recent foreign travel.
- *Examination* Usually normal. Dehydration may prompt admission.

**Investigation and management** See vomiting and diarrhoea (🕮 p.384). Advise fluid replacement. Only give antibiotics if recommended following stool culture (exception is *Giardia* diarrhoea—🕮 p.647).

**Campylobacter jejuni** Most common cause of food poisoning in the UK. Symptoms occur 2–5d after ingestion of infected food (usually milk or poultry). Malaise followed by abdominal pain and diarrhoea—often bloody. Rarely associated with arthritis. Usually clears spontaneously. If needed, treatment is with erythromycin or ciprofloxacin.

**Salmonella** Second most common cause of food poisoning in the UK. Several species cause food poisoning in man. Usually ingested in infected meat, poultry, or eggs. *Symptoms*: vomiting, diarrhoea, abdominal pain and fever—develop from 12h to 2d after ingestion. Rarely, associated with arthritis 2–3 wk after acute infection. In <1% a carrier state develops. Only use antibiotics on microbiologist advice.

**Escherichia coli diarrhoea** Many different strains of *E. coli* cause diarrhoea via a variety of mechanisms. In most cases, treatment is supportive with fluid replacement. Rarely, antibiotics may be recommended for enterohaemorrhagic strains, but use is controversial as antibiotic treatment has been linked with haemolytic uraemic syndrome.

**Cryptosporidium** Protozoan causing diarrhoeal disease. Infections are usually spread in water. Responsible for ~5% of all gastroenteritis in both industrialized and developing countries. Presents with profuse watery diarrhoea, abdominal cramp ± nausea, anorexia, fever, and malaise. Treatment is supportive. Usually symptoms last 1–2 wk (rarely >1mo). Immunocompromised patients develop profuse intractable diarrhoea which is difficult to clear and may continue intermittently for life.

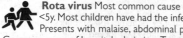 **Rota virus** Most common cause of gastroenteritis in children <5y. Most children have had the infection and are immune by 5y. Presents with malaise, abdominal pain, diarrhoea and vomiting. Common cause of hospital admission. Treatment is supportive.

**Further information**
**Health Protection Agency (HPA)** Infections: Topics A–Z: Gastrointestinal disease 🖥 www.hpa.org.uk

**Table 13.12** Common causes of gastroenteritis in the UK

| Organism/ source | Incubation | D | V | P | F | O | Food |
|---|---|---|---|---|---|---|---|
| Staph. aureus | 1–6h | ✓ | ✓ | ✓ | | ↓BP | Meat |
| B. cereus | 1–5h | ✓ | ✓ | | | | Rice |
| C. perfringens | 6–24h | ✓ | | ✓ | | | Meat |
| C. botulinum | 12–36h | | ✓ | | | Paralysis | Canned food |
| Salmonella spp | 12–48h | ✓ | ✓ | ✓ | ✓ | | Meat, eggs, poultry |
| Shigella[ND] | 48–72h | ✓ | | ✓ | ✓ | Blood in stool | Any food |
| Campylobacter | 48h–5d | ✓ | | ✓ | ✓ | Blood in stool | Milk, poultry |
| E.coli | 12–72h | ✓ | | ✓ | ✓ | Blood in stool | Food, water |
| Y. enterocolitica | 24–36h | ✓ | | ✓ | ✓ | | Milk, water |
| Giardia lamblia | 1–4wk. | ✓ | | | | | Water |
| Cryptosporidium | 4–11d | ✓ | | ✓ | ✓ | | Water |
| Listeria | | | | | | Flu–like illness, pneumonia | Milk products, pâtés, raw vegetables |
| V. para–haemolyticus | 12–24h | ✓ | ✓ | ✓ | | | Fish |
| Rotavirus | 1–7d | ✓ | ✓ | | ✓ | Malaise | Food, water |
| Small viruses | 36–72h | ✓ | ✓ | | ✓ | Malaise | Any food |
| Entamoeba histolytica | 1–4wk | ✓ | | ✓ | ✓ | Blood in stool | Food, water |
| Mushrooms | 15min–24h | ✓ | ✓ | ✓ | | Fits, coma, renal/liver failure | |
| Scrombrotoxin | 10–60min | ✓ | | | | Flushes, erythema | Fish |
| Heavy metals, e.g. zinc | 5min–2h | | ✓ | ✓ | | | |
| Red beans | 1–3h | ✓ | ✓ | | | | |

D=diarrhoea; V=vomiting; P=abdominal pain; F=fever; O=other

❶ Suspected food poisoning is a notifiable disease

 Some children may become cow's milk intolerant after a bout of gastroenteritis (📖 p.887).

# Coeliac disease

Gluten sensitivity results in inflammation of the bowel and malabsorption. Coeliac disease is a common disorder (UK prevalence 1:300, $♀:♂ \approx$ 3:1) although only a minority have clinically recognized disease. Can present at any age. Runs in families—first-degree relatives have a 1:10 chance of having coeliac disease. Peak incidence in adults is in 5th decade; in children at ~4y.

## Investigation

- Serological testing with IgA tissue transglutaminase (tTGA) if signs/symptoms listed in Table 13.13. Consider testing if associated condition or genetic predisposition. ❶ Test only if the patient has eaten some gluten in >1 meal/d for ≥ 6wk.
- Other bloods—depending on presenting features consider FBC, ESR, LFTs, $Ca^{2+}$, thyroid function tests.
- If presenting with diarrhoea, check a stool to exclude infective causes.

❶ If negative IgA tTGA, consider checking for IgA defeciency. If IgA deficient, offer IgA tTGA and/or IgA endomysial antibody (EMA) testing.

**Initial management** Refers for specialist review if:
- +ve serology
- Strong clinical suspicion of coeliac disease but -ve serology
- Unwilling to reintroduce gluten to diet to enable serological testing.

## Ongoing management

*Diet* Refer to a dietician for advice on a gluten-free diet. Prescribe adequate amounts of gluten-free products, marking the prescription ACBS. Add supplements of deficient nutrients, e.g. iron, folic acid, calcium, until well established on a gluten-free diet.

*Pneumococcal vaccination* All patients with coeliac disease have a degree of hyposplenism and are more prone to pneumococcal infection. Advise pneumococcal vaccination.

*Follow-up* Patients should be followed up every 6–12mo in a specialist clinic or by a GP under a shared care arrangement. Routine checks include: symptoms, weight and blood tests (Hb, $B_{12}$, folate, iron, albumin, $Ca^{2+}$, antigliadin or antiendomysial antibodies).

*Failure to respond to diet* The most common reason is continued ingestion of gluten (intentional or inadvertent). Re-refer to dieticians. If symptoms recur after a period of remission, re-refer to a specialist for reassessment of the diagnosis.

*Long term complications* Osteoporosis and malignancy (lymphoma or carcinoma of the small intestine). Both are virtually eliminated by adherence to a strict gluten-free diet.

## Further information

**NICE** Recognition and assessment of coeliac disease (2009)
🖫 www.nice.org.uk

**Table 13.13** Presentation of coeliac disease

| Signs and symptoms | Associated conditions | |
|---|---|---|
| Chronic/intermittent diarrhoea | *GI* | *Endocrine* |
| Failure to thrive/faltering growth in children | Dental enamel defects | Type 1 DM |
| | Mouth ulcers | Autoimmune thyroid disease |
| Persistent/unexplained GI symptoms including nausea/vomiting | Irritable bowel syndrome | Addison's disease |
| | Microscopic colitis | Amenorrhoea |
| Tired all the time | Persistent/unexplained constipation | |
| Recurrent abdominal pain, cramping or distension | Unexplained persistent ↑ in liver enzymes | *Other* |
| | | Unexplained alopecia |
| Sudden/unexpected weight ↓ | Autoimmune liver disease | Dermatitis herpetiformis |
| | | Depression or bipolar disorder |
| Unexplained iron-deficiency, or unspecified anaemia | *Musculoskeletal* | Polyneuropathy |
| | ↓ bone mineral density | Epilepsy |
| | Low-trauma fracture | Autoimmune myocarditis |
| **Genetic predisposition** | Metabolic bone disease (e.g. rickets, osteomalacia) | Chronic TTP |
| First-degree relative (parent, sibling or child) with coeliac disease | Sjogren's syndrome | Lymphoma |
| | Sarcoidosis | Recurrent miscarriage |
| Down's/Turner syndrome | | Unexplained subfertility |

---

## Advice for patients about coeliac disease
- Coeliac disease is intolerance to the protein gluten which is contained in a lot of foods.
- Cutting out *all* gluten from your diet will lead to an improvement in your symptoms and health.
- Coeliac disease is a lifelong condition. If you ever start eating gluten again, all your symptoms will return.
- Sticking to a gluten-free diet also helps you to avoid long-term problems associated with coeliac disease such as osteoporosis (thinning of the bones) or lymphoma (lymph node cancer of the bowel).

### Gluten-free diet
- Gluten is found in wheat, barley, and rye cereal products. Oats can be eaten (in moderation), but check labels carefully as oat flours and other products may also contain other cereals.
- Most processed foods contain gluten so avoid them.
- Look out for gluten in common cooking ingredients such as stock cubes, baking powder, soy sauce, and mustard powder.
- Coeliac UK provides a directory of approved products as well as recipes and tips on keeping to a gluten-free diet.
- Gluten-free products, such as bread, biscuits, and pasta, are available on prescription—ask your doctor.

## Information and support for parents and children
**Coeliac UK** ☎ 0870 444 8804 🖳 www.coeliac.co.uk

# Inflammatory bowel disease

Ulcerative colitis (UC) and Crohn's disease *(B.B. Crohn (1884–1983)—US gastroenterologist)* are collectively termed inflammatory bowel disease.

Both are chronic relapsing–remitting diseases characterized by acute non-infectious inflammation of the gut. In UC, inflammation is limited to the colorectal mucosa. Extent varies from disease limited to the rectum (proctitis) to disease affecting the whole colon (pancolitis). In Crohn's, any part of the gut from mouth to anus can be affected, with normal bowel between affected areas (skip lesions).

**Cause** Unknown. Both diseases are thought to result from an environmental trigger on genetically susceptible individuals Factors implicated (none proven) include:
- Smoking—protective against UC (95% are non-smokers or ex-smokers) but a causative factor in Crohn's disease (⅔ are smokers and smoking cessation halves the relapse rate).
- Gut flora or other infections, e.g. *Mycobacterium paratuberculosis*.
- Food constituents.

**Features** Table 13.15.

**Differential diagnosis**
- Irritable bowel syndrome
- Coeliac disease
- Anal fissure
- Gut infection, e.g. giardiasis
- Diverticulitis
- Colonic tumour
- Food-sensitive colitis (infants)
- Pseudomembranous colitis
- Ischaemic colitis
- Microscopic colitis.

**Suspected diagnosis** ~50% of severe attacks of UC are first attacks in patients who do not have a prior diagnosis. If bloody diarrhoea + fever >37.5°C or tachycardia >90bpm, admit as an acute emergency. If persistent unexplained diarrhoea lasting >4wk and/or persistent abdominal pain, refer for urgent further investigation to exclude GI malignancy and establish diagnosis.

**Table 13.14** Assessing the severity of ulcerative colitis

| Severity | Symptoms |
|---|---|
| Mild | <4 liquid stools/d |
| | Little/no rectal bleeding |
| | No signs of systemic disturbance |
| Moderate | 4–6 liquid stools/d |
| | Moderate rectal bleeding |
| | Some signs of systemic disturbance |
| | Mild disease that does not respond to treatment |
| Severe | >6 liquid stools/d |
| | Severe rectal bleeding |
| | Any systemic disturbance (↑ pulse rate >90, pyrexia >37.5°C, ↑ ESR, ↑WCC, ↓Hb <10g/dL) |
| | Signs of malnutrition (e.g. hypoalbuminaemia <35g/dL) |
| | Weight loss >10% |

**Table 13.15** Features of inflammatory bowel disease

| | UC | Crohn's disease |
|---|---|---|
| Incidence | 10–20/100 000/y | 5–10/100 000/y and increasing |
| Prevalence | 100–200/100 000 | 50–100/100 000 |
| Peak age | 40–60y (85% <60y) | |
| Gender | ♂=♀ | |
| Risk factors | Smoking is protective | Smoking is a risk factor |
| GI symptoms | Diarrhoea + blood/mucus (stool may be solid if rectal disease only)<br>Faecal urgency/incontinence<br>Tenesmus<br>Lower abdominal pain | Diarrhoea ± blood/mucus<br>Malabsorption<br>Abdominal pain (crampy)<br>Mouth ulcers<br>Bowel obstruction due to strictures<br>Fistulas (often perianal)<br>Abscesses (perianal and intra–abdominal) |
| Systemic symptoms | Tiredness and/or malaise<br>Weight ↓ or failure to thrive/grow (children)<br>Fever | |
| Associated conditions | *Joint disease:* arthritis, sacroileitis, ankylosing spondylitis<br>*Eye disease:* iritis or uveitis<br>*Skin changes:* erythema nodosum, pyoderma gangrenosum (UC > Crohn's)<br>*Liver disease:* autoimmune hepatitis (UC), gallstones (Crohn's), sclerosing cholangitis (UC > Crohn's)<br>*Miscellaneous:* thromboembolism, osteoporosis (Crohn's), amyloidosis (Crohn's) | |
| Examination | *Abdominal + rectal examination*—abdominal tenderness. Anal and perianal lesions (pendulous skin tags, abscesses, fistulas) and/or mass in the right iliac fossa are characteristic of Crohn's disease<br>*General examination*—clubbing, aphtous ulcers in the mouth (Crohn's), signs of weight loss, anaemia or hypoproteinaemia | |
| Investigation | *Blood* FBC (anaemia, ↑WCC), ESR (↑ when disease is active), U&E, Cr, LFTs (including serum albumin) In severe UC, CRP >45g/dL after 3d steroid treatment indicates high (~85%) risk for colectomy<br>*Stool:* M,C&S (including *Cl. difficile*) to exclude infection<br>*AXR* Consider to clarify extent of disease, exclude toxic megacolon (transverse colon diameter >5cm) or bowel obstruction, and/or identify proximal constipation<br>*Proctoscopy* Inflammation and shallow ulceration extending proximally from the anal margin suggests UC | |

UC and Crohn's disease are rare in childhood. Presentation is variable and can be with non-specific features (e.g. failure to thrive), GI symptoms (e.g. malabsorbtion, bloody diarrhoea, acute abdomen), or complications (e.g. arthropathy or iritis). If suspected refer for confirmation of diagnosis and specialist management.

## Management of ulcerative colitis BNF 1.5

*Assessing severity* Table 13.14, 📖 p.422.

### Active disease

- Mesalazine 2–4g daily. Topical 5-ASA derivatives are a useful adjunct if troublesome rectal symptoms.
- Add steroids (prednisolone 40mg od po + rectal preparation) if prompt response is needed or mesalazine is unsuccessful. Review frequently and ↓ dose over 8wk. Rapid withdrawal ↑ risk of relapse.
- Azathioprine is added if the patient is having recurring attacks despite mesalazine maintenance, frequent steroids (≥ 2 courses/y), disease relapses as dose of steroid is ↓, or relapse <6wk after stopping steroids. Requires regular supervision.
- Ciclosporin or infliximab (anti-TNF antibody)—consultant supervised—may be effective as acute therapy for severe steroid-refractory disease.

⚠ **Admit acutely if**
- Severe abdominal pain (especially if associated with tenderness)
- Severe diarrhoea (>8x/d.) ± bleeding
- Dramatic weight loss
- Fever >37.5°C, tachycardia >90bpm or other signs of systemic disease.

*Maintenance treatment* Follow-up in 2° care is routine. Most patients require lifelong therapy. Mainstays of treatment are 5-ASA derivatives (e.g. mesalazine 1-2g/d or balsalazide 3-6g/d). Use a rectal formulation (e.g mesalazine 1g/d PR) if disease is confined to the rectum or descending colon. Long-term treatment ↓ risk of colonic cancer by 75%. 10% are intolerant to 5-ASA derivatives—alternative is azathioprine. Treat proximal constipation with stool bulking agents or laxatives. NSAIDs can precipitate relapse so avoid.

*Surgery* Last resort—but should not be delayed if severe colitis and failing to respond to medical therapy. 20–30% of patients with pancolitis require colectomy—1:3 develop pouchitis (non-specific inflammation of the ileal reservoir) within 5y of surgery.

*Prognosis* At any time 50% are asymptomatic, 30% have mild symptoms, and 20% have moderate/severe symptoms. <5% are free from relapse after 10y. Relapses usually affect the same part of the colon.

*Complications* Table 13.16.

## Management of Crohn's disease

### Active ileal and/or colonic disease

- Treat with mesalazine 4g daily. Less effective than for UC.
- Add steroids (prednisolone 40mg od po or budesonide 9mg daily) if unresponsive to mesalazine. Review frequently and ↓ dose over 8wk. Rapid withdrawal ↑ risk of relapse. ❶ Steroids are associated with ↑ risk of severe sepsis and mortality in Crohn's disease so alternatives to steroid therapy are increasingly sought and steroid maintenance for >3mo should always be avoided.
- Elemental or polymeric diets for 4–6wk can be a useful adjunct or alternative to steroid treatment—take consultant advice.

- Other treatments (consultant supervision) include metronidazole, azathioprine, antitumour necrosis factor (infliximab or adalumimab).
- Surgery is an option if medical treatment has failed. 50% need surgery <10y after onset. Surgery is not curative and 50% will require a further operation at a later stage. After ileal resection check $B_{12}$ levels annually.

⚠ **Admit acutely if**
- Severe abdominal pain (especially if associated with tenderness)
- Severe diarrhoea (>8x/d.) ± bleeding
- Dramatic weight loss
- Bowel obstruction
- Fever/other signs of systemic disease.

❶ For disease elsewhere take specialist advice.

*Maintenance treatment* Follow up in 2° care is routine. Treatment is aimed at ↓ impact of the disease. The most effective measure is to stop smoking. Mesalazine has limited benefit. It is ineffective at doses <2g/d. Other agents used include azathioprine, methotrexate, and 2-monthly infliximab. All require consultant supervision. Treat diarrhoea symptomatically with codeine phosphate or loperamide unless it is due to active colonic disease. Colestyramine (4g 1–3x/d) ↓ diarrhoea due to terminal ileal disease/resection. NSAIDs can precipitate relapse so avoid.

*Prognosis* 75% are back to work after the first year but 15% remain unable to work long term. Complications—Table 13.16.

**Table 13.16** Complications of inflammatory bowel disease

| UC | Crohn's |
|---|---|
| *Toxic megacolon* Colon distends and may perforate. | *Intra-abdominal abscess* |
| *Colonic cancer* Risk ↑ if disease >8y, onset in childhood/adolescence, age >45y, HH of colon cancer, extensive colitis, sclerosing cholangitis. Prevention: screening with colonoscopy. Frequency depends on severity of the disease and duration of symptoms | *Intestinal stricture* Common—may require surgery |
| | *Toxic megacolon* Rare (see UC) |
| | *Bowel obstruction* |
| | *Fistula formation* |
| | *Perianal disease* |
| | *Malignancy* Large and small bowel cancer—5% 10y after diagnosis |
| *Sclerosing cholangitis* Fibrosis and stricture of intra- and extra-hepatic bile ducts. Presents with obstructive jaundice | *Osteoporosis* |
| *Psychological effects* Chronic lifelong conditions which have major impact on work and domestic life. Self-help groups can be useful ||

## Further information
**British Society of Gastroenterology** Guidelines for the management of inflammatory bowel disease in adults (2004) 🖳 www.bsg.org.uk

## Advice and support for patients
**National Association for Colitis and Crohn's disease (NACC)** ☎ 0845 130 2233 (info); 0845 130 3344 (support) 🖳 www.nacc.org.uk

# Irritable bowel syndrome

Irritable bowel syndrome (IBS) is a chronic (>6mo) relapsing and remitting condition of unknown cause with symptoms including: **A**bdominal pain or discomfort, **B**loating, and **C**hange in bowel habit

It is a diagnosis of exclusion with no confirmatory test and no cure. Extremely common. Lifetime prevalence ≥20%, although ~75% never consult a GP. ♀>♂ (2.5:1). Symptoms can appear at any age.

**Diagnosis of IBS** Abdominal pain or discomfort that is:
• relieved by defecation, *or*
• associated with altered bowel frequency or stool form.

*and* ≥2 of the following:
• altered stool passage (straining, urgency, incomplete evacuation)
• abdominal bloating (♀>♂), distension, tension, or hardness
• symptoms made worse by eating
• passage of mucus.

*Other commonly associated symptoms include* lethargy, nausea, backache and bladder symptoms.

## Differential diagnosis
• Colonic carcinoma
• Coeliac disease
• Inflammatory bowel disease (Crohn's disease or UC)
• Pelvic inflammatory disease
• Endometriosis
• GI infection
• Thyrotoxicosis.

**Investigation** A diagnosis of exclusion. How far to investigate is a clinical judgment weighing risks of investigation against possibility of serious disease. Judgment is based on age of the patient, family history, length of history, and symptom cluster.
• *Patients <40y* Check FBC, ESR, and antibody testing to exclude coeliac disease.
• *Patients >40y* Colonic cancer must be excluded for any patient with a persistent unexplained change in bowel habit—particularly towards looser stools (📖 p.389).
• *Other investigations to consider*
  • Thyroid function tests if other symptoms/signs of thyroid disease.
  • Stool samples to exclude GI infection if diarrhoea.
  • Endocervical swabs for *Chlamydia*.
  • Colonoscopy to exclude inflammatory bowel disease.
  • Laparoscopy to exclude endometriosis.

**Referral** to gastroenterology/general surgery if
• Passing blood (except if from an anal fissure or haemorrhoids)—*U*
• Abdominal, rectal, or pelvic mass—*U*
• Unintentional/unexplained weight loss—*U/S*
• Positive inflammatory markers and/or anaemia—*U/S*
• >40y with new symptoms—*U* (if age >60y)/*S/R*
• Change in symptoms, especially if >40y—*U* (if age >60y)/*S/R*
• Atypical features (i.e. not those listed above)—*U/S/R*
• Family history of bowel or ovarian cancer—*R*
• Patient is unhappy to accept a diagnosis of IBS despite explanation—*R*
*U*=urgent; *S*=soon; *R*=routine

**Treatment** Reassure. Information leaflets are helpful. Encourage effective use of leisure time and regular physical exercise.

**Diet** Encourage patients to have regular meals and take time to eat. Avoid missing meals or leaving long gaps between eating.
- Drink ≥8 cups of fluid/d, especially water. Restrict tea/coffee to 3 cups/d. ↓ intake of alcohol and fizzy drinks.
- ↓ intake of high-fibre food (e.g. wholemeal/high-fibre flour and breads, cereals high in bran, and whole grains such as brown rice).
- ↓ intake of 'resistant starch' found in processed or re-cooked foods.
- Limit fresh fruit to 3 × 80g portions/d
- For diarrhoea, avoid sorbitol, an artificial sweetener.
- For wind and bloating consider increasing intake of oats (e.g. oat-based breakfast cereal or porridge) and linseed (≤ 1 tablespoon/d).
- Up to 50% may be helped by exclusion of certain foods (especially patients with diarrhoea-—predominant disease). Diaries may help identify foods that provoke symptoms. Common candidates are dairy products, citrus fruits, caffeine, alcohol, tomatoes, gluten, and eggs. Refer to dietician for exclusion diet.

### Specific measure
- **Probiotics** Some evidence of effectiveness. Try a 4 wk trial of treatment.
- **Fibre/bulking agents** Constipation-predominant IBS. Bran can make some patients worse. Ispaghula husk is better tolerated. Laxatives are an alternative, but avoid use of lactulose.
- **Antispasmodics,** e.g. mebeverine, peppermint oil. All equally effective. If no response in a few days, switch to another —different agents suit different individuals. Once symptoms are controlled use prn dosing.
- **Antidiarrhoeal preparations,** e.g. loperamide. Avoid codeine phosphate as may cause dependence. Use prn for patients with diarrhoea— predominant disease. Use pre-emptive doses to cover difficult situations (e.g. air travel).
- **Antidepressants** There is evidence that low-dose amitriptyline, e.g. 10mg nocte, is effective. SSRIs are less effective unless the patient is overtly depressed. Withdraw if no response after 4–6wk.
- **Psychotherapy and hypnosis** Some effect in trials. Reserve for cases that have failed to respond to more conventional treatment.

**Failure to respond to treatment** Consider another diagnosis—review history and examination ± refer for further investigation.

**Prognosis** >50% still have symptoms after 5y.

### Further information
**NICE** Irritable bowel syndrome in adults: diagnosis and management of irritable bowel syndrome in primary care (2008) 🖳 www.nice.org.uk

### Advice and support for patients
**Gut Trust** ☎ 0872 300 4537 🖳 www.theguttrust.org

# Jaundice and abnormal liver function

**Jaundice** Yellow pigmentation of the tissues due to excessive bile pigment. Clinical jaundice appears when serum bilirubin >35 μmol/L.

## Causes

- ↑ *production of bilirubin (pre-hepatic jaundice)* Haemolytic anaemia, drug-induced haemolysis, malaria, Gilbert's/Crigler–Najjar syndrome.
- *Defective processing (hepatic jaundice)* Hepatitis, cirrhosis.
- *Blocked excretion (obstructive jaundice)* Gallstones, pancreatic cancer, primary biliary cirrhosis, primary sclerosing cholangitis, cholangiocarcinoma, sepsis, enlarged porta hepatis (e.g. 2° to lymphoma).

**History** Patients presenting with jaundice may have no other symptoms. General symptoms include tiredness, nausea, and pruritus. Ask about colour of the urine—dark urine suggests conjugated hyperbilirubinaemia and hepato-biliary disease.

**Examination** Mild jaundice is best seen by examining the sclerae in natural light. Look for signs of chronic liver disease and examine the abdomen for masses and hepatomegaly.

**Investigations** Initially check FBC and LFTs (Table 13.17). Further investigations depend on the results.

**Management** Treat the cause of the jaundice. Most patients (except those with Gilbert's syndrome or self-limiting viral hepatitis) will require specialist referral. Refer patients with pre-hepatic and hepatic jaundice to a hepatologist or gastroenterologist; refer patients with post-hepatic jaundice to a general or hepatobiliary surgeon.

**Neonatal jaundice** 📖 p.866.

## Abnormal liver function

*Raised AST/ALT/GGT in isolation* Liver enzymes can ↑ transiently as a result of viral infection, drugs, or alcohol. ALT tends to be more raised in viral and autoimmune hepatitis; AST tends to be more raised in patients with fatty liver; raised GGT is particularly associated with alcohol excess.

- Check medication, including herbal medicines.
- Stop alcohol.
- Repeat LFTs:
  - In 1 mo if AST/ALT are <3× upper limit of normal.
  - In 1 wk if AST/ALT is ≥3× upper limit of normal.
- If still raised, request hepatitis screen and USS, or refer to hepatology or gastroenterology depending on clinical state.
- If ALT is <2× upper limit of normal and hepatitis screen is negative:
  - If USS is normal, repeat LFTs every 3–6mo to see if abnormalities settle—may be due to drugs, alcohol, or early fatty liver disease.
  - If USS shows fatty liver and consuming excess alcohol, advise abstinence from alcohol and recheck LFTs every 3–6mo.
  - If USS shows fatty liver and alcohol consumption is within normal limits, advise weight loss and low fat diet, treat metabolic syndrome, and recheck LFTs every 3–6mo.
- In all other cases, refer for specialist opinion.

**Table 13.17** Distinguishing different types of jaundice

| | Type of jaundice | | |
|---|---|---|---|
| **Tests** | **Pre-hepatic** | **Hepatic** | **Cholestatic** |
| Bilirubin | ↑↑ | ↑↑ | ↑↑ |
| AST/ALT | Normal | ↑↑ | ↑ |
| Alk phos | Normal | ↑ | ↑↑↑ |
| Hb | ↓ | Normal | Normal |
| Jaundice | Mild, lemon yellow | May be marked jaundice | May be marked jaundice |
| Other symptoms | Urine is not darkened | Tender, enlarged liver | Enlarged liver, itching skin, pale stools |

❶ A mixed picture is common and can be confusing

**Raised bilirubin** Possible causes include:
• Hepatitis/biliary obstruction— if ALT/AST is ↑, refer for liver USS and do a hepatitis screen or refer as for jaundice.
• Haemolysis—check FBC/reticulocyte count. Refer to haematology if abnormal
• Gilbert's disease—likely if serum bilirubin is <40mmol/L and ALT/AST and RBC/reticulocytes are normal. Bilirubin levels ↑ after a fast
• If isolated ↑ bilirubin >40 mmol/L— probably still Gilbert's syndrome but refer.

**Raised alkaline phosphatase** Usually originates from liver or bone. Bone is more likely if serum $Ca^{2+}$ and phosphate are raised and GGT is normal. ↑ may be associated with any liver disease but is particularly marked in patients with biliary obstruction and primary biliary cirrhosis.

**Medications that cause raised AST/ALT**
• Most penicillins (especially co-amoxiclav) and minocycline
• Antifungals
• Statins
• Anti-epileptics
• NSAIDs
• Some herbal medicines
• Some recreational drugs.

**Statins and abnormal liver function** Statins cause a biochemical abnormality only, but do not cause liver failure and are not contraindicated in compensated liver disease. May improve fatty liver disease. Measure liver function tests pre-treatment and after 1–3mo. Thereafter measure each 6mo for 1y. Discontinue if AST/ALT ↑ and stays at >3× normal.

**Hepatitis screen** Check as appropriate:
• Hepatitis A, B, and C serology
• EBV serology
• Liver autoantibodies
• Iron studies and transferrin saturation to exclude haemochromatosis
• $\alpha_1$ antitrypsin level
• Serum copper and caeruloplasmin levels (if <40y)
• αFP
• Fasting blood glucose and lipids
• $HbA_{1c}$.

# Hepatitis

**Acute hepatitis** May be asymptomatic or present with fatigue, flu-like symptoms, fever, light stools, dark urine, and/or jaundice. *Causes:*

- Viral hepatitis e.g. HBV, HAV, EBV
- Alcohol (📖 p.186)
- Drugs (e.g. diclofenac, co-amoxiclav)
- Toxins
- Obstructive jaundice
- Other infections—malaria, Q fever, leptospirosis, yellow fever.

**Management** Check LFTs; FBC; U&E; eGFR; hepatitis serology. Treat the cause. Admit if condition is poor or rapidly deteriorating; refer for investigation if sustained abnormalities in liver function with unclear cause (📖 p.428). *Complications:* chronic hepatitis, acute liver failure.

**Hepatitis A (HAV)** Common. *Spread:* Faecal–oral route. Patients are infectious 2 wk before feeling ill. Incubation is 2–7wk (average 4wk). *High-risk groups:* travellers to high-risk areas; institution inhabitants and workers; IV drug abusers; patients with high-risk sexual practices. May be asymptomatic (especially young children) or present with fever, malaise, fatigue, anorexia, nausea/vomiting, abdominal pain, diarrhoea, tender hepatomegaly, pale stools, dark urine, and/or jaundice (70–80% adults).

**Management** Check LFTs (hepatic jaundice (📖 p.429)) and hepatitis serology—IgM antibodies signify recent infection, IgG remains detectable lifelong. Management is supportive. Avoid alcohol until LFTs are normal. Most recover in <2mo. There is no carrier state and hepatitis A does not cause chronic liver disease. After infection immunity is lifelong.

**Prevention** Vaccination is indicated for travellers to high-risk areas, people with chronic liver disease or those working in high-risk situations. Preparations available include monovalent vaccine (e.g. Havrix®), hepatitis A & B combined vaccine (Twinrix®), and hepatitis A and typhoid combined vaccine (e.g. Hepatyrix®). Passive immunization with human immunoglobulin gives protection for ≤3mo and is used for short-term travel or protecting household contacts of sufferers.

**Hepatitis E (HEV)** Similar to HAV infection. Usually acquired in developing countries. Incubation is 2–9 wk (average 40d). Diagnosis is made with serology. Treatment is supportive. There is no chronic state. Mortality in pregnancy can be as high as 20%. No vaccine exists.

**Hepatitis B (HBV)** 📖 p.740      **Hepatitis C (HCV)** 📖 p.740

**Chronic hepatitis** Hepatitis lasting > 6mo. May be asymptomatic or present with fatigue, RUQ pain, jaundice, arthralgia, signs of chronic liver disease (gynaecomastia, testicular atrophy, clubbing, palmar erythema, leuconychia, peripheral oedema, spider naevi, portal hypertension, recurrent infection, and/or complications), acute liver failure, cirrhosis, hepatocellular carcinoma. *Causes:*

- Viral hepatitis
- Alcohol—📖 p.186
- Drugs (e.g. nitrofurantoin, methyldopa, isoniazid)
- Chronic autoimmune hepatitis
- Primary biliary cirrhosis
- Wilson's disease
- Haemochromatosis
- $\alpha_1$-antitrypsin deficiency
- Sarcoidosis.

***Management*** Check LFTs, FBC, U&E, eGFR, and hepatitis screen (📖 p.429). Refer for specialist care.

**Chronic autoimmune hepatitis** Typically young women. Associated with personal/family history of autoimmune disease (e.g. RA, vitiligo). Diagnosis is confirmed with liver biopsy and autoimmune markers. Specialist management is with steroids ± immunosuppressants.

**Primary biliary cirrhosis** Slow progressive cholangio-hepatitis eventually resulting in cirrhosis. ♀:♂ ≈ 9:1. *Peak age at presentation:* 45y. *Cause:* probably autoimmune. *Associations:*

- Thyroid disease
- Sjögren's syndrome
- CREST syndrome
- Coeliac disease
- Hepatic and extra-hepatic malignancy
- Pancreatic hyposecretion.

***Presentation*** 50% are asymptomatic at presentation. *Symptoms/signs:*

- Fatigue
- Pruritus
- Arthralgia
- Osteoporosis/ osteomalacia
- Hirsutism
- Obstructive jaundice (late)
- Symptoms/signs of cirrhosis or liver failure.

***Investigation and management*** *Blood:* LFTs (↑Alk phos; ↑ALT; ↑GGT). Liver biopsy is diagnostic. Refer for specialist care. If asymptomatic, 1:3 remain symptom free—the rest develop symptoms in 2–4y. Median survival is 7–10y. Liver transplant is an option. Prognosis following transplant is good, but recurrence may occur in the transplanted liver.

**Primary haemochromatosis** Autosomal recessive condition of excess gut absorption of iron → iron deposition and damage to heart, liver, pancreas, joints and pituitary. ~1/400 people are homozygous for the condition but expression is highly variable. ♂ > ♀ (women present ~10y later). Often an incidental finding, or found by screening relatives of affected individuals (genetic testing or serum ferritin). *Symptoms/signs:*

- Tiredness
- Arthralgia/arthritis
- Skin pigmentation
- Hepatomegaly ± signs of cirrhosis
- DM
- Impotence/testicular atrophy
- Cardiomyopathy.

**Investigation and management** *Blood:* ↑ ferritin; ↑ iron; transferrin saturation >70%; total iron binding capacity ↓. Refer. Liver biopsy is diagnostic. Venesection returns life expectancy to normal.

**Secondary haemochromatosis** Iron overload from frequent transfusions, e.g. for haemolysis. Specialist management with desferrioxamine infusions to ↑ iron excretion is required.

$\alpha$**1-antitrypsin deficiency** 📖 p.433

**Wilson's disease** (hepatolenticular degeneration). Rare autosomal recessive disorder. Defective biliary copper excretion → accumulation of copper in the liver, brain, kidney, and cornea. Treatment is with penicillamine. Liver transplantation is the only treatment if presentation is with acute liver failure. *S.A.K. Wilson (1878–1937)—British neurologist.*

## Information and support for patients
**British Liver Trust** ☎ 0800 652 7330 🖥 www.britishlivertrust.org.uk
**Primary Biliary Cirrhosis Organization** 🖥 www.pbcers.org
**Wilson's Disease Association** 🖥 www.wilsonsdisease.org

# Liver failure and portal hypertension

*Jaundice is the disease that your friends diagnose.*
Aphorisms, Sir William Osler (1849–1920)

**Acute liver failure** Presents with sudden onset of severe illness.
- Jaundice.
- Hypoglycaemia.
- Hepatic encephalopathy—ranges from mild confusion and irritability through drowsiness and increasing confusion to coma.
- Haemorrhage—due to deranged clotting factors.
- Ascites—hepato-splenomegaly and ascites are not usually prominent.
- Infection.
- Nausea ± vomiting.
- ↑ BP.
- Foetor hepaticus (sweet smell on the breath).

## Causes
### In previously healthy patients
- Viral hepatitis
- Weil's disease
- Paracetamol overdose
- Halothane
- Idiosyncratic drug reactions
- Fungal/plant toxins
- Malignant infiltration

- Chemical exposure (e.g. carbon tetrachloride)
- Heatstroke
- Budd–Chiari syndrome
- Pregnancy
- Wilson's disease
- Reye's syndrome.

### In patients with chronic liver disease
- Infection
- GI bleeding
- Sedation

- Diuretics and/or electrolyte imbalance
- Alcohol binges
- Constipation.

**Management** Admit as emergency to a hepatologist/gastroenterologist unless an expected terminal event. Prognosis is poor (<60% survive).

**Cirrhosis** The liver is replaced by fibrotic tissue and regenerating nodules of hepatocytes.

## Causes
- Unknown (30%)
- Alcohol (25%)
- Viral hepatitis
- Primary biliary cirrhosis
- Haemachromatosis

- Wilson's disease
- Budd–Chiari syndrome
- Chronic active hepatitis
- $\alpha_1$-antitrypsin deficiency.

**Presentation** Variable. May be an incidental finding. *Symptoms/signs:*
- Hepatomegaly (though liver becomes small and hard in late stages)
- Spider naevi
- Dupuytren's contracture
- Palmar erythema

- Gynaecomastia
- Testicular atrophy
- Clubbing
- Xantholasma/xanthomata
- Portal hypertension
- Splenomegaly.

*Late signs* Occur when the liver can no longer compensate for the damage to it—jaundice, hepatic encephalopathy, leuconychia, and oedema (due to hypoalbuminaemia).

## Investigation
- *Blood* FBC, LFTs (may be normal until late stages), GGT, U&E, Cr, eGFR, hepatitis screen (📖 p.429)
- *Liver USS*

## Management
- Refer to gastroenterology/hepatology for expert advice.
- Treat the cause where possible.
- Avoid alcohol and refer to dietician for advice on nutrition.
- Pruritus 2° to jaundice may respond to colestyramine.
- Give influenza and pneumococcal vaccination.

## Complications
- Portal hypertension (± bleeding oesophageal varices)
- Encephalopathy
- Hepatocellular carcinoma
- Ascites (bacterial peritonitis complicates 1:4 cases—consider prophylaxis with ciprofloxacin)
- Renal failure

*Prognosis* Very variable. Half survive 5y.

$\alpha_1$—antitrypsin deficiency Autosomal recessive disorder. Defective $\alpha_1$-antitrypsin production → lung, and more rarely liver damage. Treatment with IV $\alpha_1$-antitrypsin ↓ progression of COPD. Paracetamol may protect the liver. Encourage use for minor illness. Liver transplantation may eventually be needed.

**Portal hypertension** Portal venous pressure is raised due to obstruction of the portal system before, within, or after the liver. In Western countries the most common cause is cirrhosis.
- Elevated portal venous pressure → collaterals between the portal and systemic circulation (including oesophageal varices). Usually presents with haematemesis and/or melaena from bleeding varices.
- Ascites develops if there is coexistent liver failure with hypoproteinaemia and hyperaldosteronism.
- Splenomegaly is common → thrombocytopenia and leucopenia.
- *Signs:* splenomegaly (80–90%); ascites; dilated veins around the umbilicus (rare); purpura; signs of chronic liver disease (jaundice, clubbing, spider naevi, palmar erythema, gynaecomastia, testicular atrophy; encephalopathy).
- Refer to gastroenterology/hepatology. Specialist management is essential. If GI bleeding, refer as a 'blue-light' emergency.

## Information and support for patients
**British Liver Trust** ☎ 0800 652 7330 🖳 www.britishlivertrust.org.uk
**Alpha-1** Support for patients with $\alpha_1$-antitrypsin deficiency
🖳 www.alpha-1.org.uk

# Other liver disease

**Fatty liver** Reversible condition affecting up to 1:4 adults in the UK. Large vacuoles of triglyceride accumulate in liver cells.

## Presentation

- Usually asymptomatic. >50% present as a result of investigation for abnormal LFTs (📖 p.428). Characteristic 'bright' appearance on liver USS.
- Less frequently presents with a smoothly enlarged liver or symptoms—nausea, vomiting, abdominal pain, fat embolus (may be fatal).

Broadly divides into 2 forms:

### Alcohol-associated fatty liver disease

- Defined as fatty liver disease with daily ethanol consumption >20g (♀) or 30g (♂).
- Typically serum AST and ALT ↑, but serum AST > serum ALT.
- GGT may be ↑ and Alk phos may also be ↑ but usually <2× upper limit of normal.
- Predisposes to alcoholic hepatitis and cirrhosis (irreversible).
- Abstinence from alcohol results in resolution.

### Non-alcoholic fatty liver disease (NAFLD)

- Associated with obesity (present in 35% of obese patients), insulin resistance, and metabolic syndrome (📖 p.353).
- Typically serum AST and ALT ↑ but serum ALT>serum AST.
- GGT may be ↑ and Alk phos may also be ↑ but usually <2× upper limit of normal.
- More severe disease results in non-alcoholic steato-hepatitis (NASH) and is thought to be one of the major causes of cryptogenic cirrhosis—liver failure is uncommon.
- A high proportion of patients develop DM long term.
- Treatment is with weight ↓, metformin, and/or thiazolidinediones.
- Treatment with statins is ineffective.

### Other rarer causes of fatty liver disease

- Drugs, e.g. amiodarone, tamoxifen, valproate
- Pregnancy (📖 p.821)
- Malnutrition
- Inflammatory bowel disease.

**Gilbert's syndrome** Inherited metabolic disorder causing unconjugated hyperbilirubinaemia. *Prevalence:* ~1–2%. Onset is shortly after birth, but the condition may go unnoticed for years. Jaundice occurs during intercurrent illness. ↑ bilirubin on fasting can confirm the diagnosis. Liver biopsy is normal. No treatment is required and prognosis is excellent.
*N. A. Gilbert (1858–1927)—French physician.*

**Benign tumours** Hepatomegaly ± RUQ pain or an incidental finding.

**Common types** Hepatic adenoma, fibroma, leiomyoma, lipoma, haemangioma, focal nodular hyperplasia (e.g. with cirrhosis).

**Management** Refer to gastroenterology to exclude malignancy and confirm diagnosis. Urgency depends on clinical picture and findings on USS.

**Hepatocellular cancer (HCC)** Rare in the UK (100 new cases and 100 deaths/y). Much more common in areas of the world where hepatitis B is endemic (e.g. China, India). Usually arises from regenerating nodules in a cirrhotic liver. *Peak age:* 60–70y. Intra- and extra-hepatic spread is common and occurs early.

**Presentation** In a patient with known cirrhosis:
- Fatigue
- Fever
- Anorexia and/or weight ↓
- Ascites
- Rapid deterioration in liver function
- Haemorrhage into the peritoneal cavity (often fatal)
- Budd–Chiari syndrome (occlusion of the hepatic vein resulting in jaundice, epigastric pain and shock)
- Examination may reveal an abdominal mass, hepatomegaly ± an arterial bruit over the tumour.

**Management** If suspected check αFP and refer for urgent assessment. αFP >500ng/mL in a patient with known cirrhosis is almost certainly diagnostic. The most important prognostic factors are the number and size of the liver lesions and the presence of vascular involvement. 95% of patients with cirrhosis have disease too extensive for curative surgery, or their severely compromised liver function makes radical surgery inappropriate. 50% of patients without cirrhosis have resectable tumours. Surgery may be combined with liver transplantation. Inoperable tumours may be treated with hepatic artery ligation or embolization. Tumours respond poorly to chemo- or radiotherapy.

**Overall prognosis** Patients with cirrhosis—median survival 3mo; patients without cirrhosis—median survival 1y.

**Cholangiocarcinoma** Rare adenocarcinoma of the biliary tract. May be associated with UC. Typically presents in patients >60y with jaundice, RUQ pain, and weight loss. The only effective treatment is surgery, which is only possible in ~10–20% of patients. Selected fit patients with unresectable disease may be offered palliative chemotherapy or enrolment in a clinical trial. Median survival 4–6 mo.

**Secondary tumours** The most common type of liver tumour—usually signalling late disease. *Presentation:* hard enlarged knobbly liver ± RUQ pain ± jaundice (late). If found and no history of malignancy refer to oncology/general surgery for urgent referral to find the primary.

*1° tumours commonly metastasizing to the liver* Lung, breast, large bowel, stomach, uterus, pancreas, carcinoid, lympoma, leukaemia.

### Advice and support for patients
**Cancer Research UK** ☎ 0800 226 237 🖥 www.cancerhelp.org.uk
**Macmillan Cancer Support** ☎ 0808 808 000 🖥 www.macmillan.org.uk
**British Liver Trust** ☎ 0800 652 7330 🖥 www.britishlivertrust.org.uk

# Gall bladder disease

**Gallstones** Gallstones are increasingly common. 9% of 60y olds have them and prevalence ↑ with age.

## Other risk factors
- Gender (♀ > ♂).
- Body weight—prevalence ↑ with weight; also associated with rapid weight ↓
- Race—in the USA, Native American > Hispanic > White > Black.
- Affluence.
- Pregnancy (and possibly HRT but not COC pill).
- Alcohol is protective.
- Diet—vegetarian diet is protective.

## Associated conditions
- Haemolysis
- DM
- Hypertriglyceridaemia
- Cirrhosis
- Crohn's disease
- Partial gastrectomy.

**Drugs which cause gallstones** Clofibrate (and other fibric acid derivatives); octreotide (somatostatin analogue).

**Presentation** Gallstones are blamed for many digestive symptoms—they are probably innocent in most cases. 70% of stones in the gall bladder do not cause symptoms. Common presentations—Table 13.18.

## Management of gallstones
- Advise the patient to stick to a low fat diet.
- Refer for surgical review ± further evaluation (e.g. endoscopic retrograde cholangiopancreatography (ERCP)).
- Gallstones can be removed by cholecystectomy (laparoscopic or open) or ERCP, or can be dissolved with ursodeoxycholic acid (stones < 5mm diameter—40% recur in <5y) or shattered with lithotripsy (1:3 develop biliary colic afterwards).
- Persistent digestive symptoms after surgery are common (50% after cholecystectomy) and difficult to treat.

**Gall bladder cancer** Rare. ♀ > ♂. Gallstones are a predisposing factor. Typically presents in patients >40y with RUQ pain, anorexia, weight ↓, and jaundice. Surgical resection offers the only hope of cure but disease is usually advanced at presentation. Selected fit patients with unresectable disease may be offered palliative chemotherapy or enrolment in a clinical trial. Prognosis is poor.

## Information and support for patients
**British Liver Trust** ☎ 0800 652 7330 🖥 www.britishlivertrust.org.uk

**Table 13.18** Presentation and management of gallstone disease

| | Presentation | Management |
|---|---|---|
| Biliary colic | Clear-cut attacks of severe upper abdominal pain which may radiate → back/ shoulder tip, lasting ≥30min and causing restlessness ± jaundice ± nausea or vomiting *Examination*: Tenderness ± guarding in the RUQ (↑ on deep inspiration—Murphy's sign) | *Treat* acute attacks with pethidine (50mg IM/PO) or diclofenac (50–100mg IM/PO/ PR) + prochlorperazine 12.5mg IM or domperidone 10mg PO/PR for nausea *Admit if* uncertain of diagnosis, inadequate social support, persistent symptoms despite analgesia, suspicion of complications, and/or concomitant medical problems (e.g. dehydration, pregnant, DM, Addison's disease) *Investigate* for gallstones with abdominal USS to prove diagnosis when the episode has settled *Differential diagnosis*: Any cause of acute abdomen *Treat* gallstones to prevent recurrence |
| Acute cholecystitis/ cholangitis | Pain and tenderness in RUQ/epigastrium ± vomiting *Examination*: Tenderness ± guarding in the RUQ ± fever + jaundice | *Treatment*: Broad-spectrum antibiotic (e.g. ciprofloxacin) and analgesia as for biliary colic *Admit if* generalized peritonism, diagnosis uncertain, very toxic, concomitant medical problems (e.g. dehydration, DM, Addison's disease, pregnancy), inadequate social support, or not responding to medication *Empyema* occurs when the obstructed gall bladder fills with pus. Presents with persistent swinging fever and pain. Usually requires cholecystectomy ± surgical drainage *Investigate* and follow up to prevent recurrence as for biliary colic |
| Pancreatitis | 📖 p.438 | 📖 p.438 |
| Gallstone ileus | Occurs usually after an attack of cholecystitis. A stone perforates from the gall bladder into the duodenum and impacts in the terminal ileum causing bowel obstruction | 📖 p.408 |
| Chronic cholecystitis | Vague intermittent abdominal discomfort, nausea, flatulence, and intolerance of fats | *Investigate* for gallstones with abdominal USS to prove the diagnosis *Differential diagnosis*: Reflux, IBS, upper GI tumour, PU *Refer* for treatment of gallstones |
| Jaundice | Obstructive jaundice (📖 p.428) ± RUQ pain | 📖 Table 13.17, p.428 |

# Pancreatitis

**Acute pancreatitis** Premature activation of pancreatic enzymes results in autodigestion and tissue damage. Most episodes are mild and self-limiting, but 1:5 patients have a severe attack. Overall mortality ~5–10%. May be recurrent.

**Causes** In 10% patients no cause is identified.
- **Common causes (80%)** Gallstones, alcohol.
- **Rarer causes**
  - Drugs (e.g. azathioprine)
  - Trauma
  - Pancreatic tumours
  - Post-ERCP
  - Viral infection (mumps, HIV, Coxsackie B)
  - Mycoplasma infection
  - Hypercalcaemia
  - Hyperlipidaemia
  - Pancreas divisum (normal variant in 7–8% of the white population)
  - Familial pancreatitis
  - Vasculitis
  - Ischaemia or embolism
  - Pregnancy
  - End-stage renal failure.

**Presentation**
- Poorly localized, continuous, boring epigastric pain which ↑ over ~1h. Often worse lying down ± radiation to the back (50%).
- Nausea ± vomiting.

**Examination**
- **General** Tachycardia, fever, shock, jaundice.
- **Abdominal** Localized epigastric tenderness or generalized abdominal tenderness; abdominal distension ± ↓ bowel sounds; evidence of retroperitoneal haemorrhage (peri-umbilical and flank bruising—rare).

**Management** Admit as an acute surgical emergency. Prior to transfer give analgesia with pethidine (morphine may induce spasm of the sphincter of Oddi).

**Complications** Delayed complications may present in general practice—suspect if persistent pain or failure to regain weight or appetite. Complications include:
- Pancreatic necrosis
- Pseudocyst—localized collection of pancreatic secretions
- Fistula/abscess formation
- Bleeding or thrombosis.

**Prevention of further attacks**
- Avoid factors that may have caused pancreatitis, e.g. alcohol, drugs.
- Advise patients to follow a low-fat diet.
- Treat reversible causes, e.g. hyperlipidaemia, gallstones.

**Chronic pancreatitis** Chronic inflammation of the pancreas results in gradual destruction and fibrosis of the gland ± loss of pancreatic function → malabsorption and DM.

**Cause** Alcohol is responsible for most cases. *More rarely*: familial; CF; haemochromatosis; pancreatic duct obstruction (gallstones/pancreatic cancer); hyperparathyroidism.

### Presentation
- Constant or episodic epigastric pain radiating to the back and relieved by sitting forwards.
- Vomiting
- Weakness
- Jaundice
- Steatorrhoea
- Weight ↓
- DM
- Chronic poor health.

**Management** Refer to gastroenterology. *Treatment:*
- *Diet* Low-fat, high-protein, high-calorie diet with fat-soluble vitamin supplements. Refer to dietician.
- *Pancreatic enzyme supplementation* e.g. Creon® capsules before meals. May improve diarrhoea.
- Alcohol abstinence
- *Pain control* Provide analgesia—beware of opioid abuse. Consider referral for coeliac plexus block.
- *Surgery* Pancreatectomy or pancreaticojejunostomy for pancreatic duct stricture, obstructive jaundice, unremitting pain, or weight loss.
- *Diabetes management*

**Pancreatic Insufficiency** Global ↓ function of the pancreas. *Causes:*
- *Child*—cystic fibrosis
- *Adult*—chronic pancreatitis, pancreatic tumour, pancreatectomy, total gastrectomy.

**Presentation** Malabsorption (frequent loose odorous stools ± abdominal pain), weight loss or failure to thrive, DM.

**Management** Take specialist advice. Treat the underlying cause. Treat associated DM. Suppplement digestive enzymes (e.g. with Creon®).

# Pancreatic tumours

Pancreatic cancer accounts for 3% of all malignancies causing 7000 deaths/y in the UK. 80% of cases occur in patients >60y ♂ > ♀ (3:2).

## Risk factors
- Smoking causes 25–30% of pancreatic cancers in the UK. Risk returns to non-smoker levels 10–20y after cessation.
- Chronic pancreatitis—usually related to excess alcohol.
- Type 2 (non-insulin-dependent) DM—relative risk ~1.8.
- Obesity—↑ risk by 19%.
- Genetic—5% of pancreatic cancers are hereditary. Characterized by presentation aged <30y and +ve FH.
- Occupation—cancer is ↑ among nickel workers and among workers exposed to insecticides, radiation, lead, iron, or chromium.

## Tumour characteristics
- The majority of pancreatic tumours develop in the exocrine part of the gland. 95% of tumours are adenocarcinomas. Rarely, tumours develop from the endocrine part—these have better prognosis.
- 75% arise in the head of the pancreas, 15% from the body, and 10% from the tail. Tumours arising in the head of the pancreas tend to present earlier and are easier to remove.
- Spread to local LNs occurs early, and metastatic spread to the peritoneum, liver and lungs is frequently found at presentation.

## Presentation Non-specific with:
- Gradual deterioration in health or fatigue.
- Anorexia or weight ↓.
- Pain—epigastric ± radiation → back. May be relieved by sitting forward.
- Diarrhoea/steatorrhoea due to malabsorption.
- Early satiety, dyspepsia, or nausea/vomiting (gastric outlet obstruction).
- Obstructive jaundice.
- Pancreatitis.
- New DM.
- Spontaneous venous thrombosis.

## Examination
Check for weight ↓, epigastric or left upper quadrant mass, hepatomegaly, jaundice. If jaundice is present, the gall bladder may be palpable as a small rounded mass beneath the liver.

## Management
Refer for urgent surgical assessment. Diagnosis is confirmed using a combination of USS, CT, MRI, and/or ERCP. The only potentially curative treatment for pancreatic cancer is surgery, but <15% of patients are suitable for surgery at presentation. The operation of choice is Whipple's procedure (pancreaticoduodenectomy). Surgery is associated with significant morbidity; mortality 5–15%.

## Prognosis
Those undergoing surgical resection have 5y survival of 7–25% (median survival 11–20mo), but those who survive 5y are likely to survive long term. Median survival for those with irresectable locally advanced disease is 6–11mo, and 2–6mo if metastatic disease.

**Palliative treatment** Patients with locally advanced/metastatic disease may benefit from surgical bypass of common bile duct and/or duodenal obstruction. An alternative is a biliary stent. Chemotherapy may give some survival benefit. Refer for palliative care support early.

**Endocrine tumours** In all cases specialist management is required.

*Glucagonoma* Islet cell tumour of the pancreas. Most are malignant and 90% have liver or LN metastases at presentation. 5–20% of tumours occur as part of multiple endocrine neoplasia (MEN-I) syndrome. *Presents with*:
• Attacks of hyperglycaemia (DM in >50%).
• Skin changes—sore mouth, necrolytic migratory erythema (70%—rash which starts as an erythematous rash then blisters before crusting).

• Weight ↓/cachexia (60%).
• Tendency to venous thrombosis (11%).

• Anaemia.
• Diarrhoea.
• Depression/psychosis.

*Insulinoma* Tumour of the APUD cells of the islets of Langerhans. >90% are benign. 7–8% are associated with MEN-I syndrome. Presents with episodes of hypoglycaemia, especially when exercising or fasting. ↑ appetite and frequent food intake to avoid hypoglycaemia often results in substantial weight gain.

*Somatostatinoma* Uncommon islet cell tumour. Most are large tumours (>5cm) in the head/body of the pancreas. Presents with gallstones, steatorrhoea, and DM.

❶ Extrapancreatic somatostatinomas can present in association with neurofibromatosis type I and phaeochromocytoma.

*Verner–Morrison syndrome* An intestinal vasointestinal peptide (VIP) producing tumour results in profuse watery diarrhoea → dehydration, metabolic acidosis, and ↓K⁺. Also associated with insulin resistance and impaired glucose tolerance. VIPomas account for <10% of islet cell tumours. 60% are malignant.
J.V. Verner (b.1927)—American physician; A.B. Morrison (b.1922)— American pathologist.

### Advice and support for patients
**Cancer Research UK** ☎ 0800 226 237 🖳 www.cancerhelp.org.uk
**Macmillan Cancer Support** ☎ 0808 808 0000
🖳 www.macmillan.org.uk

# Renal medicine and urology

# Creatinine, urea, and electrolytes

**Serum creatinine** Commonly ordered test to detect renal dysfunction. Rough guide to glomerular filtration rate (GFR) when corrected for age, gender, and weight—↓ in GFR is associated with ↑ in serum creatinine. Causes of an abnormal serum creatinine—Table 14.1.

**Estimated glomerular filtration rate (eGFR)** More sensitive measure than serum creatinine to assess renal function. *Calculated from:*
- Serum creatinine
- Age
- Gender, *and*
- Ethnicity—people of African Caribbean origin tend to have ↑ muscle mass so their eGFR must be multiplied by 1.21.

Changes in eGFR can be used to monitor changes in kidney function:
- Normal eGFR is >90mL/min/1.73m$^2$
- eGFR 60–90 does not indicate CKD unless additional markers of damage are present—persistent microalbuminuria, persistent proteinuria, persistent microscopic haematuria, or structural abnormality (e.g. polycystic kidneys)
- eGFR <60 indicates CKD (📖 p.448).

>  Renal function ↓ with age (approx 1mL/min/y >40y). Many elderly patients have a GFR <60mL/min which, because of ↓ muscle mass, may not be indicated by a ↑ serum creatinine. Measuring eGFR gives a better indication of renal function.

**Urea** Commonly ordered test to detect renal dysfunction. While ↓ GFR is associated with ↑ serum urea, serum urea may also vary independently of the GFR. Causes of abnormal serum urea—Table 14.1.

## Potassium

**Hyperkalaemia** High serum potassium (>5mmol/L). *Causes:* Table 14.2. Treat the cause.

⚠ Plasma potassium >6.5mmol/L needs urgent treatment.
- Check it is not an artefact, e.g. due to haemolysis inside the bottle.
- Admit for investigation of cause and treatment.

**ECG changes associated with hyperkalaemia** Tall tented T-waves; small P-wave; wide QRS complex becoming sinusoidal; VF.

**Hypokalaemia** Low serum potassium (<3.5mmol/L). Presents with muscle weakness, hypotonia, cardiac arrhythmias, cramps, and tetany. *Causes:* Table 14.2. If K$^+$ >2.5mmol/L and no symptoms, give oral potassium supplement. ❶ If the patient is taking a thiazide diuretic, hypokalaemia >3.0mmol/L rarely needs treating.

⚠ Plasma potassium <2.5mmol/L needs urgent treatment—admit.

**ECG changes associated with hypokalaemia** Small/inverted T-waves; prominent U-wave; prolonged P–R interval; depressed ST segment.

## Sodium

**Hyponatraemia** Low serum sodium (<135 mmol/L). Rarely symptomatic in general practice. May present with signs of water excess—confusion, fits, ↑BP, cardiac failure, oedema, anorexia, nausea, muscle weakness. *Causes*: Table 14.2. *Management*: treat the cause. If unwell admit for investigation.

**Hypernatraemia** Excess serum sodium (>145 mmol/L). Rare in general practice. *Presentation*: thirst, confusion, coma, fits, signs of dehydration—dry skin, ↓ skin turgor, postural hypotension, and oliguria if water deficient. *Causes*: Table 14.2. *Management*: admit for investigation.

**Table 14.1** Causes of an altered serum creatinine and urea

| ↑ creatinine (>150µmol/L) | ↓ creatinine (<70µmol/L) | ↑ urea (>6.7mmol/L) | ↓ urea (< 2.5mmol/L) |
|---|---|---|---|
| Renal disease/ renal failure | Muscular dystrophy (late stage) | Renal failure | Liver disease (↓ urea production) |
| Drugs, e.g. trimethoprim, probenecid, cimetidine, potassium-sparing diuretics | Myasthenia gravis | GI bleeding | Anabolic state |
| | | High-protein diet | High ADH levels (high GFR) |
| | | Drugs: high-dose steroids, tetra-cycline | Starvation or low protein diet |
| Large muscle bulk | | Dehydration | Pregnancy |
| Muscle breakdown, e.g. muscular dystrophy | | | |

**Table 14.2** Causes of altered serum electrolytes

| ↑ potassium (>5mmol/L) | ↓ potassium (<3.5mmol/L) | ↑ sodium (>145mmol/L) | ↓ sodium (<135mmol/L) |
|---|---|---|---|
| Renal failure | Diuretics | Fluid loss without water replacement (e.g. diarrhoea, vomiting, burns) | Diuretic excess—especially thiazides |
| Drugs, e.g. ACE inhibitors: excess K⁺ therapy; K⁺-sparing diuretics | Cushing's syndrome/steroids | Diabetes insipidus—suspect if large urine volume | Renal failure or nephrotic syndrome |
| Addison's disease | Vomiting and/or diarrhoea | Osmotic diuresis | Diarrhoea/vomiting |
| Metabolic acidosis (DM) | Conn's syndrome | Primary aldo-steronism: suspect if ↑BP, ↓K⁺, alkalosis | Fistula |
| Artefact (haemolysed sample) | Villous adenoma of the rectum | | Rectal villous adenoma |
| | Purgative or liquorice abuse | | Small bowel obstruction |
| | Intestinal fistula | | CF (p.338) |
| | Renal tubular failure | | Heat exposure. |
| | Hypokalaemic periodic paralysis—intermittent weakness lasting <72h | | SIADH (p.379) |
| | | | Water overload (e.g. polydipsia) |
| | | | Severe hypothyroidism |
| | | | Addison's disease |
| | | | Glucocorticoid deficiency |
| | | | Cardiac failure |
| | | | Cirrhosis |

# Presentation of renal disease

Renal disease may present to the GP with:
- Haematuria (📖 p.454) or proteinuria
- UTI/pyelonephritis (📖 p.456)
- Outflow tract obstruction (📖 p.462)
- Nephrotic syndrome (below)
- Nephritic syndrome (📖 p.447)
- Renal failure (📖 p.448)
- Hypertension (📖 p.252).

**Proteinuria** Normally detected with urine dipstick If +ve, repeat with another sample to exclude spurious results, and send sample for M,C&S to exclude UTI. Treat the cause where necessary. *Causes:*
- UTI
- Vaginal mucus
- DM
- ↑ BP
- Glomerulonephritis
- Pyrexia
- Pregnancy (and PET)
- Postural proteinuria—2–5% adolescents; rare >30y
- Haemolytic–uraemic syndrome
- CCF
- SLE
- Myeloma
- Drugs, e.g. gold, penicillamine
- Amyloid.

**Microalbuminuria** Albuminuria in the range 30–200mg/L. Not detectable with standard urine dipsticks. Special sticks are available for routine screening of high risk groups e.g. diabetics. *Causes:*
- *DM:* Microalbuminuria precedes frank proteinuria (📖 p.364)
- *Arteriopathy:* Microalbuminuria may be present in patients with CCF or ↑ BP. Presence of Microalbuminuria predicts ↑ risk of MI, CVA, CCF, and cardiovascular and all-cause mortality.
- *Other chronic illness:* Malignancy, COPD.
- *Acute illness:* Inflammatory bowel disease, MI, acute pancreatitis, trauma, burns, meningitis.

**Haematuria** 📖 p.454

**Glycosuria** 📖 p.352

**Nephrotic syndrome** Proteinuria >3g/24h, hypoalbuminaemia, and oedema. Often associated with ↑ cholesterol. *Causes:*
- Minimal change GN (90% children, 30% adults)
- Membranous GN
- Focal segmental glomerulosclerosis
- Membranoproliferative GN
- DM
- Amyloid
- Neoplasia
- Endocarditis
- PAN
- SLE
- Sickle cell disease
- Malaria
- Drugs (penicillamine, gold)

**Presentation** Swelling of eyelids and face; ascites, peripheral oedema, urine froth due to protein. *Nephrotic crisis:* unwell with oedema, anorexia, vomiting, pleural effusions, and muscle wasting.

**Investigation** Urine: total protein:creatinine ratio (TPCR) (24h protein and creatinine collections are no longer needed), microscopy for red cells, casts. *Blood:* U&E, creatinine, eGFR, albumin, cholesterol, FBC, ESR.

**Management** Refer all suspected cases of nephrotic syndrome to a renal physician. *Complications include:*
- Thromboembolism.
- Hypercholesterolaemia.
- Infection, especially pneumococcal—if persistent nephrotic syndrome offer vaccination.
- Hypovolaemia and renal failure.
- Loss of specific proteins e.g. transferrin (causes hypochromic anaemia which is iron resistant).

**Nephritic syndrome** Central feature is blood and protein in the urine from glomerular inflammation.
- **Causes** Glomerulonephritis (may occur after throat, ear, or skin infection with group A β-haemolytic streptococci), vasculitis.
- **Features** Oliguria, haematuria, proteinuria, fluid retention, ↑ BP, uraemia, and ↑ creatinine.
- **Management** Refer suspected cases immediately to a renal physician.
- **Risks** Hypertensive encephalopathy, pulmonary oedema, ARF.
- **Prognosis** Excellent in children; in adults some proteinuria/urine sediment may persist. CKD is rare.

**Nephrocalcinosis** Deposition of $Ca^{2+}$ in kidneys. X-ray: calcification. May cause symptoms of UTI or renal stones. *Cause:*
- **Medullary (95%)** Hyperparathyroidism, distal renal tubular acidosis, medullary sponge kidney, idiopathic calciuria, papillary necrosis, oxalosis.
- **Cortical** Serious renal disease or chronic GN.

**Pyelonephritis/UTI** 📖 p.456          **Hypertension** 📖 p.252

**Strangury** Distressing desire to pass something per urethra that will not pass, e.g. stone

**Table 14.3** Presentation of renal disease

| | GN | Interstitial disease | | | Vascular disease | | | Outflow tract obstruction |
| | | AIN | ATN | CIN | Small | Large | RVT | |
|---|---|---|---|---|---|---|---|---|
| Nephrotic syndrome | ++ | 0 | 0 | 0 | (+) | 0 | +* | 0 |
| Nephritic syndrome | ++ | (+) | 0 | 0 | (+) | 0 | + | 0 |
| Acute renal failure | + | + | ++** | 0 | + | + | (+) | ++ |
| Chronic renal failure | ++ | (+) | 0 | ++ | (+) | + | 0 | ++ |
| Pyelonephritis/UTI | 0 | 0 | 0 | 0 | 0 | 0 | + | + |
| Hypertension | (+) | (+) | 0 | (+) | (+) | (+) | 0 | + |

GN = glomerulonephritis (📖 p.450)        RVT = renal vein thrombosis (📖 p.451)
CIN = chronic interstitial nephritis (📖 p.450)    ATN = acute tubular necrosis
AIN = acute interstitial nephritis (📖 p.450)
*Renal vein thrombosis is a complication not a cause of nephrotic syndrome.
**Acute tubular necrosis is the most common cause of acute renal failure

**Patient support and information**
**UK National Kidney Federation** ☎ 0845 601 0209
🖥 www.kidney.org.uk

# Renal failure

**Oliguria** Urine output <400mL/24h. *Causes*: dehydration, cardiac failure, ureteric obstruction, renal failure.

**Acute kidney injury (AKI)** Also known as acute renal failure (ARF). ↓ renal function over hours/days ± oliguria/anuria. Refer immediately if acute ↑ in urea/ creatinine *or* ↓ in eGFR (to <60mL/min if normal in last 3mo, or ↓ of >15% over 5d) *Causes*: acute tubular necrosis (80%—due to acute circulatory compromise); renal tract obstruction (5%); GN.

**Chronic kidney disease (CKD)[N]** Also known as chronic renal failure (CRF). Slow ↓ renal function over months/years. *Causes*:

- DM
- ↑ BP
- Urinary tract obstruction
- Chronic pyelonephritis
- SLE
- ↑ $Ca^{2+}$
- Polycystic kidneys
- Glomerulonephritis
- Renovascular disease
- Interstitial nephritis
- Amyloid
- Myeloma
- PAN.

## Presentation

- *History* FH (polycystic kidneys); UTI; drugs (especially analgesics).
- *Symptoms* Often no symptoms. Nausea, anorexia, lethargy, itch, nocturia, impotence. *Later*: oedema, dyspnoea, chest pain (from pericarditis), vomiting, confusion, fits, hiccups, neuropathy, coma.
- *Signs* Pallor, 'lemon tinge' to skin, pulmonary/peripheral oedema, pericarditis, pleural effusions, metabolic flap, ↑ BP, retinopathy.

## Investigation

- *Urine* M,C&S, microalbuminuria, albumin: creatinine ratio (ACR) or TPCR, RBCs, glucose.
- *Blood* U&E, creatinine, eGFR, glucose, $Ca^{2+}$, $PO_4^{2-}$ urate, protein, FBC, ESR, serum electrophoresis. Classification—Table 14.4.
- *Renal tract USS* If progressive or advanced (stage 4/5) disease, refractory ↑ BP, haematuria, or palpable bladder/lower urinary tract signs.

## Management

- Treat reversible causes. Stop/avoid nephrotoxic drugs (e.g. NSAIDs). Consider ↓ dose of other drugs as excretion/metabolism may be impaired. ❶ Metformin should be stopped if eGFR <30mL/min.
- Monitor Cr/eGFR and dipstick urine (Table 14.4). If proteinuria, send urine for M,C&S. If no infection but proteinuria persists, test TPCR or ACR in early morning urine. If TPCR >100mg/mmol, or ACR >70mg/mmol, refer.
- Manage CVD risk. Monitor/treat ↑ cholesterol and ↑ BP (target 130/80—ACE/ARB as first-line agent). Treat DM. Smoking cessation.
- Monitor and treat anaemia and renal bone disease.

❶ If sudden ↓ in renal function (↓ eGFR of >15% between tests or >5mL/min/1.73m³ in <1y or >10mL/min/1.73m³ in <5y) suspect infection, dehydration, uncontrolled ↑ BP, metabolic disturbance (e.g. ↑ $Ca^{2+}$), obstruction, nephrotoxins (e.g. drugs). If unable to find cause, or treatment does not ↑ renal function, refer.

*Refer* to a renal physician if:
- Stage 4/5 CKD.
- Significant proteinuria (TPCR >100mg/mmol or ACR >70mg/mmol).
- Sudden ↓ in eGFR (>15%) and UTI excluded.

- Persistent microscopic haematuria and <50y (to urologist if >50y).
- Functional consequences of CKD i.e. anaemia (<11g/dL), bone disease, or refractory hypertension (>140/90mmHg on 4 agents).

**End-stage renal disease (ESRD)** 80 new patients/million population/y. Irreversible. Dialysis starts when GFR is 10–15% normal. Dialysis is needed lifelong unless a kidney transplant becomes available. Refer back to the renal unit managing the patient if you have any problems.

*Haemodialysis* Blood flows opposite dialysis fluid and substances are cleared along a concentration gradient across a semi-permeable membrane. *Problems:* pulmonary oedema; infection (HIV, hepatitis, bacteria); U&E imbalance; BP↓ or ↑; problems with vascular access; dialysis arthropathy (especially shoulders and wrists); aluminium toxicity; expense.

*Continuous ambulatory peritoneal dialysis (CAPD)* A permanent catheter is inserted into the peritoneum via a subcutaneous tunnel. ~2L dialysis fluid is introduced and kept in the peritoneum. This is changed for fresh fluid up to 5x/d at home. Does not tie the patient to a dialysis machine. *Problems:* peritonitis; catheter blockage (refer as an emergency); weight ↑; poor DM control; pleural effusion; leakage.

*Anaemia and erythropoietin* 2° anaemia due to ↓ kidney erythropoietin production is universal amongst people with ESRD. Exclude other causes. Recombinant erythropoietin is given if Hb<10.5g/dL (75%).

**Renal transplantation** Transplanted kidneys are usually sited in an iliac fossa. Median cadaveric graft survival ~8y. Closer genetic matches have better survival rates. *Problems:*

- Rejection
- Persistent ↑BP and ↑ cholesterol
- Atherosclerosis (5x ↑ risk MI death)
- Renal artery stenosis at 3–9mo post-op
- Obstruction at ureteric anastamosis
- Ciclosporin-induced nephropathy
- Infection due to immunosuppression
- Malignancy from immunosuppressants.

**Table 14.4** Classification of chronic kidney disease

| Stage | GFR mL/min | Description | Prevalence | Complications | Testing frequency |
|---|---|---|---|---|---|
| 1 | >90 | Kidney damage with normal or ↑ GFR | 3.3% | ↑ BP | Yearly |
| 2 | 60–89 | Kidney damage with mild ↓ GFR | 3% | ↑ BP | Yearly |
| 3A 3B | 45–59 30–45 | Moderate ↓ GFR | 4.3% | ↑ BP, $Ca^{2+}$ & $PO_4^{2-}$ changes, renal anaemia, LVF | 6mo |
| 4 | 15–29 | Severe ↓ GFR | 0.2% | As above + ↑ $K^+$ | 3–6mo |
| 5 | <15 | Established renal failure | 0.2% | As above + salt/ water retention | 6wk |

**Further information**
**BMA** CKD: frequently asked questions (2007) ▯ www.bma.org
**NICE** CKD (2008) ▯ www.nice.org.uk

# Kidney diseases

**Interstitial nephritis** Important cause of renal failure. Associated with inflammatory cell infiltration of the renal interstitium/tubules. Causes:
- *Acute interstitial nephritis* Idiosyncratic reaction to drugs (penicillin, NSAIDs, furosemide) or infection (*Staphylococcus, Streptococcus*).
- *Chronic interstitial nephritis* Idiopathic (most), drugs, sickle cell disease, analgesic nephropathy.

*Presentation and prognosis* Presents with AKI/CKD, raised temperature, arthralgia, eosinophilia. Patients with AKI have good prognosis. Those with CKD have gradual deterioration over time.

**Diabetic nephropathy** 📖 p.364

**Analgesic nephropathy** Caused by prolonged heavy use of analgesics (including NSAIDs). Presents with an interstitial nephritis-like picture. Associated with ↑ incidence UTI. Carcinoma of renal pelvis is a rare complication. Investigate promptly if the patient develops haematuria.

**Glomerulonephritis** Types and presentation (Table 14.5). Refer all suspected cases urgently to a renal physician.

*Terminology* Focal—some glomeruli affected; diffuse—all glomeruli affected; segmental—part of each glomerulus affected; global—all of each glomerulus affected.

**Chronic pyelonephritis** Presents as CKD or one of its complications. Probably arises from UTIs, vesico-ureteric reflux and consequent renal scarring in childhood (📖 p.876). Refer to a renal physician.

**Table 14.5** Types of glomerulonephritis

| Type | Features |
|------|----------|
| Minimal change | Most common in children. Presents with nephrotic syndrome |
| Membranous | 30% adult nephrotic syndrome. Underlying malignancy in 10% of adults. 1:3 enter remission, 1:3 are proteinuric, 1:3 progress to ESRD |
| Focal segmental glomerulosclerosis | Proteinuria or nephrotic syndrome. Seen with heroin abuse. >50% progress to CKD |
| Membrano-proliferative | 50% present as nephrotic syndrome. Associations: endocarditis, C3 nephritic factor (autoantibody), hepatitis C, measles |
| Proliferative | Presents with nephritic syndrome. Classically seen 2wk after *Strep.* infection. Prognosis is excellent |
| IgA disease (Berger's disease) | Causes recurrent haematuria in young men. Similar histological picture is seen in Henoch–Schönlein purpura (📖 p.534). 30% progress to ESRD |
| Rapidly progressive/crescentic | Presents with haematuria, oliguria, ↑BP, acute renal failure. Vigorous treatment may preserve renal function. *Causes:* anti-glomerular basement membrane disease (Goodpasture's disease), Wegener's granulomatosis, Henoch–Schönlein purpura |

**Haemolytic uraemic syndrome** Most common cause of AKD in children. Usually follows gastroenteritis. Due to *E. coli* toxin. Have a high index of suspicion in any child with bloody diarrhoea. Occasionally occurs without diarrhoea. *Other features:*

- Dehydration
- Oliguria (though may be polyuria)
- Proteinuria/haematuria
- Haematological features: anaemia, thrombocytopenia ± purpura

- CNS symptoms: irritability, drowsiness, ataxia, coma
- ↑ BP (associated with non-diarrhoeal disease).

**Management** Admit for specialist care—often including dialysis. Mortality in the acute phase is ~15%. If associated with diarrhoeal illness and the child survives the acute phase, >80% make full recovery. Poor prognostic indicators are age >5y. at onset and dialysis for >2wk. Disease in the absence of diarrhoea has poorer prognosis—most progress to CKD.

**Adult polycystic kidney disease** Autosomal dominant disease (1/1000). Cysts develop in the kidney causing gradual ↓ in renal function. Common cause of CKD. Presents with haematuria, UTI, abdominal mass (30% also have cysts in liver/pancreas), lumbar/abdominal pain, and/or ↑ BP. May be associated with mitral valve prolapse and SAH/berry aneurysms. USS shows large kidneys with multiple cysts. Refer to a renal physician if CKD 3–5. Treat infections and ↑ BP. Check family members (though cysts may not be seen <30y). 45% progress to ESRD by 60y.

**Medullary sponge kidney** Developmental abnormality of the medullary pyramids of the kidney, characterized by dilatation of renal collecting tubules. ♂ > ♀. There may be a family history. Most are asymptomatic and the condition is an incidental finding (found on 0.5% IVPs). If symptomatic, presents with UTIs, renal stones, haematuria. Refer if symptomatic. Usually prognosis is very good and most require no treatment.

**Renal vein thrombosis (RVT)** *Causes:* nephrotic syndrome (15–20% develop RVT); membranous GN (30%); acute dehydration. Presentation varies from no symptoms to severe pain and loin tenderness. Suspect in at-risk individuals if unexplained loss of renal function and RBCs in urine. Refer to a renal physician for further investigation.

**Renal artery stenosis** *Causes:* atheroma, fibromuscular hyperplasia (in the young). Presents with ↑ BP (may be severe or drug resistant); vascular disease elsewhere; abdominal bruit; ↑ Cr, ↓ eGFR and proteinuria. If bilateral or extensive, renal failure may be precipitated by dehydration, ↓ BP or drugs (ACE/ARB initiation, NSAIDS). Refer to a renal physician (if diagnosis is unsure) or vascular surgeon (if diagnosis is known).

**Alport's syndrome** X-linked or autosomal disease. Congenital sensorineural deafness, haematuria, proteinuria, and renal failure. Associated with lens abnormalities, platelet dysfunction, ↑ BP. Causes ESRD by 3rd decade in ♂; ♀ rarely develop ESRD. Renal failure does not recur after transplantation. *A.C. Alport (1880–1959)—South African physician.*

**Patient support and information**
**UK National Kidney Federation** ☎ 0845 601 0209 🖳 www.kidney.org.uk

# Renal stones

15% of ♂ and 5% of ♀ will develop a renal stone at some point; peak age 20–50y. Symptoms are not dependent on size of the stone.

## Risk factors

- Family history—↑ risk ×3. *Specific conditions*: X-linked nephrolithiasis, cystinuria, hyperoxaluria.
- Anatomically abnormal kidneys, e.g. horseshore kidney, medullary sponge kidney.
- Metabolic disease, e.g. gout, hypercalcaemia/hypercalciuria, cystinuria, renal tubular acidosis, or other acidosis (ileostomy, adenomatous polyp), oxaluria, aminoaciduria.
- Dehydration.    • Immobilization.    • Chronic UTI.

*Drugs predisposing patients to stone formation* Acetazolamide; allopurinol; aspirin; steroids; indinavir; nelfinavir; loop diuretics; probenecid; quinolones; sulphonamides; theophylline; thiazides; triamterene; antacids; calcium/vitamin D supplements; high-dose vitamin C.

**Presentation** Usually presents with pain ± nausea/vomiting. Location and type of pain gives clues about the site of the stone:

- *Loin pain*—kidney stone    • *Strangury*—bladder stone
- *Renal colic*—ureteric stone    • *Interruption of flow*—urethral stone

## Renal colic

- *Symptoms* Severe pain with waves of ↑ severity. Usually starts abruptly as flank pain which then radiates around the abdomen to the groin as stone progresses down the ureter. May be referred to testis/tip of penis in man or labia majora in women.
- *Signs* Patient is obviously in pain—usually unable to sit still and keeps shifting position to try to get comfortable (in contrast with peritonitis where patients tend to keep still). May be pale and sweaty. May be mild tenderness on deep abdominal palpation or loin tenderness though often minimal signs. If fever suspect infection.

*Other presentations* UTI, haematuria, retention, renal failure (rare).

**Differential diagnosis** Pyelonephritis; ruptured AAA; cholecystitis; pancreatitis; appendicitis; diverticulitis; obstruction; strangulated hernia; testicular torsion; pethidine addiction.

**Immediate investigations** Dipstick urine if possible. Absence of RBCs does not exclude renal colic but consider alternative diagnosis.

**Immediate management** Stones usually pass spontaneously. Give pain relief (diclofenac 75mg IM/100mg PR) ± antiemetic. Consider admission to hospital if:

- Fever    • Pregnant    • Analgesia ineffective/
- Oliguria    • Lives alone    short-lived
- Poor intake of fluid    • Uncertain diagnosis    • Symptoms >24h.

**If not admitted** Encourage ↑ fluid intake; seive urine for stones. Monitor/ review pain relief and for complications.

***Further investigations*** can wait until the next working day and include:
- ***Blood*** U&E; creatinine; eGFR; $Ca^{2+}$; $PO_4^{3-}$; alkaline phosphatase; uric acid; albumin.
- ***Urine*** M,C&S; RBCs. Consider checking 'spot' test for urine cystine, and TPCR, $Ca^{2+}$, $PO_4^{3-}$, uric acid, and sodium excretion.
- ***Radiology*** X-ray of kidneys, ureters, and bladder. 90% of renal stones are radio-opaque—only urate and xanthine stones are radio-transluscent. Renal tract USS ± IVP (if available).

**Follow-up** 50% recur in 5–7y. Give general advice on prevention of stones (Table 14.6). If investigations show any loss of renal function, renal obstruction, or remaining stones—refer to urology. Depending on composition of stones give dietary advice/refer to dietician (Table 14.6).

**Hyperoxaluria** May be 1°(autosomal recessive condition) or 2° to gut resection/malabsorption or dietary excess of spinach or vitamin C. Take specialist advice on management. Two types of 1° hyperoxaluria:
- *Type 1 hyperoxaluria* Calcium oxalate stones are widely distributed throughout the body. Presents as renal stones and nephrocalcinosis in children. 80% have chronic renal failure in <20y.
- *Type 2 hyperoxaluria* More benign but less common—nephrocalcinosis but no chronic renal failure.

**Cystinuria** Most common aminoaciduria. Usually presents with stones at age 10–30y. *Urine:* cystine ↑; ornithine ↑; arginine ↑; lysine ↑. Take specialist advice on management.

**Hypercalcaemia** 📖 p.374

❶ Hypercalciuria may occur without hypercalcaemia and is found in ~80% of patients with calcium oxalate stones.

**Table 14.6** Prevention of renal stones

| Type of stone | Preventative measures |
|---|---|
| All types | ↑ fluid intake (>3L/24h) especially in hot weather; ↓ salt intake |
| Calcium oxalate | Urinary alkalinization with potassium citrate. Avoid chocolate, tea, rhubarb and spinach, nuts, beans, beetroot; ↓citrus fruits. Bendroflumethiazide 2.5mg od may help if hypercalciuria; hyperoxaluria is treated with pyridoxine |
| Calcium phosphate | Low $Ca^{2+}$ diet; avoid vitamin D supplements. Bendroflumethiazide 2.5mg od may help if hypercalciuria |
| Staghorn/triple phosphate (calcium, magnesium and ammonium) | Associated with UTI due to *Proteus* species and urinary stasis, e.g. due to anatomical abnormality. Treat UTI with antibiotics |
| Urate | Allopurinol; urinary alkalinization with potassium citrate (pH >6.5) |
| Cystine | Urinary alkalinization with potassium citrate; d-penicillamine may be used as a chelating agent |

# Haematuria, bladder and renal cancer

**Haematuria** Blood in the urine. *Causes:* Table 14.7.
- May be frank (visible) or microscopic (up to 20% population).
- Investigate *all* cases of haematuria further.
- Check MSU for M,C&S, and blood for U&E, creatinine and eGFR. Free Hb and myoglobin make urine test sticks +ve in absence of red cells.
- Urine discoloration can result from beetroot ingestion, porphyria, or rifampicin.
- If cause is identified (e.g. sample taken when menstruating, UTI), repeat the check for blood in urine once treated/resolved.
- Refer if no cause is found. Rapid access one-stop clinics are now operated in most areas.

**Sterile pyuria** Presence of white cells in the urine in the absence of UTI. *Causes:*

- Inadequately treated UTI
- Appendicitis
- Calculi
- Prostatitis
- Bladder tumour
- Renal TB
- Papillary necrosis
- UTI with failure to culture organism
- Interstitial nephritis or cystitis
- Polycystic kidney
- Chemical cystitis, e.g. due to radiotherapy.

**Management** Initially repeat with clean-catch MSU. If finding persists refer to urology.

**Bladder cancer** *Incidence:* 1:5000; ♂:♀ ≈ 3:1. Transitional cell carcinoma (TCC) is most common in the UK—squamous cell carcinoma (SCC) is most common worldwide. Risk factors:
- Smoking (half male cases are attributable to smoking).
- Aromatic amine exposure (textile or rubber industries).
- Schistosomiasis (SCC).
- Stasis of urine.
- Chronic UTI.

**Presentation** Haematuria—painless or painful. *Less commonly:*
- Recurrent UTI.
- Frequency.
- Loin pain.
- Pelvic pain.
- Bladder outflow obstruction.

**Investigation** MSU—excludes UTI and detects sterile pyuria and/or microscopic haematuria.

**Management** Refer urgently to urology. Most urology departments have one-stop haematuria clinics offering rapid out-patient assessment of haematuria. Treatment depends on stage at diagnosis (Table 14.8).

## Wilm's nephroblastoma 📖 p.904

**Hypernephroma** Clear cell adenocarcinoma of renal tubular epithelium. *Typical age:* 50y. ♂:♀ ≈ 2:1. Spread can be local or haematogenous (bone, liver, lung—causes cannon ball metastases seen on CXR).

### Presentation
- Haematuria
- Loin pain
- Abdominal mass
- Left varicocoele
- Anaemia
- Occasionally night sweats.

**Investigations** *Urine:* RBCs. *Blood:* ↑ PCV (2%), anaemia, hypercalcaemia. *Radiology:* USS, CXR.

*Management* Refer to urology urgently. Treatment includes nephrectomy ± immunotherapy with interleukin 2. 30–50% 5y survival.

**Table 14.7** Causes and management of haematuria

| Causes of haematuria | | |
|---|---|---|
| Kidney | Stones | Infection |
| | Tumour | Glomerulonephritis |
| Ureter | Stones | Tumour (rare) |
| Bladder | UTI | Tumour |
| | Stones | Chronic inflammation |
| Prostate | Prostatitis | Tumour |
| Urethral inflammation | | |

**Management of haematuria[N]**

*Urgent referral* Patients:
• Of any age with painless macroscopic haematuria
• Aged ≥40y. with recurrent/persistent UTI associated with haematuria
• Aged ≥50 y. with unexplained microscopic haematuria
• With an abdominal mass identified clinically or on imaging that is thought to arise from the urinary tract.

*Non-urgent referral* Patients <50y with microscopic haematuria. If proteinuria, ↑ serum creatinine, or ↓eGFR, refer to a renal physician. Otherwise refer to urology.

❶ In male patients with symptoms suggestive of UTI and macroscopic haematuria, diagnose and treat the infection before considering referral. If infection is not confirmed, refer urgently.

**Table 14.8** Stage of bladder cancer, treatment, and prognosis

| Stage | Description and treatment | Prognosis |
|---|---|---|
| T1 (80%) | Disease confined to mucosa/submucosa. Treated with transurethral resection of the tumour (TURBI) ± single intravesical chemotherapy treatment. Follow-up is with regular cystoscopy | Very good— most die from other causes |
| T2 | Invasion into connective tissue surrounding the bladder Treatment is with TURBT ± radiotherapy. Follow-up as for T1 | 60% survive 5y |
| T3 | Invasion through the muscle into the fat layer. Radical cystectomy and/or radiotherapy | 40–50% 5y survival |
| T4 | Spread beyond the bladder. TURBT for local symptoms. Palliative radiotherapy ± chemotherapy. Palliative care | 20–30% 5y survival— less if para-aortic nodes are involved |

**Further information**
**NICE** Referral guidelines for suspected cancer (2005) ⌨ www.nice.org.uk

**Information and support for patients**
**Macmillan Cancer Support** ☎ 0808 808 0000 ⌨ www.macmillan.org.uk

# Urinary tract infection

Urinary tract infection (UTI) is one of the most common conditions seen in general practice, accounting for up to 6% of consultations (1 case/ average surgery). ♀ > ♂. 20% of women at any time have asymptomatic bacteriuria and 20–40% of women will have a UTI in their lifetime.

**Infecting organisms** *E. coli* (>70%), *Proteus* spp, *Pseudomonas* spp, streptococci, staphylococci.

## Risk factors

- Prior infection
- DM
- Stones
- Pregnancy
- Dehydration
- GU instrumentation
- Catheterization
- ↓ oestrogen (menopause)
- Sexual intercourse
- Diaphragm use
- GU malformation
- Urinary stasis (e.g. obstruction)
- Delayed micturition (e.g. on long journeys).

## Presentations of UTI

- **Cystitis** Frequency, dysuria, urgency, strangury, low abdominal pain, incontinence of urine, acute retention of urine, cloudy or offensive urine, and/or haematuria.
- **Pyelonephritis** Loin pain, fever, rigors, malaise, vomiting, and/or haematuria.

**Dysuria and urgency** Painful micturition due to urethral or bladder inflammation. *Causes:* UTI, urethral syndrome, inflammation (e.g. interstitial cystitis, radiation-induced cystitis), intravesical lesion (tumour, stone), atrophy (menopause).

**Frequency** Passage of urine more often than usual. *Causes:*

- UTI
- Urethral syndrome
- Detrusor instability
- Inflammation (e.g. interstitial cystitis)
- Fibrosis (e.g. post-radiotherapy)
- Atrophy (menopause)
- Neurogenic bladder (e.g. MS)
- DM
- External pressure (e.g. pregnancy, fibroids)
- Bladder tumour or stone
- Enlarged prostate
- Drugs (e.g. diuretics)
- Excessive fluid intake
- Habit.

**Initial investigation** If uncomplicated UTI in an otherwise healthy woman, test urine with a leucocyte and nitrite dipstick. If +ve treat for UTI. *Reasons to send MSU for M,C &S:*

- Unresolved infection after antibiotics
- Recurrent UTI
- Uncatheterized man with UTI
- Catheterized man or woman with symptomatic UTI
- Child (📖 p.876)
- Pregnant woman (📖 p.810)
- Suspected pyelonephritis
- Haematuria—microscopic or macroscopic—always investigate further (📖 p.454).

❶ MSUs should be taken prior to starting antibiotics and sent to the laboratory fresh.

**Further investigation** Consider further investigation with blood tests (U&E, Cr, eGFR, and/or PSA if >40y and ♂) and/or radiology (renal tract USS, KUB, ±IVP) if:

- UTI in a man
- UTI in a child (📖 p.876)
- Recurrent UTI in a woman
- Pyelonephritis

- Unclear diagnosis (e.g. persisting symptoms but negative MSU)
- Unusual infecting organism.

## Management
**Catheterized patients** 📖 p.461
**Pregnant women** 📖 p.810

**Children** 📖 p.876

### All other patients

- ↑ fluid intake (>3L/24h). Alkalinize urine (e.g. potassium citrate solution) to ease symptoms.
- Prescribe oral antibiotics, e.g. trimethoprim 200mg bd (80% organisms are sensitive). Use a 3d course for women with uncomplicated UTI and a 2wk. course for men, patients with GU malformations or immunosuppression, relapse (same organism), or recurrent UTI (different organism). Use a 14d course of a quinolone (e.g. ciprofloxacin 250–500mg bd) for patents with pyelonephritis.
- Refer to urology if any abnormalities are detected on further investigation or unable to resolve symptoms. Admission is rarely needed.

**Prevention of recurrent cystitis** Reinfection after successful treatment of infection (90%) or relapse after inadequate treatment.

- **General advice** Advise patients to urinate frequently; ↑ fluid intake; double void (i.e. go again after 5–10 min) and void after intercourse.
  - 📌 Efficacy of cranberry juice is controversial.
- **Prophylactic antibiotics** Consider prescribing either post-coitally (e.g. nitrofurantoin 50mg stat) or continuously (trimethoprim 100mg nocte or nitrofurantoin 50mg nocte).
- **Men with BPH** Finasteride and/or doxazosin ↓ incidence of UTI.
- **HRT** Topical oestrogen ↓ recurrent UTI in women of all ages.[R]
- **Vaccines** Results of large-scale trials are awaited.

**Prostatitis** 📖 p.465          **Chronic pyelonephritis** 📖 p.450

**Urethral syndrome** Symptoms of cystitis with –ve MSU. Unknown cause. Associated with cold, stress, nylon underwear, COC pill, and intercourse. Advise patients to drink fluids ++ and wear cotton underwear. Consider changing/stopping COC pill, or trying topical oestrogen if postmenopausal. Tetracyclines (e.g doxycycline 100mg bd for 14d) or azithromycin (500mg od for 6d)[R] are helpful in some patients. If not settling, refer to urology. Urethral dilatation/massage may be helpful.

**Interstitial cystitis** Predominantly affects middle-aged women. Can cause fibrosis of the bladder wall. Main symptoms—frequency, urgency, and suprapubic pain especially when the bladder is full. Often misdiagnosed as recurrent UTI. MSU—no bacteriuria. Refer to urologist for confirmation. There is no satisfactory treatment, though antispasmodics, amitriptyline and bladder stretching under GA may help some patients.

**Sterile pyuria** 📖 p.454

# Incontinence of urine

Involuntary loss of urine which is objectively demonstrable and a social or hygienic problem. 14% women aged 30–70y admitted incontinence ($\male$:$\female$ ≈ 1:2) in a MORI poll. This is probably an underestimate. 1:3 with incontinence consult at outset, 1:3 consult later, 1:3 suffer in silence. Opportunistic questioning can identify sufferers.

## Presentation

### History

- Frequency of complaint.
- Volume passed.
- Degree of incapacity.
- Whether occurs with standing/coughing/sneezing.
- Urgency/dysuria/frequency of micturition.
- Past obstetric and medical history.
- Medication.
- Mobility and accessibility of toilets.

### Examination

- *Abdominal including DRE* Enlarged bladder, masses, loaded colon, faecal impaction, anal tone.
- *Pelvic* Prolapse, atrophy, neurological deficit, retention of urine, and pelvic masses.

**Investigation** Intake–output diary (at least 3d including working and leisure days)—evaluates problem and benchmark for progress (record drinks & passage of urine). Urine—glucose, RBCs, MC&S; consider blood for U&E, eGFR, FBC if renal impairment/DM is suspected.

**Drugs that exacerbate/cause incontinence** Diuretics, antihistamines, anxiolytics, α-blockers, sedatives and hypnotics, anticholinergic drugs, TCAs.

**GP management** ● 30% have a mixed pattern. Treat according to dominant symptom. Try general measures before referring to urology/gynaecology or for urodynamic investigations.

### General measures

- Manipulate fluid intake: amount, type (avoid tea, coffee, alcohol), timing.
- Promote weight ↓.
- Alter medication e.g. timing of diuretics.
- Treat UTI and chronic respiratory conditions.
- Avoid constipation.
- Consider HRT (topical or systemic) for oestrogen deficiency.

### Nocturnal enuresis in children 🕮 p. 912

### Stress incontinence

- *Symptoms* Small losses of urine without warning throughout the day related to coughing/exercise.
- *Causes* Prostatectomy; childbirth; deterioration of pelvic floor muscles/nerves.
- *Treatment* Pelvic floor exercises (🕮 p.839) continued >3mo help 60% (taught by physiotherapists/continence advisors; leaflets available)—may be assisted by vaginal cones and/or electrical stimulation. Mechanical devices (e.g. Conveen® continence guard) help 75%.

**Urge incontinence/overactive bladder syndrome** Detrusor instability or hyperreflexia causes the bladder to contract unintentionally.
- *Symptoms* Frequency, overwhelming desire to void (often precipitated by stressful event), large loss, nocturia.
- *Causes* Idiopathic, neurological problems (stroke, MS, DM, spinal cord injury, dementia, PD), local irritation (bladder stones, bladder cancer, infection), obstruction (BPH), surgery (TURP).
- *Treatment* Try bladder training programmes—resist the urge to pass urine for increasing periods. Start with an achievable interval based on diary evidence and ↑ slowly—continue for >6wk. If bladder training is ineffective, try oxybutinin first line[N] (alternatives: darifenacin, solifenacin, tolterodine, trospium). Spontaneously remits/relapses; reassess every 3–4mo.

**Overflow** Constant dribbling loss day and night. *Causes*: BPH, prostate cancer, urethral stricture, faecal impaction, neurological (LMN lesions), side effect of medication. Treatment is aimed at relieving the obstruction (📖 p.462).

**Urinary fistula** Communication between bladder and the outside—normally through the vagina. Results in constant dribbling loss day and night. Refer to gynaecology/urology. *Causes*: congenital, malignancy, complication of surgery.

**Functional incontinence** No urological problem. Caused by other factors, e.g. inaccessible toilets/immobility, behavioural problems, cognitive deficit. Treat the cause.

**Table 14.9** Referral for incontinence problems

| Specialist continence advisor (or DN ) | Urodynamic studies | Gynaecology/urology opinion |
|---|---|---|
| Advice on aids or appliances | If type of incontinence is uncertain | GP management has failed |
| Advice on primary care management | Atypical features of incontinence | Severe symptoms |
| Patient support | After unsuccessful surgery | Concomitant gynaecological problems (e.g. prolapse) |
| | If neurological problem is suspected | Concomitant urological problems (e.g. chronic retention) |
| | | Failed incontinence surgery |
| | | Vesico-vaginal fistula |
| | | Haematuria 📖 p.454 |

**Aids and appliances** 📖 p.460

**Further information**
**NICE** Urinary Incontinence (2006) 🖥 www.nice.org.uk
**Association for Continence Advice** Advice for healthcare professionals 🖥 www.aca.uk.com

**Patient information and support**
**Bladder and Bowel Foundation** ☎ 0845 345 0165
🖥 www.bladderandbowelfoundation.org.uk

# Aids and appliances for incontinence

**Pads** Many different types. DNs or continence advisors are best aware of those available locally via the NHS. They are not available on FP10 and are supplied by local NHS trusts on a 'daily allowance' basis. This varies across the country.

**Bed covers** Absorb 1–4L of urine. Good laundry facilities are needed. If left wet, can cause skin breakdown. Available via NHS trusts.

**External catheters or sheaths** Can be prescribed on NHS prescription. Approved appliances are listed in part IXB of the UK Drug Tariff. Used for men who have intractable incontinence and who are highly physically dependent, do not have urine retention, and do not require an internal catheter. Assessment and fitting by a DN or continence adviser is essential. Used in association with drainage bag. *Types*:

- Self-adhesive, or attached with adhesive strips. Adhesive sheaths can last several days but daily changing is recommended.
- Non-adhesive. Replace non-adhesive sheaths 2–3×/d. Some are re-usable.

*Problems* Include ↑ susceptibility to UTI, sores on penis, and skin irritation due to the adhesive.

**Catheters** Can be prescribed on NHS prescription. Approved appliances are listed in part IXA of the UK Drug Tariff.

*Indwelling catheters* Only use catheters in patients who:

- have urinary retention or neurogenic bladder dysfunction
- have severe pressure sores
- have inoperable obstructions that prevent the bladder emptying
- have terminal illness
- are housebound without adequate carer support.

*Types* Only long-term Foley catheters are suitable for use in primary care. They last 3–12wk.

- Hydrogel coated, e.g. Bard (Biocath®).
- Silicone elastomer: coated latex, e.g. Bard, Rüsch (Sympacath®).
- All silicone, e.g. Coloplast, Medasil, Rüsch (Brilliant Aquaflate®).

*Catheter size* Unless specified, a 12 or 14Ch catheter is supplied. Use smallest diameter of catheter that drains urine effectively. Catheters >16Ch are more likely to cause bypassing of urine around the catheter and urethral strictures.

*Catheter length* Men require longer catheters than women. Specify 'male' or 'female' on the prescription.

*Catheter balloon* 10mL balloons are supplied unless specified otherwise. Pre-filled catheters contain sterile water which inflates the retaining balloon with water. They are more expensive but quicker to insert and there are no costs for syringes or sterile water.

*Insertion* 🕮 p.463.

*Drainage* Usually attached to a leg bag, although catheter valves are also available which allow the patient to use his/her bladder as a urine reservoir. The valve must be released every 3–4h to drain out the urine.

### Common problems

- **Leakage** Check no constipation; check catheter not blocked; try smaller gauge catheter.
- **Infection** 90% develop bacteriuria <4 wk. after insertion. Always confirm suspected UTI with MSU—only treat if symptomatic or *Proteus* spp grown. May prove difficult to eliminate. No good evidence bladder instillations help
- **Encrustation** *(50%)* Deposition of minerals and other materials from urine onto the catheter. Worse if there is infection with *Proteus* spp. May cause catheter blockage or pain changing catheter. Check pH of urine regularly in patients with problems. Citric acid patency solutions may help if pH >7.4 or a daily dose of vitamin C.
- **Inflammation** Results from physical presence of a catheter in the urethra. Exacerbated by encrustation and infection. There is no easy solution—try a different brand of catheter (e.g. hydrogel catheter rather than silicone).
- **Blockage** Change catheter. The interval of routine changes should be altered if there is regular blockage towards the end of the life of a catheter.

**Intermittent self-catheterization** Patient inserts a catheter into his/her bladder 4–5x/d to drain urine. ↓ problems of infection and blockage. Useful for neurological bladder dysfunction. *Types:*
- **Re-usable silver or stainless steel**, e.g. Malvern (Biscath®).
- **Re-usable PVC**—can be washed and re-used for 1 wk. Usually supply 5/mo.
- **Single use** Need 125–150/mo. Expensive. Only use on consultant advice.

**Collecting bags** Can be prescribed on NHS prescription. Approved appliances are listed in part IXB of the UK Drug Tariff.
- **Leg bags** Drainable bags last 5–7d. Usually 500/750mL. Larger-capacity bags are too heavy for mobile patients. A variety of attachment systems are available on prescription. Long tubes are needed to wear a bag on the calf.
- **Night drainage** *bags* Connect to night bag attachment of day bags. Single-use disposable non-draining bags are recommended. Bag hangers are not available on FP10.

**Enuresis alarms** 📖 p.913

### Further information
**NHSBSA** Electronic drug tariff
🖥 www.nhsbsa.nhs.uk/PrescriptionServices/924.aspx

### Patient advice and support
**Bladder and Bowel Foundation** ☎ 0845 345 0165
🖥 www.bladderandbowelfoundation.org.uk

# Urinary tract obstruction

**Causes of obstruction** (Figure 14.1) Obstruction may be unilateral (kidney, pelvi-ureteric junction, or ureter) or bilateral (bladder, urethra, prostate). Unilateral obstruction may present late if the other kidney remains functioning. Suspect if loin ache worsened by drinking. Confirm with USS and refer to urology. Obstructing lesions may be in the lumen (e.g. stones), in the wall (e.g. tumours), or impinging from outside (e.g. retroperitoneal fibrosis).

**Acute retention of urine** Sudden inability to pass urine → lower abdominal discomfort with inability to keep still. Differentiate from AKI. ♂ > ♀. *Risk factors:* age > 70y; symptoms of prostatism/poor urinary stream.

*Causes* Prostatic obstruction (82%); constipation; alcohol; drugs (anticholinergics, diuretics); UTI; operation (e.g. hernia repair). Rarer causes: urethral stricture; clot retention; spinal cord compression; bladder stone.

*Examination* Abdomen—palpable bladder; DRE—enlarged ± irregular prostate; perineal sensation to exclude neurological cause.

*Investigation* MSU to exclude infection. Blood for U&E, Cr, and eGFR. *Only* investigate if catheterizing in the community.

*Management* Catheterize (record initial volume drained) or refer to urology for catheterization—local policies vary. Treat infection. Refer to DN for instruction on management of the catheter. Refer to urology for further assessment and treatment.

**Chronic retention of urine** Insidious onset. *Causes:* benign prostatic hypertrophy; pelvic malignancy; CNS disease. May present as:
• Nocturnal enuresis      • Acute-on-chronic retention   • UTI
• Overflow incontinence   • Lower abdominal mass         • Renal failure.

*Examination and investigation* As for acute retention. Bladder is enlarged (may contain >1.5L) but usually non-tender.

*Management* Refer to urology for further assessment and treatment. Refer urgently or acutely if pain, UTI, or renal failure (eGFR <60mL/min). *Do not* catheterize in the community.

**Retroperitoneal fibrosis** Ureters become embedded in dense fibrous plaques in the retroperitoneal space. *Associations:*
• Drugs, e.g. methysergide    • Connective tissue disease
• Carcinoma                   • Raynauds syndrome
• Crohn's disease             • Fibrotic diseases (e.g. alveolitis).

*Presentation and management* Typically middle-aged men presenting with fever, malaise sweating, leg oedema, ↑BP, palpable mass, and acute-on-chronic renal failure. Refer for specialist care. Options include steroids and nephrostomies.

**Horseshoe kidney** Congenital abnormality. Kidneys are fused in the midline to form a horseshoe-shaped mass. The kidney may function normally or may present with obstructive nephropathy or UTIs.

**Unilateral**

**Bilateral**

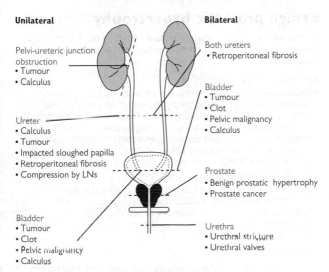

Pelvi-ureteric junction obstruction
• Tumour
• Calculus

Ureter
• Calculus
• Tumour
• Impacted sloughed papilla
• Retroperitoneal fibrosis
• Compression by LNs

Bladder
• Tumour
• Clot
• Pelvic malignancy
• Calculus

Both ureters
• Retroperitoneal fibrosis

Bladder
• Tumour
• Clot
• Pelvic malignancy
• Calculus

Prostate
• Benign prostatic hypertrophy
• Prostate cancer

Urethra
• Urethral stricture
• Urethral valves

**Fig.14.1** Causes of urinary tract obstruction

**Passing a urethral catheter** ❶ Technique learned through supervised experience. Only attempt alone if you are competent to do so.

### Prepare the equipment needed

- Sterile rubber gloves; plastic sheet to prevent spills; paper sheet to provide sterile field; cleansing materials—cotton swabs, cleansing fluid.
- Local anaesthetic/lubricating gel, e.g. 1% lidocaine+0.25% chlorhexidine.
- Catheter—usually 12Ch or 14Ch. Ensure the catheter is a long catheter if catheterizing a man (📖 p.460) and if the catheter is not pre-filled—sterile syringe +10mL of sterile water.
- Kidney dish/other receptacle to catch the urine before connecting the drainage bag; drainage tube and bag.

### Inserting the catheter

- Ensure the patient is comfortable; protect against spills with a plastic sheet; cover area with a sterile paper sheet.
- Ensure strict aseptic technique. Cleanse the penis/vulva and squeeze lubricant/local anaesthetic gel into the urethra— allow to work.
- Gently but firmly, push the catheter into the urethra. Ensure the end of the catheter is over the receptacle. When the catheter enters the bladder, urine flows into the receptacle. Inflate the balloon with sterile water (if needed) once the catheter is inside the bladder. Connect the catheter to the collecting tube and bag.
- If male, pull the foreskin over the glans again to prevent paraphimosis.

❶ If you are unable to pass a catheter, refer to urology.

# Benign prostatic hypertrophy

10–30% of men in their early 70s have symptomatic benign prostatic hypertrophy (BPH). There is no relation between size of the prostate and symptoms.

## Symptoms of prostatism

- *Obstructive* ↓ and intermittent urinary stream, double micturition, hesitancy, terminal dribbling, feeling of incomplete emptying, and straining to void. Differential diagnosis: prostatic enlargement, strictures, tumours, urethral valves, bladder neck contracture.
- *Irritative* (due to detrusor muscle hypertrophy) Urinary frequency, urgency, dysuria, and nocturia. Differential diagnosis: Enlarged prostate, UTI, polydipsia, detrusor instability, hypercalcaemia, uraemia.

## Complications 10% at presentation:

- Recurrent UTI.
- Bladder stones.
- Haematuria.
- Chronic obstruction (📖 p.462).
- Overflow incontinence (📖 p.459).
- Obstructive nephropathy.
- Acute retention of urine—with or without prior obstructive symptoms (📖 p.462).

## Assessment Table 14.10

**GP management** Studies suggest that symptoms can improve spontaneously but overall progress very slowly. 1–2%/y develop urinary retention. *Options:*

**Watchful waiting** Patients with mild to moderate symptoms at presentation with no complications of BPH and who are not severely troubled by their symptoms. Self-help includes ↓ evening fluid intake, ↓ caffeine intake, bladder retraining and prevention of constipation

**Conventional drug therapy** Those with mild to moderate symptoms who are troubled by their symptoms. *Consider:*

- α-adreceptor antagonists, e.g. Prazosin, Doxazosin. Watch for postural hypotension. ↓ symptomatic worsening.[R]
- 5-α-reductase inhibitors, e.g. finasteride. Best for patients with bulky prostates—takes up to 6mo to work. ↓ risk of urinary retention.[R]
- Combination therapy—α-adreceptor antagonist and 5-α-reductase inhibitor. ↓ progression by 66% more than either agent alone.[R]

**Alternative therapies** There is some evidence that *Serenoa repens* (saw palmetto) is beneficial. Results of a large RCT are awaited.

**Referral to a urologist** (*E*= Emergency admission; *U*=Urgent; *S*= Soon; *R*=Routine)

- Complicated BPH (e.g. acute retention)—*E/U*
- Nodular/firm prostate on DRE—*U*
- ↑ PSA (📖 p.467)—*U*
- Severe symptoms—*S*
- Failure to respond to drug therapy after 3–12mo (α-blocker) or 6–12mo (5-α-reductase inhibitor)—*R*.

**Table 14.10** Assessment of BPH

| Assessment | Comments |
|---|---|
| History | • General well-being  • Haematuria<br>• Obstructive symptoms  • Pain<br>• Polyuria and polydipsia<br>• Irritative symptoms  • Neurological symptoms<br>• Past history of urological instrumentation or STIs |
| Frequency–volume chart | Assess pattern and type of fluid consumption (e.g. alcohol/caffeine at night ↑ nocturia) |
| Symptom score (IPSS 📖 p.466) | Objectively grade symptoms giving measure of severity. IPSS scores:<br>• 0–7 mild<br>• 8–19 moderate<br>• 20–35 severe<br>General quality-of-life measurement can be used to assess impact of symptoms |
| Abdominal examination | Look for distended bladder, palpable kidneys Examine external genitalia |
| Digital rectal examination | Anal tone, size, shape and consistency of prostate (normal prostate—size of a chestnut with smooth, rubbery consistency) |
| Serum urea, creatinine and eGFR | Renal function assessment |
| MSU | Dipstick for blood and glucose; M,C&S |
| Ultrasound measurement of post-micturition residual* | |
| Maximum voiding flow rate* | <15mL/s for voided volume >100mL/s is abnormal |
| Serum PSA | High values can indicate prostate cancer (📖 p.467) |

\* May be available through open-access prostate assessment clinics

**Prostatitis** Consider acute prostatitis in all men presenting with symptoms of UTI. Treat with 4wk. course of oral antibiotic which penetrates prostatic tissue, e.g. trimethoprim 200mg bd.

## Further information
**NEJM** McConnell JD et al. The long term effect of doxazosin, finasteride and combination therapy on the clinical progression of benign prostatic hyperplasia (2003) **349**, 2387–98

# International Prostate Symptom Score

| | Not at all | Less than 1 time in 5 | Less than half the time | About half the time | More than half the time | Almost always | Your score |
|---|---|---|---|---|---|---|---|
| Over the past month, how often have you had a sensation of not emptying your bladder completely after you finish urinating? | 0 | 1 | 2 | 3 | 4 | 5 | ❏ |
| Over the past month, how often have you had to urinate again <2h after you finished urinating? | 0 | 1 | 2 | 3 | 4 | 5 | ❏ |
| Over the past month, how often have you stopped and started several times when you urinated? | 0 | 1 | 2 | 3 | 4 | 5 | ❏ |
| Over the past month, how often have you found it difficult to postpone urinating? | 0 | 1 | 2 | 3 | 4 | 5 | ❏ |
| Over the past month, how often have you had a weak urinary stream? | 0 | 1 | 2 | 3 | 4 | 5 | ❏ |
| Over the past month, how often have you had to push or strain to begin urinating? | 0 | 1 | 2 | 3 | 4 | 5 | ❏ |
| Over the past month, typically from the time you went to bed to the time you got up in the morning, how many times did you get up to urinate? | 0 | 1 | 2 | 3 | 4 | 5+ | ❏ |
| **Total IPSS score** | | | | | | | ❏ |

| | Delighted | Pleased | Mostly satisfied | Satisfied= dissatisfied | Mostly Dissatisfied | Unhappy | Terrible |
|---|---|---|---|---|---|---|---|
| If you were to live the rest of your life with your urinary condition the way it is now, how would you feel about it? | 0 | 1 | 2 | 3 | 4 | 5 | 6 |

0–7 = mildly symptomatic    8–19 = moderately symptomatic
20–35 = severely symptomatic

The International Prostate Symptom Score is reproduced from Roehrborn CG, M<sup>c</sup>Connell JD, Barry MJ et al. *Benign Prostatic Hyperplasia Guideline*, Guideline on the management of benign prostatic hyperplasia, with permission from the American Urological Association Education and Research Inc., 2003. 🖳 www.auanet.org/guidelines/bph.cfm

**Prostate-specific antigen (PSA) testing** There is considerable demand for PSA testing amongst men worried about prostate cancer. There is no prostate screening programme in the UK but men can request a PSA test. The government has introduced a PSA Informed Choice Programme. Warn patients about the poor specificity of the test before performing the test and provide information about the pros and cons of testing.

In addition, PSA is routinely measured in men with urological symptoms. Abnormal PSA is a common reason for referral to a urologist. Its sensitivity and specificity are poor.

### Pros and cons of PSA testing

*Benefits of PSA testing*
- It may provide reassurance if the test result is normal.
- It may find cancer before symptoms develop and at an early stage when treatments could be beneficial.
- If treatment is successful, the consequences of more advanced cancer are avoided.

*Downside of PSA testing*
- It can miss cancer, and provide false reassurance.
- It may lead to unnecessary anxiety and medical tests when no cancer is present.
- It might detect slow-growing cancer that may never cause any symptoms or shortened lifespan.
- The main treatments of prostate cancer have significant side effects, and there is no certainty that treatment will be successful.

### Reasons for increased PSA
- Prostate cancer
- Benign prostatic hypertrophy
- Acute or chronic prostatitis
- Physical exercise
- Acute urinary retention
- Prostate instrumentation (includes prostate biopsy, urinary catheterization and rectal examination)
- Old age.

❶ PSA may be *normal* when early prostate cancer is present.

**Performing a PSA test** Do the PSA test before doing a digital rectal examination. If that is not possible, delay the test for 1 wk. after the examination. Exclude urinary infection before PSA testing. Do NOT do a PSA test if the man has:
- A proven UTI—treat the UTI and postpone the PSA test for ≥ 1mo
- Ejaculated within 48h
- Exercised vigorously in the previous 48h
- Had a prostate biopsy <6wk ago.

### PSA cut-offs that should prompt referral

| Age (y) | Refer to urology if PSA (ng/mL) |
| --- | --- |
| 50–59 | ≥3.0 |
| 60–69 | ≥4.0 |
| ≥70 | >5.0 |

❶ Finasteride ↓ PSA by ~50%

# Prostate cancer

Prostate cancer is the sixth most common cancer worldwide. It is the second most common cancer affecting men, and 9000 men/y die from the disease in the UK. 1:6 men have clinical prostate cancer in their lifetime, and the incidence is rising.

## Classification
*Non-metastatic prostate cancer* Can be divided into:
- Clinically localized disease—cancer thought, after clinical examination, to be confined to the prostate gland.
- Locally advanced disease—cancer that has spread outside the capsule of the prostate gland but has not yet spread to other organs.

*Metastatic prostate cancer* Cancer that has spread outside the prostate gland to local, regional, or systemic LNs, seminal vesicles, or other body organs (e.g. bone, liver, brain).

## Risk factors
- *Age* Uncommon <50y; 85% of men with prostate cancer are diagnosed aged >65y.
- *Genetic* ↑ incidence if first-degree relative affected.
- *Racial* Incidence varies according to location in the world and ethnic group. Highest rates are in men of black ethnic group in the USA—lowest in Chinese men.
- *Dietary* Links are proposed between prostate cancer and low intake of fruit (particularly tomatoes) and high intake of fat, meat, and $Ca^{2+}$.

**Screening** A large-scale trial of screening for prostate cancer is under way in the UK. *Problems with screening:*
- Incidental post-mortem evidence of prostate cancer is high (~75% men >75y). Very few become clinically evident, so many more men would be found with prostate cancer by screening than would die or have symptoms of it.
- Natural history of prostate cancer is not understood—there is no means of detecting which 'early' cancers become more widespread.
- Inadequate screening tests.
- It is not clear if early treatment enhances life expectancy.
- Peak incidence of morbidity and mortality is in old age (75–79y), so potential years of life saved by screening are small.

## Screening tests
- *Prostate specific antigen (PSA)* 📖 p.467
- *Digital rectal examination (DRE)* Operator-dependent, fails to detect early prostate cancers, and lacks specificity. Annual screening in the USA and Germany has not ↓ mortality.
- *Transrectal ultrasound (TRUS)* Too expensive for widespread use.

The most effective screening regime involves rectal examination and PSA testing followed by TRUS for suspicious lesions.[S] Optimal screening interval is unknown, but serial screening does ↑ detection.

## Symptoms and signs

*Early cancer* Symptomless. Usually detected following an incidental finding of ↑ PSA. Hard nodule sometimes felt in prostate on DRE.

### Local disease

- Prostatism
- Urinary retention
- Haematuria

- Lower extremity oedema
- On rectal examination, the prostate is hard, non-tender and sulci lose definition.

### Metastatic disease

- Malaise
- Weight loss
- Bone pain
- Pathological fractures

- Spinal cord compression
- Ureteric obstruction may cause renal failure
- Signs depend on site of metastases.

**Investigation**[N] A digital rectal examination and a PSA test (after counselling) are recommended for patients with any of the following unexplained symptoms.

- Erectile dysfunction
- Haematuria
- Lower back pain
- Bone pain

- Inflammatory or obstructive lower urinary tract symptoms
- Weight loss, especially in the elderly.

**⚠** Exclude UTI before PSA testing and postpone digital rectal examination until after the PSA test is done.

### Urgent referral[N]

- Rectal examination—hard irregular prostate typical of prostate cancer. PSA result should accompany the referral.
- Rectal examination—normal prostate, but rising/raised age-specific PSA ± lower urinary tract symptoms.*
- Symptoms and high PSA levels.
- Asymptomatic men with borderline age-specific PSA results, repeat PSA after 1–3mo. If the PSA level is rising, refer the patient urgently.

*Consider discussion with specialist and patient ± carer before referral for very elderly patients/those compromised by other comorbidities.

**⚠** Referral is not needed if the prostate is simply enlarged and the PSA is in the age-specific reference range.

## Further information for GPs

**NICE** 🖳 www.nice.org.uk
- Referral guidelines for suspected cancer (2005)
- Prostate cancer: diagnosis & treatment (2008)

**Cancer Research UK** 🖳 www.cancerresearchuk.org
**National screening** 🖳 www.cancerscreening.nhs.uk

## Information for patients on PSA testing and prostate cancer

**National screening** 🖳 www.cancerscreening.nhs.uk
**Macmillan Cancer Support** ☎ 0808 808 0000 🖳 www.macmillan.org.uk
**Prostate Cancer Charity** ☎ 0800 074 8383 🖳 www.prostate-cancer.org.uk
**Prostate Cancer Support Association** ☎ 0845 601 0766
🖳 www.prostatecancersupport.co.uk

# Treatment of prostate cancer

**Symptomless local disease** Treatment is controversial. There are two arguments:

| Benefits of treatment are outweighed by risks | or | Aggressive treatment before spread is the only way to ensure cure |
|---|---|---|

The picture is further complicated as >50% of men >50y who die from other causes are found post mortem to have prostate cancer—prostate cancer kills only a small minority of men who have it. The personal and economic cost of treating men whose cancer would never have caused them any problems must be considered.

## Options

- *Watchful waiting* Monitor with PSA/rectal examination. ↑ in PSA or size of nodule triggers active treatment. At 10y follow-up <10% with moderately well-differentiated cancer will have died from their cancer. Progression rates are higher in patients with poorly differentiated cancer. Some men find the uncertainty of waiting difficult to cope with.
- *Radical prostatectomy* Has potential for cure, but in the age group most affected by prostate cancer, mortality is 1.4%. Other common complications: impotence (50%), incontinence (25%).
- *Radiotherapy* May not be effective—persistent cancer is found in 30% on biopsy. Brachytherapy (radioactive treatment in implanted seeds or wires) has proven efficacy in early prostate cancer.
- *Hormone treatment* No convincing evidence that this gives survival benefit in early disease.
- *Others* Minimally invasive treatments, e.g. cryotherapy and microwave therapy, are as yet unproven.

**Symptomatic disease** 30% 5y survival. Hormone manipulation is the mainstay of treatment and gives 80% ↓ in bone pain, PSA, or both, and a lower incidence of serious complications (e.g. spinal cord compression) if treatment starts at the time of diagnosis. *Options*:

*Luteinizing hormone releasing hormone (LHRH) analogues* e.g. goserelin. SC injection every 4–12 wk (depending on the preparation used). Testosterone levels ↓ to levels of castrated men in <2mo Side effects: impotence, hot flushes, gynaecomastia, local bruising and infection around injection site. When starting LHRH analogues, LH level initially ↑ which can cause increased tumour activity or 'flare'. Counteracted by prescription of anti-androgens (e.g. flutamide) for a few days before administration of the first dose of LHRH and concurrently for 3wk. Response in most patients lasts for 12–18 mo.

*Anti-androgens* e.g. cyproterone actetate, flutamide, bicalutamide. Anti-androgens do not suppress androgen production completely. Used to prevent side effects due to testosterone flare during initiation of LHRH analogues, as monotherapy (e.g. bicalutamide 150mg od), and in combination with LHRH analogues to produce maximum androgen blockade.

*Surgical castration* ↓ testosterone secretion permanently without the need for medication. Rarely used.

**Bony metastases** In addition to hormone therapy, local radiotherapy and corticosteroids are used for bone pain. Radioactive strontium ↓ the number of new sites of bone pain developed. Mean survival <5y.

**Hormone-resistant disease** No agreed treatment. Involve the multidisciplinary team, including urology, oncology, and palliative care. Dexamethasone 0.5mg daily or docetaxel may be helpful.

| **Factors affecting prognosis of prostate cancer** | | | | |
|---|---|---|---|---|
| **Stage** | | | | |
| *Tumour* | | *Lymph nodes involved?* | | *Metastases?* |
| T1 | Impalpable | N0 | No | M0 | No spread outside the pelvis |
| T2 | Completely within the prostate gland | N1 | 1 +ve LN <2cm diameter | M1 | Spread outside the pelvis |
| T3 | Has breached the capsule of the prostate | N2 | >1 +ve LN or 1 LN of 2–5cm diameter | | |
| T4 | Has spread within the pelvis, e.g. to bladder or bowel | N3 | Any +ve LN > 5cm diameter | | |

*Gleason score* Histological grade. Cells are graded 1–5 the less differentiated they are. The two areas of the biopsy with the highest-grade cells are added together. Low-grade tumours likely to grow slowly have low scores (2–4); high-grade tumours have high scores (7–10).

*Age* Older patients with low-grade tumours are likely to die from something other than their prostate cancer.

*PSA*
• PSA >40—high chance of nodal or metastatic spread.
• PSA >100—metastatic spread is very likely.

*Prognosis* 5y survival rates for tumour stage:
• 1 or 2—tumour confined within the prostate (65–98%)
• 3—tumour has breached the capsule of the prostate (60%)
• 4—spread to LNs, within the pelvis or elsewhere (20–30%).

**Further information**
**NICE** Prostate cancer: diagnosis and treatment (2008) 🖥 www.nice.org.uk
**Cancer Research UK** 🖥 www.cancerresearchuk.org

# Conditions of the penis

 **Posterior urethral valves** Folds of mucosa inhibit or block passage of urine, causing urethral, bladder, ureter, and renal pelvis dilatation.

**Presentation** Usually detected on antenatal USS. Can present in neonates with urinary retention or dribbling urine + distended bladder, UTI, or uraemia, or later in childhood with recurrent UTI or incontinence.

**Investigation and management** MCUG confirms diagnosis. In all cases refer to urology for surgical disruption of the valves.

**Hypospadias** 1:400 male births. The urethral meatus opens on the ventral side of the penis. There is often hooding of the foreskin and ventral flexion of the penis. Refer to urology. Treated with corrective surgery, ideally pre-school.

**Non-retractile foreskin** Usually noted by parents. May be history of recurrent balanitis. *Examination*: foreskin adherent.

**Management** Age <4y—do nothing unless recurrent balanitis. If >4y refer to paediatric surgery.

**Phimosis** Foreskin obstructs urine flow. Common in small children. Time usually obviates need for circumcision. Refer if recurrent balanitis.

**Peyronie's disease** Hard lumps in the shaft of the penis. Cause unknown. Affects 4% men >40y. 1:3 affected have pain or bending of the penis when erect. Associated with erectile dysfunction (📖 p.774). 5% have Dupytren's contracture. *F.G. de la Peyronie (1678–1747)—French physician.*

**Management** Reassurance usually suffices. No proven medical treatments. Refer to urology for surgery if pain or severe bending on erection so that intercourse is not possible.

**Paraphimosis** Foreskin is retracted then (due to oedema) unable to be replaced. Commonly occurs in catheterized patients when the catheter is changed.

**Management** Try to replace foreskin using ice packs (↓ swelling) and lubrication (e.g. K-Y Jelly®). If unable to replace the foreskin, admit for surgery.

**Balanitis** Acute inflammation of glans and foreskin. Common organisms—staphylococci., streptococci., coliforms, *Candida*. Can occur at any age. Most common in young boys when associated with non-retractile foreskin/phimosis. In elderly patients consider DM.

**Management** Oral antibiotics (e.g. flucloxacillin) or topical antifungals (e.g. clotrimazole). If recurrent or due to phimosis consider referral for circumcision.

**Balanitis xerotica et obliterans** Chronic fibrosing condition of the foreskin which may become adherent to the glans. Treatment is with topical steroid creams, e.g betamethasone 0.1%. Consider referral for circumcision.

**Trauma to the foreskin** Torn frenulum—seen after poorly lubricated intercourse or if caught in a zip. No treatment required. If recurrent, consider referral for circumcision.

**Erectile dysfunction** 📖 p.774

**Priapism** Persistent painful erection not related to sexual desire. *Cause* medication for erectile dysfunction, idiopathic, leukaemia, sickle cell disease, or pelvic tumour.

*Management* ask the patient to climb stairs (arterial 'steal' phenomenon), apply ice packs. If unsuccessful refer to A&E for aspiration of corpora. Rarely, surgery is needed.

**Erythroplasia of Queryat** Premalignant condition of glans. Moist velvety looking patches. Refer to urology. Treatment is surgical.

**Carcinoma of the penis** Squamous cell carcinoma (95%) or malignant melanoma. Usually elderly men. Rare in the UK.

*Management*[N] Refer urgently patients with symptoms or signs of penile cancer. These include:
• Progressive ulceration in the glans, prepuce, or skin of the penile shaft
• Mass in the glans, prepuce, or skin of the penile shaft

❶ Lumps within the corpora cavernosa can indicate Peyronie's disease, which does not require urgent referral.

**Penile discharge** Associated with urethritis, e.g. due to Chlamydia or gonorrhoea. Refer to GUM clinic.

**Further information**
**NICE** 🖥 www.nice.org.uk
• Improving outcomes in urological cancers (2002)
• Referral guidelines for suspected cancer (2005).

# Testicular disease

**Testicular pain** Treat the cause:
- Epididymo-orchitis
- Torsion of the testis
- Trauma and haematoma formation
- Varicocoele
- Testicular tumour (rarely painful).

**Torsion of the testis** Peak age 15–30y. Presents with sudden-onset severe scrotal pain. May be associated with right iliac fossa pain, nausea, and vomiting. *Examination*: tender hard testis riding higher than contralateral testis. Admit urgently to surgical/urology team

**Torsion of the hydatid of Morgagni** Torsion of a small embryological remnant at the upper pole of the testis. Presents in a similar way to torsion of the testis. Refer as an emergency to surgery/urology to exclude torsion of the testis.

**Epididymo-orchitis** Inflammation of the testis and epididymis due to infection. The most common viral cause is mumps. The most common bacterial infections are gonococci and coliforms. May occur at any age. Chronic infection with TB or syphilis is rare.

***Presentation*** Acute onset pain in testis; swelling and tenderness of testis/epididymis; fever ± rigors; may be dysuria and ↑ frequency.

***Management*** May be difficult to distinguish from torsion of the testis. If in doubt admit for urology/surgical opinion.

**Testicular lumps and swellings**—Figure 14.2

**Hydrocoele** Collection of fluid in tunica vaginalis. Occurs at any age.
- *1° hydrocoele*—no predisposing cause in scrotum.
- *2° hydrocoele*—reaction to pathology in testis or covering (infection, tumour, torsion). In adults presenting with hydrocoele always consider impalpable tumour beneath.

***Presentation*** Swelling in the scrotum. The examiner should be able to get above the swelling. Smooth surface; transilluminates; testis is within the swelling and not palpable separately.

***Management*** Investigation is not required in children; refer adults for USS if testis is not palpable. Options for adults:
- Conservative management, reassurance—small hydrocoeles.
- Tapping—may be suitable for large hydrocoeles where surgery is inappropriate. 2° infection and recurrence are common.
- Surgery—refer to urologist.

> Hydrocoeles in children are usually congenital. May be unilateral or bilateral. Most resolve spontaneously in the first year of life. Refer to urology if persists >1y.

**Hydrocoele of the cord** Arises in part of the processus vaginalis in the spermatic cord above the testis. Rounded lump which slips up and down the inguinal canal. No action needed.

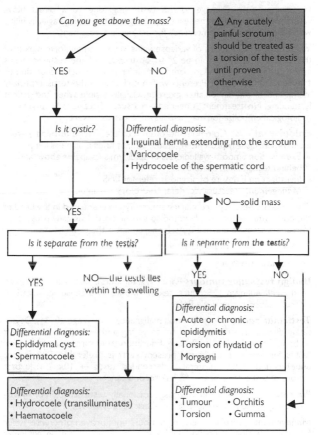

**Fig. 14.2** Diagnosis of testicular lumps

### Referral guidelines[N]

- Refer urgently patients with a swelling or mass in the body of the testis.
- Consider an urgent ultrasound in men with a scrotal mass that does not transilluminate and/or when the body of the testis cannot be distinguished.

### Further information

**NICE** ☐ www.nice.org.uk
- Improving outcomes in urological cancers (2002)
- Referral guidelines for suspected cancer (2005).
**Cancer Research UK** ☐ www.cancerresearchuk.org

**Haematocoele** Damage to the testis (e.g. due to a direct blow, vasectomy) can result in the testis rupturing and the tunica vaginalis filling with blood. Refer as an emergency for urological assessment.

**Varicocoele** Collection of varicose veins in the pampiniform plexus of the cord and scrotum. Can be 2° to obstruction of the testicular veins in the abdomen. L > R. Associated with infertility (thought to be due to ↑ temperature of testis). Presents with a dull ache in the testis, especially at the end of the day or after exercise. Usually visible when the patient is standing. No treatment is needed—reassure. Occasionally surgery or radiological embolization may help if symptoms are severe.

**Epididymal cyst** Common and often multiple. Found in middle-aged/elderly men. Usually presents when the patient finds a painless lump.
- *Examination* Smooth-walled cysts in epididymis (palpable above and behind testis), often bilateral.
- *Investigation* If unsure of diagnosis refer for USS.
- *Management:* Reassurance. Refer to urology if painful.

**Spermatocoele** Cyst containing sperm. Typically situated in the head of the epididymis—more rarely in the spermatic cord. Clinically presents in the same way as epididymal cysts. Management is the same.

**Testicular gumma** 📖 p.747

**Testicular tumours**

*Benign testicular tumours* Rare (<2% tumours). Sertoli cell adenomas; Leydig cell adenomas. Produce sex hormones and cause feminization/masculinization respectively. Refer.

*Testicular cancer* Most common malignancy in men age 20–34y. Devastating disease as sufferers tend to be young and fit and do not expect to be ill. Screening is not effective. Education to ensure men check their testes for lumps regularly and present early is preferable. *Risk factors*: undescended testes—bilateral undescended testis → 10× ↑ risk; past history of testicular cancer—4% risk second cancer.

*Presentation* Painless lump in testis; occasionally testicular pain or hydrocoele; may present with metastases—back pain/dyspnoea

*Management* Testicular lumps are tumours until proven otherwise. Refer for urgent urological opinion. USS can help diagnosis but *do not* delay referral. Definitive diagnosis is only made at biopsy. Specialist treatment depends on tumour type and extent (Table 14.11). Sperm banking is routinely offered in case of ↓ fertility due to treatment.

❶ Children conceived of men treated for testicular cancer are not at ↑ risk of congenital abnormality.

**Empty scrotum** If the scrotum has never contained a testis, it is hypoplastic. If the scrotum has contained a testis, it is normally developed but empty. *Causes of an empty scrotum:* undescended or retractile testis; surgical removal (e.g. for torsion, trauma or tumour); testicular atrophy (e.g. due to mumps or trauma); ambiguous genitalia; testicular agenesis—diagnosis of exclusion.

**Table 14.11** Types and features of testicular cancer

|  | Seminoma (60%) | Teratoma |
|---|---|---|
| *Typical age* | 30–40y | <30y |
| *Tumour markers* | None | β-HCG<br>αFP<br>LDH—correlates with volume of metastatic disease |
| *Nature of tumour* | Solid | Solid/cystic components<br>40% occur within seminomas; mixed tumours are treated like teratomas |
| *Growth speed* | Slow growing | Fast growing—can ↑2× in size in days |
| *Stage of presentation* | 90% stage 1 (tumour confined to testis) | 60% stage 1 (tumour confined to testis) |
| *Treatment* | Treated with inguinal orchidectomy + radio-therapy<br>Relapses are treated with chemotherapy<br>More advanced disease is treated with radio- or chemotherapy | Treatment of stage 1 disease is with inguinal orchidectomy and surveillance of tumour markers. 25% relapse in <18mo<br>Treatment of relapses and metastatic disease is with chemotherapy |
| *Survival* | 98% 5y survival for stage 1 disease. Overall >85% 5y survival | Prognosis depends on stage and degree of differentiation |

**Carcinoma of the scrotal skin** SCC or melanoma. Uncommon <50y. Painless lump/ulcer of the scrotal skin ± enlarged inguinal LNs. If suspected, refer urgently to urology or dermatology.

**Fournier's gangrene** Necrotizing fasciitis of the scrotal skin and/or penis. Patients are usually elderly and often have a hydrocoele. Starts as a black spot and spreads rapidly. Early diagnosis is critical to survival so, if suspected, admit as an acute urological emergency. Treatment is with surgical debridement and IV antibiotics.

**Undescended testis** Affects 2–3% of ♂ neonates, but most descend during the first year. Refer those that do not for surgical descent/fixation to avoid ↑ risk of malignancy and later infertility.

**Retractile testis** Usually young boys with active cremasteric reflex. No treatment needed.

***Examination*** Scrotum is usually well developed. Try to find the testis and milk it down into scrotum. May be found anywhere from the scrotum to the internal inguinal ring. If not found or you are unable to bring the testis down into the scrotum, assume that it is undescended.

**Information and support for patients with testicular cancer**
**Macmillan Cancer Support** ☎ 0808 808 0000 🖳 www.macmillan.org.uk
**Cancer Research UK** ☎ 0800 226 237 🖳 www.cancerhelp.org.uk

# Musculoskeletal problems

# Symptoms of musculoskeletal disease

**Bone pain** *Consider*
- *Fracture*—due to injury, stress fracture or pathological fracture.
- *Arthritis*—referred pain from affected joints.
- *Malignancy*—primary bone malignancy, haematological malignancy (e.g. multiple myeloma), or secondaries (usually from breast, prostate, lung, thyroid, kidney—more rarely, bowel, melanoma).
- *Benign bone tumour*
- *Osteomyelitis*
- *Metabolic causes*, e.g. hypercalcaemia.

## Joint pain or arthralgia
**Pain in one joint** Common. Ask:

*Is the problem articular or periarticular?*
- Articular disease (e.g. osteoarthritis) is suggested by joint line tenderness and pain at the end of the range of movement in any direction.
- Periarticular problems (e.g. ligamentous injury)—point tenderness over the involved structure, and pain exacerbated by movements.

*If articular,* is the problem inflammatory or mechanical? Look for:
- Signs of inflammation—warmth, redness, effusions. May indicate joint infection or inflammatory arthritis.
- Features of a mechanical problem—locking or catching, e.g. cartilage tear.

*If periarticular,* which structure is causing pain? Options: bursa; tendon; tendon sheath; ligament; soft tissue.

> ⚠ **Red flags** Features which should prompt early/urgent referral.
> - Inflamed joint with associated fever or constitutional disturbance—beware of infection.
> - Any joint which is 'locked' or so painful that movement is impossible.
> - Severe pain at rest or at night.
> - Pain that gets relentlessly worse over a period of days or weeks.

### Pain in multiple joints
- Differentiate between articular or periarticular disease, and whether the condition is inflammatory or not, as for pain in 1 joint. Screening with blood tests (ESR or CRP, FBC ± autoimmune profile) may help.
- Look for the pattern of disease—joint sites involved and other symptoms/signs.

*Common arthropathies* (📖 pp.520–531)
- Osteoarthritis
- Rheumatoid arthritis
- Ankylosing spondylitis
- SLE
- Reactive arthritis
- Psoriatic arthritis
- Enteropathic arthropathy
- Gout or pseudogout
- Sicca syndrome
- Malignancy.

⚠ *Red flags* Features which should prompt early/urgent referral.
- Severe systemic symptoms—high fevers, significant weight loss, or a very ill patient (suggests rheumatoid arthritis, sepsis or malignancy).
- Focal systemic signs e.g. rashes, nodules or GI disturbances.
- Severe pain and/or inability to function.

**Myalgia** Isolated myalgia can be a result of over-use or soft tissue injury. Generalized myalgia is associated with many diseases including:
- Infection
- Fibromyalgia
- Chronic fatigue syndrome
- PAN
- Wegener's granulomatosis.

**Dystonia** 📖 p.554

**Short stature** 📖 p.890

**Tall stature** 📖 p.891

**Chest deformity** 📖 p.306

---

**Children with musculoskeletal pain of unknown cause**
Take a history and examine carefully to exclude other causes. Investigate further with FBC, blood film and ESR ± X-ray if bone pain, rest pain, or persistent or unexplained back pain.[N] If no cause is found, treatment is with analgesia and reassurance. Advise to return for reassessment ± orthopaedic referral if pain worsens, continues > 6wk, changes in nature or other symptoms develop.

**Nocturnal musculoskeletal pains (growing pains)** Episodic muscular pains, usually in the legs, lasting ~30min and waking the child from sleep. Rubbing the limb brings rapid relief. There is no pain or disability in the morning. Diagnosis can be made on history if there are no associated symptoms and examination is normal. If in doubt, check FBC and ESR, which should be normal. In most cases reassurance ± analgesia are all that is needed. In resistant cases, physiotherapy may help.

**The limping child** 📖 p.499

**Further information**
**NICE** Referral guidelines for suspected cancer 🖥 www.nice.org.uk

# Neck pain

⚠ **Neck trauma** Any significant cervical trauma requires neck immobilization with a hard collar and referral to A&E for cervical spine X-rays to exclude vertebral fracture or instability that could threaten the spinal cord.

Neck pain is common (lifetime incidence 50%) and contributes to 2% of GP consultations. Prevalence is highest in middle age. Most neck pain is acute and self-limiting (within days/weeks) but 1:3 have symptoms lasting >6mo or recurring pain.

## History

- Pain—onset, site, radiation, aggravating and relieving factors, timing.
- Stiffness—timing. Continuous? Worse in the mornings?
- Deformity—e.g. torticollis. Onset, changes.
- Neurological symptoms—numbness, paraesthesiae, weakness.
- Other symptoms—weight loss, bowel/bladder dysfunction, sweats.

❶ Pain is often poorly localized and neck problems commonly present with shoulder pain and/or headache (cervicogenic headache).

## Examination

- *Look*—posture; deformity, e.g. torticollis, asymmetry of scapulae; arms and hands—wasting, fasciculation? Leg weakness?
- *Feel*—tenderness? Midline tenderness may be due to supraspinous or spinous process damage following a whiplash injury. Paraspinal tenderness ± spasm radiating into the trapezius is common with cervical spondylosis; crepitation—common with cervical spondylosis.
- *Move/measure* Normal ranges: flexion/extension—130° total range; lateral flexion—45° in each direction from a neutral position; rotation—80° in each direction from a neutral position.
- *Neurology* Weakness in the upper limbs in a segmental distribution, with loss of dermatomal sensation and altered reflexes indicates a root lesion (Table 15.1). If cervical cord compression is suspected, examine the lower limbs looking for upgoing plantars and hyper-reflexia.

**Cervical spondylosis** Degenerative disease of the cervical spine can cause pain but minor changes are normal (especially >40y) and usually asymptomatic. Pain is normally intermittent and related to activity. Examination reveals ↓ neck mobility. Severe degeneration can cause nerve root signs. Treat with analgesia ± cervical collar. X-ray only if conservative measures fail, troublesome pain, nerve root signs or the patient has psoriasis (?psoriatic arthropathy).

**Nerve root irritation or entrapment** Secondary to degeneration, vertebral displacement/collapse, disc prolapse, local tumour or abscess. Causes neck stiffness, pain in arms or fingers, ↓ reflexes, sensory loss, and ↓ power. The level of entrapment can be determined clinically (Table 15.1). Treat with analgesia ± cervical collar. X-ray cervical spine—lateral or oblique views. Refer for physiotherapy. Refer for further investigations (e.g. MRI) if conservative management fails and there is objective evidence of a root lesion.

**Table 15.1** Neurology associated with cervical nerve root entrapment

| Root | Sensory changes | Motor weakness | Reflex changes |
|------|-----------------|----------------|----------------|
| C5 | Lateral arm | Shoulder abduction/flexion<br>Elbow flexion | Biceps |
| C6 | Lateral forearm<br>Thumb<br>Index finger | Elbow flexion<br>Wrist extension | Biceps<br>Supinator |
| C7 | Middle finger | Elbow extension<br>Wrist flexion<br>Finger extension | Triceps |
| C8 | Medial side of lower forearm<br>Ring and little fingers | Finger flexion | None |
| T1 | Medial side of upper forearm | Finger abduction/adduction | None |

⚠ Refer urgently if there are signs of spinal cord compression:
- Root pain and lower motor neuron signs at the level of the lesion *and*
- Spastic weakness, brisk reflexes, up-going plantars, loss of co-ordination and sensation below the lesion.

**Spasmodic torticollis (wry neck)** Common. Sudden onset of painful stiff neck due to spasm of trapezius and sternocleidomastoid muscles. Self-limiting. Heat, gentle mobilization, muscle relaxants, and analgesia can speed recovery. A cervical collar may help in the short term but can prolong symptoms. Often caused by poor posture, e.g. computer-seating position; carrying heavy uneven loads.

**Cervical rib** Congenital condition—C$_7$ vertebra costal process enlargement. Usually asymptomatic but can cause thoracic outlet compression → hand or forearm pain, weakness or numbness, and thenar or hypothenar wasting. Radial pulse may be weak. X-ray of thoracic outlet may show cervical rib—but symptoms are sometimes due to fibrous bands that are not seen on X-ray. Refer to upper limb orthopaedic surgeon for further assessment.

**Whiplash injuries** Neck pain due to stretching or tearing of cervical muscles and ligaments due to sudden extension of neck—often due to a RTA. Pain and ↓ neck mobility typically starts several hours or days after injury. Pain may radiate to shoulders, arms, and head.

*Management* Examine carefully to exclude bony tenderness requiring X-ray. Treat with analgesia and early mobilization—collar may help initially but avoid long-term use. Recovery is often slow and 40% of patients suffer long-lasting symptoms. As a general rule of thumb, the quicker the symptoms develop, the longer they will take to disappear. Early physiotherapy, if available, can improve recovery rate. Psychological problems and medico-legal issues can affect progress.

# Low back pain

## Definitions
- *Acute low back pain* New episode of low back pain of <6wk duration. Common—lifetime prevalence 58%
- *Chronic low back pain* Back pain lasting >3mo If present >1y has poor prognosis.

## Causes of back pain Table 15.2

## History Ask:
- Circumstances of pain—history of injury; duration.
- Nature/severity of pain—pain/stiffness mainly at rest/at night, easing with movement suggests inflammation, e.g. discitis, spondylarthropathy.
- Associated symptoms—numbness, weakness, bowel/bladder symptoms.
- PMH—past illnesses (e.g. carcinoma), previous back problems.
- Exclude pain not coming from the back. (e.g. GI or GU pain).

## Examination
- Deformity, e.g. kyphosis (typical of ankylosing spondylitis), loss of lumbar lordosis (common in acute mechanical back pain), scoliosis.
- Palpate for tenderness, step deformity, and muscle spasm.
- Assess flexion, extension, lateral flexion, and rotation of the back whilst standing.
- Ask to lie down—this gives a good indication of severity of symptoms.
- In lower limbs look for muscle wasting and check power, sensory loss, and reflexes (knee jerk and ankle jerk). Assess straight leg raise (SLR)—sciatica is present if SLR on one side elicits back/buttock pain (usually ipsilateral but can be either side) compared with SLR on the other side.

## ⚠ Red flags
- <20 or >55y
- Non-mechanical pain
- Pain that worsens when supine
- Night-time pain
- Thoracic pain
- Past history of carcinoma
- HIV
- Immune suppression
- IV drug use
- Taking steroids
- Unwell
- Weight ↓
- Widespread neurology
- Structural deformity

**Management of acute pain in the community** Triage according to history and examination (Figure 15.1, 📖 p.487).

❗ **Do not X-ray routinely** X-rays require a high radiation dose and +ve findings are rare. Exceptions: young (<25y)—X-ray sacroiliac joints to exclude ankylosing spondylitis; elderly—to exclude vertebral collapse/malignancy; history of trauma; 'red flag' signs.

### For patients who do not require immediate referral
- *Explain the likely natural history* of the pain and advise to avoid bed rest and try to maintain normal activities (↓ chance of chronic pain).
- *Prescribe analgesia,* e.g. paracetamol ± NSAIDs and suggest self-help exercises.

- *Consider referral for exercise/manipulation or acupuncture[N]* Refer patients not returning to normal activities by 6wk for back exercises or manipulation to physiotherapy, chiropractic or osteopathy. Refer sooner if in a lot of pain. Consider acupuncture if available. Do not refer if there is any possible serious pathology.

**Cauda equina syndrome** Results from compression of the cauda equina below L2, e.g. by disc protrusion at L4/5. Presents with:
- Numbness of the buttocks and backs of thighs.
- Urinary/faecal incontinence.
- Lower motor neuron weakness—signs depend on level at which the cauda equine is compressed:
  - L4—loss of dorsiflexion of the foot (and toes—L4/5)
  - S1—loss of ankle reflex, plantarflexion and eversion of the foot.

*Management* Refer/admit as a neurological emergency. Rapid surgical intervention increases the chance of full motor and sphincter recovery.

**Table 15.2** Causes of back pain: Age suggests the most likely cause

|  | Causes |  |
|---|---|---|
| Age 15–30y | Postural | Fracture |
|  | Mechanical | Ankylosing spondylosis |
|  | Prolapsed disc | Spondylolisthesis |
|  | Trauma | Pregnancy |
| Age 30–50y | Postural | Discitis |
|  | Degenerative joint disease | Spondyloarthropathies |
|  | Prolapsed disc |  |
| Age >50y | Postural | Malignancy (lung, breast, prostate, thyroid, kidney) |
|  | Degenerative |  |
|  | Osteoporotic collapse | Myeloma |
|  | Paget's disease |  |
| Other causes | Referred pain | Cauda equina tumours |
|  | Spinal stenosis | Spinal infection |

**Table 15.3** Neurology associated with lumbosacral nerve root entrapment

| Root | Sensory changes | Motor weakness | Reflex changes |
|---|---|---|---|
| L2 | Front of thigh | Hip flexion/adduction | None |
| L3 | Inner thigh | Knee extension | Knee |
| L4 | Inner shin | Knee extension<br>Foot dorsiflexion | Knee |
| L5 | Outer shin<br>Dorsum of foot | Knee flexion<br>Foot inversion<br>Big toe dorsiflexion | None |
| S1 | Lateral side of foot/sole | Knee flexion<br>Foot plantarflexion | Ankle |

**Spinal cord compression in cancer patients** Affects 5% of cancer patients—70% in the thoracic region. Presentation can be subtle. Maintain a *high* level of suspicion in all cancer patients who complain of back pain, especially those with known bony metastases or tumours likely to metastasize to bone.

*Presentation*
- Often back pain, worse on movement, appears before neurology.
- Neurological symptoms/signs can be non-specific—constipation, weak legs, urinary hesitancy.
- Lesions above L1 (lower end of spinal cord) may produce upper motor neuron sign (e.g. ↑ tone and reflexes) and a sensory level.
- Lesions below L1 may produce lower motor neuron signs (↓ tone and reflexes) and perianal numbness (cauda equina syndrome).

*Management* Prompt treatment (<24–48h from first neurological symptoms) is needed if there is any hope of restoring function. Once paralysed, <5% walk again. Treat with oral dexamethasone 16mg/d and refer urgently for assessment and surgery/radiotherapy unless in final stages of disease.

**Scoliosis** Lateral curvature of the spine associated with rotation of vertebrae ± ribs or wedging of vertebrae. Early treatment of scoliosis prevents progression. Early-onset scoliosis (<8y) is responsible for cosmetic problems, pain, and cardiopulmonary disturbance. Late-onset scoliosis is less severe but also causes pain and significant deformity.

*Causes*
- Idiopathic.
- Congenital malformations of the spine (butterfly vertebra).
- Neuromuscular problems, e.g. cerebral palsy, neurofibromatosis, Friedrich's ataxia, muscular dystrophy, polio.
- Trauma → damage in vertebral growth plate and uneven growth.
- Metabolic, e.g. bone dysplasias.
- Neoplasm 1°, 2°, or as a result of radiotherapy.
- Infection—TB of spine.

*Clinical features* Difference in shoulder height; spinal curvature; difference in the space between the trunk and upper limbs. ❶ Scoliosis which disappears on bending is postural and of no clinical significance.

*Management* In all cases where scoliosis is suspected, refer for an orthopaedic opinion. If associated with pain, especially at night, consider spinal tumour and refer urgently.

**Further information**
**CKS** Guidance on lower back pain 🖥 www.cks.library.nhs.uk
**NICE** Low back pain (2009) 🖥 www.nice.org.uk

**Patient information and support**
*The Back Book* HMSO (ISBN 0017020788)
**Arthritis Research Campaign** ☎ 0870 850 5000 🖥 www.arc.org.uk

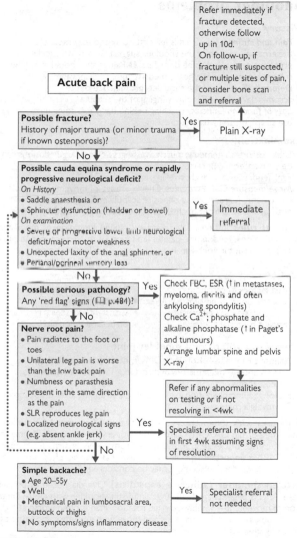

**Fig. 15.1** Triage of acute back pain

# Shoulder problems

## History

- *Pain and stiffness* Joint pain is felt anteriorly and may radiate down the arm; pain on top of the shoulder suggests acromioclavicular joint problems or cervical spine disorders. ❶ Pain in the shoulder may be referred from the neck, heart, mediastinum, or diaphragm.
- *Deformity* Swelling of the shoulder; prominence of the acromioclavicular (AC) joint; winging of the scapula
- *Loss of function* Difficulty reaching behind back, e.g. doing up bra strap), brushing hair, or dressing.

## Examination

- *Look* Posture; asymmetry; muscle wasting; swelling (large effusions can be seen anteriorly); scars.
- *Feel* Tenderness; warmth; swelling; crepitus.
- *Move/measure* Compare sides. Check—range of movement; complex movements (e.g scratching opposite scapula in 3 ways, hands behind head, arm across front of chest to top of opposite shoulder); power.

*General rules* Intra-articular disease—painful limitation of movement in all directions; tendonitis—painful limitation of movement in one plane only; tendon rupture or neurological lesions—painless weakness.

### ⚠ Red flags

- Past history of carcinoma
- Constitutional symptoms, e.g. fever, chills, or unexplained weight ↓
- Recent bacterial infection
- IV drug use
- Immune suppression
- Constant/worsening rest pain
- Structural deformity

## Causes of a stiff painful shoulder joint

- Adhesive capsulitis—1°or 2° to DM or intrathoracic pathology.
- Inflammation—inflammatory arthritis (e.g. RA, psoriatic), infection.
- Osteoarthritis.
- Prolonged immobilization, e.g. hemiplegia, strapping after dislocation.
- Polymyalgia rheumatica.

**Shoulder OA** Often occurs after a history of trauma. Less common than knee or hip OA. Often associated with crystal-induced inflammation and 2° causes of OA (e.g. gout, haemachromatosis). Imaging for synovitis (USS/MRI) is important to rule out disease that may benefit from steroid injection. Shoulder replacement may be considered in severe cases.

**Frozen shoulder (adhesive capsulitis)** Overdiagnosed in primary care. Affects patients aged 40–60y. Painful stiff shoulder with global limitation of movement—notably external rotation. Pain is often worse at night. Cause unknown but ↑ in diabetics and those with intra-thoracic pathology (MI, lung disease) or neck disease.

*Management* If not known to be diabetic, check fasting blood glucose. NSAIDs, physiotherapy and local steroid injection can all be helpful. May take >1y to recover and long-term outcome is uncertain. If restricted movements are slow to return, consider orthopaedic referral.

**Rotator cuff injury** The shoulder is the most mobile joint in the body and relies on the musculo-tendinous rotator cuff to maintain stability. Disorders of the rotator cuff account for most shoulder pain.

- *Acute tendinitis* Often caused by excessive use/trauma in patients <40y. Presents with severe pain in the upper arm. Patients hold the arm immobile and are unable to lie on the affected side. Usually starts to resolve spontaneously after a few days. In middle age can be caused by inflammation around calcific deposits—requires steroid injection.
- *Rotator cuff tears* May accompany subacromial impingement pain and is difficult to diagnose clinically unless the tear is large—suspect if impingement pain is recurrent. Refer.
- *Subacromial impingement* Pain occurs in a limited arc of abduction (60–120° *painful arc syndrome*) or on internal rotation due to acromial or ligament pressure on a damaged rotator cuff tendon. In patients <40y, associated with glenohumeral instability from generalized connective tissue laxity, or labral injury. In older patients, often due to chronic rotator cuff tendinitis or functional cuff weakness/tear.

**Investigations** X-ray may show calcification of the supraspinatus tendon in acute tendinitis and irregularities/cysts at humeral greater tuberosity if chronic cuff tendinitis.

**Treatment** Rest followed by mobilization and physiotherapy, NSAIDs and/or subacromial steroid injection (🕮 p.168). If conservative measures fail, refer for imaging, arthroscopy, and consideration for surgery.

**Shoulder dislocation** Usually due to fall on arm or shoulder—anterior dislocation is most common. Shoulder contour is lost (flattening of deltoid) and the head of the humerus is seen as an anterior bulge. Axillary nerve may be damaged → absent sensation on a patch below the shoulder. Refer to A&E for X-ray and reduction. ~30% of young patients have recurrent dislocations afterwards due to labral tear. Dislocation is associated with rotator cuff tear in ~25% of elderly patients.

**Recurrent dislocation** Usually anterior and follows trauma—but 5% recurrent dislocations are in teenagers with no trauma but general joint laxity. Refer for specialist physiotherapy and consideration of surgery.

**Acromioclavicular joint problems** Pain on the top of the shoulder or in the suprascapular area suggests a problem with the AC joint or neck. AC joint pain is usually due to trauma or OA—joint tenderness and pain are present on palpation and passive horizontal adduction. *Management:* NSAIDs ± local steroid injection.

**Fractured clavicle** 🕮 p.1107

**Cleido-cranial dysostosis** Inherited autosomal dominant condition. Part/all of the clavicle is missing and ossification of the skull is delayed—sutures remain open. Associated with short stature. No treatment.

**Rupture of the long head of biceps** Discomfort in arm on lifting and a feeling of 'something going'. A lump appears in the body of biceps muscle on elbow flexion. May be associated with other shoulder pathology. *Management:* exclude distal rupture of the tendon at the elbow. Reassure. No treatment necessary.

# Elbow problems

## History

- *Pain and stiffness* Joint pain is diffuse; pain well localized over the medial or lateral epicondyles may be due to tendinitis.
- *Deformity* Swelling? Nodules? Structural deformity?
- *Loss of function* May be limitation of flexion, extension, pronation, and/or supination. This can affect function, e.g. causing difficulty eating (cannot get hand to mouth) or with personal care.
- *Neurology* Numbness and paraethesiae distal to the elbow—particularly in the ulnar nerve distribution.

## Examination

- *Look* Carrying angle (~ 11° for ♂; 13° for ♀). Effusion may be visible either side of the olecranon. A discrete swelling over the olecranon could be RA nodule, gouty tophus, olecranon bursa, or other nodule. Check for muscle wasting.
- *Feel* Tenderness? Swellings? Warmth? If indicated test neurology and check pulses distal to the elbow.
- *Move* Active and passive movements. Compare both sides. Normal range is from 0° in full extension to 145° in full flexion. Check pronation/supination. Normal ranges are 75° and 80°, respectively.

## Tennis elbow and golfer's elbow (epicondylitis)

- *Tennis elbow* Tenderness over the lateral epicondyle and lateral elbow pain on resisted wrist extension.
- *Golfer's elbow* Tenderness over the medial epicondyle and medial elbow pain on resisted wrist pronation.

Common extensor tendon inflammation at the epicondyle. *Cause:* repeated strain. *Management:* stop trigger movements if possible. Often settles with time ± NSAIDs. Recovery is speeded by local steroid injection (📖 p.168). Physiotherapy may help, as may an epicondylar clasp.

**Dislocated elbow** Usually due to fall on outstretched hand with flexed elbow. Ulna is displaced backwards, elbow is swollen, and held in fixed flexion. May have associated fracture. Refer to A&E for reduction.

**Olecranon bursitis** Traumatic bursitis due to repeated pressure on the elbow. Pain and swelling over olecranon. Aspirate fluid from bursa—send for microscopy to exclude sepsis and gout (request polarized light microscopy). Fluid may reaccumulate—if sepsis has been excluded, inject hydrocortisone to help it settle. Refer septic bursitis for drainage.

**Ulnar neuritis** Narrowing of the ulnar grove (from OA, RA, or post fracture) causes pressure on the ulnar nerve → ulnar neuropathy. Clumsiness with the hand is often the first symptom, then weakness ± wasting of hand muscles innervated by the ulnar nerve and ↓ sensation in the little finger and medial half of ring finger. Rule out metabolic and autoimmune causes of a mononeuritis and refer for consideration of surgical decompression ± nerve conduction studies if entrapment is likely.

## Further information for patients

**Arthritis Research Campaign** ☎ 0870 850 5000 🖥 www.arc.org.uk

**Pulled elbow** Common in children <5y. Traction injury to elbow causes subluxation of radial head. Often occurs when the child is pulled up suddenly by the hand. Child will not use the arm. No clinical signs. ♂ > ♀. Left arm > right. X-rays are unhelpful.

*Management* Apply anterior pressure with the thumb on the radial head whilst supinating and extending the forearm. Immediate recovery is seen after reduction.

# Wrist and hand problems

## History
### Wrist
- *Pain/stiffness* Pain is often well localized in the wrist. Five conditions are associated with point tenderness: de Quervain's disease; old scaphoid fracture; carpometacarpal OA; Kienbock's disease (avascular necrosis of the lunate); tenosynovitis of the extensors. Wrist pain may also be associated with RA, OA, ganglia. Carpal tunnel syndrome is associated with pain in the hand.
- *Deformity* May be swelling of tendon sheaths or wrist. Bony deformity is a late feature of arthritis or secondary to trauma.
- *Function* Ask about weakness and numbness in the hand.

### Hand
- *Pain/stiffness* Pain from the hand is felt in the fingers and/or palm. A diffuse ache may be referred from the neck, shoulder, or mediastinum.
- *Deformity* May occur acutely, e.g. due to tendon rupture or slowly due to bone or joint pathology. The pattern and symmetry of joint involvement can be diagnostic.
- *Function* Good hand function is essential for everyday tasks, e.g. turning keys, doing buttons up, writing. Ask about limitations.

## Examination
### Wrist
- *Look* Symmetry; swelling; deformity (ulnar deviation, volar subluxation; rheumatoid nodules; ganglia); muscle wasting in forearm/hand.
- *Feel* Temperature; nature of any swellings; tenderness of the radiocarpal, midcarpal or distal radio-ulnar joint.
- *Move/measure* Range of movement (normal range: extension >75°, flexion >75°, pronation >75° from the vertical, supination >80° from the vertical); crepitation?
- *Neurology* Check for ulnar and median nerve function.

### Hand
- *Look* Posture of the hand; swellings (rheumatoid nodules; Heberden's and Bouchard's nodes; ganglions; tophi); nail signs, e.g. pitting of psoriasis; scars; deformity (mallet finger; swan-neck deformity; boutonnière deformity; Dupytren's contracture); ulnar deviation. If there is joint disease note distribution and whether it is symmetrical.
- *Feel* Temperature; condition of the skin, e.g. dryness, sweating; nature of swellings; muscle bulk, e.g. small muscles of the hand; tenderness.
- *Move/measure* Ask the patient to make a fist, spread his/her fingers out and then test each individual joint. Then test opposition, pinch grip, key grip, palmar grasp of ball, and practical tasks (e.g. picking up a coin).

## Fractures 📖 p.1106

**Ganglion** Smooth, firm, painless swelling—usually around the wrist. No treatment is needed unless causing local problems. May resolve spontaneously; can be drained (large bore needle)/excised, but often recurs.

**For all hand injuries** Check for:

**Nerve injury** Can occur due to trauma or lacerations of the hand or wrist. Examine sensory and motor function. Always ensure no other structures are damaged before suturing skin wounds. Refer all nerve injuries for specialist assessment and management—surgery can improve the outcome considerably in some cases. Intensive hand physiotherapy is important to regain function. *Types of nerve injury:*

• **Neurapraxia** Temporary loss of nerve conduction— often caused by pressure causing ischaemia.
• **Axonotmesis** Damage to the nerve fibre but the nerve tube is intact— the chance of successful nerve regrowth and a good recovery is high.
• **Neurotmesis** Divided nerve —lack of guidance to the regrowing fibrils gives less chance of a good recovery and a neuroma may develop.

**Median nerve damage** The median nerve controls grasp. Damage causes inability to lift the thumb out of the plane of the palm (abductor pollicus brevis failure) and loss of sensation over the lateral side of the hand.

**Ulnar nerve damage** Injury distal to the wrist causes a claw hand deformity, loss of abduction/adduction of the fingers, and sensory loss over the little finger and a variable area of the ring finger.

**Radial nerve damage** The radial nerve opens the fist—injury produces wrist-drop and variable sensory loss including the dorsal aspect of the root of the thumb.

**Tendon injury** Can occur due to attrition or lacerations of the hand or wrist. Examine hand function. Always ensure no other structures are damaged before suturing skin wounds. Extensor or flexor tendons can be affected. Refer—primary surgical repair is usually the treatment of choice.

**Vascular injury** Can occur due to trauma/lacerations of the hand or wrist. Check perfusion and temperature of fingers and examine pulses. Ensure no other structures are damaged before suturing skin wounds. Refer all vascular injuries for specialist assessment and management.

**Work-related upper limb pain** Work-related pain in the arm ± wrist, e.g. due to keyboard use. Over-use syndrome. Often termed repetitive strain injury (RSI). Diagnosis of exclusion—no physical signs. Exclude other conditions, e.g. carpal tunnel syndrome (CTS), tennis elbow.

**Management** Reassure—condition is curable. Continue work but avoid the aggravating activity; liaise with work to ensure evaluation of workstation ergonomics. Gradually reintroduce activity. Physiotherapy may help. Explore psychological and work-related issues. A multidisciplinary approach is needed. ❶ Work-related upper limb pain is a notifiable industrial disease.

☛ Existence of RSI has been challenged—rigorous assessment often reveals undiagnosed causes. A country's compensation system has a great effect on the reporting of RSI.

**Reflex sympathetic dystrophy** (algodystrophy, complex regional pain disorder). Pain ± vasomotor changes in a limb → loss of function. Most common in the hand and wrist. Usually follows trauma—but the trauma may be trivial and signs may appear weeks/months later. *Signs:* pain at rest exacerbated by movement and light touch, swelling, discolouration, temperature changes, abnormal sensitivity, sweating, and loss of function. X-ray may show osteopoenia.

**Management** Physiotherapy improves prognosis if started early, analgesia (NSAIDs). Refer to pain clinic and/or rheumatology for IV bisphosphonates (responds well if treated early) and 'mirror' therapy.

**Tenosynovitis** Inflammation of the tendon sheath—often due to unaccustomed activity (e.g. gardening). May affect extensor or flexor tendons. Pain is often worse in the morning. Presents with swelling and tenderness over the tendon sheath and pain on using the tendon. Treat with rest and NSAIDs. If not settling, an injection of steroid into the tendon sheath may help. ❶ Notifiable industrial disease if work related

**De Quervain tenosynovitis** Tenosynovitis of thumb extensor and abductor tendon sheaths. Pain over radial styloid and on forced adduction/flexion of the thumb. Treat with thumb splint ± local steroid injection. Refer if not settling. *F. de Quervain (1868–1940)—Swiss surgeon.*

**Carpal tunnel syndrome** Pain in the radial 3½ digits of the hand ± numbness, pins and needles, and thenar wasting. Due to compression of the median nerve as it passes under the flexor retinaculum. Worse at night. Symptoms are improved by shaking the wrist. *Associations:* pregnancy, hypothyroidism, obesity, and carpal arthritis.

**Investigations** Phalen's test—hyperflexion of wrist for 1min triggers symptoms; Tinel's test—tapping over the carpal tunnel causes paraesthesiae; request nerve conduction studies if diagnosis is in doubt.

**Management** GP treatment—night splints may help ± carpal tunnel steroid injection (📖 p.168). Less likely to help if age >50y or symptoms >10mo. If GP treatment fails, constant paraesthesiae and/or triggering of fingers, refer to orthopaedics for division of the flexor retinaculum.

**Kienböck's disease** The lunate bone develops patchy necrosis after acute or chronic injury. Patient is usually a young adult complaining of aching and stiffness of 1 wrist. *Examination:* tenderness in the centre of the back of the wrist ± limitation of wrist extension. X-ray is normal at first but later shows ↑ density of the lunate ± deformity. Refer for orthopaedic opinion. *R. Kienböck (1871–1953)—Austrian radiologist.*

**Osteoarthritis in the hand**
• Heberden's nodes—swellings of DIP joints. No treatment needed.
• Bouchard's nodes—swellings of PIP joints. No treatment needed.

**First carpometacarpal OA** Pain and swelling at the base of the thumb. Thumb becomes stiff. A splint or steroid injection can be helpful. If pain persists surgery may help.

**Dupuytren's contracture** Palmar fascia contracts so that the fingers (typically the right fifth finger) cannot extend. *Prevalence*: 10% ♂ > 65y (more if family history). Less common in women. *Associations*: smoking, alcohol, heavy manual labour, trauma, DM, phenytoin, Peyronie's disease, AIDS. Often simple reassurance suffices. Ultimately surgery may be needed. G. Dupuytren (1777–1835)—French surgeon.

**Trigger finger** Nodules on the tendon can occur spontaneously and in RA and DM. Most common in ring and middle fingers. The nodule can be palpated moving with the tendon. Pain and triggering (the finger is in fixed flexion and needs to be flicked straight by the other hand) occur because the nodule jams in the tendon sheath. *Management*: local steroid injection or surgery.

**Mallet finger** The finger tip droops due to avulsion of the extensor tendon attachment to the terminal phalanx (Figure 15.2). Refer for X-ray. *Management*: a plastic splint which holds the terminal phalanx in extension is worn for 6wk to help union (it must not be removed). Arthrodesis may be needed if healing does not occur.

**Gamekeeper's thumb** Forced thumb abduction causes rupture of the ulnar collateral ligament. Can occur on wringing a pheasant's neck—hence the name—or, more commonly, by catching the thumb in the matting on a dry ski slope. The thumb is very painful and pincer grip is weak. Refer—open surgical repair is the most effective treatment.

### Nail injuries

***Avulsed nail*** Protect the nail bed of an avulsed nail with soft paraffin and gauze, check tetanus status, and give antibiotic prophylaxis (e.g. flucloxacillin 250mg qds for 5d). Partially avulsed nails need removing under ring block to exclude an underlying nail bed injury—the nail is replaced to act as a splint to the nail matrix.

***Subungual haematoma*** A blow to the finger can cause bleeding under the nail—very painful due to pressure build up. Relieve by trephining a hole through the nail using a 19 gauge needle (no force required just twist the needle as it rests vertically on the nail) or a heated point (e.g. of a paper clip or cautery instrument). Of benefit up to 2d after injury.

---

**Polydactyly** Extra digits can vary from small fleshy tags to complete duplications. They may be an isolated defect or associated with syndromes. Small fleshy tags are removed in the first few months. For extra digits firmly fixed or involving tendons or joints, surgery is delayed until the child is >1y. Refer to orthopaedics or plastic surgery.

**Syndactyly** Digits may be joined by a web of skin or more firmly fused. Webbing is usually mild and treatment is for cosmetic reasons if at all. Where digits are fused, separation and skin grafting is carried out at ~4y. Refer to plastic surgery.

---

**Further information for patients**
**Arthritis Research Campaign** ☎ 0870 850 5000 🖥 www.arc.org.uk

# Hip and pelvis problems

**History** Pain on walking? Pain at rest? Hip joint pain is usually felt in the groin (Table 15.4). Referred pain is often felt in the knee. Hip disease results in ↓ walking distance, difficulty climbing stairs and getting out of low chairs

## Examination
- *Look* Watch the patient walk: hip disease → limp or waddling gait.
- *Feel* Joint tenderness is just distal to the midpoint of the inguinal ligament..
- *Move* Passive movement with the patient lying supine. Check range of movement. Pain reproduced on movement? Crepitus?
- *Measure* Hip disease is often associated with shortening of the affected leg—true leg length anterior superior iliac spine → medial malleolus; apparent leg length umbilicus → medial malleolus
- *Trendelenburg test* Ask the patient to stand on one leg and lift the foot on the contralateral side off the ground. Place your fingers on the anterior superior iliac spines. If the pelvis sags on the unsupported side (+ve Trendelenburg sign), the hip on which the patient is standing is painful or has a weak/mechanically disadvantaged gluteus medius. ❶ false +ve in 10%.

**Malignancy** Hip and pelvis are common sites for 2° malignancy. Pain is severe and unremitting, day and night. Often accompanied by weight loss. X-ray may show no abnormalities or reveal lytic or sclerotic deposits. Bone scan is diagnostic but may miss myeloma. Depending on clinical circumstances, either refer for specialist advice (oncologist, radiotherapist) or palliative care. Treat with analgesia meanwhile. High risk of pathological fracture.

**Osteoarthritis of the hip** Major cause of hip pain and disability. Incidence ↑ with age; ♂ ≈ ♀. *Predisposing factors*: past hip disease (e.g. Perthes' disease) or trauma; unequal leg length.

*Presentation* Pain may be diffuse and felt in hip region, thigh or knee. Relieved by rest in early stages of disease. *Signs*: ↓ internal rotation and abduction of hip with pain at extremes of movement; antalgic gait; eventually fixed flexion of the hip. *Investigation*: X-ray may confirm diagnosis but is often not needed. There is poor correlation between X-ray changes and pain felt.

*Management* Analgesia (e.g. regular paracetamol, NSAIDs), education, weight ↓, exercise, correction of unequal leg length. Walking stick ± shock-absorbing shoe insoles can help. Consider referral for physiotherapy (muscle strengthening exercises may ↓ pain) or to orthopaedics for consideration of hip resurfacing or replacement.

*Total hip replacement* >90% achieve good result. Most last 10–15y. *Post-op care*: risk of dislocation in first 6wk—advise to avoid crossing legs, take care with transfers, use a walking stick, no driving for 6wk. Physiotherapy is usually arranged via secondary care.

**Table 15.4** Causes of pain around the hip

| Pain | Causes |
|------|--------|
| Buttock pain | PMR, sacroilitis, vascular insufficiency, referred from back |
| Groin pain | Hip joint disease (OA, RA, Paget's, osteomalacia), fracture, osteitis pubis, hernia, psoas abscess |
| Lateral thigh pain | Trochanteric bursitis, referred pain from back, enthesitis (spondyloarthropathies), gluteus medius tear, meralgia paraesthetica, fascia lata syndrome |

---

### General advice for patients with hip osteoarthritis

- Sit in a partially reclined position when relaxing.
- Stand with weight equally distributed between both legs.
- Lift and carry weight close to the body.
- Sleep on the unaffected side with a large pillow between the knees.
- Keep your weight down.
- Exercise regularly, e.g. swimming with crawl kick (legs kept straight).
- Avoid extremes of hip motion.
- Minimize jarring and high-impact activities, e.g. contact sports like football or 'stop-and-go' sports like tennis.

**Self-help exercises ❶** It may help to have a warm bath or to apply a heat pad to the affected hip before doing these exercises.

**Knee–chest pulls** Lie on your back. Bend your hip and knee to 90°. Hold your upper shin and gently pull your knee towards your chest. Hold this position for 5 seconds and then relax back to 90°. Repeat 15–20 times every day.

**Figure-of-four stretch** Still lying on your back, put your foot beside your other knee. Gently rock your flexed knee outwards. Repeat 15–20 times each day. The higher the foot is raised, the greater the stretch.

**Straight-leg raises (strengthening the hip flexors)** Still lying on your back, bend one leg. Keep the opposite leg straight and raise it 5–10cm (3–4 inches) off the bed and hold it there for 5 seconds. Do this 15–20 times with each leg every day.

**Leg extensions (strengthening the gluteals)** Turn over onto your tummy. Raise one leg 5–10cm (3–4 inches) up off the bed and hold it there for 5 seconds. Repeat 15–20 times for each leg every day.

❶ If any of these exercises causes pain, stop and consult your doctor or physiotherapist before doing that exercise again.

⚠ These exercises are NOT suitable for patients who have had a hip replacement.

**Hip dislocation** Occurs in front seat passengers in car accidents as the knee strikes the dashboard. Reduction under anaesthetic is required.

**Greater trochanter pain (trochanteric bursitis)** Can mimic ± coexist with hip OA. May be associated with muscle weakness around the hip. *Diagnosis:* Point tenderness over the greater trochanter.

**Management** Consider local steroid injection if trochanteric bursitis is likely—though most cases are due to referred back pain. Refer to physiotherapy for exercises to strengthen hip musculature to prevent recurrence or for treatment of back problems if causing the pain.

**Fascia lata syndrome** Inflammation of the fascia lata causing pain in the lateral thigh. Often due to over-use or weak musculature around the hip. Treatment is with rest ± referral to physiotherapy.

**Hip infection** Presents with hip pain, ↓ weight, night sweats, and rigors. Be aware of infection in patients with RA, hip prosthesis, or immunocompromise. Refer for investigation. X-rays are often unhelpful—bone scan is non-specific. Admit for US-guided drainage, bed rest, and IV antibiotics.

**Avascular necrosis** May present with hip pain. Have a high level of suspicion in patients with risk factors—SLE, sickle cell disease, high alcohol consumption, pregnancy, or corticosteroids. X-ray or bone scan may confirm diagnosis but MRI is most sensitive. Specialist management is needed. Usually progresses to cause OA.

**Pubic symphysis dehiscence** Painful condition occuring in late pregnancy which may persist after delivery. The pubic symphysis separates, resulting in low abdominal pain which may be accompanied by low back pain and radiate down both thighs. Pain is constant and worse on movement. It resolves on rest. Examination reveals a soft abdomen, and obstetric examination is normal. Advise simple analgesia (paracetamol 1g qds). Rest in a semi-recumbent position when in pain. Refer for physiotherapy (especially if still a problem in the puerperium). Most resolve spontaneously within several months of delivery. Some persist and need specialist referral.

### Further information for patients
**Arthritis Research Campaign (ARC)** ☎ 0870 850 5000 🖥 www.arc.org.uk
**Steps** Support for patients with lower limb conditions and their families ☎ 01925 750271 🖥 www.steps-charity.org.uk

**The limping child**
- If a child is limping, take it seriously. Look for a problem.
- Children find it difficult to localize pain. Pain can be referred from the hip to the knee. Examine the whole limb carefully.
- Other causes of referred pain include spinal pathology, psoas spasm from GI pathology (e.g. appendicitis).
- Limping without pain is uncommon and may be due to undiagnosed congenital hip dislocation (📖 p.852).
- Do not forget local causes such as minor foot injuries, plantar foreign bodies and verrucae.

**Transient synovitis of the hip (irritable hip)** The most common reason for limping in childhood. *Peak age:* 2–10y. ♂ > ♀. The child is usually well, but complains of pain in the hip or knee and may refuse to weight-bear. Often occurs after a viral infection. Cause is unknown. Exclude septic arthritis—refer to orthopaedics. Usually resolves in 7–10d without treatment.

**Perthes' disease** Pain in the hip or knee; limp and limited hip movement developing over ~1mo. Due to avascular necrosis of the femoral head. Bilateral in 10%. *Peak age:* 4–7y (range 3–11y). ♂:♀ ≈ 4:1.

***Management*** If suspected refer for X-ray and to orthopaedics. Treatment is with rest, X-ray surveillance, bracing, and/or surgery depending on severity. Usually heals over 2–3y. Joint damage may cause early arthritis. Risk factors for poor outcome include:
- ♀
- Onset >8y
- Involvement of the whole femoral head
- Pronounced metaphyseal rarefaction
- Lateral displacement of the femoral head.

*G.C. Perthes (1869–1927)— German surgeon.*

**Slipped upper femoral epiphysis** The upper femoral epiphysis slips with respect to the femur, usually in a postero-inferior direction. Bilateral in 20%. *Incidence:* 1:100 000. *Peak age:* 10–15y. ♂:♀ ≈ 3:1. Typically affects obese underdeveloped children or tall thin boys.

***Presentation*** Pain at rest in the groin, hip, thigh, or referred to the knee; limp, and/or pain on movement; ↓ hip movements—particularly abduction and medial rotation. The affected leg may be externally rotated and shortened.

***Management*** Confirm diagnosis on X-ray (include lateral views)—shows backwards and downwards slippage of the epiphysis. Refer to orthopaedics—surgical pinning or reconstructive surgery is needed. Monitoring of the other hip is essential. Complications include avascular necrosis, coxa vara, early OA, slipped epiphysis on the contralateral side.

**Congenital dislocation/developmental dysplasia of the hip** 📖 p.852

# Knee problems

## History
- *Trauma* History of injury—ask about degree and direction of force.
- *Pain/stiffness* Attempt to distinguish well-localized mechanical pain and diffuse inflammatory/degenerative pain.
- *Deformity* Swelling? If injury, time of onset of swelling in relation to history (immediate effusion suggests haemarthrosis; post-traumatic effusions appear later). Knock knees or bow legs?
- *Function* Does the knee problem prevent any activities? How far can the patient walk? Can he/she manage stairs? Does the knee click? If so, when? Does the knee lock? If so, in what position? What provokes locking and how is it relieved? Does the knee give way? If so, when (e.g. when going downstairs, when walking on uneven ground)?

## Examination Always compare the two knees.
- *Look* Watch the patient walk. Look at the knees whilst standing—?varus/valgus deformity. Ask the patient to lie down. Note quadriceps wasting, scars, skin changes, swelling, and deformity. A space under the knee viewed laterally suggests a fixed flexion deformity. With legs extended, lift both feet off the bed to demonstrate hyperextension.
- *Feel* the quadriceps for wasting and palpate the knee for warmth. Check the joint line, collateral ligaments, tibial tubercle, and femoral epicondyles for tenderness. Palpate the popliteal fossa for Baker's cyst. Check for an effusion. Test for patellofemoral lesions by sliding the patella sideways across the underlying femoral condyles.
- *Move* With the patient lying on his/her back check active and passive range of movement. Pain reproduced on movement? Crepitus? Test the medial and lateral collateral ligaments and cruciate ligaments.
- *Measure* quadriceps diameter 18cm up from the joint line in adults.

❶ Knee pain can be referred from the hip, so examine the hip as well.

## Non-traumatic knee effusion Common causes:
- Gout.
- RA.
- Calcium pyrophosphate dihydrate disease (pseudo-gout).
- Spondylarthropathies (includes reactive arthritis).

## Investigation
- Blood: consider FBC, ESR, rheumatoid factor, anti-nuclear antibody, LFTs, bone biochemistry, and thyroid function tests.
- Drain effusion (or refer to rheumatology to drain) and send fluid for polarized light miscroscopy (for crystals) and microbiology (?infection).

## Management
- If no infection inject with long-acting steroid (□ p.166), immobilize, and advise no weight-bearing for 48h.
- Refer to rheumatology.

**Hypermobility** Occurs in children or young adults with lax joints. <½ are symptomatic. Those who have symptoms present with recurrent joint pains—mainly affecting the knees. Other symptoms include joint effusion, dislocation, ligamentous injuries, low back pain, and premature osteoarthritis. The condition is benign, and joints become stiffer with age. Treatment, when needed, is with physiotherapy. Rarely, associated with congenital disorders, e.g. Ehlers–Danlos syndrome.

**Osteoarthritis of the knee** Very common. X-ray evidence of OA is even more common. *Treatment:* education; glucosamine; analgesia (paracetamol ± NSAIDs); exercise (refer to physiotherapy). Suggest using a walking stick. Steroid injection can be helpful in some patients. If pain and disability are severe refer to orthopaedics for consideration of total or partial knee replacement. Knee replacement is a very successful procedure resulting in ↓ pain and ↑ mobility. 95% prostheses last 10y.

**Infection of the knee joint** Most commonly infected joint. *Signs:* hot, red, swollen, and painful knee. *Differential diagnosis:* Reiter's disease, gout, pseudo-gout, traumatic effusion, RA. If infection is suspected refer as an emergency to rheumatology or orthopaedics for investigation. ❶ Don't give antibiotics until the joint has been aspirated.

**Bipartite patella** Detected on X-ray. Usually asymptomatic incidental finding but can cause pain due to excessive mobility of a patella fragment. If troublesome refer for fragment excision.

> **Chondromalacia patellae** Common in teenage girls. Pain on walking up or down stairs or on prolonged sitting. *Signs:* pain on stressing the undersurface of the patella. Arthroscopy (indicated only in severe cases) reveals degenerative cartilage on the posterior surface of the patella. Treat with analgesia + physiotherapy (vastus medialis strengthening relieves pain in 80%). For persistent cases, exclude spondylarthropathy (enthesitis pain—📖 p.526) and refer to orthopaedics for arthroscopy.

**Osgood–Schlatter disease** Seen in athletic teenagers. Pain and tenderness ± swelling over the tibial tubercle. X-rays not required. Avoid aggravating activities. Usually settles over a few months. If not settling, refer to orthopaedics or rheumatology for further assessment. *R.B. Osgood (1873–1956)—US orthopaedic surgeon; C.B. Schlatter (1864–1934)—Swiss physician.*

## Bow legs and knock knees in children

- *Genu varum (bow legs)* Outward curving of the tibia usually associated with internal tibial torsion. Except in severe cases always resolves spontaneously. Severe cases raise the possibility of rickets or other rare developmental disorders—refer for orthopaedic opinion.
- *Genu valgum (knock knees)* Common amongst 2–4y olds. Innocent if symmetrical and independent of any other abnormality. Severe progressive cases suggest rickets—refer for X-ray.

**Patellar dislocation** Lateral dislocation of the patella and tearing of the medial capsule/quadriceps can occur due to trauma. More common in young people and if joint hypermobility syndrome. Patient is in pain and unable to flex knee. Refer via A&E or orthopaedics for reduction.

**Recurrent subluxation of the patella** Medial knee pain + knee 'gives way' due to lateral subluxation of the patella. Most common in girls with valgus knees. *Associations:* familial, hypermobility, high-riding patella. *Signs:* ↑ lateral patella movement and +ve apprehension test (pain and reflex contraction of quadriceps on lateral patella pressure). Refer to physiotherapy for vastus medialis exercises. If that is unhelpful, refer to rheumatology to exclude a hereditary connective tissue disorder and/or to orthopaedics for consideration of lateral retinacular release.

**Patella tendinitis** Small tear in the patella tendon causes pain. Most commonly seen in athletes. Differential diagnosis includes inferior patellar pole enthesitis (spondylarthropathies), fat-pad syndrome, anterior cartilage lesion and bursitis. Diagnosis is with USS. Treatment is with rest, NSAIDs ± steroid injection around (not into) the tendon.

**Bursitis** Prepatella bursitis (housemaid's knee) is associated with excessive kneeling. Vicar's knee (infrapatella bursitis) is associated with more upright kneeling. Avoid aggravating activity, aspirate ± steroid injection (↓ recurrence). If clinically infected refer to orthopaedics for drainage and antibiotics.

**Baker's cyst** Popliteal cyst (herniation of joint synovium) can cause swelling and discomfort behind the knee. Usually caused by a degenerative knee. Rupture may result in pain and swelling in the calf mimicking DVT. Treat underlying knee synovitis. Surgical cyst removal may be necessary if persistent problems. *W.M. Baker (1839–1896)—British surgeon.*

**Collateral ligament injury** Common in contact sports. Causes knee effusion if severe ± tenderness over the injured ligament. Collateral ligaments provide lateral stability to the knee. Normally there is <5° of movement—if >5° the ligament may be ruptured. Treat with rest, knee support, analgesia. Refer to orthopaedics if rupture is suspected.

**Cruciate ligament injury** Cruciate ligaments provide anterior–posterior knee stability.
- *Anterior cruciate tears* Occur due to a blow to the back of tibia ± rotation when foot is fixed on the ground. *Signs:* effusion and +ve draw test (with the patient supine with foot fixed and knee at 90°, apply pressure to pull the tibia forward—it should be stable; test is +ve if the tibia moves forward on the femur).
- *Posterior cruciate tears* Caused e.g. when the knee hits the dashboard in car accidents. Reverse draw test is +ve (with patient supine and knee at 90°, apply pressure to push tibia backwards—it should be stable; test is +ve if the tibia moves backward on the femur).

*Management* Refer to orthopaedics. Assessment can be difficult—refer if unsure. Plaster cast and then physiotherapy helps most (60%) but some require reconstructive surgery—consider urgent referral if keen sportsman.

**Osteochondritis dissecans** Necrosis of articular cartilage and under-lying bone. Can cause loose body formation. Cause unknown. Seen in young adults → pain after exercise and intermittent knee swelling ± locking. X-ray shows cartilage damage. Predisposes to arthritis. Refer for expert management.

**Meniscal lesions** Twisting with the knee flexed can cause medial (bucket-handle) meniscal tears and adduction with internal rotation can cause lateral cartilage tears. *Symptoms/signs:*
• Locking of the knee—extension is limited due to cartilage fragment lodging between the condyles.
• Giving way of the knee.
• Tender joint line.
• +ve McMurray's test—rotation of the tibia on the femur with flexed knee followed by knee extension causes pain and a click as the trapped cartilage fragment is released—◆ reliability of this test is debated.

*Management* Refer for MRI ± arthroscopy. Treated by removal of the torn meniscal fragment.

**Meniscal cysts** Pain + swelling over the joint line due to a meniscal tear. Lateral cysts are more common than medial. The knee may click and give way. Refer for arthroscopy removal of damaged meniscus relieves pain.

**Loose bodies in the knee** May result in locking of the knee joint in any direction of movement and/or effusion. *Causes:* OA, chip fractures, osteochondritis dissecans, synovial chondromatosis. If problematic refer for removal.

**Iliotibial tract syndrome** Pain due to inflammation of the synovium under the iliotibial tract from rubbing of the tract on the lateral femoral condyle. Seen in runners. Treat with rest, NSAIDs, specialist physiotherapy ± steroid injection.

**Shin splints** Exercise-related shin pain may be due to a stress fracture of the tibia, compartment syndrome, or periostitis. Fractures are not always seen on X-ray—bone scan is more sensitive and shows periostitis. Treat with rest and analgesia. Consider referral to sports physiotherapist.

### Further information for patients
**Hypermobility syndrome association (HMSA)** 🖳 www.hypermobility.org
**Arthritis Research Campaign (ARC)** ☎ 0870 850 5000
🖳 www.arc.org.uk
**Steps** Support for patients with lower limb conditions and their families
☎ 01925 750271 🖳 www.steps-charity.org.uk

# Ankle and foot problems

**History** Trauma; ↑ activity, e.g. walking or running a long way for the patient; feeling of instability; pain/stiffness (relation to weight-bearing; localized/diffuse); deformity (problems getting shoes, shoes wear in odd places or shoes are always uncomfortable); interference with activities.

**Examination** Compare one foot with the other.
- *Look* Watch the patient walk normally and on tiptoe. Look at the foot with the patient seated. Check for deformities, the colour of the foot, and any skin/nail changes. Check the shoes for any abnormal patterns of wear (wear is normally under the ball of the foot medially and posterolaterally at the heel).
- *Feel* Is there any tenderness? Palpate any swellings. Check pulses and skin temperature.
- *Move* Assess active and passive movements of the ankle, subtalar, mid-tarsal, and toe joints systematically. Check range of movement of joints and pain.
- *Neurology* Check sensation if patient reports any loss of sensation.

**Ankle, foot, and toe fracture** 📖 p.1106

**Achilles tendonitis** Inflammation of the Achilles tendon may be related to over-use or a spondylarthropathy. Presents as a painful local swelling of the tendon. Advise rest. NSAIDs, heel padding, physiotherapy ± steroid injection may help (never inject into the tendon). If persistent refer to rheumatology.

**Ruptured Achilles tendon** Presents with a sudden pain in the back of the ankle during activity (felt as a 'kick'). The patient walks with a limp. There is some plantar flexion, but the patient cannot raise the affected heel from the floor when standing on tip toe. A 'gap' can usually be felt in the tendon. Refer immediately for consideration of repair. The alternative is immobilization in plaster with the foot plantar flexed.

**Pes cavus** High foot arches may be idiopathic due to polio, spina bifida, or other neurological conditions. Toes may claw. Padding under the meta-tarsal heads relieves pressure. Operative treatment—soft tissue release or arthrodesis—straightens toes. Can lead to tarsal bone OA causing pain—refer for fusion.

**Foot drop** Patients trip frequently or walk with a high stepping gait. On examination, patients are unable to walk on their heels and cannot dorsi-flex their foot. Check ankle jerk. *Causes:*
- Common peroneal palsy (e.g. due to trauma)—normal ankle jerk.
- Sciatica—ankle jerk absent.
- L4, L5 root lesion—ankle jerk may be absent.
- Peripheral motor neuropathy (e.g. alcoholic)—ankle jerk weak or absent.
- Distal myopathy—ankle jerk weak or absent.
- Motor neuron disease—↑ ankle jerk.

**Club foot (talipes)** Consists of inversion of the foot, adduction of fore foot relative to hindfoot and equinus (plantar flexion).

**Positional talipes** Moulding deformity seen in neonates. The foot can be passively everted and dorsiflexed to the normal position. Treatment is with physiotherapy. Follow up to check the deformity is resolving.

**True talipes** The foot *cannot* be passively everted and dorsiflexed to the normal position. Refer to orthopaedics. Treatment is with physiotherapy, splints ± surgery.

**Flat feet (pes planus)** Low medial arch. All babies and toddlers have flat feet. The arch develops after 2–3y of walking. Persistent flat feet may be familial or due to joint laxity. If pain free, foot is mobile, and the patient develops an arch on standing on tiptoe ('flexible' foot), no action is required. If painful may be helped by analgesia, exercises, or insoles. For severe pain, hind foot fusion is an option. Refer if the arch does not restore on tiptoeing ('rigid').

### In-toe and out-toe gait

- **In-toe** Originates in the femur (persistent anteversion of the femoral neck), tibia (tibial torsion), or tibia (metatarsus varus). Does not cause pain or affect mobility. Usually resolves by age 5–6y.
- **Out-toe** Common <2y. May be unilateral. Corrects spontaneously.

**Sever's disease** Apophysitis of the heel. Peak age: 8–13y. Treated with analgesia, raising the heel of the shoe a little, calf-stretching, and avoiding strenuous activities for a few weeks.

**Osteochondritis** Table 15.5

**Syndactyly and polydactyly** p.495

**Table 15.5** Osteochondritis of the foot in children and young adults

| | Bone(s) involved | Features | Treatment |
|---|---|---|---|
| Kohler's disease | Navicular bone | Peak age: 3–5y. Presents with pain and tenderness over the dorsum of the mid-foot. X-ray—small navicular bone of ↑ density | Pain usually resolves with simple analgesia and rest |
| Freiberg's disease | Second and third metatarsal heads | Most common in teenagers and young adults. ♀ > ♂. Presents with pain in the foot on walking; the head of the metatarsal is palpable and tender. X-ray shows a wide flat metatarsal | Treatment is usually conservative with cushioning of shoes and simple analgesia. If severe refer to orthopaedics. Excision of the metatarsal head may relieve pain |

**Tender heel pad** Dull throbbing pain under the heel. Develops a few months after heel trauma. May be due to plantar fasciitis, bursitis, or tendonitis. Treat with rest and heel padding. Refer to physiotherapy— ultrasound treatment can help. Blind steroid injections into the fat pad are not recommended. In persistent cases refer to rheumatology.

**Plantar fasciitis/bursitis** Common cause of inferior heel pain, especially amongst runners. Pain is worst when taking the first few steps after getting out of bed. Usually unilateral and generally settles in <6wk Advise shoes with arch support, soft heels, and heel padding (e.g. trainers). Achilles tendon stretching exercises can help, NSAIDs, and steroid injection are also helpful. In persistent cases refer to podiatry (for fitting of an in-sole) ± orthopaedics.

**Metatarsalgia (forefoot pain)** May be due to synovitis, stress fractures, sesamoid fracture, injury, or ↑ pressure on the metatarsal heads due to mechanical dysfunction (e.g. in RA) Treat with insoles and padding under the metatarsal heads. Surgery may be helpful in RA—discuss with rheumatologist.

**Morton's metatarsalgia (interdigital neuroma)** Pain due to entrapment of the interdigital nerve between the 3rd/4th metatarsal heads. Gradual onset of sudden attacks of pain or paraesthesia during walking. Refer to orthopaedics.Treatment is with steroid injection and advice re footwear. Some need surgical excision of the neuroma. *T.G Morton (1835–1903)—US surgeon.*

**Hammer and claw toes** (Figure 15.2)
- *Hammer toes* Extended MTP joint, hyperflexed PIP joint, and extended DIP joint. Most common in 2nd toes.
- *Claw toes* Extended MTP joint, flexion at PIP and DIP joints. Due to imbalance of extensors and flexors (e.g. after polio).

If causing pain or difficulty with walking/foot wear refer for surgery.

**Hallux valgus (bunion)** Lateral deviation of the big toe at the MTP joint exacerbated by wearing pointed shoes ± high heels. A bunion develops where the MTP joint rubs on footwear. Arthritis at the MTP joint is common. Bunion pads can help, but severe deformity requires surgery.

**Hallus rigidus** Arthritis at 1st MTP joint causes a stiff painful big toe. Refer severe cases to podiatrist or orthotist for offloading or custom-made rocker-bottom foot orthoses. Resistant pain requires surgery.

**Ingrowing toe nail** Most common in the big toe. Ill-fitting shoes and poor nail cutting predispose to the nail growing into the toe skin → pain. The inflamed tissue is prone to infection. Advise re cutting nails (cut straight with edges beyond the flesh). Refer to podiatry. Treat infection with antibiotics (e.g. flucloxacillin 250–500mg qds). If recurrent infection consider referral for surgery (e.g. wedge resection of the nail).

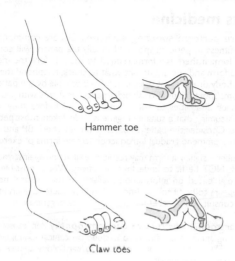

Fig. 15.2 Hammer and claw toes

Reproduced from Davies R, Everitt H, and Simon C *Musculoskeletal Problems* (2006) with permission from Oxford University Press.

### Achilles tendon stretching exercises

*Towel stretch* Sit on the floor with your legs stretched out in front of you. Loop a towel around the top of the injured foot. Slowly pull the towel towards you keeping your body straight. Hold for 15–30 seconds, then relax—repeat 10×.

*Calf/Achilles stretch* Stand facing a wall. Place your hands on the wall chest high. Move the injured heel back and with the foot flat on the floor. Move the other leg forward and slowly lean toward the wall until you feel a gentle stretch through the calf. Hold for 15–20 seconds and repeat.

*Stair stretch* Stand on a step on the balls for your feet; hold the rail or wall for balance. Slowly lower the heel of the injured foot to gently stretch the arch of your foot for 15–20 seconds.

*Toe stretch* Sit on the floor with knee bent. Pull the toes back on the injured foot until stretch across the arch is felt. Hold for 15–20 seconds and repeat.

*Frozen can roll* Roll your bare injured foot back and forth from the tip of the toes to the heel over a frozen juice can (not fizzy) or small plastic water bottle. This is a good exercise after activity because it both stretches the plantar fascia and provides cold therapy to the injured area.

### Further information

**Bandolier** Ruptured Achilles tendons—systematic review (2002)
🖳 www.medicine.ox.ac.uk/bandolier/band103/b103-5.html

### Information for patients

**British Orthopaedic Foot Surgery Society** 🖳 www.bofss.org.uk

# Sports medicine

**Fitness to perform sporting activities** GPs are commonly asked to certify fitness to perform sports. Normally the patient will come with a medical form. If there is a form, request to see it before the medical. If there is no form and you are unsure what to check, telephone the sport's governing body or the event organizer. A fee is payable by the patient.

Many gyms/sports clubs also ask older patients/patients with pre-existing conditions or disabilities to check with their GP before they will sign them on. Assuming that a suitable regime is undertaken, most people can participate. Consider the patient's baseline fitness, check BP and medications, and recommend gradual introduction to new forms of exercise.

❶ Remember—signing a form may result in legal action against you should the patient NOT be fit to undertake an activity. Where possible include a caveat, e.g. 'based on information available in the medical notes the patient appears to be fit to …, although it is impossible to guarantee this'. If unsure, consult your local LMC/medical defence organization.

⚠ **Hypertrophic obstructive cardiomyopathy** can cause sudden death during sport. It is difficult to exclude on clinical examination—if there is a FH or systolic murmur refer to cardiology before recommending new intense activity.

**Benefits of exercise** 📖 p.182

>
> **Children and sport**
> - Exercise is good for children—it stimulates development of the musculoskeletal and cardiovascular systems.
> - It should be fun and not physically or emotionally over-demanding.
> - Children are more prone to sports injuries because of continuing growth (bone growth plates are prone to damage) but are more flexible so have ↓ injury rate.
> - Children's temperature control is not as good as adults.
> - Equipment must be checked regularly to ensure that it fits.
> - Encourage warm-up and stretching exercises before sport.
> - Refer children with suspected over-use or sports injuries which do not recover rapidly with simple analgesia for specialist assessment.

**Nutrition** Recommend a normal varied diet (📖 p.176).
- *Special circumstances* Particular sports have special requirements (e.g. ↑ protein for strength athletes). Increasing muscle glycogen stores before exercise can ↓ fatigue during prolonged heavy exercise, e.g. 'carbohydrate loading'—3–4d of ↑ carbohydrate (8–10g/kg body weight) and a carbohydrate meal 3–4h before competing.
- *Fluids* Sufficient fluid during exercise is vital to good performance and health, especially in hot conditions. Rehydration fluids containing carbohydrate and electrolytes are absorbed faster than plain water.
- *Supplements,* e.g. vitamins, minerals, amino acids, carnitine, creatine. A good diet generally supplies sufficient nutrients.

**Drugs and sport** Most regulating bodies have strict codes regarding drug use. Regulations may differ between different sports.

100% ME produces an 'Anti-doping Advice Card' giving more detailed information (available from 🖳 www.100percentme.co.uk). Status of a particular medicine may be checked on the Drug Information Line ☎ 0800 528 0004.

### Prohibited classes of drugs

- *Stimulants*—e.g. amphetamine, caffeine (above 12 micrograms/mL), ephedrine, certain $\beta_2$ agonists (inhaled medication for asthma is allowed).
- *Narcotics*—e.g. morphine, diamorphine, pethidine, methadone (codeine is allowed).
- *Anabolic agents*—e.g. nandrolone, DHEA, testosterone.
- *Diuretics*—e.g. furosemide, bendroflunethiazide.
- *Hormones, hormone antagonists, and related substances*, e.g. growth hormone, erythropoietin.
- *Cannabinoids.*

### Classes of drugs subjected to restrictions

- *Alcohol and marijuana*—restricted in certain sports.
- *Local anaesthetics*—local or intra-articular injections only are allowed (provide written notification of administration)
- *Corticosteroids*—topical, inhaled, or local/intra-articular injection only are allowed (provide written notification of administration).
- *β-blockers*—restricted in certain sports.

**Drugs for pain relief** Generally paracetamol, all NSAIDs, and codeine are allowed for pain relief. Stronger opioids and drugs containing caffeine are banned. If in doubt, check on the Drug Information Line before prescribing.

**Anabolic steroid misuse** Significant problem in the UK (5% in gyms and fitness clubs). Drugs are often used in complicated regimes at high doses to ↑ lean muscle mass and ↓ body fat.

**Side effects** include ↑ cholesterol, ↑ BP, gynaecomastia, ↑ LFTs, testicular atrophy, baldness, acne and mood changes. Other drugs may be taken in conjunction with anabolic steroids to ↓ these side effects.

⚠ Doctors who prescribe or collude in the provision of drugs or treatment with the intention of improperly enhancing an individual's performance in sport risk losing their GMC registration. This does not preclude the provision of any care or treatment where the doctor's intention is to protect or improve the patient's health.

### Further information

**UK Sport** 🖳 www.uksport.gov.uk Status of a particular medicine can be checked on the Drug Information Line ☎ 0800 528 0004.

**100%ME** UK Sports athlete-centred programme providing information on drug-free sport. 🖳 www.100percentme.co.uk

# Management of sporting injuries

### Principles of managing sporting injuries

- *First aid* (**A**irway, **B**reathing, **C**irculation) refer severe injuries to A&E.
- *RICE*
  - **R**est Relative rest of affected part whilst continuing other activities to maintain overall fitness.
  - **I**ce *and analgesia* Use immediately after injury (wrap ice in a towel and use for maximum 10min at a time to prevent acute cold injury).
  - **C**ompression Taping or strapping can be used to treat (↓ swelling) and also to prevent acute sprains and strains.
  - **E**levation ↓ local swelling and dependent oedema enabling quicker recovery.
- *Confirm the diagnosis* Clinical examination, X-ray.
- *Early treatment* according to cause. Do not delay.
- *Liaise* with sports physician, sports physio, and coach if elite athlete.
- *Rehabilitation* Regaining fitness, strength, and flexibility; examine and correct the cause of the injury (e.g. poor technique, equipment).
- *Graded return to activity* Discuss with coach.
- *Prevention* Suitable preparation and training (e.g. suitable footwear, warm-up and warm-down exercises, safety equipment) can ↓ likelihood of injuries.

### Muscle injuries

- *Haematoma* within or between muscles can → dramatic whole limb bruising (due to tracking of blood) and stiffness. Treat with RICE regime; encourage movement in pain-free range.
- *Strain* (e.g. hamstring injury) Refer to physiotherapy. A 2° injury is likely if the patient returns to sport too soon.

### Ligament injuries (sprains)

- *Grade 1*—local tenderness, normal joint movement. Give NSAIDs, support strain, encourage mobilization.
- *Grade 2*—slightly abnormal joint movement. More joint protection, NSAIDs, elevate limb, encourage middle of the range movement.
- *Grade 3*—abnormal joint movement. Refer to orthopaedics.

### Groin pain in athletes Consider:

- conjoint tendon pathology (Gilmour's groin)
- symphysitis (footballers notably), *and*
- adductor tendonitis.

Liaise with a sports medicine physician or physiotherapist early.

**Over-use injuries** Incidence is increasing because of increasingly intensive training regimes, especially in young adults—even amongst amateurs.

- *Causes* Load too great for conditions, poor technique or posture, faulty or poor quality equipment.
- *Types of injury* Stress fractures, joint tenderness or effusion, ligament and tendon strains, muscle stiffness.
- *Management* Rest, NSAIDs, physiotherapy, improved training regime.

- *Prevention* Recognize and correct poor posture or technique; check equipment is appropriate and fits; warm up and stretching before exercise; gradually ↑ intensity and duration of training.

**Over-training syndrome** Poor performance, fatigue, heavy muscles, and depression due to excessive sports training or competing without sufficient rest. Usually diagnosed from history. Exclude other causes of fatigue (💷 p.536). *Management:* rest, reassurance, and alteration of training programme.

**'Scrumpox' (herpes gladiatorum)** Herpes simplex virus is very contagious and outbreaks among sporting teams are common, e.g. spread by close contact and facial stubble grazes whilst scrumming. *Treatment:* aciclovir (cream or tablets) and exclusion of infected players. Impetigo, erysipelas, and tinea barbae can be transmitted in the same way.

### Environmental factors

- *Heat cramps* Painful spasm of heavily exercised muscles (calves and feet) due to salt depletion. *Treatment:* rest, massage of affected muscle, and fluid and salt replacement (e.g. Dioralyte®).
- *Heat stroke/exhaustion* Exercising in excessive heat → salt and water depletion, dehydration, and metabolite accumulation. *Signs:* headache, nausea, confusion, incoordination, cramps, weakness, dizziness, and malaise. Eventually thermoregulatory mechanisms fail → seizures and coma. *Signs:* flushing, sweating, and dehydration. Temperature may be normal (mild cases) or ↑. *Treatment:* rest, fluid and salt replacement (e.g. Dioralyte®). Admission for IV fluids and supportive measures in severe cases.
- *Hypothermia* Ensure appropriate clothing and limit time in the cold. *Signs:* behaviour change, incoordination, clouding of consciousness. *Treatment:* remove from cold environment, wrap in blankets (including the head), and transfer to hospital. Do not use direct heat.
- *Frostbite* Freezing of the peripheries (usually feet, hands, ears, or nose). Tissues become hard, insensitive, and white. *Treatment:* gentle re-warming. Refer if significant dead tissue. Debridement is usually delayed to allow natural recovery.
- *Diving* Decompression illness is due to rapid ascent causing nitrogen dissolved in blood to form gas bubbles. Usually <1–36h after surfacing. *Presentation:* deep muscle aches, joint pains, skin pain, paraesthesia, itching and burning, retrosternal pain, cough and breathlessness, neurological symptoms. Refer suspected cases urgently to A&E.

### Further information

**British Association of Sport and Exercise Medicine** 🖥 www.basem.co.uk
*Oxford Handbook of Sports and Exercise Medicine* OUP (2006) (ISBN 0198568398)

# Bone disorders

**Osteogenesis imperfecta** Inherited condition with autosomal dominant inheritance (rarely recessive). Several types, but all have an underlying problem with collagen metabolism resulting in fragile bones that break easily. Other features include lax joints, thin skin, blue sclerae, hypoplastic teeth, and deafness. Presentation varies according to severity. May be obvious at birth or present early with fractures. Less severe cases present later and may be mistaken for NAI. Mild cases may not present until adolescence with thin bones on X-ray. Treatment is supportive.

**Osteopetrosis (marble bone disease)** Inherited condition with autosomal dominant or recessive inheritance. Dominant form presents in childhood with fractures, osteomyelitis ± facial paralysis. Recessive form is more severe, causing bone marrow failure and death. Bone marrow transplantation has been tried but is of limited success.

**Paget's disease of bone** Accelerated disorganized bone remodelling due to abnormal osteoclast activity. Affects up to 1:10 of the elderly but only a minority are symptomatic. ♂:♀ ≈ 3:1.

**Presentation** Pain—dull ache aggravated by weight-bearing (often remains at rest); deformity—bowing of weight-bearing bones especially tibia (sabre), femur, and forearm (usually asymmetrical); frontal bossing of the forehead; distinctive changes on X-ray; ↑ bone-specific Alk phos; normal $Ca^{2+}$, $PO_4$, and PTH.

**Management** Refer to rheumatology. Give analgesia. Bisphosphonates (e.g. risedronate 30mg/d for 2mo) ↓ pain and long-term complications. *Complications:* Pathological fractures; OA of adjacent joints; high-output CCF; hydrocephalus and/or cranial nerve compression → neurological symptoms (e.g. deafness); spinal stenosis; bone sarcoma (10% of those affected >10y.).

**Osteomyelitis** Infection of bone. May spread from abscesses or follow surgery. Often no primary site is found. More common in those with DM, sickle cell disease, impaired immunity, and/or poor living standards. *Organisms involved:* Staph. aureus, streptococci, E. coli, Salmonella, Proteus and Pseudomonas spp, TB. Presents with pain, unwillingness to move affected part, warmth, effusions in neighbouring joints, fever, and malaise. Blood cultures are +ve in 60%, ↑ESR/CRP, ↑WCC.

**Management** Refer suspected cases for same-day orthopaedic opinion. Diagnosis is confirmed with imaging, e.g. MRI or bone scan (X-ray changes can take days to appear). *Treatment:* is with IV, then po antibiotics (≥6wk) and surgery to drain abscesses. *Complications:* septic arthritis, pathological fracture, deformity of growing bone, chronic infection.

**Chronic osteomyelitis** Occurs after delayed/inadequate treatment of acute osteomyelitis. *Signs:* pain, fever, and discharge of pus from sinuses. Follows a relapsing/remitting course over years. Needs specialist management.

## Referral guidelines for suspected sarcoma[N]

**Refer for immediate X-ray** Any patient with suspected spontaneous fracture. If the X-ray:
- Indicates possible bone cancer, refer urgently.
- Is normal but symptoms persist, follow up and/or request repeat X-ray, bone function tests, or referral.

**Refer urgently** if a patient presents with a palpable lump that is:
- >5 cm in diameter
- Deep to fascia, fixed or immobile
- A recurrence after previous excision.
- Increasing in size
- Painful

**❶** If a patient has HIV, consider Kaposi sarcoma and make an urgent referral if suspected.

**Urgently investigate** increasing, unexplained, or persistent bone pain or tenderness, particularly pain at rest (and especially if not in the joint) or an unexplained limp. In older people, metastases, myeloma, or lymphoma, as well as sarcoma, should be considered.

**Sarcoma** is cancer of the bone or connective tissue. 1850 patients/y are diagnosed with sarcoma in the UK, and it causes 1000 deaths. There are two peaks of incidence—one in teenagers, and another in old age. Five types of sarcoma account for >80% of tumours.

**Osteosarcoma and the Ewing family of tumours** Present with aching bone pain, swelling ± pathological fracture. If X-ray is normal but symptoms persist, consider checking bone function tests, re-X-raying, discussing the patient with a specialist or referral. Treatment involves surgery and chemotherapy. Overall 5y survival is 50–80%.

**Adult soft tissue sarcoma of limb or trunk** Usually presents with a palpable lump. The most common tumours are leiomyosarcoma, liposarcoma, and synovial sarcoma. Treated with surgery ± radiotherapy (high-grade tumours). Chemotherapy is reserved for palliation.

**Kaposi's sarcoma** 📖 p.745

**Intra-abdominal sarcoma** Usually presents late. Often arises in the retroperitoneum. If possible, surgery is the main treatment. Local relapse is common and often not responsive to cytotoxic therapy.

 **Rhabdomyosarcoma** Originates from striated muscle. Usually presents in children <2y with a lump. Responds to intensive multi-modal therapy; outlook is generally good (>60% long-term survival).

## Further information
**NICE** Referral guidelines for suspected cancer (2005) 🖥 www.nice.org.uk

## Patient information and support
**Brittle Bone Society** ☎ 0800 0282 459 🖥 www.brittlebone.org
**Osteopetrosis Support Trust** 🖥 www.osteopetrosis.co.uk
**National Association for the Relief of Paget's Disease**
☎ 0161 799 4646 🖥 www.paget.org.uk
**Sarcoma UK** 🖥 www.sarcoma-uk.org

# Rickets and osteomalacia

Vitamin D deficiency causes rickets in children and osteomalacia in adults. The body needs ~10 micrograms of vitamin D daily to maintain healthy bones. The body makes its own vitamin D when sunlight falls on the skin in the summer months, but a diet with adequate vitamin D (Table 15.6) is needed to maintain the supply in the winter—especially for people who do not get out or for cultural or religious reasons are completely shielded from the sun by their clothing.

## Clinical features of rickets
- *Bone pain/tenderness*—arms, legs, spine, pelvis.
- *Skeletal deformity*—bow legs, pigeon chest (forward projection of the sternum), rachitic rosary (enlarged ends of ribs), asymmetrical/odd-shaped skull due to soft skull bones, spinal deformity (kyphosis, scoliosis), pelvic deformities.
- *Pathological fracture*.
- *Dental deformities*—delayed formation of teeth, holes in enamel, ↑ cavities.
- *Muscular problems*—progressive weakness, ↓ muscle tone, muscle cramps.
- *Impaired growth* → short stature (can be permanent).

## Clinical features of osteomalacia
- *Bone pain*—diffuse, particularly in hips.
- *Muscle weakness*.
- *Pathological fractures*.
- *Low calcium* → perioral numbness, numbness of extremities, hand and foot spasms and/or arrhythmias.

## Causes and management
*Dietary deficiency (<30 nmol/L)* Particularly in children with pigmented skin in northern climes. Give vitamin D and $Ca^{2+}$ supplements.

*Age-related deficiency (<30 nmol/L)* Vitamin D metabolism deteriorates with age and many >80y are deficient. Consider giving vitamin D (800iu/d) to all elderly >80y.

*Secondary rickets/osteomalacia* Vitamin D deficiency is due to other disease, e.g. malabsorption, liver disease, renal tubular disorders, or chronic renal failure. Treat underlying cause/supplement $Ca^{2+}$ and vitamin D.

*Vitamin D dependent rickets* Rare autosomal recessive inherited disorder resulting in an enzyme deficit in the metabolism of vitamin D. Refer for specialist care. Treated with vitamin D and $Ca^{2+}$ supplements.

*Hypophosphataemic rickets (vitamin D resistant rickets)* X-linked dominant trait resulting in ↓ proximal renal tubular resorption of phosphate. Parathyroid hormone and vitamin D levels are normal. Specialist management is needed. Treatment is with phosphate replacement ± calcitriol.

**Table 15.6** Approximate vitamin D content of common foods*

| Food | Serving | Vitamin D (micrograms) |
| --- | --- | --- |
| Margarine | 10g (½oz) | 0.8 |
| Eggs | 1 size 3 | 1.1 |
| Cheese | 60g (2oz) | 0.2 |
| Milk | 0.15L (¼ pint) | 0.05 |
| Butter | 10g (½oz) | 0.1 |
| Fortified cereals | 30g (1oz) | 0.5 |
| Herring | 100g (3½oz) | 16.5 |
| Mackerel | 100g (3½oz) | 8 |
| Sardines | 100g (3½oz) | 7.5 |
| Tinned tuna | 100g (3½oz) | 4 |
| Tinned salmon | 100g (3½oz) | 12.5 |
| Kippers | 100g (3½oz) | 13.5 |

* Recommended daily intakes: birth to 50y, 5 micrograms; 50–70y, 10 micrograms; >70y, 15 micrograms

**Table 15.7** Approximate calcium content of common foods*

| Food | Serving | Calcium (mg) |
| --- | --- | --- |
| Whole milk | 0.2L (1/3 pint) | 220 |
| Semi-skimmed milk | 0.2L (1/3 pint) | 230 |
| Hard cheese | 30g (1oz) | 190 |
| Cottage cheese | 115g (4oz) | 80 |
| Low-fat yoghurt | 150g (5oz) | 225 |
| Sardines (including bones) | 60g (2oz) | 310 |
| Brown or white bread | 3 large slices | 100 |
| Wholemeal bread | 3 large slices | 55 |
| Baked beans | 115g (4oz) | 60 |
| Boiled cabbage | 115g (4oz) | 40 |

* Recommended daily intakes: birth to 6mo, 210mg; 7mo–1y, 270mg; 1–3y, 500mg; 4–8y, 800mg; 9–18y, 1300mg; 19–50y, 1000mg; >50y, 1200mg

## Patient information and support
**Arthritis Research Campaign** Information for patients in English and five South Asian languages ☎ 0870 850 5000 🖵 www.arc.org.uk

# Osteoporosis

Lifetime risk of osteoporotic fracture is 40% in ♀ and 13% in ♂. The main morbidity and financial costs of osteoporosis relate to hip fracture where incidence ↑ steeply >70y. Treatment aims to prevent fracture.

**Definition** Osteoporosis is defined as bone mineral density >2.5 standard deviations (SD) below the young adult mean (T score of −2.5). There is ↑ relative risk of fracture 2–3× for each SD ↓ in BMD.

❶ Osteopoenia cannot be reliably diagnosed on X-ray, although vertebral fractures may be seen.

**Bone mineral density (BMD) measurement** Hip and lumbar spine BMD measurement by dual-energy X-ray absorptiometry (DEXA) scan can quantify risk of osteoporotic fracture (Figure 15.3). Follow local referral guidelines.

The report from the DEXA scan should contain information on fracture risk, management, and time interval for re-checking BMD. Generally, treatment with a bisphosphonate is started if the T score is ≤−2.5.

**Major risk factors for osteoporosis**
- Age.
- Glucocorticoid use.
- FH of maternal hip fracture aged <75y.
- Previous fragility fracture.
- Low BMI (<19 kg/m²).
- Untreated premature menopause, prolonged amenorrhoea or ♂ hypogonadism.
- Conditions associated with prolonged immobility.
- Medical disorder independently associated with bone loss, e.g. inflammatory bowel or coeliac disease, chronic liver disease, hyperthyroidism, ankylosing spondylitis, chronic renal failure, type 1 DM, RA.

**Glucocorticoid use** Steroid use is a risk factor for osteoporosis.
- Minimize steroid dose.
- Advise *all* patients taking any dose of oral steroids to take calcium/vitamin D supplements.[G]

*In addition* For patients taking oral/high-dose inhaled steroids for >3mo:
- Add a bisphosphonate for patients > 65y, *or*
- Refer patients <65y for a DEXA scan and add a bisphosphonate if T score ≤−1.5.

**Previous fragility fracture** Fracture sustained falling from ≤ standing height—includes vertebral collapse (may not be as a result of a fall). Previous fracture is a risk for future fracture. *Common fractures:*
- *Hip*—associated with ↑ mortality.
- *Wrist*—Colles' fracture
- *Spine*—Osteoporotic vertebral collapse causes pain, ↓ height, and kyphosis. Pain can take 3–6mo to settle and requires strong analgesia. Calcitonin is useful for pain relief for 3mo after vertebral fracture if other analgesics are ineffective.

### *Investigation*

- DEXA scan if <75y (Figure 15.3).
- Exclude other causes of pathological fracture, e.g. malignancy, osteomalacia, hyperparathyroidism. Check FBC, ESR, TSH, Cr, eGFR, bone, and liver function tests—all should be normal.
- Consider checking serum paraproteins/urine Bence Jones protein, bone scan, and FSH/testosterone/LH (if hormonal status unclear).

### *Management*[N]

- If ≥75y treat without DEXA once all non-osteoporotic causes of fracture have been ruled out.
- If 65-74y treat if DEXA confirms osteoporosis (*T* score ≤–2.5)
- Treat if <65y and very low BMD (*T* score ≤–3) *or* if *T* score ≤–2.5 and the patient has ≥1 additional risk factor for osteoporosis apart from age.

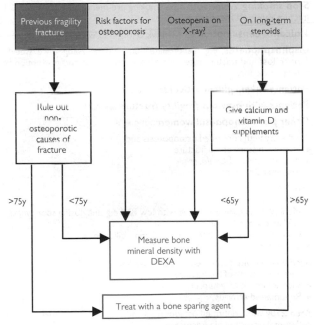

*NICE recommends that the diagnosis of osteoporosis may be assumed in women aged ≥75y if the responsible clinician considers a DEXA scan to be clinically inappropriate or unfeasible.

**Fig. 15.3** Who should have a DEXA scan?*

Reproduced from Davies R, Everitt H, Simon C, *Musculoskeletal Problems* (2006), with permission from Oxford University Press.

### Information and support for patients

**Arthritis Research Campaign** ☎ 0870 850 5000 🖳 www.arc.org.uk
**National Osteoporosis Society** ☎ 0845 450 0230 🖳 www.nos.org.uk

# Treatment options for osteoporosis

**Lifestyle advice** Provide to all at risk patients.
***Adequate nutrition***
- Maintain body weight so BMI >19kg/m².
- Advise adequate intake of calcium and vitamin D (food rich in calcium and vitamin D—Tables 15.6 and 15.7, 🔲 p.515).
- Give Ca²⁺ and/or vitamin D supplements to post-menopausal women with dietary deficiency.
- Supplement with Ca²⁺ (0.5–1g/d) and vitamin D (800u or 20 micrograms/d) if on long-term steroids, >80y, housebound, or institutionalized.

***Regular exercise*** Weight-bearing activity >30min/d ↓ fracture rate.

***Stop smoking*** Women that stop smoking pre-menopause have a 25% ↓ fracture rate post menopause.

***↓ alcohol consumption*** to <21u/wk ♂ or <14u/wk ♀.

**Bisphosphonates**, e.g. alendronate 10mg od or 70mg once weekly. ↓ bone loss and fracture rate.[C] Mainstay of treatment and prevention of osteoporosis for:

***Patients taking glucocorticoids*** 🔲 p.516

***Patients with previous fragility fracture*** 🔲 p.516

***Other postmenopausal women*** but *only* if:

*Aged <65y* with confirmed osteoporosis and:
- Parental history of hip fracture
- Alcohol intake of ≥4u/d, *or*
- Rheumatoid arthritis

*and*
- BMI <22kg/m²
- Medical conditions associated with low BMI e.g. ankylosing spondylitis, coeliac disease, Crohn's disease
- Conditions that result in prolonged immobility, *or*
- Untreated menopause.

*Aged 65–69y* with confirmed osteoporosis and:
- Parental history of hip fracture
- Alcohol intake of ≥4u/d, *or*
- Rheumatoid arthritis.

*Aged ≥70y* with confirmed osteoporosis and:
- Parental history of hip fracture
- Alcohol intake of ≥4u/d
- Rheumatoid arthritis
- BMI <22kg/m²
- Medical conditions associated with low BMI e.g. ankylosing spondylitis, coeliac disease, Crohn's disease
- Conditions that result in prolonged immobility, *or*
- Untreated menopause.

❶ If ≥2 of these risk factors are present and the woman is aged ≥75y, a DEXA scan may not be required if clinically inappropriate or unfeasible.

**Strontium ranelate,** e.g. Protelos® 2g od in water. ↑ formation and ↓ resorption of bone. Use for post-menopausal osteoporosis when bisphosphonates are contraindicated or not tolerated and severe osteoporosis. ↓ hip/vertebral fracture risk by 36–41%.

**Selective oestrogen receptor modulator (SERM),** e.g. raloxifene 60mg od—use for patients with previous fragility fracture if bisphosphonates are contraindicated/not tolerated or there is an unsatisfactory response (further fracture and/or ↓ in BMD after ≥1y treatment) with bisphosphonates. SERMS are not recommended for primary prevention of osteoporotic fracture[N].

**HRT** (📖 p.710) Postpones postmenopausal bone loss and d fractures.[C] Optimum duration of use is uncertain (>5–7y) but benefit disappears within 5y of stopping. ↑ in breast cancer and cardiovascular risk limits use.[R]

> **CSM guidance (2003)**
> * Premature menopause HRT is recommended for the prevention of osteoporosis until women reach 51y.
> * >51y HRT should not be considered first-line therapy for long-term prevention of osteoporosis. HRT remains an option where other therapies are contraindicated or cannot be tolerated, or if there is a lack of response. Risks and benefits should be carefully assessed.

**Teriparatide** Most powerful treatment for osteoporosis currently available. Consider referral for consultant initiation if other treatment options are exhausted. Given by daily injection.

**Referral** Routinely refer to endocrinology or menopause clinic (as appropriate) if:
* Premature menopause (<40y)
* Unexplained cause of osteoporosis
* Osteoporosis in a man, *or*
* Problems with management.

## Further information

**NICE** 🖳 www.nice.org.uk
* Osteoporosis—secondary prevention (2005)
* Osteoporosis—primary prevention (2008)
* Osteoporosis—assessment of fracture risk and the prevention of osteoporotic fracture in high risk individuals (in preparation).

**National Osteoporosis Society** Primary care strategy for osteoporosis and falls (2002) 🖳 www.nos.org.uk

**Royal College of Physicians** Osteoporosis: clinical guidelines for prevention and treatment (2003) 🖳 www.rcplondon.ac.uk

**CSM Guidance** Further advice on safety of HRT (12/2003) 🖳 www.mca.gov.uk

# Osteoarthritis

Osteoarthritis (OA) is the most important cause of locomotor disability. It used to be considered 'wear and tear' of the bone/cartilage of synovial joints but is now recognized as a metabolically active process involving the whole joint, i.e. cartilage, bone, synovium, capsule and muscle.

The main reason for patients seeking medical help is pain. Level of pain and disability are greatly influenced by the patient's personality, anxiety, depression, and activity, and often do not correlate well with clinical signs.

**Risk factors** ↑ age (uncommon <45y); ♀ > ♂; ↑ in black and Asian populations; genetic predisposition; obesity; abnormal mechanical loading of joint, e.g. instability; poor muscle function; post-meniscectomy; certain occupations, e.g. farming.

**Symptoms and signs** Joint pain ± stiffness, synovial thickening, deformity, effusion, crepitus, muscle weakness and wasting, and ↓ function. Most commonly affects hip, knee, and base of thumb. Typically exacerbations occur that may last weeks to months. Nodal OA, with swelling of the distal interphalangeal joints (Heberden's nodes), has a familial tendency.

**Investigations** X-rays may show ↓ joint space, cysts and sclerosis in subchondral bone, and osteophytes. OA is common and may be a coincidental finding. Exclude other causes of pain, e.g. check FBC and ESR if inflammatory arthritis is suspected (normal or mildly ↑ in OA—ESR >30 suggests RA or psoriatic arthritis).

**Management of osteoarthritis in primary care** Employ a holistic approach. Assess effect of OA on the patient's functioning, quality of life, occupation, mood, relationships, and leisure activities. Formulate a management plan with the patient which includes self-management strategies, effects of comorbidities, and regular review.

*Information and advice* Give information and advice on all relevant aspects of osteoarthritis and its management. The ARC website (🖳 www.arc.org.uk) has a wide range of information leaflets for patients. Use the whole multidisciplinary team. e.g. refer to:
• Physiotherapist for advice on exercises, strapping and splints
• OT for aids
• Chiropodist for foot care and insoles
• Social worker for advice on disability benefits and housing
• Orthopaedics for surgery if significant disability/night pain.

*↓ load on the joint* Weight reduction can ↓ symptoms and may ↓ progression in knee OA. Using a walking stick in the opposite hand to the affected hip and cushioned insoles/shoes (e.g. trainers) can also help.

*Exercise and improving muscle strength* ↓ pain and disability, e.g. walking (for OA knee), swimming (for OA back and hip but may make neck worse), cycling (for OA knee but may worsen patellofemoral OA). Refer to physiotherapy for advice on exercises especially isometric exercises for the less mobile.

## Pain control
- Use non-pharmacological methods first (activity, exercise, weight↓, footwear modification, walking stick, TENS, local heat/cold treatments).
- Regular paracetamol (1g qds) is first-line drug treatment for all OA and/or topical NSAIDS for knee/hand OA only. Topical NSAIDs have fewer side effects than oral NSAIDs—more acceptable to patients.
- Use opioids, oral NSAIDs, or COX2 inhibitors as second-line agents in addition to, or instead of, paracetamol. Use the lowest effective dose for the shortest possible time. Co-prescribe a proton pump inhibitor (e.g. omeprazole 20mg od) with NSAIDs.
- Low-dose antidepressants, e.g. amitriptyline 10–75mg nocte (unlicensed)—are a useful adjunct especially for pain causing sleep disturbance.
- Capsaicin cream can also be helpful for knee/hand OA. NICE does not recommend rubefacients for other OA.

**Aspiration of joint effusions and joint injections** Can help in exacerbations. Some patients respond well to long-acting steroid injections—it may be worth considering a trial of a single treatment. Hyaluronic acid knee injections are not recommended by NICE.

**Complementary therapies** ~60% of sufferers from OA are thought to use CAM, e.g. copper bracelets, acupuncture, food supplements, dietary manipulation. There is good evidence that chiropractic/osteopathy can be helpful for back pain, but otherwise evidence of effectiveness is scanty. Advise patients to find a reputable practitioner with accredited training who is a member of a recognized professional body and carries professional indemnity insurance.

**Glucosamine** ✿ It is controversial whether glucosamine modifies OA progression. NICE does not recommend prescription of glucosamine but patients may wish to purchase it over the counter.

**Psychological factors** have a major impact on disability from OA. Education about the disease, and emphasis that it is not progressive in most people, is important. Seek and treat depression and anxiety with screening tools (📖 p.998).

## Refer
- **To rheumatology** to confirm diagnosis if coexistent psoriasis (psoriatic arthritis mimics OA and can be missed by radiologists); to rule out 2° causes of OA (e.g. pseudo-gout, haemochromatosis) if young OA or odd distribution; if joint injection is thought worthwhile but you lack expertise or confidence to do it.
- **To orthopaedics** for joint replacement if symptoms are severe. Refer as an emergency if you suspect joint sepsis.

## Further information
**NICE** Osteoarthritis the care and management of osteoarthritis in adults (2008) 🖥 www.nice.org.uk
**Bandolier** Topical NSAIDs (2003)
🖥 www.medicine.ox.ac.uk/bandolier/band110/b110-6.html

## Information and support for patients
**Arthritis Research Campaign (ARC)** ☎ 0870 850 5000 🖥 www.arc.org.uk

# Rheumatoid arthritis

Rheumatoid arthritis (RA) is the most common disorder of connective tissue, affecting ~1% UK population. It is an immunological disease triggered by environmental factors in patients with genetic predisposition. Disease course is variable with exacerbations and remissions.

⚠ Refer all suspected cases of rheumatoid arthritis to rheumatology—early treatment with disease-modifying drugs can significantly alter disease progression. Refer urgently[N] if:
* Small joints of the hands/feet are affected
* >1 joint is affected
* There has been a delay of ≥3mo between onset of symptoms and seeking medical advice.

## Presentation
* Can present at any age—most common in middle age. ♀:♂ ≈ 3:1.
* Variable onset—often gradual but may be acute.
* Usually starts with symmetrical small joint involvement, i.e. pain, stiffness, swelling, and functional loss (especially in the hands). Joint damage and deformity occur later.
* Irreversible damage occurs early if untreated and can → deformity and joint instability.
* Other presentations: monoarthritis; migratory (palindromic) arthritis; PMR-like illness; systemic illness of malaise, pain, and stiffness.

**Symptoms and signs** Predominantly peripheral joints are affected—symmetrical joint pain, effusions, soft tissue swelling, early morning stiffness. Progression to joint destruction and deformity. Tendons may rupture. Specific features—Table 15.8

**Differential diagnosis** Diagnosis may not be easy—consider:
* Psoriatic arthritis
* Nodal OA
* SLE (especially in ♀ <50y)
* Bilateral carpal tunnel syndrome
* Other connective tissue disorders
* Polymyalgia rheumatica if >50y.

## Investigations
* Check FBC (normochromic normocytic or hypochromic, microcytic anaemia), ESR and/or CRP (↑). May have ↑platelets, ↓WCC.
* Rheumatoid factor and anti-CCP antibodies are +ve in the majority. A minority have a +ve ANA titre.
* X-rays—normal periarticular osteoporosis or soft tissue swelling in the early stages; later, loss of joint space, erosions, and joint destruction.

**Management** Multidisciplinary team approach is ideal, e.g. GP, medical and surgical teams, physiotherapist, podiatrist, OT, nurse specialist, and social worker.

***Screening for depression*** 📖 p.998

***General support*** Provision of information about the disease, treatments and support available (including equipment and help with everyday activities, self-help and carers groups, 'blue' disabled parking badges, financial support, e.g. DLA, AA—📖 p.229).

***Physical therapy*** Exercises, splints, appliances, and strapping help to keep joints mobile, ↓ pain, and preserve function.

**Table 15.8** Specific features of rheumatoid arthritis

| | |
|---|---|
| *Hands* | • Ulnar deviation of the fingers<br>• Z deformity of the thumb<br>• Swan-neck (hyperextended PIP and flexed DIP joints) and boutonnière (flexed PIP and extended MCP joints, hyperextended DIP joint) deformities of the fingers (Figure 15.4)<br>• ↓ grip strength and ↓ hand function causes disability |
| *Legs and feet* | • Subluxation of the metatarsal heads in feet and claw toes → pain on walking<br>• Baker's cysts (📖 p.502) at the knee may rupture, mimicking DVT |
| *Spine* | Especially cervical spine—causing neck pain, cervical subluxation, and atlanto-axial instability leading to a risk of cord compression. X-rays are required prior to general anaesthesia |
| *Non-articular features* | Common. Weight ↓, fever, malaise<br>• *Rheumatoid nodules* (especially extensor surfaces of forearms)<br>• *Vasculitis*—digital infarction, skin ulcers, mononeuritis<br>• *Eye*—Sjögren's syndrome, episcleritis, scleritis<br>• *Lungs*—pleural effusions, fibrosing alveolitis, nodules<br>• *Heart*—pericarditis, mitral valve disease, conduction defects.<br>• *Skin*—palmar erythema, vasculitis, rashes<br>• *Neurological*—nerve entrapment, e.g. carpal tunnel, mononeuritis, and peripheral neuropathy<br>• *Felty's syndrome*: combination of RA, splenomegaly, and leucopoenia. Occurs in patients with in long-standing RA. Recurrent infections are common. Hypersplenism → anaemia and thrombocytopoenia. Associated with lymphadenopathy, pigmentation, and persistent skin ulcers. Splenectomy may improve the neutropoenia |

**C-reactive protein (CRP)** Acute phase protein that ↑ ≤ 6h. after an acute event. Follows clinical state more rapidly than ESR (📖 p.659). Not ↑ by SLE, leukaemia, UC, pregnancy, OA, anaemia, polycythaemia, or heart failure. Highest levels are seen in bacterial infections (>10mg/L).

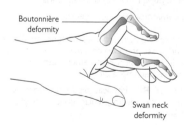

**Fig. 15.4** Boutonnière and swan neck deformities of the fingers

Reproduced from Davies R, Everitt H, Simon C, *Musculoskeletal Problems* (2006), with permission from Oxford University Press.

**Information and support for patients**
**Arthritis Research Campaign** ☎ 0870 8505 000 🖥 www.arc.org.uk
**Arthritis Care** ☎ 0808 800 4050 🖥 www.arthritiscare.org.uk

### Medication

**NSAIDs and simple analgesics**, e.g. regular paracetamol. Provide symptomatic relief but do not alter the course of disease. Patient's response to NSAIDs is individual—start with the least gastrically toxic, e.g. ibuprofen 200-400mg tds, and alter as necessary, e.g. to diclofenac 50mg tds. A modified release form at night may help early morning symptoms. If the patient has a history of indigestion/gastric problems, consider adding gastric protection, e.g. misoprostol or a PPI, or, if there is no history of CVD using a COX2 inhibitor, e.g. celecoxib 100mg bd.

**Corticosteroids** Intra-articular injections of steroids (e.g. Kenalog) can settle localized flares (e.g. knee or shoulder) and can be used up to 3×/y. in any particular joint. Depot IM injections or IV infusions (pulses) can also help settle an acute flare but offer short-term benefits with the risk of systemic side effects. Daily low-dose oral steroids help symptoms and there is some evidence that they can modify disease progression, but concerns about adverse side effects have limited use.

### Disease-modifying drugs (DMARDs)

- Methotrexate
- Sulfasalazine
- Penicillamine
- Gold
- Azathioprine
- Leflunomide
- Hydroxychloroquine
- Ciclosporin
- Cyclophosphamide
- Cytokine inhibitors (adalimumab, anakinra, etanercept, infliximab).

Use only under consultant supervision. ↓ disease progression by modifying the immune response and inflammation. Used individually or in combination, they are now started very early in the disease (i.e. first 3–6mo)— hence the need for early referral. DMARDs can take several months to show any effect. Before starting, check baseline U&E, Cr, eGFR, LFTs, FBC, and urinalysis. Side effects and monitoring—Table 15.9.

⚠ **Results requiring action**
- Total WBC <3.5 × $10^9$/L
- Neutrophils <2 × $10^9$/L
- Persistent proteinuria (>1+ ×2) or haematuria
- Platelets <150 × $10^9$/L
- LFTs (ALT/AST) >2x baseline

Discuss with rheumatologist ± stop medication.

**Surgery** Aims to relieve pain and improve function. Consideration of the risks, benefits, and most appropriate timing of surgery is vital. Common procedures include: joint fusion, replacement, and excision; tendon transfer and repair; and nerve decompression.

**Complications of RA** Physical disability, depression, osteoporosis, ↑ infections, lymphoma, cardiovascular disease, amyloidosis (10%), side effects of treatment.

### Further information

**NICE** Rheumatoid arthritis (2009) ⌨ www.nice.org.uk
**British Society for Rheumatology** Guidelines for DMARD therapy (2008) ⌨ www.rheumatology.org.uk
**BNF** ⌨ www.bnf.org
**Primary Care Rheumatology Society** ☎ 01609 774794
⌨ www.pcrsociety.org.uk

**Table 15.9** Specific disease-modifying drugs—side effects and monitoring

⚠ Before starting check baseline U&E, Cr, eGFR, LFTs, FBC, and urinalysis.

| Drug | Routine monitoring | Side effects to monitor |
|------|--------------------|--------------------------|
| Methotrexate 7.5–25 mg weekly It is common practice to give folate 5mg the day after methotrexate (i.e. weekly) as well. | FBC, U&E and LFT weekly until dose and monitoring are stable. Then monthly for at least 1y. Frequency of monitoring may be ↓ by specialist if disease/dose stable after 1y. CXR within 1y of start of treatment. Check baseline lung function if lung disease. | Ask to report symptoms/ signs of infection, especially sore throat If severe respiratory symptoms <6mo after starting, refer to A&E If MCV>105fL check $B_{12}$/folate |
| ❶ Advise patients NOT to self-medicate with aspirin or ibuprofen. Avoid alcohol | | |
| Sulfasalazine 1g bd/tds maintenance | FBC and LFT monthly for first 3mo. Then every 3mo. Urgent FBC if intercurrent illness during initiation. If stable after a year, frequency of monitoring may be ↓ by specialist. | Rash (1%) Nausea/diarrhoea—often transient Bone marrow suppression in 1–2% in the first months. If MCV>105 fL check $B_{12}$/folate |
| Intramuscular gold (Myocrisin®) 50mg monthly | FBC, and urinalysis at the time of each injection. CXR within 1y of start of treatment. | Ask patients to report: Symptoms/signs of infection— especially sore throat Bleeding/bruising Breathlessness/cough Mouth ulcers/metallic taste or Rashes |
| D penicillamine 500–750 mg/d. maintenance | FBC, urinalysis 2 weekly for 3mo, and 1wk after any ↑ dose. Then monthly. | Altered taste (can be ignored) Rash |
| Azathioprine 1.5–2.5mg/kg/d maintenance | FBC and LFT weekly for 6wk, then every 2wk until dose/ monitoring stable for 6wk. Then monthly. | GI side effects, rash, bone marrow suppression Avoid live vaccines |
| ⚠ If allopurinol is co-prescribed, ↓dose to 25% of the original. | | |
| Ciclosporin 1.25mg/kg bd maintenance | FBC and LFT monthly until dose/monitoring stable for 3mo, then every 3mo. U&E,Cr/eGFR every 2wk. until dose stable for 3mo, then monthly. Lipids 6 monthly. | Rash, gum soreness, hirsutism, renal failure ↑ Cr (if ↑ by >30% from baseline, withold and discuss with rheumatologist), ↑BP. Monitor BP |
| Hydroxychloroquine 200–400mg/d maintenance | Baseline eye check and annual check of visual symptoms and visual acuity | Rash, GI effects, ocular side effects (rare) |
| Leflunomide 10–20mg/d maintenance | FBC and LFT monthly for 6mo then, if stable every 2mo. | Rash, GI, ↑ BP, ↑ ALT Check weight and BP at each review. |

# The spondylarthropathies

A group of inflammatory rheumatic diseases characterized by predominant involvement of axial and peripheral joints and entheses (areas where tendons, ligaments, or joint capsules attach to bone). Includes:
- Ankylosing spondylitis
- Psoriatic arthritis
- Reactive arthritis and Reiter syndrome
- Behçet disease
- Arthritis accompanying inflammatory bowel disease
- Whipple's disease (📖 p.415).

Sacroiliitis and spondylitis occur with all of them, and they are all associated with the HLA B27 genotype.

**Ankylosing spondylitis (AS)** Prevalence 1:2000. ♂:♀ ≈ 2.5:1. 95% HLAB27 +ve—prevalence in a population mirrors the frequency of the HLAB27 genotype. Risk of developing AS if HLAB27 +ve ≈1:3.

**Presentation** Typically presents with morning back pain/stiffness in a young man. Progressive spinal fusion (ankylosis) leads to ↓ spinal movement, spinal kyphosis, sacroiliac (SI) joint fusion, neck hyperextension, and neck rotation. *Other features:*
- ↓ chest expansion
- Chest pain
- Hip and knee arthritis
- Plantar fasciitis and other enthesopathies
- Iritis
- Crohn's or UC
- Heart disease—carditis, aortic regurgitation, conduction defects
- Osteoporosis
- Psoriaform rashes.

**Tests**
- *Blood* FBC—normochromic or microcytic hypochromic anaemia, ↑ ESR (may be normal), rheumatoid factor is usually –ve.
- *X-ray* Initial signs are widening of the SI joints and marginal sclerosis— later SI joint fusion and a 'bamboo spine' (vertebral squaring/fusion).

**Management** Aims to ↓ inflammation, pain, and stiffness; alleviate systemic symptoms, e.g. fatigue; slow or stop long-term progression of the disease. Exercise helps back pain. NSAIDs (e.g. diclofenac 50mg tds) also help pain. Refer to rheumatologist early for confirmation of diagnosis, education, disease-modifying drugs (📖 p.525), and advice on appropriate exercise regimes to maintain mobility.

**Psoriatic arthritis** Inflammatory arthritis associated with psoriasis (~40% psoriasis patients. ♂ = ♀). 75% of patients have a pre-existing history of psoriasis before the arthropathy; in 15% the rash appears simultaneously with the joint symptoms; in 10% the arthritis precedes the skin changes. Presentation is variable. Patterns include:
- *Distal arthritis* DIP joint swelling of hands/feet, nail dystrophy ± flexion deformity. Sausage-shaped fingers are characteristic of psoriatic arthritis affecting the hand.
- *Rheumatoid-like* Polyarthropathy similar to rheumatoid arthritis (📖 p.522) but less symmetrical and rheumatoid factor is –ve.

- *Mutilans* Associated with severe psoriasis. Erosions in small bones of hands/feet ± spine. Bones dissolve → progressive deformity.
- *Ankylosing spondylitis/sacroiliitis* Usually HLA B27 +ve.

**Investigations** WBC—usually ↑; ESR/CRP—usually ↑; rheumatoid factor –ve; X-ray appearances can be diagnostic.

**Management** Education; physiotherapy; NSAIDs. Refer to rheumatology for confirmation of diagnosis, advice on management and disease-modifying drugs (🕮 p.525). Medication, e.g. methotrexate, may improve both skin and musculoskeletal symptoms.

**Reactive arthritis** Often asymmetrical aseptic arthritis in ≥1 joint. Occurs 2–6wk after bacterial infection elsewhere, e.g. gastroenteritis (*Salmonella, Campylobacter*), GU infection (chlamydia, gonorrhoea). ↑ in HLA B27 +ve individuals.

**Management** NSAIDs, physiotherapy, and steroid joint injections. Recovery usually occurs within months. A minority develop chronic arthritis requiring disease-modifying drugs. Refer to rheumatology.

**Reiter syndrome** Polyarthropathy, urethritis, iritis, and a psoriaform rash. Affects men with HLA B27 genotype. Commonly follows genito-urinary or bowel infection. Joint and eye changes are often severe. Refer for specialist management. *H.C. Reiter (1881–1969)–German public health physician.*

**Behçet disease** Multi-organ disease of unknown cause though thought to be infective. ♂:♀ ≈ 2:1. *Clinical picture:* (only some features): arthritis; ocular symptoms and signs—pain, ↓ vision, floaters, iritis; scarring painful ulceration of mouth and/or scrotum; colitis; meningoencephalitis. Refer to GUM clinic, ophthalmologist, or general physician depending on symptom cluster. Treatment is usually with steroids ± azathioprine or ciclosporin. Topical steroids may be useful for ulcers. *H. Behçet (1889–1948)—Turkish dermatologist.*

**Enteropathic spondylarthropathy** Oligoarticular or polyarticular arthritis linked to inflammatory bowel disease. Presentation is variable and includes sacroiliitis, plantar fasciitis, inflammatory spinal pains, and other enthesitides (insertional ligament/tendon inflammation). Arthritis may evolve and relapse/remit independently of bowel disease.

**Management** NSAIDs may help joint pain but aggravate bowel disease. Refer to rheumatology for confirmation of diagnosis, advice on management and disease-modifying drugs.

## Information and support for patients
**National Ankylosing Spondylitis Society (NASS)** ☎ 020 8948 9117
🖳 www.nass.co.uk
**Psoriatic Arthropathy Alliance (PAA)** ☎ 01923 672837
🖳 www.paalliance.org
**Arthritis Research Campaign** ☎ 0870 850 5000 🖳 www.arc.org.uk

# Crystal-induced arthritis

**Acute gout** Intermittent attacks of acute joint pain due to deposition of uric acid crystals. *Prevalence:* 3–8/1000. ↑ with age; ♂:♀ ≈ 5:1.

## Predisposing factors

- FH
- Obesity
- Excess alcohol intake
- High purine diet
- Diuretics
- Acute infection
- Ketosis
- Surgery
- Plaque psoriasis
- Polycythaemia
- Leukaemia
- Cytotoxics
- Renal failure.

**Presentation of acute gout** Painful swollen joint (big toe, feet, and ankles most commonly), red skin which may peel ± fever. Can be polyarticular, especially in elderly ♀. May mimic septic arthritis.

## Investigation

- **Blood** ↑ WCC; ↑ ESR; ↑ blood urate (but may be normal).
- **Microscopy of synovial fluid** Not usually required—reveals sodium mono-urate crystals on polarized light microscopy.
- **X-rays** Not usually required—show soft tissue swelling only, unless severe disease when an erosive pattern is seen.

## Management of acute gout

- Exclude infection.
- Rest and elevate joint—apply ice packs.
- NSAIDs are helpful (e.g. diclofenac 75mg bd)—caution if GI problems.
- Alternatively, if NSAIDs are contraindicated, try colchicine 500 micrograms bd increased slowly to qds until pain is relieved or side effects, e.g. nausea, vomiting, or diarrhoea (max. 6mg—do not repeat in <3d).
- Steroid joint injection e.g. methylprednisolone 80-120mg IM are also effective.

Resolves in <2wk—often after 2–7d if treated.

## Prevention of further attacks

- ↓ weight
- Avoid alcohol and purine-rich foods (e.g. offal, red meat, yeast extracts, pulses, and mussels).
- Avoid thiazide diuretics and aspirin.
- Consider prophylactic medication if recurrent attacks: Allopurinol 100–300mg daily—wait until 1mo after acute attack and co-prescribe colchicine (500 micrograms bd) or NSAID for first 1–3mo to try to avoid precipitation of another acute attack. Check serum urate level after 2mo—aim for low normal range.
- Alternatively or in addition try a uricosuric, e.g. probenecid 250–500mg bd.

---

**❶**
- Gout may be linked to ↑ risk of hypertension and coronary heart disease—screen patients.
- Refer any patient with gout and kidney stones or recurrent UTI to urology.

**Hyperuricaemia** Increased serum uric acid. *Causes:* ↑ production or ↓ excretion of urate.
- *Drugs* Cytotoxics; thiazides; ethambutol.
- ↑*cell turnover* Lymphoma; leukaemia; psoriasis; haemolysis; muscle necrosis.
- ↓ *excretion* Primary gout; chronic renal failure; lead nephropathy; hyperparathyroidism.

*In addition* associated with ↑ BP and hyperlipidaemia. Urate may be ↑ in disorders of purine synthesis, e.g. Lesch–Nyhan syndrome.

**Chronic gout** Recurrent attacks, tophi (urate deposits) in pinna, tendons, and joints, and joint damage. Refer to rheumatology.

**Calcium pyrophosphate deposition disease (CPPD)** Inflammatory arthritis due to deposition of pyrophosphate crystals. Associated with OA, hyperparathyroidism, and haemochromatosis.

*Presentation* Attacks are less severe than gout and may be difficult to differentiate from other types of arthritis. Knee, wrist, and shoulder are most commonly affected. Acute attacks can be triggered by intercurrent illness and metabolic disturbance.

*Investigation* Chondrocalcinosis may be seen on X-ray (calcification of articular cartilage). Presence of joint crystals confirms diagnosis.

*Management*
- Treat acute attacks like acute gout.
- A chronic form also occurs—frequently erosive. Refer to rheumatology for confirmation of diagnosis and advice on management and disease-modifying drugs.

⚠ **Septic arthritis** This is the most important differential diagnosis for acute gout. It is most common in children <5y old and most commonly affects the hip or knee, but septic arthritis can occur at any age and affect any joint. The patient is usually systemically unwell and holds the affected joint completely still. The joint may be swollen, hot, and tender. This is an emergency—if suspected admit. Treatment is with IV antibiotics ± surgical washout of the joint.

# Connective tissue diseases

Often difficult to diagnose. Group of overlapping diseases which affect many organs, and are associated with fever, malaise, chronic (often relapsing/remitting) course, and response to steroids.

**Systemic lupus erythematosus (SLE)** Autoimmune disease with prevalence 1:3000; ♀:♂ ≈ 9:1. ↑ in African Caribbeans and Asians. Onset 15–40y. Presentation—Table 15.10. There *must* be multisystem involvement.

**Investigations** Check an autoimmune profile—95% are antinuclear antibody (ANA) +ve. *Other immunological abnormalities:* ↑ double-stranded DNA, RhF +ve (40%), ↓ complement (C3, C4). FBC: ↓Hb, ↓WCC, ↑ESR.

**Management** Refer to rheumatology. Use NSAIDs for symptom control. Sunscreens protect skin (ACBS). Steroids are the mainstay of treatment of acute flares (always discuss with a rheumatologist). Hydroxychloroquine can improve skin and joint symptoms. Cyclophosphamide, methotrexate, and ciclosporin are also used.

⚠ Sulfonamides and hormonal contraceptives/HRT may worsen SLE.

**Drug-induced lupus** Occurs with:
- Minocycline
- Isoniazid
- Hydralazine
- Procainamide
- Chlorpromazine
- Sulfasalazine
- Losartan
- Anti-convulsants.

Remits slowly when the drug is stopped, but steroids may be needed.

**Discoid lupus erythematosus (LE)** ♀:♂≈2:1. ≥1 well-defined, red, round/oval plaques on the face, scalp or hands. Scarring may → scalp alopecia and skin hypopigmentation. Internal involvement is not a feature. Confirm with lesion biopsy. Investigate with an autoimmune profile as for SLE. Treat with potent topical steroids and sunscreen. Remission occurs in 40%. 5% develop SLE.

**Antiphospholipid syndrome** ↑ clotting tendency which may occur with SLE or alone. Associated with thrombosis, stroke, migraine, miscarriage, myelitis, MI, and multi-infarct dementia. If suspected, start aspirin 150mg od and refer to rheumatology. May need anticoagulation.

## Sjögren syndrome

- *Primary Sjögren syndrome* Under-recognized cause of fatigue and dryness of skin/mucous membranes (may present with dyspareunia). Often presents with nodal OA. Long-term, associated with lymphoma. Autoimmune profile is characteristic.
- *Secondary Sjögren syndrome* Association of any connective tissue disease (50% have RA) with keratoconjunctivitis sicca (↓ lacrimation → dry eyes) or xerostomia (↓ salivation → dry mouth).

**Management** Refer to rheumatology. Provide information/support. Use artificial tears for dry eyes. Xerostomia may respond to frequent cool drinks, artificial saliva sprays (e.g. glandosane), or sugar-free gum. Inform dentist of the diagnosis. Rashes may respond to antimalarials.
*H.S.C. Sjögren (1899–1986)—Swedish ophthalmologist.*

**Raynaud's syndrome** Intermittent digital ischaemia precipitated by cold or emotion. Fingers ache and change colour: pale → blue → red on rewarming. Usually presents <25y of age and is idiopathic. Prevalence: 3–20%; ♀>♂; often abates at the menopause; 5% develop autoimmune rheumatic disease—mainly scleroderma and SLE.

### Differential diagnosis
- *Other rheumatology conditions* Scleroderma; SLE; RA.
- *Haematology conditions* Leukaemia; polycythaemia; thrombocytosis; cold agglutinins; monoclonal gammopathy; mixed cryoglobulinaemia.
- *Drugs* e.g. β-blockers
- *Thoracic outlet obstruction*
- *Smoking/arteriosclerosis*
- *Trauma* e.g. use of vibrating tools.

**Management** keep warm—woolly socks/gloves/hats in cold weather; hand warmers; stay inside if cold. Avoid drugs that worsen symptoms, e.g. β-blockers. Stop smoking. Nifedipine 10–20mg tds, amlodipine 5mg od or fluoxetine 20mg od (unlicensed) may help. If associated/severe symptoms refer to rheumatology (urgently if critical ischaemia, e.g. ulceration/infarcts on fingers). A.G.M. Raynaud (1031 1001) French physician.

**Systemic sclerosis** Spectrum of disorders causing fibrosis and skin tightening (scleroderma). Raynaud's is usually present, ± ↑ BP, lung fibrosis, GI symptoms, telangiectasia, polyarthritis, and myopathy. Provide education/support. Treat symptoms. Early specialist referral is vital. CREST (Calcinosis of subcutaneous tissues; Raynaud's; oEsophageal motility problems; Sclerodacyly; Telangectasia) have better prognosis.

**Table 15.10** Presentation of SLE

| System | % of patients | Presenting complaints | |
|--------|---------------|------------------------|---|
| *Joints* | 95% | Arthritis | Myalgia |
| | | Arthralgia | Tenosynovitis |
| *Skin* | 80% | Photosensitivity | Hair loss |
| | | Facial 'butterfly' rash | Urticaria |
| | | Vasculitic rash | Discoid lesions |
| *Lungs* | 50% | Pleurisy | Pleural effusion |
| | | Pneumonitis | Fibrosing alveolitis |
| *Kidney* | 50% | Proteinuria | Glomerulonephritis |
| | | ↑BP | Renal failure |
| *Heart* | 40% | Pericarditis | Endocarditis |
| *CNS* | 15% | Depression | Fits |
| | | Psychosis | Cranial nerve lesions |
| | | Infarction | |
| *Blood* | 95% | Anaemia (very common) | Splenomegaly |
| | | Thrombocytopoenia | |
| *Fatigue* | 95% | | |

### Information and support for patients
**Lupus UK** ☎ 01708 731251 🖳 www.lupusuk.com
**Raynaud's and Scleroderma Association** ☎ 01270 872776
🖳 www.raynauds.org.uk
**British Sjögren's Association** ☎ 0121 455 6549 🖳 www.bssa.uk.net

# Polymyalgia and temporal arteritis

Polymyalgia rheumatica (PMR) and temporal, or giant cell, arteritis (GCA) are two clinical syndromes that are part of the same spectrum. *Key features:*
- Both PMR and GCA affect the elderly (rare <50y)
- 50% of patients with GCA also have PMR.
- 15% with PMR also have GCA.
- ♀:♂ ≈ 3:1
- Both conditions typically respond rapidly and dramatically to corticosteroids.

**Presentation** Diagnosis is clinical.
- *General symptoms* Both PMR and GCA may present with malaise, anorexia, fever, night sweats, weight loss, depression.
- *PMR—typical symptoms* Proximal symmetrical muscle pain and stiffness worse after rest (Box 15.2).
- *GCA—typical symptoms*
  - Unilateral throbbing headache, facial pain, scalp tenderness e.g. on brushing hair and/or jaw claudication.
  - Visual symptoms—amaurosis fugax, diplopia, sudden loss of vision. Before steroid treatment, 30–60% became blind.
  - Temporal artery—thickened, tender or nodular with ↓ pulsation.

**Investigation**
- *Blood* ↑ESR (usually >30) ± normocytic anaemia.
- *Temporal artery biopsy* Refer urgently if GCA is suspected. Biopsy may be −ve even in true cases due to skip lesions. Do not withhold treatment whilst waiting for biopsy, but if the patient has had steroids ≥2wk +ve biopsy is less likely.
- Exclude other diagnoses depending on symptoms, e.g. malignancy, RA, myeloma. For PMR—consider acute neck pain syndromes with referred pain, bilateral shoulder lesions, arthritis, spinal stenosis, acute discitis with referred pain, and myositis.

**Initial management** Corticosteroids prevent vascular complications, particularly blindness, and rapidly relieve symptoms (70% improvement in <1wk).
- *GCA* Prescribe prednisolone 40–60mg daily, refer urgently to ophthalmology (same day if visual symptoms) or rheumatology.
- *PMR* Prednisolone 15–20 mg od; review after 2–4d. Most patients with PMR do not need rheumatology referral. Consider referral if diagnosis is in doubt (e.g. no response to steroids, or persistently ↑ ESR/CRP despite steroid treatment) or if the patient has excessive side effects from steroids.

**Ongoing management**
- At the start of treatment give osteoporosis prophylaxis (📖 p.518) and supply with a steroid card (📖 p.316).
- Continue starting dose of prednisolone for 4wk.
- After 4wk, ↓ dose of prednisolone every 2–4wk, by 2.5mg for patients with PMR or 5mg for patients with GCA until the dose is 10mg/d.

- Once stable on 10mg/d, ↓ dose of prednisolone by 1mg every 4–6wk to 7mg/d. Stay at a maintenance dose of 7mg/d for 12mo before attempting further reduction in dose.
- If stable after 1y on 7mg of prednisolone daily, ↓ dose by 1mg/d every 6–8wk until taking 3mg/d. Thereafter ↓ by 1mg every 12wk until prednisolone is stopped.

## Monitoring and relapses
- Relapse is common.
- Check ESR/CRP with steroid dose changes.
- Do not ↑ dose of steroids if ESR/CRP rises but no worsening of symptoms.
- Recheck ESR if ↑ symptoms. Go back to the last dose that controlled symptoms, or current dose +5mg—whichever is the the lower dose. Once stable for 4wk, start tapering dose again.
- Severe relapses, and relapses once steroids have been stopped, may require dose increase back to the starting dose.

**Prognosis** Most patients require >2y of treatment. Relapse is common after stopping treatment (50% if stopped after 2y).

---

### Box 15.2 Diagnosis of PMR

A person may be regarded as having PMR if ≥3 of the following criteria are present:*
- Bilateral shoulder pain or stiffness
- Onset of illness <2wk ago
- Initial ESR >40mm/h
- Morning stiffness lasting >1h
- Age ≥65y
- Depression and/or weight loss
- Bilateral tenderness in the upper arms.

* Reproduced from Bird HA *et al.* (1979) An evaluation of criteria for polymyalgia rheumatica *Ann Rheum Dis* **38**, 434–9, with permission of BMJ Publishing Group.

---

## Patient information and support
**Arthritis Research Campaign** ☎ 0870 850 5000 🖳 www.arc.org.uk

# Vasculitis

Characterized by inflammation within or around blood vessels ± necrosis. Severity depends on size and site of vessels affected. Systemic vasculitis can be life threatening. *Causes:*
- Idiopathic (50%)
- Connective tissue disease (e.g. RA, SLE)
- Infection (e.g. rheumatic fever, infective endocarditis, lyme's disease)
- Drugs (e.g. NSAIDs, antibiotics)
- Neoplasia (e.g. lymphoma, leukaemia).

**Presentation** Variable—may be confined to the skin or systemic involving joints, kidneys, lungs, gut, and nervous system.
- *Skin signs* Palpable purpura (often painful)—usually on lower legs/buttocks.
- *Systemic effects* Fever, night sweats, malaise, weight ↓, myalgia, and arthralgia may occur in all types of vasculitis.

**Conditions** Table 15.11—many are rare

**Patient information and support**
**Arthritis Research Campaign** ☎ 0870 8505000 🖳 www.arc.org.uk
**Stuart Strange Trust** 🖳 www.vasculitis-uk.org
**European Vasculitis Study Group** 🖳 www.vasculitis.org
**Kawasaki Support Group** ☎ 024 7661 2178 🖳 www.kssg.org.uk

**Table 15.11** Vasculitic conditions

| Condition | Features | Management |
|-----------|----------|------------|
| *Erythema nodosum* | 📖 p.601 | 📖 p.601 |
| *Henoch–Schönlein purpura (HSP)* | More common in children than adults; ♂ > ♀<br>Presents with a purpuric rash over buttocks and extensor surfaces.<br>Platelet count is normal<br>Often follows a respiratory infection<br>*Other features:* urticaria, nephritis, joint pains, abdominal pain (may mimic acute abdomen) | Refer to paediatrics for confirmation of diagnosis<br>Most recover fully without treatment over a few months |
| *Polyarteritis nodosa (PAN)* | Uncommon in the UK. ♂:♀ ≈ 4:1. Peak incidence in middle age<br>Multi-system necrotizing vasculitis → aneurysms of medium-sized arteries.<br>Presents with tender subcutaneous nodules along the line of arteries, coronary arteritis, ↑BP, mononeuritis multiplex, renal failure, and gastrointestinal symptoms<br>Sometimes associated with hepatitis B | Refer to rheumatology for angiography to confirm diagnosis and for advice on management<br>Treatment is with control of ↑BP, high-dose steroids, and cyclophosphamide |

**Table 15.11** *(Continued)* Vasculitic conditions

| Condition | Features | Management |
|---|---|---|
| Churg–Strauss syndrome | Associated with asthma<br>Affects coronary, pulmonary, cerebral, and splanchnic circulations<br>Skin manifestations and mononeuritis can also occur<br>Diagnosis is based on clinical features and biopsy | Refer for specialist treatment with high-dose prednisolone ± cyclophosphamide<br>Avoid leukotriene receptor agonist drugs for control of asthma as may worsen symptoms |
| Wegener's granulomatosis | Granulomatous vasculitis<br>Any organ may be involved and symptoms/signs relate those affected, e.g. mouth ulcers, nasal ulceration with epistaxis/rhinitis, otitis media, cranial nerve lesions, lung symptoms and shadows on CXR, ↑BP, eye signs (50%)<br>Often long prodrome of 'limited Wegener's granulomatosis'—nasal stuffiness, headaches, hearing difficulties, and nose bleeds | Refer to rheumatology/general medicine for investigation<br>ANCA helps diagnostically and in disease monitoring<br>Treatment is with high-dose steroids, methotrexate, mofetil, and cyclophosphamide |
| Kawasaki's disease | Predominantly affects children <5y<br>Cause unknown<br>*Diagnosis*: Diseases with similar presentations have been excluded *and* ≥5 of:<br>• Fever for ≥5d<br>• Bilateral conjunctivitis<br>• Polymorphous rash<br>• Changes in lips/mouth: red, dry, or cracked lips; strawberry tongue; diffuse redness of mucosa<br>• Changes in extremities: reddening of palms/soles, oedema of hands/feet, peeling of skin of hands, feet and/or groin.<br>• Cervical lymphadenopathy >15mm diameter (usually single and painful)<br>↑ suspicion if poor response to anti-pyretics | If suspected refer for urgent paediatric assessment<br>Early treatment (<10d after onset) with IV immunoglobulin and aspirin ↓ incidence and severity of aneurysm formation as well as giving symptom relief<br>*Complications*: Coronary arteritis with formation of aneurysms; accelerated athero-sclerosis |

# Tiredness and chronic fatigue syndrome

**Tired all the time** Fatigue is common. 1: 400 sustained episodes of fatigue generate a GP consultation. GPs see 30 patients/y whose main complaint is fatigue and it may be a 2° symptom in many others. 2% of consultations result in 2° care referral. Almost any disease processes can cause tiredness, whether physical or psychological. Physical causes account for ~9% of cases; 75% have symptoms of emotional distress.

## Assessment
- *Onset and duration* Short history/abrupt onset suggest post-viral or DM.
- *Pattern of fatigue* on exertion relieved by rest suggests organic cause; worst in the morning and never goes suggests depression.
- *Associated symptoms*, e.g. breathlessness, weight ↓ or anorexia suggest underlying organic disease. Chronic pain may cause fatigue.
- *Sleep patterns* Early morning wakening/unrefreshing sleep suggest depression; snoring, pauses of breathing in sleep, and daytime sleepiness suggest sleep apnoea.
- *Psychiatric history* Symptoms of depression, anxiety, and stress.
- *Alcohol and medication* Including OTC and illicit drugs.
- *Patient's worries* What does the patient think is wrong?
- *Examination* Usually normal.

## Common organic causes of fatigue in general practice
- Anaemia
- Infections (EBV, CMV, hepatitis)
- DM
- Hypo- or hyperthyroidism
- Perimenopausal
- Asthma
- Carcinomatosis
- Sleep apnoea.

**Investigation** If sustained fatigue with no obvious cause, check
- **Urine** Dipstick for for protein, blood, and glucose.
- **Blood** FBC (all children should have FBC/blood film on presentation with fatigue[N]); ESR; CRP; U&E, Cr; eGFR; LFTs; $Ca^{2+}$; TFTs; random blood glucose; coeliac serology; CK.

 In addition check serum ferritin if the patient is a child/young person Do not check ferritin in adults unless FBC suggests iron deficiency.

Use clinical judgement to decide on additional tests to exclude other diagnoses (e.g. serological testing if history suggestive of infection).

**Management** Treat organic causes. In most no physical cause is found—reassure. Explaining the relationship of psychological and emotional factors to fatigue can help patients deal with symptoms. If lasts >6–12 wk and symptoms/signs of depression, consider a trial of antidepressants, e.g. sertraline 50mg od.

**Chronic fatigue syndrome (CFS, ME)** A debilitating and distressing condition. *Prevalence*: 0.2–2.6%; ♀:♂ ≈ 3:2. Cause is unknown though viral infections (~10% after EBV), immunization, chemical toxins (e.g. organophosphates, chemotherapy drugs) have all been implicated.

❶ Fatigue must have been present for ≥4mo for adults and ≥3mo for children and young people for a diagnosis of CFS to be made.

***Clinical features*** Unexplained persistent and/or recurrent fatigue of new/definite onset, not explained by other conditions and resulting in ↓ activity (often starting 1–2d after mental/physical exertion and lasting >24h) and ≥1 of:

- General malaise
- Dizziness/nausea
- Palpitations without cardiac dysfunction
- Cognitive dysfunction, e.g. impaired concentration/memory
- Tender cervical/axillary LNs without enlargement
- Physical/mental exertion makes symptoms worse
- Headaches of new type, pattern or severity
- Multi-site muscle/joint pain without inflammation
- Sore throat
- Difficulty with sleeping.

***Additional symptoms*** must not have predated fatigue. Symptoms may fluctuate or change in nature over time. Include:

- Postural dizziness
- Vertigo
- Altered temperature sensation
- Paraesthesiae
- Sensitivity to light/sound
- Palpitations
- IBS
- Food intolerance
- Fibromyalgia
- Feelings of dyspnoea
- Mood swings
- Panic attacks
- Depression.

❶ Infection/immunization, drugs, caffeine, alcohol, and stress cause setbacks.

⚠ ***Red flag symptoms that suggest another diagnosis***
- Significant weight ↓
- Localizing/focal neurological signs
- Signs/symptoms of inflammatory arthritis or connective tissue disease
- Signs/symptoms of cardiorespiratory disease
- Sleep apnoea
- Clinically significant lymphadenopathy.

***Reconsider diagnosis if none of the following are present*** Cognitive difficulties; chronic pain; post-exertional fatigue/malaise; sleep disturbance.

***Management*** Provide support and reassurance—explanation, information ± self-help groups. Avoid exacerbating factors, e.g. caffeine, alcohol. Advise graded exercise and regular limited rest periods (e.g. 30 min 4–5×/d). Treat symptoms, e.g. amitriptyline 10–50mg nocte to help sleep ± relieve headache/neuropathic pain, SSRI for depression. Refer adults if severe symptoms, or symptoms persist >6mo Specialist treatments include CBT and rehabilitation programmes.

 Children presenting with sustained fatigue of any duration with no obvious cause should *always* be referred for paediatric review.

***Prognosis*** Variable. 55% of adults have symptoms >6 mo. Risk ↑ ×3 if history of anxiety/depression. Prognosis in children is better.

### Further information
**NICE** Diagnosis and management of CFS/ME in adults and children (2007) 🖥 www.nice.org.uk

### Information and support for patients
**ME Association** ☎ 0844 576 5326 🖥 www.meassociation.org.uk
**Action for ME** ☎ 0845 123 2314 🖥 www.afme.org.uk; www.a4me.org.uk

# Miscellaneous conditions

**Fibromyalgia** Painful non-articular condition of unknown cause predominantly involving muscles. Fibromyalgia is common and often results in significant disability and handicap with inability to cope with a job or household activities. Peak age 40–50y; 90% female.

### Diagnostic criteria

• History of widespread pain (defined as pain on both left and right sides, above and below the waist, together with axial skeletal pain e.g. neck or back pain), *in combination with*
• Pain in ≥ 11 out of 18 tender sites (Figure 15.5) on digital palpation.

### Other clinical features

• Pain is worsened by stress, cold, and activity, and associated with generalized morning stiffness.
• Paraesthesiae or dysaesthesiae of hands and feet are common.
• Analgesics, NSAIDs, and local physical treatments are ineffective and may worsen symptoms.
• Sleep patterns are poor—patients tend to wake exhausted and complain of poor concentration.
• Anxiety and depression scores are high.
• Associated symptoms—unexplained headache, urinary frequency, and abdominal symptoms are common.
• Clinical findings are unremarkable.

**Investigation** Exclude other causes of pain and fatigue (e.g. hypothyroidism, SLE, Sjögren's, psoriatic arthritis, inflammatory myopathy, hyperparathyroidism, osteomalacia)—check FBC, ESR, TFTs, U&E, eGFR, $Ca^{2+}$, CK, $PO_4$, ANA, RhF, and immunoglobulins.

**Management** A multidisciplinary approach is helpful—usually accessed through a rheumatology or pain clinic. Be supportive—reassurance that there is no serious pathology, explanation, and information are vital. Low-dose amitriptyline 25-75mg nocte may help with sleep and pain. SSRI, e.g. sertraline 25–50mg od, may help anxiety, depression, and sleep—stop if no improvement after a month's trial. Graded exercise regimes can improve pain, lethargy, mood, and general malaise. Counselling and learning coping strategies can be beneficial, as can cognitive behavioural therapy if available locally. Some patients benefit from injection of hypalgesic trigger points with steroid or acupuncture to trigger points.

**Tietze syndrome** Idiopathic costochondritis. Pain is enhanced by motion, coughing, or sneezing. The 2nd rib is most commonly affected. *Examination*: marked localized tenderness. *Differential diagnosis*: muscular sprain; rarely inflammatory chest wall enthesitis/osteitis 2° to spondylarthropathy.

**Management** Explanation and reassurance that nothing serious is happening; simple OTC analgesia, e.g. ibuprofen 400mg tds. If pain persists local steroid or bipivacaine injections can be helpful. If not settling, consider referral to rheumatology.
A.Tietze (1864–1927)—German surgeon.

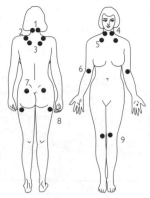

1. Insertion of nuchal muscles into the occiput
2. Upper border of trapezius mid-portion
3. Muscle attachments to upper medial border of scapula
4. Anterior aspects of the $C_5, C_7$ intertransverse spaces
5. 2nd rib space ~3cm lateral to the sternal border
6. Muscle attachments to the lateral epicondyle at the elbow
7. Upper outer quadrant of gluteal muscles
8. Muscle attachments just posterior to the greater trochanter
9. Medial fat pad of the knee just proximal to the joint line

**Fig. 15.5** Tender point sites for diagnosis of fibromyalgia

Reproduced from Davies R, Everitt H, and Simon C *Musculoskeletal Problems* (2006), with permission from Oxford University Press.

**Neuropathic arthritis** Charcot's disease is a rapidly progressive degeneration in a joint which lacks position sense and protective pain sensation. Upper limb disease is usually associated with syringomyelia. Lower limb disease is usually associated with diabetic neuropathy or cauda equina lesions. The joint may be very deformed but is usually painless. Treat the underlying condition (e.g. DM) accordingly. The joint cannot recover, but refer to orthopaedics for advice on stabilization.

**Reflex sympathetic dystrophy** 📖 p.494

**Haemophiliac arthopathy** 📖 p.668

**Patient information and support**
**Arthritis Research Campaign** ☎ 0870 850 5000 🖥 www.arc.org.uk
**Fibromyalgia Association UK** ☎ 0845 345 2322
🖥 www.fibromyalgia-associationuk.org

# Neurology

# Reflexes

Automatic responses. The reflex arc goes from the stimulus via a sensory nerve to the spinal cord and then back along a motor nerve to cause muscle contraction, without brain involvement.

**Key reflexes** (Table 16.2) Record whether absent, present with reinforcement, normal, or brisk ± clonus.

**Absent or ↓ reflex** Implies a breach in the reflex arc at:
- Sensory nerve or root, e.g. neuropathy, spondylosis.
- Anterior horn cell e.g. MND, polio.
- Motor nerve or root, e.g. neuropathy, spondylosis.
- Nerve endings, e.g myasthenia gravis, or
- Muscle, e.g. myopathy

**↑ reflex** Implies lack of higher control—an upper motor neuron (UMN) lesion, e.g. post-stroke.

**Clonus** Rhythmic involuntary muscle contraction due to abrupt tendon stretching, e.g. by dorsiflexing the ankle—associated with an UMN lesion.

**Reinforcement** Method of accentuating reflexes. Use if a reflex seems absent. Ask the patient to clench his/her teeth (to reinforce upper limb reflexes) or clench his hands and pull in opposite directions (to accentuate lower limb reflexes). This effect only lasts ~1s, so ask the patient to perform the manoeuvre simultaneously with the tap from the tendon hammer.

**Primitive reflexes** 📖 p.846

**Table 16.1** Quick screening test for muscle power

| Joint | Movement | Nerve roots | Joint | Movement | Nerve roots |
|---|---|---|---|---|---|
| Shoulder | Abduction | C5,6 | Hip | Flexion | L1–3 |
| | Adduction | C6–8 | | Extension | L4,5, & S1 |
| Elbow | Flexion | C5,6 | Knee | Flexion | L5 & S1 |
| | Extension | C7,8 | | Extension | L3,4 |
| Wrist | Flexion | C7,8 | Ankle | Dorsiflexion | L4,5 |
| | Extension | C6,7 | | Plantarflexion | S1,2 |
| Fingers | Flexion | C8 | Toes | Extensors | L5,S1 |
| | Extension | C7 | | Flexors | S2 |
| | Abduction | T1 | | | |

❶ Test proximal muscle power by asking the patient to sit from lying, pull you towards him/herself, or rise from squatting.

**Table 16.2** Key reflexes and nerve roots involved

| Reflex | Test | Expected result | Nerve roots |
|---|---|---|---|
| Jaw | Ask the patient to let his mouth open slightly. Place a finger on the chin and tap the finger with a tendon hammer | Contraction of masseters and closure of mouth | Vth cranial nerve |
| Gag | Touch the back of the patient's pharynx on each side with a spatula. If absent, ask the patient whether he can feel the spatula—if he can, then Xth nerve palsy | Contraction of the soft palate | IXth/Xth cranial nerve |
| Biceps | Tap a finger placed on the biceps tendon by letting the tendon hammer fall on it | Contraction of the biceps + elbow flexion | C5,6 |
| Supinator | Tap the lower end of the radius just above the wrist with the tendon hammer | Contraction of brachioradialis + elbow flexion | C5,6 |
| Triceps | Support elbow in flexion with 1 hand. Tap the triceps tendon with a tendon hammer held in the other hand | Contraction of triceps + elbow extension | C7,8 |
| Knee | Support the knees so relaxed and slightly bent. Let the tendon hammer fall onto the infrapatellar tendon | Contraction of quadriceps + extension of knee | L3,4 |
| Ankle | Externally rotate the thigh and flex the knee. Let the tendon hammer fall onto the Achilles tendon | Contraction of gastrocnemius + plantarflexion of the ankle | S1 |
| Abdominal | Lightly stroke the abdominal wall diagonally towards the umbilicus in each of the four abdominal quadrants. | Abdominal wall contractions. When absent can be normal or indicate UMN or LMN lesion | T7–12 |
| Cremaster | ♂ patients only. Pre-warn the patient. Stroke the superior and medial aspect of the thigh in a downwards direction | Contraction of cremasteric muscle → raising of scrotum and testis on the side stroked. Absent in UMN and LMN lesions | L1 |
| Anal | Scratch the perianal skin | Reflex contraction of the external sphincter. Absent in UMN and LMN lesions | S4,5 |
| Plantar | Pre-warn the patient. Run a blunt object up the lateral side of the sole of the foot, curving medially before the MTP joints | Flexion of big toe (if >1y old). Extension implies UMN lesion | S1 |

# Cranial nerve lesions

Cranial nerves may be affected at any point from the nerve nucleus within the brainstem to the point of innervation. Think systematically about the level of the lesion. *Potential sites:*

- Muscle
- Neuromuscular junction
- Along the course of the nerve outside the brainstem
- Within the brainstem.

Any cranial nerve may be affected by DM, MS, tumours, sarcoid, vasculitis, or syphilis and >1 nerve may be affected by a lesion. Refer according to cause (ENT, ophthalmology, neurology).

**Table 16.3** Cranial nerve lesions and their causes

| Nerve | Clinical test | Causes |
|---|---|---|
| I Olfactory | *Smell*—test each nostril for the ability to differentiate different smells | Trauma, frontal lobe tumour, meningitis |
| II Optic | *Acuity*—Snellen chart *Visual fields*—compare with your own visual fields by standing directly in front of the patient with your head at the same level as theirs *Pupils*—size, shape, reaction to light, and accommodation *Ophthalmoscopy*—darken room, dilate pupil with 1 drop tropicamide 0.5% if needed; view optic disc (?pale, swollen); follow each vessel outwards to view each quadrant; track outwards to check lens and cornea | *Monocular blindness*—lesion in one eye or optic nerve (e.g. MS, giant cell arteritis) *Bitemporal hemianopia*—optic chiasm compression, e.g. pituitary adenoma, craniopharyngioma, internal carotid artery aneurysm *Homonymous hemianopia*—affects half the visual field on the side opposite the lesion. Lesion beyond the optic chiasm, e.g. stroke, abscess, tumour |
| III | Ptosis, large pupil, eye looks down and outwards ❶ Diplopia from a 3rd nerve lesion may cause nystagmus | DM, giant cell arteritis, syphilis, posterior communicating artery aneurysm, idiopathic. If pupil normal size, due to DM or other vascular cause |
| IV | Diplopia on looking down and in; may compensate by tilting head. | Rare in isolation. May occur due to trauma to the orbit |
| V Trigeminal | *Motor*—open mouth. Jaw deviates to the side of the lesion *Sensory*—corneal reflex lost 1st. Check all 3 divisions | *Sensory*—trigeminal neuralgia (📖 p.565), herpes zoster, nasopharyngeal carcinoma *Motor*—bulbar palsy (📖 p.557), acoustic neuroma |
| VI | Horizontal diplopia on looking outwards | MS, pontine CVA, ↑ICP |

**Table 16.3** (*Continued*) Cranial nerve lesions and their causes

| Nerve | Clinical test | Causes |
|---|---|---|
| **VII**<br>Facial | Causes facial weakness and droop<br>Ask to raise eyebrows, show teeth, puff out cheeks:<br>—*LMN lesion* all one side of face affected<br>—*UMN lesion* lower ⅔ face affected only | *LMN*—Bell's palsy, polio, otitis media, skull fracture, cerebellopontine angle tumours, parotid tumours, herpes zoster (Ramsay Hunt syndrome 📖 p.546)<br>*UMN*—stroke, tumour |
| **VIII**<br>Vestibulo-auditory | *Auditory*—ask to repeat a number whispered in 1 ear whilst you block the other<br>*Vestibular*—ask about balance, check for nystagmus (📖 p.948)—ask patient to fix on finger 0.75m away—check gaze—upwards, downwards, lateral (both directions), keeping finger <30° from midline | Noise, Paget's disease, Ménière's disease (📖 p.949), herpes zoster, acoustic neuroma, brainstem CVA, drugs (e.g. furosemide) |
| **IX, X** | Gag reflex, palate moves → normal side on saying 'Aah' | Trauma, brainstem lesions, neck tumours |
| **XI** | *Trapezii*—shrug shoulders against resistance<br>*Sternomastoid*—turn head to right/left against resistance | Rare. Polio, syringomyelia, tumours near jugular foramen, stroke, bulbar palsy (📖 p.557), trauma, TB |
| **XII** | Tongue deviates to the side of the lesion | Trauma, brainstem lesions, neck tumours |

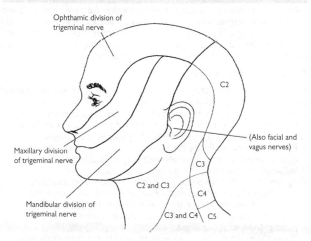

**Fig. 16.1** Cutaneous innervation of the head and neck

Reproduced from Simon C, *Neurology* (2006), with permission from Oxford University Press.

# Neuropathy

**Dermatomes and peripheral nerve distribution** Figure 16.2 (📖 p.548) and Figure 16.3 (📖 p.549)

**Mononeuropathy** Lesions of individual peripheral (including cranial) nerves. *Causes*: trauma, compression, DM, leprosy. If >1 peripheral nerve is involved, the term *mononeuritis multiplex* is used. *Causes*: DM, sarcoid, cancer, PAN, amyloid, leprosy.

## Common mononeuropathies Table 16.4

**Bell's palsy** Facial palsy without other signs. Unknown cause—possibly viral. *Peak age*: 10–40y. ♂ = ♀. *Lifetime incidence*: ~1:65. Affects left and right side of the face equally often. Usually sudden onset—may be preceded by pain around the ear. *Other possible symptoms*: facial numbness; ↓ noise tolerance; disturbed taste on the anterior part of the tongue.

**Management** ~70% recover completely; 13% have insignificant sequelae; the remainder have permanent deficit. 85% improve in <3wk—reassure. Give prednisolone (25mg bd for 10d) if <72h after onset of symptoms.[R] Protect eye—tape lid shut and pad at night; glasses in the day ± artificial tears if drying. *Refer*:
• If recovery is not starting after 3wk
• For tarsorraphy if complete or long-standing palsy
• If unacceptable cosmetic result—may benefit from plastic surgery.
C. *Bell (1774–1842)—Scottish anatomist and surgeon.*

**Ramsay Hunt syndrome (herpes zoster oticus)** Severe pain in the ear precedes facial nerve palsy. Zoster vesicles appear around the ear, in the external ear canal, on the soft palate, and in the tonsillar fossa. Often accompanied by deafness ± vertigo which are slow to resolve and may result in permanent deficit. Pain usually abates after 48h but post-herpetic neuralgia can be a problem. If detected <24h after the rash appears, treatment with antivirals (e.g. aciclovir 800mg 5×/d for 1wk) may be effective. *J. Ramsay Hunt (1872–1937)—American neurologist.*

## Morton's metatarsalgia 📖 p.506

**Autonomic neuropathy** Postural hypotension (dizziness or syncope on standing, after exercise, or after a large meal); impotence; inability to sweat; vomiting and dysphagia; diarrhoea or constipation; urinary retention or incontinence, Horner's syndrome (📖 p.308). Check BP lying and standing—a postural drop of ≥30/15mmHg is abnormal. *Causes*:
• **Primary autonomic failure** No known cause. Occurs alone or as part of multisystem atrophy. Typically middle-aged/elderly men. Onset is insidious. Survival—rarely >10y after diagnosis.
• **Ageing** 25% >74y have postural hypotension. Review medication, discourage prolonged bed rest. Often associated with disordered thermoregulation making elderly people prone to hypothermia. Exclude other disorders (e.g. DM, multisystem atrophy, drugs) before putting down to ageing alone.
• **Drugs** Common culprits—antihypertensives (e.g. thiazides), diuretics (over-diuresis), L-dopa, TCAs, phenothiazines, benzodiazepines.

- *Polyneuropathies* May occur as part of more general polyneuropathy, e.g. DM, Guillain–Barré syndrome, or alcoholic/nutritional neuropathy.
- *Other causes* Craniopharyngioma, vascular lesions, spinal cord lesions, tabes dorsalis, Chagas disease, HIV, familial dysautonomia.

**Management** Treat any underlying cause. Advise patients to stand slowly, raise the head of the bed at night, eat little and often, and ↓ carbohydrate and alcohol intake. Fludrocortisone (0.1mg/d, increasing prn) may help those most severely affected. Refer if diagnosis is unclear or simple measures are ineffective.

**Polyneuropathy** 📖 p.550

**Table 16.4** Common mononeuropathies

| Nerve involved | Nerve roots | Presentation | Common causes |
|---|---|---|---|
| Median | C5–T1 | Loss of sensation over lateral 3½ digits and palm; wasting of the thenar eminence; inability to flex the terminal phalanx of the thumb implies involvement of the anterior interosseous branch | Trauma (especially wrist lacerations), carpal tunnel syndrome (📖 p.494) |
| Ulnar | C7–T1 | Weakness and wasting of interossei muscles (weakness of abduction of fingers) and claw hand deformity. Wasting of hypothenar eminence. Sensory loss over medial 1½ fingers and ulnar side of the hand. Flexion of 4th and 5th fingers is weak if proximal lesion | Trauma or compression at the elbow (📖 p.490), trauma at the wrist |
| Radial | C5–T1 | Sensory loss is variable but always includes the dorsal aspect of the root of the thumb. Wrist drop and weak extension of thumb and fingers | Compression against the humerus, trauma |
| Sciatic | L4–S2 | Weakness of hamstrings and all muscles below the knee (foot drop). Loss of sensation below the knee laterally | Back injury, pelvic tumour |
| Common peroneal | L4–S2 | Inability to dorsiflex the foot (foot drop), evert the foot, extend the toes. Sensory loss over dorsum of the foot. | Trauma |
| Tibial | S1–S3 | Inability to stand on tiptoe, invert the foot, or flex toes. Sensory loss over sole. | Trauma or entrapment |

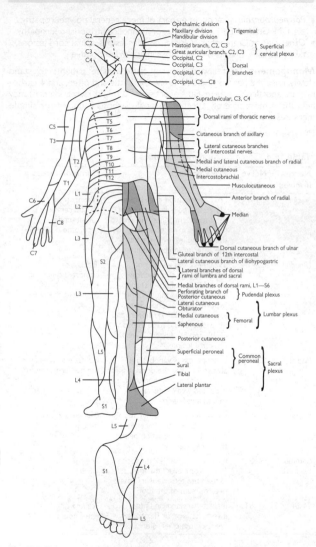

**Fig. 16.2** Dermatomes and peripheral nerve distribution—rear view

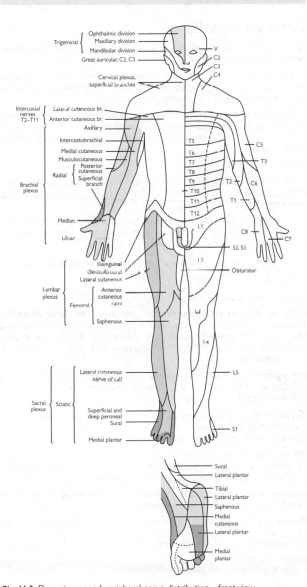

**Fig. 16.3** Dermatomes and peripheral nerve distribution—front view

# Polyneuropathy

Generalized disorder of peripheral nerves, including cranial and autonomic nerves. Distribution is bilateral, symmetrical, and widespread.

**Sensory neuropathy** presents as numbness, tingling or burning sensation often affecting the extremities first (glove and stocking distribution), or clumsiness handling fine objects (e.g. needle).

**Motor neuropathy** presents as progressive weakness or clumsiness of hands, stumbling/falls on walking, respiratory difficulty (can progress rapidly). *Examination:* wasting and weakness most marked distally; reflexes are ↓ or absent.

**Causes** Table 16.5

**Initial investigations** Exclude common causes—check blood glucose, FBC, ESR, U&E, Cr and eGFR, jLFTs, TFTs, plasma $B_{12}$, autoimmune profile, syphilis serology.

**Management** Treat cause if possible. Involve physiotherapists and OT. If sensory neuropathy care of the feet is important to minimize trauma and consequent disability. Refer if a cause is not found.

⚠ If rapid deterioration admit as acute medical emergency as ventilation may be needed.

## Specific polyneuropathies

***Charcot–Marie–Tooth syndrome (peroneal muscular atrophy)***
Presents at puberty or in early adult life and begins with foot drop and weak legs. The peroneal muscles are the first to atrophy. The disease spreads to the hands then arms. Sensation and reflexes are also ↓. Unknown cause.

*Management* Once diagnosis is confirmed treatment is supportive.
*J.M. Charcot (1825–1893) and P. Marie (1853–1940)—French neurologists; H.H. Tooth (1856–1925)—English neurologist.*

***Guillain–Barré polyneuritis*** Develops within a few weeks of surgery, flu vaccination, or infection (URTI, flu, VZ, HSV, CMV, EBV, *Campylobacter; Mycoplasma*). In 40% no precipitating event is found.

*Presentation* Ascending motor neuropathy which may advance fast. Proximal muscles are more affected than distal muscles. Trunk, respiratory muscles, and cranial nerves are commonly affected.

*Management* If suspected admit immediately to hospital as an emergency. Ventilation on ITU is frequently required.

*Prognosis* 85% make a complete or near-complete recovery. 10% are unable to walk alone at 1y. *Mortality*: 10%.
*C. Guillain (1876–1961) and J.A. Barré (1880–1967)—French neurologists.*

**Polio** 📖 p.587

***Refsum's syndrome*** Rare autosomal recessive disorder which presents in the 2nd decade or later with sensorimotor polyneuropathy, ataxia, visual, and/or hearing problems. Treatment involves dietary restriction (avoidance of chlorophyll-containing foods) and plasmapheresis.
*S. Refsum (1907–1991)—Norwegian physician.*

**Table 16.5** Causes of polyneuropathy

| | |
|---|---|
| *Inflammatory* | Gullain–Barré syndrome (mostly motor) |
| | Chronic inflammatory demyelinating polyneuropathy (CDP) |
| | Sarcoidosis |
| *Metabolic* | DM (mainly sensory) |
| | Renal failure (mainly sensory) |
| | Hypothyroidism |
| | Hypoglycaemia |
| | Mitochondrial disorders |
| *Vasculitis* | Polyarteritis nodosa |
| | Rheumatoid arthritis |
| | Wegener's granulomatosis |
| *Malignancy* | Paraneoplastic syndromes (especially small cell lung cancer) |
| | Polycythaemia rubra vera |
| *Infection* | HIV |
| | Syphilis |
| | Lyme disease |
| | Leprosy (mainly sensory) |
| *Vitamin deficiency* | Lack of $B_1$, $B_6$, $B_{12}$ (e.g. alcoholic) |
| *Inherited* | Refsum's syndrome |
| | Charcot–Marie–Tooth syndrome (mostly motor) |
| | Porphyria |
| *Toxins* | Lead (mostly motor) |
| | Arsenic |
| *Drugs* | Alcohol |
| | Cisplatin |
| | Isoniazid |
| | Vincristine |
| | Nitrofurantoin |
| | *Less frequently*: metronidazole, phenytoin |
| *Others* | Paraproteinaemias, e.g. multiple myeloma, amyloidosis |

# Walking problems

> **Walking difficulty ('off legs')** Common amongst the elderly. *Causes:*
> * *Musculoskeletal* OA or RA, osteoporotic fractures, fractured neck of femur, osteomalacia, Paget's disease, polymyalgia rheumatica.
> * *Psychological* Depression, bereavement, fear of falling.
> * *Neurological* Stroke, Parkinson's disease, peripheral neuropathy.
> * *Spinal cord compression.*
> * *Systemic* Pneumonia, UTI, anaemia, hypothyroidism, renal failure, infection, hypothermia.
>
> **Management** Treat according to cause. Refer if inadequate support at home, cause warrants admission, or no cause is found.

**Abnormal gait** Gait means manner of walking. Abnormal gait can give clues to the underlying problem.

**Abnormal movements** Normal gait is interrupted by abnormal movements, e.g. choreiform movements, athetoid movements, or hemiballismus. May indicate underlying neurological problem, e.g. cerebral palsy, Huntington's chorea

**Antalgic gait** Gait adjusts to try to minimize pain in a joint—usually OA hip. The patient leans towards the affected side and takes a rapid step on that side followed by a slower step on the contralateral side—check Trendelenburg's sign (🕮 p.496).

**Drunken gait** As its name suggests, a drunken gait is the type of gait adopted by someone who is drunk. The other major cause is a cerebellar lesion. *Features:*
* Wide-based gait or reeling gait on a narrow base.
* Feet are often raised too high and placed over carefully with the patient looking ahead.
* If a cerebellar lesion, the patient falls to the side of the lesion.

**Foot drop** Patients trip frequently or walk with a high stepping gait. On examination patients are unable to walk on their heels and cannot dorsiflex their foot. Check ankle jerk. *Causes:*
* *Common peroneal palsy,* e.g. due to trauma—normal ankle jerk
* *Sciatica*—ankle jerk absent.
* *L4, L5 root lesion*—ankle jerk may be absent.
* *Peripheral motor neuropathy,* e.g. alcoholic—ankle jerk weak or absent.
* *Distal myopathy*—ankle jerk weak or absent.
* *Motor neuron disease*—↑ ankle jerk.

**Hemiplegic gait** Style of walking seen in patients with UMN lesions. *Features:*
* Arm adducted and internally rotated, elbow flexed and pronated ± finger flexion.
* Foot is plantarflexed and the leg swings in a lateral arc.

**Frontal lesions** Marked unsteadiness—the feet appear stuck to the floor causing a wide-based shuffling gait.

**Parkinsonian gait** Seen in patients with Parkinson's disease and other causes of Parkinsonism. *Features*:
- *Shuffling gait* Short steps, with the feet barely leaving the ground, producing an audible shuffling noise. May trip over small obstacles.
- *Turning 'en bloc'* Keeping the neck and trunk rigid, and requiring multiple small steps to accomplish a turn.
- *Gait freezing* Inability to move feet. May worsen in tight, cluttered spaces or when attempting to initiate gait.
- *Festinant gait* Flexed posture as if hurrying to keep up with feet.
- *Lack of normal arm swing*.

**Scissor gait** As the name implies, the patient walks as if his/her legs were like a pair of scissors. Associated with spastic paraplegia.
- Both legs are held rigid with plantarflexion of the ankle, extension of the knee, and adduction/internal rotation of the hips.
- The patient walks on tiptoe and the knees rub together/cross during the walking cycle.
- Often accompanied by complex movements of the upper limbs to assist the walking movements.

**Sensory ataxic gait** Loss of proprioception due to peripheral neuropathy or spinal cord disease (e.g. cervical spondylosis, MS, syphilis, combined degeneration of the cord) results in an ataxic gait similar to that seen with cerebellar disease. Check Romberg's test. *Features*:
- Broad-based gait with a tendency to stamp feet down clumsily.
- Patient tends to look at feet throughout the walking cycle.
- Romberg's sign +ve.

**Waddling gait** Typically seen in patients with proximal myopathy, e.g. due to muscular dystrophy. *Other causes*: pregnancy, congenital dislocation of the hip. *Features*:
- Broad-based gait. The pelvis drops to the side of the leg being raised.
- The patient moves his/her body and hips to accommodate this, resulting in a duck-like waddle in the swing phase.
- Commonly accompanied by ↑ forward curvature of the lower spine

**Examining gait** Note abnormalities and any aids/assistance required.
- Make sure that you can see the legs well.
- Ask the patient to stand up from a chair without support. If able to do that repeat with feet together and/or with eyes closed.
- Ask the patient to stand still with feet together. If able to do that ask the patient to close his eyes and see what happens (Romberg's sign).
- Ask the patient to walk normally for ~5m, turn round and walk back.
- Ask the patient to walk heel-to-toe (testing for cerebellar disease).
- Ask the patient to stand with the feet together
  - With eyes open—testing cerebellar and posterior column function.
  - With eyes closed—testing posterior column function.
  - On toes alone—impossible with S1 lesions.
  - On heels alone—impossible if L4/L5 lesion.

# Other movement problems

**Abnormal gait** 📖 p.552

**Cramp** Painful muscle spasm. Common—especially at night and after exercise. Rarely associated with disease—salt depletion, muscle ischaemia, myopathy. Forearm cramps suggest motor neuron disease. Night cramps in the elderly may respond to quinine bisulphate 300mg nocte twice weekly.

**Dystonia** Prolonged muscle contraction producing abnormal postures or repetitive movements.
- *Spasmodic torticollis* Head is pulled to one side and held there by a contracting sternomastoid muscle. Treat with physiotherapy.
- *Blepharospasm* Involuntary contraction of the orbicularis oculi.
- *Writer's cramp* Spasm of the hand and forearm muscles on writing.

**Dyspraxia** Impairment of performance of complex movements despite preservation of ability to perform their individual components. Test by asking the patient to perform everyday tasks (e.g. ask to dress/undress), copy complex hand movements, and perform familiar sequences of movements (e.g. 'head, shoulders, knees, and toes').

*Childhood* 📖 p.914

*Adults* Most common causes are stroke or space-occupying lesion. Involve rehabilitation services and OT.
- *Dressing dyspraxia* Patient is unsure of the orientation of clothes on his/her body.
- *Constructional dyspraxia* Difficulty in assembling objects or drawing (ask to draw 5-pointed star).
- *Gait dyspraxia* Gait disorder although the lower limbs function normally—more common amongst the elderly.

**Tremor**
- *Resting tremor* Present at rest but abolished on voluntary movement. Most common cause—PD when tremor is rhythmic.
- *Intention tremor* Irregular large-amplitude tremor worse on movement e.g. reaching for something. Typical of cerebellar disease.
- *Tremors on movement* Thyrotoxicosis, anxiety, benign essential tremor (inherited), and drugs (e.g. β-agonists) cause a fine tremor abolished at rest. Alcohol and β-blockers may help.

**Asterixis** Intermittent lapses of an assumed posture. May involve arms, neck, tongue, jaw, and eyelids. Usually bilateral, absent at rest, and asynchronous on each side. *Causes:* liver failure (flapping tremor), heart failure, respiratory failure, renal failure, hypoglycaemia, barbiturate intoxication.

**Athetosis** Slow confluent, often rhythmic, purposeless movements of hands, tongue, fingers, or face. *Causes:* cerebral palsy, kernicterus.

**Chorea** Non-rhythmic jerky purposeless movements (especially hands) with voluntary movements possible in between. *Most common causes:* cerebral palsy, Huntington's chorea, Sydenham's chorea.

**Hemiballismus** Large-amplitude involuntary flinging movements of limbs. May occur after stroke, in Huntington's disease, or with high doses of L-dopa for PD.

**Myoclonus** Sudden involuntary focal or general jerks. May be normal especially if occurs when falling asleep. *Other causes:*
• Neurodegenerative disease (e.g. CJD).
• Myoclonic epilepsy.
• Benign essential myoclonus (generalized myoclonus beginning in childhood as muscle twitches; may be inherited as autosomal dominant).
• Asterixis (metabolic flap, e.g liver failure, uraemia).

*Treatment* If needed treat with sodium valproate or clonazepam.

**Tardive dyskinesia** Involuntary chewing and grimacing movements due to long-term neuroleptics (metoclopramide and prochlorperazine are also possible causes). Withdraw neuroleptic—if no improvement after 3-6mo consider tetrabenazine 25–50mg tds po.

**Tics** Brief, repeated, and stereotyped movements which are able to be suppressed voluntarily for a while. Common in children and usually resolve spontaneously. Consider clonazepam or clonidine if tics are severe.

*Gilles de la Tourette syndrome* 📖 p.909

# Speech problems

**Hoarseness** 📖 p.934

**Stammer** Disorder of rhythm and fluency of speech in which syllables, words, or phrases are repeated. ♂:♀ ≈ 4:1. *Cause*: unknown. Can result in stress and embarrassment.
- *Younger children* Often short-lived. Usually resolves spontaneously.
- *Older children/adults* Refer to speech therapy

**Dysarthria** Difficulty with articulation due to incoordination or weakness of the musculature of speech. Language is normal. Ask to repeat 'baby hippopotamus' or 'British constitution'. Treat the cause if possible; otherwise support with speech therapy and aids to communication. *Assessment and causes*: Table 16.6.

**Dysphasia** Impairment of language due to brain damage to the dominant hemisphere. The left hemisphere is dominant for 99% of right-handed people and 60% of left-handers. In most cases due to stroke or brain tumour. Rarely due to head injury or dementia.

*Classification* Table 16.7. Mixed pictures are common.

*Treatment*
- Speech therapy may or may not be helpful.
- Support, e.g. dysphasia groups.
- Aids to communication, e.g. computers, picture boards.

**Myasthenia gravis** Autoimmune disease. Antibodies to the acetylcholine receptor cause a deficit of receptors at the neuromuscular junction → muscle weakness. Antibodies are detectable in 90%. ♀:♂ ≈ 2:1. Associated with thymic tumours and other autoimmune disease, e.g. RA, SLE, hyperthyroidism. Generally follows a relapsing or slowly progressive course. If thymoma present, 5y survival ~30%.

*Presentation* Young adults with easy fatigability of muscles. Commonly affected muscles are:
- Orbital muscles causing ptosis and diplopia *and*
- Bulbar muscles causing slurring of speech—ask to count to 50.

Weakness is exacerbated by pregnancy, infection, drugs (e.g. β-blockers, opiates, tetracycline, quinine), climate change, emotion, and exercise.

*Management* If suspected, refer for confirmation by a neurologist and specialist treatment. *Treated with*:
- Anticholinesterase, e.g. pyridostigmine
- Immunosuppression with prednisolone, methotrexate, or azathioprine
- Thymectomy → remission in 30% and benefit in another 40%
- Plasmapheresis.

**Patient support**
**Myasthenia Gravis Association UK** 🖥 www.mgauk.org

**Table 16.6** Causes of dysarthria

| Cause | Characteristics |
|---|---|
| Cerebellar disease | Slurring of speech as if drunk |
| | Speech is irregular in volume and scanning in quality |
| Extrapyramidal disease e.g. Parkinson's disease | Soft, indistinct, and monotonous speech |
| Pseudo-bulbar palsy e.g. stroke (bilateral), MS, MND | Alteration of speech—typically nasal speech sounding like Donald Duck |
| | Difficulty swallowing or chewing |
| | Tongue is spastic and jaw jerk ↑ |
| Bulbar palsy e.g. MND, Guillain–Barré, alcoholic brainstem myelinolysis, 1° or 2° brainstem tumours, syringobulbia, polio, hyponatraemia | Speech—quiet, hoarse, or nasal |
| | Loss of function of tongue, muscles of chewing/swallowing ± facial muscles |
| | Flaccid fasciculating tongue |
| | Jaw jerk normal or absent |
| Palate paralysis | Nasal speech |
| | Asymmetric or absent gag reflex |
| Myasthenia gravis | 🕮 p.556 |

**Table 16.7** Assessment and classification of dysphasia

**Assessment**

*Is speech fluent, grammatical, meaningful, and apt?* If yes, dysphasia is unlikely.
*Comprehension:* Can the patient follow 1, 2 or multiple step commands?
*Repetition:* Can the patient repeat a phrase after you?
*Naming:* Can the patient name common and uncommon items?
*Reading and writing?* Usually affected too. If not, question the diagnosis of dysphasia.

| Characteristics of dysphasia | Broca's (expressive) | Wernicke's (receptive) | Conduction | Transcortical |
|---|---|---|---|---|
| Fluent? | ✗ | ✓ | ✓ | ✓ or ✗ |
| Repetition normal? | ✗ | ✗ | ✗ | ✓ |
| Understanding impaired? | ✗ | ✓ | ✗ | ✓ or ✗ |

# Fits, faints, and funny turns

Blackouts, faints, and 'funny turns' are all common presentations to general practice. The major questions which should be asked seeing an individual who has had a funny turn are:

• Is it epilepsy?
• If it is epilepsy, then what kind?
• If it is not epilepsy, then is there another serious underlying cause (e.g. heart disease)?

**History** A good history from the patient and ideally from a witness is essential in the correct diagnosis. *Ask:*

• What happened?
• When and where? Particularly, did it start during sleep?
• Were there any precipitating events?
• Were there any warning signs (e.g. aura, feeling going to faint, etc.)?
• Does the patient remember the whole episode? If not, which bits are missing and how long are the gaps?
• Did the patient lose consciousness? Quite frequently patients describe episodes of dizziness or unsteadiness/falling as 'funny turns'.
• Did the patient jerk his/her limbs? If so, was the jerking generalized or restricted to one area of the body?
• What did the patient look like during the attack? An eye witness account is helpful.
• Did anything else happen during the attack (e.g. tongue biting, incontinence)?
• What happened after the attack? Was the patient conscious straight away? Was there disorientation, drowsiness, or headache?

## Also check

• General medical history including cardiac history and history of other neurological symptoms.
• Psychiatric history—anxiety, depression, panic attacks?
• Past medical history—birth trauma, febrile convulsions in childhood, significant head injury, and/or meningitis/encephalitis.
• Family history—epilepsy.
• Substance abuse? Drugs or alcohol.

**Examination** Complete general and neurological examination. Particularly check for:

• *Skin changes* Café-au-lait spots (neurofibromatosis); adenoma sebaceum (tuberous sclerosis); trigeminal capillary haemangioma (Sturge–Weber syndrome)
• *Cardiovascular abnormalities* Heart rate and rhythm, murmurs, carotid bruits, BP.
• *Focal neurological deficits* Suggest presence of a structural neurological lesion

**Funny turns in small children** 📖 p.894

**Epilepsy** 📖 p.582

**Syncope** Abrupt and transient loss of consciousness due to a sudden ↓ in cerebral perfusion. Common—prevalence ~6% adults. It has many causes ranging from benign (vasovagal syncope) to fatal (sustained ventricular tachycardia): the prognosis depends on the cause.

**Diagnosis** A typical attack takes the following pattern:

- *Prodromal symptoms* Nausea, clammy sweating, blurring, greying and possible loss of vision, lightheadedness, dizziness and tinnitus, yawning. The collection is characteristic.
- *Anoxic phase* Loss of consciousness, pallor, sweating, pupil dilatation, tachypnoea, bradycardia. Muscle tone is ↓, causing eyes to roll up, and the patient to fall. May be accompanied by a few myoclonic jerks as the patient falls.
- *Recovery* In the horizontal position, skin colour, pulse, and consciousness usually return within seconds. ❶ If the patient is unable to fall and is kept upright a 2° anoxic seizure may occur.
- *After-effects* Confusion, amnesia, and drowsiness are not prolonged. Injury and incontinence are rare but may occur. Tongue biting is very rare.

Presyncope Is the term applied to a less severe attack with partial loss of consciousness and a near fall.

**Simple faint/vasovagal attack** Common Peripheral vasodilation, bradycardia, and venous pooling → postural hypotension. Often cause is unclear although ♀ > ♂. *Known precipitants*: fright (e.g. during venesection) or emotion. Exclude other reasons for loss of consciousness. No treatment needed—reassure.

**Dizziness and giddiness** Distinguish between true vertigo (the illusion of rotatory movement—the room spinning) and a feeling of unsteadiness or lightheadedness:

- *Vertigo* 📖 p.948
- *Imbalance* Implies difficulty in walking straight, e.g. from disease of peripheral nerves, posterior columns, or cerebellum.
- *Faintness* The feeling of being about to pass out. Associated with some seizure disorders and a variety of non-neurological conditions (e.g. postural hypotension, vasovagal fainting, hyperventilation, hypoglycaemia, arrythmias, cough syncope). Sometimes >1 element coexists.

**Hyperventilation and panic attacks** 📖 p.1116
❶ Usually history is diagnostic but occasionally seizures of temporal lobe origin may have similar symptomatology.

**Hypoglycaemia** Affects patients with DM, particularly those taking insulin or oral hypoglycaemic agents. Produces autonomic changes, e.g. pallor, sweating and tachycardia, and behavioural changes (confusion, altered personality). If action is not taken to ↑ blood sugar, coma ± fitting ensues (📖 p.1096).

**Abnormal perceptions** (e.g hallucinations) 📖 p.986

# Assessment of headache

Common presenting complaint. The skill lies in deciding which headaches are benign, needing no intervention, and which require action.

## History

- *Does the patient have >1 type of headache?* Take a separate history for each.
- *Time* When did the headaches start? New or recently changed headache calls for especially careful assessment. How often do they happen? Do they have any pattern (e.g. constant, episodic, daily)? How long do they last? Why is the patient coming to the doctor now?
- *Character* Nature and quality, site and spread of the pain. Associated symptoms, e.g. nausea/vomiting, visual disturbance, photophobia, neurological symptoms.
- *Cause* Predisposing and/or trigger factors; aggravating and/or relieving factors; family history.
- *Response* Details of medication used (type, dose, frequency, timing). What does the patient do (e.g. can the patient continue work)?
- *Health between attacks* Do the headaches go completely or does the patient still feel unwell between attacks?
- *Anxieties and concerns* of the patient.

**Examination** *In acute, severe headache,* examine for purpuric skin rash. *In all cases* check BP, brief neurological examination including fundi, visual acuity, and gait, palpation of the temporal region/sinuses for tenderness, and examination of the neck. *In young children* measure head circumference and plot on a centile chart

### ⚠ Red flags

- New/unexpected headache
- Thunderclap headache
- Aura for first time and using COC
- New onset age >50y or <10y
- New onset in a patient with a history of HIV or cancer
- Headache with atypical aura (>1h ± motor weakness)
- Progressive headache, worsening over weeks
- Associated postural change.

**Investigation** Often not needed. ESR if temporal arteritis is suspected.

**Differential diagnosis and management** Table 16.8. ↑BP may cause acute or chronic headache. Direct treatment at cause.

**Meningism** Headache, stiff neck, and photophobia. Associated with meningitis. May also be seen with encephalitis and SAH.

**Facial pain** Treat the cause. Common causes include trigeminal neuralgia, temporomandibular joint disorders, dental disorders, sinusitis, migrainous neuralgia, shingles, and post-herpetic neuralgia. No cause is found in many patients—it is then termed **atypical facial pain.** Atypical facial pain may respond to simple analgesia with paracetamol or a NSAID. If this fails, try nerve painkillers, e.g. amitriptyline nocte. Refer those with troublesome symptoms to ENT, maxillofacial surgery, or neurology.

**Table 16.8** Differential diagnosis of headache

| | Cause | Features | Management |
|---|---|---|---|
| Acute new headache | Meningitis | Fever, photophobia, stiff neck, rash, photophobia | IV or IM penicillin V and immediate admission (📖 p.1074) |
| | Encephalitis | Fever, confusion, ↓ conscious level | Immediate admission (📖 p.1074) |
| | Subarachnoid haemorrhage | 'Thunder-clap' or very sudden onset headache ± stiff neck | Immediate admission (📖 p.571) |
| | Head injury | Bruising/injury; ↓ conscious level, periods lucidity, amnesia | Consider admission (📖 p.1108) |
| | Sinusitis | Tender over sinuses ± history of URTI | 📖 p.940 |
| | Dental caries | Facial pain ± tenderness | 📖 p.930 |
| | Tropical illness | History of travel, fever | 📖 p.646 |
| Acute recurrent headache | Migraine | Aura, visual disturbance, nausea/vomiting, triggers | 📖 p.562 |
| | Cluster headache | Nightly pain in 1 eye for 2–3mo, then pain free for >1y | 📖 p.564 |
| | Exertional or coital headache | Suggested by history of association | NSAID or propranolol before attacks |
| | Trigeminal neuralgia | Intense stabbing pain lasting seconds in trigeminal nerve distribution | 📖 p.565 |
| | Glaucoma | Red eye, haloes, ↓ visual acuity, pupil abnormality | 📖 p.974 |
| Subacute headache | Temporal (giant cell) arteritis | >50y, scalp tenderness, ↑ ESR, rarely ↓ visual acuity | 📖 p.532 |
| Chronic headache | Tension type headache | Band around the head, stress, low mood | 📖 p.564 |
| | Cervicogenic headache | Unilateral or bilateral, band from neck to forehead, scalp tenderness | 📖 p.482 |
| | Medication over-use headache | Rebound headache on stopping analgesics | 📖 p.564 |
| | ↑ intracranial pressure | Worse on waking/sneezing, neurological signs, ↑BP, ↓ pulse rate | 📖 p.566 |
| | Paget's disease | >40y, bowed tibia, ↑ alk phos | 📖 p.512 |

## Further information

**British Association for the Study of Headache** Diagnosis and management of migraine and tension type headache (2007) 🖥 www.bash.org.uk

# Migraine

Migraine affects 15% of the UK population. ♂:♀ ≈ 1:3. One in three sufferers will experience significant disability as a result of their migraines at some stage of their lives. Caused by disturbance of cerebral blood flow under the influence of 5-HT.

**Clinical picture** Three common types:
- *Aura* Aura alone with no headache—visual chaos (e.g. zigzag lines, jumbling of print, dots); hemianopia; hemiparesis; dysphasia; dyspraxia; dysarthria; ataxia (basilar migraine).
- *Classical* Aura lasting 10–30 min followed by unilateral throbbing headache ± nausea/vomiting ± photophobia.
- *Episodic (common)* Unilateral throbbing headache ± nausea/vomiting ± photophobia *without* aura. Often premenstrual.

**Criteria for diagnosis if no aura** ≥5 headaches lasting 4–72h + nausea/vomiting or photo/phonophobia and ≥2 of following:

- Unilateral headache
- Pulsating headache
- Moderate/severe pain intensity
- Interferes with normal functioning
- ↑ by climbing stairs/other routine activities.

**History, examination and differential diagnosis** 📖 p.560

**Management of an acute attack**[G] Advise to rest in a quiet dark place and sleep if possible. Use a treatment ladder. Step up if 3 failures at any one step.
- *Step 1: Oral analgesic and antiemetic* Aspirin 600–900mg or ibuprofen 400–600mg ± prochlorperazine 3–6mg bd or domperidone 10mg qds.
- *Step 2: Rectal analgesic ± antiemetic* Diclofenac 100mg (maximum 200mg/24h.) + domperidone 30–60mg (maximum 120mg/24h).
- *Step 3: Specific anti-migraine drugs,* e.g. sumatriptan 50–100mg po, 20mg nasal spray, or 6mg SC. Not effective if taken before the headache develops. Stops 70–85% attacks. Start with lowest dose and ↑ as needed. Do not give if ergotamine taken <24h previously.
- *Step 4: Combinations*, e.g. sumatriptan 50mg + naproxen 500mg.

## Emergency treatment of patients at home
- Give diclofenac 75mg IM ± chlorpromazine 25–50mg IM (potent antiemetic and sedative—if not available use metoclopramide 10mg IM/IV).
- Alternatively consider 5HT₁ agonist, e.g.sumatriptan, unless 2 injections/tablets/nasal sprays already given in last 24h (or ergotamine in <24h).
- Avoid opioids (e.g. morphine, codeine, dihydrocodeine) as ↑ nausea.
- Admit if becoming dehydrated.

**Treatment of recurrence within the same attack** Repeat symptomatic treatments within their dose limitations—pre-emptively if recurrence is usual/expected. If using triptans, a 2nd dose may be effective, but repeated dosing can cause rebound headache. Naratriptan and eletriptan are associated with relatively low recurrence rates.

**Management of chronic migraine**[G] Aims to control symptoms and minimize their impact on the patient's life. Cure is not a realistic aim.

**Trigger factors** Half have a trigger for their migraine. *Consider:*
* *Psychological factors* Stress/relief of stress; anxiety/depression; extreme emotions, e.g. anger or grief.
* *Food factors* Lack of food/infrequent meals; foods containing monosodium glutamate, caffeine, and tyramine; specific foods, e.g. chocolate, citrus fruits, cheese; alcohol, especially red wine.
* *Sleep* Overtiredness (physical/mental); changes in sleep patterns (e.g. late nights, weekend lie-in, shift work, holidays); long distance travel.
* *Environmental factors* Loud noise; bright/flickering lights; strong perfume; stuffy atmosphere; VDUs; strong winds; extreme heat/ cold.
* *Health factors* Hormonal changes (e.g. monthly periods, COC pill, HRT, the menopause); ↑ BP; toothache or pain in the eyes, sinuses, or neck; unaccustomed physical activity.

**Assessing severity** Assessment scales (e.g Migraine Disability Assessment Score (MIDAS)—□ p.593) can be useful in assessing impact of symptoms on daily life and monitoring response to treatment.

**General measures** Reassure about the benign nature of migraine. Instruct about management of acute attacks. Ask to keep a diary to identify possible trigger factors and assess headache frequency, severity, and response to treatment Avoid trigger factors where possible. Give advice on relaxation techniques and stress management. Stop the COC pill if migraine starts/worsens when the pill is started, especially If focal symptoms (□ p.753). Consider prophylaxis if frequent/severe attacks.

**Prophylaxis** Consider if ≥4 attacks/mo or severe attacks. ↓ attacks by ~50%. Try a drug for 2mo before deeming it ineffective. If effective, continue for 4–6mo, then ↓ dose slowly before stopping.
* *1st line* β-blocker, e.g. atenolol 25–100mg bd, or TCA e.g. amitriptyline 10–150mg 1–2h. before bed. Start at low dose; ↑ dose every 2–4wk.
* *2nd line* Topiramate 25–50mg od/bd; sodium valproate 300mg–1g bd.
* *3rd line* Gabapentin 300mg od–800mg tds; methysergide 1–2mg tds.
* *Others* Pizotifen, clonidine, verapamil, SSRIs—limited/uncertain effect.

**Alternative therapies** Feverfew 200mg daily—some evidence of effectiveness after 6wk use.[C] Acupuncture may also be helpful.

**Menstrual migraine** Consider (for a minimum of 3 cycles):
* *NSAIDs*, e.g. mefenamic acid 500mg tds/qds from onset of menstruation to last day of bleeding.
* *Triptans*, e.g. fovatriptan for 6d. (5mg day 1, 2.5mg day 2–6) starting 2d. before expected onset of migraine.
* *Transdermal oestrogen*, 100 micrograms 3d before period and continued for 7d.
* *Women on COC pill* Running 3 packets back to back before pill break and bleed. Alternatively use an oestrogen-dominant pill, e.g. Cilest.

### Further information
**British Association for the Study of Headache** Diagnosis and management of migraine and tension type headache (2007) □ www.bash.org.uk

### Patient information and support
**Migraine Action Association** ☎ 0116 275 8317 □ www.migraine.org.uk
**Migraine Trust** ☎ 020 7462 6601 □ www.migrainetrust.org

# Other headaches

**Asssessment and differential diagnosis of headache** 📖 p.560

**Migraine** 📖 p.562

**Chronic daily headache** Prevalence 4%. Defined as any headache that occurs >15d/mo. *Common causes*: tension headache, cervicogenic headache (📖 p.482), medication overuse headache, migraine, errors of refraction (usually headache is mild, frontal, in the eyes themselves, and absent on waking). Treat the cause.

**Tension type headache** Associated with stress and anxiety and/or functional or structural abnormalities of the head or neck. Prevalence ~2%. ♀:♂ ≈ 2:1. Symptoms begin aged <10y in 15% of patients. Prevalence ↓ with age. Family history of similar headaches is common (40%), but twin studies do not suggest a genetic basis. Distinguish between episodic and chronic tension type headache:

* *Episodic* Defined as headache lasting 30 min–7d and occurring <180d/y (<15d/mo).
* *Chronic* Headaches on ≥15d/mo (≥180 d/y) for ≥6mo.

In both cases pain:

* Is bilateral, pressing, and/or tightening in quality
* Of mild or moderate intensity
* Does not prohibit activities
* Is not associated with vomiting
* Is not aggravated by routine physical activity
* Is associated with ≥ 1 of: nausea, photophobia, or phonophobia.

**Management** Reassure no serious underlying pathology. Try measures to alleviate stress—relaxation, massage, yoga, exercise. Cognitive therapy is probably effective but not widely available.[CE] Treat musculoskeletal symptoms with physiotherapy.

*Drug therapy* Analgesics are of limited value and might make matters worse (see medication over-use headache).

* *Headache <2×/wk*: simple analgesia, e.g. paracetamol, ibuprofen. Avoid codeine-containing preparations.
* *Chronic headache*: amitriptyline 25–75mg nocte may help. Stop once improvement maintained for >4–6mo.

**Medication overuse (analgesic) headache** Persistent headache may develop in patients with other causes of headache, e.g. tension headache or migraine, if they over-use the medication used to treat those conditions. Affects 1:50 adults; ♀:♂ ≈ 5:1. Implicated drugs include: ergotamine, triptans, aspirin, paracetamol, and NSAIDs.

**Management** Ask any patient complaining of chronic daily headache to give a detailed account of medication use (including OTC)—a diary to record symptoms/medication use can be helpful. Aim for the patient to withdraw from the over-used medication. Warn that symptoms may worsen initially (days 3–7) before improving. Review treatment of underlying headache.

**Cluster headaches (migrainous neuralgia)** Clusters of extremely painful headaches focused around 1 eye with associated autonomic symptoms (drooping eyelid, red watery eye, runny or blocked nose).

May occur at any age but rare <20y. ♂:♀ ≈ 6:1. More common in smokers. Pain lasts up to 1h and occurs 1–2×/d every day for 4–12wk; then disappears for 1–2y. Recurrences affect the same side. Onset is often predictable (1–2 h after falling asleep; after alcohol).

**Management** Refer for specialist advice. *Drug treatments*:
- *Acute attack* 100% oxygen (10–15L/min) for 10–20min; 5HT₁ agonists, e.g. sumatriptan (6mg SC), stop 75% of attacks in <15min.
- *Prophylaxis* Consider if attacks are frequent. More effective if initiated early at the start of a new cluster. *Options*:
  - Verapamil 80mg tds/qds.
  - Prednisolone 60–100mg od for 2–5d. with rapid tapering over 2–3wk.
  - Lithium—used as for manic depression (📖 p.1005).
  - Ergotamine 1–2mg PR—take 1 h before the attack is due. Should not be used for prolonged periods.
  - Methysergide 1–2mg tds—effective but limited by side effects. Used if other drugs are contraindicated, not tolerated, or ineffective.

**Trigeminal neuralgia** Paroxysms of intense stabbing, burning or 'electric shock' type pain lasting seconds to minutes in the trigeminal (V) nerve distribution. 96% are unilateral. Mandibular/maxillary > ophthalmic division. Between attacks there are no symptoms. Frequency of attacks ranges from hundreds/d to remissions lasting years. Pain may be provoked by movement of the face (talking, eating, laughing) or touching the skin (shaving, washing). Can occur at any age but more common >50y. ♀ > ♂. Unknown cause. Associated with MS and, in ♀, with ↑ BP.

**Management** Spontaneous remission may occur.
- Carbamazepine ↓ frequency and intensity of attacks. NNT=1.8.[C] Start at low dose, e.g. 100mg od/bd, and ↑ over weeks until symptoms are controlled. Usual dose ≈ 200mg tds. Oxcarbazepine is an alternative.
- Gabapentin ↓ frequency and intensity of attacks. Start with 300mg od. Increase according to response to maximum of 1.8g/d (divided doses).

*Refer to neurology if* <50y old; neurological deficit between attacks; treatment with carbamazepine/gabapentin fails—specialist options include lamotrigine, duloxetine, baclofen, phenytoin, or surgical intervention.

❶ >1 type of headache may coexist. 50% of migraine sufferers develop tension type headache, resulting in background pain between attacks. Consider each separately.

### Further information
**British Association for the Study of Headache** Diagnosis and management of migraine and tension type headache (2007) 🖥 www.bash.org.uk

### Patient information and support
**Organisation for the Understanding of Cluster Headaches (OUCH UK)** ☎ 01646 651 979 🖥 www.ouchuk.org
**Trigeminal neuralgia association UK** ☎ 01883 370214 🖥 www.tna.org.uk

# Raised intracranial pressure

Raised intracranial pressure (↑ICP) usually presents with increasing headache associated with drowsiness, listlessness, vomiting, focal neurology, and/or seizures. *Causes include*: 1° or 2° tumours, head injury, intracranial haemorrhage, hydrocephalus, meningitis, encephalitis, brain abscess, and cerebral oedema (2° to tumour, trauma, infection, ischaemia).

**Clinical features of ↑ICP** ⚠ If suspected, admit as an emergency.

- Drowsiness
- ↓ conscious level
- Irritability
- VI nerve palsy
- Papilloedema

- Dropping pulse
- Rising BP
- Focal neurological signs—caused by underlying pathology
- Pupil changes—constriction then dilatation

**Benign intracranial hypertension** Symptoms/signs of SOL but none is found. Usually occurs in young obese women. Cause unknown. Treated with repeat lumbar puncture, ventriculo–peritoneal shunt, diuretics, or dexamethasone. Usually resolves—but 10% recur later.

**Brain abscess** May be single or multiple. Organisms reach the brain via the blood stream, direct implantation, or local extension from adjacent sites (e.g. sinusitis). Present with ↑ ICP, focal neurological signs, systemic effects of infection, and/or local effects due to the cause. Usually features develop over 2–3wk—occasionally onset is rapid in the immunosuppressed. If suspected, admit as an emergency. Treatment is with IV antibiotics ± surgical drainage. Mortality is 20–30%. 50% of survivors have long-term neurological deficit; 30% epilepsy.

## Intracranial tumours

- *1° tumours* 70%. Classified by whether they are benign/malignant and cell type. Glioma is an umbrella term meaning tumour of nervous system origin. *Common subtypes*: astrocytoma, oligodendroglioma, glioblastoma multiforme, and ependymoma. Tumours of the meninges (*meningiomas*) and cerebral blood vessels (*cerebellar haemangioblastomas*) can also occur.
- *2° brain tumours* 30%—usually from carcinoma of breast, lung or melanoma. In 50% tumours are multiple

**Presentation** ❶ <1% of patients with headache have a brain tumour
- *↑ICP* Papilloedema 23–50% at presentation; headache 25–35%.
- *Seizures* 25–30%. Suspect in all adults who have a first seizure—especially if focal or with localizing aura. Refer for urgent assessment.[N]
- *Evolving focal neurology* Depends on the site. >50% have focal neurology at presentation. Frontal lobe lesions tend to present late.
- *False localizing signs* Caused by ↑ICP. VI nerve palsy (causing double vision) is most common because of its long intracranial course.
- *Subtle personality change* 16-20% at presentation—irritability, lack of application, lack of initiative, socially inappropriate behaviour.
- *Local effects* Skull base masses, proptosis, epistaxis.

**Differential diagnosis** Stroke; MS; head injury; vasculitis; encephalitis; Todd's palsy (📖 p.582); metabolic/electrolyte disturbance; other causes of space-occupying lesion (aneurysm, abscess, chronic subdural haematoma, granuloma, cyst).

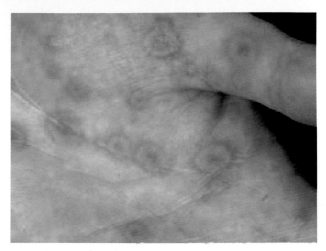

**Plate 1** Typical target lesions of erythema multiforme.

Reproduced from *Student BMJ* (2005) **13**: 265–308 with permission from the BMJ Publishing Group,

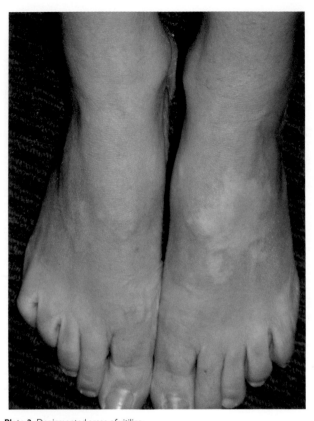

**Plate 2** Depigmented areas of vitiligo.

Reproduced with permission of the New Zealand Dermatological Society Incorporated (NZDSI) www.DermNetNZ.org

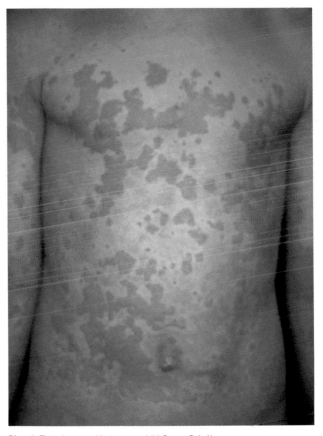

**Plate 3** Typical urticarial lesions in a child. Porter R (ed.)

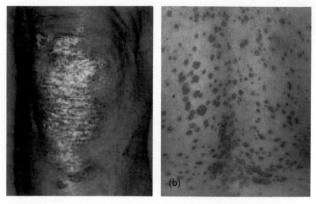

**Plate 4** Psoriasis (a) silvery scale of plaque psoriasis and (b) wide-spread rash of guttate psoriasis.

(a) and (b) Republished with permission from Dr Lyn Guentner, Professor of Dermatology, the University of Western Ontario, and SkinCareGuide.com Ltd.

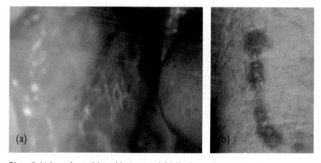

**Plate 5** Lichen planus (a) oral lesions and (b) Koebner phenomenon.

(a) Reproduced with permission of the New Zealand Dermatological Society Incorporated (NZDSI) ▣ www.DermNetNZ.org

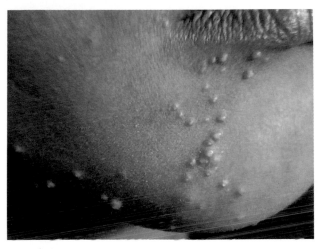

**Plate 6** Molluscum contagiosum.
Reproduced with permission of the UK Clinical Virology Network
www.clinical-virology.org

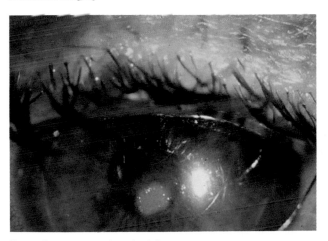

**Plate 7** Corneal abrasion: Stained with fluorescein appears green.
Reproduced with kind permission of Southampton University Hospitals Trust.

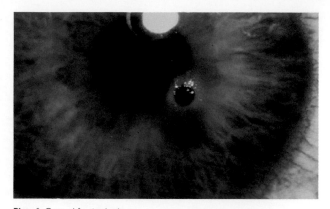

**Plate 8** Corneal foreign body.
Reproduced with kind permission of Southampton University Hospitals Trust.

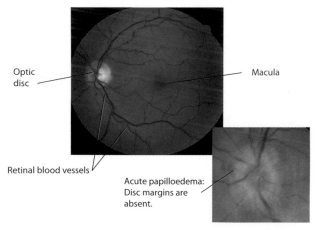

Optic disc

Macula

Retinal blood vessels

Acute papilloedema: Disc margins are absent.

**Plate 9** The normal retina and papilloedema.

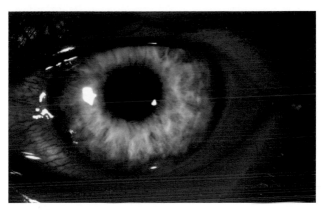

**Plate 10** Acute infective conjunctivitis.
Reproduced with kind permission of Southampton University Hospitals Trust.

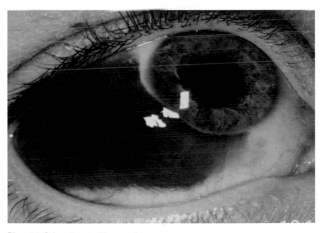

**Plate 11** Subconjunctival haemorrhage.
Reproduced with kind permission of Southampton University Hospitals Trust.

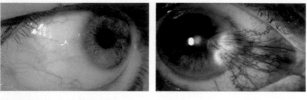

**Plate 12** Pinguecula (left) and pterygium (right).
Reproduced with kind permission of Southampton University Hospitals Trust.

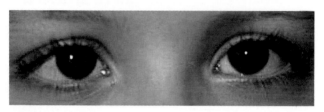

**Plate 13** Esometropic squint.
Reproduced with kind permission of Southampton University Hospitals Trust.

*Prognosis* Gliomas all have <50% 5y survival. Depending on site, meningiomas and haemangioblastomas have better prognosis.

### △ Referral guidelines for suspected brain tumour[N]

*Refer urgently* patients in whom a brain tumour is suspected with:
- Symptoms related to the CNS, including:
  - Progressive neurological deficit
  - New-onset seizures
  - Headaches
  - Mental changes
  - Cranial nerve palsy
  - Unilateral sensorineural deafness.
- Headaches of recent onset accompanied by features suggestive of raised intracranial pressure, e.g.
  - Vomiting
  - Drowsiness
  - Posture-related headache
  - Pulse-synchronous tinnitus

  *or* accompanied by other focal or non-focal neurological symptoms, e.g. blackout, change in personality or memory.
- A new qualitatively different unexplained headache that becomes progressively severe.
- Suspected recent-onset seizures.

*Consider urgent referral* in patients with rapid progression of:
- Subacute focal neurological deficit.
- Unexplained cognitive impairment, behavioural disturbance or slowness, or a combination of these.
- Personality changes confirmed by a witness and for which there is no reasonable explanation even in the absence of the other symptoms and signs of a brain tumour.

*Consider non-urgent referral* or discussion with specialist for unexplained headaches of recent onset:
- Present for ≥ 1mo.
- Not accompanied by features suggestive of ↑ intracranial pressure.

**Hydrocephalus** Dilatation of the cerebral ventricles and accumulation of CSF. May be:
- *Communicating* Due to ↓ reabsorption of CSF. *Causes:* post-meningitis; SAH (80% develop some degree of hydrocephalus); trauma; neoplastic infiltration in the subarachnoid space.
- *Non-communicating* CSF flow is blocked due to an obstruction within the ventricles. Due to congenital malformations, tumour, brain abscesss, SAH, meningeal scarring due to meningitis, or cranial trauma.

*Presentation and management* In infants presents with macrocephaly (📖 p.891), convulsions, developmental delay, and/or spasticity. In adults presents with ↑ ICP. Refer for urgent neurological assessment.

❶ All patients with a CSF shunt should have pneumococcal vaccination.

### Further information
**NICE** (2005) Referral guidelines for suspected cancer 🖥 www.nice.org.uk

### Information and support for patients
**Brain & Spine Foundation** ☎ 0808 808 1000 🖥 www.brainandspine.org.uk

# Intracranial bleeds

**Haemorrhagic stroke** 📖 p.570

**Subarachnoid haemorrhage (SAH)** Spontaneous bleeding into the subarachnoid space. Incidence 15/100 000. ♀ > ♂. Peak age 35–65y Frequently fatal. *Causes:*

- No cause (15%)
- Rupture of congenital berry aneurysm (70%)
- Arteriovenous malformation (15%)
- Bleeding disorder
- Mycotic aneurysm 2° to endocarditis (rare).

*Risk factors* Smoking, alcohol, ↑ BP, lack of oestrogen (less common premenopause). Berry aneurysms may run in families and are associated with polycystic kidneys, coarctation of the aorta, and Ehlers–Danlos syndrome.

## Presentation

- Typically presents as a sudden devastating headache—'thunderclap headache'—often occipital
- Rarely (6%) preceded by a 'sentinel headache' representing a small leak ahead of a larger bleed.
- Vomiting and collapse with loss of consciousness ± fitting ± focal neurology follow.

*Examination* May be nothing to find initially. Neck stiffness takes 6h to develop. In later stages:

- Papilloedema
- Retinal and other intraocular haemorrhages
- Focal neurology
- ↓ level of consciousness.

*Action* If suspected, admit immediately as a medical emergency. Only 1:4 admitted with suspected SAH turn out to have one. In most no cause for the headache is found.

**Subdural haemorrhage** Bleeding is from bridging veins between cortex and venous sinuses, resulting in accumulation of blood between the dura and arachnoid. *Causes:* trauma (may be trivial), idiopathic.

*Risk factors* Age, alcohol, falls, epilepsy, anticoagulant therapy.

*Presentation* Often insidious and history may go back several weeks.

- Fluctuation of conscious level (35%)
- Physical and intellectual slowing
- Sleepiness
- Headache
- Personality change
- Unsteadiness on feet
- Slowly evolving stroke (e.g. hemiparesis)
- Symptoms/signs of ↑ICP.

*Differential diagnosis* Stroke, cerebral tumour, dementia.

*Action* If suspected, admit as a medical emergency for further investigation. Evacuation of clot is possible even in very elderly patients and often results in full recovery.

**Extradural haemorrhage** Blood accumulated between the dura and bone of the skull. Usually occurs after head injury.

*Presentation* Deterioration of level of consciousness after head injury which initially produced no loss of consciousness, or after initial post-injury drowsiness has resolved. This 'lucid' interval may last anything from a few hours to a few days. May be accompanied by worsening headache, vomiting, confusion ± focal neurological signs.

*Action* If suspected, admit as an emergency for further investigation. Early evacuation of clot carries excellent prognosis. Outlook is less good if coma pre-op.

# Acute stroke

Clinical syndrome typified by rapidly developing signs of focal or global disturbance of cerebral functions, lasting >24h or leading to death, with no apparent causes other than of vascular origin. Common and devastating condition—most common cause of adult disability in UK. Half of all strokes occur in people >70y.

## Causes

- *Cerebral infarction* (~70%) Atherothrombotic occlusion or embolism. *Sources of embolism*: left atrium (AF) or left ventricle (MI or heart failure). Ischaemia causes direct injury from lack of blood supply.
- *Intracerebral or subarachnoid haemorrhage* (~19%) Haemorrhage causes direct neuronal injury and pressure exerted by the blood results in adjacent ischaemia.
- *Rare causes* Sudden ↓ BP, vasculitis, venous-sinus thrombosis, carotid artery dissection.

## Risk factors

- Age
- ↑BP
- DM
- AF
- Previous stroke or TIA
- MI
- Artificial heart valves
- Hyperviscosity syndromes
- Smoking
- Alcohol
- Obesity
- Low physical activity.

## Presentation

- *History* Sudden onset of CNS symptoms or stepwise progression of symptoms over hours or days.
- *Examination* Conscious level may be ↓ or normal; neurological signs (including dysphagia and incontinence); BP; heart rate and rhythm; heart murmurs; carotid bruits; systemic signs of infection or neoplasm.

**Differential diagnosis** Decompensation after recovery from previous stroke (e.g. due to infection, metabolic disorder); SOL—1° or 2° cerebral neoplasm; cerebral abscess; trauma—subdural haematoma, traumatic brain injury; epileptic seizure; migraine; MS.

**Acute management** Admit all patients who have suffered an acute stroke to hospital. Treatment of stroke in a stroke unit →↓ mortality and morbidity.[C] Thrombolysis early after stroke results in better outcome, so do not delay referral until the patient is seen. If stroke is suspected, admit directly to hospital by emergency ambulance.

⚠ Do not give aspirin prior to admission.

**Transient ischaemic attack (TIA)** History is as for stroke but recovery takes place within 24h of initial symptoms. Patients with a history of TIA have a 20% risk of stroke in the following month with highest risk in the first 72h. Risk can be predicted using the ABCD2 scoring system (Table 16.9).

## Management of TIA

- Admit if >1 TIA in less than a week. Consider admission/same day specialist assessment if the patient falls into a high risk group.
- If not admitting, once all symptoms have stopped, start aspirin 75mg od. Check blood for FBC, ESR, U&E, Cr, eGFR, lipids, and glucose. Consider clotting screen ± thrombophilia screeening if FH thrombosis. Check ECG and CXR.

- Start treatment for risk factors, e.g. advise to stop smoking, start antihypertensives if ↑ BP.
- Refer for assessment and further investigation to a specialist service, e.g. neurovascular clinic. Specialist investigations include: CT or MRI scan to confirm diagnosis, carotid dopplers if carotid artery territory symptoms; echocardiogram if recent MI, CCF/LVF, or murmur.

**Amaurosis fugax** Form of TIA resulting from emboli passing through the retina. Causes brief loss of vision for a matter of minutes 'like a curtain'. Management is as for TIA.

**Subarachnoid haemorrhage** 📖 p.568

**Secondary prevention of stroke** 📖 p.572

**Rehabilitation** 📖 p.206 and p.590

**Table 16.9** ABCD2 scoring system predicts future risk of stroke

| ABCD2 | Feature | Score |
|---|---|---|
| Age | <60y | 0 |
| | ≥60y | 1 |
| BP | Systolic ≥ 140 and/or diastolic ≥ 90 | 1 |
| Clinical features | Unilateral weakness | 2 |
| | Speech disturbance without weakness | 1 |
| | Other | 0 |
| Duration | ≥1h | 2 |
| | 10–59min | 1 |
| | <10min | 0 |
| Diabetes | Patient is diabetic | 1 |
| | Patient is not diabetic | 0 |

**Scoring**
High risk: 6–7 points—8.1%; 2d risk of stroke—(21% of patients)
Medium risk: 4–5 points—4.1%; 2d risk of stroke—(45% of patients)
Low risk: 0–3 points—1%; 2d risk of stroke—(34% of patients)

Reprinted from Johnston SC, Rothwell PM, Nguyen-Huynh MN et al. Validation and refinement of scores to predict very early stroke risk after transient ischaemic attack (2007) **369**: 283–92, with permission from Elsevier.

## Further information
**Royal College of Physicians** National clinical guidelines for stroke (2004) 🖥 www.rcplondon.ac.uk
**NICE** Stroke: The diagnosis and acute management of stroke and TIA (2008) 🖥 www.nice.org.uk

## Patient information and support
**Stroke Association** ☎ 0845 3033 100 🖥 www.stroke.org.uk
**Different Strokes** ☎ 0845 130 7172 🖥 www.differentstrokes.co.uk
**Speakability** ☎ 0808 808 9572 🖥 www.speakability.org.uk

# Management after stroke

**After stroke** Stroke is a family illness. 40% of carers suffer psychological distress starting <6wk after discharge. Involve carers/families. Provide information/support. Address psychosocial issues and physical disability.

- Monitor and reassess frequently. Continue follow-up even when specialist services have finished. Stroke is a long-term problem. Monitor secondary prevention measures. Refer for more specialist rehabilitation if there is any deterioration in function.
- Aids/appliances can help. Patients/carers may be entitled to benefits.
- Concordance—after stroke most patients are prescribed ≥1 drug to ↓ risk of further stroke, but some have memory loss or problems opening containers. Provide verbal and written information about medicines and help with packaging, e.g. non-childproof tops.

**Screening for depression** 🕮 p.998

**Secondary stroke prevention** Patients with a past history of stroke or TIA/amaurosis fugax have a 30–43% risk of recurrent stroke within 5y. Prevention focuses on ischaemic/embolic events which account for the majority of strokes. Preventative strategies include:

### Lifestyle advice

- Stopping smoking (🕮 p.184).
- Regular exercise (🕮 p.182).
- Diet and achieving a satisfactory weight (🕮 pp.176–181).
- Reducing salt intake—↓ salt of 3g/d → ↓ in stroke risk of 13%.
- Avoiding alcohol excess—predisposes to both ischaemic and haemorrhagic stroke through effects on BP (🕮 pp.186–189).

**Antiplatelet drugs** Start all patients not taking warfarin, who have suffered a non-haemorrhagic stroke (confirmed on CT/MRI) or TIA, on aspirin (75–300mg od) as soon as possible after the event. Aspirin ↓ long-term risks of cardiovascular events by a quarter. Dipyridamole 200mg bd can be used in addition to aspirin (effects are additive). Clopidogrel 75mg od is an alternative for those intolerant of aspirin.

### Warfarin

- *1° prevention* Patients with potential causes of cardiac thromboemboli should be anticoagulated with warfarin. This includes patients with rheumatic mitral valve disease, prosthetic heart valves, dilated cardiomyopathy, and AF associated with valvular heart disease or prosthesis. Only anticoagulate patients with non-valvular AF if annual risk of stroke is >3% (Table 16.10). If <3% start aspirin instead.
- *2° prevention* Anticoagulate all patients who have suffered a stroke or TIA and have persistent or paroxysmal AF, or a major source of cardiac embolism, with warfarin. Start >14d after stroke and only if haemorrhagic stroke has been excluded. Target INR 2–3.

### Hypertension management

- Systolic and diastolic BP independently predict stroke. Risk escalates with increasing BP. A 5–6mmHg ↓ BP reduces risk by >30%.

- National Stroke Guidelines recommend treatment with a combination of a thiazide diuretic and ACE inhibitor. Aim to keep systolic BP <140 mmHg and diastolic BP <85mmHg (<130/80mmHg if diabetic).
- After stroke (but not after TIA) defer treating hypertension until >2wk after the event as ↑ BP may be physiological response—lowering BP decreases perfusion of the brain and may be harmful.

### Cholesterol

- *1° prevention* A 22% ↓ in cholesterol using a statin → a 30% ↓ in stroke in individuals with no past history of stroke/TIA. Treat if patients meet criteria for coronary prevention (☐ p.264).
- *2° prevention* All patients with a history of CVD should be treated with a statin regardless of baseline cholesterol. National Stroke Guidelines suggest treatment with a statin, e.g. simvastatin 40mg od, if total cholesterol is >3.5mmol/L unless contraindicated.

**Carotid stenosis and carotid endarterectomy** Carotid endarterectomy ↓ mortality if carotid stenosis is symptomatic. Benefits ↓ as the degree of stenosis gets less—no evidence of benefit if <30% stenosis.
- *Patients without history of stroke/TIA* 2% annual risk of stroke so surgery is controversial   in general risks outweigh benefits.
- *Patients with a history of stroke/TIA* Referral for carotid endarterectomy/carotid artery stenting should be considered if >70% carotid artery stenosis and no severe disability.

**Table 16.10** Non-valvular AF and stroke

| Risk group | Annual risk of stroke | | |
| --- | --- | --- | --- |
| | Untreated | Aspirin | Warfarin |
| **Very high** | 12% | 10% | 5% |
| Previous ischaemic stroke or TIA | | | |
| **High** | 5–8% | 4–6% | 2–3% |
| Age >65y and ≥1 other risk factor. (↑BP, DM, heart failure, LV dysfunction) | | | |
| **Moderate** | 3–5% | 2–4% | 1–2% |
| Age >65y, no other risk factors | | | |
| Age <65y, other risk factors | | | |
| **Low** | 1.2% | 1% | ~0.5% |
| Age <65y, no other risk factors. | | | |

Consider warfarin treatment for all patients in the very high, high, and moderate risk groups. In all cases weigh the benefit of treatment against potential harms (e.g. bleeding risk if not compliant/unreliable about taking medication) and treatment preference. Target INR 2–3.

### Further information
**Royal College of Physicians** National clinical guidelines for stroke (2004) ☐ www.rcplondon.ac.uk

### Patient information and support
**Stroke Association** ☎ 0845 3033 100 ☐ www.stroke.org.uk

# Parkinsonism and Parkinson's disease

**Parkinsonism** Syndrome of:
- *Tremor* Coarse tremor, most marked at rest, 'pill-rolling'.
- *Rigidity* Limbs resist passive extension throughout movement—*lead-pipe rigidity*—and juddering on passive extension of the forearm or pronation/supination—*cogwheel rigidity*.
- *Difficulty in initiating movement.*
- *Slowness of movement* Mask-like or expressionless face, ↓ blink rate, ↓ fidgeting, ↓ peristalsis.
- *Abnormal gait* Small steps—*shuffling gait*—and flexed posture as if hurrying to keep up with feet—*festinant gait.*
- *Micrographia* Small hand writing.

## Causes
- Parkinson's disease (PD)
- Other neurodegenerative diseases, e.g. Alzheimer's disease, multisystem atrophy
- Following encephalitis
- Drugs, e.g. haloperidol, chlorpromazine, metoclopramide
- Toxins, e.g. CO poisoning
- Trauma
- Normal pressure hydrocephalus.

***Treatment of drug-induced parkinsonism*** If possible, stop the implicated drug. If on an antipsychotic for schizophrenia do not stop treatment, but add an antimuscarinic (e.g. procyclidine 2.5mg tds). Consider switching to an atypical antipsychotic drug—take specialist advice.

**Steel–Richardson–Olszewski syndrome** Parkinsonism accompanied by absent vertical gaze and dementia. Due to progressive supranuclear palsy. J.C. Steel, J.C. Richardson and J.Olszewski—*Canadian neurologists.*

**Parkinson's disease (PD)** Incurable progressive degenerative disease affecting the dopaminergic neurons of the substantia nigra in the brainstem → deficiency of dopamine and relative excess of acetylcholine transmitters. *Cause:* unknown. *Lifetime risk:* ~1:40. ♂ = ♀. *Peak age at onset:* ~65y but 5–10% patients are diagnosed when <40y old. Prevalence ↑ with age. *J. Parkinson (1755–1824)—English physician.*

❶ A quarter of those diagnosed with PD in life have another cause of their symptoms at autopsy.

***Management*** Aims to:
- ↓ symptoms and ↑ quality of life
- ↓ rate of disease progression
- Limit side effects of treatment.

*Screening for depression* 📖 p.998

***Referral*** Refer all patients to a specialist with an interest in Parkinson's disease for confirmation of diagnosis, advice on management, and to access a multidisciplinary specialist rehabilitation team.

***Rehabilitation*** Liaise closely with the specialist rehabilitation team:
- General principles 📖 p.206
- Specific issues 📖 p.590

***Drug treatment*** (BNF 4.9) Corrects imbalance of transmitters but not the underlying process. Rarely achieves complete control of symptoms.

5–10% respond poorly to treatment. Treatment for PD should be consultant initiated and is not usually started until symptoms cause significant disruption of daily activities. *Options*:

*Dopamine receptor agonists*, e.g. bromocriptine, pergolide. Often used alone as 1st-line treatment. ↑ dose gradually according to response and tolerability. Withdraw gradually. Can also be used in association with L-dopa to ↓ off times and motor impairment.

⚠ Bromocriptine, pergolide, cabergoline, and lisuride have been associated with pulmonary, retroperitoneal, and pericardial fibrosis.
• Check CXR ± spirometry, ESR, and creatinine before starting.
• Monitor for dyspnoea, persistent cough, chest pain, cardiac failure, abdominal pain or tenderness.

*Levodopa (or L-dopa)* Precursor of dopamine. ↑ dopamine levels within the substantia nigra. Start with low dose and ↑ in small steps—aim to keep final dose as low as possible and a compromise between ↑ mobility and dose-limiting side effects (involuntary movements, psychiatric effects). Optimum dose interval varies between individuals.
• Only effective for PD. Not effective for patients with parkinsonism due to other degenerative brain disease or drugs. Improves bradykinesia and rigidity > tremor.
• Often given with a co drug (carbidopa or benserazide) which prevents peripheral breakdown of L-dopa to dopamine but does not cross the blood–brain barrier (e.g. sinemet, madopar).
• With time there is ↓ response and troublesome side effects appear:
  • *On–off effect*—fluctuation between periods of exaggerated involuntary movements and periods of immobility
  • *End-of-dose effect*—duration of benefit after each dose reduces
  • Abnormal involuntary movements ↑.

*Other drugs*
• *Monoamine oxidase B inhibition*, e.g selegiline. Used in severe PD in conjunction with L-dopa to ↓ end-of-dose effect. Early use may postpone onset of treatment with L-dopa.
• *Amantadine* Improves bradykinesia, dyskinesias, tremor, and rigidity. Introduce and withdraw slowly.
• *Inhibition of enzymatic breakdown of dopamine*, e.g. entacapone, tolcapone. For patients suffering from end-of-dose effect.

**Surgery** A small propotion of carefully selected patients benefit from 'deep brain stimulation' (DBS).

**Driving** 📖 p.130          **Carers** 📖 p.222

## Further information
**NICE** Parkinson's disease: diagnosis and management in primary and secondary care (2006) 🖥 www.nice.org.uk

## Patient advice and support
**Parkinson's Disease Society** ☎ 0808 800 0303
🖥 www.parkinsons.org.uk

# Multiple sclerosis

Multiple sclerosis (MS) is a chronic disabling neurological disease due to an autoimmune process of unknown cause. Characterized by formation of patches of demyelination ('plaques') throughout the brain and spinal cord. There is no peripheral nerve involvement.

It is the most common neurological disorder of young adults with a lifetime risk of 1:1000. Peak age of onset is 20–40y. ♀:♂ ≈ 2:1. There is a marked geographical variation—prevalence ↑ with latitude.

**Presentation** Depends on the area of CNS affected. Take a careful history—although a patient usually presents with a single symptom, history may reveal other episodes that have gone unheralded. Isolated neurological deficits are never diagnostic. The hallmark of MS is a series of neurological deficits distributed in time and space not attributable to other causes. Predominant areas of demyelination are optic nerve, cervical cord, and periventricular areas.

## Common features

- Pain on eye movement (optic neuritis)
- Visual disturbance—↓, blurring or double vision
- ↓ balance
- ↓ coordination
- Sensory disturbance (e.g. numbness, tingling)
- Pain (e.g. trigeminal neuralgia)
- Fatigue
- Depression
- Transverse myelitis (📖 p.580)
- Problems with speech (e.g. slurred or slow)
- Bladder problems (e.g. frequency, urgency, incontinence)
- Constipation
- Sexual dysfunction (e.g. impotence)
- Cognitive changes (e.g. loss of concentration, memory problems)
- Dysphagia.

❶ Symptoms may be worsened by heat or exercise.

## Prognosis

- *Benign MS* (10%) Retrospective diagnosis. The patient has a few mild attacks and then complete recovery. There is no deterioration over time and no permanent disability.
- *Relapsing–remitting MS (RRMS)* 85% of patients. Episodes of sudden ↑ in neurological symptoms or development of new neurological symptoms with virtually complete recovery after 4–6wk.. With time remissions become less complete and residual disability accumulates.
- *Secondary progressive MS (SPMS)* After ~15y 65% of the patients with relapsing–remitting disease begin a continuous downward progression which may also include acute relapses.
- *Primary progressive MS (PPMS)* 10% of patients. Steady progression from the outset with increasing disability.

**Management** If suspected, refer to neurology for confirmation of diagnosis and support from the specialist neurological rehabilitation team.

*Disease-modifying drugs* ↓ frequency and/or severity of relapses by ~30% and slow course of the disease. Options are β-interferon (for RRMS and SPMS) and glatiramer (for RRMS only). Prescription must be consultant led under the NHS risk-sharing scheme (Table 16.11).

**Table 16.11** Indications for β-interferon and glatiramer[N]

|  | β-interferon | Glatiramer |
|---|---|---|
| **Age** | ≥18y | ≥18y |
| **Contraindications** | No contraindications | No contraindications |
| **Walking distance** | *RRMS* Can walk ≥ 100m without assistance  *SPMS* Can walk ≥ 10m without assistance | *RRMS* Can walk ≥ 100m without assistance |
| **Relapses** | *RRMS* ≥2 clinically significant relapses in the last year  *SPMS* Minimal ↑ in disability due to gradual progression and ≥2 disabling relapses in the past 2y | *RRMS* ≥ 2 clinically significant relapses in the last year |
| **Stop if** | • Intolerable side effects  • Pregnant or planning pregnancy  • ≥2 disabling relapses within a year  • Inability to walk (± assistance) persisting ≥ 6mo  • 2° progression with observable ↑ in disability over 6mo | • Intolerable side effects  • Pregnant or planning pregnancy  • ≥2 disabling relapses within a year  • Inability to walk (± assistance) persisting ≥ 6mo  • 2° progression |

**Natalizumab** Monoclonal antibody for treatment of highly active relapsing–remitting MS despite treatment with β-interferon, or rapidly evolving severe relapsing–remitting MS. Prescription must be consultant led. Associated with a ↑ risk of opportunistic infection and progressive multifocal leucoencephalopathy (PML). If new/worsening neurological symptoms/signs refer to neurology immediately to exclude PML.

**Immunization** Offer influenza vaccination to all MS patients.

**Acute relapses** Treat episodes causing distressing symptoms or ↑ limitation with high-dose steroids, e.g. methylprednisolone 500mg–2g od po for 3–5d. Alternatively, refer for high-dose IV steroids. Refer to specialist neurological rehabilitation if residual deficit, or if frequent relapses.

**Management of symptoms and disability** Liaise closely with the specialist neurological rehabilitation team.
• Screening for depression 📖 p.998
• General principles of rehabilitation 📖 p.206
• Common neurological rehabilitation problems 📖 p.590.

## Further information
**NICE/RCP** Diagnosis and management of multiple sclerosis in primary and secondary care (2004) 🖥 www.nice.org.uk
**MS Society** A guide to MS for GPs and primary care teams (2006) 🖥 www.mssociety.org.uk

## Patient advice and support
**MS Society** ☎ 0808 800 8000 🖥 www.mssociety.org.uk

# Motor neuron disease and CJD

**Motor neuron disease (MND)** is a degenerative disorder of unknown cause affecting motor neurons in the spinal cord, brainstem, and motor cortex. Prevalence in the UK ~ 4.5/100 000 population ♂:♀ ≈ 3:2. Peak age of onset ~60y. 10% have FH. There is *never* any sensory loss.

**Patterns of disease** There are 3 recognized patterns of MND:
- *Amyotrophic lateral sclerosis (ALS)* (50%)—combined LMN wasting and UMN hyper-reflexia.
- *Progressive muscular atrophy* (25%)—anterior horn cell lesions affecting distal before proximal muscles. Better prognosis than ALS.
- *Progressive bulbar palsy* (25%)—loss of function of brainstem motor nuclei (LMN lesions) resulting in weakness of the tongue, muscles of chewing/swallowing, and facial muscles.

**Clinical picture** Combination of progressive upper and/or lower motor neuron signs affecting >1 limb or a limb and the bulbar muscles.

## Symptoms and signs

- Stumbling (spastic gait, foot-drop)
- Tiredness
- Muscle wasting
- Weak grip
- Weakness of skeletal muscles
- Cramp
- Fasciculation of skeletal muscles

- Fasciculation of the tongue
- Difficulty with speech (particularly slurring, hoarseness or nasal or quiet speech)
- Difficulty with swallowing
- Aspiration pneumonia.

❶ MND *never* affects eye movements (cranial nerves III, IV, VI).

**Management** Refer to neurology for exclusion of other causes of symptoms and confirmation of diagnosis. MND is incurable and progressive. Death usually results from ventilatory failure 3–5y after diagnosis.

## Drug therapy

- Riluzole (50mg bd) is the only drug treatment licensed in the UK.
- Evidence suggests it extends life or time to mechanical ventilation for patients with ALS. It may also slow functional decline.[N]
- It should be initiated by a specialist with experience of MND.[N]
- Monitoring of liver function is essential—monthly for the first 3mo, then 3 monthly for 9mo, then annually thereafter.

## Support

- Involve relevant agencies early, e.g. DN, social services, carer groups, self-help groups.
- Apply for all relevant benefits (💷 p.224).
- Screen for depression (💷 p.998).
- Discuss the future and the patient's wishes for the time when they become incapacitated with patient and carer(s).
- Regular review to help overcome any new problems encountered is helpful for patients and carers.

*Symptom relief*
- *Spasticity*—baclofen, tizanidine, botulinum toxin.
- *Drooling*—propantheline 15–30mg tds po or amitriptyline 25–50mg tds po.
- *Dysphagia*—blend food, discuss NG tubes/PEG (📖 p.591).
- *Depression*—common. Reassess support; consider drug treatment and/or counselling.
- *Joint pains*—analgesia
- *Respiratory failure*—discuss tracheostomy/ventilation. Weigh pros and cons of prolongation of life versus prolongation of discomfort.
- *Palliative care* 📖 pp.1026–1043.

**Creutzfeldt–Jakob disease (CJD)** (human spongiform encephalopathy). Fatal degenerative brain disease due to a rogue form of brain protein or 'prion'. *Types:*
- *Sporadic or classical* Most common form in the UK (~50 cases/y). Rare <40y. Median duration of symptoms 3–4mo. *Cause:* unknown.
- *Variant* Affects younger people than classical CJD and duration is longer, lasting a median of 14mo. *Cause:* transmitted by ingestion of nervous tissue in beef infected with bovine spongiform encephalitis or 'mad cow disease'. Compensation may be available to families.
- *Iatrogenic* Cases associated with treatments using human growth hormone and human dura mater grafts. Rarely associated with corneal grafts or contaminated instruments used in surgery.
- *Familial prion disease* ~20–30 families in the UK are affected with a version of CJD passed from generation to generation in an autosomal dominant pattern. Median duration of symptoms from onset is 2–5y.

**Presentation** Long incubation (>25y in some cases). Clinical features vary according to the areas of brain most affected but are always rapidly progressive. *Common features:* personality change; psychiatric symptoms; cognitive impairment; neurological deficits (sensory and motor deficits, ataxia); myoclonic jerks, chorea, or dystonia; difficulty with communication, mobility, swallowing, and continence; coma and death.

**Differential diagnosis** Dementia, depression, MS, MND, SOL.

**Management** There is no simple diagnostic test and often families feel frustrated by early misdiagnosis. Refer to neurologist if suspected. Treatment is supportive. Palliative care 📖 pp.1026–1043.

**General principles of rehabilitation** 📖 p.206

**Common neurological rehabilitation problems** 📖 p.590

**Further information**
**NICE** Riluzole for motor neurone disease (2004) 🖥 www.nice.org.uk

**Patient advice and support**
**Motor Neurone Disease Association** ☎ 08457 626262
🖥 www.mndassociation.org
**Brain and Spine Foundation** ☎ 0808 808 1000
🖥 www.brainandspine.org.uk

## Spinal cord conditions

Spinal cord injury tends to affect young people, especially young men. It is devastating and the GP and primary care team are a vital part of the ongoing support network. *Causes:* trauma (42% falls, 37% RTAs); herniated disc; transverse myelitis; tumour; abscess.

**Quadriplegia and tetraplegia** Caused by spinal cord injury above the 1st thoracic vertebra. Usually results in paralysis of all four limbs, weakened breathing, and an inability to cough and clear the chest.

**Paraplegia** Occurs when the level of injury is below the 1st thoracic nerve. Disability can vary from the impairment of leg movement, to complete paralysis of the legs and abdomen up to the nipple line. Paraplegics have full use of their arms and hands.

### Incomplete spinal cord injuries

- *Anterior cord syndrome* Damage is towards the front of the spinal cord, leaving the patient with loss or ↓ ability to sense pain, temperature, and touch sensations below the level of injury. Pressure and joint sensation may be preserved.
- *Central cord syndrome* Damage is in the centre of the spinal cord. Typically results in loss of function in the arms, but some leg movement may be preserved ± some control of bladder/bowel function.
- *Posterior cord syndrome* Damage is towards the back of the spinal cord. Typically leaves the patient with good muscle power, pain and temperature sensation, but difficulty coordinating limb movements.
- *Brown-Séquard syndrome* Damage is limited to one side of the spinal cord resulting in loss or ↓ movement on the injured side but preserved pain and temperature sensation, and normal movement on the uninjured side but loss or ↓ in pain and temperature sensation. *C.E. Brown-Séquard (1817–1894)—French neurologist/physiologist.*

**Cauda equina lesion** The spinal cord ends at $L_1/L_2$ at which point a bundle of nerves travels downwards through the lumbar and sacral vertebrae. Injury to these nerves causes partial or complete loss of movement and sensation. There may be some recovery of function with time.

**Transverse myelitis** Inflammation of the spinal cord at a single level. Symptoms develop rapidly over days/weeks and include limb weakness, sensory disturbance, bowel and bladder disturbance, back pain, and radicular pain. Recovery generally begins within 3mo but is not always complete. *Causes:*

- Idiopathic (thought to be auto-immune mechanism)
- Autoimmune disease e.g. SLE, Sjögren's syndrome, sarcoidosis
- Infection
- MS
- Vaccination
- Malignancy
- Vascular, e.g. thrombosis of spinal arteries, vasculitis 2° to heroin abuse, spinal AV malformation.

*Management* Depending on severity of symptoms, admit as an acute medical emergency or refer for urgent neurological opinion.

**Syringomyelia** Tubular cavities (syrinxes) form close to the central canal of the spinal cord. As the syrinx expands, it compresses nerves within the spinal cord. Most common in patients with previous spinal injury—though may be years before. Typically presents with wasting and weakness of hands and arms, and loss of temperature and pain sensation over trunk and arms (cape distribution). *Action*: refer to neurology.

**General principles of rehabilitation** 📖 p.206

**Common neurological rehabilitation problems** 📖 p.590

**Specific problems associated with spinal cord injury**

*Autonomic dysreflexia (hyper-reflexia)* Reflex sympathetic over-activity causing flushing and ↑ BP which may be severe. Only occurs in patients with lesions above T$_{5/6}$. Usually triggered by discomfort below the level of the lesion. Presentation is with pounding headache, sweating, and flushing or mottling above the level of the lesion.

*Action* Sit the patient up and remove any obvious cause, e.g. pain, bladder distension, constipation. Give GTN spray (1–2 puff s/ling) or nifedipine 5–10mg capsule broken sublingually. If not settling, admit to hospital.

**Loss of temperature control** Most people with complete spinal cord injuries do not sweat below the level of the injury and many quadriplegics cannot sweat above the injury either (even though they may sweat due to autonomic dysreflexia). With loss of ability to sweat or vasoconstrict within affected dermatomes, careful control of environmental conditions becomes essential to avoid hypothermia or overheating. In hot weather advise cooling with wet towels applied to the skin.

*Infertility* Many ♂ patients suffer infertility due to:
- Failure of ejaculation
- Retrograde ejaculation
- Thermal damage due to sitting in a wheelchair → poor quality sperm
- Chronic infection of prostate and seminal vesicles (common)
Refer for specialist advice.

*Bowel/bladder function* Both bladder and bowel function are reflex actions that we learn to override as children. If the lesion is above the level of this reflex pathway (T$_{12}$ for bowel and T$_6$ for bladder function), automatic emptying will still occur when the bladder or bowel is full—though there is no control. If the lesion is below this level, there is no emptying reflex. Bladder–bowel care programmes reflect this. Useful leaflets are available from the spinal injuries association.

**Spasticity** 📖 p.591  **UTI** 📖 p.456

**Pressure sores** 📖 p.617  **Depression** 📖 p.998

**Patient advice and support**
**Spinal Injuries Association** ☎ 0800 980 0501 🖥 www.spinal.co.uk
**Brain and Spine Foundation** 🖥 www.brainandspine.org.uk
**Transverse Myelitis Association** 🖥 www.myelitis.org.uk
**Ann Conroy Trust (syringomyelia and associated conditions)**
☎ 01788 537676 🖥 www.theannconroytrust.org.uk

# Epilepsy

Epilepsy is a group of disorders in which fits or seizures occur as a result of spontaneous abnormal electrical discharge in any part of the brain. They take many forms, but usually take the same pattern on each occasion for a given individual. Prevalence 5–10/1000. 5% of those >21y old having their first fit have cerebral pathology (10% age 45–55y).

**Epilepsy in children** 📖 p.896

**Management of a fitting patient/status epilepticus** 📖 p.1066

**Management after first fit** 60% adults who have one fit will never have another (90% if EEG is normal).

⚠ Refer *all* patients with a first suspected seizure for urgent (within 2wk) assessment by a neurologist with training and expertise in epilepsy to exclude underlying causes (e.g. tumour) and receive clear guidance on medication, work, and driving.[N]

**Classification of seizure types** is important, as these have implications for management and prognosis:

- *Partial seizures* The seizure is limited to one area of the brain only. Termed 'simple' if no impairment of consciousness (previously called focal or Jacksonian epilepsy) and 'complex' if consciousness is impaired (previously called psychomotor or temporal lobe epilepsy). Partial seizures may become generalized.
- *Generalized seizures* The whole brain is involved. Consciousness is usually but not always impaired. There are 6 major types: tonic–clonic (grand mal); absence (petit mal); myoclonic; tonic; clonic; and atonic.

❶ Some people have seizures that cannot be classified in this way.

**Todd's palsy** Focal CNS signs (e.g. hemiplegia) following an epileptic seizure. The patient seems to have had a stroke but recovers in <24h.

**Causes of epilepsy in adults** A cause is found in more than two-thirds of people with epilepsy. The most common causes are:

- Cerebrovascular disease
- Cerebral tumours
- Genetic, congenital, or hereditary conditions
- Drugs, alcohol, and other toxic causes
- Head trauma (including surgery)
- Post-infective causes (e.g. meningitis, encephalitis).

**Assessment** Table 16.12

**Screening for depression** 📖 p.998

**Long-term management of epilepsy** 📖 p.584

**Epilepsy and pregnancy** 📖 p.827

**Mortality** Death rate is ↑ ×2–3. Deaths are related to underlying condition, accidents, SUDEP, or status epilepticus.

*Sudden unexplained death in epilepsy (SUDEP)* Probably due to central respiratory arrest during a seizure. Minimize risk by optimizing seizure control and being aware of potential consequences of night seizures.

**Table 16.12** Summary of points to cover during assessment

| History | | |
|---|---|---|
| Background | • Previous head injury<br>• Alcohol/drug abuse<br>• Meningitis or encephalitis | • Stroke<br>• Febrile convulsions<br>• Family history of epilepsy |
| Provoking factors | • Sleep deprivation<br>• Alcohol withdrawal | • Flashing lights |
| Prodrome/aura | *Prodrome*—precedes fit. May be a change in mood or behaviour noticed by the patient or others<br>*Aura*—part of the seizure that precedes other manifestations. Odd sensations, e.g. déjà-vu (odd feeling of having experienced that time before), strange smells, rising abdominal sensation, flashing lights | |
| Features of the attack | *Eye witness report* if available—colour of the patient, movement, length of fit, circumstances, after-effects<br>*Memories of the patient* Memories of the event and/or first memories after the event; frequency of attacks; relationship to sleep, menses, etc. | |
| Residual symptoms after the attack | • Bitten tongue<br>• Incontinence of urine/faeces (not specific for epilepsy)<br>• Confusion<br>• Headache<br>• Aching limbs or temporary weakness of limbs (Todd's palsy) | |
| **Examination** | | |
| Neurological examination | • Fever, photophobia, neck stiffness, or petechial rash?<br>• Any residual deficit<br>• Focal neurology<br>• Signs of ↑ICP (📖 p.566) | |
| General examination | • BP, heart sounds, heart rhythm and rate<br>• Signs of systemic illness | |
| **Investigations (first fit only)** | | |
| | • ECG<br>• Blood for U&E, Cr, eGFR, LFT, Ca²⁺, FBC, ESR | |

**Differential diagnosis**

| | |
|---|---|
| • Vasovagal syncope | • Normal phenomenon (e.g. déjà-vu) |
| • Psychogenic non-epileptic attacks (pseudo-seizures) | • Cardiac arrythmias |
| • Tics | • Other cardiac disorders (e.g. aortic stenosis, HOCM) |
| • Panic attack | • TIA |
| • Hypoglycaemia | • Migrainous aura |

## Further information

**NICE** 🖥 www.nice.org.uk
• The epilepsies: the diagnosis and management of the epilepsies in adults and children in primary and secondary care (2004)
• Referral guidelines for suspected cancer (2005).

## Patient advice and support

**Epilepsy Action** ☎ 0808 800 5050. 🖥 www.epilepsy.org.uk

# Management of epilepsy

After a new diagnosis of epilepsy, patients are investigated and started on any medication under specialist care. The neurologist and GP then share care. Regular GP review, at least annually, is essential.

**Education** Epilepsy is a diagnosis causing alarm and fear. Education is important. Find out how much the patient (and family) understand about epilepsy and what information they have. Acknowledge their distress at diagnosis and answer their questions. Provide information on:
- What to expect—fits are controlled with drugs in 80%.
- What to do during an attack.
- Driving (📖 p.132) and work—stop driving and notify DVLA and motor insurance company. Inform employer. Do not work at heights or with/ near dangerous machinery.
- Avoiding risks—avoid cycling in traffic; only swim if lifeguard present.
- Importance of concordance with medication.
- When drug withdrawal may be considered if fit free.

Good leaflets are available from Epilepsy Action. Self-help and support groups can be helpful.

**Drug therapy** (BNF 4.8.1) NICE recommends drug treatment after the 2nd seizure except in specific circumstances. Drug choice is a specialist decision. ❶ Patients on anticonvulsants are entitled to free prescriptions.

**Withdrawal of drug therapy** Consider if fit free for 2–3y. Decision to the stop *must* be the patient's. Balance problems/inconvenience of drug-taking against risks of fits. Refer to neurology for supervision of drug withdrawal. 59% of adults with grand mal epilepsy stay fit free for 2y.

*Seizure recurrence is more likely if* generalized tonic–clonic seizures, myoclonic epilepsy or infantile spasms, taking >1 drug for epilepsy, ≥1 seizure after starting treatment, duration of treatment >10y, fit free <5y.

⚠ Advise patients not to drive during withdrawal of epileptic medica-tion or for 6mo afterwards.

**Surgery** Increasingly used for intractable partial seizures, hemi-epilepsy, and epilepsy with focal EEG and/or radiological features.

**Ketogenic diet** Effective in some patients with refractory epilepsy—take specialist advice.

**At review** Review the patient's individual careplan. Record any fits and precipitating causes, drug concordance (frequency of repeat prescriptions) and side effects, if fit free >2y (depending on the type of epilepsy), and then discuss the possibility of withdrawing medication if appropriate.

**Re-refer** For review by a neurologist if:
- Control is poor or drugs are causing unacceptable side effects.
- Seizures have continued despite medication for >2y, or on 2 drugs.
- Pointers to a previously unsuspected cause for the fits appear.
- Concurrent illness (physical or psychiatric) complicates management.
- For pre-conceptual advice or to discuss withdrawal of medication.

**Table 16.13** Commonly used drugs in epilepsy Stress the importance of concordance. Start at a low dose and ↑ dose until fits are controlled or side effects occur. Use monotherapy wherever possible—2 drugs ↑ toxicity and side effects. Polytherapy offers no advantage over monotherapy for 90% of patients. Prescribe by brand name—generic prescribing may lead to changing of brand. Changing brand carries 10% risk of worsening of seizure control.

| | | Ethosuximide | Sodium valproate | Carbamazepine | Lamotrigine | Phenytoin |
|---|---|---|---|---|---|---|
| **Type of epilepsy** | Absence | ✓ | ✓ | | | ✓ (unlicensed) |
| | Myoclonic | ✓ | ✓ | | ✓ | |
| | Tonic clonic | | ✓[1] | ✓ | ✓ | ✓ |
| | Partial ± 2° generalized | | ✓ | ✓ | ✓ | ✓ |
| **Adult starting dose** | | 500mg od | 300mg bd | 100–200mg od or bd | 25mg od for 2wk[2] | 100mg od |
| **Incremental dose** | | 250mg/d at weekly intervals | 200mg/d at 3 day intervals | 100mg/d at weekly intervals | From starting dose to 50mg od for 2 wk then ↑ by 50mg/d at weekly intervals | 100mg/d at weekly intervals |
| **Usual daily dose** | | 1–1.5g od | 500mg–1g bd | 200–1200mg | 100–200mg | 200–500mg |
| **Common/important side effects** | | Blood dyscrasias,[3] nausea, sedation, vomiting, dizziness, ataxia. | Pancreatitis, liver toxicity,[4] blood dyscrasias,[3] sedation, tremor; weight ↑, hair thinning, ankle swelling. | Blood dyscrasias,[3] rash,↓ liver toxicity,[4] nausea, sedation, diplopia, dizziness, fluid retention, ↓Na.[5] | Blood dyscrasias,[3] rash, fever; influenza-like symptoms, drowsiness or worsening of seizure control | Blood dyscrasias,[3] rash, drowsiness, ↓memory, gum hyperplasia, nystagmus, diplopia, tremor, dysarthria, ataxia |

1. Drug of choice for primary syndromes of generalized epilepsy.
2. Starting dose is different if used in association with other epileptics—see BNF.
3. Check FBC if bruising, mouth ulcers or symptoms of infection (sore throat, fevers).
4. Warn about symptoms of liver disease—check LFTs soon after starting and at review.
5. Monitor U&E at regular review.
⚠ Sodium valproate is teratogenic.

# Muscle disorders

**Symptoms** Muscle weakness, fatiguability. Pain at rest suggests inflammation—pain on exercise, ischaemia, or metabolic myopathy.

**Signs** Look for associated systemic disease.
• Myotonia—delayed muscular contraction after relaxation, e.g. on shaking hands.
• Local muscular tenderness or firm muscles—may be due to infiltration of muscle with connective tissue or fat.
• Fasciculation—spontaneous, irregular, and brief contractions of part of a muscle—suggests LMN disease (e.g. MND).
• Lumps—tumours are rare. Lumps may be due to tendon rupture, haematoma, or herniation of muscle through fascia.

**Muscular dystrophies** Group of genetic disorders characterized by progressive degeneration and weakness of some muscle groups.

 *Duchenne's muscular dystrophy* Sex-linked recessive inheritance means almost always confined to boys. 30% of cases are due to spontaneous mutation. Investigation shows markedly ↑ CK (>40× normal). Presents typically at ~4y with progressively clumsy walking. Few survive to >20y old. Refer for confirmation of diagnosis and ongoing specialist support. Genetic counselling is important. *G.B.A. Duchenne (1807–1875)—French neurologist.*

*Patient information and support*
**Muscular dystrophy campaign** ☎ 0800 652 6352
🖥 www.muscular-dystrophy.org

**Myotonic disorders** Characterized by myotonia.

*Dystrophia myotonica* Most common myotonic disorder. Autosomal dominant inheritance. Presents from 20–30y with weakness of hands, legs, and face, and myotonia. Wasting of the face gives a haggard appearance. Associated with cataract, frontal baldness in men, atrophy of testes/ovaries, cardiomyopathy, endocrine abnormalies (e.g. DM), and mental impairment. Most die in middle age of intercurrent illness. Refer to confirm diagnosis, and for advice on management/genetic counselling.

*Patient information and support*
**Dystonia Society** ☎ 0845 458 6322 🖥 www.dystonia.org.uk

**Toxic myopathies** Certain drugs can cause myopathy including:

• Alcohol
• Labetalol
• Cholesterol lowering drugs (including the statins)

• Steroids
• Chloroquine
• Zidovudine
• Vincristine

• Ciclosporin
• Cocaine
• Heroin
• PCP.

*Management* Stop the implicated drug immediately. If symptoms do not resolve, refer for confirmation of diagnosis and management advice.

**Acquired myopathy of late onset** Often a manifestation of systemic disease, e.g. thyroid disease (especially hyperthyroidism), carcinoma, Cushing's disease. Investigate to find the cause. Treat the cause if found else refer for further investigation.

**Polymyositis** Insidious symmetrical proximal muscle weakness due to muscle inflammation. Dysphagia, dysphonia, and/or respiratory muscle weakness may follow. 25% have a purple rash on cheeks, eyelids, and other sun-exposed areas (*dermatomyositis*) ± nailfold erythema. CK levels are ↑. Associated with malignancy in 10% of patients >40y. Refer.

## Poliomyelitis[ND]

***Acute polio*** *Spread*: droplet or faeco-oral. *Incubation*: 7d. Presents with 2d flu-like prodrome, then fever, tachycardia, headache, vomiting, stiff neck, and unilateral tremor ('pre-paralytic stage'). 65% who experience the pre-paralytic stage go on to develop paralysis (myalgia, LMN signs ± respiratory failure). *Management*: supportive—admit to hospital. <10% of those developing paralysis die. Permanent disability may result.

### Prevention
* *1° immunization in babies and children <10y* Three doses of the 5-part vaccine (DTaP/IPV/Hib) protecting against polio, diphtheria, whooping cough, tetanus, and *Haemophilus influenza*, each 1mo apart—usually at 2mo, 3mo, and 4mo. If schedule is disrupted, resume where stopped.
* *Booster doses in children* 1 dose of 4 part vaccine (DTaP/IPV) protecting against polio, diphtheria, whooping cough, and tetanus >3y after the 1° course (usually pre-school) and another dose of 3-part vaccine (Td/IPV) against tetanus, diptheria, and polio 10y later (age 13–18y).
* *1° immunization in children >10y and adults* 3 doses of 3-part vaccine (Td/IPV) each 1mo apart. Booster doses are required 3y and 10y after the primary course.
* *Booster doses for travel* Not required unless at special risk, e.g. travelling to endemic/epidemic area or healthcare workers. Boosters of Td/IPV are then given every 10y.

***Late effects of polio*** 20–30y after initial infection some patients develop new symptoms often triggered by a period of immobilization.
* ↑ muscle weakness and fatigue.
* Pain in muscles and joints.
* Respiratory difficulties (particularly in those who spent some time in an iron lung ventilator)—may present with symptoms relating to sleep.

Once other causes are excluded, treatment is supportive.

**Motor neuron disease** 📖 p.578

**Myasthenia gravis** 📖 p.556

**Lambert–Eaton syndrome (or myasthenic syndrome)** Occurs in association with small cell carcinoma of the lung or rarely autoimmune disease. Differs from myasthenia gravis by tendency to hyporeflexia. Autonomic involvement is common. Proximal limb muscles/trunk are most commonly involved. Specialist treatment is essential. *L.M. Eaton (1905–58) and E.H. Lambert (b.1915)—US neurologists/neurophysiologists.*

# Other neurological syndromes

## Neurofibromatosis

### *von Recklinghausen's disease (type 1 neurofibromatosis: NF1)*

Autosomal dominant trait. Criteria for diagnosis: ≥2 of:

- ≥6 café-au-lait patches (flat coffee-coloured patches of skin seen in 1st year of life, increasing in number and size with age) >5mm (prepubertal) or >15mm (postpubertal).
- ≥2 neurofibromas:
  - Dermal neurofibromas—small violaceous skin nodules which appear after puberty.
  - Nodular neurofibromas—subcutaneous firm nodules arising from nerve trunks (may cause paraesthesiae if compressed) or a plexiform neurofibroma which appears as a large subcutaneous swelling.
- Freckling in axilla, groin, neck base, and submammary area (women). Present by age 10y.
- ≥2 Lisch nodules—nodules of the iris only visible with a slit lamp.
- Distinctive bony abnormality specific to NF1, e.g. sphenoid dysplasia.
- First-degree relative with NF1.

***Management*** Ongoing specialist management is essential.

***Complications*** affect 1:3 patients:

- Mild learning disability
- Short stature
- Macrocephaly
- Nerve root compression
- GI bleeding or obstruction
- Cystic bone lesion
- Scoliosis

- Pseudoarthrosis
- ↑ BP (6%)—due to renal artery stenosis or phaechromocytoma
- Malignancy (5%)—optic glioma or sarcomatous change of neurofibroma
- Epilepsy (slight ↑).

*F.D. von Recklinghausen (1833–1910)—German pathologist.*

***Type 2*** Much rarer than type 1. Autosomal dominant inheritance.

***Diagnosis*** One of:

- Bilateral vestibular schwannoma (acoustic neuroma—sensorineural hearing loss, vertigo ± tinnitus).
- First-degree relative with NF2 *and either* a unilateral vestibular schwannoma *or* ≥1 neurofibroma, meningioma, glioma, Schwannoma, or juvenile cataract.

***Management*** Screen at-risk patients with annual hearing tests. Once diagnosis is made, specialist neurosurgical management is needed.

***Complications*** Schwannomas of other cranial nerves, dorsal nerve roots, or peripheral nerves; meningioma (45%); other gliomas (less common).

**Restless legs syndrome (Ekbom syndrome)** The patient (who is usually in bed) is seized by an irresistible desire to move his/her legs in a repetitive way accompanied by an unpleasant sensation deep in the legs. Sleep disturbance is common, as is +ve FH. *Cause:* unknown.

## Management

- Exclude drug causes. Common culprits: β-blockers, $H_2$ antagonists, neuroleptics, lithium, TCAs, anticonvulsants.
- Exclude peripheral neuropathy or ischaemic rest pain.
- Iron deficiency (with or without anaemia) is associated in 1:3 sufferers so check FBC and serum ferritin.
- Also check U&E, Cr, eGFR, fasting blood glucose, and TFTs.
- Try non-drug measures first—reassurance, information, walking/ stretching, warmth, relaxation exercises, massage.
- Licensed drugs—ropinirole (250 micrograms nocte for 2d, then 500 micrograms nocte for 5d, then 1mg nocte for 1wk, then increase by 500 micrograms /wk to usual dose of 2mg nocte as needed) and pramipexole (88 micrograms 2–3h before bed, double every 4–7d as needed to usual dose of 350 micrograms/d).
- Refer if severe symptoms or diagnosis is in doubt.

*K.A. Ekbom (1907–1977)—Swedish neurologist.*

### Patient support

**Restless leg syndrome foundation** ▢ www.rls.org

**Wernicke encephalopathy** Thiamine deficiency causing nystagmus, ophthalmoplegia, and ataxia. Other eye signs, e.g. ptosis, abnormal pupillary reactions, and altered consciousness or confusion, may also occur. Consider in any patient with symptoms and a history of alcoholism.

**Management** Refer for confirmation of diagnosis. Meanwhile start thiamine 200–300mg od po to prevent irreversible Korsakoff's syndrome. In severe cases admit as a medical emergency. *K. Wernicke (1848–1904)— German psychiatrist.*

**Korsakoff syndrome** ↓ ability to acquire new memories. May follow Wernicke encephalopathy and is due to thiamine deficiency. Confabulation to fill gaps in memory is a feature. *S.S. Korsakoff (1853–1900)—Russian neuropsychiatrist.*

**Gilles de la Tourette syndrome** ▢ p.909

**Huntington disease (chorea)** Autosomal dominant trait. Testing can identify affected individuals before symptoms occur. Pre-conceptual and antenatal testing is available and should be offered to any couple with a family history on either the mother or the father's side. Presents with movement abnormalities (e.g. hemichorea and rigidity) and dementia. Memory is relatively spared compared to cognition. Refer for expert advice. *G. Huntington (1851–1916)—US physician.*

**Friedreich's ataxia** The most common inherited ataxia (autosomal recessive). Prevalence—1:50 000. Presents in adolescence with progressive gait and limb ataxia, loss of proprioception, pyramidal weakness, and dysarthria. Extra-neurological involvement includes hypertrophic cardiomyopathy (most patients) and DM (10%). Treatment is supportive. Most patients become chairbound within 15y and die in the 4th or 5th decade from cardiac or pulmonary complications. *N. Friedreich (1825–1882)—German neurologist.*

# Neurological rehabilitation problems

**New symptoms or limitations** Consider:
• Is it due to an unrelated disease (e.g. change in bowel habit in someone who has had a stroke might indicate bowel cancer)?
• Is it due to an incidental infection (e.g. UTI, chest infection)?
• Is it due to a relapse (e.g. acute relapse in MS, TIA, or further stroke in a stroke patient)?
• Is it due to a side effect of treatment (e.g. acute confusion, involuntary movements or the on–off effect in a patient with PD)?
• Is it part of a gradual progression (e.g. in MS, MND, brain tumour)?

Treat any cause of deterioration identified. If no cause is found, consider re-referring for specialist review and/or referring to the multidisciplinary rehabilitation team involved with the patient.

### General principles of rehabilitation 📖 p.206

**Fatigue** Consider and treat factors that might be responsible:
• Depression
• Chronic pain
• Disturbed sleep
• Poor nutrition.

**Action** Review support, diet, and medication; encourage graded aerobic exercise; consider a trial of amantadine 200mg/d to improve symptoms.[N]

**Depression and anxiety** Common. Diagnosis can be difficult. Standardized questionnaires, e.g. PHQ-9 (📖 p.999), are helpful for screening.

**Action** Give opportunities to talk about the impact of the illness on lifestyle. Jointly identify areas where positive changes could be made, e.g. referral to day care to widen social contact. Consider referral for counselling or to a self-help/support group. Consider antidepressant medication and/or referral to psychiatric services.

**Emotionalism** If the patient cries (or laughs) with minimal provocation, consider emotionalism—impairment in the control of crying. Reassure.

**Sexual and personal relationships** Problems are common. Useful information sheets are available at 🖥 www.outsiders.org.uk

**Communication problems** Speech therapy assessment is vital. Consider support via dysphasia groups and communication aids, e.g. simple pointing board (take advice from speech therapy and OT).

**Poor vision** Refer to an optician in the first instance. If corrected vision is still poor refer for ophthalmology review.

**Respiratory infections** Common. Treat with antibiotics unless in terminal stages of disease. Advise pneumococal and influenza vaccination.

**Venous thromboembolism** Common but clinically apparent in <5%. Ensure adequate hydration and encourage mobility. Consider use of aspirin 75–150mg od and compression stockings if immobile. Prophylactic anticoagulation does not improve outcome.

**Motor impairment** Aim to maintain physical independence:
- Involve physiotherapy—often only 2–3 visits are needed.
- Involve OT—a task-oriented approach is used (e.g. learning how to dress). Can also supply/advise on aids and appliances, e.g. Velcro fasteners, wheelchairs, adapted cutlery, etc.
- Refer for social services OT assessment if aids, equipment, or adaptations are needed for the home.
- Refer for home care services as necessary.
- Give information about driving (📖 pp.130–133) and/or employment (📖 p.126) where appropriate.

**Spasticity ± muscle and joint contractures** Treat with physiotherapy (usually involving exercise ± splinting) ± drugs. Anti-spasticity drugs include dantrolene (25mg od), baclofen (5mg tds or rarely through a pump), and tizanidine (2mg od). Botulinum toxin can be directed at specific muscles. Refer via the specialist rehabilitation team.

**Pain** Most pain arises from ↓ mobility. *Other causes include:* premorbid disease (e.g. osteoarthritis); central pain due to neurological damage, and neuropathic pain.

***Action*** Chronic pain, especially central pain, may respond to TCAs. Peripheral pain may respond to simple analgesia + physiotherapy. Other options are TENS and local joint injection. Use of cannibinoids for relief of pain/muscle spasm in MS is currently under assessment. Refer patients with intractable pain to specialist pain clinics.

**Bladder problems**
- *UTI* If suspected check urine dipstick ± send MSU for M,C&S and start antibiotics. If >3 proven UTIs in 1y refer to specialist incontinence service or urology for further assessment.
- *Incontinence* 📖 pp.458–461.
- *Nocturia* Desmopressin 100–400 micrograms po or 10–40 micrograms intranasally may be helpful.
- *Urgency* Modify environment (e.g. provide commode); try anticholinergic (e.g. tolterodine 2mg bd or oxybutinin 5mg tds). If not settling, refer for specialist assessment.

**Bowel problems**
- *Dysphagia* Common. Fluids are more difficult to swallow than semi-solids. Formal assessment by trained staff is essential. Feeding through NG tube or percutaneous endoscopic gastrostomy (PEG) may be needed long or short term—in terminal disease (e.g. MND) weigh provision of nutrition against prolongation of poor-quality life.
- *Constipation* Difficulty with defecation or bowel opening <2×/wk— ↑ fluid intake and ↑ fibre in diet. If no improvement use po laxative ± regular suppositories/enemas.
- *Incontinence* Exclude overflow due to constipation.

**Skin breakdown** *Prevented by:* positioning, mobilization, good skin care, management of incontinence, pressure-relieving aids (e.g. special mattresses/cushions). Involve community nursing services.

# Neurological assessment scales

**Modified Barthel ADL index\*** Measure of physical disability used widely to assess behaviour relating to activities of daily living for stroke patients or patients with other disabling conditions. It measures what patients do in practice. Assessment is made by anyone who knows the patient well.

| **Bowels** | **Transfer (bed to chair and back)** |
|---|---|
| 0= Incontinent or needs enemas | 0= Unable, no sitting balance |
| 1= Occasional accident (1×/wk) | 1= Major help (1 or 2 people), can sit |
| 2= Continent | 2= Minor help (verbal or physical) |
| | 3= Independent |
| **Bladder** | **Mobility** |
| 0= Incontinent or needs enemas | 0= Immobile |
| 1= Occasional accident (1×/wk) | 1= Wheelchair independent (including corners) |
| 2= Continent | 2= Walks with the help of 1 person (physical or verbal help) |
| | 3= Independent (may use aid) |
| **Grooming** | **Dressing** |
| 0= Needs help with personal care | 0= Dependent |
| 1= Independent (including face, hair, teeth, shaving) | 1= Needs help—can do ~½ unaided |
| | 2= Independent (including buttons, zips, laces, etc.) |
| **Toilet use** | **Stairs** |
| 0= Dependent | 0= Unable |
| 1= Needs some help | 1= Needs help (verbal or physical) |
| 2= Independent | 2= Independent |
| **Feeding** | **Bathing** |
| 0= Unable | 0= Dependent |
| 1= Needs help, e.g. cutting | 1= Independent (bath or shower) |
| 2= Independent | |

## Score

- <15—usually represents moderate disability.
- <10—usually represents severe disability.

\*Reproduced from Mahoney FI, Barthel DW. Functional evaluation: the Barthel Index (1965), *Maryland State Medical Journal* **14**: 61–65. Used with permission.

**Migraine Disability Assessment Score (MIDAS)** Used to assess the impact of migraine symptoms on lifestyle.

*Instructions* Please answer the following questions about ALL the headaches you have had over the last 3mo. If you did not do the activity in the last 3mo, write 0.

| | |
|---|---|
| 1. On how many days in the last 3mo did you miss work or school because of your headache? | ☐ days |
| 2. On how many days in the last 3mo was your productivity at work or school ↓ by ≥½ because of your headaches? *(Do not include days you counted in question 1 where you missed work or school)* | ☐ days |
| 3. On how many days in the last 3mo did you not do household work* because of your headache? | ☐ days |
| 4. On how many days in the last 3mo was your productivity in household work ↓ by ≥½ because of your headaches? *(Do not include days you counted in question 3 where you did not do household work)* | ☐ days |
| 5. On how many days in the last 3mo did you miss family, social, or leisure activities because of your headaches? | ☐ days |
| **MIDAS score**                                **TOTAL** | ☐ days |
| A. On how many days in the last 3mo did you have a headache? *(If a headache lasted more than 1 day, count each day)* | ☐ days |
| B. On a scale of 0–10, on average how painful were these headaches? *(0 = no pain at all, and 10 = pain as bad as can it be)* | ☐ |

*Unpaid work such as housework, shopping and caring for children and others

Questions A and B measure the frequency of the migraine and the severity of pain. They are not used to reach the MIDAS score, but provide extra information helpful for making treatment decisions.

### Interpreting the MIDAS score

| I | Score 0–5 | Minimal/infrequent disability | Tend to have little or no treatment needs. Can often manage with OTC medication. If infrequent severe attacks may require triptan |
|---|---|---|---|
| II | Score 6–10 | Mild/infrequent disability | May require medication for acute attacks, e.g. NSAID ± antiemetic or triptan |
| III | Score 11–0 | Moderate disability | Will need medication for acute attacks. Consider prophylaxis. |
| IV | Score ≥21 | Severe disability | Consider other causes for headaches, e.g. tension type headache |

The Migraine Disability Assessment Score is reproduced with permission from Dr Joshua Liberman, on behalf of Caremark, Inc.

# Dermatology

# Changes in skin colour and skin eruptions

**Pallor** Non-specific sign which may be racial, familial, or cosmetic. Pathology suggested includes anaemia, shock, Stokes–Adams attack, vasovagal faint, myxoedema, hypopituitarism, and albinism.

**Hypo- and hyperpigmentation** 📖 p.602

**Erythema** 📖 p.600

**Linear lesions** *Consider:*
- Koebner phenomenon (lesions arise in area of injury, e.g. in scratches)—occurs in psoriasis, eczema, lichen planus
- Linear urticaria
- Self-inflicted trauma—dermatitis artefacta
- Reaction to garden plants—psoralen-induced phytophotodermatitis
- Impetigo—may spread along scratch marks
- Herpes zoster—at the edge of a dermatome.

**Ring-shaped lesions** *Consider:*
- Psoriasis
- Fungal infection, e.g. ringworm
- Granuloma annulare
- Discoid eczema
- Erythema multiforme
- Basal cell carcinoma
- Urticaria
- Pityriasis rosea
- Lichen planus
- Burns (especially on a child—may be non-accidental injury)
- Orf.

**White patches** Consider all causes of patchy hypopigmentation.
- Vitiligo.
- After inflammation: cryotherapy, eczema, psoriasis, morphoea.
- Pityriasis alba: white post-inflammatory patch on a child's face—no treatment needed.
- Exposure to some chemicals: substituted phenols, hydroquinone.
- Certain infections: pityriasis versicolor.
- Tuberous sclerosis.
- Halo naevus (pale area around a mole).
- Piebaldism (from birth—associated with a white forelock).
- Extensive hyperpigmentation, e.g. chloasma—the patches of normal skin may appear hypopigmented.

**White spots** *Consider:*
- Pustules/whiteheads, e.g. due to acne, folliculitis, or rosacea.
- Molluscum contagiosum: white spots with a pearl-like appearance.
- Milia: small white spots usually on upper arms/face of children—resolve spontaneously.

**Brown spots** *Consider:*
- Freckles
- Moles
- Lentigos—like freckles but darker and not affected by sunlight
- Melanoma
- *Café au lait* spots— >5 associated with neurofibromatosis
- Basal cell carcinoma
- Seborrhoeic warts
- Senile keratoses
- Dermatofibroma
- Systemic disease
- Addison's
- Acanthosis nigrans
- Haemochromatosis.

## Scaling
- *Silvery scaling on the surface of red patches*—psoriasis
- *Fine scaling accompanied with rash*—pityriasis
- *Coarse, scaly skin with no rash*—ichthyosis.

**Yellow crusting** Usually due to staphylococcal infection (impetigo)

**Telangectasia** Dilated distal venule/arteriole (spider naevus). *Causes:*
- *Congenital*, e.g. hereditary haemorrhagic telangectasia
- *Venous disease in the leg*, e.g. venous stars
- *Rosacea*—facial
- *Excess oestrogen*, e.g. liver disease, COC pill, pregnancy
- *Skin atrophy*, e.g. ageing skin, radiation dermatitis, topical steroids.

**Spider naevi** Small red lesions (barely visible—0.5cm diameter) in superior vena cava distribution, i.e. on arms, neck, and chest wall. Large arteriole with numerous small vessels radiating from it giving the appearance of a spider—hence the name. Pressure applied to the central arteriole (e.g. with a pointed object) causes blanching of the whole lesion. >2 spider naevi is abnormal. *Causes:*
- Cirrhosis—most frequently, alcoholic.
- Oestrogen excess—usually in association with chronic liver disease.
- Rheumatoid arthritis—rarely.
- Viral hepatitis (transient).
- Pregnancy—usually appear during the 2nd–5th months and disappear in the final trimester

**Blisters** 📖 p.598

**Subcutaneous nodules** *Consider:*
- Rheumatoid arthritis
- Xanthelasma
- Neurofibroma
- Granuloma annulare
- Sarcoid
- Polyarteritis.

**Purpura** Blue-brown discoloration of the skin due to bleeding within it. Petechiae are small dot-like purpura, whilst ecchymoses are more extensive. Treat the cause. *Causes:*
- *Idiopathic*, e.g. idiopathic pigmented purpura (brownish punctate lesions on the legs).
- *Vessel wall defects* Vasculitis, paraproteinaemia, infection (e.g. meningococcal meningitis, septicaemia, glandular fever), ↑ intravascular pressure (e.g. venous disease).
- *Clotting defects* Abnormal platelet function, thrombocytopenia, anticoagulant therapy, coagulation factor deficiency.
- *Defective dermal support* Dermal atrophy (e.g. ageing, steroids, disease), scurvy (vitamin C deficiency).

> ⚠ *Referral of patients with purpura*
> - Admit unwell patients with new purpura/petechiae as an emergency
> - Refer well children/young adults with unexplained petechiae immediately to be seen the same day[N]
> - For well older adults with unexplained bruising, bleeding, or purpura, check FBC, blood film, clotting screen, and ESR/viscosity/CRP[N]

# Itching and blistering of the skin

**Itching** In any patient presenting with pruritus or itch, ask: *Are there skin lesions present?*

***Skin lesions present*** Search for unexcoriated lesions. Investigations are not usually needed. Exceptions are patch testing for contact dermatitis and skin biopsy for dermatitis herpetiformis. *Causes:*

- Urticaria
- Contact dermatitis and allergies to food and drugs
- Prickly heat.
- Skin infestations, e.g. scabies, pediculosis, insect bites
- Infections—viral, e.g. chickenpox; fungal
- Dermatitis herpetiformis
- Lichen planus
- Senile atrophy
- Psychological causes*.

*Excessive excoriation causes lichenification of the skin.

***Skin lesions absent*** Large differential diagnosis. Look for pallor, jaundice, weight ↓, LN enlargement, and abdominal organomegaly. Investigate as necessary—consider urinalysis (dipstick and MSU), FBC, ESR, serum ferritin, LFTs (including alkaline phosphatase), U&E, Cr and eGFR, glucose, serum $Ca^{2+}$, TFTs, and CXR. If still undiagnosed—refer. *Causes:*

- Hepatic—obstructive jaundice, pregnancy
- Endocrine—DM, thyrotoxicosis, hypothyroidism, hyperparathyroidism
- Renal—chronic renal failure
- Haematological—polycythaemia rubra vera, iron deficiency, leukaemia, Hodgkin's disease
- Malignancy—any carcinoma
- Drug allergies
- Psychological—obsessive states, schizophrenia
- Rare causes—diabetes insipidus, roundworm infection.

**Blisters** Type of blister depends on level of cleavage of the skin—subcorneal or intra-epidermal blisters rupture easily, sub-epidermal blisters are much tougher. *Causes:*

- *Subcorneal* Pustular psoriasis (📖 p.622), bullous impetigo (📖 p.630).
- *Intra-epidermal* Eczema (📖 pp.612–616), HSV (📖 p.632), VZ—chickenpox (📖 p.650) or shingles (📖 p.651), pemphigus, friction
- *Subepidermal* Cold or heat injury (burns—📖 p.1110), pemphigoid, dermatitis herpetiformis, linear IgA disease.
- *Other* Insect bites (may cause cleavage at any level).

**Pemphigoid**[G] Autoimmune disorder.

- *Bullous pemphigoid* Usually affects the elderly. An urticarial reaction may precede onset of blistering. Large, tense blisters arise on red or normal skin on the limbs, trunk and flexures. Oral lesions in 20–30%. May be localized to one site e.g. lower leg. *Differential diagnosis:* pemphigus, dermatitis herpetiformis, linear IgA disease.
- *Cicatricial pemphigoid* Mainly affects mucous membranes in the eyes/ mouth. Scarring results in visual loss. Refer to ophthalmology.
- *Pemphigoid gestationis* Rare but characteristic bullous eruption associated with pregnancy. Remits after delivery but often recurs in subsequent pregnancies.

**Management** Refer to dermatology for skin biopsy and confirmation of diagnosis. Treatment is usually with oral steroids (prednisolone 30–60mg daily initially, reducing as symptoms improve). Other treatments include antibiotics and nicotinamide, azathioprine or other immunosuppressants.

**Prognosis** Self- limiting in 50%—steroids are often stopped after ~2y.

**Pemphigus[G]** Uncommon autoimmune disorder affecting skin and mucous membranes. Affects adults (peak incidence 30–70y). *Cause:* 90% have detectable circulating autoantibodies. Associated with other autoimmune disorders, e.g. myasthenia gravis.

**Presentation** 50% present with oral lesions. Suspect in anyone presenting with mucocutaneous erosions/blisters. Flaccid superficial blisters then appear—sometimes months later—over scalp, face, back, chest, and flexures. As blisters are fragile they burst early and the condition may present as crusted erosions. Untreated, the condition is progressive.

**Management** Refer to dermatology. Treatment is with high-dose systemic steroids or other immunosuppressive agents. Treatment is continued long term although occasional remissions occur. Before treatment with steroids three quarters of patients died in <4y. Now excess morbidity and mortality are due to side effects of treatment.

**Dermatitis herpetiformis** Closely related to coeliac disease (📖 p420) 2–5% of patients with coeliac disease have dermatitis herpetiformis. ♂>♀ (2:1), *Peak incidence:* 3rd/4th decade. Consists of itchy vesicular skin rash on elbows (extensor surface), knees, buttocks, and scalp which are often broken by scratching to leave excoriations. Associated with small intestinal enteropathy but symptoms of GI malabsorption are uncommon. *Differential diagnosis:* scabies, eczema, linear IgA disease.

**Management** Refer to dermatology. Responds to withdrawal of gluten, although may take up to 1y. Controlled in the interim with dapsone or sulfapyridine.

**Epidermolysis bullosa** A group of genetically inherited diseases characterized by blistering on minimal trauma. Range from being mild and trivial to being incompatible with life. Most common is *simple epidermolysis bullosa* (autosomal dominant)—blistering is caused by friction, is mild, and is limited to hands and feet. Patients are advised to avoid trauma.

**Linear IgA disease** Rare condition of blisters and urticarial lesions on the back and extensor surfaces. Refer to dermatology. Responds to dapsone.

### Further information
**Electronic Dermatology Atlas** 🖥 www.dermis.net
**British Association of Dermatologists** 🖥 www.bad.org.uk
- Guidelines for the management of pemphigus vulgaris (2003)
- Guidelines for the management of bullous pemphigoid (2002)

# Erythema

Erythema is redness of the skin—usually due to vasodilation. It may be localized (e.g. pregnancy—on the palms) or generalized (e.g. drug eruption, viral exanthema).

⚠ **Erythroderma** Inflammatory dermatosis affecting >90% skin surface. Rare, but systemic effects are potentially fatal. ♂:♀ ≈ 2:1. Typical patient is middle-aged or elderly. Patchy erythema becomes universal in <48h. Accompanied by fever, shivering, and malaise. 2-6d later scaling appears. The skin is hot, red, itchy, dry, and thickened, and feels tight. Hair and nails may be shed. Admit as an acute medical emergency.

*Causes* Eczema (40%); psoriasis (25%); lymphoma (15%); drug eruption (10%); other skin disease (2%); unknown (8%).

**Flushing** 📖 p.605

**Palmar erythema** Reddening of the palms associated with pregnancy, liver disease, and polycythemia.

**Livedo reticularis** Marbled patterned cyanosis of the skin. If not reversible by warming, investigate the cause. Treat the cause. *Causes:* physiological (e.g. cold); vasculitis (e.g. SLE); hyperviscosity

**Chilblains** Inflamed and painful purple-pink swellings on fingers, toes, or ears. Appear in response to cold. ♀ > ♂. Advise warm housing/clothing, gloves, and woolly socks. In severe cases oral nifedipine may help.

 **Erythema ab igne** Reticulate pigmented erythema due to heat-induced damage. Common in the elderly—especially from sitting in front of the fire or using hot water bottles to alleviate pain. Explain the cause. Resolves spontaneously.

**Erythema multiforme** Immune mediated disease characterized by target lesions on hands and feet (Plate 1). *Causes:*
• *Idiopathic* (50%)
• *Infective*—streptococcal, HSV, hepatitis B, mycoplasma
• *Drugs*—penicillin, sulphonamide, barbiturate
• *Other*—SLE, pregnancy, malignancy.

*Presentation* Target lesions (red rings with central pale or purple area) on hands and feet. New lesions appear for 2–3wk. Frequently oral, conjunctival, and genital mucosa are affected—if severe termed *Stevens–Johnson syndrome*.

*Differential diagnosis* Toxic erythema; toxic epidermal necrolysis; Sweet's disease; urticaria; pemphigoid.

*Management* Identification and removal of the underlying cause. Mild cases resolve spontaneously and require symptomatic measures only. Admit if extensive involvement.

**Erysipelas, cellulitis, scalded skin syndrome** 📖 p.631

**Erythema nodosum** Tender erythematous nodules 1–5cm diameter on extensor surfaces of limbs (especially shins) ± ankle and wrist arthritis ± fever. ♀:♂≈3:1. Resolves in <8wk, non-scarring. No treatment needed.

**Associations** 20% of cases are idiopathic with no associations

- Streptococcal infection
- Drugs, e.g. oral contraceptives, sulphonamides
- Acute sarcoidosis
- Inflammatory bowel disease — UC, Crohn's
- Malignancy
- TB.

**Rosacea** Chronic inflammatory facial dermatosis characterized by erythema and pustules. Most common in middle age (30–50y) and in fair-skinned people of Northern European descent. ♀>♂ (~3:2). *Cause:* Unknown—although possible associations with the face mite *Demodex folliculorum*, *Helicobacter pylori* infection, and migraine headaches.

**Presentation** Earliest symptom is flushing. Erythema, telangectasia, papules, pustules ± lymphoedema affect cheeks, nose, forehead, and chin. Exacerbated by sunlight and topical steroids.

**Aggravating factors** Sun exposure (61%); emotional stress (60%); hot weather (53%); alcohol (45%); spicy foods (43%); exercise (39%); cold weather or wind (36–38%); hot baths (37%); hot drinks (36%); cosmetics/skin care products (24%).

**Complications** Rhinophyma (bulbous appearance of nose); eye involvement—blepharitis and conjunctivitis.

**Differential diagnosis** Acne (lacks comedones and older age group); contact dermatitis; SLE; photosensitive eruptions; seborrhoeic dermatitis.

*Management*

- Avoid triggers
- Antibiotics—repeated treatment is usually needed over many years with prolonged courses of topical or systemic antibiotics (e.g. metronidazole 0.75% gel bd or oral tetracycline 1g daily, decreasing to 250mg od after 3wk and continuing for 2–3mo).
- Refer to dermatology if rhinophyma, ocular complications, or failure to respond to treatment in general practice.

**Lyme disease** *Cause: Borrelia burgdorferi. Spread:* transmitted by ticks—usually from deer or sheep. Presents with erythema migrans (75%—red macule/papule on upper arm, leg or trunk 3-32d after a tick bite which expands to form a ring with central clearing; diameter can be up to 50cm; further smaller lesions then develop elsewhere); flu-like illness; lymphadenopathy ± splenomegaly; arthralgia. Symptoms are typically intermittent and changing. Complications include neurological abnormalities, aseptic meningitis, myocarditis, and arthritis.

*Management* Confirm diagnosis with serology. Treatment is usually with doxycycline or erythromycin—take microbiology advice. ☛ Treatment with antibiotics after a tick bite but before symptoms have arisen is controversial.

*Removal of ticks* 📖 p.1104

# Pigmentation disorders

**Hypopigmentation** Lack of skin pigmentation. May be:
- *Generalized*—albinism, phenylketonuria, hypopituitarism
- *Patchy*—vitiligo, tuberous sclerosis, morphoea, pityriasis alba, or after inflammation (e.g. post-cryotherapy, 2° to eczema or psoriasis), infection (e.g. pityriasis versicolor), or exposure to chemicals (substituted phenols, hydroquinone).
- *Around a mole*—halo naevus

**Hyperpigmentation** Excess skin pigmentation. May be:
- *Genetic*—racial, freckles, neurofibromatosis, Peutz–Jegher syndrome
- *Due to drugs*—amiodarone (blue-grey pigmentation of sun-exposed areas), psoralens, minocycline (blue-black pigmentation in scars and buccal mucosa), chloroquine (blue grey pigmentation of face and arms), chlorpromazine (grey pigment in sun-exposed sites), cytotoxics
- *Endocrine*—Addison's disease, chloasma, Cushing's syndrome
- *Nutritional*—excess ingestion of carrots (carotinaemia), malabsorption
- *Post-inflammatory*—varicose eczema, lichen planus, systemic sclerosis
- *Other*—benign naevi, malignant melanoma, chronic renal failure (lemon yellow), liver disease (jaundice), acanthosis nigricans

**Freckles and lentigines**
- *Freckles* are small, light brown macules, typically facial, which darken in the sun. They are common, particularly in redheads, and develop in childhood. Require no treatment.
- *Lentigines* are also brown macules but are more scattered and do not darken in the sun. Most common in elderly sun-exposed skin. Respond to cryotherapy.

**Chloasma** Patterned macular symmetrical facial pigmentation, usually involving the forehead and/or cheeks, ♀>>♂. Peak age 20–40y. Affects dark skins more than fair skins.

**Risk factors** Pregnancy (usually fades after delivery); taking the COC pill or depot contraceptives (may be slow to fade when stopped); use of cosmetics, perfumes, or deodorant soap.

**Management** Reassurance is normally all that is needed. *Consider:*
- Stopping hormonal contraception
- Avoid irritating the skin with strong soaps/abrasive cleaners
- Sunscreens may prevent chloasma becoming more pronounced
- Bleaching creams: apply only to affected areas bd—may help some but requires application for >6mo to have any effect
- Rarely, patients are so worried about their appearance that camouflage cosmetics are warranted
- Laser resurfacing: mixed results—refer for expert advice

**Vitiligo** Plate 2. Affects 1% of the population. ♂ = ♀. *Peak age of onset:* 10–30y. *Cause:* autoimmune; 30% have a family history. *Associations:* pernicious anaemia, Addison's and thyroid disease.

**Presentation** May be precipitated by injury or sunburn. Presents as sharply defined white macules which contain no melanocytes. Often symmetrical distribution. *Most common sites:* hands, wrists, knees, neck, face around eyes and mouth.

**Differential diagnosis** Post-inflammatory hypopigmentation, chemical exposure.

**Management** Prognosis is variable—some develop a few lesions which remain static; some progress to larger depigmented areas; some even repigment. There is no cure. Advise use of sunscreens for affected areas (ACBS prescription); camouflage cosmetics (refer to Red Cross for advice on application, ACBS prescription). In severe cases refer for dermatology opinion —high-dose steroids or PUVA may help.

**Albinism** *Prevalence:* 1/20 000. Rare genetic syndrome (autosomal recessive inheritance) in which the melanocytes are unable to produce skin, hair, or eye pigment. Patients have white hair, pale skin, pink eyes, poor sight, photophobia, and nystagmus. Several different varieties exist.

**Management** Strict sun avoidance, sunglasses, sunscreens; refer any skin lesions for biopsy (↑ risk squamous cell carcinoma).

**Morphoea (localized scleroderma)** ♀: ♂ ≈ 3:1. Localized bands of sclerosis on the skin. Pathologically distinct from lesions of systemic sclerosis. Internal disease is not associated. *Cause:* unknown—may follow trauma. Presents with round/oval plaques of induration and erythema which become shiny and white, eventually leaving atrophic hairless pigmented patches. Affects trunk/proximal limbs. No established treatment—topical steroids are often tried. Usually spontaneously resolves in a few months.

**Further information**
**Electronic dermatology atlas** 🖳 www.dermis.net

# Hair and sweat gland problems

**Hair loss or alopecia** May be diffuse or localized, scarring or non-scarring. Treatment is according to cause. *Differential diagnosis:*

- *Diffuse non-scarring* Male pattern baldness (repsonds to minoxidil but hair loss returns as soon as stopped); hypothyroidism; iron deficiency; malnutrition; hypopituitarism; hypoadrenalism; drug-induced.
- *Localized non-scarring* Alopecia areata; ringworm; traumatic; hairpulling; traction; SLE; secondary syphilis.
- *Scarring* Burns; radiation; shingles; tertiary syphilis; lupus erythematosus; morphoea; lichen planus.

**Alopecia areata[G]** Chronic inflammatory disease affecting the hair follicles ± nails (~10%). Presents as patches of hair loss usually on the scalp but can affect any hair-bearing skin. 20% have a family history.

*Management* Investigation is usually unnecessary. If mild hair loss, reassure and monitor hair loss; more severe cases refer to dermatology. Treatment options include topical/local injection/systemic steroids and contact immunotherapy. ~40% recover in <1y; 20% lose all scalp hair—recovery in these cases is unusual (<10%).

**Hirsutism** 📖 p.350

**Hypertrichosis** Excess hair in non-androgenic distribution—usually face and trunk. Mostly drug induced (e.g. phenytoin, ciclosporin A, minoxidil). If not, investigate to find other causes: malnutrition, anorexia nervosa, porphyria cutanea tarda, malignancy. If a cause cannot be found, treat symptomatically with electrolysis, bleaching, waxing ± depilatories.

*Local hypertrichosis* Can be associated with topical steroid usage, be over a melanocytic naevus, or associated with spina bifida occulta.

**Hidradenitis suppurtiva** Unpleasant chronic inflammatory condition of sweat glands in axilla, groin, and perineum. Nodules, abscesses, cysts, and sinuses form → scarring. Treat with topical antiseptics (e.g. chlorhexidine), systemic antibiotics ± surgical drainage/excision.

**Hyperhidrosis** Sweating, or perspiration, is normal and essential for temperature control. The amount people sweat varies enormously. Usually sweating can be controlled with shop-bought antiperspirants and is only excessive when it cannot be controlled and interferes with the patient's quality of life. Excessive sweating may be focal or generalized.

*Generalized hyperhidrosis* Most likely to occur 2° to other medical conditions. Where possible treat the cause.

- *Physiological*—after and during exercise; hot humid conditions; emotional response (e.g. anxiety).
- *Infection*—can occur with any bacterial or viral infection. Consider malaria if recent history of travel.
- *Non-infective*—menopause; thyrotoxicosis; phaeochromocytoma; lymphoma; leukaemia.

*Management* If no cause is found, β-blockers (e.g. propranolol 40mg od/bd) or SSRIs (e.g. fluoxetine 20mg od) may be effective (unlicensed).

**Focal hyperhidrosis** Usually a 1° condition—mainly affects the axillae, palms, soles of feet, and/or face. Affects ~5% of the population. Onset is typically in the teenage years. Distressing and socially disabling.

• *Advice for patients:* avoid clothing made of Lycra, nylon, or other man-made fibres and tight clothing; wear colours that do not show the sweat, e.g. white, black; use emollient washes/moisturizers rather than soap; identify trigger factors for sweating (e.g. alcohol, crowded rooms) and avoid those situations.

• Treat topically with 20% aluminium chloride (e.g. Anhydrol Forte®). Apply to clean skin at night—wash off in morning. ↓ frequency of application as symptoms subside. Treat local irritation with topical steroid, e.g. hydrocortisone 1%. Absorbent dusting powder may help axillary/plantar sweating.

• Consider a trial of drug therapy with β-blockers (e.g. propranolol 40mg od/bd) or SSRIs (e.g. fluoxetine 20mg od) (both unlicensed uses)

• Refer to dermatology or vascular surgery if not responding.

*2° care treatments include*

• *Iontophoresis*—for palmar/foot hyperhidrosis. A mild electric current is passed through the skin whilst immersed in a warm water bath. Multiple sessions are needed initially; then treatments every 6wk–6mo.

• *Botulinum toxin injections*—for isolated excess sweating of the axillae/groins. ↓ sweating. Lasts 4–12mo then repeat injections are needed.

• *Endoscopic transthoracic sympathectomy (ETS)*—99% effective for palmar hyperhidrosis; 80% effective for axillary hyperhidrosis; 70% effective for facial flushing, blushing, or sweating. Expect compensatory hyperhidrosis elsewhere (usually the small of the back).

**Flushing** Erythema due to vasodilation. Common and usually benign. Tends to affect face, neck, and upper trunk. *Cause:*

• *Physiological,* exertion, heat

• *Emotion,* e.g. anger, anxiety, embarrassment

• *Foods,* e.g. spices, chillis, alcohol

• *Endocrine,* e.g. menopause, Cushing's syndrome

• *Drugs,* e.g. morphine, tamoxifen, danazol, GnRH analogues, clomifene, nitrates, calcium-channel blockers

• *Dermatological,* rosacea (unknown mechanism); contact dermatitis

• *Inflammatory,* SLE; dermatomyositis

• *Infection,* e.g. slapped cheek syndrome (fifth disease); cellulitis/erysipelas

• *Tumour:* pancreatic tumours, medullary thyroid cancer, carcinoid, phaeochromocytoma.

**Management** Treat cause if possible (e.g. avoid alcohol, HRT). Embarrassing flushing may be helped with propranolol (e.g. 40mg od/bd) or clonidine (e.g. 50 micrograms bd). If severe and disabling and no response to conservative measures, consider referral for surgery as for hyperhidrosis.

#### Further information

**British Association of Dermatologists** Guidelines for the management of alopecia areata (2003) 🖳 www.bad.org.uk

#### Patient information

**Hairline International** 🖳 www.hairlineinternational.com

# Nail changes

Nail changes may be due to nail disease or indicate other dermatological or systemic disease.

## Assessment
- *Take a history*—duration, initial changes, evolution of changes, other systemic or local symptoms, family history, drug and alcohol history, occupation, hobbies.
- *Examine*—colour, shape, extent and pattern of involvement; consider examination/investigation for other skin or systemic disease (guided by history and appearance of nails).

**Table 17.1** Nail changes: description and cause

| Change | Description of nail | Differential diagnosis |
|---|---|---|
| Colour | Black transverse bands | Cytotoxic drugs |
| | Blue | Cyanosis<br>Antimalarials<br>Haematoma |
| | Blue-green | *Pseudomonas* infection |
| | Brown | Fungal infection<br>Cigarette staining<br>Chlorpromazine<br>Gold<br>Addison's disease |
| | Brown 'oil stain' patches | Psoriasis |
| | Brown longitudinal streak | Melanocytic naevus<br>Malignant melanoma<br>Addison's disease |
| | Red streaks, 'splinter haemorrhages' | Infective endocarditis<br>Other vasculitic disease<br>Trauma |
| | White spots | Trauma to the nail matrix |
| | White transverse bands | Heavy metal poisoning |
| | White/brown half-and-half nails | Chronic renal failure |
| | White (leuconychia) | Hypoalbuminaemia (e.g. associated with cirrhosis) |
| | Yellow | Psoriasis<br>Fungal infection<br>Jaundice<br>Tetracycline<br>Yellow nail syndrome (defective lymph drainage, nails grow very slowly, may be associated with pleural effusion) |
| Brittle | Nails break easily—usually at the distal end. | Effect of water and detergent, iron deficiency, hypothyroidism, digital ischaemia. |

**Table 17.1** (*Continued*) Nail changes: description and cause

| Change | Description of nail | Differential diagnosis |
|---|---|---|
| *Clubbing*<br><br>⚠ Refer any patient with unexplained clubbing for urgent CXR[N] | Loss of angle between nail fold and plate<br>Bulbous finger tip<br>Nail fold feels boggy | *Respiratory*: bronchial carcinoma (not small cell); chronic infection; fibrosing alveolitis; asbestosis<br>*Cardiac*: SBE; congenital cyanotic heart disease<br>*Other*: inflammatory bowel disease (Crohn's > UC); thyrotoxicosis; biliary cirrhosis; congenital; AV malformation |
| *Koilonychia* | Spoon-shaped nails | Iron deficiency anaemia<br>Lichen planus<br>Repeated exposure to detergents |
| *Onycholysis* | Separation of nail from the nail bed | Psoriasis<br>Fungal infection<br>Trauma<br>Thyrotoxicosis<br>Tetracyclines |
| *Pitting* | Fine or coarse pits in the nail bed | Psoriasis<br>Eczema<br>Alopecia areata<br>Lichen planus |
| *Beau's lines* | Transverse grooves | Any severe illness which affects growth of the nail matrix |
| *Ridging* | Transverse | Beau's lines<br>Eczema<br>Psoriasis<br>Habit tic dystrophy (thumb > other finger nails due to habitual rubbing/picking at the cuticle)<br>Chronic paronychia |
|  | Longitudinal | Lichen planus<br>Darrier's disease (keratosis follicularis—genetic disorder appearing in adolescence mainly affecting skin/nails) |
| *Nail fold telangectasia* | Dilated capillaries and erythema at the nail fold | Connective tissue disorders |
| *Tumours of the nail fold* | Benign | Viral warts<br>Myxoid (mucus) cysts (treat with steroid injection or cryotherapy)<br>Periungual fibroma (associated with tuberous sclerosis—appear at puberty) |
|  | Malignant | Melanoma<br>Squamous cell carcinoma |

# Sunlight and the skin

**Skin conditions worsened by sunlight** HSV (cold sores); lupus erythematosus (LE); porphyria; rosacea; vitiligo.

**Skin conditions improved by sunlight** Acne; atopic eczema; pityriasis rosea; psoriasis (10% get worse).

**Skin cancer** 📖 p.628

**Sunburn** 📖 p.1111

**Solar keratosis** Single or multiple discrete scaly hyperkeratotic rough-surfaced areas over sun-exposed sites (e.g. dorsum of hands; head, and neck). Occasionally occurs on lower lip. More common with fairer skin types. May regress spontaneously or be pre-malignant.

*Management* Removal by cryotherapy, currettage, excision biopsy or application of fluorouracil cream (apply thinly od/bd for 3–4wk) or diclofenac gel (apply thinly bd for 2–3mo). Advise patients to wear sunblock daily; avoid sun exposure by covering up, and wear a hat with a brim.

*Complications* Malignant change; cutaneous horn development (treat with excision or curretage).

**Solar elastosis** Sun-exposed skin is yellow, thickened, and wrinkled. No treatment. Advise to avoid sun exposure and wear sunblock.

**Drug-induced photosensitivity** Drugs may produce a light eruption in exposed areas by either dose-dependent or allergic mechanisms. The reaction produced varies according to the drug. *Common examples are:* amiodarone, chlorpropamide, furosemide, griseofulvin, phenothiazines, sulphonamides, tetracyclines, thiazides, nalidixic acid, coal tar, and plant-derived psoralens.

**Plant-induced photodermatitis** Photocontact dermatitis similar in appearance to contact dermatitis due to other agents (📖 p.614) results from local sensitization of the skin by contact with psoralens from plants, e.g. carrots, celery, fennel, parsnip, common rue, giant hogweed. Oils used in perfumes derived from plants (e.g. oil of bergamot) may also contain psoralens.

**Polymorphic light eruption** Pruritic papules, plaques ± vesicles appear in sun-exposed areas ~24h after exposure. Most common photodermatosis. ♀:♂ ≈ 2:1. *Cause:* unknown. *Management:* sunscreens and avoidance of sun exposure (sit in the shade, long sleeves, trousers, broad-brimmed hat); a short course of PUVA in the spring may help severe cases—refer to dermatology. *Differential diagnosis:* photoallergic contact dermatitis; drug-induced photosensitivity; LE.

**Solar urticaria** Rare. Wheals appear within minutes of sun exposure. *Differential diagnosis:* porphyria. *Management:* sunscreens, avoidance. Refer to dermatologist if disabling.

**Actinic prurigo** Rare. Starts in childhood. Papules and excoriations on sun-exposed sites. *Management:* sunscreens and avoidance. Refer to dermatology for confirmation of diagnosis and advice on further management.

**Pellagra** Dietary deficiency of nicotinic acid. May give photosensitive dermatitis in association with dementia and diarrhoea. Treatment of underlying deficiency alleviates symptoms.

**Porphyria** A group of rare, mostly inherited, metabolic disorders. Porphyrins are important in the manufacture of haemoglobin. Deficiency of enzymes in the porphyrin pathway results in build up of intermediary metabolites which are toxic to skin and nervous system. All require specialist management by either a general physician or a dermatologist. The main porphyrias are:

- *Acute intermittent porphyria* Intermittent attacks precipitated by many drugs. *Presentation:* fever, GI symptoms (vomiting, abdominal pain—can be severe); neuropsychiatric symptoms (hypotonia, paralysis, fits, impaired vision, peripheral neuritis, odd behaviour—even psychosis); *no* skin features. Urine may go deep red on standing.
- *Porphyria cutanea tarda* Most common porphyria. Typically occurs in male alcoholics with liver damage. Presents with sun-induced sub-epidermal blisters on hands which scar. *Management:* avoidance of alcohol and aggravating drugs (e.g. oestrogens); venesection; chloroquine.
- *Erythropoietic protoporphyria* Autosomal dominant; starts in childhood; red blistering eruption leaving scars on hands and nose.
- *Variegate porphyria* Autosomal dominant. Common in South Africa. Skin signs are like porphyria cutanea tarda, but abdominal pain and neuropsychiatric symptoms resemble acute intermittent porphyria

## Further information

**British Association of Dermatologists** Guidelines for the management of actinic keratoses (2007) ▣ www.bad.org.uk

## Patient information

**British Association of Dermatologists** Patient leaflet on polymorphic light eruption ▣ www.bad.org.uk

# Treatment of skin conditions

Skin conditions are usually treated with topical creams and lotions. Consider the vehicle as well as the active ingredient. In primary care the choice is usually between creams and ointments.
- *Creams*—emulsions of oil and water. Well absorbed into the skin, less greasy and easier to apply than ointments.
- *Ointments*—greasy preparations suitable for chronic dry lesions

Other alternatives include applications, gels, lotions, and pastes.

**Emollients** (BNF 13.2.1), e.g. aqueous cream, white soft paraffin. Useful for all dry or scaling disorders to soothe, smooth, and hydrate the skin—apply in the direction of hair growth. Effects are short-lived—advise frequent application even after improvement occurs.
- Severity of the condition, patient preference, and site of application guide choice of emollient. Some ingredients rarely cause sensitization (Box 17.1)—suspect if an eczematous reaction occurs.
- Preparations such as aqueous cream and emulsifying ointment can be used as soap substitutes for handwashing and in the bath. Addition of an emollient bath oil, e.g. Oilatum® or Balneum®, may also be helpful.
- Avoid preparations containing an antibacterial unless infection is present or a frequent complication.
- Using a preparation with added urea, e.g. Balneum Plus® or Eucerin®, may improve hydration for scaling conditions or in elderly patients.

**Topical corticosteroids** (BNF 13.4)
- Used to suppress inflammatory conditions of the skin, e.g. eczema, when other measures such as emollients are ineffective. Use the least potent preparation which is effective (Table 17.2). Apply a thin layer od/bd to affected areas only.
- Creams are suitable for moist or weeping lesions and ointments for dry, lichenified, or scaly lesions or where a more occlusive effect is wanted. Lotions may be useful when minimal application to a large or hair-bearing area is needed or for the treatment of exudative lesions.
- Inclusion of urea or salicylic acid ↑ penetration of the corticosteroid.

*Cautions and contraindications* Topical steroids:
- Are of no value in the treatment of urticaria
- Are contraindicated for rosacea and not recommended for acne
- May worsen ulcerated or secondarily infected lesions
- Should not be used indiscriminately for pruritus—they will only be of benefit if inflammation is causing the itch
- Should not be used long term (>7–14d) on the face (and keep away from eyes) or for children.

Use potent or very potent corticosteroids only under specialist supervision.

❶ For perioral inflammatory lesions use hydrocortisone 1% for ≤7d or, if infected (e.g. angular cheilitis), hydrocortisone + miconazole cream.

⚠ Potent topical or systemic steroids used to treat patients with psoriasis can result in rebound relapse, development of generalized pustular psoriasis, and/or local and systemic toxicity.

## Box 17.1 Ingredients that may cause skin sensitization

| | |
|---|---|
| Beeswax | Hydroxybenzoates (parabens) |
| Benzyl alcohol | Imidurea |
| Butylated hydroxyanisole | Isopropyl palmitate |
| Butylated hydroxytoluene | N-(3-chloroallyl)hexaminium chloride |
| Cetostearyl alcohol (including acetyl and stearyl alcohol) | (quaternium 15) |
| Chlorocresol | Polysorbates |
| Edetic acid (EDTA) | Propylene glycol |
| Ethylenediamine | Sodium metabisulphite |
| Fragrances | Sorbic acid |
| | Wool fat/related substances including lanolin |

**Table 17.2** Topical corticosteroid preparation potencies

| Potency | Examples |
|---|---|
| Mild | Hydrocortisone 0.1–2.5%, Dioderm®, Efcortelan®, Mildison® |
| | –with antimicrobials Canesten® HC, Fucidin® H, Timodine® |
| | –with crotamiton Eurax-Hydrocortisone® |
| Moderate | Betnovate®-RD, Eumovate®, Synalar® 1 in 4 dilution |
| | –with antimicrobials Trimovate® |
| | –with urea Alphaderm®, Calmurid® HC |
| Potent | Betamethasone valerate 0.1%, Betacap®, Betnovate®, Diprosone®, Elocon®, Locoid®, Propaderm®, Synalar® |
| | –with antimicrobials Aureocort®, Betnovate®-C or -N, Fucibet® |
| | –with salicylic acid Diprosalic® |
| Very potent | Dermovate®, Halciderm® Topical, Nerisone Forte® |
| | –with antimicrobials Dermovate®-NN |

**Table 17.3** Quantities of emollients and corticosteroids to prescribe

| Area affected | Emollient* | | Topical steroid** |
|---|---|---|---|
| | Cream/ointment | Lotion | |
| Face/neck | 10–30g | 100mL | 15–30g |
| Both hands | 25–50g | 200mL | 15–30g |
| Scalp | 50–100g | 200mL | 15–30g |
| Both arms | 100–200g | 200mL | 30–60g |
| Both legs | 100–200g | 200mL | 100g |
| Trunk | 400g | 500mL | 100g |
| Groins/genitalia | 15–25g | 100mL | 15–30g |

* Amounts are for an adult for twice daily application for 1wk.
** Amounts are for an adult for once daily application for 2wk.

❶ One fingertip unit (distance from the tip of the adult index finger to the first crease ≈ 500mg) of steroid cream is sufficient to cover an area twice the size of the flat adult palm.

# Atopic eczema

Affects 15–20% of schoolchildren and 2–10% of adults—usually starts <6mo of age, and by 1y 60% of those likely to develop eczema will have done so. Associated with other atopic conditions, e.g. asthma, hay fever. Remission occurs by 15y of age in 75%, although some relapse later.

**Differential diagnosis** Scabies; ringworm; rare syndromes (e.g. Wiskott–Aldrich syndrome); dermatitis herpetiformis.

**Presentation** Waxing and waning itchy condition:

>
> - **Infants** Itchy vesicular exudative eczema on face ± hands often with 2° infection. May cause sleep disturbance due to itch. > ½ are free of eczema by 18 mo.
> - **Children >18mo** Involves antecubital and popliteal fossae, neck, wrists, and ankles. Lichenification, excoriation, and dry skin are common. Face may be erythematous and have typical infra-orbital folds. Loss of self-esteem, behaviour and sleep problems are common.

- **Adults** The most common manifestation is irritant hand dermatitis in someone with a past history of atopic eczema (📖 p.614). A small number continue to have generalized atopic eczema. May interfere with employment and social activities. Exacerbated by stress.

**Diagnosis** Itchy skin *plus* ≥ 3 of:

- Itching in skin creases
- History of asthma or hay fever
- Onset in the first 2y of life
- Generally dry skin
- Visible flexural eczema.

**Assessment** Ask about:
- Family (²/₃) and personal history of atopy and eczema
- Onset and distribution of the disease
- Aggravating factors (e.g. pets, irritants such as soaps/detergents or allergens)
- Sleep disturbance due to itching/rubbing
- Impact on quality of life (school work, career, social life)
- Previous treatments (including dietary restrictions), expectations of treatment, and other medications being taken (e.g. steroids for asthma).

⚠ **Eczema of the nipple** Suspect cancer (Paget's disease of the breast). Refer urgently to breast surgeon if no response to topical treatment[N].

## Complications

- **Skin thickening and scaling**
- **Bacterial infection** 2° infection (usually with *Staph. aureus*) commonly causes exacerbations and may not be seen as obvious infection. Bacterial infection is suggested by presence of crusting or weeping, or sudden deterioration of eczema.
- **Viral infection** ↑ susceptibility to infection, e.g. with viral warts and molluscum contagiosum. *Eczema herpeticum*—propensity to develop widespread lesions with HSV and VZ—may require admission and IV aciclovir.
- **Cataracts** Rarely occur in young adults with very severe eczema.
- **Growth retardation** Children with severe eczema, cause unknown. A growth chart should be kept for children with chronic severe eczema.

## Management
- Explain the condition; educate and provide verbal and written information on stepped approach to care and management of flares.[N]
- Advice: loose cotton clothing; avoid wool (exacerbates eczema); avoid excessive heat; keep nails short; gloves in bed.
- If a specific irritant is identified (e.g. house dust mite, pets), avoid.

### Specific treatment
- **Emollients** e.g. aqueous cream, bath emollients—use regularly on skin and as soap substitutes—even if skin is clear. May need to try several to find one that suits. Ideally should be applied 3–4×/d to moist skin. Ensure enough is supplied. Addition of an antipruritic substance (e.g. lauromacrogol) to the emollient may help break the scratch–itch cycle. Addition of an antiseptic to bath emollient may d bacterial infection.
- **Topical steroids** Prescribe the least potent strength that is effective. Use od or bd. Ointments are preferable on dry scaly eczema; creams on wet exudative eczema. Emollients ↓ steroid requirement.
- **Antibiotics** For infected eczema—topical (alone or in combination with a steroid) or oral (e.g. flucloxacillin or erythromycin 250mg qds for 2 wk) Take a swab if antibiotic treatment is ineffective.
- **Oral steroids** Rescue therapy while waiting for an urgent consultant opinion. Only use short courses, e.g. prednisolone 20–30mg od for 5d.
- **Topical immunosuppressants**, e.g. tacrolimus—on consultant advice.
- **Antihistamines** Sedative antihistamines given nocte ↓ desire to itch, e.g. promethazine, hydroxyzine.
- **Bandages:** Excoriated or lichenified eczema—ichthammol (Icthaband®) or zinc and calamine (Calaband®). Bandages can be applied at night on top of steroid ointment. Refer to dermatology.
- **Wet wrapping** Can be used for exudative eczema—Tubigrip bandage or tubular gauze soaked in emollient is applied and covered with a dry bandage. Refer to dermatology.
- **Dietary manipulation** Few (<10%) benefit. Egg and milk are the most common allergens. Advise dietician supervision to avoid malnutrition.

**Referral** (E=Emergency admission; U=Urgent; S=Soon; R=Routine)
- Infection with disseminated HSV (eczema herpeticum)—E
- Severe eczema resistant to treatment. Additional secondary care treatments include phototherapy and immunosuppressive agents—U
- Infection which cannot be cleared in primary care—U
- Severe social/psychological problems due to eczema—S
- Treatment requires excessive amounts of topical steroids—S
- Failure to control symptoms in primary care—R
- Patient/family might benefit from additional advice on application of treatments (e.g. bandaging techniques)—R
- Patch testing required if contact dermatitis suspected—R
- Dietary factors are suspected (refer direct to dietician)—R

### Further information
**NICE** Atopic eczema in children (2007) ▢ www.nice.org.uk

### Patient information and support
**National Eczema Society** ☎ 0800 089 1122 ▢ www.eczema.org

# Other eczemas

**Contact dermatitis<sup>G</sup>** Precipitated by an exogenous agent which is:
- *Irritant* (e.g. water, abrasives, chemicals, detergent) *or*
- *Allergen* (e.g. nickel—10% ♀, 1% ♂; chrome; rubber).

Clinical presentation is often indistinguishable. More common in patients with a past history of atopic eczema. In some patients contact dermatitis may be an industrial disease (☐ p.118). *Differential diagnosis:* endogenous eczema, psoriasis, fungal infection.

**Presentation** Affects any part of the body—site and knowledge of occupation, hobbies, sports, etc. help elucidate cause.
- *Acute* Itchy erythema and skin oedema ± papules, vesicles, or blisters.
- *Chronic* Lichenification, scaling, and fissuring.

**Management**
- *Identification of the allergen or irritant* Consider referral for patch testing (☐ p.682).
- *Exclusion of the offending allergen or irritant from the environment* May be impossible. There is some evidence that nickel avoidance diets can help patients with nickel sensitivity.<sup>G</sup> Nickel testing kits are available from dermatology departments.
- *Hand care* See Table 17.4.
- *Emollients* help skin to recover—apply frequently.
- *Topical steroids* help but are secondary to avoidance measures.

**Pompholyx**
- Sago-like intensely itchy vesicles on the sides of fingers ± palms/soles.
- No associated atopic eczema or contact dermatitis.
- Young adults. More common in warm weather. Frequently recurrent.
- Treatment: emollients, topical steroids (some need potent steroids).
- Treat any infection with oral antibiotics.
- In severe cases refer to dermatology for wet dressings.

**Varicose eczema** ☐ p.616

**Discoid (nummular) eczema**
- Middle-aged/elderly patients. ♂>♀. Unknown cause.
- *Presentation*: intensely itchy, coin-shaped lesions on limbs. Tend to be symmetrical. May be vesicular or chronic and lichenified
- *Differential diagnosis*: tinea corporis; contact dermatitis.
- *Management*: often clears spontaneously after a few weeks but tends to recur. If treatment is needed, use a moderate or potent topical steroid. 2° infection is common—treat with topical/systemic antibiotics.

**Asteatotic eczema (eczema craquelé)**
- *Risk factors*: ↑ age; over-washing; dry climate; hypothyroidism; diuretics.
- *Presentation*: dry itchy eczema with fine crazy-paving pattern of fissuring and cracking of the skin of the limbs.
- *Management*: treat with emollients—occasionally a mild topical steroid is required.

**Seborrhoeic dermatitis** Chronic scaly eruption affecting scalp, face, and/or chest. *Differential diagnosis:* psoriasis, rosacea, contact dermatitis, fungal infection. Five patterns:

- *Scalp and facial involvement* Most common in young men. Excessive dandruff, itchy scaly erythematous eruption affecting sides of the nose, eyes, ears, hairline. May be associated blepharitis.
- *Petaloid* Dry scaly eczema over the pre-sternal area.
- *Pityrosporum folliculitis* Erythematous follicular eruption with papules/pustules over the back.
- *Flexural* Most common in the elderly. Axillae, groins, and submammary areas. Moist intertrigo. Associated with 2° candida infection.
- *Infantile* 🕮 p.891.

*Treatment*

- *Facial, truncal, and flexural involvement* Imidazole + hydrocortisone. *Pityrosporum* folliculitis may respond to itraconazole 200mg od for 7d or fluconazole 50mg od for 2 wk.
- *Scalp lesions* Ketoconazole or coal tar shampoo. In resistant cases apply 2% sulphur + 2% salicylic acid cream several hours before shampooing.
- Recurrence requiring repeated treatment is common.

**Dandruff** is exaggerated physiological exfoliation of fine scales from an otherwise normal scalp. More severe forms merge with seborrhoeic dermatitis and treatment is the same.

**Lichen simplex chronicus** Area of lichenified eczema due to repeated rubbing or scratching. May be due to habit or stress. *Treatment:* topical steroids, weak tar paste, and tar-impregnated bandages.

**Table 17.4** Hand care

| | |
|---|---|
| Hand washing | Use warm water and substitute soap with emollient, e.g. aqueous cream; dry with a clean cotton towel—avoid paper towels or drying machines |
| Avoidance | Avoid handling hair preparations (including shampoos), other detergents, household or industrial cleaning fluids, raw vegetables (e.g. peeling potatoes, tomato juice), fruits (e.g. peeling oranges), or raw meat |
| Protection | If performing any task where hands would get wet, or any of the substances listed above are being handled, wear cotton gloves under PVC gloves. Wear gloves for dusty work or in the cold |
| Medication | Use emollients frequently throughout the day (e.g. aqueous cream). If necessary apply a thin layer of steroid ointment od/bd |

**Further information**
**British Association of Dermatologists** Guidelines for the management of contact dermatitis (2009) 🖳 www.bad.org.uk
**Electronic dermatology atlas** 🖳 www.dermis.net

**Patient information and support**
**National Eczema Society** ☎ 0800 089 1122 🖳 www.eczema.org

# Varicose eczema and leg ulcers

## Venous (stasis, varicose) eczema
- Middle-aged/elderly patients. ♀>♂.
- Associated with underlying venous disease.
- *Early signs* Capillary veins and haemosiderin deposition around the ankles and over prominent varicose veins.
- *Later signs* Eczema ± lipodermatosclerosis (fibrosis of the dermis and subcutaneous tissue) ± ulceration.
- *Management* Treat with emollients ± mild or moderate steroid ointment and compression hosiery. Treat venous disease (📖 p.296) or ulceration on its own merits.

**Leg ulcer** Painful and debilitating condition affecting 1% of the adult population and 3.6% of those >65y.

*Cause* >90% are due to arterial disease, venous disease, or neuropathy. *Other causes:* trauma, obesity, immobility, vasculitis (rheumatoid arthritis, SLE, PAN), malignancy, osteomyelitis, blood dyscrasias, lymphoedema, self-inflicted.

## Common sites
- *Arterial* Shin, toes, over pressure points (under heel, over malleoli).
- *Venous* Above medial or lateral malleoli of the ankle.
- *Neuropathic* Sole of foot, over pressure points.

## History Ask about:
- Duration of ulceration.
- Pain—painful unless neuropathic when often painless.
- Mobility.
- Past history of ulceration, DVT, or varicose vein surgery.
- History of trauma to the limb.
- Systemic disease—DM, peripheral vascular disease, RA, etc.

## Examination
- *Ulcer* Position; evidence of infection; surrounding callus—typical of neuropathic ulcers; evidence of tracking to involve the bones of the foot.
- *Leg* Pulses; varicose veins, and/or signs of venous hypertension—haemosiderin pigmentation, varicose eczema, atrophie blanche (white lacy scars), lipodermatosclerosis; sensation—↓ when peripheral neuropathy, range of joint movement.

## Investigation
- Bloods—FBC, ESR, VDRL, blood glucose.
- Ankle–brachial pressure index (📖 p.239).
- Swab for M,C&S if any signs of cellulitis/infection.
- Diabetic ulcers—if signs of infection, X-ray foot to exclude osteomyelitis.

## Management
- *Arterial ulcers* Refer to vascular surgery.
- *Diabetic foot ulcers* Refer to a specialist diabetic foot team.

- *Venous ulcers* If ABPI >0.8, can be managed in the community with graduated compression bandaging (elastic bandages applied in multiple layers over a non-adherent dressing). Change dressings 1–2×/wk. Keep skin under the bandage moist with simple emollients and treat surrounding eczema with topical steroids. Give analgesia. Encourage walking, weight ↓ if obese, and elevation of the leg when resting. 65–70% heal in < 6mo.

## Referral
- *Non-healing ulcers or ulcers of uncertain cause*—dermatology.
- *ABPI <0.8*—vascular surgery.
- *Varicose veins*—vascular surgery; 60% may benefit from vein surgery.

**Prevention of recurrence** 5y recurrence rate is 40%—graduated compression hosiery ↓ recurrence. Below-knee class 2 stockings are adequate for most and can be prescribed with NHS prescription, but are difficult to apply especially with arthritic hands. Applicators are available and can be obtained on NHS prescription, via the OT or bought from specialist disability shops.

## Complications
- Infection—treat with systemic antibiotics only if rapidly advancing ulcer edge, cellulitis, or systemic symptoms.
- Lymphoedema.
- Contact dermatitis—topical medicaments and dressings. Consider referral for patch testing if suspected.
- Malignant change—squamous cell cancer (rare). Refer for biopsy to confirm diagnosis.

**Pyoderma gangrenosum** Starts as a pustule/inflamed nodule which breaks down to form an ulcer, which may expand rapidly. The ulcer has a purplish margin and surrounding erythema. Usually on trunk/lower limbs. Refer to dermatology.

*Causes* UC (50% of patients with pyoderma gangrenosum have UC); Crohn's disease; RA; Behçet's syndrome; multiple myeloma and monoclonal gammopathy; leukaemia.

---

**Bed sores or pressure ulcers**
- Due to pressure necrosis of the skin. Immobile patients are at high risk, especially if frail ± incontinent.
- If at risk refer to the DN for advice on prevention of bed sores— protective mattresses and cushions, incontinence advice, advice on positioning and movement.
- Warn carers to make contact with the DN if a red patch does not improve 24h after relieving the pressure on the area. Treat aggressively and admit if not resolving.

---

## Further information
**The Circulation Foundation** 🖥 www.circulationfoundation.org.uk
**Tissue Viability Society** 🖥 www.tvs.org.uk
**NICE** Pressure ulcer management (2005) 🖥 www.nice.org.uk

# Urticaria and angio-oedema

**Urticaria** (hives or nettle rash). Common condition affecting 1 in 6 at some time. Consists of superficial itchy swellings of the skin or *weals* (Plate 3). Weals come and go during an attack, giving the appearance of a shifting rash.

**Angio-oedema** Deeper longer-lasting swellings that are painful rather than itchy. Commonly affect eyes, lips, genitalia, hands, and/or feet. May affect bowel (abdominal pain, nausea, vomiting, diarrhoea) or airway (tongue swelling, shortness of breath, wheeze). If airway compromise, consider anaphylaxis.

**Anaphylaxis** 📖 p.1068.

**Classification** 1 in 10 patients have angio-oedema alone; 4 in 10 have urticaria and angio-oedema; half present with urticaria alone.

*Ordinary or idiopathic* Spontaneous weals ± angio-oedema. Cause unknown. *Triggers include:* stress, overheating, drugs, alcohol, viral infections (particularly children). Individual weals last 2–24h. May be:
- *Acute* <6 wk of continuous activity.
- *Chronic* ≥6 wk of continuous activity—affects 1–5/1000. May remit/relapse. Relapses are triggered by illness, stress, drugs, alcohol, or hormonal changes (e.g. menstruation). 50% resolve in 3–5y; 1:5 persist >10y. Severe impact on quality of life—14% develop depression.
- *Episodic* (acute intermittent or recurrent activity). Symptoms last hours/days but recur over months/years. Treated like chronic urticaria

*Physical* Induced by a specific physical stimulus. Except for delayed pressure urticaria, weals last <1h. Avoiding the stimulus prevents attacks.
- *Mechanical* Delayed pressure urticaria (weals develop in 2–6h and fade over 48h); symptomatic dermographism; vibratory angio-oedema.
- *Thermal* Cholinergic urticaria (induced by sweating); cold contact urticaria; localized heat urticaria.
- *Other* Aquagenic urticaria (contact with water); solar urticaria; exercise-induced anaphylaxis.

*Contact* Caused by allergens (e.g. nuts, shellfish, milk, eggs, penicillin, insect stings, latex) or chemicals (e.g. drugs—opioids, aspirin, NSAIDs; radio-contrast media; food additives—azo-dyes, preservatives). Weals last <2h. Refer for allergy testing if specific allergen is suspected.

*Urticarial vasculitis* Suspect if relentless rather than self-limiting urticaria, individual weals last >24h, lesions are burning/painful rather than itchy, and/or lesions leave scaling, bruising, purpura, or petechial haemorrhages. *Other associated features:* joint pains, fever and/or malaise. Refer. Diagnosis is confirmed by skin biopsy. Specialist treatment is with steroids and/or other immunosuppressive agents.

*Angio-oedema alone* Swellings last <3d. *Causes:* idiopathic; drug-induced (ACE inhibitors, ARBs, NSAIDs); $C_1$ esterase inhibitor deficiency.

*Autoimmune* Urticaria, pyrexia, and malaise + disease-specific features. Hereditary or acquired (e.g. SLE). Treat the cause.

**Associations** Autoimmune thyroid disease is ↑2× in patients with chronic ordinary urticaria. Children/adolescents with chronic urticaria have ↑ prevalence of coeliac disease.

**Management of acute urticaria** Treatment is not needed if the episode is mild. If symptomatic treatment is needed:

• Try antihistamines—non-sedating for daytime symptoms (e.g. cetirizine, fexofenadine) ± sedative if interferes with sleep (e.g. chlorphenamine, hydroxyzine). If one antihistamine is ineffective, try another.
• Topical menthol 1% cream is an alternative/adjunct to antihistamines.
• If severe symptoms, consider short-course steroids (e.g. prednisolone 40mg od for 3–5d.). If rebound symptoms occur after stopping, seek specialist advice. Do not give repeat courses of steroids except with specialist advice.

**Management of chronic urticaria** Check FBC, ESR, and TFTs. Assess severity and impact on day-to-day life. Identify potential causes. Advise to avoid non-specific aggravating factors, e.g. overheating, stress, alcohol, and aspirin/codeine (and NSAIDs if aspirin-sensitive). Prescribe antihistamines as for acute urticaria. If these measures do not control symptoms, refer.

*Other treatments* Usually specialist initiated—include $H_2$ receptor antagonists (e.g. cimetidine, ranitidine); antileukotrienes (e.g. montelukast). Unlicensed indications—response is highly variable.

### Management of angio-oedema

• If anaphylaxis is suspected, give adrenaline and admit (🕮 p 1068).
• If any airway compromise, admit—even if anaphylaxis is not suspected.
• If a decision is made not to admit, treat as for acute urticaria and monitor carefully for airway compromise.
• Refer to an allergy clinic/immunology, unless taking ACE inhibitors. If taking an ACE inhibitor, stop and only refer if symptoms continue or recur >3mo after stopping.

**$C_1$ esterase inhibitor deficiency (hereditary angio-oedema)** Due to deficiency of $C_1$ esterase inhibitor. Autosomal dominant—usually presents in puberty with episodes of angio-oedema without weals. ↓ $C_4$ level suggests the diagnosis. Emergency treatment is with hospital admission for fresh frozen plasma or $C_1$ inhibitor concentrate infusion. Maintenance therapy (usually with anabolic steroids or tranexamic acid—consultant supervision only) is necessary only for patients with symptomatic recurring angio-oedema or related abdominal pain.

---

 **Urticaria pigmentosa (cutaneous mastocytosis)** Appears in infancy (usually <2wk old). Dark freckle-like lesions on the face, limbs, or trunk become urticarial when the skin is rubbed. No treatment is needed—clears spontaneously in childhood.

---

### Further information

**British Association of Dermatologists** Guidelines for evaluation and management of urticaria in adults and children (2007) 🖥 www.bad.org.uk
**BSACI** Guidelines for the management of chronic urticaria and angio-oedema (2007) *Clinical and Experimental Allergy* **37**, 631–50.

## Acne

Chronic inflammatory condition characterized by comedones, papules, pustules, cysts, and scars. Acne vulgaris is common and affects >80% of teenagers. *Peak age:* 18y; ♂ = ♀.

**Cause** Complex—androgen secretion results in ↑ sebum excretion; pilosebaceous duct blockage (producing comedones); colonization of the duct with *Proprionobacterium acnes* bacteria and release of inflammatory mediators. Inflammatory acne is the result of the host response to the follicular *Propionibacterium acnes*.

### Rarer causes

- Endocrine—PCOS, Cushing's, virilizing tumours
- Squeezing—*acne excoriée*
- Aromatic industrial chemicals—*chloracne*
- Cosmetics
- Drugs—systemic steroids, androgens, topical steroids
- Infantile—faces of male infants; cause unknown
- Physical occlusion, e.g. under a violinist's chin.

**Presentation** Spots on face, neck ± back and chest. Examination reveals blackheads (dilated pores with black plug of keratin = comedones) and whiteheads (small cream-coloured dome-shaped papules); red papules; pustules ± cysts. There may be scarring from old lesions. Burrowing abscesses and sinuses with scarring (*conglobate acne*) are seen in severe cases. Scars may become keloidal.

**Differential diagnosis** Rosacea (📖 p.601), bacterial folliculitis—often coexists (📖 p.631).

**Classification** Severity of acne is often overestimated by the patient and minimized by the doctor. Four main types:

- Purely comedonal (non-inflammatory)
- Mild papular
- Scarring papular
- Nodular or scarring acne.

**Management** *Aims to:* ↓ number of lesions, prevent scarring, ↓ the psychological impact of the condition.

- *Misconceptions* Explain:
  - Acne is not a disease of poor hygiene. The black tip of a comedone is oxidized sebum, not dirt.
  - Diet is not associated with acne.
- *General measures* Wash with soap and water twice daily. Apply a moisturizer (e.g. aqueous cream) after washing.
- *Medication* See Table 17.5. Warn patients that any treatment takes weeks → months to work fully and is usually continued for months/ years; reassess progress every 2–3 mo and continue treatment until new lesions stop developing.

**Complications** Acne is not a trivial disease—it can cause scars (both skin and emotional) that last a lifetime. Anxiety, social isolation, and lack of self-confidence are common.

**Table 17.5** Treatment of acne (BNF 13.6)

|  | Description | Management |
|---|---|---|
| Mild acne | Open and closed comedones and some papules | Topical treatment applied to the whole area (not just the spots):<br>*Benzoyl peroxide* applied bd—start at lowest strength and build up as needed.<br>*Topical retinoids* (e.g. isotretinoin)—apply low-strength preparation every 2–3 nights initially and build up strength and frequency as tolerated—warn patients they should avoid the sun. Retinoids cause erythema and scaling in most patients which settle with time and acne may worsen for the first few weeks of treatment.<br>*Topical antibiotics*—resistance is increasing; use only in combination with benzoyl peroxide or if benzoyl peroxide has failed. Avoid if using oral antibiotics. |
| Moderate acne | More frequent papules and pustules with mild scarring | Try topical treatment first.<br>If not working after 4–8wk try either:<br>*Long-term oral antibiotics* (e.g. tetracycline 500mg bd) for a minimum of 8wk or,<br>For girls, *an anti-androgen* for >6mo (e.g. cyproterone acetate in co-cyprindiol—also contraceptive).<br>❶ Topical preparations may be used simultaneously with systemic therapy |
| Severe acne | Nodular abscesses → more widespread scarring | As for moderate acne.<br>If ineffective, or relapses rapidly after antibiotics are stopped, refer to dermatology for consideration of oral retinoid treatment.<br>Oral retinoids are teratogenic. |

⚠ Oral and topical retinoids are teratogenic do not prescribe to a woman of childbearing age unless using adequate contraception. Oral tetracyclines may also cause birth defects.

**Referral to dermatology** (*U*=Urgent; *S*=Soon; *R*=Routine)
• Acne fulminans: seen in adolescent males, severe acne is associated with fever, arthritis and vasculitis—*U*
• Severe acne or painful deep nodules or cysts which could benefit from oral isotretinoin—*S*
• Severe social/psychological sequelae—*S*
• At risk of/developing scarring despite primary care remedies—*R*
• Poor treatment response—*R*
• Suspected underlying cause for acne (e.g. PCOS—📖 p.723)—*R*

**Perioral dermatitis** Papules and pustules which appear around the mouth and chin of a woman who has used topical steroids. Treat with oral tetracycline as for acne.

**Further information**
**BMJ** Webster G.F. *Acne vulgaris* (2002) **325**: 475–9.

# Psoriasis

Chronic non-infectious inflammatory skin condition characterized by well-demarcated erythematous plaques topped by silvery scales. Epidermal cell proliferation rate is ↑ ×20 and turnover time ↓ from 28 to 4d. Affects ~2% Caucasian population (less in other races). Presents at any age—mean 28y; rare < 8y ♂=♀. Presentation—Table 17.6

**Cause** Genetic (polygenic inheritance; 35% have a family history; there is a 25% probability that a child with one parent with psoriasis will be affected—60% chance with two). Environmental factors trigger disease.

## Precipitating factors

- Trauma (Koebner phenomenon)
- Infection
- Drugs, e.g. β-blockers, NSAIDs, lithium, chloroquine
- Alcohol
- Sunlight—aggravates psoriasis in 10%
- Psychological stress.

**Management** >50% experience a lack of self-confidence. Social or psychological problems are common. Be supportive. Explain the condition and treatment options. Advise on self-help groups.

**Drug treatment** (BNF 13.5). Frequent emollients ±
- **Salicylic acid** ↓ surface scale. Available as Lassar's paste (apply bd) or together with dithranol (Psorin® scalp gel or ointment) or coal tar (e.g. Sebco® scalp ointment).
- **Coal tar** Anti-inflammatory and anti-scaling properties. The thicker the patch the stronger the preparation required.
- **Vitamin D analogue** (e.g. calcipotriol, tacalcitol). Plaque/scalp psoriasis—effective and no unpleasant smell or staining of clothing.
- **Dithranol** Plaque psoriasis—apply to lesion only. Stains.
- **Topical retinoids** (e.g. tazarotene). Mild/moderate plaque psoriasis.
- **Mild topical steroids** Can be used for flexural, facial, or scalp psoriasis.

❶ Plaques can become inflamed and/or aggravated on starting topical treatments, after prolonged use of topical steroids or if steroids are stopped suddenly.

**Referral** (E=Emergency; U=Urgent; S=Soon; R=Routine)
- Generalized pustular or eythrodermic psoriasis—E
- Patient's psoriasis is acutely unstable—U
- Widespread guttate psoriasis (to benefit from early phototherapy)—U
- Severe social or psychological sequelae—S
- Rash is so extensive as to make self-management impractical—S
- Rash is in a sensitive area (e.g. face, hands, feet, genitalia) and the symptoms are troublesome—S
- Time off work/school and interfering with employment/education—S
- For management of associated arthropathy—S
- Rash fails to respond to primary care management—R.

**Additional secondary care treatment options** Phototherapy and PUVA; oral retinoids; cytotoxic and immunosuppressive thearapy; specialist nursing services.

**Table 17.6** Patterns of psoriasis

| Pattern | Features |
|---|---|
| Erythroderma | Inflammatory dermatosis affecting >90% skin surface (📖 p.600). Admit. |
| Generalized pustular | Rare but serious. Unwell with fever and malaise. Sheets of small sterile yellowish pustules develop on an erythematous background and spread rapidly. Admit. |
| Plaque (Plate 4a) | Most common form. Well-defined disc-shaped plaques involving the knees, elbows, scalp, hair margin, or sacrum. Plaques are usually red and covered with waxy white scales which may leave bleeding points if detached. Plaques may be itchy. *Differential diagnosis*: psoriasiform drug eruption; hypertrophic lichen planus. |
| Scalp psoriasis | Very common. May be confused with dandruff, but generally better demarcated and thicker scales. |
| Guttate (Plate 4b) | Acute symmetrical raindrop lesions on trunk/limbs. Most common in adolescents/young adults—may follow streptococcal throat infection. *Differential diagnosis*: pityriasis rosea. |
| Flexural | Affects axillae, submammary areas, and natal cleft. Plaques are smooth and often glazed. Most common in elderly patients. *Differential diagnosis*: flexural candidiasis. |
| Nail | Nail bed is affected in 50%. Fingernails > toenails. Thimble pitting, onycholysis, and oily patches (oily brownish-yellow discoloration of the nail bed, often adjacent to onycholysis). Associated with arthropathy. Treatment is difficult. *Differential diagnosis*: fungal nail infection. |
| Palmoplantar pustulosis | Yellow-brown sterile pustules on palms or soles. |
| Napkin psoriasis | Well-defined eruption in nappy area of infants. |

**Arthropathy** ~40% psoriasis patients. ♂ = ♀.
- **Distal arthritis** DIP joint swelling of hands/feet ± flexion deformity.
- **Rheumatoid-like** Polyarthropathy similar to rheumatoid arthritis (📖 p.522) but less symmetrical; rheumatoid factor is –ve.
- **Mutilans** Associated with severe psoriasis. Erosions in small bones of hands/feet ± spine. Bones dissolve → progressive deformity.
- **Ankylosing spondylitis/sacroiliitis** Usually HLA B27 +ve (📖 p.526).

**Management** Education; physiotherapy; NSAIDs. Refer to rheumatology for confirmation of diagnosis, advice on management, and disease-modifying drugs.

#### Further information
**British Association of Dermatologists** Recommendations for the initial management of psoriasis (2006) 🖥 www.bad.org.uk

#### Patient information and support
**Psoriasis Association** ☎ 0845 676 0076 🖥 www.psoriasis-association.org.uk
**Psoriatic Arthropathy Alliance** 🖥 www.paalliance.org

# Lichen planus, pityriasis, and keratinization disorders

**Lichen planus** Very itchy, polygonal, flat-topped papular lesions 2–5mm diameter, of unknown cause, affecting flexor surfaces, palms/soles, mucous membranes (two-thirds of cases—usually buccal), and genitalia in a symmetrical pattern. *Koebner phenomenon* (lesions occur in the line of damaged skin due to a scratch) is exhibited (Plate 5b). Papules may have a surface network of white lines (Wickham's striae). Initially papules are red but become violaceous. Papules flatten over a few months to leave pigmentation or occasionally become hypertrophic. Two-thirds of cases occur in the 30–60y age group. ♂ = ♀.

*Differential diagnosis* Lichenoid drug eruption; psoriasis.

*Variants*
- *Annular* (10%): commonly on glans penis.
- *Atrophic*: rare, associated with hypertrophic lesions.
- *Bullous*: blistering is rare.
- *Follicular*: may occur with typical lichen planus or just affect the scalp.
- *Hypertrophic*: plaques may persist for years.
- *Mucous membrane* (Plate 5a): alone or with skin changes.

*Complications* Nail involvement (10%)—longitudinal pitting and grooving; scalp—scarring; alopecia. Malignant change—◉ it is controversial whether oral lichen planus can undergo malignant transformation. If it can, risk is low (<2% over 10y). NICE recommends that patients with confirmed oral lichen planus are monitored for oral cancer as part of routine dental examination[N].

*Management* Self-limiting in most patients. Moderate → high potency topical steroids provide symptomatic relief. Oral lesions can be treated with triamcinolone in dental paste, or hydrocortisone pellets. Rarely, oral lesions are a reaction to mercury amalgam fillings—removing the fillings and replacing them with other materials may solve the problem. Refer to dermatology if:

- Diagnosis is in doubt
- Extensive involvement
- Potentially scarring nail dystrophy
- Resistant to topical treatment.

Specialist treatment involves oral steroids ± PUVA.

*Prognosis* Half are clear in <9mo; 15% have continuing symptoms >18mo; 20% have a further attack.

**Lichen planus-like drug eruptions** Recorded after treatment with:
- Thiazide diuretics
- Tolbutamide
- Penicillamine
- Isoniazid
- Phenothiazines
- Streptomycin
- Tetracycline
- Gold
- Quinine
- Chloroquine.

Resolution after withdrawal of drug is often slow.

**Lichen sclerosus** 📖 p.729

**Pityriasis rosea** Acute self-limiting disorder most commonly affecting teenagers and young adults. *Cause:* unknown. Generalized eruption is preceded by the herald patch—a single large oval lesion 2–5cm in diameter. Several days later the rash appears, consisting of many smaller lesions mainly on the trunk but also on upper arms and thighs. Lesions are oval, pink, and have a delicate 'collarette' of scale. May be asymptomatic or cause mild/moderate itch. Treatment does not speed clearance. Topical steroid may relieve itch. Fades spontaneously in 4–8wk.

**Pityriasis (tinea) versicolor** Chronic, often asymptomatic, fungal infection of the skin (*Pityrosporum orbiculare*). Common in humid/tropical conditions. In the UK often affects young adults and teenagers. On untanned white skin appears as pinkish-brown oval or round patches with a fine superficial scale. In tanned or darker skin patchy hypo-pigmentation occurs. Involves trunk ± proximal limbs.

*Management* Topical imidazole antifungal (e.g. clotrimazole cream) or topical selenium sulphide shampoo to all affected areas at night, washed off the following morning (repeated ×2 at weekly intervals). For resistant cases, try a systemic antifungal, e.g. fluconazole 50mg od for 1wk. Recurrences are common. Hypopigmentation may take some time to clear.

**Pityriasis alba** Finely scaled white patches on face or arms. Affects children/young adults. Associated with atopy. Usually no treatment is required. Resolves spontaneously over months or years. If severe refer to dermatology for confirmation of diagnosis. Treatment for severe cases is with topical steroids and/or PUVA.

**Callosities** Painless localized thickenings of the keratin layer—protective response to friction/pressure. *Management:* keratolytics, e.g. 5–10% salicylic acid ointment or 10% urea cream; attention to footwear.

**Corns** Painful. Develop at areas of high local pressure on the feet, e.g. where shoes press on bony protrusions. *Management:* attention to footwear, keratolytics, cushioning (e.g. corn pads). Occasionally surgery may be indicated if deformity of the foot causes recurrent corns.

**Ichthyosis** Inherited disorders characterized by dry scaly skin. Most common form is *ichthyosis vulgaris*: prevalence 1/300, autosomal dominant. Small branny scales on extensor aspects of limbs and back. Mild and often undiagnosed. *Management:* topical emollients ± bath additives. Severe cases require dermatology advice.

**Keratoderma** Hyperkeratosis of palms and soles. *Tylosis* is diffuse hyperkeratosis of the palms and soles. It is usually inherited (autosomal dominant) but rarely may be associated with oesophageal cancer. Acquired keratoderma occurs in women around the menopause and patients with lichen planus. Treat with keratolytics, e.g. 10% urea cream.

**Keratosis pilaris** Common, sometimes inherited condition. Small horny plugs on the upper thigh, upper arm, and face. Associated with icthyosis vulgaris. Keratolytics (e.g. 10% urea cream) improve symptoms.

## Further information
**Electronic dermatology atlas** ▣ www.dermis.net

## Patient information and support
**Ichthyosis Support Group** ▣ www.ichthyosis.co.uk

# Benign skin tumours

**Naevus** Benign proliferation of ≥1 normal constituent of the skin. The most common type is the melanocytic naevus or 'mole'. Most develop in childhood and adolescence. *Features:*

- *Congenital* Present at birth in 1% Caucasians (less in darker-skinned races). Usually large (>1cm diameter). ~5% risk of malignancy.
- *Junctional* Flat, round/oval, brown/black, 2–10mm diameter. Common sites: soles, palms, genitalia.
- *Intradermal* Dome-shaped papule/nodule commonly on the face or neck. May be pigmented.
- *Compound* <10mm diameter, smooth surface, variable pigmentation.
- *Blue* Blue-coloured solitary naevus usually found on extremities—especially hands and feet.
- *Halo* Found in children or adolescents. White halo of depigmentation surrounds the naevus which then disappears. Associated with vitiligo.

**Differential diagnosis** Freckle, lentigo, seborrhoeic wart, haemangioma (may be pigmented), dermatofibroma, pigmented BCC, malignant melanoma.

**Management** Patients usually present if worried about a mole. Any change merits serious attention. *Reasons for excision biopsy:*

- Concern about malignancy (📖 p.628)
- ↑ risk of malignant change (e.g. congenital naevi)
- Cosmetic reasons
- Repeated inflammation
- Recurrent trauma.

Most areas now have specialist 'mole clinics' for assessment and excision of suspicious lesions. Otherwise refer for urgent dermatology assessment if malignancy is suspected.

**Seborrhoeic wart (senile wart, basal cell papilloma)** Common >60y. Often multiple—most commonly on trunk. Warty nodules, usually pigmented, 1–6cm in diameter, with a 'stuck-on' appearance. Pieces of the wart can be picked off. *Cause:* unknown.

**Management** Reassurance. If removal is required, cryotherapy, curettage, shave biopsy, and excision biopsy are all effective.

**Skin tags** Common. Small pedunculated polyps found in axillae, groin, neck, or on the eyelids.

**Management** Reassurance. Cosmetic removal can be achieved by snipping across the skin tag with scissors, cryotherapy, or diathermy.

**Sebaceous cyst (epidermal cyst)** Common. Round or oval, keratin-filled firm cysts, 1–3cm in diameter, within the skin. Usually a punctum is seen on the surface.

**Management** Reassurance. Treat any complicating bacterial infection with oral antibiotics (e.g. flucloxacillin 250mg qds). Excision is curative.

**Milia** Small white raised spots (1–2mm in diameter) usually on the face (upper cheeks and eyelids). Most common in children but can occur at any age. No treatment is required.

**Dermatofibroma** Common ($\female$ > $\male$; young adult > elderly) and usually asymptomatic. Firm (sometimes pigmented) nodule 5–10mm in diameter which may occur following an insect bite or minor trauma. *Most common site:* lower legs.

*Management* Excision biopsy of symptomatic or diagnostically doubtful lesions.

**Lipoma** Common. Benign tumours of fat. Present as soft masses in the subcutaneous tissue. Often multiple; most common on trunk, neck, and upper extremities. Removal by excision is rarely necessary.

**Keloid scars** Proliferation of connective tissue presenting as firm smooth nodules/plaques in response to trauma. A scar is termed hypertrophic if changes are limited to the scar, but keloid if it extends beyond the limit of the original injury. *Most common sites:* upper back, chest, ear lobes. More common in negroid races (2nd–4th decades).

*Management* Refer to dermatologist or plastic surgeon—treated by injection of steroid into the scar, cryotherapy, or topical silicone gel sheeting.

**Pyogenic granuloma** Bright red/blood-crusted nodule which bleeds easily Typically develops at the site of trauma (e.g. small cut) and enlarges rapidly over 2–3wk. *Most common site:* finger. Usually occurs in children/ young adults *Differential diagnosis:* malignant melanoma.

*Management* Excision biopsy to exclude malignancy.

**Keratoacanthoma** Rapidly growing nodular tumour (<2cm in diameter) of sun-exposed skin of face/arms. A central keratin plug may fall out to leave a crater. Heals spontaneously over several months leaving a scar. Differential diagnosis: SCC.

*Management* Excision biopsy or curettage and cautery.

**Chondrodermatitis nodularis** Small, painful nodule in the upper rim of the pinna. Most common in elderly men. Due to inflammation of the cartilage. Refer for excision.

**Campbell de Morgan spot (cherry angioma)** Small bright red papules on the trunk in middle-aged/elderly patients. Usually requires no treatment. *Campbell de Morgan (1811–1876) English surgeon.*

**Further information**
Electronic dermatology atlas ▢ www.dermis.net

**Patient information**
**British Association of Dermatologists** Patient information leaflets on: seborrhoeic warts, keratoacanthoma, dermatofibroma, pyogenic granuloma ▢ www.bad.org.uk

# Skin cancer

⚠ **Sun safety code** 80% of skin cancer is preventable.
- Take care not to burn.
- Cover up with loose cool clothing, a hat, and sun glasses.
- Seek shade during the hottest part of the day.
- Apply high-factor sunscreen (≥ SPF 15) to sun-exposed body parts.
- Take special care to protect children in the sun.

**Cutaneous malignant melanoma** In the UK: 9000 new cases/y; 1800 deaths/y. Incidence is rising. ♀:♂ ≈ 2:1. Particularly common in Caucasians. Frequently metastasizes. May present with metastasis. *Types:*
- *Superficial spreading* 70% UK cases. ♀ > ♂. Most common site: lower leg in ♀ (50%); back in ♂. Macular lesion with variable pigmentation.
- *Nodular* 20% UK cases. ♂ > ♀. Most common on trunk. Pigmented nodule grows rapidly and may ulcerate.
- *Lentigo* A lentigo maligna arises in sun-damaged skin (usually on the face) and melanoma develops many years afterwards within it. Most common >60y, especially if outdoor occupation.
- *Acral lentiginous* 35–60% melanoma in black-skinned populations. Affects palms, soles, nail beds. Often detected late. Poor prognosis.

*Causes* 30% of malignant melanomas arise out of pre-existing moles, but risk of change in a benign mole (except dysplastic or congenital naevus) is small. *Risk factors:* sun exposure; genetic (10% have family history); multiple benign moles (>50 of >2mm diameter); congenital naevus; previous malignant melanoma; immunosuppression; fair skin type (red hair, blue eyes, and burns easily).

*Management* Encourage patients to report changes in moles early. Use the 7-point checklist (Box 17.2) to identify changes needing referral.

*Refer* suspicious lesions for urgent dermatology assessment ± wide excision. Best chance of cure comes with complete excision. Chemotherapy/radiotherapy are of little benefit but laser therapy and immunotherapy with interferon/interleukin 2 are now commonly used.

*Prognosis* Relates to tumour depth at presentation. 5y survival: <1mm deep, 95–100%; >4mm deep, 50%.

**Squamous cell carcinoma (SCC)** 20% of skin cancer in the UK. Most common >55y ♂>♀. May metastasize (10%). Usually develops in light-exposed sites, e.g. face, neck, hands. May start within an actinic (solar) keratosis (🕮 p.608), or *de novo* as a nodule which progresses to ulcerate and form a crust.

*Causes* Chronic sun damage, X-ray exposure, chronic ulceration and scarring (aggressive SCC may develop at the edge of chronic ulcers), smoking pipes and cigars (lip lesions), industrial carcinogens (tars, oils), wart virus, immunosuppression, genetic.

*Management* Refer urgently to dermatology. Treated with surgical excision ± LN biopsy. Large lesions may require skin grafting. Radiotherapy is an alternative for large lesions in elderly patients.

---

**Box 17.2 The 7-point check list for moles** Score 2 points for any major feature and 1 point for any minor feature. Lesions scoring ≥3 points are suspicious—refer.

*Major signs*
- Change in size—increase in size
- Irregular colour
- Irregular shape—irregular border, asymmetry, elevation.

*Minor signs*
- ≥7mm diameter
- Inflammation
- Oozing, including crusting/bleeding
- Change in sensation, including symptoms of minor irritation or itch.

❶ One feature is enough to prompt referral if high level of suspicion. For low-suspicion lesions, monitor for change over 8wk.

---

**Basal cell carcinoma (rodent ulcer, BCC)** Most common form of skin cancer—accounts for >75% of skin cancer in the UK. Locally invasive but rarely metastasizes. Tends to occur in middle-aged/elderly patients. May be multiple and appears mainly on light exposed areas—most commonly the face. 3 main types (all can be pigmented):
- **Nodular** Most common—starts as small pearly nodule. May necrose centrally leaving a small crusted ulcer with pearly rolled edge.
- **Cystic.**
- **Multicentric** Plaque-like, large, superficial ± central depression.

**Causes** Sun exposure, X-ray irradiation, chronic scarring, genetic predisposition, arsenic ingestion.

**Management** Complete excision is ideal. Refer routinely—if low risk to GPwSI working in a community skin cancer clinic; if uncertain or any high risk features, to dermatology. High risk features:
- Site—nose/paranasal folds, scalp/temples, lips
- Size —>2cm
- Previously treated lesion
- Immunosuppression
- Genetic disorder associated with BCC, e.g. Gorlin's syndrome

**Prognosis** Recurrence rate is 5% at 5y for all modalities of treatment. Development of new BCC at other sites is common.

**Bowen's disease** Intra-epidermal carcinoma. Common—typically occurs on the lower leg in elderly women. Lesions are pink/slightly pigmented scaly plaques (<5cm diameter) and may be solitary or multiple. Risk factor: exposure to arsenicals. Transformation to SCC is rare. Biopsy confirms diagnosis. Treatment is with cryotherapy, curettage or excision. *J.T. Bowen (1857–1941)—US dermatologist.*

**Kaposi sarcoma** 📖 p.745

**Further information**

**British Association of Dermatologists** 🖥 www.bad.org.uk
- Guidelines for the management of BCC (2008)
- Guidelines for management of Bowen's disease (2006)
- Multiprofessional guidelines for the management of the patient with primary cutaneous squamous cell carcinoma (2009)
- UK guidelines for the management of cutaneous melanoma (2002)

**NICE** Improving outcome for people with skin tumours including melanoma: The Manual (2006) 🖥 www.nice.org.uk

# Bacterial skin infection

> **Impetigo** Superficial skin infection due to *Staph. aureus*. A thin-walled blister ruptures easily to leave a yellow crusted lesion. May occur anywhere—most common on face. *Differential diagnosis:* HSV, fungal infection, e.g. ringworm. Lesions spread rapidly and are contagious. Avoid spreading to other children—no sharing of towels, face flannels, etc.; some schools prohibit attendance until lesions are cleared.
> - *Localized cases* Treat with topical antibiotics (e.g. fusidic acid cream).
> - *Widespread infection* Treat with oral flucloxacillin or erythromycin.
>
> **Scalded skin syndrome** Acute toxic illness usually of infants. Characterized by shedding of sheets of skin. May follow impetigo. Admit as a paediatric emergency. Requires IV antibiotics.

### Boils and carbuncles

- *Boil (furuncle)* Acute infection of a hair follicle, usually with *Staph. aureus*. A hard tender red nodule surrounding a hair follicle becomes larger and fluctuant after several days. Occasionally associated with fever ± malaise. Later may discharge pus and a central 'core' before healing; may leave a scar. *Predisposing factors:* usually absent—DM, HIV, obesity, blood dyscrasias, immunosuppressive drugs.
- *Carbuncle* Swollen painful area discharging pus from several points. Occurs when a group of hair follicles become deeply infected, usually with *Staph. aureus*. May be associated with fever ± malaise. *Predisposing factors:* malnutrition, cardiac failure, drug addiction, severe generalized dermatosis, prolonged steroid therapy, DM.

### Management

- *Lesions that are non-fluctuant* Apply moist heat to relieve discomfort, help localize the infection, and promote drainage.
- *Associated fever/surrounding cellulitis or lesion on the face* Treat with oral antibiotics, e.g. flucloxacillin 250mg qds for 7d; erythromycin 250mg qds is an alternative if allergic to penicillin.
- *Lesions that are large but localized, painful, and fluctuant* Consider incision and drainage. Admission may be needed if young or uncooperative child, or the boil is in a sensitive area, e.g. genital region, face, neck, axilla, breast. Do not attempt incision and drainage in the surgery if you are not confident. Afterwards treat with oral antibiotics until inflammation resolves.
- *Admit* if not settling with primary care treatment.
- *If recurrent or chronic* Take swabs for culture from lesions and carrier sites (nose, axilla, and groin); treat carrier sites with topical antibiotic (e.g. Naseptin® qds for 10d). Advise improved hygiene and use of antiseptics in bath (e.g. chlorhexidine); consider long-term antibiotics (e.g. erythromycin 250–500mg od).

**Acute paronychia** Infection of the skin and soft tissue of the proximal and lateral nail fold, most commonly caused by *Staph. aureus*. Often originates from a break in the skin or cuticle as a result of minor trauma, e.g. nail biting. Skin and soft tissue of the proximal and lateral nail fold are red, hot, and tender; nail may appear discoloured/distorted. Treat in the same way as a boil.

**Staphylococcal whitlow (felon)** Infection involving the bulbous distal pulp of the finger following trauma or extension from an acute paronychia. The finger bulb is red, hot, oedematous, and usually exquisitely tender. Onset of pain is rapid and there is swelling of the entire finger pulp. *Differential diagnosis:* herpetic whitlow (🕮 p.633). *Management:* admit for drainage and antibiotics.

**Folliculitis** Inflammation of the hair follicles caused by infection (usually *Staph. aureus*), physical injury, or chemical irritation. Classified as superficial or deep by the depth of involvement of the hair follicle. Presents as pustules in hair-bearing areas, e.g. legs, beard area. *Risk factors:* obesity, DM, occlusion from clothing, topical steroid use. *Differential diagnosis:* Pityrosporum folliculitis (🕮 p.615).

**Management** Exclude DM; treat with topical antiseptic, or if resistant topical or systemic antibiotics (e.g. fusidic acid cream or oral flucloxacillin). *If recurrent or chronic:* Treat as for recurrent boils.

**Wound infection** Suspect if a wound becomes painful. Look for swelling, erythema, wound tenderness ± pus. *Risk factors:*

• Malnutrition   • Carcinomatosis   • Infection near the site of incision
• DM             • Steroid therapy  • Contamination of the wound.

**Management** If pus is present send a swab for M,C&S:
• If the wound is indurated and infection localized to the wound suspect staphylococcal infection. Treat with flucloxacillin 250–500mg qds (or erythromycin 250–500mg qds if penicillin allergy)
• If there is cellulitis around the wound suspect streptococcus. Treat with penicillin V 250–500mg qds or erythromycin 250–500mg qds.
• If foul smell, suspect anaerobes—treat with metronidazole 400mg tds.

Give adequate analgesia; dress the wound frequently; review regularly; allow pus to drain. If a surgical wound, refer back to the operating surgeon if simple measures are ineffective.

**Necrotizing fasciitis** Acute and serious infection. Usually occurs in otherwise healthy individuals after surgery/trauma (often minor). Ill-defined erythema + high fever. Rapidly becomes necrotic. *Management:* emergency admission for IV antibiotics ± surgical debridement.

**Erysipelas and cellulitis** Acute infection of the dermis. Preceded by systemic symptoms—fever, 'flu-like' symptoms. Usually affects face or lower leg. May be an obvious entry wound. Appears as a painful tender reddened area with a well-defined edge. Often the area is swollen and may blister. *Differential diagnosis:* angioedema, contact dermatitis, gout.

**Management** Oral penicillin V 250–500mg qds or erythromycin for 7–14d. Severe infections may require hospital admission for IV antibiotics. Recurrent infections (>2 episodes at one site) require prophylactic long-term penicillin (e.g. penicillin V 250mg od or bd) and attention to potential entry portals (e.g. tinea pedis). Complications include lymphangitis ± permanent damage to lymph drainage, glomerulonephritis (🕮 p.450), or guttate psoriasis (🕮 p.623).

# Viral skin infection

**Systemic viral infections** 📖 p.650

**Viral warts** Common and benign. Due to infection of epidermal cells with human papilloma virus (HPV); >50 types identified. The virus is transmitted by direct contact. Immunosuppressed patients are particularly vulnerable.

**Genital warts** 📖 p.746

**Common warts** Dome-shaped papules with papilliferous surface. Usually >1. Most common on hands but may affect other areas. In children 30–50% disappear spontaneously in <6mo.

**Plantar warts (verrucas)** On soles of feet. Common in children. Pressure makes them grow into the dermis. Often painful. Characterized by dark punctate spots on the surface (may need to pare callus off to see). Warts group together to form mosaics.

**Plane warts** Smooth flat-topped papules, often slightly brown in colour. Most common on face and backs of hands. Usually >1. Manage as for common/plantar warts. Eventually resolve spontaneously. May show Koebner phenomenon.

***Treatment of common, plantar, and plane warts*** Table 17.7

**HPV vaccination** 📖 p.747

---

 **Molluscum contagiosum** Most common in pre-school children.
- DNA pox virus infection spread by contact, including towels. Presents as discrete pearly pink umbilicated papules 1–3mm in diameter. If squeezed, papules release a cheesy material
- Lesions are multiple and grouped, usually on the trunk, face, or neck.
- Untreated lesions resolve spontaneously after several months.
- In the older child, removal by expressing the contents with forceps, curettage or cryotherapy is possible but usually unnecessary.

---

**Orf** Solitary, red, rapidly growing papule <1cm diameter, often on hand. Evolves into a painful purple pustule. Patients usually have had close contact with sheep (e.g. vet, farmer). Incubation period ~6d. Resolves spontaneously in 2–4wk. Complications include infection (treat with topical/systemic antibiotics); erythema multiforme; lymphangitis.

**HIV infection** 📖 p.744

**Herpes simplex virus (HSV) infection** HSV is transmitted by direct contact with lesions. Lesions may appear anywhere on the skin or mucosa but are most frequent around the mouth and on the lips, conjunctiva, cornea, and genitalia. Diagnosis is usually clinical.

***Primary herpes infection of the mouth (stomatitis)*** May be asymptomatic and go unnoticed. After a prodromal period (generally <6h) of tingling, discomfort, or itching, small tense vesicles appear on an erythematous base. These burst to form multiple small painful mouth ulcers. Infection may be accompanied by systemic symptoms, e.g. fever, malaise, and tender lymph nodes.

***Management*** Give symptomatic relief—try analgesic mouthwashes (e.g. Difflam®); healing occurs within 8–12d. If seen <48h after onset of symptoms, prescribe oral antivirals (e.g. aciclovir 200mg 5×/d). If unable to take fluids and becoming dehydrated, admit for IV fluids.

***Recurrent infection (cold sores)*** After initial infection, HSV remains dormant in the nerve ganglia. Recurrent eruptions can occur, precipitated by overexposure to sunlight, febrile illnesses, physical or emotional stress, or immunosuppression. The trigger stimulus is often unknown. Recurrent disease is generally less severe and more localized. Treat with aciclovir cream 5% 5×/d if needed (available OTC).

***Herpetic whitlow*** Swollen, painful, and erythematous lesion of the distal phalanx, results from inoculation of HSV through a skin break or abrasion and is most common in health workers.

***Neonatal herpes*** 📖 p.716

***Genital herpes*** 📖 p.746

**Table 17.7** Treatment of viral warts (not genital warts)

| Treatment option | Examples | Notes |
| --- | --- | --- |
| Topical salicylic acid | Salactol® Duofilm® Bazuka® | Avoid use on the face or in patients with atopic eczema. Ensure dead skin is pared off daily before reapplication. |
| Cryotherapy | Liquid nitrogen | May cause blistering and be painful for several days after treatment. |
| Curettage/cautery | | Useful for solitary warts on the face. Warts may recur. |

⚠ Refer immunosuppressed patients for specialist advice on management.

---

❶ **Cryotherapy and cautery for warts** Cryotherapy and cautery are painful. Cryotherapy may also cause scarring. Only consider:
- If the wart/verruca is not resolving spontaneously after >3mo of topical treatment *and*
- If the patient really wants treatment and is able to understand the nature and side effects of treatment.

---

**Further information**

**British Association of Dermatologists** Guidelines for the management of cutaneous warts (2001) 🖥 www.bad.org.uk

# Fungal infection

Two major groups of fungal skin infections are seen in the UK.

**Candidiasis** A virtually uniform commensal of the mouth and GI tract which produces opportunistic infection. *Risk factors:* moist opposing skin folds; obesity; DM; neonates; pregnancy; poor hygiene; humid environment; wet work occupation; use of broad-spectrum antibiotic. Presentation— Table 17.8.

**Dermatophyte infection** Tinea denotes fungal infection. Common. Affects skin, hair, or nails. Skin scrapings or nail clippings may confirm diagnosis. Presentation—Table 17.9.

**General measures for prevention of fungal infections** Keep body folds separated and dry (e.g. with dusting powder) and minimize hot and humid conditions (e.g. advise open footwear).

## Management of fungal infections

### Topical treatment
- **Genital lesions** Imidazole cream or pessaries.
- **Nail infections** If confined to 1 or 2 nails, consider using a lacquer or paint (e.g.amorolfine lacquer 1–2×/wk for durations stated in the BNF.
- **Skin lesions** Imidazole cream, spray, or powder; terbinafine cream.

**Table 17.8** Presentation of candidiasis

| Presentation | Symptoms | Differential diagnosis |
|---|---|---|
| Genital infection 'thrush' 📖 p.735 | ♀ >> ♂. Itchy sore vulvovaginitis ± white plaques on mucous membranes and cheesy discharge. Men develop a similar clinical picture | Psoriasis; lichen planus; lichen sclerosus; other causes of vaginal discharge |
| Intertrigo | Reddened moist, glazed area in the submammary, inguinal, or axillary folds. In wet workers may occur between digits. Patients may notice skin changes or present with itch | Psoriasis; tinea cruris; seborrhoeic dermatitis; bacterial skin infection |
| Oral | Sore mouth; poor feeding in infants. Most common in babies, patients with poor oral hygiene, or the elderly with false teeth. White plaques visible on buccal musosa which can be wiped off ± angular stomatitis | Lichen planus; epithelial dysplasia |
| Nappy candidiasis | Babies in the nappy area | 📖 p.901 |
| Chronic paronychia | Often seen in wet workers. Presents with chronic nail fold inflammation. | Bacterial infection; chronic eczema |
| Systemic candidiasis | Occurs in immunosuppressed individuals (e.g. HIV, malignancy). Red nodules may appear on the skin | |

**Table 17.9** Dermatophyte infections

| Tinea | Affects | Presentation | Differential diagnosis |
|-------|---------|--------------|------------------------|
| Corporis Ringworm | Trunk or limbs | Single/multiple plaques with scaling and erythema especially at the edges. Lesions enlarge slowly and clear centrally (hence 'ringworm'). | Discoid eczema; psoriasis; pityriasis rosea |
| Cruris 'Jock itch' | Groin ♂ > ♀ Common in athletes | Associated with T.pedis. Involves upper thigh (+ scrotum rarely). Red plaque with scaling especially at the edge. | Intertrigo; candidiasis; erythrasma |
| Pedis 'Athlete's foot' | Feet ♂ > ♀ Young > old | Itchy, maceration between toes. Risk factors: swimming; occlusive footwear; hot weather. | Contact dermatitis; psoriasis; pompholyx |
| Capitis | Hair and scalp | Defined inflamed scaly areas ± alopecia with broken hair shafts. | Alopecia areata; psoriasis; seborrhoeic eczema |
| Unguium | Nails —prevalence ↑ with age Rare in children Toenails > fingernails | Begins at distal nail edge and progresses proximally to involve the whole nail. Eventually results in thickening, yellowing, and crumbling of the nail plate. T.pedis often coexists. | Psoriasis, trauma, candidiasis |

- **Mouth lesions**—remove tongue deposits with a toothbrush by brushing 2x/d. Treat with oral pastilles, suspensions or gels (e.g. nystatin, miconazole). If false teeth advise to place imidazole gel on the teeth before insertion and sterilize overnight with dilute hypochlorite solution (e.g. Milton®).

**Systemic treatment** Use for recurrent, extensive, systemic, or resistant infection, and nail or scalp infection. Examples:

- **Oral, mucocutaneous or systemic candidiasis,** e.g. oral fluconazole 50mg od for 1-2wk. Higher doses/prolonged therapy may be needed if immunosuppressed (seek specialist advice).
- **Genital candidiasis** Single oral dose of 150–200mg fluconazole.
- **Dermatophyte infection** Oral terbinafine (250mg od) or itraconazole (100–200mg od). Warn about possible side effects.
- **Nail infection** Consider if topical treatment is unsuccessful or >2 nails involved. Confirm diagnosis with nail clipping mycology before treatment. Consider treating with oral terbinafine or pulsed itraconazole—treat at dosage and for durations recommended in the BNF (5.2).

# Infestations

 **Head lice** Most common in children age 4–11y (♀ > ♂) but may occur in anyone. Contrary to popular belief lice infest clean as often as dirty hair. Adult lice are about the size of a sesame seed, brownish grey in colour, and wiggle their legs. Only adults are contagious. Spread by close head–head contact. Lice do not jump/fly and do not stay viable away from a host.

**Symptoms/signs** Normally asymptomatic. Detected by contact tracing of other cases or routine inspection at home or school. Occasionally present as itchy scalp. Presence of 'nits' (egg shells—white dots attached to hair), eggs, or dead lice indicate past infection—a moving louse must be found to confirm active infection.

**Detection** After washing hair, apply conditioner and comb with fine-tooth detector comb (available from pharmacy). In at-risk groups, e.g. schoolchildren, repeat weekly. Lice are removed by the comb and seen trapped in its teeth.

## Management
- *Prophylactic preparations*—no evidence of effectiveness.
- *Dimeticone* Lotion or spray. Coats head lice and interferes with water balance in lice by preventing the excretion of water. Advise to rub into dry hair and scalp in the evening, allow to dry naturally, then shampoo off the next morning. Repeat after 7d.
- *Insecticides*—effective. Four types: malathion, phenothrin, permethrin (all available OTC but NHS prescriptions are often sought), and carbaryl (prescription only). Malathion and phenothrin/permethrin are used as 1st/2nd line; carbaryl reserved for 3rd line. Apply according to manufacturer's instructions using 2 applications, 7d apart. Check wet conditioned hair with a detector comb before the 1st application, then every 2d until 3d after 2nd application. Supply enough for 2 applications. Shampoos are not effective—use lotions, liquids, or cream rinses.
- *Mechanical clearance* (wet-comb conditioned hair with a fine tooth comb until all lice are removed and repeat at 3–4d intervals for 2wk). Alternative to insecticides but requires motivation.
- *Other methods of treatment*—electric combs, aromatherapy (tea tree oil), herbal treatments. No evidence supporting their use.
- *Contact tracing*—all cases. Trace close contacts over the past month.

**Reinfestation/resistance to treatment** If lice have not cleared there are 3 possible reasons:
- *Reinfestation*—lice found are large adults only. Ask patient to check close contacts again. Re-treat with a different insecticide.
- *Incorrect use of insecticide/mechanical clearance*—lice at mixed stages of development will be seen. Check procedure with the patient and make sure instructions are understood. Repeat treatment with a different insecticide.
- *Resistance to insecticide*—lice are seen at all stages of development. Re-treat with another product.

**Crab lice** 📖 p.747

**Scabies** The scabies mite (*Sarcoptes scabei*) is ~0.5mm long and spread by direct physical contact. Average infection consists of 12 mites. Symptoms appear 4–6 wk after infection.

**Presentation** Intense itching. Examination reveals burrows (irregular, tortuous, and slightly scaly <1cm long) on sides of fingers, wrists, ankles, and nipples. May form rubbery nodules on genitalia. Itching results in excoriations. Untreated infection becomes chronic.

**Differential diagnosis** Lichen planus; dermatitis herpetiformis; papular urticaria; eczema.

**Management** Treat with scabicide e.g. malathion lotion. Apply according to manufacturer's instructions. All close contacts need treatment (which may result in all occupants of a residential home being treated). Apply to whole body including scalp, neck, face, ears; ensure finger/toe webs are covered and brush lotion under ends of finger/toe nails. Re-apply if hands are washed with soap <8h after application and after 1wk. Advise patients to launder all worn clothing and bedding after application. Itching may persist for some time after elimination of infection—use oral antihistamines for symptomatic relief.

**Complications** 2° infection (treat with topical or systemic antibiotics).

# Skin changes associated with internal conditions

**Table 17.10** Systemic conditions associated with skin changes

| Condition | Associated skin changes |
|---|---|
| Addison's disease | Pigmentation, vitiligo. |
| Cushing's disease | Pigmentation, hirsutism, striae, acne, truncal obesity, moon facies, buffalo hump. |
| Diabetes mellitus | <ul><li>*Diabetic dermopathy*—depressed pigmented scars on the shins.</li><li>*Necrobiosis lipoidica*—shiny atrophic yellowish-red plaques on the shins. Affects <1% diabetics but limited to those with DM or who will later develop DM.</li><li>*Granuloma annulare*—palpable annular lesions on hands, feet, or face. Only rarely associated with DM. Fades spontaneously in <12mo. Differentiate from ringworm.</li><li>*Xanthoma* (see hypercholesterolaemia)</li><li>*Fungal infection* (📖 p.634)</li><li>*Neuropathic ulcers* (📖 p.368)</li></ul> |
| Drug eruptions | Common. Withdrawal of the offending drug usually results in clearance of the eruption in <2wk. Simple emollients ± topical steroids may ease symptoms in the interim. Occasionally patients with severe reactions may require admission for supportive treatment until effects of the drug wear off.<br>*Stevens–Johnson syndrome* (erythema multiforme—📖 p.600) |
| Hyperlipidaemia | *Xanthoma:* yellowish lipid deposits in the skin. May be eruptive (like a rash), tendinous, plane (palmar creases), tuberous (knees, elbows).<br>*Xanthelasma:* yellowish plaques on eyelids. Not always associated with hyperlipidaemia. |
| Inflammatory bowel disease | |
| Crohn's disease | Perianal abscess, sinus or fistula; erythema nodosum, Sweet's disease (dark red plaques on face, arms, and legs), clubbing. |
| Ulcerative colitis | Pyoderma gangrenosum, erythema nodosum, Sweet's disease (see Crohn's disease), clubbing. |
| Liver disease | Pruritus, spider naevi, erythema, white nails, pigmentation, xanthomas (see hypercholesterolaemia). |
| Malabsorption | Dry itchy skin, ichthyosis, eczema, oedema. |

**Table 17.10** (*Continued*) Systemic conditions associated with skin changes

| | |
|---|---|
| Malignancy | *Acanthosis nigricans*—rare epidermal thickening and pigmentation in flexures and neck. Associated with GI malignancy. |
| | *Mycosis fungoides*—lymphoma that evolves in the skin. Slowly progressive becoming systemic only in terminal stages. May resemble psoriasis or eczema in early stages. |
| | *Paget's disease of the nipple* (📖 p.696) |
| | *Skin secondaries*—most commonly breast, GI, ovary, lung or haematological |
| | *Lymphoedema* (📖 p.1039) |

*Other conditions occasionally associated with malignancy*—flushing, generalized pruritus, hyperpigmentation, ichthyosis, dermatomyositis, erythroderma, hypertrichosis, pyoderma gangrenosum, superficial thrombophlebitis, tylosis.

| | |
|---|---|
| Malnutrition | *Iron deficiency*—alopecia, koilonychia, itching. |
| | *Scurvy*—bleeding gums, woody oedema, perifollicular oedema. |
| | *Protein deficiency*—pigmentation, dry skin, oedema, pale brown/orange hair. |
| | *Pellagra*—light-exposed dermatitis, pigmentation. |
| Neurofibromatosis | 📖 p.588 |
| Pregnancy | Pigmentation, spider naevi, abdominal striae, pruritus, pruritic urticarial papules and plaques of pregnancy (PUPP) (1:240 pregnancies), pemphigoid gestationis (rare). |
| Sarcoidosis | Nodules, plaques, erythema nodosum, dactylitis, lupus pernio (dusky-red infiltrated plaques on nose ± fingers). |
| Thyroid disease | |
| Hypothyroidism | Alopecia, coarse hair, dry, puffy brownish yellow skin. |
| Thyrotoxicosis | Pink soft skin, hyperhydrosis, alopecia, pigmentation, onycholysis, clubbing, pretibial myxoedema (raised erythematous plaques on shins—topical steroids may help) |
| Tuberous sclerosis | *Adenoma sebaceum*—red/yellow fibromatous plaques, usually around nose. |
| | *Periungual fibroma*—pink fibrous projections under nail folds. |
| | *Ash-leaf macules*—white oval macules. Best seen under Wood's light. |
| | *Shagreen patches*—yellowish naevi with cobblestone surface. Found on the back. |

## Infectious diseases covered in other sections

# Infectious disease

# Immunization

**Immunity can be induced in two ways**

- *Active immunity* Induced using inactivated or attenuated live organisms or their products. Act by inducing cell-mediated immunity and serum antibodies. Generally long-lasting.
- *Passive immunity* Results from injection of human immunoglobulin. The protection afforded is immediate but lasts only a few weeks.

**Storage of vaccines** Follow manufacturers' instructions. Do not store vaccines in the door of a vaccine fridge and make sure there is a maximum and minimum thermometer in the fridge. Record readings regularly and discard vaccines if not stored at the correct temperature.

**Administration of vaccines** Only suitably trained GPs/nurses should give immunizations. Check immunization is needed and the patient is fit. Check consent has been obtained and that immunizations are the correct ones and in date. Ensure resuscitation facilities are available. Record vaccine expiry date/batch number. Reconstitute vaccine (if necessary) and give according to manufacturer's instructions. Record date and site in the medical notes.

>  **Childhood immunization** In the UK, routine vaccinations for the under-fives are usually done in the GP surgery. Routine vaccinations for older children are normally done through the school health service. Schedule for childhood immunizations—Table 18.1.

**Adult immunization**

*Influenza and pneumococcal vaccination* Available as a directed enhanced service—existing practices do not have preferred provider status. Additional payments are available through the Quality and Outcomes Framework for ensuring that at-risk patients receive vaccination.

*Other necessary vaccinations* Can be provided as an additional service. Opting out incurs a 2% ↓ in global sum. A list of eligible vaccinations and terms of eligibility is available on the BMA website (🖳 www.bma.org.uk). Travel vaccinations that do not fall into these criteria can be administered as a private service.

**Contraindications to vaccination** For specific contraindications to individual vaccinations consult the Green Book. General rules:

- *Acute illness* Delay until fully recovered. Minor ailments without fever or systemic upset are not reasons to postpone immunization.
- *Severe local reaction to previous dose* Extensive area of redness/ swelling that involves much of the antero-lateral surface of the thigh or a major part of the circumference of the upper arm.
- *Severe generalized reaction to a previous dose* Fever ≥39.5°C <48h after vaccination; anaphylaxis, bronchospasm, laryngeal oedema, and/or generalized collapse; prolonged unresponsiveness; prolonged high-pitched or inconsolable screaming for >4h; convulsions or encephalopathy <72h after vaccination.

**Contraindications to live vaccines** BCG; measles; mumps; oral typhoid; rubella; yellow fever. *Do not* give live vaccines:

• to pregnant women
• to immunocompromised patients—those on high-dose steroids for >1wk (>1mg/kg/d prednisolone for children or ≥40mg/d for adults), if haematological malignancy, if radiotherapy/chemotherapy in the last 6mo, or if another immunodeficiency syndrome
• <3wk after another live vaccine (but two live vaccines may be given together at different sites), *or*
• with immunoglobulin (from 3wk before to 3mo after).

**❶** Patients with HIV may have live vaccine except BCG and yellow fever.

**Vaccine damage payments** Only payable if a patient is >80% impaired by a vaccination given within the NHS. Apply to the Vaccine Damage Payments Unit, Palatine House, Lancaster Road, Preston PR1 1HB ☎ 01772 899944 🖥 www.dwp.gov.uk Recipients receive a lump sum.

**Table 18.1** UK schedule of childhood immunization

| Disease (vaccine) | Age | Comment |
|---|---|---|
| Tuberculosis (BCG) | High-risk neonates | 1 injection |
| Diphtheria/tetanus/pertussis/ *Haemophilus influenzae* type b/ inactivated polio (D IaP/IPV/Hib) | 2, 3, and 4mo | Primary course (3 doses, a month between each dose) |
| Pneumococcal vaccine | 2, 4, and 13mo | Primary course |
| Meningococcus type C (men C) | 3, 4, and 12mo | Primary course |
| *Haemophilus influenzae* type b (Hib) | 12mo | Booster dose |
| Measles/mumps/rubella (MMR) | 13mo | 1st dose |
| Diphtheria/tetanus/acellular pertussis/ inactivated Polio (DTP/IPV) | 3y 4mo–5y (3y after completion of 1° course) | Booster dose |
| Measles/mumps/rubella (MMR) | 3y 4mo–5y | 2nd dose |
| Tetanus/low-dose diphtheria (Td/IPV)/inactivated polio | 13–18y | Booster dose |
| HPV vaccination | 12–13y (♀ only) | 3 doses over >6mo |

### Further information

**DH** The Green Book: Immunization Against Infectious Disease.
🖥 www.dh.gov.uk/greenbook
**Health Protection Agency (HPA)** Information on vaccines and vaccination schedules and on notifications of infectious diseases.
🖥 www.hpa.org.uk

### Patient information

**Immunisation** 🖥 www.immunisation.org.uk

# Symptoms, signs, and notification of infectious disease

Specific symptoms and signs of infection depend on the infecting organism and organs affected. For example, a chest infection will cause respiratory symptoms, a urine infection urinary tract symptoms. Symptoms suggesting an infectious cause include:

**Lymphadenopathy** Palpable enlargement of the LNs.

### Benign causes
- *Infective*—bacterial (pyogenic, TB, brucella); fungal; viral (EBV, CMV, HIV); toxoplasmosis; syphilis.
- *Non-infective*—sarcoid; connective tissue disease (rheumatoid arthritis); skin disease (eczema, psoriasis); drugs (phenytoin); berylliosis.

**Malignant causes** Lymphoma, CLL, ALL, metastases.

### Management
*Adults* Refer immediately for urgent investigation if:
- Rapidly growing.
- Non-tender, firm/hard LN >3cm in diameter.
- LNs associated with other unexplained signs of ill-health (night sweats, weight loss, persistent fever).
- LNs associated with other sinister signs, e.g. petechial rash (same day assessment), suspected head or neck tumour.
- Enlarged supraclavicular nodes in the absence of local infection.

Most enlarged LNs are reactive LNs—suggested by a short history, soft tender mobile lump, and concurrent infection. If there are no sinister features, give these 2 wk to settle. If not settling, check FBC, ESR ± EBV screen. Refer lymphadenopathy >1cm diameter persisting for >6wk for urgent further investigation.

---

*Children* Refer to paediatrics urgently, particularly if there is no evidence of local infection, if ≥1 of:
- Non-tender, firm/hard LN.
- LN >2cm diameter.
- Progressively enlarging LNs.
- LNs associated with other signs of ill health (e.g. fever, weight loss).
- Enlarged axillary nodes in the absence of local infection or dermatitis.
- Supraclavicular node involvement.

Investigate with FBC and blood film if generalized lymphadenopathy.

---

**Rigors** Shaking episodes (sometimes violent) associated with sudden rise in fever.

**Night sweats** Consider TB, lymphoma, leukaemia, solid tumour (e.g. renal carcinoma), menopause, anxiety states.

**Fever in children under the age of 5** 📖 p.872

**Pyrexia/fever** Oral temperature raised above 37.5°C. Normal range varies according to where measured (Table 18.2). *Common causes*:

**Infection** By far the most common cause in general practice:
- Viral infection (e.g. EBV, URTI, influenza)
- UTI
- Chest infection
- Tonsillitis
- Otitis media
- Sinusitis
- Cholecystitis
- Cellulitis

❶ Do not forget tropical diseases, e.g. malaria in patients returning from abroad. Think of TB and SBE—especially in high-risk patients.

**Cancer** Lymphoma, leukaemia, solid tumours (e.g. hypernephroma).

**Immunogenic causes** Connective tissue disease and autoimmune disease (e.g. RA, SLE, PAN, polymyalgia rheumatica), sarcoidosis.

**Thrombosis** DVT, PE                **Drugs** e.g. antibiotics

**Table 18.2** Normal temperature as measured in different locations

| Place of measurement | Normal range |
|---|---|
| Oral | 35.5–37.5°C (95.9–99.5°F) |
| Rectal | 36.6–38.0°C (97.9–100.4°F) |
| Axillary | 34.7–37.3°C (94.5–99.1°F) |
| Ear | 35.8–38.0°C (96.4–100.4°F) |

**Pyrexia of unknown origin** Defined as a fever (either intermittent or continuous) which has lasted for >3wk and for which no cause has been found. Re-check history. Re-examine carefully. Check FBC, EBV screen (depending on age of the patient), ESR, CRP, LFTs, amylase, urine (M,C&S), viral titres, blood cultures, and CXR. If cause does not become obvious refer urgently for further investigation.

**Notifiable diseases (^ND)** Notification of certain diseases is required under the Public Health (Control of Disease) Act 1984 and Public Health (Infectious disease) Regulations 1988. Notification is made to the local authority's medical officer for environmental health (who also provides forms for notification purposes). A fee is payable. *Diseases included*:
- Acute encephalitis
- Acute poliomyelitis
- Anthrax
- Cholera
- Diphtheria
- Dysentery
- Food poisoning
- Leprosy
- Leptospirosis
- Malaria
- Measles
- Meningitis (all types)
- Meningococcal septicaemia
- Mumps
- Ophthalmia neonatorum
- Paratyphoid fever
- Plague
- Rabies
- Relapsing fever
- Rubella
- Scarlet fever
- Smallpox
- Tetanus
- Tuberculosis
- Typhoid fever
- Typhus fever
- Viral haemorrhagic fever
- Viral hepatitis
- Whooping cough
- Yellow fever.

**Further information**
**NICE** Referral guidelines for suspected cancer(2005) ⬚ www.nice.org.uk

# Illness in returning travellers

⚠ In all returned travellers who present unwell consider imported disease in addition to the usual differential diagnosis. Tropical medicine is a specialized field. If unsure seek expert advice by telephone or admit the patient.

**History** *Ask about*:

- Symptoms
- Areas travelled to (including brief stopovers)
- Duration of travel
- Immunizations received prior to travel

- Malaria prophylaxis
- Health of members of the travel party
- Sexual contacts whilst abroad
- Medical treatment received abroad

**Examination** Full examination. Particularly check for fever, jaundice, abdominal tenderness, chest signs, rashes, lymphadenopathy.

**Investigations** Depend on symptoms and examination findings. Consider: FBC, thick and thin blood films for malaria, LFTs, viral serology, blood culture, stool culture (ensure it is fresh), MSU.

**Fever** *Consider*:

**Malaria[ND]** 2000 cases/y are notified in the UK. Easy to miss.

- *Symptoms* Malaria is a great mimic and can present with virtually any symptoms. Usually consists of a prodrome of headache, malaise, myalgia, and anorexia followed by recurring high fevers, rigors, and drenching sweats—lasting 8–12h. at a time.
- *Examination* May be normal—look for anaemia, jaundice ± hepatosplenomegaly.
- *Investigation* In all cases of fever in patients who have returned from a malarial endemic area, even if the plane just landed there and they did not get off, send a thick and thin film for malaria.
- *Management* Admit for further investigation and treatment if:
  - Very unwell
  - Unable to check a thick and thin film (e.g. presentation at a weekend or out of hours)
  - Thick and thin film +ve
  - Persistent fever despite –ve thick and thin film.

**Falciparum malaria** Caused by *Plasmodium falciparum*. Accounts for ~½ UK cases—it may not present for up to 3mo after return from a malarial area. Can be fatal in <24h, especially if it occurs in pregnant women or small children (<3y). *Complications*: cerebral malaria (80% deaths), hypogly-caemia, renal failure, pulmonary oedema, splenic rupture, disseminated intravascular coagulation, death.

**Benign malaria** Caused by *P. vivax*, *P. ovale*, and *P. malariae*. May cause illness up to 18mo after return. All have very low mortality. Relapse may occur at intervals after initial infection as parasites lie dormant in the liver (*P. vivax* and *P. ovale*) or blood (*P. malariae*).

**Typhoid[ND] and paratyphoid[ND]** Caused by *Salmonella typhi* and *Salmonella paratyphi* ~200 cases/y are notified in the UK.
- *Spread* by the faeco-oral route.
- *Incubation* 3d—3wk.
- *Symptoms* Usually presents with malaise, fever, headache, cough, constipation (or diarrhoea), nose bleeds, bruising, and/or abdominal pain.
- *Examination* Pyrexia, relative bradycardia, rose-coloured spots on the trunk (40%), splenomegaly, CNS signs (coma, delirium, meningism).
- *Management* Admit for further investigation and treatment with antibiotics.
- *Prognosis* 10% die if untreated, <0.1% if treated. 1% become chronic carriers after infection.

**Traveller's diarrhoea** 50% of travellers experience some diarrhoea. Most cases last 4—5d; 1—2% last >1mo In all cases send a fresh stool sample for M,C&S at first presentation, noting on the form areas visited. Consider the usual causes for diarrhoea (📖 p.384) and gastroenteritis (📖 p.418). In addition consider:

**Cholera[ND]** Caused by Gram –ve bacterium *Vibrio cholerae*.
- *Spread* by faeco-oral route.
- *Incubation* Few hours–5d.
- *Presentation* Profuse watery stools, fever, vomiting, rapid dehydration.
- *Management* Admit. Requires expert treatment with rehydration ± antibiotics.

**Giardiasis** Common flagellate protozoan. Infection is suggested by an incubation period ≥2wk; watery stool with flatus++ (explosive diarrhoea), no fever. Stool microscopy may be –ve. If suspected treat with metronidazole. Rapid response is diagnostic.

**Amoebic dysentery[ND]** May begin years after infection. Diarrhoea begins slowly, becoming profuse and bloody ± fever ± malaise. Diagnosis is confirmed by microscopy of fresh stool. Take specialist advice on management

**Sexually transmitted diseases** 📖 pp.736–747

**HIV** 📖 p.742      **TB** 📖 p.334

**Hepatitis A** 📖 p.430      **Meningitis** 📖 p.1074

**Hepatitis B and C** 📖 p.740

**Further information**
**Health Protection Agency (HPA)** Topics A–Z: Malaria, Giardia, Cholera. 🖥 www.hpa.org.uk

# Infections in immunocompromised patients

Infections in patients whose host defence mechanisms are compromised range from minor to fatal. They are often caused by organisms that normally reside on body surfaces.

**Opportunistic infections** Infections from endogenous microflora that are non-pathogenic or from ordinarily harmless organisms. Occur if host defence mechanisms have been altered by:

- Age
- Infection
- Burns
- Neoplasms
- Metabolic disorders
- Irradiation
- Foreign bodies
- Corticosteroids
- Immunosuppressive or cytotoxic drugs
- Diagnostic or therapeutic instrumentation.

The precise character of the host's altered defences determines which organisms are likely to be involved. These organisms are often resistant to multiple antibiotics.

## Organisms commonly involved

- Non-pathogenic streptococci
- E.coli
- Herpes viruses
- CMV
- Cryptococcal infection
- Toxoplasmosis
- Mycobacteria
- Pneumocystis
- Candida.

**Management** Expert care is always required—refer promptly to the consultant responsible for the patient.

## Prophylaxis

**Antibiotics** Used for prevention of:
- Rheumatic fever and bacterial endocarditis
- TB and meningitis in exposed patients
- Recurrent UTIs and otitis media
- Bacterial infections in granulocytopenic patients
- Pneumocystis in AIDS patients.

⚠ Watch for signs of superinfection with resistent organisms.

## Active immunization

- **Influenza vaccine** Give annually—see 📖 p.331 for list of indications.
- **Haemophilus influenzae type b vaccine** For asplenic/hyposplenic patients—children should complete routine Hib vaccinations. Individuals immunized in infancy who then become asplenic should receive one booster dose aged >1y. Unimmunized adults and children >10y should receive a single dose of Hib.
- **Meningococcal vaccine** Give to close contacts of patients with type A or C meningococcal meningitis. In some cases given to patients with immunosuppression—take specialist advice.
- **Pneumococcal vaccine** Single dose—give to chronically ill, asplenic, and elderly patients, and those with sickle cell and HIV disease. Booster doses are not required except for patients with asplenia or nephrotic syndrome when a booster should be given after 5–10y.

- *Hepatitis B vaccine* Give to patients who repeatedly receive blood products as well as to medical and nursing personnel and others at risk.

**Passive immunization** Can prevent or ameliorate herpes zoster (VZ-Ig), hepatitis A and B, measles, and cytomegalovirus infection in selected immunosuppressed patients. If a patient is in contact with any of these diseases, ask advice from the consultant looking after the patient or a consultant in communicable disease control.

**Immunoglobulin administration** Effective for patients with hypogammaglobulinaemia. Given on a regular basis by IV infusion.

**Asplenic patients** All asplenic patients (or functionally asplenic patients, e.g. patients with sickle cell disease) are at ↑risk of bacterial infection. Ensure patients have:
- *Vaccinations* Hib, pneumococcal, influenza, and in some cases meningococcal vaccine. If possible vaccinations should be given >2wk prior to splenectomy.
- *Prophylactic antibiotics* Oral penicillin continuously until age 16y or for 2y post-splenectomy, whichever is longer.
- *Stand-by amoxicillin* To start if symptoms of infection begin.
- *Patient-held card* Alerting health professionals to infection risk.

⚠
- Warn patients about severe malaria and other tropical infections
- Admit to hospital if infection develops despite prophylactic measures

Patient cards and information sheets are available to download from the Department of Health website 🖥 www.dh.gov.uk. Patients should also be encouraged to wear a Medic-Alert bracelet or necklace.

**HIV** 📖 p.744

# Childhood viral infections

 **Table 18.3** Common childhood viral infections

| Condition | Duration | Main symptoms |
|---|---|---|
| Measles[ND] | 10d | *Incubation:* 10–14d.<br>*Early symptoms:* fever, conjunctivitis, cough, coryza, LNs.<br>*Later symptoms:* koplik's spots (tiny white spots on bright red background found on buccal mucosa of cheeks), rash (florid maculopapular appears after 4d—becomes confluent).<br>*Complications:* bronchopneumonia, otitis media, stomatitis, corneal ulcers, gastroenteritis, appendicitis, encephalitis (1/1000 affected children), subacute sclerosing panencephalitis (rare). |
| Rubella[ND] (*German measles*) | 10d | *Incubation:* 14–21d.<br>*Symptoms:* mild and may pass unrecognized. Fever, LNs (including suboccipital nodes), pink maculopapular rash which lasts 3d.<br>*Complications:* birth defects if infected in pregnancy, arthritis (adolescents), thrombocytopenia (rare), encephalitis (rare). |
| Mumps[ND] | 10d | *Incubation:* 16–21d.<br>*Symptoms:* subclinical infection is common. Fever, malaise, tender enlargement of one or both parotids ± submandibular glands.<br>*Complications:* aseptic meningitis, epididymo-orchitis, pancreatitis. |
| Chickenpox | 14d | *Incubation:* 10–21d (infectious 1–2d before rash appears and for 5d afterwards).<br>*Symptoms:* rash ± fever. Spots appear in crops for 5–7d on skin and mucus membranes and progress from macule → papule → vesicle, then dry and scab over.<br>*Complications:* eczema herpeticum (📖 p.612), encephalitis (cerebellar symptoms most common), pneumonia, birth defects, neonatal infection (📖 p.806). |
| Roseola infantum | 4–7d | Child <2y<br>*Symptoms:* high fever, sore throat, and lymphadeno-pathy; macular rash appears after 3–4d when fever ↓ |
| Erythema infectiosum (*5th disease/ slapped cheek*) | 4–7d | Parvovirus infection<br>*Symptoms:* erythematous maculopapular rash starting on the face ('slapped cheeks'), reticular, 'lacy' rash on trunk and limbs, mild fever, arthralgia (rare)<br>Contact with parvovirus in pregnancy—📖 p.804 |
| Hand, foot, and mouth disease | 5–7d | Coxsackie virus infection<br>*Symptoms:* oral blisters/ulcers, red-edged vesicles on hands and feet, mild fever. |

**Management** For all the infections listed in Table 18.4, management is supportive with paracetamol, fluids ± antibiotics for 2° infection. Teething gels may sooth mouth lesions in hand, foot, and mouth disease. Admit if any serious complications develop.

### Prevention of measles, mumps, and rubella

• Measles, mumps, and rubella (MMR) vaccination consists of live attenuated measles, mumps, and rubella viruses. Vaccine viruses are not transmitted. MMR is routinely given to all children after their first birthday and again pre-school. Re-immunization is needed if given to children <1y. Children with chronic illness (e.g. CF) are at particular risk from measles and should be immunized. Malaise, fever, and rash are common ~1wk after immunizations and last 2–3d. Advise on fever prevention.

• Attenuated rubella vaccine is given to girls aged 10–14y who have not received MMR and non-pregnant women who lack immunity to rubella. Check rubella status at any opportunity in women of child-bearing age and vaccinate any women not immune. Advise women to avoid pregnancy for 3mo after vaccination. If lack of immunity is detected on routine antenatal screening, vaccinate after delivery.

☞ Scientific opinion is strongly in favour of there being no link between MMR vaccination and either autism or inflammatory bowel disease, but ↓ public confidence in MMR has resulted in ↓ vaccination uptake, risk of measles outbreaks, and debate over the use of single vaccines.

### Prevention of chickenpox

• Chickenpox (varicella) immunization (two doses 4–8wk apart) is recommended for non-immune healthcare workers who have direct patient contact. Those with a definite history of varicella infection can be considered immune—antibody test the others. Vaccination is contraindicated if pregnant or immunocompromised.

• Non-immune immunosuppressed patients, pregnant women, or neonates (📖 p.806) with significant exposure to chickenpox/shingles, should receive zoster immunoglobulin (VZ-Ig) <3d after contact. Check antibody levels if immune status is unknown.

**Shingles** Re-activation of latent chickenpox virus. Contacts may develop chickenpox but shingles cannot be acquired by exposure to chickenpox. Infectious until all lesions have scabbed.

• *Incidence*: 1:25 Any age—more common if immunocompromised.

• *Presentation*: unilateral pain precedes a vesicular rash by 2–3d. Crops of vesicles appear over 3–5d and are in the distribution of ≥1 adjacent dermatomes. The affected area is usually hyper-aesthetic—pain may be severe. Lesions scab over and fall off in <14d.

• *Management*: disease is usually mild in children, so treat as for chickenpox. Oral aciclovir (or similar) is only effective if initiated <48h after onset of the rash. If immunocompromised admit for IV antivirals.

**Complications** Post-herpetic neuralgia (rare in children); dissemination to other areas (occurs in immunosuppressed patients—admit for IV aciclovir); eye involvement—refer urgently to ophthalmology (📖 p.967); Ramsay Hunt syndrome (📖 p.546).

# Streptococcal and staphylococcal infections

**Streptococcal infection** Several groups are pathogenic to humans—A, B, C, G, D, and *Viridans* streptococci.

### Presentation

- Pharyngitis
- Tonsillitis
- Wound/skin infections
- Septicaemia
- Scarlet fever
- Pneumonia
- Rheumatic fever
- Glomerulonephritis
- Neonatal sepsis
- Postpartum sepsis
- Endocarditis
- Septic arthritis
- Pneumonia
- UTI
- Dental caries.

**Investigation** Diagnosis is usually clinical. Evidence of infection can be obtained by measuring changing antibody response to infection (ASO titres). ASO titres ↑ in ~80% infections. Wound swabs are +ve if infection is on the skin and throat swabs may be +ve in pharyngitis/tonsillitis.

**Treatment** Most streptococci are sensitive to penicillin (e.g. penicillin V 250–500mg qds for 7–10d) although resistance is increasingly common.

**Pneumococcal infection** There are > 85 types of *S.pneumoniae*. Pneumococci are carried in the noses and throats of half the population. In most people they are harmless. Spread is by droplet infection.

### Presentations

- Pneumonia
- Acute otitis media
- Sinusitis
- Meningitis
- Endocarditis,
- Septic arthritis (rare)
- Peritonitis (rare).

**Treatment** Amoxicillin 250–500mg tds for 7d (erythromycin in allergic individuals). Resistance to penicillin in the community is still low.

**Vaccination** Routine vaccination is now being offered as part of the childhood immunization schedule. In addition, offer to high-risk patients (Box 18.1). Ineffective in children <2mo. In children aged 2mo–5y, give conjugate vaccine initially and then polysaccharide vaccine after 2y. Booster doses are not needed except for patients with asplenia or nephrotic syndrome, when give booster after 5–10y.

> **Box 18.1  High-risk patients for pneumococcal infection**
> *Those:*
> - ≥ 65y of age
> - With asplenia/functional asplenia, e.g. splenectomy, sickle cell
> - With immune deficiency due to disease (e.g. lymphoma, Hodgkin's disease, multiple myeloma, HIV) or treatment (e.g. chemotherapy, prolonged systemic steroids)
> - With chronic heart disease, lung disease (e.g. asthma, COPD), renal disease (or nephritic syndrome) or liver disease
> - With coeliac disease
> - With cochlear implant
> - With DM requiring insulin or oral hypoglycaemic drugs *and/or*
> - With CSF shunts or other conditions where leakage of CSF fluid can occur.

**Scarlet fever** Gp.A haemolytic streptococcus infection.
- *Incubation*: 2–4d.
- *Presentation*: fever, malaise, headache, tonsillitis, rash (fine punctate erythema sparing face), 'scarlet' facial flushing, strawberry tongue (initially white turning red by 3rd/4th day).
- *Treatment*: penicillin V 250 –500mg qds for 10d.
- *Complications*: rheumatic fever (📖 p.284); acute glomerulonephritis.

**Staphylococcal infection** Usually *Staph. aureus*—occasionally *Staph. epidermidis*. Carried in the nose of ~30% of healthy adults. Antibiotic-resistant strains are common.

### Presentation
- Breast abscess/mastitis
- Abscesses/faruncles/carbuncles
- Septicaemia
- Endocarditis
- Wound infection
- Osteomyelitis/septic arthritis
- Pneumonia—especially patients with COPD, Influenza, or receiving corticosteroids or immunosuppressive therapy
- Neonatal infections—usually appear <6wk after birth (pustular or bullous skin lesions on neck, axilla or groin).

**Management** Antibiotics (usually flucloxacillin or erythromycin 250–500mg qds for 7–10d), abscess drainage where appropriate, and general supportive measures. Where possible obtain specimens for culture before instituting or altering antibiotic regimens

**Methicillin-resistant *Staph. aureus* (MRSA)**[N] MRSA acts in exactly the same way as any other *Staph. aureus*—it is carried harmlessly in most but occasionally causes a range of infections. It is only different because of its multiple resistance to antibiotics. Often contracted in hospital.
- ↓ tendency for multiple resistance by prudent use of antibiotics.
- Wash hands thoroughly with an appropriate antibacterial preparation if they appear soiled.
- If hands appear clean, wash with an alcoholic rub between each and every patient contact.
- Follow local policies for management of patients who are known to be infected with or carry MRSA.

**Toxic shock syndrome** Caused by staphylococcal exotoxin.
- *Risk factors* Tampon use; postpartum; staphylococcal wound infection; influenza; osteomyelitis; cellulitis.
- *Presentation* Sudden-onset high fever, vomiting, diarrhoea, confusion, and skin rash. May progress to shock ± death.
- *Management* Admit as a medical emergency—mortality 8–15%.

### Further information
**DH** Winning ways: working together to reduce healthcare associated infection in England (2003) 🖥 www.dh.gov.uk
**NICE** Infection control, prevention of healthcare-associated infection in primary and community care (2003) 🖥 www.nice.org.uk
**Health Protection Agency (HPA)** Topics A–Z: Streptococcal infections, *Staphylococcus aureus* 🖥 www.hpa.org.uk

# Other bacterial infections

**Haemophilus influenzae** 99% of infections are due to type b. Rare <3mo then incidence rises reaching peak incidence at 10–11mo Thereafter incidence declines until the age of 4y after which infection is rare. *Presentation*:

- Meningitis—60% (permanent neurological sequelae, 8–11%; death, 5%)
- Epiglottitis—15%
- Septic arthritis
- Pneumonia
- Septicaemia—10%
- Cellulitis
- Pericarditis.
- Osteomyelitis

**Management** Admit patients with severe infections. Organisms are often penicillin resistant and treatment is usually with IV cefotaxime.

**Prevention** Vaccination is routinely offered to all children (📖 p.643). In addition offer one-off vaccination to all unimmunized asplenic patients (preferably 2wk prior to splenectomy) and HIV +ve patients.

**Clostridium infections** Anaerobic spore-forming bacilli found in dust, soil, vegetation, and GI tracts of humans and animals. 25–30 species cause disease in humans. *Presentations*:

- Food poisoning—*C. perfringens*
- Pseudomembranous colitis—overgrowth of *C. difficile* following antibiotic therapy. Presents with bloody diarrhoea. Treated with vancomycin or metronidazole if toxin is isolated from stool
- Botulism—caused by toxin released by *C. botulinum* which is ingested in contaminated food Presents with neurological symptoms and warrants immediate admission for antitoxin.
- Wound infections—*C. perfringens* causes cellulitis which may → gas gangrene, septicaemia ± death. Admit for IV antibiotics.
- Tetanus.

**Tetanus (Lockjaw)^ND** 50 cases/y in UK. Incubation: 2–50d. *C. tetani* infects contaminated wounds that may be trivial, the uterus postpartum (maternal tetanus), or newborn umbilicus (tetanus neonatorum). Tetanus toxin → generalized or localized tonic spasticity ± tonic convulsions. Suspect in any patient who has not been immunized who develops muscle stiffness/spasm several days after suffering a skin wound or burn.

**Management** If suspected, admit for specialist care. Treatment is with antitoxin, wound debridement, and general support. Effects may last several weeks. Mortality—40%.

> ⚠ **Tetanus-prone injuries** Any burn/wound sustained >6h before surgical treatment of that wound *or* any burn or wound that:
> - Has a significant amount of dead tissue within it
> - Is a puncture-type wound
> - Has had contact with soil/manure likely to harbour tetanus organisms
> - Is clinically infected.

**Prevention** Tetanus vaccine:
- *Primary immunization*: three doses of vaccine each 1mo apart. If the schedule is disrupted, the course should be resumed from where it was stopped as soon as possible.

- *Booster doses in children* One dose >3y after the 1° course of immunization (usually given pre-school) and another 10y later (usually given on leaving school).
- *Booster doses in adults* 10y after the primary course and again 10y later. Probably gives lifelong protection. If an adult has received >5 doses in total, further routine boosters are not recommended.
- *Open wounds* 📖 p.1103.

**Diptheria**[ND] Caused by *Corynebacterium diptheriae*. Rare in the UK since routine immunization. Spread by droplet infection, contact with articles soiled by an infected person. *Incubation:* 2–5d.

**Presentation** In countries where hygiene is poor cutaneous diptheria is the predominant form. Elsewhere, characterized by an inflammatory exudate which forms a greyish membrane in the respiratory tract (may cause respiratory obstruction). *C.diptheriae* secretes a toxin which affects myocardium, nervous and adrenal tissues.

**Management** Admit for antitoxin and IV erythromycin. Patients may be infectious for up to 4wk but carriers shed *C.diptheriae* for longer.

**Prevention** Vaccination—part of the routine childhood vaccination programme in the UK (📖 p.643). In addition, give booster dose to people in contact with a patient with diptheria or carrier, or before travel to epidemic or endemic areas.

**Pseudomonas aeruginosa** Common and serious pathogen. Treatment is difficult because of multiple antibiotic resistance. Always send a specimen for culture and sensitivity if suspected.
- In immunocompetent patients may cause UTI, wound infections (particularly leg ulcers—gives a characteristic greenish colouring), osteomyelitis, and skin infections (e.g. otitis externa).
- In immunocompromised patients and patients with CF, it is a common cause of pneumonia and septicaemia.

**Enterobacteria** Examples include:

- *Salmonella*
- *Shigella*
- *Escherichia*
- *Klebsiella*
- *Enterobacter*
- *Proteus*
- *Morganella*
- *Providencia*
- *Yersinia*

Some are normal gut commensals. Others are pathogenic causing:
- Diarrhoea and intra-abdominal infections including peritonitis and hepatobiliary infections.
- UTI—often *E. coli*; *Proteus* species are associated with bladder stones.
- Septicaemia and/or meningitis—*E.coli* is the most common cause of meningitis in neonates.
- Chest infection—*Klebsiella* may cause a severe form of pneumonia.
- Endocarditis—rare.

Organisms are usually sensitive to co-amoxiclav and/or trimethoprim. Severe infection requires admission to hospital for IV antibiotics.

**Further information**
**Health Protection Agency (HPA)** Topics A–Z: Haemophilus influenzae, Pseudomonas, Clostridium, Tetanus, Diphtheria 🖳 www.hpa.org.uk

# Haematology and immunology

# Full blood count and ESR

The most commonly requested blood test is the full blood count (FBC). It gives information on:

- *Red blood cells*—red cell count, packed cell volume (haematocrit), mean cell volume (MCV), haemoglobin (Hb), and mean cell haemoglobin concentration (MCHC)
- *White blood cells*—white cell count and the proportion of each of its components (neutrophils, lymphocytes, monocytes, eosinophils, and basophils)
- *Platelets*—number of platelets.

## Red blood cells

*Anaemia* 📖 p.660                          *Polycythaemia* 📖 p.677

### Mean cell volume (MCV)

- *Low MCV* (microcytic, <80fL): *Most common cause*: iron deficiency anaemia. Confirm by showing that serum ferritin is ↓. *Rarer causes*: thalassaemia (suspect if MCV is 'too low' for the level of anaemia); congenital sideroblastic anaemia (very rare).
- *High MCV* (macrocytic, >100fL): Vitamin $B_{12}$/folate deficiency; alcohol; liver disease; drugs (e.g. iron, azathioprine, zidovudine); haemolysis; pregnancy; hypothyroidism; marrow infiltration; myelodysplasia.

**White cells** Normal white cell count is $4–11\times10^9$/L. Reasons for individual components to be ↑ or ↓ are summarized in Table 19.1.

## Platelets

**Thrombocytopoenia** ↓ platelets (<$150\times10^9$/L). *Causes:*

- ↓ *production* Marrow failure; megaloblastic anaemia.
- ↓ *survival* Idiopathic thrombocytopoenic purpura; viruses; disseminated intravascular coagulation; drugs (e.g. penicillin, sulphonamides, NSAIDs, furosemide, acetazolamide); SLE; lymphoma; thrombotic thrombocytopoenic purpura; hypersplenism; genetic disease.
- *Platelet aggregation* Heparin (5% patients).

**Thrombocythaemia (thrombocytosis)** ↑ platelets(>$400\times10^9$/L). *Causes:*

- *Essential thrombocytosis*—rare.
- *Reactive* (2°) thrombocytosis. Due to infection, malignant disease, acute or chronic inflammatory disease, pregnancy, or iron deficiency; after splenectomy or following haemorrhage.

❶ ~50% with unexplained thrombocytosis have a malignancy.

**Pancytopoenia** Reduction in red cells, white cells, and platelets. *Causes:*

- Aplastic or megaloblastic anaemia
- Bone marrow infiltration or replacement e.g. by lymphoma, leukaemia, myeloma, 2° carcinoma, myelofibrosis
- Hypersplenism
- Disseminated TB
- SLE
- Paroxysmal nocturnal haemoglobinuria.

**Erythrocyte sedimentation rate (ESR)** Rate of fall of red cells in a column of blood. A measure of the acute phase response—the pathological process may be infective, immunological, malignant, ischaemic, or traumatic. ESR ↑ with age; ♀>♂. ❶ ↑ in patients with severe anaemia.

**Plasma viscosity** Measure of the acute phase response—pathological process may be infective, immunological, malignant, ischaemic, or traumatic. ♂=♀; ↑ slightly with age; unaffected by the level of Hb.

**Table 19.1** Differential diagnosis for white cell count changes

| White cell type Normal range (percentage) | Causes of increased count | Causes of decreased count |
|---|---|---|
| Neutrophils 2.0–7.5×10⁹/L (40–75%) | Bacterial infection<br>Physical injury, e.g. trauma, burns, surgery<br>Inflammation, e.g. PMR, RA<br>Myocardial infarction<br>Pregnancy<br>Malignancy: leukaemia, disseminated malignancy<br>Drugs, e.g. steroids | Viral infections, e.g. mumps, hepatitis, influenza<br>Drugs, e.g. carbimazole, cytotoxics<br>Hypersplenism<br>B₁₂ or folate deficiency<br>Bone marrow failure |
| Lymphocytes 1.5–4.9×10⁹/L (20–15%) | Viral infection, e.g. EBV, early HIV, hepatitis, rubella<br>Other infections: whooping cough, toxoplasmosis<br>CLL and ALL<br>❶ Large numbers of abnormal ('atypical') lymphocytes are characteristically seen with EBV infection | Drugs, e.g cytotoxics, steroids<br>Burns/surgery<br>Influenza<br>SLE<br>Uraemia<br>Marrow infiltration<br>HIV infection |
| Monocytes 0.2–0.8×10⁹/L (2–10%) | Chronic bacterial infections (e.g. TB, SBE)<br>Autoimmune disorders | N/A |
| Eosinophils 0.04–0.44×10⁹/L (1–5%) | Atopic disease including asthma (80%)<br>Parasitic infections (8%)<br>Haematological malignancy (2.5%)<br>Allergic/atopic skin conditions (2%)<br>Solid tumours (2%)<br>GI disease (inflammatory bowel disease, coeliac) 1.5%<br>Lung disease (1%)<br>Connective tissue disease (0.5%) | N/A |
| Basophils 0.01–0.1×10⁹/L (<1%) | CML/myeloproliferative disease<br>Hypothyroidism<br>Drugs, e.g. oestrogen | N/A |

# Anaemia: diagnosis and initial investigation

**Anaemia** A lack of sufficient red blood cells and thus haemoglobin (♂: Hb <13g/dL; ♀: Hb <12g/dL or <11g/dL if pregnant). Results if there is:
- ↓ *red cell production*—defective precursor proliferation and/or maturation
- ↑ *loss or rate of destruction*—bleeding or haemolysis
- ↓ *tissue requirement for oxygen*—in practice, hypothyroidism.

**Presentation** Patients who become anaemic slowly may remain asymptomatic for a long time. As anaemia progresses, pallor, exertional dyspnoea, tachycardia, palpitations, angina (especially if past history of coronary artery disease), night cramps, and cardiac bruits appear. Ultimately, with severe anaemia high-output cardiac failure may develop.

❶ *Pallor* may indicate anaemia but is a very non-specific sign which may also be racial, familial, or cosmetic. *Other causes of pallor*: shock, Stokes–Adams attack, vasovagal faint, myxoedema, hypopituitarism; albinism.

**Initial investigation of anaemia** Table 19.2

**Management** Treat the cause—if no cause for anaemia is found, refer for specialist investigation.

**Table 19.2** Investigation and differential diagnosis of anaemia

| MCV | Causes | Further investigations |
|---|---|---|
| *Low* <80fL | Iron deficiency Thalassaemia Haemoglobinopathy Anaemia of chronic disorder | Blood film Ferritin Hb electrophoresis (if indicated) Reticulocyte count Rectal examination Faecal occult blood test |
| *Normal* | Acute blood loss Haemolysis Anaemia of chronic disorder Uraemia Haemoglobinopathy Marrow failure | Blood film Reticulocyte count Hb electrophoresis (if indicated) Ferritin Serum $B_{12}$ (+intrinsic factor levels if ↓) Serum and red cell folate Renal function Serum bilirubin |
| *High* >100fL | Folate deficiency $B_{12}$ deficiency Alcohol Liver disease Thyroid disease Myelodysplasia | Blood film Serum $B_{12}$ (+intrinsic factor levels if ↓) Serum and red cell folate Liver function Thyroid function tests |

**Vitamin B$_{12}$ deficiency** Vitamin B$_{12}$ is found in liver, kidney, fish, chicken, meats, and dairy products. Absorption takes place by active and passive mechanisms. The latter are dependent on intrinsic factor, a protein produced by gastric parietal cells.

***Presentation*** Deficiency may be an incidental finding or present with anaemia, sore mouth (glossitis, angular cheilosis, and/or mouth ulcers), and/or neurological features (peripheral neuropathy, optic atrophy, subacute combined degeneration of the cord or rarely psychosis).

*Causes of deficiency*
- *Inadequate dietary intake*, e.g. vegans. Give dietary advice and/or dietary supplements.
- *Malabsorption* After gastrectomy (total or partial) or ileal resection; pernicious anaemia—treat with regular doses of parenteral vitamin B$_{12}$ (hydroxocobalamin IM: initially 1mg on alternate days for 1–2wk, then 0.25mg weekly until blood count is in the normal range; maintenance dose is 1mg every 2–3mo).

**Pernicious anaemia** Caused by severe lack of intrinsic factor 2° to gastric atrophy. *Risk factors*: FH, other autoimmune disease (e.g. vitiligo, hypothyroidism), premature greying, blood groups A and HLA3. Long term, patients have ↑ risk of stomach cancer. Intrinsic factor antibodies (either blocking or binding antibodies) are diagnostic. *Treatment*—see B$_{12}$ deficiency. Check FBC, B$_{12}$, and TFTs annually.

**Folate deficiency** Folate is found in highest concentrations in liver and yeast, but is also present in spinach, other green vegetables, and nuts.

***Presentation*** Deficiency may be an incidental finding or presents with symptoms and signs of anaemia ± polyneuropathy or dementia. Always check serum B$_{12}$ as deficiencies may coexist.

*Causes of deficiency*
- *Inadequate dietary intake* Common, e.g. old age, poor social conditions, malignancy, anorexia, excess alcohol.
- *Malabsorption* Coeliac disease, Crohn's disease, partial gastrectomy, tropical sprue, lymphoma, diabetic enteropathy.
- *Excess use* Pregnancy, lactation, prematurity, ↑ cell turnover (e.g. malignancy, haemolysis).
- *Drugs* Anticonvulsants, trimethoprim.

***Management*** In all cases, treat the cause. Supplement folate with folic acid 5mg od for 4mo. If malabsorption, may need ↑ dose to 15mg od. For prophylaxis in chronic haemolytic states or for renal dialysis, up to 5mg od long-term is used (take advice).

⚠ **Folate supplements in pregnancy** Advise women to take supplements from planning pregnancy to 12wk gestation to prevent neural tube defect. *Dose*: to prevent first occurrence, 0.4mg od; to prevent recurrence or if on anticonvulsants, 5mg od.

# Iron deficiency anaemia

Iron deficiency anaemia is the most common form of anaemia in the UK. (prevalence 2–5% among adult men and post-menopausal women). It is a common cause of gastroenterology referral (4–13% of referrals).

**Causes ❶** More than one cause may be present.
- *GI blood loss* Aspirin/NSAID use (10–15%); colonic carcinoma (5–10%); gastric carcinoma (5%); benign gastric ulceration (5%); angiodysplasia (5%); oesophagitis (5%); oesophageal carcinoma (1–2%)
- *Malabsorption* Coeliac disease (4–6%)—may be the presenting feature; post-gastrectomy; gut resection
- *Non-GI blood loss* Menstruation (20–30%); blood donation (5%); haematuria (1%); epistaxis
- *Other* Pregnancy; lactation; premature infants; deficient diet.

## Management
- Treat the underlying cause where possible.
- Give oral iron supplements, e.g. ferrous sulphate 200mg bd. Iron may cause constipation and turn stools black. If ferrous sulphate 200mg bd is not tolerated, try a lower dose or alternative preparation, e.g. ferrous fumarate. Ascorbic acid (250–500mg bd with the iron preparation) may enhance iron absorption.
- Hb should ↑ by 1g/dL/wk—confirm response to treatment 2–3wk after starting. Continue treatment for 3mo after correction of the iron deficiency to allow replenishment of the iron stores.

⚠ Asymptomatic colonic and gastric carcinoma may present with iron deficiency anaemia—seeking and excluding these conditions is a priority.
- Refer urgently for gastroscopy/specialist opinion if dyspepsia and iron deficiency anaemia.[N]
- Refer urgently for suspected lower GI cancer if Hb <11g/dL in a man or <10g/dL in a non-menstruating woman.[N]

*Failure to respond to iron supplements* Consider continuing bleeding, non-compliance with iron tablets, or that oral iron is not absorbed, diagnosis is incorrect, or anaemia is mixed.

*Follow-up* Once normal, monitor Hb, MCH, and MCV every 3mo for 1y and then annually. Give further iron supplements if Hb, MCH, or MCV fall below normal levels. Only investigate further if unable to maintain Hb in this way.

**Iron deficiency without anaemia** Proven by low serum ferritin (hypoferritinaemia). 3× as common as iron deficiency anaemia but there is a very low prevalence of GI malignancy in this group (<1% of post-menopausal women and men). Investigate as in Figure 19.1. In all cases give iron supplements to replenish iron stores.

## Further information
**NICE** Referral guidelines for suspected cancer (2005) ▣ www.nice.org.uk
**British Society of Gastroenterology** Guidelines for the management of iron deficiency anaemia (2005) ▣ www.bsg.org.uk

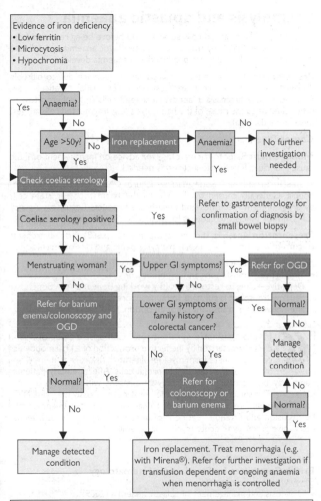

**Fig.19.1** Investigation and management of iron deficiency

Reproduced in modified form from Guidelines for the Management of Iron Deficiency Anaemia, May 2005, with permission from the British Society of Gastroenterology.

# Haemolysis and aplastic anaemia

**Haemolysis** Normal red cells survive 120d before being removed from the circulation—mainly by the spleen. In haemolytic anaemia red cells are destroyed faster than they are produced and anaemia develops.

**Presentation** Anaemia often accompanied by jaundice due to bilirubin released when the red cells are destroyed. FBC: ↓Hb; ↑ reticulocytes. Film shows polychromasia ± abnormal-shaped cells (e.g. spherocytes) or other clues as to the cause of the haemolysis (e.g. fragmented cells suggest mechanical damage).

**Causes** Table 19.3

**Management** Refer to haematology for advice on management or if the cause is unclear. Rarely, splenectomy is needed.

**Aplastic anaemia**<sup>G</sup> Bone marrow failure. Characterized by pancytopoenia. Generally caused by damage to the haematopoietic stem cells by drugs (inform Medicines and Healthcare Products Regulatory Agency 📖 p.148) or toxins. No cause is found in 50%.

**Presentation** Anaemia, thrombocytopenia (📖 p.668) and neurtropenia (recurrent infection). FBC reveals pancytopoenia and lack of reticulocytes.

**Management** Refer urgently to haematology. Treatment is:
- *Supportive*—transfusions and antibiotics, *or*
- *Definitive*—aims to restore a healthy working bone marrow. Bone marrow transplant is curative. Immunosuppressive therapy is an alternative when transplant is not an option.

> **Myelodysplastic syndromes**<sup>G</sup> Comprise a group of disorders characterized by ineffective production of ≥1 haemopoietic cell line. Differs from myeloproliferative disorder as there is no invasion of normal marrow by abnormal cells. Affects elderly patients and may be discovered incidentally or present with anaemia and/or bleeding. The spleen may be palpable but is never grossly enlarged. FBC and blood film are diagnostic. Refer to haematology—treatment is with transfusion and prompt treatment of infection ± chemotherapy. Tends to evolve gradually to acute myeloid leukaemia (¾ in <2y).

## Further information
**British Committee for Standards in Haematology**
🖥 www.bcshguidelines.com
- Diagnosis and management of aplastic anaemia (2009)
- Diagnosis and management of hereditary spherocytosis (2004)
- Diagnosis and management of adult myelodysplastic syndromes (2003)

## Patient information and support
**Aplastic Anaemia Trust** 🖥 www.theaat.org.uk

**Table 19.3** Causes of haemolytic anaemia

| Cause | Examples |
|---|---|
| **Congenital** | |
| *Membrane abnormalities* | Hereditary spherocytosis or elliptocytosis. |
| *Haemoglobin abnormalities* | Abnormal Hb, e.g. sickle cell anaemia (📖 p.667) |
| | Defective synthesis, e.g. thalassaemia (📖 p.666) |
| *Metabolic abnormalities* | Glucose-6-phosphate dehydrogenase (G6PD) or pyruvate kinase deficiency |
| **Acquired** | |
| *Immune* | Autoimmune (warm or cold); isoimmune (e.g. transfusion reaction; haemolytic disease of the newborn (📖p.818)) or drug induced |
| *Hypersplenism* | Malaria, lymphoma, RA, portal hypertension |
| *Red cell fragmentation* | Artificial heart valves |
| *Activated complement* | Paroxysmal nocturnal haemoglobinuria |
| *Secondary* | Renal disease, liver disease |
| *Miscellaneous* | Infections (e.g. malaria), burns, chemicals, toxins, drugs |

# Haemoglobinopathy

## Screening

- *Antenatal screening* (📖 p.798) for sickle cell disease and
  α-thalassaemia is offered to all pregnant women in the UK. Ideally should
  take place at <10wk gestation. If the mother is a carrier, the father can be
  tested and consideration given to antenatal testing for the foetus.
- *Neonatal blood spot screening* (📖 p.849) for sickle cell disease is
  currently offered to all babies in England.

❶ These screening tests will lead to many more people being aware of
their carrier status.

**Thalassaemia** Common in populations from Africa, the Middle East,
the Mediterranean, Indian subcontinent and South East Asia. Results from
↓ production of either the α (α-thalassaemia) or β (β-thalassaemia) globin
chains of haemoglobin. Two main types of each are recognized:
- $\alpha^o$ and $\beta^o$ thalassaemia: no gene product is produced.
- $\alpha^+$ and $\beta^+$ thalassaemia: α and β chains but produced at ↓ rate.

## β-thalassaemia

- Defective β-chain production → excess α-chain synthesis.
- Excess α chains precipitate in red cell precursors causing their
  destruction in bone marrow and spleen → proliferation of marrow,
  bony deformity (mongoloid facies, bossing of skull, thinning of long
  bones), and progressive splenomegaly.
- Homozygotes develop profound anaemia from 3mo of age and without
  repeated transfusions would die in <1y.
- Children who receive repeated transfusions grow and develop
  normally but iron accumulates. Treatment is with desferrioxamine
  infusions to ↑ iron excretion, but iron still accumulates and death is
  usual in the 2nd/3rd decade due to iron overload.

*Management* If suspected in an infant refer urgently to paediatrics.
Specialist ongoing care is essential. Consider referring family members for
genetic counselling.

## α-thalassaemia

- The homozygous state for $\alpha^o$ thalassaemia is associated with fetal
  death at ~38wk (Barts hydrops).
- Haemoglobin H results from inheritance of $\alpha^o$ from one parent and
  $\alpha^+$ from the other. Patients are moderately anaemic with splenomegaly
  and have haemoglobin H (4 β chains combined with a haem molecule)
  in their red cells. Specialist management is needed.

**Asymptomatic patients** Heterozygotes for α- and β-thalassaemia and
homozygotes for $\alpha^+$-thalassaemia are usually asymptomatic. Patients may
have mild anaemia with hypochromic and microcytic red cells.

❶This anaemia can be confused with iron deficiency but ferritin is normal
and it does not respond to iron supplements.

### Patient information and support
**UK Thalassaemia Society** ☎ 020 882 0011 🖥 www.ukts.org

**The sickling disorders** Most common amongst people originating from areas in which malaria is endemic: Africans (1–2% newborns) and certain Mediterranean, Middle Eastern, and Indian populations. Varieties:

• Heterozygous state for haemoglobin S (sickle cell trait—AS).
• Homozygous state (sickle cell anaemia/disease—SS).
• Heterozygous states for haemoglobin S and haemoglobins C,D, E or other structural variants.
• Combination of haemoglobin S with any form of thalassaemia.

**Mechanism** Haemoglobin S undergoes liquid crystal formation as it becomes deoxygenated, causing sickling of affected blood cells. The effect of sickling is to shorten survival of red cells → haemolytic anaemia, and cause aggregation of the sickled cells, which in turn leads to:

• Tissue infarction, resulting in pain and/or tissue damage, e.g. stroke (10% of children with sickle cell anaemia have a stroke and half of those have recurrent strokes), and/or
• Sequestration in the liver, spleen, or lungs, producing sudden and profound anaemia.

**Diagnosis** FBC and film—chronic anaemia with sickling on film. Confirm diagnosis with haemoglobin electrophoresis.

**Sickle cell trait** Patients with <40% haemoglobin S have no symptoms unless they are subjected to anoxia, e.g. anaesthesia.

**Sickle cell anaemia** Low Hb level (typically 8–9g/dL) with high reticulocyte count, although generally patients compensate well. Illness is due to complications arising as a result of acute exacerbations or 'crises' and by the effects of recurrent tissue damage due to microinfarction over a long period of time. Prognosis is variable. In Africa, children usually die in <1y. In the UK, patients frequently survive into adulthood (average survival 42–48y). Most common cause of death is infection.

**Management** There is no medication to prevent sickling.

• Treat as if hyposplenic—give Hib and pneumococcal vaccination, annual influenza vaccination ± prophylactic antibiotics (🕮 p.649). All children should receive prophylactic penicillin (erythromycin if allergy).
• Advise patients to avoid cold and maintain adequate hydration. Warn about the dangers of anaesthetics (a Medic Alert bracelet is helpful).
• Treat infection early.
• Give analgesia (including opioids if needed) for painful crises—admit if severe.
• Admit if significant crisis of any sort (e.g. stroke, dyspnoea, acute abdomen, aplastic anaemia).
• Refer for early management of long-term complications (e.g. renal failure, epilepsy).

**Further information**
**British Committee for Standards in Haematology**
🖥 www.bcshguidelines.com
• Significant haemoglobinopathies: guidelines for screening and diagnosis (2009)
• Management of the acute painful crisis in sickle cell disease (2003)

**Patient information and support**
**Sickle Cell Society** ☎ 020 896 17795 🖥 www.sicklecellsociety.org

# Bleeding and clotting disorders

**Coagulation tests** (sodium citrate tube; false results if under-filled)
- *Prothrombin time (PT)* Prolonged by coumarins (e.g. warfarin), vitamin K deficiency, liver disease.
- *Thrombin time* ↑ in heparin treatment, DIC, or afibrinogenaemia.
- *INR* Ratio of time the sample takes to clot to time taken by a control sample.

## The pupuras

*Vascular purpuras* result from damage to the vessel wall. *Due to*:
- Infection (e.g. meningococcal septicaemia, EBV)
- Immune dysfunction (e.g. Henoch–Schönlein purpura)
- Vitamin C deficiency
- Ageing (senile purpura)
- Local stasis or ↑ venous pressure (e.g. varicose veins)
- Drug reaction (e.g. steroid-induced purpura)

*Thrombcytopoenic purpura* Pupura is related to the level of the platelet count. Bleeding is inevitable if platelet count ↓ to <5–10×10⁹/L.
- *Non-immune thrombocytopoenic purpura* Results from conditions that damage the bone marrow, e.g. aplastic anaemia (📖 p.664), leukaemia (📖 p.674), myeloproliferative disorders (📖 p.676), CLL (📖 p.676), multiple myeloma (📖 p.672).
- *Immune thrombocytopoenic purpura* Usually idiopathic (ITP). May be associated with SLE, transfusions, or drug reactions (e.g. heparin).

### Idiopathic thrombocytopoenic purpura (ITP)
- *In children* Self-limiting disorder often occurring after a viral illness. The child is purpuric with a platelet count of <10×10⁹/L. Despite this, severe bleeding is rare. *Management*: refer to paediatrics as an emergency. Often no specific treatment is needed.
- *In adults* Chronic relapsing illness. Insidious onset with haemorrhage and bruising. Platelet count is ↓. Ask about drug history (particularly thiazides, quinine, or digoxin). Look for evidence of SLE or lymphoma. Examine for presence of an enlarged spleen. Refer to haematology.

*Impaired platelet function* May occur with any haematological malignancy resulting in bleeding, even if the platelet count is normal.

**Clotting factor deficiencies** Genetic deficiencies of every clotting factor have been described—the majority are rare. Acquired clotting factor deficiencies are common, e.g. vitamin K deficiency in newborns (📖 p.846), anticoagulation (📖 p.670), liver disease.

*Haemophilia* 2 common forms: haemophilia A (factor VIII deficiency) and haemophilia B (factor IX deficiency, Christmas disease). Sex-linked recessive disorders. ♂>>♀. *Prevalence*: 90/million population (haemophilia A); 16/million population (haemophilia B).

*Classification* Carrier (♀ heterozygotes, >25% clotting factor activity); mild (5–25% clotting factor activity); moderate (2–5% clotting factor activity); severe (50% haemophiliacs, ≤ 1% clotting factor activity).

*Clinical features* Bleeding → joints or muscles is often delayed following trauma. If untreated, results in permanent damage. Pressure effects occur if bleeding takes place into a confined space, e.g. intracranial bleed. Severity of bleeding is related to levels of clotting factors.

*Management* All haemophiliacs should be followed up under the care of a specialist haemophilia centre. Prenatal and antenatal screening is available—refer to genetics. Treatment can be 'on demand' or 'prophylactic'.

• *On-demand treatment*: Transfusion of factor VIII or IX preparation as soon as possible after bleeding has started—most administer it to themselves—and symptomatic treatment of bleeds, e.g. rest, analgesia ± physiotherapy for bleeds into muscles/joints.
• *Prophylactic*: Prevents bleeds and their consequences. Agents used:
  • Tranexamic acid—prevents bleeding after minor surgical procedures for patients with mild haemophilia/carriers with symptoms.
  • Desmopressin—stimulates production of factor VIII (not factor IX). Prevents bleeding in patients with mild/moderate haemophilia A.
  • Factor VIII or IX—factor VIII 3×/wk; factor IX 2×/wk.

*Problems with treatment*
• *Inhibitors*: 25% of patients have antibodies to factor VIII or IX products. Treated with IV factor VIIa or, in children, through an 'Immune tolerization programme' of daily administration of factor VIII/IX.
• *Infection from blood products*: ~1500 UK haemophiliacs have been infected with HIV through contaminated blood products—more with hepatitis B and C. Whenever possible genetically engineered 'recombinant' products are used rather than blood products.

**von Willebrand's disease** Autosomal dominant deficiency of a clotting factor (vW factor). ♂ = ♀. *Prevalence*: 1% of population. Most are mildly affected with easy bruising, nose bleeds, and/or menorrhagia. Severe cases may bleed into joints. *FBC*: normal platelets; clotting screen: ↑ bleeding time. Refer to haematology. Mild cases are managed with tranexamic acid, desmopressin, and/or COC pill (for menorrhagia). In severe cases may need treatment with vW factor. No recombinant form available yet. *E.A. von Willebrand (1870–1939)—Finnish physician.*

**Thrombophilia**[G] ↑ tendency to clot. due to variety of inherited defects in natural anticoagulants (e.g. protein S) and clotting factors (e.g. factor V Leiden) Screening is useful in high-risk individuals, if knowing a person is affected will affect management. Consider referral to haematology for screening (ideally after discussion with a haematologist) if:

• Venous thromboembolism <40y
• Arterial thrombosis <30y
• Recurrent thromboembolism
• FH of thrombophilic abnormality
• Clear FH of venous thrombosis.

Patients may need short-term prophylaxis with anticoagulants at times of risk (e.g. surgery, pregnancy) or, rarely, long-term anticoagulation.

**Further information**
**British Committee for Standards in Haematology** Diagnosis and management of heritable thrombophilia (2001) ▱ www.bcshguidelines.com

**Patient information and support**
**Haemophilia Society** ☎ 0800 018 6068 ▱ www.haemophilia.org.uk

# Anticoagulation

**Heparin in the community** Only use on specialist advice. Usually SC low-molecular-weight heparin (LMWH) is chosen as it does not need daily monitoring.

**Warfarin** Antagonizes the effects of vitamin K to ↓ clotting tendency. Indications and target INRs—Table 19.4.

***Initiation of warfarin*** Most patients are anticoagulated in hospital (e.g. after MI) or in the community under consultant supervision (e.g. DVT). If there is no urgency for initiation (e.g .chronic AF), start warfarin in the community (Table 19.5). Check baseline blood sample for FBC, clotting screen, renal and liver function tests. Complete a DH oral anticoagulant booklet for the patient to carry. Take patient/carer through the educational points in the booklet. Ensure they understand the local monitoring system. Advise to take warfarin at the same time each day.

***Monitoring*** (Table 19.6) If there is a change in clinical state monitor more frequently until steady state is re-established.

**Table 19.4** Indications for warfarin and target INRs

| Indication | INR (range) |
| --- | --- |
| **Long-term anticoagulation** | |
| Mechanical prosthetic heart valves—first generation | 3.5 (3.0–4.0) |
| Prophylaxis of recurrent DVT/PE—occurring on warfarin | 3.5 (3.0–4.0) |
| Mechanical prosthetic heart valves—second generation | 3.0 (2.5–3.5) |
| Antiphospholipid syndrome | 3.0 (2.5–3.5) |
| Rheumatic mitral valve disease | 2.5 (2.0–3.0) |
| AF due to valve disease, congenital heart disease, or thyrotoxicosis | 2.5 (2.0–3.0) |
| Non-valvular AF + medium/high stroke risk (□ p.572) | 2.5 (2.0–3.0) |
| Dilated cardiomyopathy | 2.5 (2.0–3.0) |
| Prophylaxis of recurrent DVT/PE—occurring off warfarin | 2.5 (2.0–3.0) |
| Inherited thrombophilia with previous episode of thrombosis | 2.5 (2.0–3.0) |
| **For 6mo after the event** | |
| First PE or proximal vein DVT and no persistent risk factors | 2.5 (2.0–3.0) |
| **For 3mo after the event** | |
| First calf DVT and no persistent risk factors | 2.5 (2.0–3.0) |
| Mural thrombus post MI | 2.5 (2.0–3.0) |
| **Others** | |
| Cardioversion—anticoagulate 3wk before to 4wk after the procedure | 2.5 (2.0–3.0) |
| Inherited thrombophilia—no previous thrombosis: anticoagulate for high-risk activities, e.g. surgery | 2.5 (2.0–3.0) |

**Table 19.5** Dose regime for starting warfarin in the community

| INR on day 5 | Dose on days 5–7 | INR on day 8 | Dose from day 8 | Instructions: |
|---|---|---|---|---|
| ≤1.7 | 5mg | ≤1.7 | 6mg | • Give warfarin 5mg od for 4d then check INR. |
| | | 1.8–2.4 | 5mg | • Adjust dose as in table. |
| | | 2.5–3 | 4mg | • Recheck INR on day 8 and adjust dose as in table. |
| | | >3 | 3mg for 4d | • Thereafter check INR weekly (unless 4d interval stated) and adjust dose accordingly until dose is stable in the target range. |
| 1.8–2.2 | 4mg | ≤1.7 | 5mg | |
| | | 1.8–2.4 | 4mg | |
| | | 2.5–3 | 3.5mg | |
| | | 3.1–3.5 | 3mg for 4d | |
| | | >3.5 | 2.5mg for 4d | |
| 2.3–2.7 | 3mg | ≤1.7 | 4mg | **⚠ High INR** |
| | | 1.8–2.4 | 3.5mg | *INR ≥8 (lower if other risk factors for bleeding)*—admit to hospital even if not bleeding. |
| | | 2.5–3 | 3mg | |
| | | 3.1–3.5 | 2.5mg for 4d | |
| | | >3.5 | 2mg for 4d | *INR >3.7 and <8*—omit warfarin 1–2d and recheck INR. Restart when INR <5 and retitrate dose. |
| 2.8–3.2 | 2mg | ≤1.7 | 3mg | |
| | | 1.8–2.4 | 2.5mg | |
| | | 2.5–3 | 2mg | |
| | | 3.1–3.5 | 1.5mg for 4d | |
| | | >3.5 | 1mg for 4d | |
| 3.3–3.7 | 1mg | ≤1.7 | 2mg | |
| | | 1.8–2.4 | 1.5mg | |
| | | 2.5–3 | 1mg | |
| | | 3.1–3.5 | 0.5mg for 4d | |
| | | >3.5 | omit for 4d | |
| >3.7 | 0mg | <2 | 1.5mg for 4d | |
| | | 2–2.9 | 1mg for 4d | |
| | | 3–3.5 | 0.5mg for 4d | |

Reproduced from Oates A et al. (1998) A new regime for starting warfarin therapy in outpatients, *British Journal of Clinical Pharmacology* **46**: 157–61, with permission of Wiley-Blackwell.

**Table 19.6** Warfarin therapy: recall periods during maintenance therapy

| INR | Recall interval and action |
|---|---|
| 1 high INR ⚠ If INR>8—admit | Recall 7–14d. Stop treatment for 1–3d (max 1wk in prosthetic valve patients) and restart at a lower dose. |
| 1 low INR | ↑ dose and recall in 7–14d. |
| 1 therapeutic INR | Recall 4wk. |
| 2 therapeutic INRs | Recall 6wk (maximum interval if prosthetic heart valve). |
| 3 therapeutic INRs | Recall 8wk* |
| 4 therapeutic INRs | Recall 10wk* |
| 5 therapeutic INRs | Recall 12wk* |

* Except prosthetic heart valves where maximum recall interval is 6wk.

⚠ Warfarin is a dangerous drug. In every case weigh up the pros and cons of prescribing.

# Haematological malignancy

⚠ **Suspected haematological malignancy** May present with non-specific symptoms/signs. Have a high level of suspicion.

### Immediate referral
- FBC/blood film reported as acute leukaemia
- Suspected spinal cord compression
- Suspected renal failure due to myeloma.

### Urgent referral to a team specializing in blood cancers
Persistent unexplained splenomegaly.

### Investigations
Combinations of the following symptoms/signs warrant examination and further investigation with FBC, blood film, and ESR (or CRP/plasma viscosity) ± referral to a team specializing in haematological malignancy.
- Drenching night sweats and/or fever
- Weight loss
- Generalized itching—in addition check U&E, Cr, eGFR, TFTs, LFTs
- Breathlessness—in addition check CXR
- Unexplained bleeding/bruising/purpura and/or symptoms suggesting anaemia
- Recurrent infections
- Persistent bone pain—in addition check X-ray, U&E, Cr and eGFR, liver profile, bone profile, and PSA (in men)
- Alcohol-induced pain
- Abdominal pain
- Splenomegaly—refer if persistent
- Fatigue—repeat FBC, blood film, and ESR at least once if condition remains unexplained and does not improve
- Lymphadenopathy—if present ≥6wk, LNs are increasing in size, LN >2cm in size, widespread lymphadenopathy, or associated weight ↓, night sweats and/or splenomegaly, consider further investigation, discussion with specialist, and/or referral.

**Multiple myeloma** Age usually >50y. 3750 new cases/y in the UK and 2500 deaths. A mutant B lymphoid clone is present. The proliferating cells grow mainly in the bone marrow where they cause infiltration, localized tumours, and bone erosion. Main sites of myeloma involvement are: skull, spinal column, thoracic cage, pelvis, and proximal long bones.

### Presentation
- Infection, e.g. chest infection
- Anaemia and/or bleeding
- Bone pain ± tenderness, particularly back, pelvis, femur
- Pathological fracture
- Hypercalcaemia
- Renal failure
- Hyperviscosity syndrome (CNS features, e.g. blurred vision, altered consciousness, confusion)
- Amyloidosis (heart, tongue, carpal tunnel).

## Investigation
- *FBC*—anaemia; *blood film*—rouleaux formation.
- *ESR* ↑↑.
- *Renal function*—↑ Cr; ↓ eGFR.
- *$Ca^{2+}$*—frequently ↑.
- *Serum electrophoresis*—paraprotein band.
- *Urine electrophoresis*—Bence Jones protein.
- *X-ray*—erosive lesions in skull, ribs, pelvis. Fractures and vertebral collapse are common.

**Management** Refer urgently to haematology. Specialist management depends on symptoms and whether there is tissue/organ damage.
- **Asymptomatic disease** Patients are usually monitored closely and treatment starts if symptoms or tissue/organ damage develop
- **Symptomatic disease** Treatment is with melphalan or combination chemotherapy, and steroids. Biological agents (bortezomib and/or interferon) may prolong effects of chemotherapy. Bisphosphonates are used to prevent and treat hypercalcaemia and bone pain. Bone pain may also respond to radiotherapy. Renal failure may require dialysis. Hyperviscosity may require plasmapheresis. Intensive chemotherapy + bone marrow/stem cell transplant is an option for younger fit patients.
- **Relapsed disease** Patients who have gone into remission almost always relapse at some point. If relapse is >6mo after initial treatment the patient is usually retreated with the same chemotherapy. Otherwise an alternative regime is used. The role of thalidomide and bortezomib in treatment of relapse is under evaluation.

**Prognosis** Overall 5y survival is 23%. However, for patients <70y who are fit enough to undergo intensive treatment, 5y survival more than doubles to 50%.

## Monoclonal gammopathy of undetermined significance (MGUS)
Presence of monoclonal paraprotein band in isolation with no other features of myeloma or other lymphoproliferative disease. Present in 1% >50y age and 5% if >80y. Usually found incidentally. Most remain stable but ~1%/y progress to myeloma or other haematological malignancy.

### Management
- Discuss with haematology/refer to exclude myeloma.
- Monitor clinical symptoms and check FBC, ESR, U&E, Cr and eGFR, and Ca, immunoglobulins, and electrophoresis at 3mo, 6mo, and then annually.
- Advise patients to re-attend promptly if new symptoms (e.g. back pain) develop.

## Further information
**NICE** Referral guidelines for suspected cancer (2005) 🖥 www.nice.org.uk
**British Committee for Standards in Haematology**
🖥 www.bcshguidelines.com
- Guidelines for the investigation of newly detected M-proteins and the Management of Monoclonal Gammopathy of Undetermined Significance (MGUS) (2009)
- Guidelines on the diagnosis and management of multiple myeloma (2005/6)

# Acute leukaemia

Clonal malignant disorders (from a single cell) affecting all age groups.

**Acute lymphoblastic leukaemia (ALL)** Abnormal proliferation in the lymphoid progenitor cells (Figure 19.2). Incidence is 1–4/100 000 population/y. ♂ > ♀. *Usual age range:* 2–10y with a peak at 3–4y. Accounts for 85% of childhood leukaemia. Incidence then falls with increasing age, apart from a secondary peak at ~40y.

**Acute myeloid leukaemia (AML)** Abnormal proliferation of a myeloid progenitor cell (Figure 19.2). There are at least 7 different subtypes. Most common leukaemia of adulthood with incidence of ~1.5/100 000 population/y. Incidence ↑ with age. Median age at presentation ~60y. ♂ = ♀. Risk factors include smoking (1:5 cases), previous chemotherapy or radiotherapy, and exposure to radiation. Children with Down's syndrome are more likely to develop AML.

**Presentation** Short history (weeks). Syptoms/signs arise from:
**Bone marrow failure** Anaemia—pallor, lethargy, dyspnoea; neutropoenia—infections of the mouth, throat, skin, fever; thrombocytopenia—spontaneous bruising, menorrhagia, bleeding from wounds, bleeding of gums or nose bleeds

**Organ infiltration** Superficial lymphadenopathy (>50%); hepatosplenomegaly (70%); bone pain (ALL only); skin infiltration (AML only); testicular enlargement; respiratory symptoms 2° to mediastinal LNs; gum hypertrophy; unexplained irritability/behaviour change/↓ performance.

**Differential diagnosis** Infections, e.g. EBV; other blood conditions, e.g. aplastic anaemia, ITP, myelodysplasia; other malignancies, e.g. lymphoma, neuroblastoma, metastatic disease; rheumatoid arthritis.

## Investigation
- *FBC* Normal or ↓ Hb and platelets; WCC <1×10⁹/L to >200×10⁹/L.
- *Blood film* Is abnormal with presence of blast cells.
- *Renal function* Renal impairment if leucocyte count is very high.
- *CXR* May show mediastinal mass and/or lytic bone lesions.

**Initial management** Refer for same-day specialist opinion if:
- Abnormal blood count reported as needing urgent investigation.
- Petechiae/pupura/spontaneous bleeding.
- Fatigue in a previously healthy individual if accompanied by generalized lymphadenopathy and/or hepatosplenomegaly.*
- Any other suspicious symptoms/signs.

* Children with an abdominal mass should always be referred for same-day assessment.

**Specialist management** Once diagnosis is confirmed, treatment is coordinated in specialized centres and involves intensive supportive care together with systemic chemotherapy and radiotherapy ± bone marrow transplant. For patients with ALL, treatment includes maintenance therapy for 2y to help maintain remission. Prognosis—Table 19.7.

### Short-term side effects of treatment
- *Treatment side effects* Most chemotherapeutic agents have pronounced side effects, e.g. nausea, vomiting, hair loss, neuropathy.

- *Immunosuppression* Any fever in a neutropoenic child or adult must be taken seriously and immediately referred back to the unit in charge of care. Likewise, any chickenpox contact must be referred immediately for consideration of administration of VZ-Ig, or measles contact for administration of measles Ig.

**Long-term side effects of treatment** Heart—cardiomyopathy, arrythmias; lung—fibrosis; endocrine system— growth delay, hypothyroidism, infertility; kidney—↓ eGFR; secondary malignancies—may appear after many years; psychological effects.

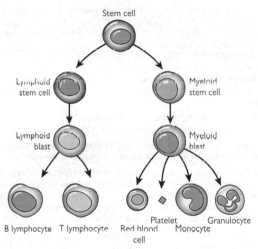

**Fig.19.2** Blood cell production

Reproduced with permission from CancerHelp UK, the patient information website of Cancer Research UK: 🖳 www.cancerhelp.org.uk

**Table 19.7** Prognosis of acute leukaemia

|  | Overall 5y survival |
| --- | --- |
| Childhood ALL | 80% |
| Adult ALL | 40% (80% achieve remission) |
| AML age <55y | 40–60% |
| AML age >55y | 20% |

**Information and support for patients and carers**
**Leukaemia Research Fund** ☎ 020 7405 0101 🖳 www.lrf.org.uk
**Children with Leukaemia** ☎ 020 7404 0808 🖳 www.leukaemia.org.uk
**CLIC and Sargent** ☎ 0800 197 0068 🖳 www.clicsargent.org.uk

# Chronic leukaemia and myeloproliferation

**Chronic lymphocytic leukaemia (CLL)** Occurs in the elderly accounting for 40% leukaemias in that age group. Closely related to small lymphocytic lymphoma (📖 p.679). 70–80% of all diagnoses follow FBC done for another reason. Otherwise presents with widespread painless lymphadenopathy often noted over a period of months/years. *Examination*: check for lymphadenopathy, splenomegaly ± hepatomegaly.

**Investigation** ↑ lymphocyte count (>$5\times10^9$/L). Blood film—small lymphocytes, many of which are disrupted to form 'smear'cells.

**Management** Refer to haematology or discuss with a haematologist depending on age and clinical state of the patient. Once diagnosis has been confirmed, well patients with low levels of lymphocytosis are often managed in primary care with regular FBC and clinical review (at least every 6mo). Treat infections promptly. Refer for treatment if:
• Symptomatic disease (fevers, sweats, weight ↓)
• Lymphadenopathy and/or hepatosplenomegaly
• Rising lymphocyte count (↑ >50% in 2mo or doubling time of <6mo)
• Anaemia or thrombocytopoenia.

*Specialist treatment* Chemotherapy/radiotherapy. Splenectomy is indicated for massive symptomatic splenomegaly and refractory cytopoenia.

❶ The term 'leukaemia' provokes fear in many. Explain the diagnosis of CLL, its benign nature in many, and that prognosis can be >10y.

**Chronic myeloid (granulocytic) leukaemia** *Peak age*: 30–60y. Chance finding in 20%. Otherwise presents with non-specific symptoms, e.g. weight ↓, lassitude, gout, anaemia. Splenomegaly is common—may present with abdominal pain, digestive symptoms or pleuritic pain due to splenic infarction. Rarely bleeding due to abnormal platelet function.

**Investigation** *FBC*: ↑ WCC (usually >$50\times10^9$/L) ± anaemia.
*Blood film:* bone marrow pre-cursors of myeloid cells (blasts).

**Management** Refer urgently to haematology. Treatment is determined by phase of the disease.
• *Chronic* (90% at diagnosis) <10% of cells in the bone marrow are immature blasts. Treatment of choice is imatinib (Glivec®) which has dramatically improved prognosis in recent years.
• *Accelerated* 10–30% of cells in the bone marrow are immature blasts. Treatment is with chemotherapy ± bone marrow/stem cell transplant, or dasatinib (unless not previously treated with imatinib).
• *Blast* (also called acute phase, blast crisis) >30% of cells in the bone marrow are immature blasts—treated with chemotherapy

**Myeloproliferative disorders** Proliferation of ≥1 of the haemopoietic components of the bone marrow. Includes:
• Chronic myeloid leukaemia
• Primary proliferative polycythaemia
• Essential thrombocythaemia
• Myelofibrosis.

**Polycythaemia** Increase in the number of circulating red cells. May be 1° (PPP) or 2°. Secondary polycythaemia may be:
- *Appropriate* High altitude, chronic lung disease (e.g. COPD), cardiovascular disease with a right → left shunt, heavy smoking, ↑ affinity for haemoglobin (familial polycythaemia) *or*
- *Inappropriate* Due to excess erythropoietin, e.g from renal tumour, hepatocellular tumour, or massive uterine fibroid.
❶ Hb may also appear ↑ if dehydrated—concentration effect.

**Primary proliferative polycythaemia (PPP)** Also known as polycythaemia rubra vera and erythrocytosis. Haematological malignancy resulting in overproduction of red cells. *Age range:* most >50y.

*Presentation* Non-specific symptoms/signs:
- Night sweats
- Dusky cyanotic hue with red face
- Itching (especially provoked by water, e.g. after a bath)
- Splenomegaly (70%) ± hepatomegaly
- Headaches, dizziness, vertigo, and/or tinnitus
- Gout—due to high red cell turnover
- Peptic ulceration (5–10%)
- Thrombosis and haemorrhage—due to abnormal platelet function and hyperviscosity.

*Investigation* May be diagnosed incidentally following FBC done for other reasons—↑Hb (usually >20g/dL) + haematocrit (>0.52 for ♂; >0.48 for ♀) sustained for >2mo.

*Management* Refer urgently to haematology. Hb level is ↓ by regular venesection ± cytotoxics. Aspirin ↓ risk of thrombosis. Slowly progressive, and survival for 10–20y is not unusual; 10–20% eventually transform to acute myeloid leukaemia; 1:3 to myelofibrosis.

**Essential thrombocythaemia** Rare disorder. Patients have ↑ risk of both thrombosis and haemorrhage due to abnormal platelet function. FBC—platelet count is persistently >600×10⁹/L. WCC is normal or ↑; Hb is ↑ or ↓. Refer urgently to haematology. Treatment is usually with hydroxycarbamide or interferon. May eventually transform to AML.

**Myelofibrosis (myelosclerosis)** Progressive accumulation of fibrous tissue in the bone marrow cavity replacing normal marrow. Haemopoietic function is taken over by the spleen/liver. Patients are usually elderly and present with symptoms of anaemia, malaise, fever ± gout. The spleen is massively enlarged. FBC—↓ Hb. *Blood film*—immature erythroid cells (normoblasts) and myeloid cells (metamyelocytes/myelocytes). Red cells are teardrop shaped. Refer urgently to haematology. Median survival is 2–3y, but many live much longer. 5–10% transform to AML.

**Further information**
**British Committee for Standards in Haematology**
🖳 www.bcshguidelines.com
- Diagnosis and management of chronic lymphocytic leukaemia (2004)
- Diagnosis and management of adult myelodysplastic syndromes (2003)

**Patient information and support**
**Leukaemia Research Fund** ☎ 020 7405 0101 🖳 www.lrf.org.uk

# Lymphoma

Cancer of the lymphatic system. Two main types.

**Non-Hodgkin's lymphoma (NHL)** Derived from malignant transformation of lymphocytes—85% B cells. Usually develops in LNs but can arise in any tissue. *Incidence:* 10 000 cases/y in the UK (4% cancers), causing 4500 deaths/y. ♂ = ♀. 69% occur in patients >60y.

**Presentation** May be detected incidentally on CXR (mediastinal mass) or present with painless peripheral lymphadenopathy; abdominal mass (nodal or spleen); weight ↓; night sweats/unexplained fevers. Other symptoms are dependent on site, e.g. neurological symptoms if CNS involvement; pleural effusion; skin lesions.

**Investigation** *FBC*—may be normal if no bone marrow involvement; monospot—perform in all patients <30y with persistent lymphadenopathy to exclude EBV; *ESR*—usually ↑; *LFTs*—abnormal if liver involvement.

**Initial management** Consider discussion with a haematologist, urgent referral for LN biopsy, or urgent referral to haematology if:
- Lymphadenopathy present ≥ 6wk
- LNs are increasing in size or LN >2cm in size
- Widespread lymphadenopathy
- Lymphadenopathy + weight ↓, night sweats and/or splenomegaly
- Any other suspicious symptoms/signs.

**Specialist treatment** is based on histology and stage. Treatment options include a wait-and-see approach for low-grade lymphomas, radiotherapy, chemotherapy, bone marrow transplant, monoclonal antibody therapy (rituximab), and/or immunotherapy.

**Prognosis** varies widely between different types of NHL and the age of the patient. Younger fitter patients with less widespread disease do better. Overall 5y survival is 51% with 45% surviving 10y.

**Hodgkin's lymphoma** 1200 cases/y in the UK. *Peak age ranges:* 15–35y (>50% occur <40y) and 50–70y. Derived from B lymphocytes. Two types of Hodgkin's lymphoma are recognized.
- *Classical* (95%)—Reed Sternberg cells present.
- *Nodular lymphocyte predominant* (5%)—'popcorn' cells present

**Presentation** Painless lymphadenopathy (70–95% have affected cervical LNs at diagnosis), weight ↓, night sweats/unexplained fevers, pruritus. The spleen is involved in 30% → splenomegaly.

**Investigation and management** As for NHL.
**Prognosis**
- *Early stage disease* (Ann Arbor stage 1/2—affected lymph tissue is confined to one side of the diaphragm): 80% 10y survival.
- *Late stage disease* (Ann Arbor stage 3/4—affected lymph tissue both sides of diaphragm and/or extralymphatic tissue involvement): 60% 5y survival.

*T. Hodgkin (1798–1866) English physician/pathologist.*

**Information and support**
Lymphoma Association ☎ 0808 808 5555 🖥 www.lymphomas.org.uk

**Table 19.8** Features of common type of NHL

| Type | Features |
|---|---|
| **High-grade NHL** | |
| Diffuse large B cell (DLBCL) | 20% of NHL (including childhood). For adults peak age=70y. |
| | Presents with rapidly enlarging lymphadenopathy. Extranodal involvement is common. 10% have bone marrow involvement at presentation. |
| Anaplastic large cell | Two forms. Both originate from T cells or unknown cells |
| | *Systemic form* Affects children/young adults. ♀>♂. Usually presents at a late stage and with systemic symptoms. |
| | *Cutaneous form* 5% NHL. Affects adults (peak age 61y). Presents with reddish-brown skin nodules or ulceration ± regional LN involvement (25%). |
| Burkitt's lymphoma | Affects children—30–40% childhood lymphoma. ♂>♀. B-cell lymphoma. Two varieties. Endemic variety is more common in Africa and associated with EBV infection. Peak age 5–10y. Sporadic variety occurs worldwide and affects slightly older children. |
| | Presents with bulky central nodal disease ± extranodal (typically abdomen), bone marrow, and/or CNS involvement. |
| **Low grade NHL** | |
| Follicular | Affects adults. B cell origin. Three types divided according to the ratio of small to large cells. |
| | Usually presents with disseminated disease. 50% present with bone marrow involvement. May transform to DLBCL. |
| Small lymphocytic | 4–5% NHL. Median age 60y. Clinically/morphologically identical to CLL (📖 p.676). Distinguished by degree of lymph tissue vs. blood/bone marrow involvement. |
| | Presents with diffuse lymphadenopathy and some blood/bone marrow involvement. 10–20% transform to CLL. 3% to DLBCL. |
| Mantle cell | 5% NHL. Affects adults usually >50y. ♂>♀ (4:1). Although classified as low grade, behaves and is treated as high grade. |
| | Usually presents with widespread disease involving LNs, bone marrow (60–90%), peripheral blood, and spleen. Poor prognosis. |
| Marginal zone | B-cell origin. Three distinct types. |
| | *Nodal* 1-3% NHL. Presents with localized lymphadenopathy. |
| | *Splenic* <1% NHL. Affects adults. Presents with massive splenomegaly and blood/bone marrow involvement without lymphadenopathy. |
| | *Mucosa associated (MALT)* 10% NHL. May be associated with inflammation (e.g. *H.pylori* infection and gastric MALT; Hashimoto's thyroiditis and thyroid MALT). 70% have localized disease on presentation. Symptoms depend on the organ involved |
| Lympho-plasmacytic | 1.5% NHL. Also called Waldenstrom's macroglobulinaemia. B-cell lymphoma. Average age at presentation is 63y. |
| | Often presents late with lymphadenopathy, splenomegaly, and bone marrow involvement. May spread to the lung or GI tract. Usually associated with paraproteinaemia (IgM). |

# Immune deficiency syndromes

A group of diverse conditions caused by immune system defects and characterized clinically by ↑ susceptibility to infections.

⚠ Consider an immunodeficiency disorder in anyone with infections that are unusually frequent, severe, resistant or due to unusual organisms.

**History** Ask about:
- Family history: immune deficiency, early death, similar disease, autoimmune illness, early malignancy.
- Adverse reaction to immunization or viral infection.
- Splenectomy, tonsillectomy, or adenoidectomy.
- Prior prophylactic antibiotic or immunoglobulin therapy.

**Primary immunodeficiency** Since many 1° immunodeficiencies are hereditary or congenital, they appear initially in infants and children. ~80% of those affected are <20y old and, owing to X-linked inheritance ♂>>♀. Genetic screening is available for some conditions. Refer all suspected cases to paediatrics/immunology.

*Classification* > 70 primary immunodeficiencies have been described. They are classified into 4 groups depending on which component of the immune system is deficient:
- B cells
- T cells
- Phagocytic cells
- Complement.

*Prevalence* Selective IgA deficiency (usually asymptomatic) occurs in 1:400 people. All other primary immune deficiencies are rare. Excluding IgA deficiency, ½ of affected patients have B-cell deficiency, 30% have T-cell deficiency, 18% have phagocytic deficiencies, and 2% have complement deficiency.

*Presentation* Table 19.9 lists some of the more common immune deficiencies. All immune deficiencies present with increased tendency to infections. Type of infection varies according the component of the immune system involved.

**Secondary immunodeficiency** Impairment of the immune system resulting from illness (including drug therapy, e.g. with cytotoxics or steroids) or removal of the spleen in a previously normal person. Often reversible if the underlying condition or illness resolves. 2° immunodeficiencies are common—most prolonged serious illness interferes with the immune system to some degree. Treat the cause.

**Asplenia and splenectomy** 📖 p.649

**Infection in the immunocompromised** 📖 p.648

**Information and support for patients**
**Immune Deficiency Foundation** 🖥 www.primaryimmune.org

**Table 19.9** Immune deficiency syndromes

| Type | Syndrome | Clinical details |
|------|----------|------------------|
| B-cell deficiency<br><br>Prone to infection with Gram +ve organisms (e.g. streptococci) | Selective IgA deficiency and IgG subclass deficiencies | Variable symptoms with most only mildly affected. When more severely affected, early treatment of infection may be required |
| | Congenital X-linked hypogamma-globulinaemia and Common variable immunodeficiency | Not inherited—cause unknown<br>↓ immunoglobulins<br>Treatment is with IV immunoglobulin<br>↑ risk of leukaemia/lymphoma |
| T-cell deficiency<br><br>Prone to viral, fungal, and opportunist infections | DiGeorge's syndrome | Defect on chromosome 22 → absent/hypoplastic thymus (and ↓ T cells), absent parathyroid glands ± cardiac and/or facial abnormalities<br>• Mild (80%)—treated supportively.<br>• Severe—requires thymus/bone marrow transplant |
| | HIV | 📖 p.744 |
| Combined B- and T-cell deficiency | Severe combined immunodeficiency | Autosomal or X-linked recessive<br>Absence of both T-cell and B cell immunity<br>Presents <6mo old with frequent infections.<br>Treatment is with bone marrow transplant.<br>Untreated most die at <1y. |
| | Ataxia telangectasia | Autosomal recessive<br>Selective IgA deficiency or hypogamma-globulinaemia and T-cell dysfunction<br>Characterized by telangectasia, cerebellar ataxia, and recurrent chest infections<br>Treatment is supportive<br>↑ risk of leukaemia/lymphoma |
| | Wiskott–Aldrich syndrome (partial combined immunodeficiency syndrome) | X-linked recessive.<br>↑IgA and IgE; normal or ↓ IgG; ↓ IgM<br>Presents with eczema, thrombocytopoenia and recurrent infections<br>Treatment is with bone marrow transplant—rarely survive beyond teens without ↑ risk of leukaemia/lymphoma |
| Phagocytic deficiency<br><br>Prone to staphylo-coccal and Gram –ve infections | Chronic granulomatous disease | X-linked ($^2/_3$) or autosomal recessive<br>Phagocyte dysfunction<br>Usually presents <6mo of age with fungal pneumonia, lymphadenopathy, hepatosplenomegaly and/or osteomyelitis<br>Treatment is supportive with prophylactic antibiotics and early treatment of infections |
| | Agranulocytosis | Usually caused by drugs e.g. carbimazole<br>Absence of neutrophils<br>Sudden onset of fever ± rigors, sore throat, mouth ulcers, headache and malaise → septicaemia<br>If suspected check urgent FBC and/or admit |

# Allergies

*One man's meat is another man's poison.*

Allergic diseases result from an exaggerated response of the immune system to external substances. Affects 1:6 of the British population—and is increasing. Allergic problems include:

- Asthma 📖 p.316
- Occupational asthma 📖 p.344
- Eczema 📖 p.612–614
- Anaphylaxis 📖 p.1068
- Urticaria 📖 p.618
- Rhinitis 📖 p.940
- Conjunctivitis 📖 p.964
- Food intolerance 📖 p.683.

## Assessment

- Age
- Symptoms—past and present, main problem, frequency and severity, seasonal/perennial, provoking factors
- Impact on lifestyle—time off work/school, sleep
- Occupation/hobbies
- Treatment—past and present
- Home environment—pets, damp, dust, smoking
- Allergies in the past
- Family history of allergic illness
- Examination will depend on main symptoms (e.g. asthma, 📖 p.316).

## Investigation

***Skin prick testing*** Identifies IgE sensitivity to common allergens, allowing diagnosis or exclusion of atopy. An alternative is measurement of serum IgE levels. In most places this is a 2°care procedure though a pilot study has shown it is feasible in general practice. Patients should avoid using antihistamines before skin prick testing.

***Patch testing*** Identifies substances causing contact allergy. A battery of allergens on discs are applied to the skin (usually on the back) and stuck in place with tape. The skin response is then monitored. Only done in specialist allergy or dermatology clinics.

## Management

***Allergen avoidance*** For patients with anaphylaxis may be lifesaving.
- ***Pets*** Exclude the offending animal
- ***Pollens*** Keep windows shut (including car windows); wear glasses/ sunglasses; avoid grassy spaces; fit a pollen filter on the car.
- ***Foods/drugs*** Avoid the food/drug; avoid hidden exposure (check labels carefully); inform any school/ clubs a child attends; take food with you wherever possible; record drug allergies in medical notes.

***House dust mite*** Evidence that anti-house-dust-mite measures are effective in the relief of asthma and eczema is not strong. Measures focus on the bedroom. Advise that the room should be ventilated regularly; encase mattresses, pillows, and duvets in mite-proof covers (leave in place 6mo); wash bedclothes at 60°C every 1–2wk; use a vacuum cleaner with an adequate filter; remove bedroom carpet; ↓ soft toys to a minimum and wash frequently/put in the freezer to kill house dust mites.

*Medication* See individual conditions.

*Referral to specialist allergy clinic*
- For investigation and management of anaphylaxis
- If the diagnosis of allergy is in doubt
- Food allergy
- Occupational allergy
- Urticaria in which allergic aetiology is suspected
- For consideration of immunotherapy.

**Bee/wasp sting allergy** Accounts for ~4 deaths/y in the UK. May result in a local or generalized reaction of varying severity. Intensity of reaction is also variable—because someone has had one bad reaction they will not necessarily have another. Treat local or mild generalized reactions with antihistamine. Supply patients with more severe reactions with an EpiPen® and teach them, and close contacts, to use it. Refer to an allergy clinic for consideration of desensitization.

**Food allergy** Affects 1.4% of the adult population and 5–7% of children. Types of adverse reaction to foods include:
- Type I food allergy—acute allergy e.g. acute peanut allergy.
- Type IV food allergy—delayed, e.g. milk causing eczema.
- Non-allergic food intolerance:
    - Pharmocological, e.g. tyramine in red wine or cheese may provoke migraine.
    - Metabolic, e.g. lactase deficiency.
    - Toxic, e.g. reaction to preservative rather than food.
- Food aversion—symptoms non-specific and unconfirmed by blinded food challenge.

A limited number of foods are responsible for the vast majority of cases of true food allergy—nuts (especially peanuts), wheat, eggs, fish, shellfish, and cows' milk.

*Management* Avoid offending food; refer to allergy clinic for confirmation of diagnosis and dietary advice; supply EpiPen® (and teach to use) in the interim if anaphylactic reaction.

**Patient information and support**
**Allergy UK** ☎ 01322 619898 ▣ www.allergyuk.org
**Anaphylaxis Campaign** ☎ 01252 542029 ▣ www.anaphylaxis.org.uk
**Medic Alert Foundation** Supply Medic Alert bracelets ☎ 0800 581 420
▣ www.medicalert.org.uk
**Medi-Tag** ☎ 0121 212 1616 ▣ www.hoopers.org/mediset.htm

## Breast awareness

Breast awareness means knowing what your breasts look and feel like normally. Evidence suggests that there is no need to follow a specific or detailed routine such as breast self-examination, but you should be aware of any changes in your breasts.

### The breast awareness 5-point code

1. Know what is normal for you.
2. Know what changes to look and feel for.
3. Look and feel.
4. Report any changes to your GP without delay.
5. Attend for routine breast screening if you are aged 50 or over.

### Changes to be aware of

- *Size*—if one breast becomes larger or lower.
- *Nipples*—if a nipple becomes inverted (pulled in) or changes position or shape.
- *Rashes*—on or around the nipple.
- *Discharge*—from one or both nipples.
- *Skin changes*—puckering or dimpling.
- *Swelling*—under the armpit or around the collarbone (where the lymph nodes are).
- *Pain*—continuous, in one part of the breast or armpit.
- *Lump or thickening*—different to the rest of the breast tissue.

**What should I do if I notice a change?** If you do notice a change in your breasts, see your GP as soon as you can. Your GP may ask you to come back at a different time in your menstrual cycle, or send you to a breast clinic for a more detailed examination.

❶ Remember that most breast changes are not cancer, even if they need follow-up treatment or further investigation.

### Further information

Breast cancer care ⌨ www.breastcancercare.org.uk
NHS Cancer Screening 'Be breast aware' leaflet and other information
⌨ www.cancerscreening.org.uk/breastscreen/breastawareness.html

# Breast disease

# Breast symptoms

## Urgent referral of patients with breast disease[N]

*Urgent referral* (to be seen in <2wk) is always required for:

### Lump
- Any age with a discrete hard lump with fixation ± skin tethering.
- Any age with a past history of breast cancer presenting with a further lump or other suspicious symptoms.
- Aged ≥30y with a discrete lump that persists after the next period, or presents after menopause.
- Aged <30y
  - With a lump that enlarges
  - With a lump that is fixed and hard
  - In whom there are other reasons for concern such as family history.

### Nipple changes
- Unilateral eczematous skin or nipple change that does not respond to topical treatment.
- Nipple distortion of recent onset.
- Spontaneous unilateral bloody nipple discharge.

### *Consider a non-urgent referral* if
- The woman is aged <30y and has a lump which has no suspicious features and is not enlarging.
- Breast pain and no palpable abnormality when initial treatment fails and/or symptoms persist (use of mammography is not recommended).

⚠ In patients presenting with symptoms and/or signs suggestive of breast cancer, investigation prior to referral is not recommended.

## Breast lump

*History* Age (malignancy is rare <30y); how and when noticed; relationship to menstrual cycle; changes in shape or size since noticed; pain; nipple discharge; pregnancy and breastfeeding; family history; current medication (in particular contraceptive pill or HRT).

*Examination* With the woman seated with arms at her sides, above her head, and pressing on her hips, look at the size and shape of the breasts, skin contour, and skin and nipple changes. Seat the woman at 45° supported on a couch. Ask her to place the hand on the side being examined behind her head. Ask the woman to point to or find the lump. Palpate each quadrant of the breast with a flat hand. Check the tail of the breast in the axilla. Examine both breasts. If a lump is found, assess shape, size, surface, edge, consistency, mobility, and attachments. Check local LNs in axilla and supraclavicular region and for hepatomegaly.

### Differential diagnosis
- Breast cancer (📖 p.694)
- Fibroadenoma (📖 p.690)
- Breast cyst (📖 p.690)
- Mammary duct ectasia/periductal mastitis (📖 p.691)
- Haematoma or fat necrosis (📖 p.690)
- Phyllodes tumour (📖 p.690)
- Intraductal pailloma (📖 p.691)
- Lipoma or sebaceous cyst.

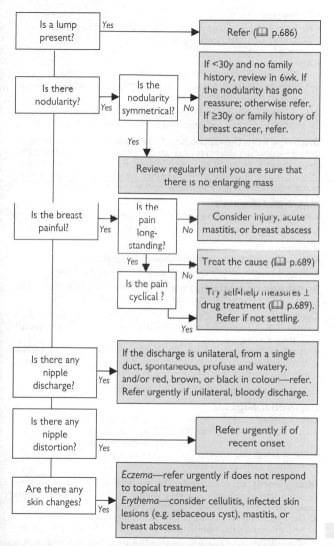

**Fig. 20.1** Algorithm for management of breast symptoms

## Management
- *No lump* Reassure. Educate the woman about breast awareness (📖 p.684). Consider reviewing in 6wk.
- *Discrete lump* Refer
- *Asymmetrical nodularity*
  - <30y with FH of breast cancer or ≥30y—non-urgent referral.
  - <30y and no family history—review in 6wk. If the nodularity has gone, reassure; otherwise refer.

❶ Any patient being referred with a breast lump will be concerned about the possibility of breast cancer, even though most will not have cancer.

**Discharge from the nipple** 90% of premenopausal women can express milky multiple-duct discharge. Ask about colour, quantity and whether the discharge is unilateral or bilateral. Examine to check for lumps. Note colour/quantity of discharge and whether the discharge is coming from multiple ducts or a single duct and is spontaneous or expressed.

## Differential diagnosis
- Physiological (e.g. pregnancy)
- Duct ectasia (📖 p.691)
- Breast cancer (📖 p.694)
- Intraductal papilloma (📖 p.691).

## Management
- Refer urgently if unilateral spontaneous bloody discharge.
- Refer if >50y or features suggesting pathological cause (Table 20.1).

**Breast pain or mastalgia** Most common in women aged 30–50y. Use a pain chart for >2mo to distinguish cyclical from non-cyclical pain.

**Cyclical breast pain** Common—~²/₃ of women >35y have cyclical mastalgia which causes distress or interferes with lifestyle. Symptoms are often long-standing. *Features*
- Usually bilateral although may not be the same intensity in both breasts
- Pain is generally felt over the lateral side of the breast, increases from mid-cycle onwards, and is relieved by menstruation.

Examination may reveal tenderness ± areas of nodularity/lumpiness.

## Differential diagnosis
- Physiological
- Duct ectasia/periductal mastitis (📖 p.691)
- Breast cancer (📖 p.694)
- Sclerosing adenosis (📖 p.690)
- Mastitis (📖 p.691)
- Breast abscess (📖 p.691)
- Referred pain (e.g. cervical root pressure)

## Management of mild/moderate cyclical pain 85% of patients.
Reassure that breast pain is a very *unusual* symptom of breast cancer. Explain the hormonal basis of symptoms. *Consider:*
- *Diet*—reducing saturated fats and caffeine may help.
- *Support*—advise the woman to try wearing a soft support bra at night.
- *OTC medication*—try simple analgesia (e.g. paracetamol) and/or NSAID. Some women also find oil of evening primrose (gamolenic acid) is effective, but it may take 4mo to work.
- *Changing/stopping hormonal contraceptives or HRT*

**Management of severe cyclical pain** Defined as pain for >7d/mo for >6mo which interferes with lifestyle. 15% of patients. Try measures for management of mild/moderate cyclical pain first. If they fail, consider:

- *Danazol*—100mg tds for 3–6mo. Start on day 1 of the menstrual cycle. Acne, weight gain, menorrhagia, and muscle cramps are common side effects. Withdraw if virilization.
- *Bromocriptine*—1–1.25mg nocte increased slowly to 2.5mg bd. Acts in <2mo but associated with pulmonary, retroperitoneal, and pericardial fibrotic reactions (CSM advises checking CXR and blood for ESR and Cr + eGFR prior to treatment, and monitoring for dyspnoea, persistent cough, chest pain, cardiac failure, and abdominal pain/tenderness). May also cause hypotensive reactions and/or sleepiness—warn not to drive or operate machinery if affected.
- *Tamoxifen* (unlicensed)—20mg on days of the cycle when symptoms are predicted. Common side effects include hot flushes and vaginal discharge. Associated with ↑ risk of DVT. Advise patients to report sudden breathlessness or unilateral calf pain. Also associated with endometrial changes including hyperplasia, polyps, and cancer. Advise patients to report menstrual irregularities, abnormal discharge, and/or pelvic pain/pressure.
- *LHRH analogues* (e.g. goserelin)—only used in specialist settings.

Drug treatment helps ~80% of women. Review treatment after 3–6mo and continue if necessary. After stopping, symptoms recur in about half, but are often less severe. Refer if treatment fails.

**Non-cyclical breast pain** Pain which is either continuous or intermittent but with no relationship to the menstrual cycle. Treat the cause. Ask if the pain is localized or diffuse.

- *Well-localized/point-specific*—consider breast cyst, breast abscess, mastitis, breast cancer (rarely presents with pain), chest wall causes (e.g. costochondritis).
- *More generalized*—usually referred pain. Consider nerve root pain, post-herpetic neuralgia, lung disease.

**Eczema of the nipple** Suspect underlying breast cancer. Refer for specialist assessment if no response to topical treatment (☐ p.694).

**Further information**

NICE Referral guidelines for suspected cancer (2005) 🖥 www.nice.org.uk

**Table 20.1** Features of nipple discharge which suggest physiological or pathological cause

| Physiological cause likely | Pathological cause likely—refer |
|---|---|
| Bilateral | Unilateral |
| Multiple ducts | Single duct |
| On expression only | Spontaneous |
| Green, milky | Red, brown, black |
| Stains only | Profuse and watery |

# Benign breast disease

Most breast complaints are benign and have a physiological basis. Despite this, most women with breast complaints 'assume the worst' when a new problem is discovered. In most cases reassurance that there is nothing sinister underlying their symptoms is all that is required.

**Mastalgia** 📖 p.688

**Fibroadenoma** An aberration of normal lobular development. Peak age 16–24y. 3 types: common, giant (>5cm diameter), and juvenile (adolescent girls). Present with a discrete, firm, non-tender, and highly mobile lump ('breast mouse'). Account for 13% of breast lumps.

*Management* Refer for confirmation of diagnosis—urgently if ≥30y, any personal/family history of breast cancer, or any sinister features (📖 p.686). Diagnosis is confirmed with a combination of USS, mammography, and fine-needle aspirate/core biopsy. If the lump is large (>4cm), the fibroadenoma is excised. In other groups, reassurance is usually all that is needed. 95% of fibroadenoma do not enlarge after diagnosis and 25% ↓ in size or disappear with time.

❶ Fibroadenomas may calcify in older women and give a characteristic appearance in mammograms

**Sclerosing adenosis** Benign condition resulting from over-proliferation of the terminal duct lobules. It can cause recurring pain and/or result in a small firm lump in the breast. Often detected incidentally on mammography as a calcified 'stellate' abnormality. Always refer for confirmation of diagnosis. Treatment is symptomatic.

**Phyllodes tumour** Peak age 40–50y. 3 types—benign (most common); borderline malignant (uncommon), and malignant (rare).

*Presentation and management* Presents with a breast lump. Refer for confirmation of diagnosis through a combination of USS, mammography, and fine-needle aspirate/core biopsy. Treatment is always surgical with wide excision of the lump. Recurrence may occur.

**Fat necrosis** Usually history of injury ± bruising. As bruising settles, scarring results in a firm lump in the breast ± puckering of the skin. Most common in women with large breasts. Always refer to a breast surgeon for triple assessment (USS, mammography + fine-needle aspiration/core biopsy). Once diagnosis is confirmed, no treatment is needed. The lump often disappears spontaneously.

**Breast cyst** Benign and fluid-filled. Cysts may be of any size, single, or multiple. Most common >35y. Usually pre-menopausal women but may occur in post-menopausal women taking HRT. Presents as a firm rounded lump which is not fixed and not associated with skin changes/skin tethering.

*First breast cyst* Refer for exclusion of malignancy—urgently if ≥30y, FH of breast cancer, or other suspicious features. Diagnosis is confirmed with aspiration and/or USS and/or mammography.

*Past history of breast cysts* 30% of patients who have had a breast cyst develop another at a later date. If the lump is accessible, it is reasonable to attempt aspiration. There is no need to send aspirated fluid for cytology if the fluid is *not* bloodstained and the lump completely resolves. Refer if the fluid aspirated is bloodstained, the lump does not disappear completely, the cyst refills, aspiration fails, or cytology reveals malignant or suspicious cells

⚠ Do not attempt aspiration if you have not been trained to do so as there is a small but significant risk of pneumothorax.

**Galactocoele** Milk-containing cyst which arises during pregnancy. Refer any new lump arising in pregnancy to a breast surgeon. Repeated aspiration may be needed. Resolves spontaneously.

**Duct ectasia** Occurs around the menopause. Ducts become blocked and secretions behind stagnate. Presents as discharge from ≥1 duct which may be bloodstained ± breast lump ± nipple retraction ('transverse-slit' appearance) ± breast pain.

**Management** Refer for confirmation of diagnosis—urgently if lump and/or bloodstained nipple discharge and/or nipple retraction. Usually no treatment is needed, although surgery may be required to confirm diagnosis, if discharge is troublesome, or to evert the nipple.

**Periductal mastitis** Infected subareolar ducts. Affects younger women than duct ectasia with peak age 32y. Presents with breast tenderness ± inflammation in the areolar area. May also have nipple discharge and/or retraction and/or an associated inflammatory mass/abscess.

**Management** Treat with antibiotics, e.g. co-amoxiclav 250/125 tds. Advise smokers that smoking can slow the healing process. If an abscess is present, refer for drainage. Refer if any residual inflammation or masses following treatment to exclude cancer. If recurrent infection, refer for consideration of surgery to remove the blocked duct

*Mastitis in lactating women* 📖 p.836

**Intraductal papilloma** Benign wart-like lump that forms within a duct just behind the areola. Perimenopausal women are more likely to have a single intraductal papilloma; younger women often have >1. May be bilateral. Presents with nipple discharge which may be bloodstained ± a subareolar lump/nodule (30%). Refer for confirmation of diagnosis—urgently if lump and/or bloodstained discharge. Usually excised.

**Breast abscess** Usually occurs in a lactating breast following mastitis; occasionally in a non-lactating breast in association with indrawn nipple, mammary duct ectasia, or local skin infection. Presents with gradual onset of pain in one breast segment with hot tender swelling of the affected area.

**Management** Refer for surgical assessment. May be treated with repeated aspiration under ultrasound guidance or surgical incision and drainage.

**Mammary duct fistula** Fistula between a mammary duct and the skin. Usually a complication of a breast abscess. Refer for surgical excision.

# Breast cancer screening

In the UK there has been a national screening programme for breast cancer since 1988 (Table 20.2). The aim of the programme is to detect breast cancer at an early stage in order to ↑ survival chances (stage I tumours—5y survival 84%; stage IV tumours—5y survival 18%).

**Breast awareness** Trials of self-examination have not ↓ mortality. Instead, less formal 'Breast Awareness' is advocated (📖 p.684).

## Screening test

***Women >50y*** Two-view mammographic screening is currently available to women aged 50–70y every 3y. This is soon to be extended to women aged 47–73y. Older women can also request screening every 3y. Screening detects 85% of cancers in women aged >50y (60% of which are impalpable) and ~70–80% screening-detected cancers have good prognosis. Screening more frequently does not ↓ mortality.[R] Organization of breast cancer screening in the UK—Figure 20.2.

***High-risk women <50y*** Women with a family history of breast cancer may be at ↑ risk of breast cancer themselves (Figure 20.3, 📖 p.695) and may benefit from earlier screening and/or genetic screening.
* All raised/high-risk women aged 40–49y should be offered annual two-view mammography
* Women known to have a genetic mutation should be offered annual MRI surveillance—from 20y if TP53 mutation, and from 30y if BRCA1/2 mutation.
* MRI surveillance should also be offered to women aged 30–39y with 10y risk >8%, women aged 40–49y with 10y risk >20%, and at-risk women aged 40–49y with a dense breast pattern on mammography.

**Interval cancers** Cancer occurring in the interval between screens. Can occur through failure to detect a cancer at screening or as a result of a new event after screening took place. In the 1st year after screening 20% breast cancers are interval cancers. This ↑ to ~60% in the 3rd year.

**Acceptability of screening** 81% of women find mammography uncomfortable but 90% return for subsequent screens. GPs have an important role—sending personalized invitations for screening to women from their GPs increases uptake rates.[R]

**Anxiety due to screening** False-positive results cause anxiety as well as prompting further invasive investigations. Anxiety levels in women recalled and then found to be disease free are higher in the year after the recall appointment than in women who receive negative results at screening.

## Further information

**NHS Breast Screening** 🖥 www.cancerscreening.org.uk
**NICE** Familial breast cancer (2006) 🖥 www.nice.org.uk

**Information for patients** 🖥 www.cancerscreening.org.uk
* Breast Screening—the Facts
* Over 70? You are still entitled to breast screening.

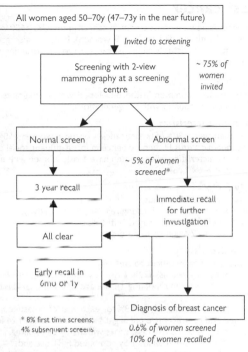

**Fig. 20.2** Organization of breast cancer screening in the UK

**Table 20.2** Pros and cons of breast cancer screening

| Benefits | Adverse effects |
|---|---|
| • Earlier diagnosis<br>• Improved prognosis and lower mortality<br>• Less radical and invasive treatment needed<br>• Reassurance for those with –ve results. | • Discomfort and inconvenience of screening<br>• Radiation risks of screening (very small)<br>• Reassurance to those women who have false –ve results<br>• Reassurance to those who develop an interval cancer and possibly later presentation due to false sense of security<br>• Anxiety and adverse effects of further investigation for those with false +ves<br>• Overdiagnosis of minor abnormalities that would never develop into breast cancer<br>• Earlier knowledge of disease and overtreatment for those for whom, despite early diagnosis, the prognosis is unchanged. |

# Breast cancer

Breast cancer is now the most common cancer in the UK: >100 women/d are diagnosed with the disease (1 in 9 women). Men can also get breast cancer but it is rare. Virtually all breast cancers are adenocarcinoma (85% ductal, 15% lobular)

## Risk factors

**Geography** More common in the developed world—migrants assume the risk of the host country within 2 generations.

### Personal characteristics

- *Age*—↑ with age—~80% of breast cancers occur in women >50y.
- *Socio-economic status* Higher incidence in more affluent social classes.
- *Physical characteristics* Taller women have ↑ risk; women with denser breasts have 2–6× ↑ risk.

### Lifestyle factors

- *Obesity* ↑ risk post menopause.
- *Physical activity* 30% ↓ risk if taking regular physical activity.
- *High fat diet* Probably associated with ↑ risk.
- *Alcohol* ↑ risk by 7%/unit consumed/d.

### Reproductive history

- *Early menarche or late menopause*↑ risk.
- *Pregnancy* ↑ parity → ↓ risk (32% ↓ risk in women reporting 3 births compared with women reporting 1); late age when first child is born ↑ risk.
- *Breastfeeding* ↓ relative risk by 4.3% for each year of breastfeeding.
- *Combined oral contraceptive pill* Slight ↑ risk (relative risk 1.24 for current users)—excess risk disappears within 10y of stopping.
- *HRT* Risk ↑ by 6 cases/1000 after 5y combined HRT use and 19 cases /1000 after 10y use. Risk for combined oestrogen and progesterone preparations is greater than oestrogen-only preparations. HRT also ↓ sensitivity of mammography.

### Other past medical history

- *Past history of breast disease* Ductal or lobular carcinoma in situ, florid hyperplasia, and papilloma with fibrovascular core all ↑ risk.
- *Ionizing radiation* Exposure ↑ risk.

**Family history** Referral algorithm—Figure 20.3
- *One first-degree relative with breast cancer (mother or sister)* Risk ↑ 2×, but 95% of women with breast cancer have no family history
- *Several family members with early onset breast cancer* Refer for genetic screening—BRCA1 and BRCA2 genes account for 2–5% of all breast cancers.

❶ Family relationships:
- *First-degree relative*—mother, father, sister, brother, daughter, son.
- *Second-degree relative*—grandparents, grandchildren, aunt, uncle, niece, nephew, half-sister, half-brother.

**Breast cancer screening** 📖 p.692.

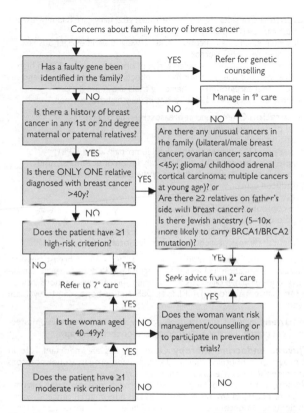

### High risk criteria
**Female breast cancer**
1x 1st degree relative + 1x 2nd degree relative diagnosed < average age of 50y
2x 1st degree relatives diagnosed < average age of 50y
1x 1st degree relative with bilateral breast cancer where first primary diagnosed at <50y
?3x 1st/2nd degree relatives

**Male breast cancer**
1x 1st degree relative

**Breast and ovarian cancer**
1x 1st/2nd degree relative with breast cancer + another with ovarian cancer (1 must be 1st degree relative)

### Moderate risk criteria
**Female breast cancer**
1x 1st degree relative <40y
1x 1st degree relative + 1x 2nd degree relative diagnosed > average age of 50y
2x 1st degree relatives diagnosed > average age of 50y

**Fig. 20.3** Referral of women with family history of breast cancer[N]

**Prevention** Consider referral to secondary/tertiary care if family history of breast cancer (📖 p.694)
- Lifestyle measures—↓ alcohol intake; ↓ weight; avoid exogenous sex hormones (e.g. HRT); breast feed.
- Chemoprophylaxis—Tamoxifen ↓ risk of breast cancer by 40% in high risk women but use is limited by side effects (thromboembolism and endometrial carcinoma)—other drug trials are in progress.
- Prophylactic surgery—↓ risk by 90% in very high risk women.

**Presentation** Often found at breast screening (📖 p.692).
Clinical presentations include:
- Breast lump (90%)
- Breast pain (21% present with painful lump; pain alone <1%)
- Nipple skin change (10%). Any red scaly lesion or eczema around the nipple suggests *Paget's disease of the breast*—intraepidermal intraductal cancer.
- Family history (6%)
- Skin contour change (5%)
- Nipple discharge (3%)
- Rarely presents with distant metastases, e.g. bone pain
- In the elderly, may present with extensive local lesions.

**Management** Refer for urgent assessment (<2wk) to a breast surgeon. Specialist investigation includes mammography, USS ± fine-needle aspiration, or core biopsy. If diagnosis is confirmed, further investigations include tumour markers and/or CT/MRI, liver USS, and/or bone scan to evaluate spread.

**Treatment** Includes surgery (lumpectomy ± axillary clearance, mastectomy), endocrine therapy, radiotherapy, and/or chemotherapy.

*Adjuvant endocrine therapy* Oestrogen has an important role in the progression of breast cancer. Oestrogen and progesterone receptors determine the response to endocrine therapy.
- *Tamoxifen* ↑ survival of patients with oestrogen receptor +ve tumours (60% tumours) of any age but rarely causes endometrial cancer—warn patients to report any untoward vaginal bleeding. Continue tamoxifen for ≥5y—take advice from a specialist prior to stopping.
- *Anastrozole, letrozole and exemestane*—block synthesis of oestrogen. Superior efficacy when compared with tamoxifen for postmenopausal women with hormone-sensitive early breast cancer and first choice drug for postmenopausal women with advanced breast cancer. Continue for ≥5y—take advice from a specialist prior to stopping.
- *Trastuzumab* Monoclonal antibody directed against HER2, a receptor found in 1:5 breast cancers. Affects division and growth of breast cancer cells. Treatment option for women with early HER2 +ve cancer at high risk of recurrence and women with advanced HER2 +ve breast cancer. Administered IV every 3 wk for 1y.

❶ Optimum treatment regimes for breast cancer change regularly and there are regional variations. Many women will be asked to participate in clinical trials to answer important questions about best treatments.

**Prognosis** 72% of women diagnosed now will live 10y; 64% live ≥ 20y.
- Recurrence is most likely <2y after treatment—late recurrences do occur but the longer since diagnosis, the less the chance of recurrence.
- Prognosis for a given individual depends on age (best prognosis if 50–69y), stage of disease (Table 20.3), grade of tumour, and oestrogen receptor status (oestrogen receptor –ve tumours have poorer prognosis).
- Women living in affluent areas have better survival rates than those in deprived areas.

**Psychological impact of breast cancer** Depression, anxiety, marital, and sexual problems are common. Be sensitive. Discuss possibilities of reconstructive surgery or breast prostheses as appropriate. Refer to specialist breast care nurse for support and advice.

**Lymphoedema** 📖 p.1039

**Table 20.3** Classification of breast cancer stage

| Stage | TNM equivalent | Features |
|---|---|---|
| In situ | Tis N0 M0 | Non-invasive |
| I | T1 N0 M0 | ≤2cm diameter<br>No LNs affected<br>No spread beyond breast |
| II | T0–2 N1 M0 or<br>T2/3 N0 M0 | 2–5cm diameter and/or LNs in axilla involved<br>No evidence of spread beyond axilla |
| III | T0-2 N2 M0 or<br>T3 N1/2 M0 or<br>T4 any N M0 or<br>Any T N3 M0 or | >5cm diameter<br>LNs in axilla involved<br>No evidence of spread beyond the axilla |
| IV | Any T/N M1 | Any-sized tumour<br>LNs in axilla may be affected<br>Distant metastases |

**Sentinal lymph node biopsy** Prognosis and decisions about adjuvant treatment are based on knowledge of the axillary node status. The only way to assess that is to remove nodes surgically and look at them under the microscope. Axillary node clearance can result in lymphoedema and decreased arm function. Sentinel node biopsy is the removal of the key or sentinel LN in patients undergoing surgery for early breast cancer to accurately predict the state of nodal disease in the remaining axillary LNs. Radical axillary surgery to clear the axillary nodes can then be reserved for the 20–40% with a +ve sentinel LN biopsy.

**Further information**
**NICE** Familial breast cancer (2006) 🖳 www.nice.org.uk

**Information and support for patients**
**Breakthrough breast cancer** ☎ 08080 100 200 🖳 www.breakthrough.org.uk
**Breast Cancer Care** ☎ 0808 800 6000 🖳 www.breastcancercare.org.uk

# Gynaecology

# The menstrual cycle

A good working understanding of the menstrual cycle is essential to understand its endocrine disorders and their management. One menstrual cycle lasts from the start of one period until the day before the start of the next. The average length of a cycle is 28d, but anything from 24 to 35d is common. The menstrual cycle is split into 4 (Figure 21.1).

## Follicular or proliferative phase

*Hormone changes* Levels of oestrogen and progesterone, are low. There is ↓ negative feedback on the pituitary as a result; thus follicle-stimulating hormone (FSH) levels ↑. FSH stimulates follicle development in the ovary. The developing follicles then produce oestrogen.

### Changes within the reproductive organs

- *Ovaries*—follicles develop. One follicle becomes dominant.
- *Uterus*—lining thickens (proliferates).
- *Vagina*—tends to be drier with thicker mucus.

**Ovulation** Occurs halfway through a cycle (~14d. after the start of the period). The dominant follicle ruptures and an egg is released into the fallopian tube. The follicle fills with blood after rupturing and there may be brief pain—*Mittelschmerz*. The egg travels along the Fallopian tube into the uterus, and may be fertilized if the woman is sexually active and not using contraception.

## Secretory or luteal phase

*Hormone changes* After ovulation, the ruptured follicle forms the corpus luteum (yellow body), and secretes oestrogen and progesterone.

### Changes within the reproductive organs

- *Ovaries*—corpus luteum forms. If pregnancy does not occur the corpus luteum begins to degenerate ~4d prior to menstruation.
- *Uterus*—progesterone causes the lining of the uterus to alter so that it is ready to receive a fertilized egg. The endometrium becomes oedematous and more vascular, and the glandular component becomes coiled and tortuous.
- *Vagina*—mucus becomes thinner, more watery, and slippery. It becomes thicker again towards the next period as progesterone ↓.
- *Other changes*—progesterone may cause 'water retention', breast tenderness, and mood changes.

**Periods (menstruation)** With the regression of the corpus luteum, oestrogen and progesterone levels ↓. There is necrosis, bleeding, and sloughing of the endometrium, resulting in a period or menstruation. Periods begin aged 11–16y and continue until the menopause—usually between 45 and 55y. Bleeding can last from 1 to 8d (average 5d) and is generally heaviest in the first 2d. Blood loss in each period is ~20–60mL (>80mL is associated with anaemia). Some period pain is common and normal.

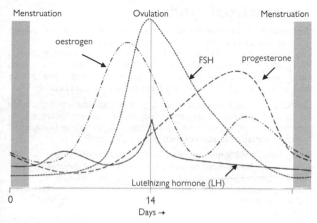

Fig. 21.1 Hormone changes throughout the menstrual cycle

**Prolonged menstruation** Bleeding for >5–6d/cycle. Most loss occurs in the first 3d. Long periods do not equate to ↑ menstrual loss, so prolonged menstruation *per se* does not need investigation. Frequently goes with menorrhagia—📖 p.706.

### Postponing menstruation
- *Combined oral contraceptive (COC) pill*—started ≥1mo before and continued throughout the time the withdrawal bleed should have occurred (two packets back-to-back without a break). The withdrawal bleed will occur after the second packet is finished.
- *Combined oral contraceptive patch*—can be used for 6wk without a patch-free break to postpone a period.
- *Norethisterone*—5mg tds starting 3d before the anticipated onset of menstruation. Menstruation will occur 2–3d after stopping the norethisterone.

### Odd colour/smell of menstrual blood No known associations.

### Post coital and intermenstrual bleeding
- *Post-coital bleeding (PCB)* Non-menstrual bleeding occuring after sexual intercourse. Always consider cervical pathology (📖 p.724). Other possible causes include infection, vaginal pathology, and trauma.
- *Intermenstrual bleeding (IMB)* Vaginal bleeding at any time during the menstrual cycle other than mestruation. May be physiological or indicative of cervical pathology (📖 p.724). Other possible causes include drugs (e.g. POP or other progestogenic contraceptive, COC, tamoxifen), pregnancy, infection, and other gynaecological tumours.

⚠ Always perform a full pelvic examination. If suggestive of cervical cancer refer urgently (<2wk) for gynaecology opinion. Do not wait for a smear result. Consider urgent referral if persistent intermenstrual bleeding but normal examination.

# Premenstrual syndrome

Most women of reproductive age notice some symptoms/bodily changes in the days/weeks leading up to their periods. These changes resolve, or ↓ significantly, during the period. They are termed premenstrual tension (PMT) or premenstrual syndrome (PMS) if they occur on a regular basis and are severe enough to interfere with quality of life. >95% women have some symptoms but <1:5 seek help. Debilitating symptoms occur in 5%.

**Cause** Underlying mechanism is not fully understood but is thought to be due to the hormonal changes that occur after ovulation affecting neurotransmitters in the brain. Premenstrual symptoms can also be precipitated by giving exogenous hormones such as the COC or HRT.

**Symptoms** >100 symptoms described. The most common are:
- Psychological—nervous tension, mood swings and/or irritability (when severe termed **premenstrual dysphoric disorder** (PMDD))
- ↑ weight and abdominal bloating
- Breast tenderness
- Headache.

**Management** Aims to alleviate symptoms. Usually symptoms return when treatment is stopped.
- Take a history of symptoms and ask the patient to keep a diary to establish cyclical nature.
- If mild/moderate symptoms, try lifestyle/dietary modification first:
  - Make allowances on days when symptoms are likely to be worst
  - Wear loose clothes if feeling bloated
  - Ensure adequate sleep and take regular exercise
  - Eat regularly—some find that small frequent meals help; avoid sweet snacks between meals; make sure diet is low in fat/salt, caffeine and alcohol, and contains plenty of fruit/vegetables and complex carbohydrate (e.g. bread, pasta, rice, potatoes)
  - ↓ fluid intake or eat diuretic foods (e.g. strawberries, water melon, aubergines, prunes, figs, parsley) to ease fluid retention
  - OTC remedies may help (Table 21.1).
- Consider drug therapy (Table 21.1) if symptoms are severe or do not respond to diet and lifestyle measures. Base choice on symptoms.
- For all treatments try a 3–6mo trial. Ask women to keep a symptom diary. Follow-up—the first treatment may not work.
- If primary care management is ineffective, refer to gynaecology/ psychiatry for specialist management.

**❶** Because of side effects, oestrogen patches and gonadotrophin-releasing hormone analogues are usually only used by specialists for severe or resistant PMS/PMDD.

**Further information**
**RCOG** Management of premenstrual syndrome (2007) ⌨ www.rcog.org.uk

**Information and support for patients and their partners**
National Association for Premenstrual Syndrome ☎ 0870 777 2178
⌨ www.pms.org.uk

**Table 21.1** Treatment of premenstrual tension

| Treatment | Effective? | Notes |
|---|---|---|
| **Hormonal manipulation** | | |
| COC[G] | ✓ | First-line treatment. The RCOG recommends combined new gerneration pills e.g. Yasmin® or Cilest®—given cyclically or continuously. |
| Low dose oestrogen[G] | ✓ | Second-line treatment. Use 100 mcgm oestradiol patches. To avoid giving unopposed oestrogen, combine with duphaston 10mg from day 17–28 or IUS if the uterus in intact. |
| GNRH analogues[R] | ✓ | Reserved for specialist care. Usually given in combination with add-on HRT. |
| **Antidepressants** | | |
| SSRIs[G] | ✓ | ↓ physical as well as psychological symptoms. First-line treatment that can be given continuously or just in the luteal phase (days 15–28). |
| **Other drugs** | | |
| Diuretics[CE] | ✓ | Spironolactone is effective for bloating/breast tenderness. Many women prefer 'natural' diuretics e.g Waterfall® though there is no evidence of effectiveness. |
| NSAIDs[CE] | ✓ | Particularly helpful for pre-menstrual pain and to ↓ menstrual bleeding. |
| **Surgery** | | |
| Hysterectomy + oophorectomy[G] | ✓ | Curative. Most women require HRT/ testosterone replacement afterwards. |
| **Complementary therapies** | | |
| Oil of evening primrose[S] | ✓/✗ | May help breast tenderness. Can cause fits in patients with epilepsy. |
| Vitamin B6[G] | ✓ | Most studies suggest effective—advise women to take 10mg/d. High doses (>100mg/d) may cause reversible peripheral neuropathy. |
| Chaste-tree berry (Vitex agnus-castus)[S] | ✓ | Evidence of effectiveness is generally positive—can cause menstrual irregularity. |
| Magnesium supplements[G] | ✓ | Evidence of effectiveness is generally positive. Used in the pre-menstrual phase. |
| Calcium supplements[S] | ✓ | ↓ symptoms including breast tenderness and swelling, headaches, migraine, and abdominal cramps. |
| Exercise[CE] | ✓ | High-intensity exercise improves symptoms > low-intensity exercise. |
| Cognitive therapy[CE] | ✓ | Evidence that effective. Effects are smaller and slower than SSRI—but more long-lasting. |
| Relaxation/ Reflexology[R] | ✓/✗ | Conflicting evidence—can do no harm. |

# Amenorrhoea

**Oligomenorrhoea** Infrequent periods. Manage as for amenorrhoea.

**Primary amenorrhoea** No 2° sexual characteristics or menstruation by age 14y with growth failure *or* no menstruation by age 16y when growth and sexual development is normal. *Causes:*
- *Outflow abnormalities* Mullerian agenesis, transverse vaginal septum, androgen insensitivity (androgen insensitivity syndrome 📖 p.893), imperforate hymen.
- *Ovarian disorders* PCOS; gonadal dysgenesis due to chromosomal abnormalities e.g. Turner's syndrome—❶ gonads may have malignant potential.
- *Pituitary disorders* Prolactinoma (📖 p.378).
- *Hypothalamic disorders* Kallman's syndrome.

**Secondary amenorrhoea** Absence of menses for ≥6 mo in a previously menstruating woman. *Causes:* Figure 21.2.

**History** Always consider the possibility of pregnancy
- *Symptoms*
  - Galactorrhoea—30% prolactinomas
  - Weight change
  - Hirsutism
  - Life crisis or upset, e.g. exams, bereavement
  - Level of exercise—gymnasts are frequently amenorrhoeic
  - Sweats and/or flushes
  - Cyclical pain.
- *Family history* of premature menopause or late menarche.
- *Drug history* particularly contraceptives, e.g. injectable progestogens.
- *Past history* of chemo- or radiotherapy or gynaecological surgery.

## Examination
- *Weight and height*—common if BMI <19kg/m$^2$.
- *External genitalia*—structural abnormality, virilism.
- *Vaginal examination*—including cervical smear if overdue.
- *Pelvic examination*—ovarian masses, uterine size.
- *General examination*—2° sexual characteristics, hirsutism, ↓ weight, systemic disease.
- *Visual fields and retinal examination*

❶ Replace vaginal and pelvic examination with pelvic USS in young girls.

## Investigation
- *Blood*—serum prolactin; TFTs; FSH/LH; karyotype if phenotypical abnormality; serum testosterone if LH high, hirsutism, or virilism.
- *USS pelvis* if structural abnormality or PCOS suspected.

**Management** Treat the cause:

*Contraception*
- Injectable progestogens—periods usually return within a year.
- Other hormonal methods—look for another cause.

*Weight* Investigate and treat reasons (e.g. anorexia). Encourage weight ↑. If no response refer to gynaecology.

*Physical exercise* Explain the reason for the amenorrhoea—many refuse to cut their activity levels, so consider HRT/COC pill to protect bone density.

*Stress* Reassure. Treat any psychiatric problems—periods should return spontaneously. Set a limit for return (e.g. another 3–4mo). If periods do not return consider referral as there may be another cause.

### Endocrine
- Thyroid dysfunction—treat hyper- or hypothyroidism.
- Hypothalamic causes—after 6mo there is ↑ risk of coronary heart disease and osteoporosis. Consider use of HRT or COC pill.
- Hyperprolactinaemia—refer to gynaecology or endocrinology.

### Gynaecological
- Premature menopause (📖 p. 709)
- PCOS (📖 p.723).

**Cause not found** Refer to gynaecology.

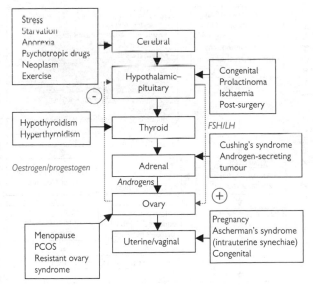

**Fig. 21.2** Causes of secondary amenorrhoea

### Further information
Monga A, Baker PN (eds) *Gynaecology by Ten Teachers* (2006) Hodder Arnold, London. ISBN: 0340816627.

# Menorrhagia

Menorrhagia (heavy periods) is defined as menstrual loss ≥80mL/mo 10% meet this criterion but 1:3 feel their loss is excessive. Ask about number of tampons or pads used daily, use of double protection to prevent leaks, flooding, and clots to gauge bleeding. Ask how periods affect life and activities. A menstrual diary may help. *Assessment:* Figure 21.3.

**Differential diagnosis** Physiological bleeding or dysfunctional uterine bleeding (50%). *Other causes:*

- Fibroids
- Congenital uterine abnormality, e.g. bicornuate uterus
- Pelvic infection
- Endometriosis
- Endometrial/cervical polyps
- Presence of IUCD
- Endometrial carcinoma
- Bleeding tendency
- Hormone-producing tumours.

❶ Hyper- or hypothyroidism, DM, prolactin disorders, adrenal, kidney, or liver disease, and some medications can also cause menstrual disturbance

**Dysfunctional uterine bleeding (DUB)** Excessive menstrual loss in the absence of any detectable abnormality.

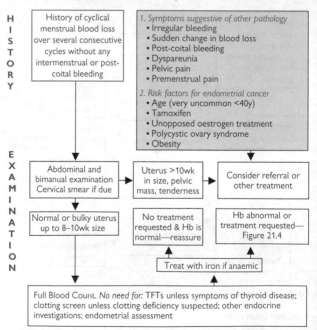

**Fig. 21.3** Assessment of menorrhagia in primary care

Reproduced from NICE Guidance on Heavy Menstrual Bleeding (2007), with permission from the National Collaborating Centre for Women's and Children's Health.

***Management*** (Figure 21.4) *Treatment may fail if:* high blood loss; low pre-treatment loss; other uterine pathology; lack of concordance. *2° care management:* assessment of endometrium; IUS; surgery—endometrial resection and ablation, myomectomy, hysterectomy ± oophorectomy.

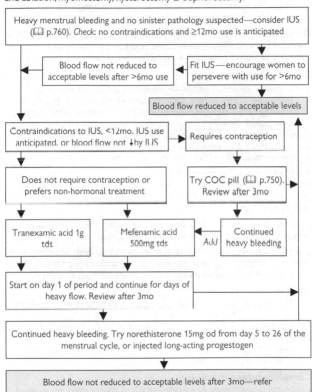

Heavy menstrual bleeding and no sinister pathology suspected—consider IUS (▢ p.760). *Check:* no contraindications and ≥12mo use is anticipated

Blood flow not reduced to acceptable levels after >6mo use

Fit IUS—encourage women to persevere with use for >6mo

Blood flow reduced to acceptable levels

Contraindications to IUS, <12mo. IUS use anticipated, or blood flow not ↓ by IUS

Requires contraception

Does not require contraception or prefers non-hormonal treatment

Try COC pill (▢ p.750). Review after 3mo

Tranexamic acid 1g tds

Mefenamic acid 500mg tds

*Add* Continued heavy bleeding

Start on day 1 of period and continue for days of heavy flow. Review after 3mo

Continued heavy bleeding. Try norethisterone 15mg od from day 5 to 26 of the menstrual cycle, or injected long-acting progestogen

Blood flow not reduced to acceptable levels after 3mo—refer

Fig. 21.4 Medical management of menorrhagia in primary care

Reproduced from NICE Guidance on Heavy Menstrual Bleeding (2007), with permission from the National Collaborating Centre for Women's and Children's Health

### △ Management of very heavy bleeding

- Resuscitate as necessary—admit if shocked. D&C in the acute situation can ↓ haemorrhage by 75–80%.
- Stop bleeding with progestogen, e.g. norethisterone 5mg tds for 10d. Effective in 24–48h. A lighter bleed follows on stopping. Alternatively, consider tranexamic acid (1g tds for 4d) to ↓ bleeding.
- Correct anaemia and refer for gynaecology assessment.

### Further information

**NICE** Heavy menstrual bleeding (2007) ▣ www.nice.org.uk

# The menopause

From the Greek *men* (month) and *pausis* (halt). Menopause occurs when menstruation stops. Average age in the UK ~50y. Smoking brings it forwards by ~2y. Impact on a woman's life varies and depends on cultural, health, and social factors.

**Diagnosis** >12mo amenorrhoea with no other cause in ♀ >50y *or* >24mo amenorrhoea in ♀ <50y. The *climacteric* refers to the time as the ovaries fail, when production of oestrogen ↓ over a number of years.

## Period changes

- *Changes in menstrual pattern*—common in the years before the menopause. Typically cycle shortens after 40y by up to 7–10d. Cycle then lengthens—periods may occur at 2–3mo intervals until stopping.
- *Dysfunctional uterine bleeding*—common leading up to the menopause but investigate post-menopausal, very heavy, painful, irregular, intermenstrual, or post-coital bleeding.
- *Late menstruation (>54y)*—investigate as ↑ risk of malignancy.

**Psychological symptoms** Controversial. Some studies report that depression/anxiety are more common; others find no association. Depression is multifactorial—consider social, physical, and cultural factors before resorting to HRT as a solution.

**Flushes and sweats** 80% have flushes during the menopause—20% seek help. Often associated with palpitations.

*Lifestyle changes* Exercise (↓ flushes by ~50%), deep breathing exercises, cool ambient temperature, wearing natural fibres (e.g. cotton), stress ↓, avoiding trigger foods/drinks (e.g. spicy foods, caffeine, alcohol).

## Drug treatments

- HRT—flushes are controlled successfully with oestrogen in the form of HRT (📖 p.710) in most women.
- SSRIs/SNRIs (e.g. fluoxetine 20mg od, unlicensed) ↓ flushes in >50%.
- Norethisterone (5mg od) and megestrol acetate (40mg od) ↓ flushes in >80%. Megestrol acetate may cause vaginal bleeding on withdrawal.
- Clonidine—no more effective than placebo.

## Complementary therapies

- Natural progesterone from yams—trials of effectiveness are awaited.
- Black cohosh eases hot flushes—long-term effects are unknown.
- Red clover may help—studies have mixed results. Avoid with warfarin.
- Foods containing phyto-oestrogens (e.g. soy foods) may be helpful and are unlikely to be harmful.
- Dong quai, evening primrose oil, vitamin E, and ginseng are no better than placebo. Avoid kava—it is linked to cases of serious liver damage.

**Sexual dysfunction** Vaginal dryness and atrophy are common. Manage with systemic or topical oestrogen. Loss of libido post-menopause (especially after surgical removal of the ovaries) responds to administration of androgens, e.g. testosterone implants in combination with HRT, until libido is re-established.

**Urinary problems** Common—incontinence, nocturia, and urgency. Stress incontinence does not respond to HRT but topical oestrogen may improve outcome of surgery. Recurrent UTIs in older women ↓ with use of topical vaginal oestrogen.

**Ischaemic heart disease** Risk is ↑ 2× after the menopause but there is no evidence to support use of HRT for 1° or 2° prevention of IHD.

**Osteoporosis** Consider HRT to prevent osteoporosis in premature menopause (📖 p.519). In older women, HRT is now *not* recommended as first-line treatment of osteoporosis unless there are other reasons for prescribing the HRT.

**Could the symptoms be due to another cause?** *Exclude*:
- Physical illness, e.g. thyroid disease, anaemia, DM, chronic renal disease.
- Side effects of medication, e.g. $Ca^{2+}$ antagonists cause flushing.
- Social problems or psychiatric illness—depression screening questionnaires can be helpful.

**Is the diagnosis in doubt?** *Check FSH/LH*:
- Following hysterectomy with conservation of ovaries.
- If amenorrhoea age <45y or
- If having regular bleeds due to cyclical HRT/COC pill. Check at the beginning of a packet (oestrogen phase) or end of the pill-free week, respectively. The COC/HRT can ↓FSH/LH. To make a more accurate assessment, stop the preparation and check FSH levels 6 and 12 wk after stopping. FSH >30IU/L and amenorrhoea suggests the woman is post-menopausal.

❶ It is unnecessary to check FSH/LH in other groups. FSH/LH levels may be normal in the perimenopause.

**Premature menopause** Menopause in a woman <40y old. Associated with ↑ all-cause mortality and ↑ risk of osteoporosis and cardiovascular disease. *Causes*:
- Idiopathic.
- Radiotherapy and/or chemotherapy.
- Surgery—bilateral oophorectomy → instant menopause; hysterectomy without oophorectomy can also induce premature ovarian failure.
- Infection—TB and mumps.
- Chromosome abnormalities—particularly the X chromosome.
- Autoimmune endocrine disease, e.g. DM, hypothyroidism, Addison's.
- FSH receptor abnormalities.
- Disruption of oestrogen synthesis.

*Management* Usually HRT is recommended until the average age of menopause, i.e. 50y.

### Information and support for patients
**British Menopause Society**
🖥 www.thebms.org.uk
**The Daisy Network** (premature menopause) 🖥 www.daisynetwork.org.uk

# Hormone replacement therapy (HRT)

Short-term use of HRT is recommended for the relief of symptoms related to oestrogen deficiency peri- and post-menopausally, e.g. flushes/sweats. Carefully balance risks against benefits for each individual.

**Contraindications** Cancer of the breast or endometrium; thromboembolic disease (including AF); liver disease where LFTs have failed to return to normal. In women with past history of liver disease, gallstones, or taking liver-enzyme-inducing drugs, consider transdermal therapy. ❶ Stop HRT 4–6wk prior to surgery—restart after full mobilization.

## Particular indications
- Early menopause—consider alternatives if prescribing for osteoporosis prevention alone. Continue until age 50y.
- Hysterectomy before menopause even if ovaries are conserved—~1:4 have early menopause.
- Second-line treatment of osteoporosis (📖 p.518).

**Choice of preparation** (BNF 6.4.1.1). Start with low dose and provide 3mo supply. Tablets, patches, gels, and implants are available:
- *For women without a uterus*—give oestrogen alone unless past history of endometriosis (endometrial foci may remain despite hysterectomy, so consider addition of a progestogen).
- *For women with an intact uterus*—progestogen is required for the last 12–14d of the cycle to prevent endometrial proliferation. Alternatively use a continuous oestrogen and progestogen preparation (not suitable in the perimenopause or <12mo after last menstrual period).

**Tibolone (Livial®)** Oestrogenic, progestogenic, and weak androgenic action. Use in the same way as continuous combined HRT.

**Topical vaginal preparations** Oestrogen pessaries, creams, or rings. For vaginal dryness/ atrophic vaginitis. Use is limited to 3–6mo if uterus is present. Consider prescribing a progestogen if given for longer periods or higher doses are used. Investigate abnormal bleeding.

## Things to do before starting HRT

**History** Why does the woman want to start HRT? What are her expectations of treatment? Has she had a hysterectomy? If not, ask about bleeding pattern. Investigate abnormal bleeding prior to starting HRT.

*Other points to cover*
- Risk factors for osteoporosis, DVT, and CVD; FH of breast cancer.
- Contraceptive requirement—HRT does not provide contraception. If <50y, the COC (📖 p.750) may provide contraception and alleviate menopausal symptoms
- Drug history—previous experience of HRT; Levothyroxine (may need to ↑ dose of thyroxine when start HRT—check TFTs); steroids (HRT ↓ effectiveness of steroids); anti-epileptics (↑ elimination of oestrogen).

**Examination** Check: BP; weight; breasts (check no lumps, demonstrate breast self-examination techniques); smear is up to date; consider examination for prolapse /vaginal abnormalities if symptoms.

**Starting HRT** Explain the pros and cons of HRT (Table 21.2). Support with health promotion information, e.g. about smoking cessation, breast cancer screening programme. Review after 3mo. Check BP and weight. ↑ dose if symptoms are not controlled. *Common side effects:*

- *Oestrogen related*—fluid retention, breast enlargement and tenderness, nausea, headaches.
- *Progestogen related*—headache, ↑ weight , bloating and depression (↓ by changing to a preparation with a less androgenic progestogen, e.g. dydrogesterone or medroxyprogesterone)

**Bleeding** may be erratic for the first 2–3mo in patients taking cyclical HRT but should occur after the progestogen supplement in subsequent cycles. Continuous combined preparations may cause spotting for up to 12mo. If bleeding continues >12mo, investigate to exclude endometrial abnormality and consider changing to a cyclical preparation.

**Once established on HRT** Review every 6–12mo and if any problems. Check BP, weight, breasts, symptoms, and bleeding pattern. Re-assess risks and benefits. HRT is needed for <5y for vasomotor symptoms. When stopping, withdrawal flushes may be distressing—stop in cold weather and half dose for 1mo first. *Reasons to stop immediately:*

- Severe chest pain
- Sudden breathlessness/cough with bloodstained sputum
- Unexplained severe pain in calf
- Severe stomach pain
- Hepatitis, jaundice, liver enlargement
- BP >160mmHg systolic and/or >100mmHg diastolic
- Detection of a risk factor, e.g. DVT, stroke
- Prolonged immobility after surgery or leg injury
- Serious neurological effects, e.g. severe headache, motor or sensory deficit, first epileptic seizure.

**Table 21.2** Risks and benefits of HRT

| Risks | Short-term benefits | Long-term benefits |
|---|---|---|
| ↑ Breast cancer (RR 1.43*) <br> ↑ DVT (RR 1.45**) <br> ↑ Stroke (RR 1.15**) <br> ↑ Gallbladder disease <br> ↑ ovarian cancer if using oestrogen-only HRT for >5y <br> No ↓ risk of CHD—may ↑ risk in the first year of use | Alleviation of menopausal symptoms eg flushes/sweats/ vaginal dryness <br><br> ↓ recurrent UTIs | ↓ Osteoporosis <br> ↓ Colorectal cancer <br><br> ❶ HRT does not prevent coronary heart disease or protect against ↓ in cognitive function and should not be prescribed for these purposes. |

*Relative risk in women aged 50–64y using combined HRT for 5y.
**Relative risk in women aged 60–69y taking combined HRT for 5y.

**Further information**
**RCP (Edinburgh)** Consensus conference on HRT: Final consensus statement (2003) ⊞ www.rcpe.ac.uk/esd/consensus/hrt_03.html

**Information and support for women**
**British Menopause Society** ⊞ www.thebms.org.uk

# Pelvic pain

**History** Allow the woman to tell her story. Ask about the pain—site; severity; onset (? pregnant); character/timing/pattern (e.g. relationship to menstrual cycle or sexual intercourse, exacerbating/relieving factors); other associated features. Bowel/bladder symptoms? Past history—ectopic pregnancy, pelvic infection or surgery, psychological symptoms.

**Examination** Abdominal, pelvic, and vaginal examination—including rectal examination if indicated and cervical smear if overdue. Normal pelvic and vaginal examination makes a gynaecological cause unlikely.

**Investigation** Consider: *urine*—pregnancy test, M,C&S, dipstick for protein, RBCs, nitrites and leucocytes; *blood*—FBC, CRP; *radiology*—pelvic USS if gynaecological cause is suspected.

**Management** Consider possible causes—Table 21.3.
- *Acute pelvic pain* Admit unless cause is clear and ectopic pregnancy can be excluded.
- *Chronic pelvic pain* Pain for ≥ 6mo. Affects 1:6 women. Decide whether the cause is gynaecological—patients usually have dyspareunia and pain may be cyclical. If suspected gynaecological cause and pelvic USS is normal, refer for laparoscopy. If GI pain is likely, consider referral for colonoscopy. ❶ May be due to a combination of factors.

**Dyspareunia** Pain on intercourse. 10% women admit sexual intercourse usually causes discomfort. It may be *superficial* (felt around the introitus) or *deep* (felt deep inside). There is a psychological element in most cases (a vicious circle of pain leading to fear of intercourse which exacerbates symptoms). Address both physical and psychological aspects.

*Superficial dyspareunia* Examine if possible but do not insist. Treat cause. If no specific treatment, try lidocaine gel. *Causes:*
- *Vulval*—vulvitis—atrophic, infective (candida, HSV); dystrophy; neoplasm; lichen sclerosis
- *Vaginal*—vaginismus (☐ p.772); lack of lubrication; vaginitis (atrophic, infective); congenital (imperforate hymen, atresia); surgery (e.g. painful episiotomy scar); contracture (atrophy, or after surgery/radiotherapy).
- *Urethral*—urethritis; urethral caruncle; urethral diverticulum.

*Deep dyspareunia* *Causes:* endometriosis; pelvic inflammatory disease; retroverted uterus; ovarian cancer (rarely). Examine; treat any cause found, otherwise refer for further investigation. If no cause is found or cause is untreatable, pain can be ↓ by limiting penetration. Often becomes a chronic problem.

**Mittelschmerz** Mid-cycle pain which occurs around the time of ovulation. Reassure. No action needed.

**Dysmenorrhoea** (painful periods). >½ of all pre-menopausal women have some degree of pelvic discomfort around the time of their period and up to 1:10 find period pain significantly interferes with lifestyle.

**Table 21.3** Causes of pelvic pain

| Gynaecological | | Non-gynaecological | |
|---|---|---|---|
| **Acute** | **Chronic** | **Acute** | **Chronic** |
| Ectopic pregnancy | Endometriosis | Appendicitis | Irritable bowel syndrome |
| Infection | Adhesions | Cystitis | Musculoskeletal |
| Endometriosis | Fibroids | Neurological | Psychological[*] |
| Torsion of fibroid | Ovarian cyst | Colitis | Bowel or bladder cancer |
| Dysmenorrhoea | Venous | Psychological[*] | Neurological |
| Ovarian cyst (torsion, bleeding or rupture) | congestion | | |
| | Pelvic inflammatory disease | | |

*Psychological causes of pelvic pain do occur but be careful not to dismiss organic symptoms as psychological. Psychological pain may be a consequence of and perpetuate physical pain. Diagnosis is one of exclusion.

**Primary dysmenorrhoea** No underlying pelvic pathology. Tends to start 6–12mo after menarche when ovulatory cycles are established. Presents with lower abdominal cramps ± back ache which occur in the first 1–2d. of each period. May be associated with GI disturbance e.g. diarrhoea/vomiting. Young women (<20y) with no other symptoms do not require examination unless pathology is suspected. Perform a full abdominal and pelvic examination if older woman or atypical features.

**Treatment** NSAIDs, e.g. mefenamic acid (500mg tds), ibuprofen (200–400mg tds)—effective in 80–90%—start when bleeding starts; COC pill—effective in 80–90%. ❶ 10–20% do not respond, consider a missed cause.

**Secondary dysmenorrhoea** Underlying pathology. *Causes:*
- Endometriosis/adenomyosis
- Chronic pelvic infection
- IUCD
- Endometrial polyps
- Cervical stenosis
- Submucous fibroid
- History of pelvic/abdominal surgery
- Intrauterine adhesions (Asherman's syndrome)
- Psychosexual problems.

Starts later than teenage years, or may present as a change in pattern, type, or intensity of usual pain. Pain can last throughout the period and start just before. Often associated with deep dyspareunia ± other associated symptoms, e.g. abnormal bleeding, vaginal discharge.

**Assessment** Abdominal, vaginal speculum and bimanual pelvic examination. Look for tethered /fixed uterus, uterine tenderness, masses, thickening in the posterior fornix (associated with dyspareunia and endometriosis), and/or endocervical polyps. Do a cervical smear if overdue/cervical abnormality, and endocervical swabs (including chlamydia) if infection is suspected; consider pelvic USS.

**Management** Treat underlying cause; otherwise refer for further investigation (e.g. laparoscopy, hysteroscopy).

**Pelvic venous congestion** Chronic pelvic pain due to dilation and congestion of the pelvic veins. Presents with chronic pelvic pain. Refer to exclude PID and endometriosis. Once confirmed, treatment is with progestogens (e.g. medroxyprogesterone 30mg od for 6mo) or GnRH analogues (e.g. goserelin 3.6mg monthly for 6mo). Symptoms often recur following treatment.

# Endometriosis and adenomyosis

**Endometriosis** Presence of tissue histologically similar to endometrium outside the uterine cavity and myometrium. Most commonly found in the pelvis but can occur anywhere. Affects 10–15% of women presenting with gynaecological symptoms. Ovarian deposits may result in *chocolate cysts* or *endometriomas*.

**Risk factors** Age; family history; heavy periods; frequent cycles. ❶ Oral contraceptives and pregnancy are protective.

**Theories of pathogenesis**
- **Reflux and implantation** Menstrual loss flows backwards through Fallopian tubes into the pelvis where it implants into the peritoneum and continues to grow under the influence of oestrogen.
- **Transformation/induction** Peritoneal tissue transforms into endometrium either under the influence of ovarian steroids or as a result of factors released when menstrual loss refluxes into the peritoneum.
- **Mechanical transplantation** Endometrium transplanted from one location to another (e.g. during surgery) will grow at the new site.
- **Vascular ± lymphatic spread** Thought to explain distant deposits, e.g. lungs, brain.

**History**
- Pelvic pain: cyclical ± non-cyclical, dyspareunia, dysmenorrhoea (spasmodic dysmenorrhoea is highly predictive of endometriosis).
- Menorrhagia.
- Infertility.

**Examination** Abdominal, speculum and bimanual pelvic examination looking for pelvic tenderness, pelvic mass, and/or fixation of the uterus. Occasionally tender nodules can be felt on the utero-sacral ligaments.

**Investigation** Refer to gynaecology for laparoscopy/transvaginal USS. MRI may also be useful.

❶ Laparoscopic findings of endometriosis are common and extent often does not correlate with severity of symptoms. Only treat if symptomatic.

**Management**
*Infertility* Refer for specialist opinion (📖 p.770).
- If tubal damage—reconstructive surgery or IVF.
- If no tubal damage—laparoscopic ablation may improve fertility.

*Pain and bleeding*
- Cyclical pain and/or heavy periods—NSAID (e.g. ibuprofen 400mg tds prn from first day of period.
- IUS ↓ endometriosis pain with symptom control maintained >3y.
- If a woman is not trying to conceive and there is no evidence of a pelvic mass, try a progestogen (e.g. norethisterone 10 –15mg/d for at least 4–6 mo starting on day 5 of the cycle—if spotting occurs ↑ dose to 20–25mg/d and ↓ once bleeding has stopped) or continuous COC (3 or 4 packets without a break, then 7d break).
- If symptoms are not controlled—refer.

### Specialist treatments
- *Medical options* include continuous COC pill, gestrinone, and GnRH agonists (e.g. goserelin) ± HRT (↓ side effects and bone demineralization). Side effects can be troublesome.
- *Surgical options* include laparoscopy or laparotomy with ablation of lesions and division of adhesions, tubal surgery, hysterectomy. Laparoscopic ablation of mild endometriosis may improve fertility.

❶ For all forms of specialist treatment there is a 15–20% recurrence rate. If relapse in <6mo, treatment has failed and an alternative form of treatment should be tried. If relapse in >6mo, consider the condition to have relapsed and repeat treatment.

**Psychological support** Many women will have had pain for years. Often there is delay in diagnosis of the cause, and frequently they have been told it is psychosomatic. Be sympathetic and supportive and use a cooperative strategy for management.

**Adenomyosis** Usually affects multiparous premenopausal women aged >35y. Caused by extension of endometrial tissue and stroma into the uterine myometrium. May coexist with endometriosis (15%) but a separate entity.

**Presentation** May be asymptomatic. Dysmenorrhoea (pain often peaks towards the end of menstruation), dyspareunia, and menorrhagia. On examination, the uterus may be symmetrically enlarged and tender.

**Management** No treatment needed if asymptomatic. Refer for further investigation of symptoms. MRI may confirm diagnosis, but diagnosis is often only confirmed on histology after hysterectomy. Treatment is usually surgical with hysterectomy ± bilateral salpingo-oophorectomy. Medical treatment with GnRH analogues is a short-term option but symptoms return once withdrawn unless the woman has reached the menopause in the interim.

### Further information
**RCOG** The investigation and management of endometriosis (2006) 🖥 www.rcog.org.uk

### Information and support for patients
**Endometriosis UK** ☎ 0808 808 2227 🖥 www.endo.org.uk
**Pelvic Pain Support Network** 🖥 www.pelvicpain.org.uk

# Prolapse

**Prolapse** Pelvic organs sag into the vagina due to poor pelvic muscle tone and weakness of pelvic ligaments. Affects 12–30% of multiparous and 2% of nulliparous women. Good obstetric practice ↓ risk. Risk is ↑ by:

- Childbirth
- Menopause
- Coughing and straining
- Congenital connective tissue disorders.

**Terminology** Named according to the organs involved
- Cystocoele—bladder bulges into the vagina.
- Urethrocoele—urethra bulges into the vagina.
- Rectocoele—rectum bulges into the vagina.
- Enterocoele—loops of intesting bulge into the vagina.
- Uterine—uterus descends into the vagina.

Uterine prolapse is further classified by degree (Figure 21.5). The most dependent portion of the prolapse is assessed whilst straining.

**Presentation** Dragging sensation, feeling of 'something coming down', or a 'lump'. Symptoms are only present when upright, i.e. whilst awake, and become worse if standing for a long time, coughing, or straining.

**Associated symptoms** Stress incontinence (📖 p.458), difficulty of defecation, recurrent cystitis, frequency of micturition, and/or dyspareunia depending on structures involved. In severe cases renal failure may occur due to ureteric kinking.

**Examination/investigation** In left lateral position with Sims speculum, ask the patient to bear down and watch the vaginal walls. Exclude pelvic mass by bimanual examination. Dipstick urine ± send for M,C&S.

**Management** Choice of treatment depends on patient preference, general health, degree of prolapse, severity of symptoms, and wish to preserve fertility and sexual activity. *Options include:*
- *Lifestyle measures* Weight ↓; smoking cessation.
- *General measures* Treatment of coexisting conditions exacerbating prolapse, e.g. chronic cough due to COPD or asthma, constipation, menopause/atrophic vaginitis.
- *Physiotherapy* Pelvic floor exercises (📖 p.839). Refer to specialist physiotherapy if simple self-help techniques fail.
- *Ring pessary* Useful for those too frail for surgery, women who have symptoms but do not want surgery or as a temporary measure whilst awaiting surgery. Change pessary every 4–6mo. *Shelf pessaries* may be useful for women who cannot retain a ring pessary—consider referral.
- *Surgery* Refer to gynaecology if the woman is fit for surgery and symptoms are of sufficient severity to warrant operation *and/or* incontinence *and/or* recurrent UTI. Surgical options include repair operations (anterior or posterior colporrhaphy), colpo/vaginal suspension, and hysterectomy (vaginal or abdominal).

**Uterine retroversion** 20% women have a retroverted retroflexed uterus. May be difficult to palpate bimanually—push on the cervix to antevert. Rarely, may fail to lift out of the pelvis during pregnancy, causing discomfort and urinary retention—refer (treated with catheterization).

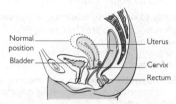

Normal position
Bladder
Uterus
Cervix
Rectum

**1st degree prolapse**—the cervix remains in the vagina

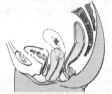

**2nd degree prolapse**—the cervix protrudes from vagina on coughing/straining

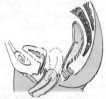

**3rd degree (procidentia)**—uterus lies outside the vagina and may ulcerate

**Fig. 21.5** Degrees of uterine prolapse.

Figure 21.5 is reproduced with permission (copyright EMIS and PIP, 2007) from 🖳 www.patient.co.uk where you can find comprehensive free, up-to-date health information provided by GPs to patients during consultations.

### Fitting a ring pessary

• Measure the approximate size required manually—the distance between posterior fornix and pubic bone can be measured roughly against the index finger.
• Soften the ring in hot water and lubricate it well.
• Insert the ring into the posterior fornix and tuck it above pubic bone.
• Change the pessary every 4–6mo. Inspect the vagina for damage (e.g. ulceration) before inserting the new ring.

#### Potential problems

• *Discomfort*—ring may be too big or atrophic vaginitis.
• *Infection*—remove, clear infection, then try again.
• *Ulceration*—remove, allow to heal, consider alternatives or reinsert when fully healed.
• *Expulsion*—ring may be too small, pelvic musculature inadequate, or retropubic rim unsuitable.

# Uterine problems

**Post-menopausal bleeding (PMB)** Perform a full pelvic examination, including speculum examination of the cervix, for all patients presenting with PMB. *All* women with PMB require referral.

***Refer urgently to a team specializing in gynaecological cancer***
- All patients with PMB who are NOT taking HRT. If taking HRT, stop HRT for 6wk and refer if ongoing/recurrent PMB.
- All patients taking tamoxifen with PMB.
- Endometrial thickness >4mm on USS.

***Differential diagnosis*** Atrophic change (most common), endometrial hyperplasia, endometrial polyps, endometrial malignancy (10% referred), cervical malignancy, uterine sarcoma.

***Pelvic or abdominal mass*** Refer urgently for USS if palpable abdominal/pelvic mass that is not obviously uterine fibroids and not of GI/urological origin. If USS is suggestive of cancer, or urgent USS is not available, refer urgently.

## Congenital abnormalities of the female genital tract
- *Duplication of the cervix and/or uterus, vaginal septum; bicornuate uterus (of varying degrees)* Caused by failure of fusion of the paramesonephric ducts. Usually found incidentally. May cause problems in pregnancy or with contraception (especially IUCD). Refer for advice.
- *Imperforate hymen* May cause cryptmenorrhoea which presents as 1° amenorrhoea (📖 p.704). Refer for surgical release if suspected.
- *Ambiguous genitalia* 📖 p.893    • *Cervical incompetence* 📖 p.814

**Fibroids (uterine leiomyoma)** Benign tumours of the smooth muscle of the myometrium affecting 1:5 women. Often multiple. Oestrogen dependent so regress post-menopause. Named by location:
- Pedunculated
- Intramural (centrally in myometrium)
- Cervical
- Subserosal (bulge into peritoneum)
- Submucosal (bulge into endometrium)
- Separate from uterus, especially in broad ligament from embryonal remnants

***Risk factors*** Nulliparity, obesity, FH of fibroids, African origin.

***Presentation*** Usually asymptomatic. May cause:
- *Pelvic pressure/discomfort* and/or backache.
- *Menorrhagia*—usually submucous fibroids distorting endometrial cavity.
- *Pain*—torsion (pedunculated fibroid), degeneration. *Red degeneration* may occur in pregnancy (pain, fever, and local tenderness).
- *Urinary symptoms*—may press on the bladder → ↑ frequency or a feeling of incomplete emptying or difficulty passing urine.
- *Infertility*—may act as a 'natural IUCD'.
- *Problems in pregnancy*—abnormal lie and ↑ risk of postpartum haemorrhage. Risk of miscarriage is not ↑.
- *Bulky uterus* ± pelvic mass felt abdominally.

Pelvic USS is diagnostic. Check FBC if menorrhagia. ❶ Calcified fibroids may be an incidental finding on X-ray.

**Management** If asymptomatic/mild symptoms—monitor growth by USS or bimanual pelvic examination after 6–12mo. Other options:

- *Medical*—COC pill ↓ menstrual loss; GnRH analogues (maximum use 6mo due to risk of osteopoenia), and selective progesterone receptor modulators (e.g. asoprisnil) cause fibroid shrinkage.
- *Surgical*—uterine artery embolization; myomectomy (removal of fibroids only); hysteroscopic resection; hysterectomy.

**Endometrial proliferation** Oestrogen causes endometrial proliferation; progesterone causes endometrial maturation; shedding follows withdrawal of oestrogen and progesterone (📖 p.700). If oestrogen is given alone, the endometrium proliferates unchecked, resulting in irregular heavy bleeding, polyps, and ↑ risk of endometrial carcinoma. Caused by anovulatory cycles or administration of unopposed oestrogen.

**Endometrial cancer** In the UK ~6000 women each year are diagnosed with endometrial cancer (4% of all female cancers). It is predominantly a disease of post-menopausal women with 93% of cases diagnosed in women >50y (peak age 61y). *Risk factors:*

- Age
- Obesity
- Nulliparity
- Late menopause
- DM
- Drugs—unopposed oestrogen, tamoxifen
- Granulosa cell ovarian tumour
- FH—breast, ovary, or colon cancer
- Previous pelvic irradiation.

Risk is ↓ with current or past use of the COC pill and/or progestogens.

**Presentation** PMB (>90%)—any woman presenting with PMB has endometrial carcinoma until proven otherwise. Pre-menopausally tends to occur in overweight women and present with continual bleeding. Rarely detected on routine cervical smear.

**Management** Refer any PMB to gynaecology for further investigation. Assessment comprises transvaginal USS to look at endometrial thickness ± endometrial sampling with pipelle or hysteroscopy.

**Treatment** TAH and BSO ± radiotherapy, progestogen therapy and/or chemotherapy depending on stage and differentiation of the tumour. Survival depends on the age of the patient and stage/grade of the tumour. Stage I disease—85% 5y survival; stage IV—25% 5y survival.

**Endometritis** Acute infection of the endometrium. Uncommon amongst pre-menopausal women. Usually occurs after surgery (including IUCD insertion) or childbirth. Presents with fever, lower abdominal pain, uterine tenderness, and/or purulent discharge (may be bloodstained). Take high vaginal/endocervical swabs for M,C&S (including chlamydia).

**Management** Treat with antibiotics, e.g. doxycycline 100mg bd for 14d + metronidazole 400mg bd for 1wk or azithromycin 1g stat for chlamydia. *Pyometra* is a complication (uterine cavity fills with pus)—suspect if fails to clear and refer to gynaecology urgently.

#### Further information
**NICE** Referral guidelines for suspected cancer (2005) 🖳 www.nice.org.uk
**SIGN** Investigation of postmenopausal bleeding (2002) 🖳 www.sign.ac.uk

# Ovarian disease

**Pelvic or abdominal mass** Refer urgently for USS if palpable abdominal/pelvic mass that is not obviously uterine fibroids and not of GI/urological origin. If USS is suggestive of cancer, or urgent USS is not available, refer urgently.

**Ovarian cancer** Ovarian cancer is difficult to diagnose. In patients with vague non-specific unexplained abdominal symptoms such as:
- Bloating
- Constipation
- Abdominal pain
- Back pain
- Urinary symptoms.

Carry out an abdominal palpation. Also consider a pelvic examination.

**Ovarian tumours** May be solid or cystic. In women of reproductive age, >80% are benign. The remainder are borderline or malignant. In post-menopausal women, the proportion of malignant ovarian tumours rises to ~50%. Classified according to tissue of origin:
- Tumours of surface epithelium—60% (Table 21.4).
- Germ cell tumours—15–25%.
- Gonadal stromal tumours—5–10%
- Metastatic (from breast, stomach, colon, or genital tract)—5–10%.

*Presentation* Early tumours are often asymptomatic and may be an incidental finding on pelvic examination done for another reason (e.g. when doing a cervical smear) or on USS. Symptoms include:
- Non-specific—weight ↓/cachexia, constipation, early satiety, fatigue.
- Abdominal pain—rapid expansion of tumour, rupture, torsion, infection, or bleeding.
- Abdominal distension/bloating—tumour or ascites.
- Pressure effects, e.g. urinary retention/ urinary frequency, prolapse.
- Menstrual disturbance.
- Endocrine effects due to hormone production by tumour.

*Management* If suspected, refer for urgent USS.
- If USS is suggestive of ovarian cancer, check CA125 and refer urgently to gynaecology (to be seen in <2wk).
- If pre-menopausal, refer any cysts with multilocular or solid elements, cysts >8 cm diameter, or cysts <8 cm which fail to regress in <6 wk.
- If post-menopausal—refer any cyst/ovarian mass.

**Simple, physiological, or functional cysts** Common and often incidental finding on USS in *pre-menopausal* women. May cause pain due to tension within the cyst, rupture, torsion, or bleeding into the cyst.
- *Follicular cyst* An ovarian follicle fails to rupture in the course of follicular development and ovulation. Unilocular and can reach a diameter of 10cm. Usually regress during the subsequent cycle.
- *Luteal cyst* Forms if there is excessive bleeding into the corpus luteum. May be tender, cause abdominal pain (sometimes acute abdomen), and delay the next period.

*Management* As for ovarian tumour.

**Chocolate cyst/endometrioma** 📖 p.714

**Table 21.4** Tumours of surface epithelium

| Type of tumour | Subtype | 10y survival |
|---|---|---|
| Serous<br>Peak age 30–40y;<br>20–50% of ovarian tumours; 30% bilateral | Benign serous cystadenoma—60% of serous tumours; 25% all benign ovarian tumours | 100% |
| | Borderline serous cystadenoma—10% of serous tumours | 90–95% |
| | Malignant serous cystadenocarcinoma—35–50% of serous tumours; bilateral in 40–60%; 40–50% of all malignant ovarian tumours; 85% have spread outside the ovaries at the time of diagnosis; >50% are >15cm diameter at diagnosis | 15% |
| Mucinous<br>Can be very large; often multilocular; often contain viscid mucin—if burst can cause pseudo-myxoma peritonei (mucin-secreting cells are spread throughout the peritoneum) | Benign mucinous cystadenoma—Peak incidence aged 30–50y; 80% of mucinous tumours; bilateral in 5–10%; 20–25% of all benign ovarian tumours | 100% |
| | Borderline mucinous cystadenoma—10% mucinous tumours; bilateral in 10% | 90–95% |
| | Malignant mucinous cystadenocarcinoma—Peak age 40–70y; 10% of mucinous tumours; bilateral in 15–30%; 5–10% of all 1° ovarian cancers; average diameter at diagnosis ~16cm | 34% |

*Endometrioid*
Peak age 50–60y; 30–50% bilateral; benign tumours are rare; malignant tumours account for 20–25% of all malignant ovarian neoplasms; 30% coexist with endometrial cancer; 10% coexist with endometriosis

*Clear cell (mesonephroid)*
5 % bilateral; 5–10% of all malignant ovarian neoplasms; 25% coexist with endometriosis; associated with hypercalcaemia

*Brenner (transitional cell)*
Rare—2–3% of all ovarian tumours; >90% are benign. If malignant have poor prognosis; <5% are bilateral; associated with mucinous cystadenoma and cystic teratoma in 1:10 cases

*Undifferentiated carcinoma*
<10% epithelial neoplasms; no histological features that characterize it

---

**Ovarian cysts in children** Unusual. Refer any ovarian cysts >2cm found in a pre-menarchal child for further assessment.

**Meigs syndrome** Benign ovarian fibroma with pleural effusion. *J.V. Meigs (1892–1963), US obstetrician/gynaecologist.*

**Ovarian hyperstimulation** Iatrogenic condition resulting from over-stimulation of the ovaries during infertility treatment.
- *Mild* >10% of patients receiving gonadotrophin therapy. Abdominal pain/swelling ± vomiting/diarrhoea. Manage with rest and simple analgesia, e.g. ibuprofen or paracetamol prn.
- *Severe* 1% of patients receiving gonadotrophin therapy. Abdominal pain/distention, vomiting/diarrhoea, ascites, pleural effusion, and/or venous thrombosis. Admit.

# Ovarian cancer and polycystic ovaries

**Pelvic or abdominal mass** Refer urgently for USS if palpable abdominal/pelvic mass that is not obviously uterine fibroids and not of GI/urological origin. If USS is suggestive of cancer, or urgent USS is not available, refer urgently.

**Ovarian cancer** Ovarian cancer is difficult to diagnose. In patients with vague non-specific unexplained abdominal symptoms such as:
- Bloating
- Constipation
- Abdominal pain
- Urinary symptoms
- Back pain

Carry out an abdominal palpation. Also consider a pelvic examination.

**Epithelial ovarian cancer (EOC)** 90% of ovarian cancers. ~7000 cases are diagnosed each year in the UK (2.5% of all cancers) and ovarian cancer accounts for 6% of ♀ deaths. Incidence is rising. *Risk factors*:
- *Age*—peak age 50–70y; 85% ovarian cancers occur in ♀ >50y.
- *Family history*—↑ risk is associated with mutations in BRCA1/2 and hereditary non-polyposis colorectal cancer (HNPCC) genes (but only 10% of ovarian cancers occur in women carrying these mutations). Women may consider prophylactic surgery (bilateral oophorectomy).
- *Nulliparity*—OR = 2.42 compared with women with ≥ 4 children.
- *Infertility* -OR for women trying to conceive for >5y is 2.67 compared with women trying to conceive for <1y (*not* due to infertility drugs).
- *Obesity* may ↑ risk.

**Protective factors** Pregnancy—the more pregnancies, the lower the risk; COC pill ↓ risk by ~60%—protective effect is maintained >20y after the COC pill has been discontinued; breastfeeding—may ↓ risk by 20%; tubal ligation—↓ risk by 30–70%; hysterectomy—may ↓ risk.

**Prevention** Ovarian cancer fulfils some criteria for population screening. Two large trials of screening currently under way in the UK.

**Presentation and primary care management** See ovarian tumours (📖 p.720). In the UK, ~80% of patients with ovarian cancer have had symptoms for <4wk before seeing their GP.

**Treatment** Specialist management is with laparotomy ± adjuvant treatment with chemotherapy dependant on stage of disease. Radiotherapy may be used for palliation. *Prognosis*: Stage I—73% 5y survival; stage IV (distant metastases—40% new diagnoses)—16% 5y survival.

**Germ-cell tumours** e.g. mature teratoma (ovarian dermoid cyst), immature teratoma, dysgerminoma, endodermal sinus tumour (yolk sac tumour), mixed germ cell tumour. Peak incidence in early 20s. Most are unilateral. Associated with ↑ AFP and ↑ β-HCG (both are used as tumour markers). Prognosis is good with the majority being cured.

**Sex-cord stromal tumours** e.g. granulosa cell tumours, thecomas, fibromas, Sertoli/Leydig cell tumours. Usually present early with symptoms of hormone production, e.g. precocious puberty, PMB, or virilism. Granulosa cell tumours are associated with endometrial hyperplasia and carcinoma.

**Polycystic ovarian syndrome (PCOS)** or *Stein–Leventhal syndrome*.
Disrupted hormone cycling together with enlarged ovaries with multiple cysts. Up to 1:3 pre-menopausal women have polycystic ovaries on USS—1:3 of these women have PCOS. Cause is unknown—often there is a family history. Diagnosis requires presence of ≥2 of:
- Oligomenorrhoea and/or anovulation
- Hyperandrogenism –clinical and/or biochemical
- Polycystic ovaries—defined as the presence of ≥12 follicles in each ovary measuring 2–9mm in diameter and/or ovarian volume >10cm3.

**Symptoms and signs** May be asymptomatic or have ≥1 of:
- Menstrual irregularity—oligomenorrhoea or amenorrhoea (affects ~67% of women with PCOS. More common in women with BMI ≥30kg/m$^2$), dysfunctional uterine bleeding
- Anovulatory infertility
- Central obesity
- Acne
- Hirsutism
- Male pattern baldness.

**Investigations**
- **USS ovaries** >12 cysts 2–9mm in diameter (string of pearls sign).
- **Blood**—ideally take blood during the first week after menstruation. Normal FSH, ↑ LH (>10iu/L—LH:FSH ratio ↑ from 1:1 to 2–3:1), ↑ testosterone (> 2.5nmol/l –if >4.8 nmol/L exclude other causes of androgen hypersecretion, e.g. tumour, Cushing's syndrome), ↓ sex hormone binding globulin (SHBG).

**Complications** Insulin resistance/impaired glucose tolerance— 2× ↑ incidence of DM; ↑ CVD risk factors—central body fat distribution, obesity, ↑ BP, ↑ triglycerides, ↓ HDL cholesterol—3× ↑ risk of stroke/TIA; ↑ endometrial cancer risk.

**Management** In all cases, encourage weight ↓ and exercise.
- If oligomenorrhoeic consider progestogens to induce a withdrawal bleed every 2–3mo to ↓ risk of endometrial hyperplasia.
- Consider COC pill to regulate menstruation (though may induce DM). COC pills with anti-androgen (e.g. co-cyprindiol) may ↓ acne/hirsutism.
- Consider offering annual fasting blood glucose check—particularly if obese (BM± >30), FH of DM or aged >40y. Screen pregnant women with PCOS for gestational DM with a glucose tolerance test at <20 wk gestation.
- Clomifene can be used to induce ovulation (📖 p.770).
- Metformin (unlicensed) may be helpful for insulin sensitivity, menstrual disturbance. Also used for infertility if clomifene has failed.
- Hirsutism (📖 p.350).

**Further information**
NICE Referral guidelines for suspected cancer (2005) 🖥 www.nice.org.uk
RCOG Long term consequences of polycystic ovary syndrome (2007) 🖥 www.rcog.org.uk

**Further information and support for patients**
Ovacome ☎ 0845 371 0554 🖥 www.ovacome.org.uk
CancerHelp ☎ 0808 800 4040 🖥 www.cancerhelp.org.uk
Macmillan Cancer Support ☎ 0808 808 0000
🖥 www.macmillan.org.uk
Verity Support for women with PCOS 🖥 www.verity-pcos.org.uk

# Conditions of the cervix

**Refer urgently (to be seen in <2wk )** to gynaecology:
- If clinical features of cervical cancer. Do not perform a cervical smear before referral or delay referral due to previous −ve smear.
- All patients with post-menopausal bleeding who are not taking HRT.
- Patients on HRT with persistent or unexplained post-menopausal bleeding after cessation of HRT for 6wk.
- All patients taking tamoxifen with post-menopausal bleeding

**Consider urgent referral** if persistent intermenstrual bleeding and negative pelvic examination.

**Refer urgently for USS** if palpable abdominal/pelvic mass that is not obviously uterine fibroids or not of GI/urological origin. If urgent USS is not available or USS is suggestive of cancer, make an urgent gynaecology referral.

**Perform a full pelvic examination,** including speculum examination of the cervix, for patients with:
- Alterations in menstrual cycle
- Intermenstrual bleeding
- Post-coital bleeding
- Post-menopausal bleeding
- Vaginal discharge.

**Cervical intra-epithelial neoplasia (CIN)** Pre-malignant change of the cervical epithelium. The majority of these changes are found in women <45y (peak incidence 25–29y). CIN is a histological diagnosis resulting from biopsy—usually following an abnormal smear.
- CIN 1—mild/moderate dysplasia. Nuclear atypia confined to basal third of the epithelium
- CIN 2—nuclear atypia in basal two-thirds of the epithelium.
- CIN 3—severe dysplasia/carcinoma *in situ*. Full-thickness epithelial nuclear abnormalities.

❶ CIN 1 may revert to normality. Any stage can progress to cervical cancer, but more likely if CIN 3.

*Treatment* Depends on stage. Ranges from local ablation (diathermy, laser diathermy, cold coagulation) through large loop excision of the transformation zone (LLETZ) and cone biopsy to hysterectomy.

**Cervical cancer** In the UK, 2800 women each year are diagnosed with cervical cancer (2% of all ♀ cancers). Almost exclusively occurs in women who are/have been sexually active. Two peaks of incidence—women in their late 30s and 70s/80s. 80% are squamous cell cancer; the remainder are adenocarcinoma. Incidence is dropping probably due to the cervical cancer screening programme and changes in sexual practices.

*Risk factors*
- Social class
- Smoking
- Early age of 1st intercourse
- Early age of 1st pregnancy
- Multiple sexual partners
- HPV infection (types 16, 18, 31, 33)
- History of dyskaryosis
- Method of contraception (↓ with barrier methods; ↑ if >5y COC use)
- Immunosuppression, HIV.

***Presentation*** May be found on routine cervical screening. Symptoms include post-coital, intermenstrual, post-manopausal bleeding and/or offensive vaginal discharge. Speculum examination may reveal cervical ulceration/ mass or a cervix that bleeds easily.

***Management*** Refer urgently to gynaecology. Treatment is with surgery ± radiotherapy depending on the stage of the disease:
- ***Stage 1*** Micro-invasive cancer (A) or cancer confined in the cervix (B)—65% women present at stage 1. 5y survival ~70–95%.
- ***Stage 2*** Invasion into the upper third of the vagina (A) or parametria (B) but not to the pelvic side wall. 5y survival ~60–90%.
- ***Stage 3*** Extension to lower third of the vagina (A) or pelvic side wall (B). 5y survival ~30–50%.
- ***Stage 4*** Tumour involving bladder/rectum (A) or extrapelvic spread (B). 5y survival ~20–30%.

**Cervical erosion/ectropion** Physiological. An erosion or ectropion is the area of columnar epithelium visible within the vagina when the squamo-columnar junction moves down the cervix at times of high oestrogen exposure (e.g. pregnancy, COC pill, puberty). Only treat if:
- Abnormal cervical smear *or*
- Symptoms are causing problems, e.g. post-coital or inter-menstrual bleeding or excess discharge—refer to gynaecologist for cautery. If using the COC pill, consider switching to an alternative.

**Nabothian cysts** Mucus retention cysts on cervix. Usually asymptomatic. Need no treatment. Refer for cautery if troublesome discharge.

**Cervicitis** Presents with vaginal discharge. Speculum examination shows mucopurulent discharge, and inflamed, friable cervix. *Causes*: chlamydia (50%), gonococcus, and HSV. Treat the cause (📖 p.738).

**Cervical polyps** Develop from the endocervix and protrude into the vagina through the external os. Usually asymptomatic, although there may be ↑ vaginal discharge and the lowest part of the polyp may ulcerate and bleed causing intermenstrual, postmenopausal, and/or postcoital bleeding. The vast majority are benign.

***Treatment*** Avulsion (send for histology). Cauterize base with a silver nitrate stick if possible. Frequently recur. If postmenopausal, intermenstrual, or postcoital bleeding, refer to gynaecology.

**Cervical incompetence** 📖 p.814

**Further information**
**NICE** Referral guidelines for suspected cancer (2005) 🖥 www.nice.org.uk
**Cancer Research UK** Cervical cancer statistics
🖥 www.cancerresearchuk.org/cancerstats

**Information and support for patients**
**Cancer Research UK (CancerHelp)** ☎ 0808 800 4040
🖥 www.cancerhelp.org.uk
**Macmillan Cancer Support** ☎ 0808 808 0000
🖥 www.macmillan.org.uk

# Cervical cancer screening

Screening prevents ~1000–4000 deaths/y in the UK from squamous cell cancer of the cervix.

**Liquid-based cytology** In the UK, the traditional Papanicolou smear (Pap smear) has been replaced by liquid-based cytology. The sample is collected in a similar way but, rather than smearing the sample from the spatula onto a slide, the head of the spatula, where the cells are lodged, is broken off into a small vial containing preservative fluid, or rinsed directly into the preservative fluid. This method ↓ the number of inadequate smears taken as cervical cells can be examined even if the sample is contaminated with blood, pus, or mucus.

**Taking a smear** Ensure adequate training—poor smear-taking misses 20% of abnormalities. Courses are available—update skills every 3y. Give all women information about the test, condition being sought, possible results of screening, and their implications.

**Timing** Avoid menstruation if possible (note on the request form if unavoidable). Ideal time is mid-cycle. Routine bimanual examination is unnecessary—only do if clinically indicated (e.g. painful/heavy periods).

**Screening interval** A smear test is routinely offered to all women age 25–64 y who are sexually active. There is no upper age limit for the first smear. Frequency of screening depends on age:
- **25–49y** 3 yearly screening interval
- **50–64y** 5 yearly screening interval
- **>65y** Only screen those who have not been screened since age 50y or have had recent abnormal tests.

**Organization of the cervical screening programme** Practices undertaking cervical screening must:
- Provide information to eligible women to allow them to make an informed decision about taking part in the programme.
- Perform the cervical screening test (and ensure staff are properly trained and equipped to perform the test).
- Arrange for women to be informed about the results of their tests.
- Ensure that results are followed up appropriately.
- Maintain records of tests carried out, results, and follow-up.

**HPV testing** Infection with human papillomavirus (HPV) 16, 18, 31, and 33 is associated with CIN/cervical cancer. 99.7% of cervical cancers contain HPV DNA and women with HPV infection are 70× more likely to develop high-grade cervical abnormalities. A pilot of HPV testing is being conducted within the UK cervical screening programme.

**Further information**
**NHS Cervical Screening** 🖳 www.cancerscreening.org.uk
**Cancer Research UK** Cervical screening
🖳 www.cancerresearch.org.uk/cancerstats

**Information for patients**
Cervical screening—the facts 🖳 www.cancerscreening.org.uk

**Table 21.5** Interpretation of smear results and action

| Result | Meaning | Action |
|---|---|---|
| Normal | No nuclear abnormalities. | Place on routine recall. |
| Inadequate (~9% conventional smears; ~2% with liquid-based cytology) | Insufficient material present or poorly spread/fixed. Vision of cells obscured by debris. | Repeat the smear as soon as convenient. After 3 consecutive inadequate results, refer for colposcopy. |
| Borderline dyskaryosis (5–10% smears are borderline or mild) | Some nuclear abnormalities but not clear whether these changes represent dyskaryosis. | Repeat smear every 6mo. Most changes will have reverted to normal. After 3 consecutive normal smears, return to normal recall. If abnormality persists 3 times, or worsens, refer for colposcopy. If in a 10y period there are 3 borderline or more severe results, refer for colposcopy. |
| Mild dyskaryosis (5–10% smears are borderline or mild) | Nuclear abnormalities indicative of low-grade CIN. | Repeat smear every 6mo. Most changes will have reverted to normal. After 3 consecutive normal smears, return to normal recall. If abnormality persists ×2, refer for colposcopy. If in a 10y period there are 3 mild or more severe results, refer for colposcopy. If CIN1 is confirmed on colposcopy, management options are to watch and wait (3 normal smears 6mo apart are needed before return to normal recall) or treat.* |
| Moderate dyskaryosis (1% smears) | Nuclear abnormalities reflecting probable CIN2 | Refer to colposcopy. If CIN is confirmed on colposcopy, treat.* |
| Severe dyskaryosis or worse (0.6% smears) | Nuclear abnormalities reflecting probable CIN3 | Refer to colposcopy or (rarely) make referral to gynaecological oncologist if invasive carcinoma is suspected. If CIN is confirmed on colposcopy, treat.* |

**Other possible abnormalities seen on cervical smear**

- Dyskaryotic glandular cells—refer for colposcopy.
- Atrophic—common in peri/post-menopausal women. No action.
- Endometrial cells—may be normal if IUCD in situ, hormonal treatment, or 1st half of 28d cycle. Otherwise, discuss with laboratory. Refer if reported as abnormal.
- Inflammatory changes—common finding. Take chlamydial, endocervical, and high vaginal swabs. Treat as necessary.
- Trichomonas, candida, or changes associated with HSV infection—treat trichomonas or candida. Discuss any new diagnosis of HSV with the patient.
- Actinomyces—associated with IUCDs (🕮 p.762).

*Following treatment women with high grade disease (CIN2, CIN3 and cGIN) require a smear at 6mo and 12mo then annually for at least 9y. Women treated for low-grade disease require a smear at 6mo, 12mo and 24mo.

# Vaginal and vulval problems

**Refer urgently (to be seen in <2wk ) to gynaecology** if unexplained vulval lump or vulval bleeding due to ulceration.

**For patients with vulval pruritus or pain** A period of 'treat, watch, and wait' is reasonable. Actively follow up until symptoms resolve or a diagnosis is confirmed. If symptoms persist, refer to gynaecology—urgency of referral depends on symptoms and concern about cancer.

## Symptoms/signs
- Vaginal discharge/infection (📖 p.734)
- Vulval ulceration—genital ulcers (📖 p. 733)

*Vulval itching (pruritus vulvae)* Treat the cause. *Causes:* infection (e.g. candida, HSV, warts, threadworms, pubic lice, scabies); atrophic vulvitis; vulval dystrophy; vulval carcinoma; generalized causes of pruritus.

*Vulval lumps* Common and usually benign.
- *General causes* Sebaceous cyst; varicose veins; haematoma; benign skin tumour (lipoma, papilloma ec.); malignant skin tumour (1° or 2°).
- *Specific causes* Bartholin's gland cyst/abscess; urethral caruncle; endometriosis; carcinoma of the vulva; inguinal hernia; hydrocoele of the canal of Nuck.

**Atrophic vaginitis** Vaginal soreness, dyspareunia, and occasional spotting. On examination, the vagina looks pale and dry. Treat with topical oestrogens for up to 3mo or consider other HRT. ❶ Refer any post-menopausal bleeding for further assessment (📖 p.718).

**Vaginal cysts** May arise from remnants of the mesonephric ducts (anterolaterally) or occasionally after healing following surgery or episiotomy (posterior, lower third).Usually no treatment is needed. If symptomatic or large, refer to gynaecaology for assessment ± removal.

**Benign vaginal tumours** Benign leiomyomas or fibromyomas are common. Refer for surgical removal.

**Vaginal intra-epithelial neoplasia (VAIN)** Multifocal. Occurs in upper third of vagina. Usually occurs in association with CIN (📖 p.724). May be asymptomatic or present with post-coital staining or abnormal vaginal discharge. Treatment is by local ablation.

**Vaginal cancer** Rare. Affects women >70y. 90% are squamous cell cancer—the rest clear cell (associated with *in utero* exposure to stilboestrol), 2° tumour or sarcoma. Presents with postmenopausal bleeding. Treated with surgery (early stages) and/or radiotherapy. Refer all women with postmenopausal bleeding for gynaecology assessment (📖 p.718).

**Urethral caruncle** Postmenopausal prolapse of the posterior urethral wall. Reddened area involving the posterior margin of the urethral opening. Usually asymptomatic. Rarely bleeds or causes dyspareunia. Treat with topical oestrogen. Refer for surgery if symptoms persist.

**Bartholin's gland swellings** Obstruction of the duct of a Bartholin's gland → cyst formation. Presents as painless vulval swelling. If infected, an abscess forms presenting as a painful tender red vulval lump. Leave cysts to resolve spontaneously. Abscesses may resolve with antibiotics (if early)

or discharge themselves. If not, admit for surgery (marsupialization).
*C. Bartholin (1655–1738), Danish anatomist.*

**Vulval dystrophy** Associated with small risk of malignant change (<5%).
Presents with vulval itching and/or soreness. Changes do not extend into
the vagina. *Classification:*

- *Hypoplastic (lichen sclerosus)* Peak age 45–60y. Most common vulval
  dystrophy. 25% have a family/personal history of autoimmune disease
  e.g. vitiligo, thyroid disease. Vulval skin looks atrophic ± white plaques
  (leukoplakia). 20% have white patches elsewhere on the body, but often
  these are asymptomatic.
- *Hyperplastic* Usually affects postmenopausal women. There are
  multiple, symmetrical, thickened, hyperkeratotic lesions on the vulva.

**Management** Treat with topical steroids—e.g. clobetasol proprionate
ointment od for 1mo, then alternate days for 1mo, then 2x/wk for 1mo.
Refer to gynaecology/dermatology for biopsy if uncertain of diagnosis, no
improvement with steroid treatment after 1mo, residual symptoms after
3mo or other lesions develop (e.g. vulval lump, other skin changes, or
ulceration). Symptoms may recur after treatment has stopped.

**Vulval intraepithelial neoplasia (VIN)** (*Bowen's disease* or carcinoma
*in situ*) May be associated with other genital tract neoplasia (e.g. CIN
□ p.724). Presents with abnormal-looking vulval skin (pinky white ±
altered texture) ± white patches ± itch There is some overlap between
vulval dystrophy and VIN. Diagnosis is histological following skin biopsy:

- **VIN 1** Thickened epidermis—atypia confined to basal third of the
  epithelium.
- **VIN 2** Nuclear atypia in the lower half of the epithelium
- **VIN 3** Carcinoma *in situ*—full-thickness nuclear atypia.

**Management** Refer all patients with abnormal-looking vulval skin (without
candidal infection or other obvious cause) to gynaecology for skin biopsy
and treatment. Treatment depends on site, histology, and extent — includes
observation with regular biopsies, surgery, cryocautery, laser vaporization,
or topical chemotherapy.

**Vulval carcinoma[G]** Rare. Mainly affects elderly women (>70y). Most
are squamous cell carcinoma; others are melanoma, basal cell carcinoma,
Bartholin's gland carcinoma, and adenocarcinoma. The majority occur
on the labia and spread to local LNs. Present early with chronic pruritus
vulvae (>2:3), vulval lump, or ulcer. Refer for confirmation of diagnosis.
Treatment is surgical—5y survival rate ~95%.

## Further information

**NICE** Referral guidelines for suspected cancer (2005) ▣ www.nice.org.uk
**British Association for Sexual Health and HIV (BASHH)** National
guidelines on the management of vulval conditions (2007) ▣ www.bashh.org
**British Association of Dermatologists** Guidelines for the management
of lichen sclerosus (2002) ▣ www.bad.org.uk
**RCOG** Management of vulval cancer (2006) ▣ www.rcog.org.uk

## Information and support for patients

**National Lichen Sclerosus Support Group** ▣ www.lichensclerosus.org
**CancerHelp** ☎ 0808 800 4040 ▣ www.cancerhelp.org.uk

# Sexual health and contraception

# Assessment of sexual health

Good communication skills are particularly important for clinicians when discussing sexual health problems and may improve health outcomes. Ensure a comfortable, private and confidential environment.

**General assessment** Objectives are to:
- Establish a constructive relationship with the patient to enable patient and doctor to communicate effectively, and serve as the basis for any subsequent therapeutic relationship.
- Determine whether the patient has a sexual health problem and, if so, what that is.
- Find out (where possible) what caused that problem.
- Assess the patient's emotions and attitudes towards the problem. Be aware of signs of anxiety/distress. Recognize non-verbal cues.
- Establish how it might be treated

**History** Use open questions at the start, becoming directive when necessary—clarify, reflect, facilitate, listen. Ask about:

*Presenting complaint* Chronological account and concerns. If appropriate, ask about:
- *Vaginal or urethral discharge*
- *Dysuria/other urinary symptoms*
- *Dyspareunia—pain on intercourse* (□ p.712)
- *Erectile dysfunction* (□ p.774)
- *Genital skin problems—soreness, itching, ulceration, warts*
- *Peri-anal/anal symptoms*
- *Other symptoms*, e.g. pelvic/abdominal/groin pain, deformity of the penis, haematospermia (blood in the ejaculate), retrograde ejaculation.

*Past medical history*
- Similar symptoms—for suspected sexually transmitted infections (STIs), ask about previous STI, date of diagnosis, and treatment.
- Obstetric history for women.
- Urological problems and treatments or pelvic surgery.
- Chronic medical problems—endocrine; cardiovascular; DM.
- Medical treatment abroad—in certain countries may be associated with ↑ HIV/hepatitis risk.
- HIV testing/hepatitis B vaccination history.

*Drugs*
- Prescription drugs, e.g. drugs associated with erectile dysfunction
- Illicit drugs—may be associated with erectile dysfunction, and history of injecting drug misuse is associated with ↑ hepatitis/HIV risk.
- Allergies

**Sexual history** Current sexual partner (person with whom the patient had last sexual intercourse) and other recent sexual partners. If appropriate, ask about:
- Nature of relationship with partner—long-term partner; casual partner who could/could not be traced; paid-for partner.
- Gender of partner.

- Nature of intercourse—oral, vaginal, anal.
- Contraception? Method used. Does the patient use a condom (male or female) regularly and consistently? Did it remain in place and intact?
- For women, establish date of LMP, cycle length, and regularity.
- Symptoms in partner?

**❶** For suspected STI, ask about all partners within the previous 3mo or incubation period of the suspected infection (if longer). If no partners are reported, note the last time the patient had sexual intercourse.

### Social history

- Smoker?
- Alcohol consumption
- Travel abroad—if suspected STI, ask whether the patient had sexual intercourse abroad other than with their travelling partner, and with whom.

### Attitudes and beliefs

- How does the patient see the problem?
- What does he/she think is wrong?
- How does he/she think his/her partner views the situation?
- What does the patient want you to do about it?

**Examination** Examine the external genitalia and perianal area. Check groins for lymphadenopathy if STI is suspected. For women, perform bimanual pelvic and vaginal speculum examination. Consider digital rectal examination if indicated.

⚠ Explain the need for the examination of all patients. Offer a suitably medically qualified chaperone. Record if a chaperone is declined.

### Action

- Summarize the history back to the patient and give an opportunity for the patient to fill in any gaps.
- Check that the patient has no other concerns.
- Draw up a problem list and outline a management plan. Further investigations and interventions are guided by the findings on history and examination—so a good history and examination are essential.
- Set a review date.

**Genital ulcers** *Causes:* genital herpes, primary syphilis, Behçet's syndrome. If history of foreign travel, partner from abroad, or doubt about diagnosis refer to the GUM clinic.

### Further information

**British Association for Sexual Health and HIV** National Guidelines for consultations requiring sexual history taking (2006) 🖥 www.bashh.org

### Patient information about sexual health

**Family Planning Association (FPA)** 🖥 www.fpa.org.uk
**Department of Health** Sexual Health Line ☎ 0800 567 123 (24h); Sexwise (for under 19s) ☎ 0800 28 29 30

# Vaginal discharge

All women have some vaginal discharge. Physiological discharge is white, becoming yellow on contact with air. Amount varies considerably and is affected by menstrual cycle, sexual activity, use of the COC pill, age, stress, and pregnancy. 5 causes account for 95% of cases presenting to GPs:

- Excessive normal secretions
- Bacterial vaginosis
- *Candida albicans*
- Cervicitis (gonococcal, chlamydial or herpetic)
- *Trichomonas vaginalis*.

❶ Discharge is only abnormal when it is different from a woman's normal discharge.

## Rarer causes

- Cervical ectropion
- IUCD
- Cervical polyp
- Fistula
- Chemical vaginitis—avoid perfumed or disinfectant bath additives.
- Foreign body (e.g. retained tampon)—remove and treat with metronidazole 400mg tds for 7d.
- Necrotic tumour (rare).

## History Ask about:

- *Symptoms*—vaginal discharge (itchy, offensive, colour, duration), vulval soreness and irritation, lower abdominal pain, dyspareunia, heavy periods, intermenstrual bleeding , fever, vulval pain.
- *Sexual history*—recent sexual contact with new partner, multiple partners, presence of symptoms in partner, worries about sexually transmitted disease.
- *Medical history*—pregnancy, diabetes mellitus, recent antibiotics.
- *Attempts at self-medication*.

**Examination** Abdominal, bimanual pelvic and vaginal speculum examination. Look for lower abdominal tenderness, tenderness on bimanual palpation, cervical erosion or contact bleeding, discharge, warts, or ulcers.

**Management** High vaginal swab for culture and endocervical swabs for gonorrhoea and chlamydia; opportunistic cervical smear if needed. If herpes infection is suspected—viral swab (or if unavailable refer to GUM). Treat the cause. If unclear refer to GUM or gynaecology.

**Bacterial vaginosis (BV)** Vaginal flora are changed from *Lactobacillus* species to anaerobes. Not sexually transmitted. Affects 10–40% of pre-menopausal women—~½ are asymptomatic. *Associated with*:

- ↑ risk of preterm delivery (and ↓ risk if treated)
- Development of PID and endometritis following abortion or birth
- Infection post-hysterectomy.

### Presentation

- *History* Grey/white, thin, offensive discharge; no vulval soreness.
- *Examination* Discharge; cervix looks normal.

*Investigation* High vaginal swab—M,C&S

***Management*^G** Without treatment, 50% remit spontaneously. Cure rate with all methods is ~85%. There is no benefit from treating the woman's partner.

*Treatment*
- Treat with metronidazole po (400mg bd for 5–7d or 2g as a single dose).
- Alternatively treat with clindamycin 2% cream 5g nocte pv for 1wk.
- Recurrent infection—•~ suppressive therapy using metronidazole 400mg bd for 6d to cover each period or metronidazole 0.75% gel 2×/wk pv for 4–6mo are used but evidence of effectiveness is lacking.

**Candidiasis** Fungal infection ~20% of patients are asymptomatic.

***Predisposing factors***
- Cushing's or Addison's disease
- DM
- Pregnancy
- Immunosuppression
- Steroid treatment
- Vaginal trauma
- Broad-spectrum antibiotics
- Radiotherapy/chemotherapy
- Tight-fitting synthetic underwear

**History** Well; pruritus vulvae; superficial dyspareunia; thick, creamy non-offensive discharge.

**Examination** Discharge (cottage cheese); sore vulva which may be cracked or fissured.

**Investigation** Usually unnecessary. Confirm diagnosis if infection persists or recurs by sending a swab from the anterior fornix for M,C&S.

***Management*^G** Only treat if symptomatic.
- Try clotrimazole pessaries—cure rate ~90%.
- Alternative is oral fluconazole 150mg stat, repeated after 3d if severe infection. Contra-indicated in pregnancy or lactation—83% cure rate.
- Sexual transmission is minimal and there is no benefit from treating the partner unless overt infection.
- Benefits of ingestion or topical application of live yoghurt are not clear, although it is probably not harmful.

***Recurrent infection*^G** Advise loose, cotton underwear and avoidance of soaps, perfumes or disinfectants in the bath. Consider vulval emollients to treat associated dermatitis. If ≥4 documented episodes (≥2 confirmed with microbiology) in a year, treat with fluconazole 150mg every 3d × 3, then 150mg weekly for 6mo.

**Sexually transmitted infections** □ p.736

**Further information**
**British Association of Sexual Health and HIV (BASHH)**
🖳 www.bashh.org
- Management of bacterial vaginosis (2006)
- Management of vulvovaginal candidiasis (2007).

**Information for patients**
**Women's Health** 🖳 www.womens-health.co.uk
**Family Planning Association (FPA)** 🖳 www.fpa.org.uk

# Sexually transmitted infection

GPs are frequently presented with symptoms/signs either presented directly or found incidentally (e.g. when doing a cervical smear) which may indicate sexually transmitted infection (STI). The easiest (and often best) option is to refer suspected cases to genito-urinary medicine (GUM) clinics. Sometimes the patient is reluctant to go and 40% of referrals never attend, so it is still necessary for GPs to know how to prevent, diagnose, and treat STI themselves.

**Contact tracing** Best done by GUM clinics. If a patient refuses to go, then provide him/her with a letter to give to contacts stating the disease he/she has been in contact with, treatment given, and suggesting contacts visit their local GUM clinic promptly.

**Use of GUM clinics** In general refer patients:
- Who require contact tracing
- If counselling is needed (e.g. first attack HSV, HIV)
- If diagnosis is still unclear after investigation
- For confirmation of diagnosis (e.g. HSV)
- If specialist treatment is required (e.g. treatment of genital warts).

**Prevention of STIs** NICE recommends:
- Identification of high-risk patients opportunistically in general practice, e.g. at new patient checks, when attending for travel advice.
- One-to-one structured discussions with individuals at high risk of STIs lasting 15–20 min. Structured on the basis of behaviour change theories to ↓ risk-taking.

*High-risk groups* Include patients with STIs, men who have had sex with other men, people who have come from/visited areas of high HIV prevalence, substance/alcohol misuse, early onset of sexual activity, unprotected sex and frequent change of/multiple partners

*Young people from vulnerable groups* (e.g. from disadvantaged backgrounds, in/leaving local authority care, low educational attainment) should be offered one-to-one sessions aimed at educating them about sexual health and contraception.

*Chlamydia screening* A screening programme for the under 25s is currently in operation in the UK (🔲 p.738).

*Vaccination* A vaccine targeting the most common forms of HPV causing cervical cancer is now available in the UK. The target population is girls aged 12–14y before they become sexually active (🔲 p.747), but potentially any sexually active woman could benefit.

*Prevention of HIV* 🔲 p.742

*Vaginal discharge* 🔲 p.734

**Acute pelvic inflammatory disease (PID)** May be asymptomatic. Peak age 15–25y. >10% develop tubal infertility after 1 episode; 50% after 3 episodes. Risk of ectopic pregnancy ↑ ×10 after a single episode. Only 70% of those with acute PID clinically, have diagnosis confirmed on laparoscopy. Most cases of PID are associated with STI (usually chlamydia (50%) or gonorrhoea). In 20% no cause is found.

### History

- Fever >38° C and malaise
- Acute pelvic pain (usually bilateral) and deep dyspareunia
- Dysuria
- Abnormal vaginal bleeding—heavier periods, intermenstrual and/or postcoital bleeding
- Purulent vaginal discharge.

**Examination** Pyrexia, bilateral lower abdominal tenderness, vaginal discharge, cervical excitation, and adnexal tenderness.

### Investigations *Consider*

- *Swabs*—HVS and endocervical swab for M,C&S and chlamydia screen.
- *Blood*—FBC (may show leucocytosis),↑ ESR/CRP.

**Management** Admit if very unwell, pregnant, or if ectopic pregnancy or other acute surgical emergency cannot be excluded. *Otherwise*:

- Advise rest and sexual abstinence, provide analgesia.
- Treat with ofloxacin 400mg bd and metronidazole 400mg bd for 14d. Alternative is ceftriaxone 250mg IM as a single dose, followed by oral doxycycline 100mg bd and oral metronidazole 400mg bd for 14d.
- If the patient has an IUCD consider removal, but only if symptoms are severe. If removed, advise re alternative contraception and emergency contraception if sexual intercourse <7d ago.
- Arrange contact tracing via GUM clinic.
- If no improvement after 48h, admit; if slow recovery consider referral for laparoscopy to exclude abscess formation.

**Chronic PID** Due to inadequately treated acute PID. Presents with pelvic pain, dysmenorrhoea, dyspareunia (1:5) ± menorrhagia. *Examination*: lower abdominal/pelvic tenderness, cervical excitation ± adnexal mass. Screen for chlamydia and gonorrhoea (🕮 p. 738). A –ve result does not exclude diagnosis. If chronic pelvic pain with no obvious cause, refer to gynaecology. Once diagnosis is confirmed treatment options include long-term antibiotics or surgery.

**Urethritis** Inflammation of the male urethra. Multifactorial condition primarily sexually acquired. Mucopurulent cervicitis is the female equivalent. Characterized by discharge and/or dysuria although may be asymptomatic (found when a swab is taken following contact tracing). Treat the cause. Classified by the organisms grown:

**Gonococcal urethritis** *N. gonorrhoea* is identified on urethral swab. Treat as for gonorrhoea (🕮 p.738).

**Non-gonococcal urethritis** The most common organisms identified are: Chlamydia (30–50%), Ureaplasmas (10%), Mycoplasma genitalium (10%) and Trichomonas vaginalis (1–17%). In 20–30% no organism is isolated. First-line treatment is with azithromycin 1g stat. If persistent/recurrent symptoms treat with azithromycin 500mg stat, then 250mg od for 4d and metronidazole 400mg bd for 5d.

### Further information

**NICE** Preventing sexually transmitted infections and reducing under-18 conceptions (2007) 🖳 www.nice.org.uk

**RCOG** Management of acute pelvic inflammatory disease (2009) 🖳 www.rcog.org.uk

**British Association for Sexual Health and HIV** National guidance on the management of non-gonococcal urethritis (2008) 🖳 www.bashh.org

# Chlamydia, gonorrhoea, and trichomonas

**Chlamydia** Major cause of pelvic pain and infertility in women.

**Screening** Chlamydia is a preventable cause of infertility, ectopic pregnancy, and pelvic inflammatory disease. Screening using urine testing or self-taken swabs ↓ prevalence and incidence of pelvic inflammatory disease.[5] The DH has implemented a National screening programme, initially aimed at young people aged 16–24y in England. Self-test kits are available through GP surgeries, sexual health/contraception clinics, and community venues (e.g. schools). Similar programmes are being considered in the rest of the UK.

**Presentation in men** Usually asymptomatic. May have urethritis. Send urethral swab or first catch urine sample for nucleic acid amplification test (NAAT) to confirm diagnosis.

**Presentation in women**
- *History* >70% are asymptomatic. *Symptoms*: vaginal discharge (30%); postcoital or intermenstrual bleeding; pelvic inflammatory disease (10–30% (📖 p. 736)); dysuria.
- *Examination* Mucopurulent cervicitis; hyperaemia and oedema of the cervix ± contact bleeding; tender adnexae; cervical excitation.
- *Investigation* Send cervical or vulvo-vaginal swab ± first catch urine sample for NAAT to confirm diagnosis. Urine samples are used for screening asymptomatic women.

 **Presentation in neonates** Conjunctivitis, pneumonia, pharyngitis, otitis media—1:3 affected mothers have affected babies.

**Management**
- Doxycycline 100mg bd for 1wk or erythromycin 500mg qds for 14 d; azithromycin 1g po as a single dose is an alternative which ensures compliance.
- During pregnancy /breastfeeding use erythromycin 500mg qds 2wk.
- Affected neonates—seek specialist advice.
- Consider supplying home-testing kits to patients at high risk of STIs.

**Gonorrhoea** *Transmission*: ~1:5 exposures (♂); 1:2 exposures (♀).

**Presentation in men** 50% acute infections are asymptomatic. May present with urethritis, prostatitis, urethral stricture, skin lesions, or septic arthritis. Send urethral ± rectal swabs for M,C&S to confirm diagnosis.

**Presentation in women** Infection may cause pelvic inflammatory disease, abscess of Bartholin's gland, miscarriage, or preterm labour. Send endocervical swab for M,C&S to confirm diagnosis. Taking rectal and urethral swabs ↑ sensitivity.

 **Presentation in neonates** Ophthlamia neonatorum. Purulent discharge from the eyes of an infant <21d old. Send swabs for M,C& S.

### Management[G]

- Ceftriaxone 250mg IM as a single dose. Alternatives are 1×400mg cefixime po or 1×500mg ciprofloxacin (if organism sensitive and not pregnant).
- Re-culture 3–7d after treatment. Contact tracing is essential (refer to GUM clinic)
- *Affected neonates.* Treat with hourly ofloxacin eye drops. Refer for urgent ophthalmology opinion as cornea may perforate.

## Trichomonas vaginalis (TV)

**Presentation in men** 15–50% are asymptomatic. May have dysuria and/or urethral discharge. Take urethral swab and first void urine sample for M,C&S.

**Presentation in women** 10–50% are asymptomatic. *Symptoms:*
- Vaginal discharge (25%)—copious, mucopurulent yellow, smelly discharge. May be frothy.
- Vulvo-vaginal soreness/itching
- Dysuria.

Examination shows typical 'fishy' yellow-white discharge, vaginal inflammation, and strawberry cervix. Send a swab from the posterior fornix at the time of speculum examination for M,C&S. May also be detected on cervical smear.

### Management[G]

- Advise patients to avoid sexual intercourse until they and their partner(s) have completed treatment and follow up.
- Metronidazole po (400mg bd for 5–7d. or 2g stat)—timidazole 2g stat is a suitable alternative.
- Consider referral to GUM clinic for contact tracing.
- Resistant TV—try higher dose metronidazole: 400mg tds po + 1g od pr for 7d, or metronidazole 2g od for 3–5d. High dose timidazole 2g bd for 2wk ± topical vaginal timidazole is an alternative.

## Further information

**British Association of Sexual Health and HIV (BASHH)**
⌨ www.bashh.org
- Management of *Chlamydia trachomatis* genital tract infection (2006)
- Management of gonorrhoea in adults (2005)
- Management of *trichomonas vaginalis* infection (2007)

**National Chlamydia Screening programme (NCSP)**
⌨ www.chlamydiascreening.nhs.uk

**Information sheets** Available from ⌨ www.patient.co.uk, ⌨ www.fpa.org.uk and ⌨ www.ssha.info

# Hepatitis B and C

**Hepatitis B (HBV)** Common. Endemic in much of Asia and the Far East. The virus has 3 major structural antigens: surface antigen (HBsAg), core antigen (HBcAg), and e antigen (HBeAg). Spread is via infected blood, sexual intercourse, mother to newborn baby, or human bites. Incubation period is 6–23wk (average 17wk).

**High-risk groups** Patients who are/have:

- Injecting drug users
- Many sexual partners
- Adopted children from high/ intermediate risk countries
- Foster parents
- Close family contacts of a case/ carrier
- Receiving regular blood/ blood products and their carers
- Chronic renal/liver disease
- Prison inmates
- At risk due to their occupation, e.g. healthcare workers
- Staff/residents of residential accommodation for individuals with mental handicap
- Travelling to high/intermediate-risk areas
- Babies born to mothers who are chronic carriers of hepatitis B/ have had acute hepatitis B in pregnancy.

**Presentation** May be asymptomatic or present with fever, malaise, fatigue, arthralgia, urticaria, pale stools, dark urine, and/or jaundice.

**Investigation** LFTs (hepatic jaundice—↑ bilirubin, ↑ ALT/AST, ↑ Alkaline phosphatase), hepatitis serology (Figure 22.1).

- HBsAg is present from 1 to 6mo post-exposure. If present >6mo after the acute episode defines carrier status.
- HBeAg—present from 6wk to 3mo after acute illness. Indicates high infectivity.
- Anti-HBs antibodies appear >10mo after infection and imply immunity.

**Management** In all cases advise patients to avoid alcohol. Refer for specialist advice. Treatment is supportive for acute illness. Chronic hepatitis is treated with interferon and lamivudine with varying success.

**Prognosis** ~85% recover fully; 10% develop carrier status; 5–10% develop chronic hepatitis—may lead to cirrhosis and/or liver carcinoma. Fulminant hepatitis and death are rare (<1%).

**Prevention** Advise patients re 'safe sex'. Immunize high-risk groups. Give passive immunization with human immunoglobulin to non-immune high-risk contacts of infected patients.

❶ *Hepatitis immunization of injecting drug misusers* If not already infected/ immune, or close contact of someone already infected, use a rapid regime— immunization at 0, 7, and 21d, and booster after 12mo.

**Hepatitis C (HCV)** Common. Spread is usually via contact with infected blood (causing post-transfusion hepatitis) but can pass from mother to baby. Not easily spread through sexual contact. In 10% no source of infection is found. Incubation is 2–25wk (mean 8wk).

**Risk factors** Blood transfusion; healthcare work; IV drug abuse; haemodialysis; infant of infected mother (5% risk); multiple sexual partners.

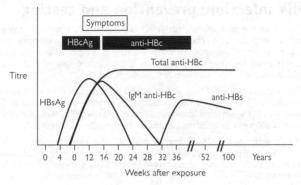

(a) Acute hepatitis B infection with recovery

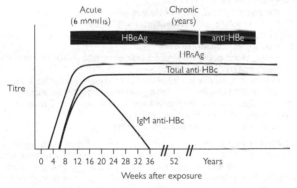

(b) Acute hepatitis B infection with progression to carrier state

**Fig. 22.1** Hepatitis B serology

Reproduced with permission of the US Centers for Disease Control and Prevention.

***Presentation and management*** As for HBV. Anti-HCV antibody is detectable 3–4mo post-infection. Refer for expert advice. Avoid alcohol. Half develop chronic infection; 5% cirrhosis, and 15% of those hepatoma.

### Further information

**British Association for Sexual Health and HIV** National guideline on the management of viral hepatidides (2008) ⌨ www.bashh.org
**Health Protection Agency (HPA)** ⌨ www.hpa.org.uk
**UK Clinical Virology Network** ⌨ www.clinical-virology.org
**Department of Health** The Green Book ⌨ www.dh.gov.uk

### Information for patients

**British Liver Trust** ☎ 0800 652 7330 ⌨ www.britishlivertrust.org.uk

# HIV infection: prevention and testing

Human immunodeficiency virus (HIV) is a retrovirus infecting T-helper cells bearing the CD4 receptor. Worldwide, the HIV epidemic continues, but prophylaxis and treatment are improving prognosis in developed countries where treatment is available. It is estimated that ~1:3 of those infected in the UK are unaware of their diagnosis.

**Transmission** Risk of transmission is ~1:1000 exposures. Transmission is sexual (60–70%)—heterosexual intercourse in 50% cases, or due to IV drug abuse (3%), infected blood products, mother → child (90% HIV infections in children), or accidental exposure (e.g. needle-stick injuries).

❶ HIV antibodies can take 3mo to develop after HIV infection, so HIV tests may miss those infected in the early stages of their disease. Consider repeating if infection may have occurred <3mo prior to testing. If in doubt, arrange a second test 3mo after the first. HIV antibody testing gives no indication of disease progression.

## Prevention of HIV infection
- Promotion of safe sex and ↓ IV drug abuse and needle-sharing.
- Consider prophylaxis if sexual contact with an infected individual (or high-risk individual if HIV status unknown) <72h before presentation—take advice from GUM clinic.
- Screening blood donors—seroconversion can take up to 3mo so there is still a small risk of transmission.
- Prevention of transmission from mother to child—risk can be ↓ to <5% by treatment with zidovudine given to the mother antenatally, during delivery, and to the neonate for first 6wk, elective Caesarean section, and advising against breastfeeding.
- Trials of HIV vaccines are in advanced stages.

***Accidental exposure*** (e.g. needle stick injury) Exposure is significant if the source is HIV +ve, the material is blood or another infectious body fluid (semen, amniotic fluid, genital secretions, CSF), and exposure is caused by inoculation (risk transmission 1:300 if HIV +ve source) or by a splash onto a mucus membrane (risk of transmission 1:3000).

⚠ *Immediate action* Irrigate site of exposure with running water. Establish potential risk of HIV—history of HIV infection and (if possible) blood sample from the source and victim. Refer to A&E immediately for instigation of HIV prevention policy.

## When should an HIV test be offered?
- Symptoms/signs of HIV disease (do not delay for HIV test if urgent specialist assessment is needed)
- Routine screening (e.g. antenatal, conditions associated with HIV such as TB, lymphoma, hepatitis B/C, syphilis or other STIs);
- Patient request, or
- Identified risk and never tested/further risk since last test:
  - Current/former infected sexual partner or sexual partner from a high prevalence area for HIV (e.g. sub-Saharan Africa, India)
  - Current/former sexual partner who is/was an injecting drug user.

- Patient is from a high prevalence area for HIV (though take careful history as may be at no risk at all).
- Anal/oral sex between men (oral sex < anal sex).
- Multiple sexual partners.
- Personal history of STI, rape, or injecting drug use.
- Surgery, blood transfusion, or other risk-prone procedure in high-risk country.

## Checklist of points to cover when arranging HIV testing

- Is the test best done in primary care? Would it be better for the patient to be referred to a GUM clinic where specialist counselling services and additional support may be available?
- Has the patient received pre-test counselling?
- Are repeat tests required?
- Should other tests be offered at the same time as HIV testing, e.g. hepatitis B/C testing, testing for chlamydia or syphilis?
- Has the patient given clear consent for all the tests proposed?
- Does the patient need hepatitis B immunization (🕮 p. 740)?
- How can the patient be contacted?
- Has an appointment been arranged for the patient to be given the result face to face?
- Has the patient a supply of condoms and lubricant to prevent new risk?

## Giving the result

*If the result is negative* Consider whether the patient needs a follow-up test in 3mo. Provide health promotion information about minimizing risk of HIV infection in future.

*If the result is positive* Give the result early in the consultation.
- Explain the result and its implications for the patient and his partner.
- Emphasize the positive aspects of knowing the diagnosis.
- Try to arrange specialist referral before the patient attends so that the patient can be given a time and date for specialist follow-up.
- Give the patient time to talk through feelings and fears.
- Talk about support available, e.g. friends/family, support organizations.
- Provide literature about HIV and patient support organizations.
- Arrange follow-up to maintain the link with primary care.

## Further information

**British Association of Sexual Health and HIV (BASHH)**
🖥 www.bashh.org
- National guidelines on HIV testing (2008)
- Guideline for the use of post-exposure prophylaxis for HIV following sexual exposure (2006).

**British HIV Association** Management of HIV infection in pregnant women and the prevention of mother-to-child transmission of HIV (2005) 🖥 www.bhiva.org

**RCOG** Management of HIV in pregnancy (2004) 🖥 www.rcog.org.uk

## Information and support for patients with HIV and carers

**NAM Aidsmap** 🖥 www.aidsmap.com
**National AIDS Helpline** ☎ 0800 567 123 (24h helpline)
**Terrence Higgins Trust** ☎ 0845 1221 200 🖥 www.tht.org.uk

# HIV infection: clinical disease

**Primary HIV** Many patients (about half) who are infected with HIV have no initial symptoms. Possible symptoms:

- Usually presentation in patients with symptoms is with a glandular fever-like syndrome of fever, fatigue, myalgia/arthralgia ± lymphadenopathy. Consider HIV as a differential diagnosis of glandular fever that is not confirmed on testing.
- More specific symptoms include a blotchy rash affecting the trunk and orogenital/perianal ulceration.
- Rarely, presents with acute neurological symptoms (aseptic meningitis, transverse myelitis, encephalitis) or diarrhoea.
- FBC may show atypical lymphocytes.
- Rarely, CD4 count drops acutely and conditions associated with immunosuppression (e.g. oral candidiasis or shingles) may occur.

⚠ If you think a patient has primary HIV infection, seek urgent advice from a specialist. HIV tests can be negative <3mo after infection.

**Early HIV** Follows seroconversion. Plasma viral load ↓ to a plateau. Level of the plateau is prognostic—'fast progressors' have high plateau levels and 'slow progressors' have low plateau levels. Most patients are asymptomatic. Symptoms if present include night sweats or generalized lymphadenopathy.

**Advanced HIV** Accompanied by immunosuppression, or *acquired immune deficiency syndrome* (AIDS) if CD4 count <200cells/mm³. Patients are at risk from opportunistic infection (e.g. pneumococcal infection, TB, CMV, *Pneumocystis jiroveci* (formerly known as PCP), toxoplasmosis, and cryptosporidial diarrhoea) and AIDS-associated malignancies (e.g. Kaposi sarcoma, lymphoma)—Table 22.1. Pneumocystis pneumonia may be the presenting feature of HIV infection.

**Death** Can be due to multiple causes, including chronic incurable systemic infections, malignancies, neurological disease, wasting and malnutrition, and multisystem failure.

**Management** Specialist treatment is essential.

- *Antiviral drugs* A combination of antiviral drugs is usual—highly active anti-retrovirus therapy (HAART). Adherence to therapy is essential to avoid resistance. Treatment failure requires switching or increasing therapy.
- *Prophylaxis against opportunistic infection* Prophylactic antibiotics are used to prevent *Pneumocystis*, toxoplasmosis, and *Mycobacterium avium* for patients with low CD4 counts.
- *Psychological support* Because of the stigma attached to HIV infection, patients and carers often lack the support offered by the community for most other serious illness.

**Kaposi sarcoma** Purple papules or plaques on skin or mucosa of any organ. Metastasizes to lymph nodes. Two types:
- Endemic—occurs in central Africa. Peripheral lesions, good response to chemotherapy
- Associated with AIDS or transplant patients—commonly skin or pulmonary lesions; lymphatic obstruction predisposes to cellulitis. If suspected get expert help.

*M.K.Kaposi (1837–1902), Hungarian dermatologist.*

**Table 22.1** CD4 counts and HIV-related problems

| CD4 count (cells/µL) | Risk of opportunistic infection | Risk of HIV-associated tumours |
|---|---|---|
| >500 | Minimal/none | Very small ↑ risk |
| 200–500 | Little risk unless falling rapidly, except TB | Small ↑ risk |
| <200 | ↑ risk of serious opportunistic infection, e.g.<br>• *Pneumocystis* pneumonia<br>• Toxoplasmosis<br>• Oesophageal candida | Increasing risk |
| <100 | Additional risk of:<br>• *Mycobacterium avium intracellulare*<br>• Cytomegalovirus | High risk and increasingly aggressive disease |

First reproduced in Madge S, Matthews P, Singh S *et al.* (2004, revised 2005) HIV in Primary Care. London: Medical Foundation for AIDS and Sexual Health (MedFASH)

## Further information
**Medical Foundation for AIDS and Sexual Health** HIV in primary care (2004, revised 2005) 🖥 www.medfash.org.uk
**British HIV Association** HIV Treatment Guidelines (2006) 🖥 www.bhiva.org

## Information and support for patients with HIV and carers
**NAM Aidsmap** 🖥 www.aidsmap.com
**National AIDS Helpline** ☎ 0800 567 123 (24h helpline)
**Terrence Higgins Trust** ☎ 0845 1221 200 🖥 www.tht.org.uk

# Other sexually transmitted infections

**Genital herpes** HSV is transmitted by direct contact with lesions. Lesions may appear anywhere on the skin or mucosa, but are most frequent around the mouth and on the lips, conjunctiva, cornea, and genitalia.

***Presentation of primary infection*** May be asymptomatic. If symptomatic, history and examination are diagnostic in 90% of cases. Presents with multiple painful genital ulcers on a red background ± inguinal lymph nodes <1wk after sexual contact. Lesions crust over then heal. Untreated lasts 3–4wk. *Complications*: urinary retention, aseptic meningitis.

## Management

- Refer to GUM if diagnosis is uncertain and for contact tracing.
- Treat with aciclovir if presents within the first 5d of symptoms starting and while new lesions are still forming (↓ duration, symptoms, and complications).
- Analgesia, ice packs and salt baths may help. 5% lidocaine ointment gives symptom relief but use with caution as may cause sensitization.
- Advice: barrier methods of contraception (risk of transmission in monogamous relationships—10%/y).
- If pregnant obtain specialist advice.

 **Neonatal infection** Presents at age 5–21d with vesicular lesions around the presenting part or, rarely, systemic infection. Usually babies of women with no history of genital HSV. Refer as a paediatric emergency.

**Recurrent infection** Reactivation of latent virus. Less severe than 1° infection. Neonatal transmission rates are low (<3%)—elective Caesarean section for those with active recurrences at term is controversial. Consider suppressive therapy if ≥6 attacks/y, e.g. aciclovir 400mg bd. Usually initiated under consultant supervision. If breakthrough occurs, ↑ dose of antiviral, e.g. aciclovir 400mg tds.

**Genital warts** Caused by human papilloma virus (HPV). Usually sexually transmitted and >25% have concomitant STIs. Disease may be clinical (found on examination) or subclinical (changes associated with infection detected on smear). In women CIN (📖 p.724) is related to infection with HPV types 16 and 18, but 90% of genital warts are caused by HPV types 6 or 11.

***Presentation in women*** Often asymptomatic but may be associated with itching or vaginal discharge. Warts are usually seen on the vulva or introitus. Warts enlarge during pregnancy.

***Presentation in men*** Warts are usually found on the penis or perianally.

***Management of clinical warts*** Treatment does not eradicate the virus but removes lesions. Barrier contraception is needed for at least 3mo after the warts are gone. Treatment options in primary care:

- *Podophyllotoxin*—suitable for home treatment of unkeratinized genital warts and licensed for a 4wk course. Avoid in pregnancy. Apply 2x/d for 3d, followed by a 4d rest. This cycle is repeated 4-5x. *Side effects*: soreness/ulceration of the genital skin—advise to discontinue treatment.

- *Imiquimod* (Aldara®) Can be used at home for keratinized or non-keratinized warts. Avoid in pregnancy. Apply 3×/wk. On each occasion wash off 6–10h later. Continue for up to 16wk. Avoid unprotected intercourse after application. Can weaken latex condoms.

*Alternatives* (usually in specialist settings): trichloroacetic acid, excision, cryotherapy, electrosurgery.

---

 **Human papilloma virus (HPV) vaccination** HPV vaccines are aimed at preventing infection with strains causing cervical cancer. Currently vaccines target strains 16 and 18, which account for ~70% of HPV-related cancer cases, ± strains 6 and 11. Vaccination in the UK is targeted at girls before the age at which they become sexually active (12–14y). Cervical screening in adulthood will still be necessary as the vaccine does not protect against all strains causing cervical cancer.

---

**Pubic lice** Pubic (or crab) lice are similar to head lice and may be sexually transmitted. All hairy areas (including eyelashes, eyebrows, and pubic and axillary hair) can be affected. Carbaryl (unlicensed), phenothrin, and malathion are all effective. Apply an aqueous solution to all parts of the body and rinse off after 12h. Repeat after 7d.

**Scabies** 📖 p.637

**Syphilis** Caused by *Treponema pallidum*. Rare in the UK but incidence is increasing. *Incubation*: 9–90d. In all cases refer for specialist care. Contact tracing is essential. 4 stages:
- *Primary syphilis* Chancre at the site of contact.
- *Secondary syphilis* Systemic symptoms 4–8wk after chancre—fever, malaise, generalized lymphadenopathy, anal papules (conylomata lata), rash (trunk, palms, soles), buccal snail track ulcers, alopecia.
- *Tertiary syphilis* 2–20y after initial infection—gummas (granulomas) in connective tissue, e.g. testicular gumma.
- *Quarternary syphilis* Cardiovascular or neurological complications. *Investigation*: blood for VDRL or TPHA.

## Further information
**British Association of Sexual Health and HIV (BASHH)**
🖳 www.bashh.org
- Management of genital herpes (2007)
- Management of *Phthirus pubis* (2007)
- Management of scabies (2007)
- Management of syphilis (2008)
- Management of genital warts (2007).
**Health Protection Agency (HPA)** 🖳 www.hpa.org.uk
**UK Clinical Virology Network** 🖳 www.clinical-virology.org

## Information for patients
**Family Planning Association (FPA)** 🖳 www.fpa.org.uk
**Herpes Association** ☎ 0845 123 2305 🖳 www.herpes.org.uk

# Summary of contraceptive methods

80% of women receive contraceptive advice and treatment through their GP. A sexually active woman has an 85% chance of becoming pregnant in <1y without contraception and ~1:3 pregnancies are unplanned.

**Contraceptive services** Provided by practices as an additional service. If a practice 'opts out' the global sum is ↓ by 2.4%. Intrauterine devices may be fitted as a *national enhanced service*. Payment is available for fitting the device and a further payment is for annual review.

**Choice of method** There is no ideal method of contraception. *Consider*: the woman's personal preference, age, lifestyle/cultural aspects, medical history, and risk of sexually transmitted disease. ❶ Prescriptions for contraceptives are free of charge for all women.

**Before providing contraception** Provide information that will enable the woman to choose a method and use it effectively (Table 22.2). Exclude pregnancy. A woman is probably not pregnant if she has not had unprotected sexual intercourse since her last period, has been using a reliable method of contraception correctly, or is <7d after the start of a normal period, <4wk postpartum, <7d post-termination or miscarriage, or fully breastfeeding, amenorrhoeic, and <6mo postpartum. If in doubt, do a pregnancy test ≥3wk after the last unprotected sexual intercourse.

## Emergency contraception

***<72h (3d) after unprotected intercourse*** Use a single dose of levonorgestrel 1.5mg—available OTC and on prescription. Efficacy: 0–24h, 95% efficacy; 25–48h, 85%; 49–72h, 58%. Possible pitfalls:
- *Vomiting <3h after taking levonorgestrel*—give a replacement dose. If an antiemetic is required, prescribe domperidone.
- *Enzyme-inducing drugs*, e.g. anti-epileptics, St. John's wort—efficacy may be ↓. Consider a copper IUCD or ↑ dose of levonorgestrel to 3mg (1.5mg immediately and 1.5mg 12h later—unlicensed).

❶ There is no evidence that treatment with levonorgestrel harms the fetus.

***<5d after unprotected intercourse*** Insertion of a copper IUCD before implantation. Progestogen-containing IUCDs are not suitable for this purpose. Failure rate <1%.

***All women*** Advise to return if abdominal pain, if next period is overdue or abnormally light/heavy, or if needs further contraceptive advice.

**Sexually transmitted infections** Discuss transmission of STIs with all women when providing contraception. Advise high-risk groups to use barrier methods in addition to hormonal methods of contraception.

## Contraception for special groups
- *Teenagers* 📖 p.768
- *Women >35y* 📖 p.769
- *Women with epilepsy* 📖 p.755
- *After termination of pregnancy or miscarriage* 📖 p.766
- *Postpartum* 📖 p.835

## Further information
**FFPRH** Emergency contraception (2006) 🖥 www.ffprhc.org.uk

**Table 22.2** Summary of contraceptive methods

| Method of contraception | % unintended pregnancy* | Advantages | Disadvantages |
|---|---|---|---|
| Sterilization (♂) | 0.05 (1:2000) | No contraindications<br>Single procedure | Difficult to reverse<br>Post-operative complications |
| Sterilization (♀) | 0.5 (1:200) | No contraindications<br>Single procedure | Requires general anaesthetic and rarely results in laparotomy<br>Post-operative complications<br>Difficult to reverse<br>↑ risk ectopic pregnancy |
| Implanon (Single capsule upper arm) | 0.05 | Lasts 3y<br>Immediately reversible | Needs training to insert and remove<br>Can cause irregular bleeding<br>Progestogenic side effects |
| Progestogen-containing intrauterine system (IUS) (e.g. Mirena) | 0.1 | Lasts 5y<br>↓ bleeding, ectopic pregnancy risk, dysmenorrhoea<br>Endometrial protection | May cause erratic bleeding<br>Progestogenic side effects |
| Combined oral contraceptive (COC) | 0.3 (8) | Regular cycle and lighter periods<br>↓ dysmenorrhoea<br>Cycle control | Compliance<br>Side effects<br>↑ risk breast cancer, thromboembolism |
| Progestogen-only pill (POP) | 0.3 (8) | Few side effects and contraindications. | Compliance<br>Irregular bleeding<br>Progestogenic side effects |
| Intrauterine contraceptive device (IUCD) | 0.6 (0.8) | Lasts ≥ 5y<br>No systemic effects | Heavy periods<br>No protection from pelvic inflammatory disease or ectopic pregnancy |
| Injectable progestogen (e.g. Depo-Provera) | 0.3 (3) | Avoids pill taking<br>↓ bleeding and can help PMS<br>↓ risk of ectopic pregnancy, endometrial cancer | Menstrual irregularity<br>Weight gain<br>Unpredictable return of fertility<br>↑ risk osteoporosis |
| Barrier methods (condoms, diaphragm) | 2 (32) | Barrier to transmission of STIs | User-dependent<br>Allergy |
| Natural methods | 1 (27) | No contraindications or side effects | Teaching required<br>High failure rate |

*Failure rates stated are with perfect use. Rates in parentheses are with typical use.

# Combined contraception

Contraceptives containing an oestrogen and progestogen are available as pills—the combined oral contraceptive pill (COC)—and patches (Evra®).

**COC pill** Most COC pills come in packets of 21 pills. The woman takes the entire packet, starting on the first day of her cycle, and then has a 7d 'pill-free' break before starting the next packet. Pills vary by:

**Oestrogen content** Ranges from 20 to 40 micrograms.
- *Low-strength preparations* Choose if risk factors for circulatory disease but COC is not contraindicated, or if oestrogenic side effects.
- *Standard strength preparations* Contain ethinylestradiol 30 or 35 micrograms. Use for most women.
- *Phased preparations* Dose of oestrogen/progestogen varies through the cycle. Try for women who do not have withdrawal bleeding or have breakthrough bleeding with monophasic products.
- *Every day (ED) preparations* 21 active pills and 7 'inactive' pills to cover the 'pill-free' week. Taken continuously. Can help women who find remembering to start a new packet difficult.

**Progestogen type** COC pills containing:
- *Levonorgestrel or norethisterone.* Suitable for most women. Choose for first-time COC pill users.
- *Desogestrel (Marvelon®), norgestimate (Cilest®), or gestodene (Femodene®)* Consider if women have side-effects with other progestogens, e.g. acne, headache, depression, weight ↑, breast symptoms, breakthrough bleeding. ❶ Desogestrel and gestodene are associated with ↑ risk of venous thromboembolism.
- *Drospirenone (Yasmin®)* has anti-androgenic and anti-mineralocorticoid activity.
- *Cyproterone acetate (Dianette®)* Licensed for treatment of acne, not for contraception, but does provide contraception. Use for 3–4mo after resolution of symptoms. Associated with 4× ↑ risk of venous thromboembolism compared with COC containing levonorgestrel.

**Contraceptive patch (Evra®)** 20 micrograms ethinylestradiol and norelgestromin in a transdermal patch. Alternative if compliance with daily pill-taking is problematic. Apply patch on day 1 of the cycle; change patch on days 8 and 15; remove third patch on day 22; then apply new patch after a 7d 'patch-free' interval to start the subsequent cycle.

## Risk is greater than benefit if
- Aged >35y and a smoker *or* age >50y and non-smoker.
- BMI >39kg/m² (if >30kg/m² ↑ risk DVT/PE—consider alternatives).
- BP is consistently >140mmHg systolic and/or 90mmHg diastolic.
- PMH of cardiovascular disease (IHD, CVA, peripheral vascular disease), ≥2 risk factors for arterial disease or complicated valvular heart disease (pulmonary hypertension, risk of AF, SBE)
- PMH of venous thromboembolism or >1 risk factor for venous thromboembolism.
- DM—if vascular complications or present for > 20y.
- Focal migraine (Figure 22.2, 📖 p.753).

**Table 22.3** Risks and benefits of combined contraception

| Disease | Rates/100 000 women | Relative risk with COC use |
|---|---|---|
| **Risks** | | |
| Coronary artery disease | 1500 | Non-smoker— no ↑ Smoker—>20×↑ risk |
| Stroke | 100 | 2×↑ in ischaemic stroke—no ↑ in haemorrhagic stroke Smoker (>15 cigarettes/d)—7×↑risk ischaemic stroke |
| Venous thrombo-embolism | 5 | 3×↑ with norethisterone/levonorgestrel-containing COCs 5×↑ with gestodene/desogestrel-containing COCs |
| Breast cancer | 2000 (up to age 50y) | Any small ↑ in risk disappears <10y after stopping the COC pill |
| Cervical cancer | 11 | Small ↑ after 5y use Risk 2× ↑ after 10y use |
| **Benefits** | | |
| Ovarian cancer | 22 | Halving of risk lasting ≥10y |
| Endometrial cancer | 15 | Halving of risk lasting ≥10y |

Reproduced with permission from the Faculty of Family Planning and Reproductive Health Care

**Venous thromboembolism** Use with caution and avoid gestodene/desogestrel COCs if 1 risk factor is present; avoid if >1:
- **FH of venous thromboembolism** in first-degree relative <45y* or known prothrobotic coagulation abnormality (e.g. factor V Leiden or antiphospholipid antibodies).
- **Obesity**—BMI >30kg/m². Avoid if BMI >39kg/m².
- **Long-term immobilization** Avoid if bed bound or leg in a cast.
- **Varicose veins** Avoid during sclerosing treatment or where definite history of thrombosis.

**Arterial disease** Use with caution if one risk factor; avoid if >1:
- **FH of arterial disease** in first-degree relative <45y. Avoid if patient has hypercholesterolaemia/hypertriglyceridaemia
- **DM** Avoid if complications present or present >20y
- **Hypertension** BP >140/90 mmHg—avoid if >160/100 mmHg
- **Smoking** Avoid if smoking ≥40 cigarettes/d.
- **Age** Avoid if >50y or if >35y and smokes.
- **Obesity** Avoid if BMI >39kg/m².
- **Migraine**—Figure 22.2, 🕮 p.753.

* Refer for thrombophilia screen.

❶ Investigate any undiagnosed vaginal bleeding before starting combined contraception.

- Female malignancy—breast cancer, genital cancer.
- Hormone-related problems in pregnancy, e.g. hydatidiform mole, pruritus, cholestasis, pemphigoid gestationis, otosclerosis
- Fully breastfeeding <6mo postpartum.
- Liver disease—acute hepatitis until LFTs are normal, liver adenoma, gallstones. Take specialist advice for other liver diseases.
- Porphyria.

## Before starting combined contraception

- Take a history—medical, sexual health, medications, and lifestyle. Use with caution if history of depression, inflammatory bowel disease, or sickle cell disease. If hyperprolactinaemia, seek specialist advice.
- Consider a routine thrombophilia screen if FH of DVT/PE in a first-degree relative aged <45y or multiple family members, and/or check cholesterol/triglycerides if FH of arterial disease in a first-degree relative <45y or multiple family members.
- Check BP.
- Education—discuss side effects/risks of combined contraception, STIs, cervical smears, smoking, weight control. Give directions on use.

**Starting combined contraception** Contraceptive effect is immediate if started:
- On day 1–3 of the cycle.
- At the end of the third week postpartum.
- <7d after miscarriage/TOP at <20wk gestation.
- Changing COC pill variety or to patch—start the new pill/patch omitting the 7d break (or 'inactive' tablets if taking ED preparation).
- On day 1 of the cycle and changing from POP (if switching to the combined patch use additional contraception for 7d).

❶ In all other cases use additional contraception for the first 7d.

**Follow-up** 3mo after starting or changing combined contraceptive—earlier if complications. Once established, review every 6–12mo. At follow-up assess risk factors and side effects; give health education, e.g. smoking cessation advice, information about STIs; check BP.

**Missed pills** In all cases, advise women to take the most recent missed pill as soon as it is remembered, and use the remaining pills at the usual time (this may entail taking 2 tablets in 1 day).
- If ≤2 × 30 or 35 micrograms, or 1 × 20 micrograms ethinylestradiol pill has been missed—no additional contraception is needed.
- If ≥3 × 30 or 35 micrograms, or ≥2 × 20 micrograms ethinylestradiol pill has been missed, advise to use condoms or abstain from sex until pills have been taken for 7d in a row. In addition:
  - If pills are missed in week 1 (days 1–7)—consider emergency contraception (📖 p.748) if unprotected sex in the pill-free interval or week 1.
  - If pills are missed in week 3 (days 15–21)—advise to finish the pills in the current pack and start a new pack the next day, omitting the pill-free break.

**Missed patches** See BNF 7.3.1.

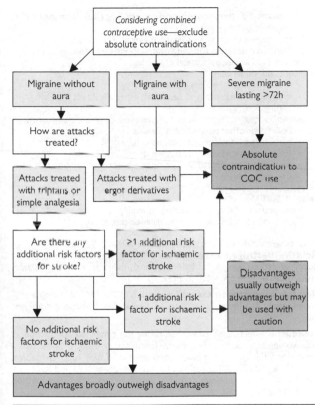

⚠ Ask women to report ↑ in headache frequency or onset of focal symptoms when using any combined contraceptive. If new focal symptoms, discontinue immediately and, if not typical of migraine aura and last >1h, admit.

**Fig. 22.2** Migraine and combined contraceptive use

Reproduced with permission from the *British Journal Family Planning* (1998) **24**:54–60.

**Long journeys and DVT** Women taking combined contraceptives are at ↑ risk of DVT during travel involving long periods of immobility (>5h). Advise women:
- To drink plenty of non-alcoholic fluids.
- To keep their legs moving whilst sitting, or walk up and down the aisle.

Graduated compression hosiery is available for purchase OTC and does ↓ risk of DVT.

⚠ **Reasons to stop combined contraception immediately** (pending investigation if needed):
• Sudden severe chest pain (even if not radiating to left arm).
• Sudden breathlessness (or cough with bloodstained sputum).
• Unexplained severe pain in calf of one leg.
• Acute abdominal pain.
• Serious neurological effects including:
  • unusual severe prolonged headache, especially if first time or getting progressively worse, or
  • sudden dysphasia, partial or complete loss of vision, disturbance of hearing, or other perceptual disorders
  • bad fainting attack or unexplained collapse
  • first unexplained epileptic seizure
  • weakness, motor disturbances, or numbness affecting one side or one part of body.
• Hepatitis, jaundice, liver enlargement.
• BP >160/100mmHg.
• Prolonged immobility after surgery or leg injury.
• Detection of a risk factor/contraindication (🕮 p.750).

**Short-term side effects** Usually resolve within 2–3 cycles.
*Relative oestrogen excess* Breast tenderness (3.6%); nausea (1.5%); dizziness; cyclical weight ↑; bloating; vaginal discharge without infection. Use a more progestogen-dominant pill.

*Relative progestogen excess* Depression (3.9%); PMT; dry vagina; sustained weight ↑; ↓ libido; lassitude; acne. Use a more oestrogen-dominant pill.

*Headache* Affects 2.9% of women taking the combined contraception. Ask women to report ↑ in headache frequency or onset of focal symptoms when taking any combined contraceptive. If new focal symptoms, discontinue immediately and, if not typical of migraine aura and lasts >1h, admit. If headaches continue, consider switching brand/alternative method of contraception.

*Breakthrough bleeding* Most common in the first few months of combined contraceptive use—after six cycles affects 1.1% of women (spotting affects 3.3% of women). If no vomiting/diarrhoea and no missed pills, breakthrough bleeding does not indicate ↓ efficacy. If breakthrough bleeding persists:
• Check for gynaecological causes—exclude STI (especially chlamydia); examine cervix; check smear is up to date and take smear if overdue; exclude pregnancy.
• Check compliance—any missed pills? (breakthrough bleeding may start 2–3d after a missed pill); any diarrhoea/vomiting?

↑ oestrogen content of COC pill if on low-dose preparation. If problem persists, change progestogen. If still persists ↑ progestogen and/or try phased preparation.

**Long-term risks/benefits** Table 22.3, 🕮 p.751.

**Drug interactions** Many drugs affect efficacy of combined contraceptives. These broadly fall into 2 categories:
- *Hepatic enzyme inducing drugs,* e.g. antibacterials; rifamycins (rifampicin, rifabutin); St John's Wort; anticonvulsants (phenytoin, carbamazepine, oxcarbazepine, phenobarbital, primidone, topiramate); griseofulvin; antivirals (nelfinavir,nevirapine, ritonavir); modafinil.
- *Broad-spectrum antibiotics* interfere with absorption by affecting gut flora (e.g. amoxicillin, tetracyclines).

## Management
- *<3wk course of a non-enzyme-inducing broad-spectrum antibiotic* e.g. amoxicillin Does *not* affect the contraceptive patch. If taking the COC pill, use additional contraception during the course and for 7d afterwards. Omit the pill-free interval if the 7d runs beyond the end of the packet. Omit the inactive tablets if using an FD preparation.
- *Short course (<7d) of enzyme-inducing drug*—advise additional barrier contraception whilst taking the enzyme-inducing drug and for 4wk after stopping it. Omit pill/patch-free week or inactive tablets if using an ED preparation.
- *Longer course of enzyme-inducing drug*—advise alternative method of contraception, e.g. intrauterine device.

*Long-term antibiotics*
- If long-term antibiotics are prescribed, additional barrier precautions are needed for the first 3wk with omission of the pill-free weeks.
- Additional precautions are unnecessary if a woman starting a COC pill has been on a course of antibacterials for ≥ 3wk.
- If the antibiotic type is changed or dose is ↑, an additional barrier method is required for 3wk with omission of the pill-free week

*Antibiotics that do NOT affect pill efficacy*— erythromycin, co-trimoxazole, sulphonamides.

*Anticonvulsants that do NOT affect pill efficacy*—sodium valproate; lamotrigine (but seizure frequency may ↑ when combined contraception and lamotrigine are used together and side effects of lamotrigine may ↑ when combined contraception is stopped).

**Diarrhoea and vomiting** Does *not* affect the contraceptive patch. If a woman vomits <2h.after taking a COC pill or has very severe diarrhoea, assume the COC pill has not been absorbed and treat as missed pill (☐ p.752).

**Surgery** Combined contraceptives should be discontinued and alternative contraceptive arrangements made (e.g. Depo injection, barrier methods) 4wk before major elective surgery and all surgery to the legs or surgery which involves prolonged immobilization of a lower limb. Restart the combined contraceptive on the first day of the next period occurring ≥2wk after full mobilization.

## Further information
**Family Planning Association (FPA)** ☎ 0845 122 8690 ☐ www.fpa.org.uk
**Faculty of Family Planning and Reproductive Healthcare**
☐ www.ffprhc.org.uk

# Progestogen-only contraceptives

Progestogen-only contraceptives thicken cervical mucus, ↓ endometrial receptivity, and inhibit ovulation. They ↓ risk of pelvic infection and can be used when oestrogen is contraindicated.

## Contraindications to all progestogen-only methods

- Undiagnosed abnormal PV bleeding.
- Hormone-dependent tumour (women with a past history of breast cancer may use the POP after 5y if no evidence of current disease).
- Porphyria.
- Liver adenoma/severe liver disease.
- Current or high risk of arterial disease.
- Pregnancy.
- ↑ HCG due to trophoblastic disease.

**Progestogen-releasing intrauterine device** (intrauterine system, Mirena®) 🕮 p.760

**Progestogen-only pill (POP or 'mini-pill')** (BNF 7.3.2.1) Oral POPs are a suitable alternative for women for whom oestrogen-containing pills are contraindicated:

- Older women.
- Heavy smokers.
- Women with past history/predisposition to venous thromboembolism.
- Patients with hypertension, valvular heart disease, DM or migraine
- Breastfeeding women <6mo-post partum. ❶ Delay until ≥3wk postpartum to avoid risk of heavy bleeding.

*Choice of POP* 5 brands are currently available in the UK:

- Etynodiol 500 micrograms—Femulen®
- Norethisterone 350 micrograms—Micronor® or Noriday®.
- Levonorgestrel 30 micrograms—Norgeston®.
- Desogestrel 75 micrograms—Cerazette®. Consider if compliance problems, history of ectopic pregnancy or ovarian cysts (desogestrel has a stronger ovarian suppressive effect than other POPs), and/or weight >70kg.

## Side effects

- Higher failure rate than COC pills.
- Menstrual irregularities—oligomenorrhoea, menorrhagia, amenorrhoea. Examine to exclude a pathological cause ± do a pregnancy test. Menstrual irregularities tend to resolve with long-term use. If necessary, consider changing progestogen or ↑ to 2 pills/d (unlicensed).
- ↑ risk of ectopic pregnancy. If a patient presents with abdominal pain, treat as an ectopic pregnancy (🕮 p.813) until proven otherwise.
- Others—nausea and vomiting; headache; dizziness; breast discomfort; depression; skin disorders; disturbance of appetite; weight changes; changes in libido.
- *Long term*—small ↑ risk breast cancer. Risk reverts to normal <10y after stopping the POP.

### Starting the POP

- *No previous hormonal contraception* Start on day 1 of cycle—no additional contraception needed
- *Changing from a COC* Start the day following completion of the course of COC without a break (omitting the 'inactive' pills if ED preparation)—no additional contraception needed.
- *After childbirth* Start any time >3wk postpartum (↑ risk of breakthrough bleeding if started earlier). Does not affect lactation. No additional contraception needed.
- *If weight >70kg* Consider desogestrel or prescribing 2 tablets/d of one of the other POPs (unlicensed).

**Directions for taking the POP** Take one tablet every day with no pill-free breaks. Take each tablet at the same time each day (>4h before usual time for intercourse to give maximum protection)—if delayed >3h (>12h for desogestrel) treat as missed pill

**Missed pills** If a pill is missed or delayed >3h (>12h for desogestrel), continue taking the POP at the usual time and use additional barrier methods for 2d.

⚠ Give emergency contraception if ≥1 POPs have been missed or taken >3h late (>12h late for desogestrel) and unprotected intercourse has occurred in the 2d following this.

**Diarrhoea/vomiting** Continue taking the POP but use an additional barrier method during the episode and for 2d afterwards.

**Interactions with other drugs** Efficacy of POPs is not affected by anti-bacterials that do not induce liver enzymes. Efficacy is ↓ by enzyme-inducing drugs (📖 p.755)—advise women to use an additional barrier or alternative contraceptive method during treatment and for >4wk afterwards.

**Follow-up** Review patients 3mo after starting the POP or changing from COC pill—earlier if complications. Once established, review every 6–12mo—assess risk factors and side effects; give health education, e.g. smoking cessation advice, information about STDs; check BP.

**Injectable progestogens** (BNF 7.3.2.2) Useful if oestrogen-containing preparations are contraindicated or compliance is a problem. Failure rate is <4/1000 women over 2y.

### Advantages

- Can be used to age 50y if no other risk factors for osteoporosis.
- ↓ ectopic pregnancy, functional ovarian cysts, and sickle cell crises.
- ↓ risk of endometrial cancer. Provides endometrial protection as part of HRT regime (unlicensed).
- May alleviate premenstrual syndrome and ↓ menorrhagia.

### Disadvantages

- May ↓ bone density in first 2–3y of use. Consider DEXA scan in older women if result would influence choice.
- Can mask natural menopause.
- May be a delay in return of fertility of up to 1y on stopping.

- Can cause menstrual disturbance. If troublesome give next injection early (8–11wk after the previous injection for Depo) or add oestrogen if no contraindications.
- Other side effects, e.g. weight ↑ (up to 2–3kg), mood swings, acne

⚠CSM advice about Depo-Provera®
- In all women, weigh benefits of use for >2y against risks.
- In women with risk factors for osteoporosis, consider a method of contraception other than Depo-Provera®.
- In adolescents, Depo-Provera® should only be used only when other methods of contraception are inappropriate.

**Depo-Provera®**—medroxyprogesterone acetate 150 mg/ml.
- Give 1 × 1mL by deep IM injection into the buttock/lateral thigh or deltoid up to day 5 of the cycle. Do not rub the injection site afterwards.
- If given after day 5, check the woman is not pregnant and provide and advise an additional method for 7d.
- Postpartum: delay until >6wk after childbirth. If not breastfeeding, first dose can be given <5d after childbirth but may cause heavy bleeding.
- Repeat every 12wk. If interval is >12wk and 5d, see Table 22.4.

**Noristerat®**—norethisterone enantate 200mg/ml. Warm first, then give 1 × 1mL by deep IM injection into the gluteal muscle before day 6 of the cycle or immediately after childbirth (avoid breastfeeding if baby has jaundice requiring treatment). Do not rub the injection site afterwards.
May be repeated once only after 8wk. Unlicensed if repeated further.

**Interactions** Effectiveness is not ↓ by antibacterials that do not induce liver enzymes. Effectiveness of Noristerat® (but not Depo-Provera®) is ↓ by enzyme-inducing drugs—advise additional contraception whilst taking these drugs and for 4wk after stopping *or* alternative method.

**Progestogen implant** (BNF 7.3.2.2) One implant is currently available in the UK. Implanon® is a semi-rigid rod (40mm × 2mm) releasing 30–40 micrograms/d of etonogestrel. The rod is inserted subdermally into the lower surface of the upper arm before day 6 of the cycle. If inserted after day 5, check that the woman is not pregnant and use an additional method for 7d.

**Advantages** Lasts 3y and once inserted no compliance required; can be used for women at risk of ectopic pregnancy; no effect on bone density; once removed, fertility returns immediately to normal

**Disadvantages** A minor operation is needed for insertion/removal. Special training is needed and complications of minor surgery can occur (e.g. infection, scarring). ↓ efficacy with liver-enzyme-inducing drugs—advise additional method for duration of treatment and 4wk afterwards, or alternative contraception if enzyme-inducing drugs are being used long term. Cannot be used as part of HRT regime. May cause menstrual disturbances—exclude other causes. Treat with oestrogen (Marvelon® contains the same progestogen), additional progestogen or NSAID. Other side effects include acne, mood swings, breast tenderness, change in libido—treat symptoms as needed.

**Table 22.4** Late Depo-Provera® guidelines

| Timing of Depo-Provera® | Has un-protected sex occurred? | Can the injection be given? | Is emergency contra-ception needed? | Are condoms or abstinence advised? | Should a pregnancy test be done? |
|---|---|---|---|---|---|
| Up to 12wk and 5d since date of previous injection | N/A | Yes | No | No | No |
| When an injection is overdue | No | Yes | No | Yes—for the next 14d* | No |
| | Yes— but only in the last 3d | Yes—or give Cerazette® for 21d | Yes | Yes—for the next 14d* | Yes—21d later |
| | Yes—but only in the last 3–5d | Yes—or give Cerazette® for 21d | Yes—offer copper IUD | No | Yes—21d later |
| | Yes—>5d previously | No | No | Yes—for 21d until pregnancy test is confirmed negative and for a further 14d* after giving Depo injection | Yes—at initial presen-tation and 21d later |

◆ *WHO/FFPRH recommendations state that injections of Depo-Provera® can be given up to 14wk and Noristerat® can be given up to 10wk after the previous injection without the need for additional barrier contraception. These guidelines also state that, when needed, additional contraception is only necessary for 7d.

## Further information
**NICE** Long-acting reversible contraception (2005) ▢ www.nice.org.uk
**Faculty of Family Planning and Reproductive Healthcare**
▢ www.ffprhc.org.uk
- Progestogen-only pills (2009)
- Progestogen-only injectable contraception (2009)
- Progestogen-only implants (2008)

## Patient information
**Family Planning Association** ☎ 0845 122 8690 ▢ www.fpa.org.uk

# Intrauterine devices

**Intrauterine contraceptive device (IUCD)** (BNF 7.3.4) Plastic carrier wound with copper wire/fitted with copper bands. Suitable for older parous women, as second-line contraception in young nulliparous women, or for emergency contraception. Acts by inhibiting fertilization, sperm penetration of the cervical mucus, and implantation. Pregnancy rate with IUCDs containing 380 mm² copper is < 20/1000 over 5y.

**Intrauterine system (IUS)** (BNF 7.3.2.3) The progestogen-only intrauterine system (Mirena®), releases levonorgestrel 20 micrograms/24h directly into the uterine cavity. It acts by preventing endometrial proliferation, thickening cervical mucus, and suppression of ovulation (some women and some cycles). Licensed uses include:
- Contraception—particularly suitable for women with heavy periods.
- Primary menorrhagia—menstrual bleeding is d significantly in 3–6mo.
- Prevention of endometrial hyperplasia during oestrogen therapy.

**Emergency contraception** 📖 p.748

**Choice of devices**—Table 22.5

## Contraindications
*IUCD only* Allergy to copper; Wilson's disease; heavy/painful periods.

### IUCD and IUS
- Pregnancy or <4wk postpartum.
- Current or high risk of STI or pelvic inflammatory disease (includes severe immunosuppression)—a woman should not have an IUCD/IUS fitted <3mo after treatment of a pelvic infection. Following treatment of STI suitability depends on ongoing risk.
- Undiagnosed uterine bleeding.
- Distorted uterine cavity.
- Current endometrial, ovarian, or cervical cancer, or trophoblastic disease.
- Anticoagulation. Caution—use another method if possible.

## Advantages
*IUCD only* No systemic side effects; does not mask the menopause; if fitted in a woman of >40y can remain in the uterus until menopause

### IUS only
- ↓ menorrhagia/dysmenorrhoea.
- ↓ risk of pelvic inflammatory disease, particularly younger age groups.
- ↓ risk of ectopic pregnancy compared with IUCD.
- If 45y and amenorrhoeic, can be left in situ for 7y for contraception (unlicensed)—change after 4y if using IUS for endometrial protection.

### IUCD and IUS
- Long-lasting and can be used until the menopause (Table 22.5).
- Once fitted, no compliance is needed.
- Easily and immediately reversible by removal.
- Can be used for women who are breastfeeding, obese, or have concurrent illness—migraine, venous thromboembolism, DM, cardiovascular disease (or ↑ risk of cardiovascular disease), or women

taking long-term hepatic-enzyme-inducing drugs (e.g. anticonvulsants, antivirals).
• Can be used for HIV +ve women, but screen for STIs first and advise condom use.

## Disadvantages and problems

### IUCD only

• *Ectopic pregnancy* Risk (0.02/100 woman-years) is higher than if using a hormonal contraceptive method but not compared with women using no contraception at all. If pregnancy occurs, ↑ risk of ectopic pregnancy (1:20). Consider ectopic pregnancy in any woman with an IUCD presenting with abdominal pain.
• ↑ *dysmenorrhoea/menorrhagia* Most common reason for discontinuation. Exclude infection and malposition. Exclude other gynaecological causes. Treat with NSAID or tranexamic acid, or consider changing to IUS.

### IUS only Progestogenic side effects:

• Changes in pattern/duration of menstrual bleeding (spotting/prolonged bleeding) are common—warn women prior to insertion. Bleeding usually becomes light/absent within 3–6mo of insertion.
• Mastalgia, mood changes, change in libido→ usually resolve in <6mo.
• Ovarian cysts—usually resolve spontaneously. Monitor with USS.
• Cannot be used for emergency contraception.

**Table 22.5** Intrauterine devices currently available in the UK.

| Device | Licence | Uterine length | Comment |
|---|---|---|---|
| Flexi-T 300® | 5y | >5cm | Easy insertion |
| GyneFix® | 5y | Any | Frameless. Special training needed for insertion. ↓ expulsion if fitted correctly |
| Load 375® | 5y | >7cm | |
| Multiload Cu375® | 5y | 6–9cm | |
| Nova-T 380® | 5y | 6.5–9cm | Small insertion diameter |
| T-Safe Cu380A® | 8y | 6.5–8cm | Gold standard |
| TT 380 Slimline® | 10y | >7cm | Easy insertion |
| UT 380 Short or Standard® | 5y | Short— <7cm Standard— >7cm | |
| Mirena® | 5y (4y if being used to prevent endometrial hyperplasia) | >6.5cm | Intrauterine system releasing levonorgestrel 20 micrograms/24h. Does *not* contain copper. |

## *IUCD and IUS*

- *Fitting and removal* requires specialist training and can be uncomfortable for the woman.
- *Expulsion/malposition*—risk of expulsion is ≈1:20. Usually occurs <3mo after insertion. Teach women to feel for threads after each period. If threads cannot be felt, advise other contraception until checked by health professional (Figure 22.3)
- *Perforation of the uterus*—risk <1:1000.
- *Pelvic inflammatory disease* ↑ risk of infection <21d after insertion. Related to existing carriage of STIs. It is good practice to screen for STIs, and treat infection, prior to insertion.
- *Actinomyces-like organisms (ALOs) on cervical smear* Assess to exclude pelvic infection. If no signs of pelvic infection, offer choice to leave device *in situ* or change it. If symptomatic discuss antibiotic treatment with microbiology and refer to GUM/gynaecology for further management.
- *Intrauterine pregnancy* Confirm intrauterine pregnancy with USS. Remove device at <12wk gestation whether or not the woman intends to continue the pregnancy. If pregnancy is >12wk or no threads are visible, refer to obstetrics/gynaecology.

**Insertion** Special training is required. The Faculty of Family Planning and Reproductive Health Care run a training scheme (☎ 020 7724 5669 🖥 www.ffprhc.org.uk). Accreditation must be updated every 5y. IUS/IUCDs may be inserted:

- < 7d after onset of menstruation—tail end of a period is the optimum time; heaviest days of a period are best avoided.
- At any other time in the cycle if replacement IUS/IUCD. If first device, and not in the first 7d of the cycle, ensure not pregnant and advise additional method for 7d.
- Immediately after TOP/miscarriage or >4wk postpartum (unlicensed <6wk postpartum), irrespective of the mode of delivery.[N]
- Always consider pre-screening for STI (especially chlamydia) ± antibiotic prophylaxis, e.g. azithromycin 1g stat prior to insertion. Advise women to contact a doctor if any sustained pain is experienced in the first 3wk after insertion.

⚠ **Cervical shock** Rare complication of IUD insertion. Presents with pallor, sweating, and bradycardia. Immediately tip the woman head down with legs raised. If symptoms/bradycardia persist, give 0.6mg atropine IV.

⚠ **Women with epilepsy** ↑ risk of seizure at the time of cervical dilation—ensure emergency drugs are available.

**Follow-up** Review after first period, then annually. Ask about periods, pelvic pain, vaginal discharge, and discomfort to partner. Perform pelvic examination to check threads.

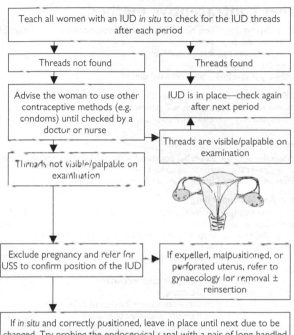

Fig. 22.3 Missing intrauterine device threads

Reproduced from Sadler et al., Women's Health (2007) with permission from Oxford University Press.

## Removal

- If pregnancy desired—remove at any time.
- If pregnancy is not desired—remove after establishing a hormonal method or use barrier methods/abstinence for ≥7d prior to removal. If urgent removal is necessary, provide emergency contraception if mid-cycle and intercourse has occurred in the previous 7d (📖 p.748).
- Menopause—remove after 1y amenorrhoea if aged >50y or after 2y amenorrhoea if aged <50y. If there is difficulty removing the device, try again after a 5d course of oestrogen.

## Further information

**FFPRHC** Intrauterine contraception (2007) 🖥 www.ffprhc.org.uk
**NICE** Long-acting reversible contraception (2005) 🖥 www.nice.org.uk

## Patient information

**Family Planning Association** ☎ 0845 122 8690 🖥 www.fpa.org.uk

# Other contraceptive methods

**Sterilization** There are no absolute contraindications to sterilization of men or women, provided that:
- They make the request themselves
- They are of sound mind *and*
- They are not acting under external duress.

⚠ If there is any question of a person not having the mental capacity to consent to a procedure that will permanently remove their fertility, the case should be referred to the courts for judgment.

## Method
- *Women*—laparoscopic tubal occlusion with clips or rings. Usually done under general anaesthetic as a day case.
- *Men*—vasectomy. Usually done under local anaesthetic as a day case.

## Pre-referral counselling
- Alternative long-term contraceptive methods (include sterilization of partner as an alternative).
- Reversibility—sterilization is intended to be permanent. Reversal is only 50–60% successful.
- Post-procedure pregnancy rate ('failure rate'—1:200 for women, 1:2000 for men).
- ↑ risk of ectopic pregnancy post tubal occlusion.
- Risk of operative complications.
- Effect on long-term health—no proven long-term risks.
- Need for contraception before and after operation:
  - *Women:* other contraception until first post-procedure period
  - *Men:* other contraception until two consecutive semen analyses, 2–4wk apart and ≥8wk after the procedure show azoospermia.

❶ All counselling should be supported by accurate impartial information.

⚠ Take additional care when counselling:
- People <30y.
- People without children.
- People taking decisions during pregnancy.
- People taking decisions in reaction to a loss of relationship.
- People at risk of coercion by their partner, family, or health or social welfare professionals.

**Condoms** Give protection against STIs. Male and female versions. Encourage to use a condom with spermicide, or prescribe separate spermicidal cream/pessaries. Advise about emergency contraception in the event of an accident. Certain lubricants (e.g. petroleum jelly, baby oil, and oil-based vaginal/rectal preparations) can ↓ effectiveness. Water-based lubricants are safe (e.g. K-Y® Jelly).

**Vaginal diaphragms or caps** (BNF 7.3.4) Flat metal spring, coiled metal rim, or arcing spring diaphragms are available. Motivation is crucial.

- Fitting must be performed by a doctor or nurse trained to fit diaphragms. Arcing diaphragms are useful when the cervix is posterior or there is mild prolapse.
- After fitting, a woman should practice inserting, wearing, checking the diaphragm is over the cervix, and removing the diaphragm for >1wk using another form of contraception.
- Spermicides must always be used in combination with diaphragms and the diaphragm must be left *in situ* for at least 6h after intercourse.
- Some vegetable/mineral oil-based lubricants (e.g. petroleum jelly, baby oil) can damage caps. Water-based lubricants are safe.

**Follow-up** Check fit and comfort after ~1wk and again discuss the routine for use, especially the importance of spermicide. See after 3mo and then annually, but more frequently if there are difficulties, if there is a weight change of >4kg, if the woman has a baby, or after pelvic surgery. Prescribe a new diaphragm yearly.

**Cervical/vault caps** (BNF 7.3.4) Attach by suction. Otherwise used in the same way as a diaphragm. Useful for women with poor muscle tone, absent retropubic ledge, or recurrent cystitis when using a diaphragm.

**Spermicides to use in combination with caps or condoms** (BNF 7.3.3) Gygel®.

**Avoidance of intercourse during times of fertility** 3 methods of estimating time of ovulation are used.

- Urine testing—a commercial kit (Persona®) is available OTC.
- Temperature—taken orally in the morning before drinking/getting up (thermometer available on FP10). ↑ 0.2–0.4°C indicates progesterone release from the corpus luteum. Unprotected intercourse can take place only from the third day of the ↑ until the next period.
- Mucus texture (Billing's method)—texture of vaginal secretions is felt between finger and thumb daily. Prior to ovulation the mucus becomes profuse and slippery; then abruptly changes to being thicker and more tacky. No unprotected intercourse from the day the mucus becomes more profuse until 3d after it becomes tacky. Patients with cycles >28d or <28d must vary timings.

**Coitus interruptus** Penis is withdrawn prior to ejaculation.

**Further information**

Family Planning Association ▣ www.fpa.org.uk
**Faculty of Family Planning and Reproductive Healthcare** Male and Female Condoms (2007) ▣ www.ffprhc.org.uk
**Royal College of Obstetricians and Gynaecologists** Male and female sterilisation (2004) ▣ www.rcog.org.uk

**Patient information**

Fertility UK ▣ www.fertilityuk.org
Family Planning Association ☎ 0845 122 8690 ▣ www.fpa.org.uk

# Termination of pregnancy

**Legal constraints** The Human Fertilization/Embryology Acts 1967 and 1990 govern termination of pregnancy (TOP) in the UK. Termination is allowed at <24wk gestation if it:

• ↓ risk to the woman's life.
• ↓ risk to the mother's physical/mental health (90% of TOPs are carried out under this clause).
• ↓ risk to the physical/mental health of the mother's existing children.
• The baby is at serious risk of being physically or mentally handicapped.

There is no upper time limit if there is:

• Real risk to the mother's life
• Risk of grave permanent injury to the mother's physical or mental health *or*
• The baby would be born seriously physically or mentally handicapped.

TOPs >24wk can only be carried out in NHS hospitals. 99% of TOPs take place <20wk Those taking place >20wk are usually performed when fetal abnormality is found on USS (or amniocentesis) or if pregnancy is concealed in the very young.

## Procedure

• *Medical* Oral mifepristone followed 1–3d later by vaginal prostaglandin.
• *Surgical* suction termination <15wk; dilatation and evacuation >15wk.

**Follow-up** In many areas post-procedure follow-up is undertaken by the GP. Worrying symptoms are:

• Excessive blood loss
• Pain *and/or*
• High temperature.

Assess, consider the possibility of infection, and treat if reasonably well—admit if worried.

❶ Check anti-D has been given if needed (📖 p.818) and chosen method of contraception has been started.

## Complications

• Infection
• Haemorrhage
• Uterine perforation
• Cervical trauma
• Failed procedure and ongoing pregnancy
• Psychological sequelae.

❶ There is no association between TOP and subsequent infertility or miscarriage/pre-term delivery.

## Contraception post termination or miscarriage <24wk

• *Combined pill/patch, POP, progestogen injection/implant* Start on the day of surgical or second part of medical abortion. No additional method required. If started >7d after abortion, an additional method is required for 7d (combined pill/patch or progestogen injection/implant) or 2d (POP).
• *IUCD or IUS* Insert at time of surgical or second part of medical abortion. No additional method required. Otherwise delay insertion to 4wk post-abortion—use another method in the interim.

## The role of the GP

• The earlier in pregnancy an abortion is performed, the lower the risk of complications. General practice is often the first stage of the referral procedure—have arrangements which minimize delay.
• Termination of pregnancy, especially for 'social' reasons, is a difficult ethical area for many GPs. We do not sit in moral judgement. Whatever your views, be sympathetic and if not prepared to refer yourself, arrange for the patient to see someone who will as soon as possible.
• Confirm pregnancy if unsure. Assess dates by bimanual palpation or arrange dating USS.
• Counselling—unbiased counselling to allow a woman to reach a decision she feels is right for her. This is an important decision she will have to live with for the rest of her life. Why does she want a termination? Has she considered alternatives? Does her partner/parents know? What are their views?
• Ideally the woman should be given some time once she has all the information to make her decision (e.g. follow-up in a few days). Offer a let out clause—she can always change her mind right up until the time of the procedure and you will support whatever decision she makes.
• Consider signing form HSA1.
• Discuss contraception after TOP (Ideally do this before TOP so it can be started immediately after).
• Arrange follow-up after the procedure.

## Further information

**RCOG** The care of women requesting induced abortion (2004)
🖳 www.rcog.org.uk

## Information and support for women considering termination of pregnancy

**Marie Stopes International** ☎ 0845 300 8090 🖳 www.mariestopes.org.uk
**British Pregnancy Advisory Service (BPAS)** ☎ 0845 730 40 30
🖳 www.bpas.org
**Brook Advisory Centres** (patients <25y only) ☎ 0800 802 1234
🖳 www.brook.org.uk
**Antenatal Results and Choices (ARC)** Supports parents faced with termination for fetal abnormality ☎ 0207 631 0285 🖳 www.arc-uk.org

# Teenagers and women over 35

## Contraception for the under 16s

***Sexual health problems*** >½ have sexual intercourse under the age of 16y. Those who have intercourse early are at ↑ risk of early pregnancy, STI, and cervical cancer. Worries about sexuality can add to the pressure for some. Sensitive support, clear guidance, and accurate information about contraception, sexuality, and STI are helpful. Remember to offer chlamydia screening (📖 p.738) to the under 25s.

***Teenage pregnancy*** The UK has the highest teenage pregnancy rate in Western Europe. Not all are unplanned. Pregnant teenagers need information and non-judgmental support to help them reach a decision whether or not to continue with the pregnancy

***Providing contraception to the under 16s*** In England and Wales, a doctor is allowed to give contraceptive advice and treatment to a girl aged <16y without parental consent if it is in her best interest that such advice/ treatment is given, and she:
- Has sufficient maturity to understand the moral, social, and emotional implications of treatment
- Cannot be persuaded to inform her parents
- Is very likely to begin, or continue, sexual intercourse with or without contraception
- Is likely to suffer if no contraceptive advice or treatment is given.

Usual principles of confidentiality apply. In particular, adolescents judged to be competent can withhold permission for parents to have access to medical information about them and request to be seen alone without a parent.

❶ Ensure that confidentiality is not breached when appointments are booked (e.g. for emergency contraception) and when telephoning about results, appointments, or prescriptions.

### Choice of contraceptive method
- Condoms are adolescents' most commonly used form of contraception but have a relatively high failure rate. Suggesting their use in addition to another form of contraception helps prevent STIs.
- The combined oral contraceptive (COC) pill is the most suitable method of contraception for the under 16s. Poor compliance can be a problem and leads to a relatively high failure rate.
- Progestogen implants/injectables—reliable alternative to COC pill. Offer long-acting reversible contraception to all teenagers. ❶ The CSM advises that, in adolescents, medroxyprogesterone acetate (Depo-Provera®) should only be used when other methods of contraception are inappropriate. May ↑ osteoporosis risk (use alternative if other risk factors and try not to use >2y), menstrual irregularity, and ↑ weight.
- The progestogen-containing intrauterine contraceptive device (IUS) is less likely to cause pelvic inflammatory disease and ectopic pregnancy than other IUCDs but can be difficult to insert in a young woman.
- The 'morning after pill' (Levonelle®) is not suitable as regular contraception, but is valuable in preventing unwanted pregnancy. Provide information on availability and ability to make an urgent appointment.

*Do's and don'ts*
- *Don't* insist on vaginal examination or taking a smear unless there is a problem that necessitates it.
- *Do* discuss the merits of delaying sexual intercourse until older.
- *Do* stress the need for protection against STI.
- If prescribing the COC pill for dysmenorrhoea or cycle control in young women, *do* explain its use for contraception too.

## Information and support for teenagers

**Brook Advisory Service** Contraceptive advice and counselling for teenagers ☎ 0808 802 1234 🖳 www.brook.org.uk

**Sexwise** For under 19s ☎ 0800 28 29 30

**Teenage Health Freak** 🖳 www.teenagehealthfreak.org

**Contraception for women >35y** Fertility ↓ with age. A woman is postmenopausal and therefore not fertile 2y after her last menstrual period if she is <50y and 1y after her last menstrual period if she is >50y. Contraception can be discontinued >55y.

❶ An FSH level >35iu/L is suggestive of menopause. Confidence with which it can be interpreted ↑ with age, length of time the woman has experienced menopausal symptoms, and duration of amenorrhoea.

**Combined oral contraceptive** Non-smokers with no risk factors for CVD or breast cancer can use the COC until 50y. Consider using lower-dose (20 micrograms oestrogen) preparation and/or one with lipid-friendly progestogen (e.g. gestodene, desogestrel). Helps menopausal and menstrual symptoms, and bone density. ↑ FSH at the end of the pill-free week is suggestive of menopause.

**Progestogen-only pill** Can be continued to 55y and used as the progestogen component of HRT—but three POPs a day are needed for endometrial protection (unlicensed use and no data for desogestrel). Does not interfere with FSH levels.

**Injectable progestogen** Can be used up to 50y in women not at risk of osteoporosis (though CSM advises that benefits of using injectable medroxyprogesterone acetate for >2y should be evaluated against risks of ↓ bone density). Helps menstrual disturbance. Masks the menopause.

**Progestogen implant** Cannot be used as part of HRT regime. Masks the menopause.

**IUS (Mirena®)** Helps menorrhagia. Licensed for endometrial protection (can be used as part of an HRT regime). Masks the menopause.

**IUCD** Does not mask the menopause. Copper intrauterine devices fitted in women >40y may remain in the uterus until post-menopause.

## Further information

**Family Planning Association (FPA)** ☎ 0845 122 8690 🖳 www.fpa.org.uk

**FFPRH** Contraception for women aged over 40 years (2005) 🖳 www.ffprhc.org.uk

**World Health Organization (WHO)** 🖳 www.who.int
- Selected Practice Recommendations for Contraceptive Use (2004)
- Medical eligibility criteria for contraceptive use (2004).

# Infertility

Failure to conceive after 1y regular unprotected sexual intercourse in the absence of known reproductive pathology. Affects ~1 in 5 couples.

**Pregnancy rates** The normal rate of pregnancy in the first year is 20–25% per cycle. 84% of couples conceive after 1y of unprotected intercourse (17 in every 20 couples); 92% conceive after 2y (19 of every 20 couples); after 3y, the pregnancy rate is still ~25%/y.

## Causes of infertility

- Ovulatory dysfunction ~30%
- Pelvic disease ~20%
- Male factor ~20%
- Unknown ~30%.

**Initial approach** Most couples tend to present at about 1y. Where possible, see the couple together. This shows mutual commitment and initiates ongoing couple-centred management.

*Couple* Ask about:

- Length of time trying to conceive.
- Frequency of and/or difficulties with sexual intercourse, e.g. psychosexual problems, physical disability. Includes excessive travelling which may limit optimal coital timing and indirectly affect fertility.

*Women* Ask about:

- Previous pregnancies—children, miscarriages, same/different partner?
- Menstrual cycle—length of cycle (normal cycle is 21–35d duration), changes in cervical mucus through the cycle, ovulatory discomfort?
- Past gynaecological history—cervical smears, previous pelvic surgery, sexually transmitted disease/pelvic inflammatory disease, PCOS.
- Past medical history—systemic or debilitating disease, e.g. thyroid dysfunction, DM, inflammatory bowel disease, anorexia nervosa.
- Drug history—chemotherapy, phenothiazines, cannabis, NSAIDs
- Lifestyle—occupation (exposure to pesticides?), smoking, alcohol, excessive exercise, stress.

*Men* Ask about:

- Previous children, same/different partner?
- PMH—mumps, other testicular disease, STI
- Any systemic or debilitating diseases?
- Drug history—sulfasalazine, nitrofurantoin, tetracycline, cimetidine, ketoconazole, colchicine, allopurinol, α-blockers, tricyclic antidepressants, MAOI, phenothiazines, propranolol, chemotherapy, anabolic steroids, cannabis, cocaine.
- Social history—occupation (exposure to pesticides, X-rays, solvents, paints, chemicals from smelting or welding), smoking, alcohol, excess exercise, stress, social or occupational factors which might cause testicular hyperthermia.

*Adverse factors* Age (♀ only—fertility ↓ significantly from mid-30s), BMI <19 (♀ only) or >29 (♂ and ♀), smoking (↓ fertility by ~ 1/3), excess alcohol (♂ only), excess caffeine (>2 cups of coffee/d, ♀ only).

**Examination** Consider pelvic/genital examination.

**GP investigations** Perform investigations if no pregnancy after a year of trying to conceive— sooner if aged >35y.

### Female
- Rubella status.
- Chlamydia serology—indicator of possible tubal disease.
- Mid-luteal progesterone—check on day 21 of the menstrual cycle for a woman with a 28d cycle. Adjust timing if longer/shorter cycle. Can only be accurately interpreted after the next period as aims to 'catch' the progesterone peak 7d before the next period. Normal value (>30nmol/L) signifies ovulation.
- FSH/LH—check on day 1–5 of the menstrual cycle.
- Consider TFTs if symptoms/signs of thyroid disease, or prolactin—if galactorrhoea or any suggestion of pituitary tumour

**Male** Sperm problems affect ~1.5 couples. Semen analysis is important even if the man already has children. If the first test is abnormal, advise loose trousers and underwear, and repeat after 3mo or as soon as possible if grossly abnormal ❶ Abnormal sperm do not fertilize ova

*Instructions for producing a semen sample for analysis* No sex for 2d beforehand and no more than 7d since last sex (may affect motility). Masturbate into labelled sterile pot without use of condoms/jellies. Keep the sample warm (e.g inside pocket) and deliver to the laboratory within 2h. Hand over directly to a member of laboratory staff if possible.

**Referral** Local protocols vary. Generally refer after 18mo of failure to conceive despite regular intercourse. Refer sooner if abnormal history, examination, or investigations, e.g.
- *Female* Age >35y; amenorrhoea/oligomenorrhoea; previous pelvic inflammatory disease or STI
- *Male* Previous genital pathology or urogenital surgery; varicocoele; significant systemic illness

### Possible treatments GPs may need to continue to prescribe
- Clomifene—ovarian stimulation, treatment for oligospermia.
- Tamoxifen—may be prescribed to women intolerant of clomifene.
- Metformin—used as an adjunct to clomifene in overweight women with PCOS who fail to respond to clomifene alone.
- Gonadotrophins, dopamine agonists (e.g. bromocriptine).

**Counselling** Consider early referral for specialist counselling. Access through national support groups and at local specialist fertility centres. Useful contacts:
- British Infertility Counselling Association 🖳 www.bica.net
- British Fertility Society 🖳 www.britishfertilitysociety.org.uk

### Further information
**RCOG** Fertility: assessment and treatment of people with fertility problems (2004) 🖳 www.rcog.org.uk

### Advice and information for patients
**National Fertility Association (ISSUE)** ☎ 0800 008 7464
🖳 www.issue.co.uk

# Sexual problems

Sexual problems may have a physical or psychological basis but *all* develop a psychological aspect in time. Both partners have a problem in ~30% cases. Be supportive—your response will determine whether the patient receives appropriate help.

### Assessment

- *History of the problem* What is the problem? If new, when did it start? Why consult now? What outcome does the patient want? Is the patient complaining or is his/her partner?
- *Sexual history* Details of sex education; attitude towards sex; past history of sexual problems (or lack of problems).
- *Medical history* Chronic disease; psychiatric problems; current medication.
- *Social history and recent life events.*
- *Examine* genitalia for abnormalities or tenderness—helpful but do not insist as it may scare the patient away.

**❶** *Always consider psychological aspects* Poor self-image; anger or resentment—relationship/financial difficulties, children, parents, work stress; ignorance or misunderstanding; shame, embarrassment or guilt—view that sexuality is 'bad', sexual abuse; anxiety/fear about sex—fear of closeness, vulnerability, letting go, and failure.

**Lack of sexual interest** Usually needs specialist help. Often there are underlying psychological difficulties which may relate specifically to sex, e.g. previous child abuse, or a general psychological disorder. Women frequently lose interest around the menopause or after operations (especially mastectomy or hysterectomy), or if their partner's performance repeatedly leads to frustration (e.g. impotence). Both sexes lose interest if depressed or after traumatic events.

**Vaginismus** Usually apparent at vaginal examination—severe spasm of the vaginal muscles and adduction of thighs. May be detected incidentally when undertaking routine procedures, e.g. cervical smear Try to find the root cause. *Common causes:*

- Fear of the unknown.
- Past history of rape, abuse, or severe emotional trauma.
- Defence mechanism against growing up.

*Management* Desensitize simple cases by encouraging the women to examine herself, and also encourage the partner to be confident enough to insert a finger into the vagina. If no success, refer.

**Orgasmic problems in women** *Consider:*

### Physical reasons

- Drugs— major tranquillizers, antidepressants.
- Neurological disease.
- Pelvic surgery—recognized complication of hysterectomy.

### Psychological reasons

- *Women who have never achieved an orgasm* may have psychological reasons. Give 'permission' for the woman to investigate her body's own responses further by masturbation or vibrator. When she has learnt how to relax, encourage her to tell her partner and incorporate caressing into their usual lovemaking.
- *Women who have lost the ability to achieve orgasm* may need counselling, especially about current relationship or loss of self-image.

**Dyspareunia** 📖 p.712          **Erectile dysfunction** 📖 p.774

**Premature ejaculation** Ejaculation sooner than either partner wishes. With practice men can learn to delay ejaculation. The stop–start technique may be effective: when during caressing or intercourse a man feels he is close to climax he should stop being stimulated and relax for 30sec; stimulation can then recommence until he is close to climax again, when the relaxation is repeated. If this fails, the woman should squeeze the penis at the base of the glans between finger and thumb during relaxation phases. Consider referral for sex therapy if no improvement.

**Delayed ejaculation** May be a sign of long-standing sexual inhibition. Often patients can ejaculate by masturbation, but not intravaginally. Explore anxiety and guilt feelings. Use a strategy like that for psychogenic erectile dysfunction (📖 p.776). If that fails, refer for psychosexual counselling.

**Retrograde ejaculation** Semen passes into the bladder rather than the urethra—complication of TURP or bladder neck incision. May also occur as a result of spinal injury or DM. The patient can usually achieve an orgasm but there is no ejaculate or the volume of the ejaculate is ↓. Urine may be cloudy after having sex. Confirm diagnosis with urine microscopy (excess sperm in urine). Unless infertility is a problem, no treatment is required.

**Haematospermia** Blood in the ejaculate. Common causes include urogenital infection and minor urethral trauma, but often no cause is found. If persistent, underlying pathology is more likely. Ask about other symptoms, e.g. discharge, pain, dysuria. Examine the external genitalia and perform DRE to assess the prostate. Check MSU and semen analysis ± urethral swab (including chlamydia) if any urethral discharge/high risk of STI. Check PSA and urine cytology if patient is aged >40y. If persists and no cause is found, refer to urology.

### Further information about specialist doctors/therapists
**British Association for Sexual and Relationship Therapy**
☎ 020 8543 2707 🖥 www.basrt.org.uk
**Institute of Psychosexual Medicine** 🖥 www.ipm.org.uk

### Information for patients
**Brown P, Faulder C** Treat Yourself to Sex (1989) Penguin, Harmondsworth. ISBN: 0140110186.

# Erectile dysfunction

50% men aged 40–70y experience inability to obtain/maintain sufficient rigidity of the penis to allow satisfactory sexual performance. 90% are too embarrassed to seek help—always ask. Incidence ↑ with age.

## Organic causes (80%)

- **Cardiovascular** CHD ↑ incidence × 4—more likely to have multi-vessel than single-vessel coronary artery disease; peripheral vascular disease; hypertension—incidence ↑ × 2.
- **DM** incidence ↑ × 3. >35% of diabetic men have erectile dysfunction.
- **Neurological** e.g. pelvic surgery, spinal injury, multiple sclerosis.
- **Side effects of prescription drugs** (see below): consider changing medication if onset of erectile dysfunction is within 2–4wk of initiation of drug therapy, e.g. thiazides.
- **Smoking** (incidence ↑ × 2), **alcohol or drug abuse**.
- **Peyronie's disease** (📖 p. 472).
- **Testosterone deficiency or hyperprolactinaemia**.

## Psychogenic causes

- Performance anxiety
- Depression or stress
- Relationship failure
- Fear of intimacy.

## Drugs causing impotence

- Antihypertensives (especially thiazides)
- Antidepressants (e.g. SSRIs)
- Major tranquillizers
- Anti-androgens
- Finasteride
- Cimetidine.

**History** Ensure that the presenting problem is erectile dysfunction and not other sexual difficulties; identify risk factors; distinguish psychogenic from organic causes (Table 22.6). ❶ Many with organic impotence develop a psychogenic component which perpetuates symptoms.

## Examination and investigation

- Testosterone insufficiency—genitals (small/absent), breasts ↑, ↓ beard growth (↓ frequency of shaving). Measure serum testosterone, FSH/LH ± prolactin if suspected.
- Peripheral vascular disease—peripheral pulses.
- Psychological distress—mental state.
- Check BP, and blood for fasting lipid profile and glucose.

**Table 22.6** Is erectile dysfunction organic or psychogenic?

|  | Psychogenic origin | Organic origin |
|---|---|---|
| *Onset sudden or gradual?* | Sudden onset | Gradual onset |
| *Consistent loss of erections?* | Inconsistent response | Consistent failure |
| *Does the patient ever wake up with an erection?* | Early morning erections | Loss of early-morning erections |
| *Does the patient want to have intercourse?* | Relationship problems | Normal libido |
| *Age?* | Usually <60y | Usually >60y |

**Table 22.7** Treatment options for erectile dysfunction

| Treatment | Notes |
|---|---|
| **Oral drugs** | |
| Phosphodiesterase type 5 inhibitors, e.g. sildenafil[S] | Effective for 70%. Use prn before intercourse (see Table 22.8). Only use 1×/d. Avoid if patient has unstable angina, recent stroke, or MI. **Do not** give a nitrate within 24h of use. |
| Apomorphine | 2–3mg prn 20min before sexual activity. |
| Yohimbine[S] | Herbal remedy available OTC. 10–30mg od is effective. May cause insomnia. |
| **Local drug treatments** | |
| Intraurethral or intracavernosal alprostadil | Intra-urethral preparation effective for 40% and intracavernosal preparation for 80% patients. Used prn. Requires some manual dexterity. Takes ~10min. to work. Penile pain is common. Prolonged erection and priapism results in ~1%. Advise patients to seek medical help if erection >4h. |
| **Mechanical devices** | |
| Vacuum devices | 80% effective. The penis is placed in the device and air withdrawn mechanically sucking blood into the penis. Erection is maintained by placing a constriction band around the base of the penis. |
| Penile prosthesis | Last resort. Inflatable or rigid. Major complication is infection. |
| **Others** | |
| Androgen supplements | Ineffective unless documented hypogonadism. Only use with specialist advice. Exclude prostatic cancer first and do annual PSA measurement during treatment. |
| Psychotherapy | Effective for 60%. Time consuming and expensive but may avert the need for drugs and give permanent resolution. |

---

### ● Andropause/male menopause

From ~30y, testosterone levels ↓ by ~10 % every decade. At the same time, sex binding hormone globulin (SHBG) level ↑, which ↓ the amount of bio-available testosterone further. Andropause is associated with low bio-available testosterone levels. ~30% of men in their 50s develop symptoms.

**Presentation** ↓ sex drive, emotional, psychological, and behavioural changes, ↓ muscle mass and muscle strength, ↑ upper and central body fat, osteoporosis and back pain, ↑ cardiovascular risk.

**Management** If suspected, check total testosterone and SHBG ± FSH/LH and prolactin. If hypogonadism is confirmed, refer for specialist management with testosterone replacement.

**GP management** Counsel the couple about the problem, its possible causes, and management (Table 22.7 📖 p.775 and Figure 22.4)
- Advice on lifestyle—↓ smoking and alcohol. Weight loss and ↑ exercise for obese underactive patients improves both sexual function and cardiovascular health.
- Discuss pros and cons of available drug treatment. Phosphodiesterase type 5 inhibitors (PDE5s) (Table 22.8) are the mainstays of treatment—titrate dose to effect (most diabetics need the maximum dose); warn the patient he may need 8 attempts before a satisfactory erection occurs; side effects include headache, flushing and acid reflux.
- Review progress—adjust dosage, consider other treatment options (intra-urethral/intracavernosal alprostadil, vacuum devices) or treatment for psychosexual problems and/or referral.

**Referral** Options:
- *Urologist* If the patient has never had an erection, has a severe vascular problem, lack of success of treatment in general practice, or severe psychological distress due to erectile dysfunction.
- *Endocrinologist* Hormone abnormalities (e.g. ↓ androgen, ↑ prolactin)—treatment does not always restore potency.
- *Psychiatrist/psychosexual counsellor* Age <40y and no evidence of organic cause; psychosexual problem.

**Psychogenic erectile dysfunction** Treatment in general practice is appropriate for couples who do not wish to be referred.
- See the couple together.
- Recommend a manual, e.g. *Treat Yourself to Sex* (P. Brown, C. Faulder, Penguin, 1989 ISBN: 0140110186).
- Forbid sexual intercourse.
- Explain that stroking should progress slowly from non-genital to genital—if anxiety occurs, go back one step.
- Progress until erection is achieved.
- Give permission for intercourse (if not already achieved).
- If unsuccessful refer to a psychosexual counsellor.

⚠ All men >25y with erectile dysfunction should be screened for cardiac risk factors and signs or symptoms of vascular disease.

❶ NHS prescriptions for erectile dysfunction are available **only** for men:
- treated for prostate cancer; with kidney failure, spinal cord injury, DM, MS, spina bifida, Parkinson's disease, polio, severe pelvic injury; or who have had radical pelvic surgery or a prostatectomy.
- already receiving drug treatment for impotence on 14.9.98.
- through specialist services for men suffering severe distress due to erectile dysfunction.

Endorse FP10/GP10 with SLS.

**Further information**
**British Heart Foundation Factfile** Drugs for erectile dysfunction (6/2005). Available from 🖥 www.bhf.org.uk

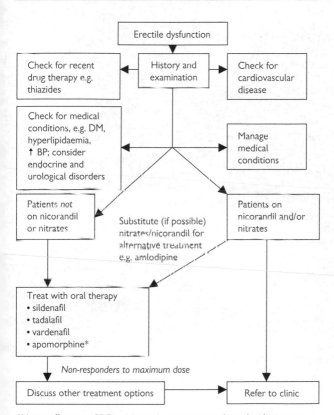

*Not as effective as PDE5 inhibitors but not contraindicated with nitrates

**Fig. 22.4** Algorithm for management of erectile dysfunction

Reproduced with permission from the British Heart Foundation Factfile: Drugs for erectile dysfunction (6/2005) 🖳 www.bhf.org.uk

**Table 22.8** PDE5 inhibitors and action times

| Drug | Onset of action in min (peak action) | Duration of action in h | Doses |
|------|--------------------------------------|-------------------------|-------|
| Sildenafil | 20–30 (60) | 4–6 | 25–50–100mg |
| Tadalafil | 60–120 (120) | 36–48 | 10–20mg |
| Vardenafil | 20–30 (60) | 4–6 | 5–10–20mg |

⚠ PDE5 inhibitors are contraindicated for patients taking nicorandil or nitrates.

Table 22.8 is reproduced from British Heart Foundation Factfile: Drugs for erectile dysfunction (6/2005) available from 🖳 www.bhf.org.uk

# Pregnancy

# Pre-conception and early pregnancy counselling

The aim of pre-pregnancy care is to give a woman enough information for her pregnancy to occur under the optimal possible circumstances. *Areas to cover are:*

**Smoking** ↓ovulation, ↓sperm count, ↓sperm motility.

Once the woman is pregnant, smoking:
- ↑ miscarriage rate (×2) and risk of ectopic pregnancy
- ↑ risk of placenta praevia and placental abruption
- ↑ risk of premature rupture of membranes and pre-term delivery
- ↑ risk of cleft deformities
- ↑ perinatal mortality and ↓ birth weight (by an average of ~200g).

Once the baby has delivered, smoking is associated with:
- ↑ rate of cot death
- ↑ chest infections and otitis media in children.

27% of pregnant women are smoking at the time of delivery Explain risks and advise on ways to stop (📖 p.184).

**Alcohol** Fetal alcohol syndrome (triad of growth restriction, CNS involvement, and facial deformity) is rare and tends to occur in babies of heavy drinkers, especially those who binge drink. Effects of smaller quantities of alcohol are less clear but even 1 drink/d is associated with a small ↓ in growth and intellect. Miscarriage rates are ↑ in moderate drinkers. Current advice is to avoid alcohol in pregnancy.

**Illicit drugs** Cannabis (used by 5% of mothers) is possibly associated with poorer motor skills in children and strongly linked with cigarette smoking—discourage. If taking other illicit drugs, refer for specialist care.

**Diet** See Healthy eating tips for women.

**Folate supplementation** ↓ risk of neural tube defect (open spina bifida, anencephaly, encephalocoele) by 72%.
- *If no previous neural tube defects*—0.4mg od when pregnancy is being planned and for 12wk after conception.
- *If personal or family history of neural tube defect, mother is on anti-epileptic medication, has coeliac disease, is diabetic, or previous child affected*—advise 5mg od from the time the pregnancy is being planned until 13wk after conception.

Only ~1:3 women take folic acid prior to conception. Effect of starting in early pregnancy is unevaluated. Supplements can be prescribed are available via the Healthy Start programme (together with vitamin C and D supplements) or are available OTC from chemists/supermarkets. Introduction of flour fortified with folic acid has recently been approved.

## Other supplements
- *Vitamin D* DH recommends 10 micrograms (400iu)/d but limited evidence for general use. Consider for women from the Indian subcontinent, coeliacs, and those on heparin.
- *Iron* Do not routinely offer—for most, side effects outweigh benefits (📖 p.820).

**Healthy eating tips for women** Eat a variety of foods including:

- Plenty of fruit and vegetables—at least 5 portions per day.
- Plenty of starchy foods, e.g. bread, pasta, rice, or potatoes.
- Protein-rich foods, e.g. lean meat, chicken, fish, eggs, beans, lentils.
- Fibre, e.g. whole-grain bread, pasta or rice, fruit, and vegetables.
- Dairy foods containing calcium, e.g. milk, cheese, and yoghurt.

*Folic acid (folate)* reduces risk of conditions such as spina bifida. Take folic acid supplements (400micrograms) every day from stopping contraception until 12 weeks pregnant. Eat foods containing folate, e.g. green vegetables, brown rice, fortified bread, and cereals

*Iron* Eat iron-rich foods, e.g. red meat, beans, lentils, green vegetables, fortified cereals. Fruit, fruit juice and vegetables help with iron absorption.

*Avoid*

*Pâté and some unpasteurized dairy products* All pâtés (including vegetable), Camembert, Brie, other ripened soft cheeses, and blue cheese may contain *Listeria* which causes miscarriage, stillbirth, and infections in newborn babies.

*Raw or undercooked meat, eggs, and ready meals* Risk of food poisoning.
- Wash your hands after handling raw meat.
- Keep raw meat separate from foods ready to eat.
- Only eat well-cooked meat—hot right through with no pink bits left.
- Only eat eggs cooked until white and yolk are solid. Shop mayonnaise and mousses are safe but avoid home-made dishes containing raw egg.
- Ensure ready meals are piping hot all the way through.

*Liver products and vitamin A supplements* Too much vitamin A can harm a baby's development. Avoid eating liver (and liver products, e.g. pâté) and supplements containing vitamin A or fish liver oils.

*Some types of fish* Eat 2 or more portions of fish per week (including 1 of oily fish—mackerel, sardines, fresh (not canned) tuna or trout) but:
- Avoid shark, swordfish, or marlin and limit tuna to 2 steaks or 4 cans weekly. Mercury in these fish can harm a baby's nervous system.
- Only eat 1 or 2 portions of oily fish per week
- Avoid raw shellfish as they can cause food poisoning

*Alcohol and caffeine* Avoid alcohol. High caffeine levels can cause miscarriage or low birth weight. There is caffeine in coffee, tea, chocolate, cola, and some 'high-energy' drinks. You can drink 4 cups of coffee, 6 cups of tea, or 8 cans of cola daily.

**Gardening and changing cat litter** Toxoplasmosis can harm an unborn baby's nervous system and/or cause blindness. The parasite which causes it is found in meat, cat faeces, and soil. Wear gloves when gardening or changing cat litter and wash your hands afterwards.

**Contraception** Women contemplating pregnancy are usually still using contraception. Discussion about how to stop/what to expect may be helpful (e.g. injectables, IUCD).

**Sexual intercourse** Not known to be harmful during pregnancy.

**Chronic disease** Review of pre-existing medical conditions with referral for expert advice where necessary.
- Diabetes mellitus—refer for specialist diabetic review and change women taking sulphonylureas or metformin to insulin (📖 p.826).
- Epilepsy—refer for specialist review of medication (📖 p.827).
- Heart disease—refer for specialist advice if situation is not clear.
- Genitourinary disease (e.g. HIV, genital warts, bacterial vaginosis)— refer for treatment/advice on mode of delivery if necessary (📖 p.808).

**Review of medication** Drug handling by the body is altered during pregnancy and drugs can cause damage to the developing fetus.
- Discontinue known teratogens prior to conception.
- Advise patients to avoid OTC medication unless they have checked safety with their doctor or midwife.
- Avoid prescribed medication as much as possible—few medicines have proven safety in pregnancy. If prescribing, use only well-known and tested drugs at the smallest possible doses, and only when benefit to the mother outweighs risk.

### Problems in previous pregnancies
- Recurrent miscarriage (📖 p.814).
- Cervical incompetence (📖 p.814).
- Congenital abnormalities/inherited disorders—pre-pregnancy counselling and detailed advice on genetic screening for high-risk pregnancies is available via regional genetics services.

**Rubella status** If rubella status is unknown, suggest that it is checked. Rubella infection in early pregnancy carries a high chance (40–70%) of deafness, blindness, cardiac abnormalities, or multiple fetal abnormalities (📖 p.804). If the woman is susceptible to rubella infection, suggest immunization with avoidance of pregnancy for 3mo afterwards (live vaccine). Re-check rubella status 3mo after immunization.

**Work/benefits** Discussion of benefits available during pregnancy (Table 23.1) and employment law (📖 p.790) is necessary so that women can avoid possible hazards at work, attend for antenatal care, and plan their maternity leave from early in pregnancy.

### Discussion of antenatal care and screening available
- Brief discussion of antenatal screening and antenatal care procedures (📖 p.784) allows women to investigate their choices in pregnancy at their leisure.
- Brief discussion about miscarriage and possibility of infertility allows women to be more confident about asking for help if problems with conception/early pregnancy occur.

### Further information on maternity rights and benefits
Citizens Advice Bureau 🖳 www.adviceguide.org.uk

**Table 23.1** Benefits available to pregnant women

| Benefit | Eligibility | How to apply | Benefits gained |
|---|---|---|---|
| Statutory Maternity Pay (SMP) | • Worked for the same employer for 26wk into the 15th wk before the baby is due.<br>• Pregnant at (or have had the baby by) the 11th wk before the baby is due.<br>• Earning ≥ NI lower earnings limit in the relevant period. | • Inform employer at least 28d before starting leave.<br>• Mat B1 form. | Paid for up to 39wk (Maternity Pay Period (MPP))—can start any time from 11th wk before the baby is due until the week of birth.<br>• 1st 6 wk—90% average earnings<br>• 6–26 wk—90% of usual earnings or £123.06/wk—whichever is lower. |
| Maternity Allowance (MA) | • Employed/self-employed for ≥26wk in the 66wk preceding the baby's due date (test period)<br>• Average weekly earnings of ≥£30/wk for at least 13wk of the test period.<br>• Do not qualify for SMP (e.g. changed jobs, become unemployed, self employed). | Apply > 26/40 and within 3mo of date MA due to start. Need:<br>• Form MA1 (available from jobcentre plus offices, employer or DWP ⊠ www.dwp.gov.uk<br>• MATB1 and, if employed,<br>• Form SMP1 from employer. | Paid for 39wk (Maternity Allowance Period (MAP))—can start any time from 11th week before the baby is due until the day after birth.<br>90% of usual earnings or £123.06/wk—whichever is lower. |
| Sure Start Maternity Grant | • From 11wk before baby is due to <3mo after birth/adoption<br>• Claiming income support or income-based JSA or ESA, Child Tax Credit at a higher rate than the maximum family element, or Working Tax Credit with a disability or severe disability element | Form SF100 from social Jobcentre Plus offices. | £500 payment |
| Health in pregnancy grant | All pregnant women are eligible. Claim ≥25wk | Claim on HiPG form available from midwife or ☎ 0845 366 7885 | One-off payment of £190 |

### Other benefits
• *Free prescriptions/dentistry:* available to all mothers while pregnant and for 1y after the expected date of delivery. Claim using form FW8.
• Women claiming income support, income-based JSA or ESA, or child tax credit may be able to claim *free milk and vitamin supplements* if >10wk pregnant. Claim online at ⊠ www.healthystart.nhs.uk or ☎ 0845 607 6823.
• *Employment and Support Allowance (ESA) and income support* may be available for women unable to claim SMP or MA—◫ Table 5.1, ◫ p.104.
• All parents responsible for the upbringing of a child are eligible for Child Benefit, ◫ p.845. All children born after 2.9.2002 are entitled to a £250 voucher to set up a Child Trust Fund. The child can access the fund after the age of 18y.

# Antenatal care

### Objectives of good obstetric care
- To provide a safe outcome for the mother and baby with the minimum of avoidable complications.
- To make the birth experience as satisfying as possible for the mother and her family.
- To make optimal use of available resources.

Pregnancy is a risky business for both mother and baby. Every year women die as a result of pregnancy—the most common causes are eclampsia, haemorrhage, pulmonary embolism, and infection.

**Maternity services** Provided by practices as an additional service, i.e. most practices are expected to provide routine antenatal care and post-natal care to mothers and babies from birth (or discharge from 2° care) until the 14th day after delivery, with the exception of intrapartum care and the neonatal check. Payment is included in the global sum. If a practice 'opts out', the global sum is ↓ by 2.1%.

*Intrapartum care* Intrapartum care and neonatal checks can be pro-vided to women by GPs at home or in GP maternity units as a *national enhanced service*. One payment is payable for each woman who receives intrapartum care and a further payment for each neonatal check.

### Definitions
- *Gravity*—number of pregnancies a woman has had (at any stage).
- *Parity*—number of pregnancies resulting in delivery >24 wk gestation (or live births <24 wk).
- *Primipara, multipara*—woman who has been delivered of a child for the first time (primipara) or second or subsequent time (multipara).

**Pregnancy tests** Detect urinary β-hCG. +ve from first day of missed period until ~20wk gestation. Remains positive for ~5d. after miscarriage/termination or fetal death.

**Antenatal care** The first antenatal appointment should be offered as early into pregnancy as possible. Further appointments for healthy women should be offered at 16, 28, 34, 36, 38, and, if not already delivered, 41wk. Additionally, healthy nulliparous women should be offered appointments at 25, 31, and 40wk. Provide additional appointments as needed for high-risk women.

**First antenatal visit** The primary function of this visit is to identify those women needing additional care. As there is so much information to be collected/discussed, consider a longer appointment or 2 appointments.

### History
- This pregnancy—LMP, usual cycle, fertility problems, contraception, desirability of pregnancy, any problems so far.
- Estimated date of delivery (EDD)—Figure 23.1.
- Past pregnancies—outcome and complications of previous pregnancies. Past/current medical history—illness (including psychiatric illness), drugs, allergies, varicose veins, abdominal/pelvic surgery.
- Family history—↑ BP, DM, congenital/genetic abnormality, twins.
- Social history—smoking, alcohol consumption, illicit drugs, support at home, work, housing, financial problems.

| Date of first day of last menstrual period | | | | | | Month → | | | | | |
|---|---|---|---|---|---|---|---|---|---|---|---|
| Day ↓ | Jan | Feb | Mar | Apr | May | Jun | Jul | Aug | Sep | Oct | Nov | Dec |
| 1 | 8/10 | 8/11 | 6/12 | 6/1 | 5/2 | 8/3 | 7/4 | 8/5 | 8/6 | 8/7 | 8/8 | 7/9 |
| 2 | 9/10 | 9/11 | 7/12 | 7/1 | 6/2 | 9/3 | 8/4 | 9/5 | 9/6 | 9/7 | 9/8 | 8/9 |
| 3 | 10/10 | 10/11 | 8/12 | 8/1 | 7/2 | 10/3 | 9/4 | 10/5 | 10/6 | 10/7 | 10/8 | 9/9 |
| 4 | 11/10 | 11/11 | 9/12 | 9/1 | 8/2 | 11/3 | 10/4 | 11/5 | 11/6 | 11/7 | 11/8 | 10/9 |
| 5 | 12/10 | 12/11 | 10/12 | 10/1 | 9/2 | 12/3 | 11/4 | 12/5 | 12/6 | 12/7 | 12/8 | 11/9 |
| 6 | 13/10 | 13/11 | 11/12 | 11/1 | 10/2 | 13/3 | 12/4 | 13/5 | 13/6 | 13/7 | 13/8 | 12/9 |
| 7 | 14/10 | 14/11 | 12/12 | 12/1 | 11/2 | 14/3 | 13/4 | 14/5 | 14/6 | 14/7 | 14/8 | 13/9 |
| 8 | 15/10 | 15/11 | 13/12 | 13/1 | 12/2 | 15/3 | 14/4 | 15/5 | 15/6 | 15/7 | 15/8 | 14/9 |
| 9 | 16/10 | 16/11 | 14/12 | 14/1 | 13/2 | 16/3 | 15/4 | 16/5 | 16/6 | 16/7 | 16/8 | 15/9 |
| 10 | 17/10 | 17/11 | 15/12 | 15/1 | 14/2 | 17/3 | 16/4 | 17/5 | 17/6 | 17/7 | 17/8 | 16/9 |
| 11 | 18/10 | 18/11 | 16/12 | 16/1 | 15/2 | 18/3 | 17/4 | 18/5 | 18/6 | 18/7 | 18/8 | 17/9 |
| 12 | 19/10 | 19/11 | 17/12 | 17/1 | 16/2 | 19/3 | 18/4 | 19/5 | 19/6 | 19/7 | 19/8 | 18/9 |
| 13 | 20/10 | 20/11 | 18/12 | 18/1 | 17/2 | 20/3 | 19/4 | 20/5 | 20/6 | 20/7 | 20/8 | 19/9 |
| 14 | 21/10 | 21/11 | 19/12 | 19/1 | 18/2 | 21/3 | 20/4 | 21/5 | 21/6 | 21/7 | 21/8 | 20/9 |
| 15 | 22/10 | 22/11 | 20/12 | 20/1 | 19/2 | 22/3 | 21/4 | 22/5 | 22/6 | 22/7 | 22/8 | 21/9 |
| 16 | 23/10 | 23/11 | 21/12 | 21/1 | 20/2 | 23/3 | 22/4 | 23/5 | 23/6 | 23/7 | 23/8 | 22/9 |
| 17 | 24/10 | 24/11 | 22/12 | 22/1 | 21/2 | 24/3 | 23/4 | 24/5 | 24/6 | 24/7 | 24/8 | 23/9 |
| 18 | 25/10 | 25/11 | 23/12 | 23/1 | 22/2 | 25/3 | 24/4 | 25/5 | 25/6 | 25/7 | 25/8 | 24/9 |
| 19 | 26/10 | 26/11 | 24/12 | 24/1 | 23/2 | 26/3 | 25/4 | 26/5 | 26/6 | 26/7 | 26/8 | 25/9 |
| 20 | 27/10 | 27/11 | 25/12 | 25/1 | 24/2 | 27/3 | 26/4 | 27/5 | 27/6 | 27/7 | 27/8 | 26/9 |
| 21 | 28/10 | 28/11 | 26/12 | 26/1 | 25/2 | 28/3 | 27/4 | 28/5 | 28/6 | 28/7 | 28/8 | 27/9 |
| 22 | 29/10 | 29/11 | 27/12 | 27/1 | 26/2 | 29/3 | 28/4 | 29/5 | 29/6 | 29/7 | 29/8 | 28/9 |
| 23 | 30/10 | 30/11 | 28/12 | 28/1 | 27/2 | 30/3 | 29/4 | 30/5 | 30/6 | 30/7 | 30/8 | 29/9 |
| 24 | 31/10 | 1/12 | 29/12 | 29/1 | 28/2 | 31/3 | 30/4 | 31/5 | 1/7 | 31/7 | 31/8 | 30/9 |
| 25 | 1/11 | 2/12 | 30/12 | 30/1 | 1/3 | 1/4 | 1/5 | 1/6 | 2/7 | 1/8 | 1/9 | 1/10 |
| 26 | 2/11 | 3/12 | 31/12 | 31/1 | 2/3 | 2/4 | 2/5 | 2/6 | 3/7 | 2/8 | 2/9 | 2/10 |
| 27 | 3/11 | 4/12 | 1/1 | 1/2 | 3/3 | 3/4 | 3/5 | 3/6 | 4/7 | 3/8 | 3/9 | 3/10 |
| 28 | 4/11 | 5/12 | 2/1 | 2/2 | 4/3 | 4/4 | 4/5 | 4/6 | 5/7 | 4/8 | 4/9 | 4/10 |
| 29 | 5/11 | | 3/1 | 3/2 | 5/3 | 5/4 | 5/5 | 5/6 | 6/7 | 5/8 | 5/9 | 5/10 |
| 30 | 6/11 | | 4/1 | 4/2 | 6/3 | 6/4 | 6/5 | 6/6 | 7/7 | 6/8 | 6/9 | 6/10 |
| 31 | 7/11 | | 5/1 | | 7/3 | | 7/5 | 7/6 | | 7/8 | | 7/10 |

Dates are given in the format day/month

❶ As a rough guide, EDD = date of LMP + 1 year +7 days – 3 months

**Fig. 23.1** Expected date of delivery calculator

### Examination
- Check weight and calculate BMI—low BMI ↑ risk of pre-eclampsia, IUGR, and pre-term delivery; high BMI is associated with pre-eclampsia.
- Listen to heart and lungs, check BP, and examine abdomen.
- Fetal heart with a sonic aid per abdomen from 12–14 wk gestation.
- Fundus can be felt per abdomen from 12wk.

### Investigations
- Offer early USS for dating purposes at 11–13wk 6d gestation ± nuchal translucency measurement (📖 p.796).
- Arrange routine anomaly scan at 18–20wk 6d gestation. If the placenta extends across the internal cervical os, arrange USS at 32wk.
- Check blood for Hb, blood group, rhesus status, and red cell antibodies; syphilis/rubella serology, HBsAg/HIV with pre-test counselling; sickle test and/or Hb electrophoresis.
- MSU for protein and bacteriuria.
- Discuss and offer antenatal screening (Figure 23.2, and 📖 p.794) for all women.

### Education
- Health promotion (📖 p.790)
- Social security benefits (📖 p.783)
- Employment rights (📖 p.790)
- Free prescriptions and dental care (📖 p.139)
- Antenatal/parentcraft classes
- Local services (e.g. aquanatal classes, yoga for pregnancy)
- Choice of place of delivery and options available (📖 p.792)
- Procedure for antenatal care—Figure 23.3 (📖 p.789)
- Travel and limitations (📖 p.791).

**Certification** Supply form FW8 which allows application for free prescriptions and dental care at the first antenatal appointment. Provide Mat B1 form at 20wk and Health in Pregnancy Grant form at 25wk.

### Information
- Offer *Screening Tests and Your Baby* (order from 🖳 www.screening.nhs.uk/anpublications) to all pregnant women.
- Offer *The Pregnancy Book* to all first-time pregnant women (order on ☎ 0870 155 54 55).
- Offer *Emma's Diary* to all pregnant women (order from RCGP on ☎ 01628 640892). Contains information about pregnancy and vouchers.

**Discussion** Worries about pregnancy or social situation—ask specifically about domestic violence.

**Follow-up visits** Ask about problems and untoward symptoms. Provide the neonatal bloodspot screening leaflet at ~28wk.

### Routine checks
- BP
- Oedema
- Urine for protein
- Fundal height (from 24/25 wk)
- Fetal heart sounds
- Fetal lie and presentation (from 36wk).

❶ Primiparous women are aware of movements from ~20wk but multiparous women often feel movements earlier.

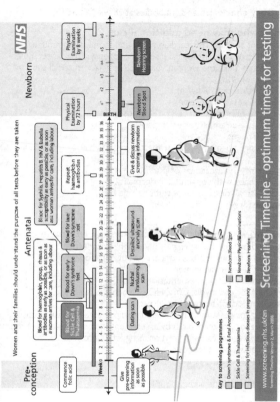

**Fig. 23.2** NHS Antenatal screening timeline

Reproduced with permission from the NHS Antenatal Screening Programme

*Laboratory checks* Hb and antibodies at 28 wk (📖 p.819).

## Women who may need additional care
- Conditions such as: ↑BP; cardiac, renal, endocrine, autoimmune, psychiatric, or haematological disorders; epilepsy; DM; cancer; HIV.
- Factors that make the woman vulnerable, e.g. lack of social support.
- Age ≥40y or ≤18y.
- BMI ≥35kg/m² or <18 kg/m².
- Previous Caesarean section
- Severe pre-eclampsia, HELLP, or eclampsia.
- Previous pre-eclampsia or eclampsia.
- ≥3 miscarriages.
- Previous pre-term birth, mid-trimester loss, stillbirth, or neonatal death.
- Previous psychiatric illness or puerperal psychosis.
- Previous baby with congenital abnormality.
- Previous small or large for gestational age baby.
- Family history of genetic disorder.

---

## Interventions that are *not* part of routine antenatal care
- Repeated maternal weighing—only weigh if clinical management is likely to be influenced, e.g. concern about nutrition.
- Breast or pelvic examination.
- Iron or vitamin D supplementation.
- Screening for chlamydia, CMV, HCV, Group B *Streptococcus*, toxoplasmosis, or bacterial vaginosis.
- Screening for gestational DM, including dipstick testing for glycosuria.
- Screening for pre-term birth by assessment of cervical length (either by USS or vaginal examination) or using fetal fibronectin.
- Formal fetal movement counting.
- Antenatal electronic cardiotocography.
- USS >24wk.
- Umbilical or uterine artery doppler USS.

---

## Further information
**NICE** 🖥 www.nice.org.uk
- Antenatal care: routine care for healthy pregnant women (2008)
- Maternal and fetal nutrition (2007).

**NHS Fetal anomaly screening programme**
🖥 www.fetalanomaly.screening.nhs.uk

## Information and support for pregnant women
**National Childbirth Trust (NCT)** ☎ 0300 3300 770/2
🖥 www.nctpregnancyandbabycare.com
**Birth Choice UK** 🖥 www.birthchoiceuk.com
**Mothers 35 plus** 🖥 www.mothers35plus.co.uk
**Emma's Diary** 🖥 www.emmasdiary.co.uk
**NHS Scotland** 🖥 www.readysteadybaby.org.uk

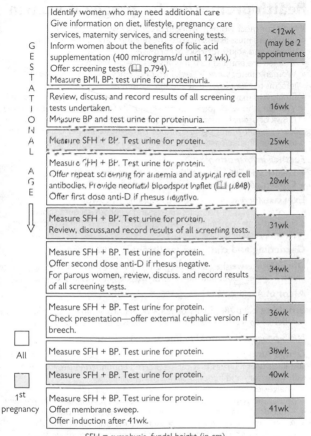

| | | |
|---|---|---|
| G E S T A T I O N A L A G E ⟱ | Identify women who may need additional care<br>Give information on diet, lifestyle, pregnancy care services, maternity services, and screening tests.<br>Inform women about the benefits of folic acid supplementation (400 micrograms/d until 12 wk).<br>Offer screening tests (📖 p.794).<br>Measure BMI, BP; test urine for proteinuria. | <12wk (may be 2 appointments |
| | Review, discuss, and record results of all screening tests undertaken.<br>Measure BP and test urine for proteinuria. | 16wk |
| | Measure SFH + BP. Test urine for protein. | 25wk |
| | Measure SFH + BP. Test urine for protein.<br>Offer repeat screening for anaemia and atypical red cell antibodies. Provide neonatal bloodspot leaflet (📖 p.848)<br>Offer first dose anti-D if rhesus negative. | 28wk |
| | Measure SFH + BP. Test urine for protein.<br>Review, discuss, and record results of all screening tests. | 31wk |
| | Measure SFH + BP. Test urine for protein.<br>Offer second dose anti-D if rhesus negative.<br>For parous women, review, discuss. and record results of all screening tests. | 34wk |
| | Measure SFH + BP. Test urine for protein.<br>Check presentation—offer external cephalic version if breech. | 36wk |
| All | Measure SFH + BP. Test urine for protein. | 38wk |
| | Measure SFH + BP. Test urine for protein. | 40wk |
| 1st pregnancy | Measure SFH + BP. Test urine for protein.<br>Offer membrane sweep.<br>Offer induction after 41wk. | 41wk |

SFH = symphysis–fundal height (in cm)

❶ Reassess the need for additional care of pregnant woman at each visit.

**Fig. 23.3** Algorithm of antenatal care

Figure 23.3 is adapted from NICE 🖥 www.nice.org.uk

---

### ⚠ Symptoms suggesting serious pregnancy complications

- Abdominal pain
- Vaginal bleeding
- Clear vaginal loss
- Severe headache
- Blurred vision
- Persistent itch
- Changed/↓ fetal activity

# Health promotion for pregnant women

**Work** For most women, work in pregnancy is safe. By law:
- Employers must assess risks to the health/safety of the pregnant woman and adjust for risks accordingly.
- Women are entitled to time off work for antenatal care.
- Women cannot work >33wk into pregnancy unless the woman's GP informs her employer that she may continue.
- Employers may not require/allow return to work <2wk after childbirth.
- Women who work for an employer qualify for 52wk of maternity leave (26wk of ordinary maternity leave and 26wk of additional maternity leave). Employment rights continue throughout this period. Women can apply for flexible/part-time working hours on return to work.

*Further information*
- **Health and Safety Executive** 🖳 www.hse.gov.uk/mothers
- **Citizen's Advice Bureau** 🖳 www.adviceguide.org.uk

**Exercise** Moderate exercise is safe and healthy. Avoid:
- Contact sports, high-impact sports, and vigorous racquet sports.
- Scuba diving—possible link with fetal birth defects and may cause fetal decompression disease.

**Gardening and changing cat litter** 📖 p.781.

**Diet** Normal weight gain in pregnancy is 7–8kg. Do not routinely weigh unless worries about nutrition and/or weight. *Foods to avoid*—📖 p.781.

**Alcohol** Avoid alcohol—📖 p.780.

**Smoking** 📖 p.780. Stress benefits of quitting at any stage. Halving the number of cigarettes smoked results in an average 92g ↑ in birth weight.

*NHS pregnancy smoking line* ☎ 0800 169 9169

**Drugs** Advise women to avoid unnecessary medicines (including OTC) and illicit drugs. Drugs that can be started/continued in pregnancy, if clinically necessary and benefits outweigh risks, include:

- Analgesics: codeine-based preparations, paracetamol
- Antacids and ranitidine
- Antibiotics: except tetracyclines; avoid trimethoprim in 1st trimester and at term
- Hormones: levothyroxine insulin
- Laxatives
- Low-dose aspirin (75mg)
- Antiemetics: cyclizine, prochlorperazine, metoclopramide, domperidone
- Antihistamines: chlorphenamine
- Antihypertensives: methyldopa, nifedipine, labetalol, doxazosin
- β-agonists: salbutamol, ipratropium, terbutaline
- Inhaled steroids.

*Drugs to discontinue or change in pregnancy*
- NSAIDs—except low-dose aspirin.
- Warfarin—may need to continue if prosthetic heart valves. Liaise with obstetrician as may need to change to LMWH.
- Antibiotics—tetracycline, doxycycline.
- Antihypertensives—ACE inhibitors, angiotensin receptor blockers.
- Retinoids e.g. isotretinoin.

*Other information on drugs in pregnancy* BNF (Appendix 4) and National Teratology Information Service ☎ (0191) 232 1525

**Complementary therapies** Use as little as possible.
- *Avoid*—oil of evening primrose (possible ↑ in PROM).
- *No benefit*—raspberry leaf tea[R] (but probably no risk either).
- *Possibly beneficial*— ginger,[R] P6 acupressure,[R] and acupuncture[C] for nausea and vomiting; moxibustion[C] for breech presentation; acupuncture[C] for backache/pelvic pain; acupuncture[R] for insomnia.
- *No/limited evidence*—St John's wort, hypnosis, aromatherapy.

**Travel**
- *Car* Seatbelt should go above and below—*not across*—the bump.
- *Air* Check specific requirements of carrier. Most airlines will not accept pregnant women >32wk (rarely 36wk, with a doctor's letter).

⚠ Travel involving long periods of immobility (>5h) is associated with ↑ risk of venous thromboembolism Advise women to drink plenty of non-alcoholic fluids, keep their legs moving whilst sitting or walk up and down the aisle, and purchase graduated compression hosiery OTC.

***Travel abroad*** Best time to travel is in second trimester. Travel to high-risk areas is best postponed/cancelled. Avoid travel to places at altitudes >2500m (↑ risk of IUGR/pre-eclampsia).

***Vaccines*** Assess risk–benefit ratio on an individual basis.
- *Avoid live vaccines*—BCG, cholera, measles, mumps, rubella, varicella, smallpox, Japanese encephalitis. ❶ Inadvertent administration has not been shown to cause harm.
- *Inactivated vaccines* Can be given if needed (best after first trimester)—hepatitis A and B, influenza (consult consultant physician), meningococcal (only if significant risk of infection), inactivated polio (normally avoid), rabies, tetanus/diphtheria, yellow fever (avoid unless high risk).

***Malaria*** Travel to malaria areas is best avoided. If unavoidable take precautions to avoid mosquito bites (📖 p.175). Chloroquine and proguanil can be used in usual doses in pregnancy. Give folic acid 5mg od with proguanil. Consider mefloquine for travel to chloroquine-resistant areas. Avoid Malarone® and doxycycline.

***Contaminated food/water*** Risk of listeriosis, toxoplasmosis, and hepatitis E. Avoid travel to hepatitis E areas: ~20% death rate in third trimester. Severe diarrhoea may be harmful to the fetus.

***Insurance for travel*** Ensure adequate cover. Most companies insure pregnant women to 28wk, some to 32wk. In Europe the European Health Insurance Card (EHIC) (📖 p.45) provides free emergency medical care. It does not cover costs of transport or repatriation.

The UK has reciprocal agreements with some other countries for urgently needed medical treatment. Countries and services available are listed on the DH travel advice website (🖥 www.dh.gov.uk). Proof of British nationality or UK residence is needed.

# Who should deliver where?

Since the publication of *Changing Childbirth*, all those offering maternity care must give women choices about type of care, place of care and birth, and the information to make those choices 'avoiding personal bias or preference'. Who delivers where ultimately depends on the choice the woman makes (Table 23.2). *Options*:

- Consultant unit.
- Midwife or GP/midwife unit integral with/attached to a consultant unit.
- 'Isolated unit'—distant from a specialist unit and manned by midwives or midwives and GPs.
- Home (~1% of deliveries in the UK).

**Legal position of GPs** GPs are often fearful of litigation if they accept a woman for delivery outside a specialist unit. Even women with no risk factors can run into problems—rapid intervention to save life is needed in ~5% of deliveries. Because of the low numbers of deliveries most GPs attend, they perceive that they lack expertise, which compounds this worry. Changes in the organization of out-of-hours cover and the time commitment to the GP entailed in home deliveries (and inadequate remuneration for that time) mean that GP-attended home deliveries are uncommon.

## The legal position is that

- GPs are responsible only for their own acts or omissions.
- Midwives are accountable for their own actions and decisions.
- The GP only becomes responsible for a woman's care in labour when the midwife attending seeks his/her advice. The GP is then bound by terms and conditions of service to offer advice (either over the telephone or by attending), whether or not the woman had been accepted for maternity care.
- If an accident occurs, the GP would be judged against standards of a colleague of similar skills and training, not a specialist obstetrician.

## Duties of the GP

- Provision of impartial advice about available services locally.
- Discussion of the available options in a way to enable the woman to make an informed choice.
- Making arrangements for provision of care.

**Specialist unit vs. community-based care** Although perinatal and maternal death rates have ↓ as the proportion of hospital births has ↑ in the UK, no evidence exists that hospital is the safest place for healthy women to have low-risk births. In other countries (e.g. the Netherlands) there is some evidence to the contrary. For women with pre-existing illness or high-risk births either advise to deliver in a consultant unit or refer to obstetrics for discussion of place of delivery.

⚠ If a woman decides to deliver away from a specialist unit, she should be informed of the facilities and levels of skill and expertise available, and facilities and specialist services that are available in a specialist unit but are *not* available in the community or a midwife/GP led unit. Record the discussion in her notes.

**Table 23.2** Reasons why women choose home or hospital births

| Home birth | Hospital birth |
| --- | --- |
| To avoid intervention (31%) | Safety (81%) |
| More in control in familiar surroundings (25%) | Previous hospital birth (6%) |
| Previous home birth (11%) | |
| More relaxed at home (10%) | |
| Fear of hospitals (10%) | |
| Continuity of care with midwife (4%) | |

## Advise to deliver in a consultant unit

### At booking if
- Pre-existing medical disorders— epilepsy, DM, cardiac, renal, respiratory, hepatitis B, HIV, active genital herpes, IV drug abuse, history of major gynaecological surgery, or known uterine abnormality.
- Familial disorder with a high risk of transmission.
- ↑BP.
- Height <150cm and primigravida.
- Weight at first examination <50kg or >100kg.
- Past obstetric history of:
  - Perinatal death
  - Rhesus iso-immunization
  - Pre-eclampsia or eclampsia
  - Ante-partum haemorrhage
  - IUGR
  - Caesarean section
  - Postpartum haemorrhage
  - Retained placenta
  - Inverted uterus
  - Shoulder dystocia.

### If any of the following develop during pregnancy
- Polyhydramnios
- Malpresentation
- Antepartum haemorrhage
- Prolonged pregnancy (>40wk+10d)
- Pre-term labour <37wk
- Suspected IUGR
- Pregnancy induced ↑BP
- Multiple pregnancy.

## Refer to obstetrics to discuss place of delivery if
- Primigravida <18y and >35y or ≥para 5.
- Excessive maternal weight ↑.
- Failure of engagement of the head near term in a primigravida.
- Past history of prolonged labour, large baby, subfertility, or cone biopsy.

⚠ Other rarer medical or obstetric conditions may require specialist advice—if in doubt refer.

## Further information
**NICE** 🖳 www.nice.org.uk
- Antenatal care: routine care for healthy pregnant women (2008)
- Intrapartum care (2007).

**RCOG** Home Birth 🖳 www.rcog.org.uk

# Screening in pregnancy

Most women undergo some form of screening before/during pregnancy aiming to identify, prevent, and treat actual or potential problems (Figure 23.2, 📖 p.787). Offer women and their partners unbiased information verbally and in writing regarding screening and diagnostic tests, the meaning and consequences of both, what to expect in terms of results, and further options for management. The right to accept or decline should be made clear, and the decision recorded in the antenatal notes.

GPs need to be aware of techniques of prenatal diagnosis to:
• Identify all women who might benefit from genetic counselling and/or early assessment by the obstetrician, *and*
• Counsel patients about the accuracy and risk of prenatal diagnosis.

**Pre-pregnancy genetic screening** There are many inherited diseases. Refer couples before pregnancy if they request referral or have factors which put them at high risk of having a baby with a genetic disorder. Warn couples that most tests give no absolute 'yes' or 'no' but are a risk assessment. ❶ The Family Origin Questionnaire (available from 🖥 www.sickleandthal.org.uk) identifies those at risk of carrying a haemoglobinopathy. A blood test establishes carrier status and risk to the baby.

**Basic screening tests** Blood and urine tests—many women are not aware that these tests have been done, let alone their purpose or results. Ensure women are given information about the reasons for, significance of, and results of routine tests, and record in the notes that permission has been given to do them. Usual tests are:
• Hb estimation(📖 p.820)
• Blood group
• Antibody screening (📖 p.818)
• Combined screen (📖 p.796)
• Haemoglobinopathy screening (📖 p.798)
• MSU for M, C & S (📖 p.810)
• Urine dipstick for proteinuria (📖 p.798)
• Rubella susceptibility
• HIV status (📖 p.798)
• Syphilis status (📖 p.810)
• Hepatitis B status (📖 p.809)

❶ Rubella immune status is not strictly a screening test for this pregnancy but does identify susceptible women (~2.5%) so that postpartum vaccination can protect *future* pregnancies.

## Ultrasound scan (USS)
• *Early USS* Offer to all pregnant women at 11–13wk 6d for accurate gestational age assessment.
• *High-resolution 'anomaly' scan* Offer at 18–20wk 6d to detect fetal structural abnormalities. Detection rates vary according to the abnormality, e.g. subtle heart anomalies are less likely to be detected than gross CNS anomalies.

**Chorionic villus sampling (CVS)** Used to detect genetic/metabolic abnormality in high-risk pregnancies. Performed from 11wk gestation. The developing placenta is sampled per abdomen with USS guidance.
• *Advantages:* undertaken earlier than amniocentesis to allow termination of affected pregnancies at an earlier stage.
• *Risks:* 2% miscarry; limb defects (rare).

**Amniocentesis** Sampling of amniotic fluid via transabominal needle under USS guidance >15wk gestation. Carries a 1% miscarriage risk. Amniocentesis is offered:
• If a high risk result is obtained following first/second trimester screening for Down's syndrome
• If the women has had a previous pregnancy affected by fetal anomaly
• If there is a strong family history of an inherited disorder.

**Fetoscopy** Fibreoptic visualization of the foetus. Carried out from ~18wk. Enables detection of external abnormalities, foetal blood sampling, and organ biopsy. Foetal loss rate ~4%.

### Risk factors that warrant pre-pregnancy genetic screening

*Personal or family history of genetic abnormality,* e.g.
• Cystic fibrosis
• Down's syndrome
• Sickle cell disease
• β-thalassaemia
• Haemophilia
• Fragile X syndrome
• Duchenne and other muscular dystrophies
• Huntington's chorea
• Polycystic kidneys

*High-risk ethnic groups*
• African Caribbean origin—sickle cell anaemia
• Indian subcontinent, Far East, Southern Europe—thalassaemia
• Ashkenazi Jew--Tay–Sachs disease

*Older women* Risk of Down's syndrome ↑ (📖 p.796)

*Consanguinous couples* First-degree cousins who have a baby together have ↑ risk of congenital malformations in their offspring.

### Routine antenatal screening is NOT recommended for

*Vaginal/genital infections*
• Bacterial vaginosis
• Chlamydia
• Group B streptococcus
• Genital herpes

*Other infections*
• Cytomegalovirus
• Hepatitis C
• HTLV-1
• Toxoplasmosis

*Genetic conditions*—refer for screening if a family member is affected
• Cystic fibrosis
• Familial dysautonomia
• Fragile X

*Others*
• Domestic violence
• Gestational diabetes
• Pre-term labour
• Thrombocytopenia
• Thrombophilia

### Further information for women
*Screening tests and your baby* Order from:
🖥 www.screening.nhs.uk/anpublications

**Down's syndrome** The most common single cause of learning difficulty in children of school age. *Incidence*: 1.2/1000 live births. Incidence ↑ with age of the mother (Table 23.3).

⚠ The UK National Screening Committee has recommended all pregnant women, irrespective of age, should be offered screening for Down's syndrome.

**Screening tests** (Table 23.4) should detect >75% of Down's syndrome pregnancies, with a screen positive rate of <3%. Women screening positive, are then investigated further, with CVS or aminocentesis.

**Combined test** Performed in the first trimester of pregnancy. Screening test of choice as it aids early diagnosis and can be completed in one stage without the need for reattendance. It produces a single estimate of the woman's risk of having a child with Down's syndrome using a combination of:
• Material blood tests—for hCG and pregnancy associated paraprotein A (PAPP-A), *and*
• Nuchal translucency (NT)—USS measurement of the translucency of the nuchal fold in the neck of the foetus.

**Integrated test** Requires women to attend at least twice for screening Women must wait until tests from *both* attendances have been processed before they receive a final risk calculation result.
• First attendance (11–13wk 6d gestation)—NT test and PAPP-A
• Second attendance (15–20wk gestation)—α-fetoprotein (AFP), hCG, unconjugated oestriol (uE$_3$), and Inhibin A.

❶ This screening test can be performed without NT testing if NT testing is not available, when it is known as the **serum integrated test.**

**Quadruple test** For women booking later in pregnancy (~15%). Between 15–20wk gestation, maternal blood is tested for AFP, hCG, unconjugated uE$_3$, and Inhibin A.

**Test results** The result is expressed as a risk assessment (e.g. 1:300 at term) or as a +ve or −ve result. A +ve result will well vary with the test performed:
• Combined test–risk >1:150 at term
• Integrated, serum integrated or quadruple test–risk >1:200 at term.

All women with +ve results should be referred promptly for counselling about further investigation and pregnancy options.

**Spina bifida** USS at 18–20wk 6d gestation detects 90–95% open neural tube defects and 100% anencephaly.

**Tay Sachs disease** Genetic condition carried by 1:25 Ashkenazi Jews. Offer genetic screening *whether or not* there is a family history. Offer screening for other diseases commonly carried in this population. (e.g. Gaucher's disease, familial dysautonomia, cystic fibrosis, Canavan's disease) *only* if there is a familial history.

**Table 23.3** Levels of risk of having a Down's syndrome pregnancy in relation to a woman's age

| Age (y) | Risk as a ratio | Percentage risk |
|---------|-----------------|-----------------|
| 20 | 1:1500 | 0.066 |
| 30 | 1:800 | 0.125 |
| 35 | 1:270 | 0.37 |
| 40 | 1:100 | 1.0 |
| ≥45 | ≥1:50 | 2.0 |

Reproduced with permission from Cuckle HS et al. (1987) Estimating a woman's risk of having a pregnancy associated with Down's syndrome using her age and serum alpha-fetoprotein level. Br J Obstet Gynaecol, **94**, 387–402.

**Table 23.4** Summary of screening tests for Down's syndrome pregnancy

| Gestation | 11wk–13wk 6d | 15–20wk |
|-----------|--------------|---------|
| Recommended tests | Combined test<br>• NT<br>• hCG<br>• PAPP A | Quadruple test<br>• AFP<br>• hCG<br>• uE$_3$<br>• inhibin A |
| | Integrated test<br>• NT<br>• PAPP-A | • AFP<br>• hCG<br>• uE$_3$<br>• inhibit A |

❶ All test results are adjusted for age and gestation.

## Information and support for patients

**Antenatal results and choices (ARC)** ☎ 0207 631 0285 🖳 www.arc-uk.org
**Department of Health** *Testing for Down's Syndrome in Pregnancy* booklet—available from 🖳 www.dh.gov.uk
**The Genetics Interests Group** ☎ 020 7704 3141 🖳 www.gig.org.uk
**Down's syndrome Association** ☎ 0845 230 0372
🖳 www.downs-syndrome.org.uk
**Association for spina bifida and hydrocephalus (ASBAH)**
☎ 0845 450 7755 🖳 www.asbah.org
**Tay sachs and Allied Disease Association** ☎ 01473 404 156

**Antenatal HIV testing** HIV testing is now offered as a routine part of antenatal screening in the UK.

*Benefits of screening* Without intervention, ~20% of babies born to mothers infected with HIV will become infected with HIV themselves. Administration of zidovudine to HIV-infected women from 28–32wk into pregnancy until and including labour, and to the baby for the first 4–6wk of life, together with delivery by Caesarian section and avoiding breast-feeding, ↓ risk of transmission to ~2%.

❶ All pregnant women who are HIV +ve should be screened for genital infection (chlamydia, gonorrhoea, and bacterial vaginosis) as early as possible in pregnancy and at around 28wk as co-infection is common in certain subgroups of these women and can ↑ rate of mother-to-child transmission, as well as adversely affecting the pregnancy itself. Also check hepatitis B and C serology unless already done.

**Haemoglobinopathies** Antenatal screening, performed as early in pregnancy as possible (<10wk gestation[N]), is now offered in the UK. In England, screening policy depends on prevalence of sickle cell disorders:
- *High prevalence areas*—all women are offered screening for sickle cell, thalassaemia and other haemoglobin variants
- *Low prevalence areas*—all women are offered screening for thalassaemia using standard red blood cell indices. In addition, the Family Origins Questionnaire (available from 🖥 www.sickleandthal.org.uk) is used to assess the risk of either the woman or her partner being a carrier for sickle cell and other haemoglobin variants. Those in identified high risk groups are offered laboratory testing.

Women identified as being a carrier (having a trait), or having the disorder, should be referred promptly for specialist counselling. Their partners should be offered screening. Follow local guidelines for management in pregnancy and the puerperium.

**Placenta praevia** Because most low-lying placenta detected at the routine 18–20wk anomaly scan will resolve by the time the baby is born, only women with placenta praevia extending over the internal cervical os should be offered another transabdominal scan at 32wk. If this is unclear, a transvaginal scan should be offered.

**Pre-eclampsia** At first contact, assess the pregnant woman's level of risk for pre-eclampsia. Risk factors for developing pre-eclampsia are:
- Nulliparity
- Age ≥40y
- Family (e.g. mother, sister) or past history of pre-eclampsia
- BMI ≥35 or <18kg/m$^2$ at first contact
- Multiple pregnancy
- Pre-existing vascular disease e.g. hypertension, DM.

Consider ↑ frequency of BP monitoring in pregnancy for these women, although optimum frequency of BP checks is unclear. Whenever BP is measured, check a urine sample at the same time for proteinuria.

⚠ Warn pregnant women of the symptoms of advanced pre-eclampsia:
- Headache.
- Problems with vision, e.g. blurring or flashing before the eyes.
- Bad pain just below the ribs.
- Vomiting.
- Sudden swelling of face, hands, or feet.

If a pregnant woman experiences any of these symptoms, she should seek advice from a doctor or midwife as soon as possible.

**Psychiatric illness** Ask about family history of perinatal mental illness, and if the woman has a current or past history of psychiatric illness. At first contact and booking, screen all women for depression (📖 p.821). Refer women with a current or past history of serious psychiatric disorder for psychiatric assessment during the antenatal period.

## Further information
**NICE** 🖳 www.nice.org.uk
- Antenatal care: routine care for the healthy pregnant woman (2008)
- Antenatal and postnatal mental health: clinical management and service guidance (2007)

**RCOG** Amniocentesis and chorionic villus sampling (2005)
🖳 www.rcog.org.uk

**British HIV Association** Management of HIV infection in pregnant women and the prevention of mother-to-child transmission of HIV (2005)
🖳 www.bhiva.org

**National Screening Committee** 🖳 www.screening.nhs.uk/an
- Antenatal and newborn screening programme
- Model of best practice (2008)

## Information and support for patients
**Antenatal results and choices (ARC)** ☎ 0207 631 0285
🖳 www.arc-uk.org
**Perinatal Institute** 🖳 www.preg.info
**Genetics Interests Group** ☎ 020 7704 3141 🖳 www.gig.org.uk
**Sickle Cell Society** ☎ 020 8961 7795 🖳 www.sicklecellsociety.org
**UK Thalassaemia Society** ☎ 020 8882 0011 🖳 www.ukts.org

# Common symptoms in pregnancy

**Abdominal pain** 🕮 p.1098

**Backache** Affects 60% of pregnant women—usually from the second trimester onwards and worse in the evenings. May interfere with sleep/activities. Encourage light exercise (unless contraindicated, e.g. pre-eclampsia)—special land- and water-based classes are run for pregnant women. Treat with simple analgesia, physiotherapy ± massage.

**Bleeding** 🕮 p.812

**Breast soreness** Most common early in pregnancy. Good support bras are essential (can be purchased from specialist clothing stores). Nipples enlarge and darken at ~12wk.

**Carpal tunnel syndrome** Affects ~28% of pregnant women (🕮 p.494). Reassure that it usually resolves after pregnancy. Night splints may help. If severe consider steroid injection. Diuretics do not help. If it does not resolve after pregnancy, refer for orthopaedic assessment.

**Constipation** Affects up to 40% of pregnant women. ↑ fluid and fibre intake. If necessary use a bulk-forming laxative, e.g. ispaghula husk. Avoid bowel stimulants as they ↑ uterine activity.

**Cramp** Leg cramp affects 1:3 in late pregnancy. Worse at night. Raising the foot of the bed by 20cm (e.g. 1–2 bricks under the bed) can help.

**Fatigue**
- *Early pregnancy* Almost universal symptom. Reaches peak at 12–15wk Advise rest and adjustment of lifestyle. Reassure.
- *Late pregnancy* Due to ↑ physical effort needed to do everyday tasks and sleep deprivation. Check not anaemic; otherwise reassure.

**Haemorrhoids** Affect 8% of women in the third trimester. May be associated with itching, pain, and bleeding. Advise ↑ fibre intake. Treat prolapse with ice packs and replacement. Topical haemorrhoid applications are commonly used but lack evidence of safety or efficacy.

**Headache** Usually tension headache. Check BP and urine for protein to exclude pre-eclampsia (🕮 p.824). Treat with rest and analgesia. Migraine may ↑ or ↓ in pregnancy.

**Heartburn** Affects 70% of women in the third trimester. Reassure not harmful. Advise low-fat bland food, small portions, and frequent meals. Avoid eating late at night if worse at night, and consider raising the head of the bed (1–2 bricks under the bed). Avoid gastric irritants, e.g. caffeine. Antacid preparations (e.g. magnesium trisilicate) are helpful if lifestyle modifications are ineffective but may worsen constipation.

⚠ Pre-eclampsia can present with epigastric pain—check BP and urine for protein—if epigastric/right upper quadrant pain unresponsive to simple antacids, refer for same-day assessment even if BP is normal and no/trace proteinuria (🕮 p.825).

**Hypotension** Common symptom of early pregnancy. Check no bleeding. Advise to avoid standing suddenly and avoid hot baths.

**Insomnia** Avoid drug treatment. Reassure. Relaxation techniques and mild physical exercise prior to sleep can help.

**Itching/pruritis** 📖 p.802

**Nausea and vomiting** >80% from 4–6wk. About half vomit. Occurs at any time of day ('morning' sickness in <20%) and made worse by odours associated with preparation/sight of food. If severe, exclude multiple pregnancy, trophoblastic disease and UTI. Symptoms usually improve by 14–16wk, although they persist in some.

**Management** Reassure—normal part of pregnancy. Adjust lifestyle, e.g. ask partner to do the shopping. Advise frequent small meals—avoid greasy/spicy foods; eat foods you can face (varies). Maintain fluid intake—small amounts frequently. Self-help measures include ginger[CE] and P6 acupressure[CE]. If severe/disabling consider antiemetics[CE] (e.g. cyclizine 50mg tds). Suppositories are an effective method of administration if po route is not tolerated. If dehydrated or >2–5kg weight loss (*hyperemesis gravidarum*—1% of pregnancies) admit for rehydration.

**Peripheral paraesthesia** Abnormalities of sensation (e.g. tingling, pins and needles) of hands/feet are common. Reassure. Symptoms usually resolve after delivery. Carpal tunnel syndrome 📖 p.494.

**Skin changes** Pigmentation (e.g. linea nigra), spider naevi, abdominal striae, chloasma/merasma, palmar erythema. *Skin rashes* 📖 p.802.

**Sweating and feeling hot** Common. Check apyrexial. If apyrexial, reassure normal in pregnancy. If pyrexial, look for a source of infection.

**Swelling** Fluid retention affects 80%—ankles, hands/fingers, face. If severe/sudden ↑ in oedema, exclude pre-eclampsia (check BP, dipstick urine for protein).

**Symphysis pubis dysfunction** 3%. Symphysis separates causing discomfort/pain in lower abdomen/pelvic area radiating to lower back, upper thighs, and perineum. Pain is constant and worse on movement, and resolves on rest. Treat with simple analgesia. Consider referral to physiotherapy for pelvic support belt or elbow crutches. Advise rest in a semi-recumbent position when in pain. Generally resolves after delivery, but if persists, refer to orthopaedics.

**Urinary frequency** Check MSU—UTI is common in pregnancy and associated with premature delivery (📖 p.810).

**Varicose veins** Cause aching legs, fatigue, itch, and ankle/foot swelling. If ankles are swollen, exclude pre-eclampsia (check BP, dipstick urine for proteinuria). Elevate legs when sitting, provide support stockings, and encourage walking/discourage standing still. Complications include thrombophlebitis—treat with ice packs, elevation, support stockings, and analgesia—and DVT (📖 p.823). If veins do not settle <2–3mo after delivery consider referral for surgery.

**Vaginal discharge** Usually ↑ in pregnancy. Investigate if smelly, itchy, sore, or associated with dysuria.

# Pruritus and rashes in pregnancy

**Contact with rashes in pregnancy** Many pregnant women have young children and contact with children with rashes is common. Management—Figure 23.4

**Presentation with itching** If a woman presents with itching, look for a rash. If there is *no* rash consider:
- *Hepatic causes* Pruritus gravidarum or recurrent cholestasis of pregnancy affects 2–20/100 pregnancies and sometimes runs in families. Usually begins in the 3rd trimester, reaching a peak in the last month.
  - Frank jaundice—rare. Refer urgently to an obstetrician.
  - No jaundice—check LFTs. Refer to obstetrics if abnormal. Otherwise treat with moisturizers (e.g. aqueous cream) ± oily calamine. Antihistamines do not help.

Pruritus gravidarum disappears after delivery but recurs in subsequent pregnancies (40–50%) and with the COC pill.
- *Endocrine causes* DM, thyrotoxicosis, hypothyroidism—consider checking fasting blood glucose and TFTs.
- *Renal causes* Chronic renal failure—check U&E and Cr.
- *Haematological causes* Iron deficiency—check FBC and ferritin.
- *Drug allergies*.
- *Psychological causes* Obsessive states, schizophrenia.

❶ If no cause is found and the problem persists, refer.

**Presentation with a rash** Consider:
- Common skin diseases, e.g. eczema, psoriasis, urticaria.
- Skin changes specific to pregnancy.
- Infectious causes:
  - Rubella
  - Parvovirus B19
  - Chickenpox/shingles
  - Measles
  - Enterovirus infection
  - EBV
  - CMV
  - Syphilis
  - Streptococcal infection
  - Meningococcal infection.

## Itchy rashes specific to pregnancy
- *Abdominal striae* may itch.
- *Pruritic urticarial papules and plaques of pregnancy* (**PUPPP**) 1:240 pregnancies. Occurs in first/multiple pregnancies or if excessive weight gain in pregnancy. Intensely itchy rash usually confined to lower abdomen/buttocks; appears at >35wk gestation. Treat with calamine and/or topical steroids. Clears spontaneously <6wk (often days) after delivery. No recurrence in subsequent pregnancies.
- *Pemphigoid gestationis* Rare. Starts in mid-pregnancy and appears as a generalized intensely itchy rash. Refer for specialist management. May recur in subsequent pregnancies and with the COC pill.
- *Impetigo herpetiformis* Rare. Starts in the third trimester. Mild itch. Systemically unwell. Refer. Remits after delivery, but may recur in later pregnancies.

**Investigation of pregnant women with rash illness** Figure 23.5, 📖 p.805

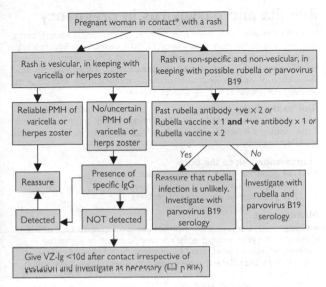

Give VZ-Ig <10d after contact irrespective of gestation and investigate as necessary (📖 p 806)

\* Contact is defined as being in the same room (e.g. house, classroom, or 2–4 bed hospital bay) for ≥ 15min or face-to-face contact

**Fig. 23.4** Investigation of pregnant women in contact with non-specific non-vesicular rash, vesicular rash, or known cases of rubella, parvovirus, varicella, or herpes zoster.

Reproduced in modified format with permission of the Health Protection Agency, Centre for Infection Immunisation Department 🖳 www.hpa.org.uk
For up-to-date advice and current Health Protection Agency (HPA) guideline on rash in pregnancy please consult the HPA website at 🖳 www.hpa.org.uk

### ⚠ At booking

- Enquire if the woman has had chickenpox and/or shingles in the past. If not, advise her to make urgent contact if she develops a chickenpox-type rash or has contact with chickenpox or shingles.
- Advise the woman to inform the midwife/GP urgently if she develops any rash during pregnancy or has contact with anyone who has a rash.

# Rubella and parvovirus in pregnancy

**Rubella** Presents with fever, LNs (including suboccipital nodes), and a pink maculopapular rash which lasts 3d. 50% of mothers infected with rubella are asymptomatic. Incubation is 14–21d. Once infected, patients are infectious from 7d before the rash appears until 7d after. Asymptomatic re-infection of women who have received vaccination can also occur, so serology is essential in all pregnant rubella contacts.

**Risk to the baby** Abnormalities that can occur include cataract, deafness, cerebral palsy, mental retardation, microcephaly, and micropthalmia. If the mother is infected with rubella at >20wk gestation, infection does not affect the baby.

**Transmission risk to the baby**
- *<11wk gestation*—90% have adverse outcome.
- *11–16wk gestation*—20% have adverse outcome.
- *>16wk gestation*—minimal risk of deafness only.

**Management**
- Contact with a non-vesicular rash or rubella—Figure 23.4, 📖 p.803.
- Presentation with a non-specific non-vesicular rash or suspected rubella infection—send blood for serology for rubella and parvovirus B19 (Figure 23.5). Refer if proven infection. After further investigation and discussion of risks, women infected with rubella at <20wk may be offered termination of pregnancy.

**Parvovirus B19 infection** Febrile illness often accompanied by tenderness of the joints/arthritis affecting hands, wrists and knees—usually lasts 1–2wk. There may be a fine rash over the trunk and extremeties. Infectious from 10d before rash appears. Incubation period 13-18d.

**Parvovirus B19 in pregnancy** ~50% of young women in the UK are not immune. Risk of infection in pregnancy ~1:400. Risk of a non-immune mother contracting the infection from a child who has fifth disease (slapped cheek) is ~50%.

**Risk to the baby** If infection is at <20wk gestation, there is a 9% ↑ miscarriage rate. 3% (14–56 babies/y in the UK) develop hydrops fetalis >3wk after infection, due to anaemia—half of those babies die. There are no long-term effects from an infection which does not cause miscarriage or hydrops.

**Transmission rate to the baby** Depends on gestation at the time of infection. There is no treatment to prevent transmission.
- *<4wk gestation*—there is no transmission.
- *From 5–16wk gestation*—transmission rate 8–15%.
- *>16wk gestation*—transmission rate is 25–70% increasing with gestation.

## *Management*

- Contact with a non-vesicular rash or parvovirus—Figure 23.4, 📖 p.803.
- Presentation with a non-specific non-vesicular rash or suspected parvovirus infection—send blood for serology for rubella and parvovirus B19 (Figure 23.5). Refer if proven infection. USS surveillance is started 4wk after onset of illness or seroconversion and then every 1–2 wk until 30wk. If there are any signs of hydrops fetalis on USS, the mother is referred to a regional centre for consideration of intrauterine transfusion. Early transfusion ↑ chances of the baby's survival.

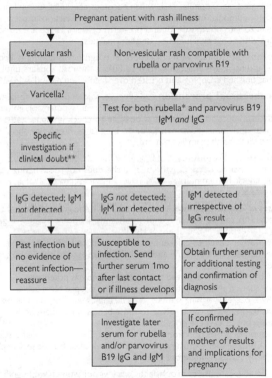

\* Irrespective of past testing or immunization
\*\*Confirm by detection of varicella virus, antigen, or DNA in vesicle fluid.

**Fig. 23.5** Investigation of pregnant women with a rash illness.

Reproduced in modified format with permission of the Health Protection Agency, Centre for Infection, Immunisation Department: 🖳 www.hpa.org.uk

For up-to-date advice and current HPA guideline on rash in pregnancy, please consult the HPA website at: 🖳 www.hpa.org.uk

# Other rash illnesses in pregnancy

**Cytomegalovirus (CMV)** More frequent cause of birth defect than rubella in the UK (5/1000 live births)—10% develop handicap. The fetus is most vulnerable when infection occurs in early pregnancy. Maternal disease may be asymptomatic or a mild flu-like illness. Occasionally there is a rash. No effective prevention strategy.

**Measles** Rare in the UK since introduction of routine MMR vaccination for children. Presents with coryza, lymphadenopathy, conjunctivitis, and disseminated maculopaular rash which becomes confluent. Complications include pneumonia, otitis media, and encephalitis. Infection in pregnancy can lead to intrauterine death and pre-term delivery. There are no associations with congenital infection or abnormalities.

**Chickenpox** Contact with chickenpox in pregnancy is common. People with chickenpox are infectious from 2d before the rash appears until the rash has finished cropping and crusted over. Incubation period is 14–21d.

*Pre-conceptual prevention* An effective chickenpox vaccine is available in the UK. There is no UK policy to screen women for immunity to varicella infection, however it is possible to check immune status and vaccinate non-immune women prior to pregnancy. Pregnancy should be avoided for 3mo after immunization.

*Exposure in pregnancy* If the mother has definitely had chickenpox there is no risk to herself or the baby. If she does not recall having chickenpox, check her immunity—80% have antibodies from silent infection (Figure 23.5, 🕮 p.805).

*In cases of 'at-risk' exposure* Arrange for VZ-Ig to be given to mother and/or baby. This can be lifesaving and significantly ↓ disease severity if given ≤10d after exposure. Babies are at risk if:
- The mother develops chickenpox from 7d before to 7d after delivery
- The mother is not immune and the baby is exposed to chickenpox <7d after birth.
- The baby has been exposed to chickenpox and has potentially inadequate transfer of maternal antibodies—e.g. pre-term babies <28wk, babies weighing <1000g at birth, babies who have had blood transfusions. VZ-Ig can be given to these babies without antibody testing, but test where possible.
- Duration of protection from VZ-Ig is limited. Give second dose if still at risk and further exposure occurs and ≥3wk since first dose. Check antibody status again before giving 2^nd dose.

☛ Some advocate use of prophylactic aciclovir for women with significant additional risk factors, e.g. immunosupression, smokers, women who did not receive early VZ-Ig, or those in the 2^nd half of pregnancy.

## Infection in pregnancy

*Risk to the mother* Chickenpox infection complicates 2–3/1000 pregnancies. Chickenpox pneumonia is more common (10%) and can be severe (1:1000 mortality).

*Risk to the baby* Rates of transmission are higher later in pregnancy (~50% >36 wk; 5–10% <28wk). Infection:

- *<20wk* —causes miscarriage. Fetal varicella syndrome affects 1–2%—segmental skin defects/scarring, limb hypoplasia ± paresis, low birth weight, microcephaly, neurological abnormalities (e.g. hypotonia, eye defects). It may occur up to 28 wk gestation.
- *20–37wk* —intrauterine infection or death shingles in childhood.
- *1wk before–1wk after delivery.* All babies should be given VZ-Ig. Onset 4d before delivery to 2d after delivery carries a 20% risk of over-whelming neonatal infection—these babies should be given aciclovir in addition to VZ-Ig. Seek specialist advice.

*Management* If clinical doubt, confirm infection by detection of varicella virus, antigen, or DNA in vesicle fluid (Figure 23.5, 🕮 p.805). Treat with aciclovir 800mg 5×/d po for 1wk or valaciclovir 1g tds po for 1 wk if presents <24h after the rash appears and the mother is >20wk gestation. Monitor daily. If <28 wk gestation, refer for detailed USS 5wk after infection to exclude fetal varicella syndrome.

*Admit if*
- Chest symptoms
- Neurological symptoms other than headache
- Haemorrhagic rash or bleeding
- Severe disease—dense rash/numerous mucosal lesions
- Significant immunosuppression e.g. HIV +ve.

*Consider admission if*
- Pregnancy approaching term
- Bad obstetric history
- Smoker
- Chronic lung disease
- Poor social circumstances
- Unable to monitor the woman closely, e.g homeless, traveller.

*Refer for urgent hospital assessment if* no deterioration but
- Fever persists, *or*
- Cropping of the rash continues >6d.

❶ Warn pregnant women with chickenpox to avoid contact with anyone potentially at risk of developing severe chickenpox, especially other pregnant women or neonates.

## Rash infections that cause no harm to the fetus
- Epstein–Barr virus (EBV).
- Enteroviruses—Coxsackie virus A, B; echovirus; enterovirus 68-71—cause diseases such as hand, foot, and mouth. Some enteroviruses can cause severe neonatal infection and prophylactic immunoglobulin may be necessary—seek specialist advice.

## Further information
**Health Protection Agency (HPA)** Guidance on the management of rash illness and exposure to rash illness in pregnancy (2008) 🖥 www.hpa.org.uk
**RCOG** Chickenpox in pregnancy (2007) 🖥 www.rcog.org.uk

# Other infections in pregnancy

**Bacterial vaginosis** Present in ~10% of pregnant women—asymptomatic in half. Associated with ↑ pre-term birth (×2). There is no screening policy in the UK, but if detected:
• Treat with metronidazole po—400mg bd for 7d or 2g stat.
• An alternative is clindamycin 2% cream 5g nocte PV for 1wk.

❶ Treatment may not lower the risk to the pregnancy.

**Chickenpox** 📖 p.806

**Chlamydia** ~1:20 pregnant women have Chlamydia infection. During pregnancy, Chlamydia infection is associated with IUGR, pre-term birth, and low birth weight. It can also pass to the baby during delivery, causing eye and/or chest infections. Postpartum, Chlamydia can cause womb infection. Treatable if detected (📖 p.738)—follow-up with swabs to confirm eradication. Refer any affected neonates for expert advice.

**Screening** As part of the National Chlamydia Screening Programme, women <25y can ask for Chlamydia self-test kits at a variety of healthcare and community settings. Otherwise there is no evidence of cost effectiveness of routine antenatal screening for sexually transmitted diseases.

**Coughs, colds, and flu** Little threat to the pregnancy itself. *Advise:* fluids, paracetamol, rest, and TLC. Inhaled decongestants are safe, but avoid cough linctus and OTC composite preparations. Treat any 2° infections as needed.

**Cytomegalovirus (CMV)** 📖 p.806          **Enteroviruses** 📖 p.807

**Genital herpes**[G] Affects ~10% of the UK population (diagnosis made in 1:3). Risk is greatest if the primary attack occurs at >34wk gestation. Secondary attacks are much less of a problem. Risks include:
• Passing the infection to the baby at the time of delivery
• Early labour
• IUGR (1° infection only).

❶ Elective Caesarean section is advised at term if a 1° attack occurs during pregnancy at >28wk gestation. It is controversial if Caesarean section is preferable if there is an active 2° attack at the time of labour.

**Gonorrhoea** <1:1000 pregnancies. Can pass to the baby during delivery, causing eye infections. Treat if detected—📖 p.738. Refer affected infants urgently for expert advice. Follow-up with swabs to confirm eradication.

**Group B streptococcus (GBS)**[G] Bacterium carried in the vagina by >1:4 pregnant women (20% of non-pregnant women). Usually harmless but if transmitted to the baby during delivery can cause neonatal septicaemia, pneumonia, or meningitis.

***Prevention of neonatal infection*** A screening programme to detect women carrying GBS infection during pregnancy (at 35–37wk) is under consideration, but at present treatment with IV antibiotics during labour is advised in 'high-risk' scenarios only:

• Early labour <37 wk.
• Prolonged (>18h) or early (<37wk) rupture of the membranes.
• GBS detected in urine in pregnancy.
• If the woman has a temperature >37.8°C during labour.
• If a previous baby has been affected with the condition (10× ↑ risk).

❶ If found incidentally during pregnancy, there is no evidence that treatment is effective. Give antibiotics during labour.

**Hepatitis B** Prevalence of HBsAg in pregnancy is up to 1% (depending on geographical area). Women are routinely offered screening for hepatitis B infection in pregnancy. Transmission to the baby occurs during labour (up to 30% of infants of women seropositive for HBsAg and 90% of infants of women seropositive for both HBsAg and HBeAg). Infants infected are at high risk (~90 %) of becoming chronic carriers and of developing chronic liver disease ± premature death.

**Postnatally** Refer infected women for hepatology assessment. Infected mothers should not donate their milk.

**Immunization** Give hepatitis B vaccine as soon as possible after birth to babies born to carrier mothers with addition of immunoglobulin (HBIG) if the mother carries the hepatitis B e antigen or had acute HBV infection during pregnancy. 85–95% effective in preventing neonatal hepatitis B infection. Further doses of vaccine are required at 1 and 2mo of age, and a booster dose at 1y at the same time as follow-up testing.

**Hepatitis C** Prevalence in pregnant women is 0.14–0.8%. Except when initial infection of the mother occurs during pregnancy (when transfer rate is much higher), transmission rate to the fetus is 5%. To date there is no evidence that HCV can be transferred to the child by breastfeeding. Infants at risk can be screened for HCV infection at 12mo (RNA screen) or 18–24mo (HCV antibody test). The majority of infants who acquire HCV infection via their mothers develop chronic hepatitis. Treatment is with interferon and achieves viral clearance rates of 40%.

**HIV** Prevalence of HIV among pregnant women in UK varies from 0.04% to 0.4% depending on geographical area. Up to 50% of infants of HIV seropositive mothers are pre- or perinatally infected with HIV, accounting for 90% of HIV infections in childhood. Risk can be ↓ to <5% by giving zidovudine to the mother antenatally and during delivery, and to the neonate for first 6wk, together with elective Caesarean section and advice against breast feeding. A detailed fetal anomaly scan is important if there is first-trimester exposure to anti-viral treatment (including folate antagonists) as possible ↑ risk of congenital abnormality.

❶ There is a theoretical concern about mother–child transmission with invasive prenatal diagnosis. For those with advanced HIV, defer until the end of the first trimester.

***Antenatal HIV testing*** 📖 p.798

**Fetal abnormalities include** wide-set eyes, short nose, patulous lips, 'box' forehead, and growth failure. However, diagnosis is usually made between 6mo and 2y of age when the child presents with lymphadenopathy, recurrent or opportunistic infections, failure to thrive, or progressive encephalopathy. Expert advice is needed throughout pregnancy and for neonatal follow-up.

**Listeriosis** Rare. May occur in epidemics. Infection of the mother is usually via infected food, e.g. pâté, soft cheese, milk. Detection is with blood cultures. Suspect if unexplained fever >48h and refer for expert advice.

*Maternal symptoms* Fever, shivering, myalgia, headache, sore throat, cough, vomiting, diarrhoea, vaginitis.

*Consequences* Miscarriage (may be recurrent), stillbirth, premature labour, transmission to the fetus (in second/third trimester). Infection in the newborn infant manifests in pneumonia ± meningitis.

*Prevention* See Box 23.1

**Malaria** Serious complications are more common in pregnancy (cerebral malaria has 50% mortality). Suspect in any pregnant woman who has a fever and has recently visited an infected area. Seek immediate expert advice.

**Measles** 📖 p.806     **Parvovirus B19** 📖 p.804

**Rubella** 📖 p.804

**Syphilis** Prevalence 0.07%. About 70–100% of pregnant mothers with primary untreated syphilis transmit the disease to the fetus (1:3 die *in utero*). Risk of transmission is ~40% in the early latent phase, and ~10–15% in the late latent phase. Neurological abnormalities as a result of congenital syphilis include encephalopathy and sensorineural deafness. Treatment ↓ risk of transmission by >98%. Refer for specialist assessment if +ve result on routine testing. ❶ +ve result is NOT specific to syphilis.

**Thrush** More common in pregnancy. Not harmful to the fetus. Requires treatment only if causes troublesome itching, soreness or discharge. *Treatment*: Imidazole pessaries for 1wk optimally.

**Toxoplasmosis** Caused by a parasite found in raw meat and cat faeces. Up to 90% of women have had not toxoplasmosis before pregnancy and ~2:1000 will catch it during pregnancy. 30–40% pass it to their fetus. Infection may result in miscarriage, stillbirth, growth problems, blindness, hydrocephalus, brain damage, epilepsy, or deafness. Risk of transmission to the fetus is related to gestation at the time of infection: third trimester, ~70%; first trimester, ~15%. If infection is suspected, refer for specialist advice. Prevention—see Box 23.1.

**Urinary tract infections** 1:25 women develop UTI in pregnancy. If suspected, send MSU to confirm diagnosis and start antibiotics immediately (e.g. cefalexin 250mg qds). Recurrent UTIs in pregnancy should be investigated — consider USS or IVU >12wk after delivery.

***Screening for UTI*** Routine screening with MSU for UTI is offered at booking. 2–5% of pregnant women have asymptomatic bacteriuria, defined as pure growth of $>10^5$ organisms/mL—one in three will develop symptomatic infection (acute cystitis, pylonephritis) if left untreated. Both untreated bacteriuria and frank UTI are associated with pre-term delivery and IUGR. Treat for at least 1wk with suitable antibiotic (avoid trimethoprim). Check MSU following treatment to ensure infection has cleared.

---

**Box 23.1 Advice for pregnant women on prevention of toxoplasmosis and listeriosis**

- Only eat well cooked meat.
- Wash hands, cooking utensils, and food surfaces after preparing raw meat.
- Keep raw meat and cooked foods on separate plates.
- Wash all soil from fruit and vegetables before eating.
- If possible get someone else to clean cat litter or use gloves and wash hands afterwards.
- Use gloves when gardening and wash hands afterwards.

---

**Further information**

**NICE** Antenatal care: routine care for the healthy pregnant woman (2008) ▣ www.nice.org.uk

**RCOG** ▣ www.rcog.org.uk
- Management of genital herpes in pregnancy (2007)
- Prevention of early onset neonatal group B streptococcal disease (2003)

**National Screening Committee** Antenatal and newborn screening programme ▣ www.screening.nhs.uk/an

**Information for patients**

**Department of Health** *Hepatitis B: how to protect your baby* ▣ www.dh.gov.uk

**Group B Streptococcus Support** ▣ www.gbss.org.uk

# Bleeding in early pregnancy

**Bleeding up to 14wk into pregnancy** Bleeding in early pregnancy occurs in 1 in 4 pregnancies. *Causes:*

- Bleeding in normal pregnancy—largest group.
- Miscarriage.
- Ectopic pregnancy.
- Trophoblastic disease.
- Non-obstetric conditions, e.g. friable cervix, polyp, cervical neoplasia.

⚠ Any sexually active woman presenting with abdominal pain and vaginal bleeding after an interval of amenorrhoea has an ectopic pregnancy until proven otherwise.

## Assessment

- Take a history of pain and bleeding—pain preceding bleeding suggests ectopic pregnancy is more likely. Have any products of conception been passed? ❶ Clots/products can be difficult to distinguish.
- Check LMP and pregnancy test result (do a test if a pregnancy test has not been done).
- Check pulse (>100bpm suggests shocked), BP, and temperature (? toxic).
- Abdominal examination—guarding, peritonism, and/or unilateral tenderness suggest ectopic pregnancy
- Pelvic examination—with the advent of early pregnancy assessment units (EPAUs), the necessity for pelvic examination is debatable. If performed, assess uterine size, cervix. Is the cervix open? (A closed cervix admits only one fingertip in a multiparous woman.) Is there any other cause for the bleeding?

**Initial management** If severe bleeding and/or pain, shocked, or toxic, admit to gynaecology as an emergency. If shocked, give syntometrine® 1mL IM and try to gain IV access. Otherwise, refer to the EPAU, if available, to check site and viability of pregnancy. USS is the definitive test of viability of pregnancy: at 5wk gestation, sac ± yolk sac is seen on scan; at 6wk a fetal pole and fetal heart beat are usually seen (occasionally not seen until 7wk). Blood group and rhesus status are also checked at the EPAU (📖 p.818).

### ⚠ Rhesus-negative women

**Bleeding <12wk gestation** Anti-D is not required for:
- Threatened miscarriage unless heavy or repeated bleeding and/or abdominal pain or
- Complete miscarriage where there is no medical or surgical uterine evacuation.

❶ If there is any clinical doubt, give anti-D.

**Bleeding >12wk gestation, ectopic pregnancy and/or medical/surgical evacuation of the uterus at any gestation** Give anti-D immunoglobulin (250iu IM if gestation <20wk) within 72h of bleeding, *whether or not the pregnancy is lost* (📖 p.818).

**Complications of bleeding** Significant sub-chorionic haematoma is associated with ↑ risk of premature rupture of membranes and IUGR—refer early for specialist antenatal care.

**Bleeding in early normal pregnancy** Often termed *threatened miscarriage*. If fetal heart is seen on USS, there is ~97% chance of the pregnancy continuing to progress. There is no evidence that rest or abstinence from sex improves outcome.

**Ectopic pregnancy**[G] A fertilized egg implants outside the uterine cavity—95% in a Fallopian tube. Incidence ~1:100 pregnancies.

### Risk factors

- Pelvic inflammatory disease (single episode ↑ risk ×7)
- Previous ectopic pregnancy (11%)
- IUCD (14%)
- Infertility (15%)
- Tubal surgery
- Age
- Smoking
- POP

### History

- **Abdominal pain** (97%). Unilateral or bilateral, often starts before bleeding, may radiate to shoulder tip, ↑ on passing urine/opening bowels
- **Amenorrhoea** (absent in 25%). Peak incidence after 7wk amenorrhoea.
- **Irregular vaginal bleeding** (79%) Described as 'prune juice' but may be fresh blood; usually not heavy. May pass decidual cast.

**Examination** Shock in 15–20%; abdominal tenderness ± rebound or guarding (71%); pelvis—enlarged uterus, adnexal mass, and/or cervical excitation.

**Management** Admit immediately for further investigation. Resuscitate before admission as needed. Hospital management may be expectant (watch and pregnancy resolves spontaneously), medical (methotrexate), or surgical (laparotomy or laparoscopic surgery). Offer early USS in future pregnancies to confirm pregnancy is intrauterine.

**Complications** Death if undetected; infertility (pregnancy rate post ectopic pregnancy is 66% with 10% having a further ectopic pregnancy).

### Psychological effects of early loss of pregnancy 📖 p.815

### Patient advice and support
**Ectopic Pregnancy Trust** ☎ 020 7733 2653 🖥 www.ectopic.org

### Miscarriage

Also termed spontaneous abortion. Occurs in 1:5 pregnancies—80% at <12 wk gestation. *Risk factors*:

- Maternal age
- BMI>29kg/m$^2$—if >32kg/m$^2$, risk is ↑ by 30%
- Smoking
- Excess alcohol

### Causes

- Fetal abnormality (50%)
- Multiple pregnancy
- Uterine abnormality—fibroids, polyps, congenital abnormality, cervical incompetence (📖 p.814—late second- trimester miscarriages).
- Systemic disease—renal, autoimmune, or connective tissue disease, particularly SLE, PCOS, DM, systemic infection.
- Drugs—cytotoxics, stilboestrol.
- Placental vascular abnormalities.

## Classification
- *Complete miscarriage* History of bleeding. No products of conception in the uterus. Provide psychological support.
- *Incomplete miscarriage* Bleeding. Products of conception remain in the uterus but there is no fetal heart—usually admitted for evacuation of retained products of conception (ERPC). Some women prefer a 'watch and wait' approach—at 3d 86% will be complete.
- *Missed (or delayed) miscarriage* No bleeding. Usually discovered when no heart beat is seen on routine antenatal scan. Treatment is with ERPC. A 'watch and wait' approach is possible, but at 4 wk only 66% are complete and associated with longer bleeding.

Medical management with prostaglandin analogues ± antiprogesterone priming is an alternative to ERPC and is offered in some units.

**❶** There is no evidence that abstinence from pregnancy for a time after miscarriage is helpful—fertility may ↑ immediately after miscarriage.

*Rhesus-negative women* 📖 p.812

## Complications
- *Early* Perforation of the uterus, retained products of conception, infection. Treat with antibiotics if infection is suspected (e.g. doxycycline 100mg od). Re-refer/readmit if shock, pain, heavy bleeding, or bleeding is not settling.
- *Later* Uterine synechiae (Asherman's syndrome), cervical incompetence (see below), psychological sequelae.

## Patient advice and support
**Miscarriage Association** ☎ 01924 200799
🖥 www.miscarriageassociation.org.uk

**Recurrent miscarriage** ≥3 miscarriages (1–2% couples). Check:
- Age—incidence of recurrent miscarriage ↑ with age.
- How many miscarriages? Confirmed pregnancies (not just late, heavy periods)? All with the same partner? What gestation? The more miscarriages, the lower the chance of successful pregnancy.
- Infertility treatment? 25–30% of women who miscarry.
- Past medical history—gynaecological problems (cervical instrumentation, PCOS); systemic disease.
- Family history—recurrent miscarriage, thrombosis/thrombophilia.

**Management of recurrent miscarriage** Refer for further investigation. No cause is found in half those referred. They have a 70% chance of successful pregnancy. Other causes include:
- *Cervical incompetence* Diagnosis is usually made on the basis of history of suggestive symptoms in past pregnancies—≥1 late second-trimester or early third-trimester miscarriage (usually painless leaking of liquor or gradual painless dilatation of the cervix). Refer all women with past history for early obstetric review. Treatment is with cervical cerclage—a stitch is placed high up around the cervix to keep it closed, e.g. Shirodkar suture. The stitch is removed at ~37 wk and labour ensues rapidly if the diagnosis was correct.
- *Antiphospholipid antibodies* (15%). Treatment with low-dose aspirin and LMWH from 6 to 34 wk improves outcome.
- *Chromosomal abnormality in one parent* (3-5%).

## Trophoblastic disease[G]

*Hydatidiform mole* Benign tumour of trophoblast containing 46 chromosomes, all of paternal origin, and no fetal material. Moles may become invasive and penetrate the uterus and/or metastasize to the lungs. 1:30 go on to develop choriocarcinoma. Presents with:

- Bleeding in early pregnancy ± exaggerated symptoms of pregnancy
- Rarely, symptoms of metastatic spread (haemoptysis, pleurisy)
- Uterus is usually large for dates and no fetal heart can be heard
- USS has a typical appearance
- Blood—↑↑ serum β-hCG.

Refer urgently to gynaecology. If mole is confirmed, women are followed up by specialist centres. Incidence in further pregnancies ~1:120. Pregnancy is not advised for 1y after mole—investigate with early USS and β-hCG estimation. COC pill is contraindicated.

*Partial mole* Benign tumour of trophoblast containing 69 chromosomes, one maternal and two paternal sets, with some fetal tissue. Treat as for mole. No ↑ risk choriocarcinoma.

*Choriocarcinoma* Malignant tumour of trophoblast which follows molar (and rarely normal) pregnancy, often many years after. Presents with vaginal bleeding and/or metastases (shadows on CXR, dyspnoea haemoptysis). Treated with chemotherapy—prognosis is excellent. Pregnancy is possible after 2y free from disease.

### Patient advice and support

**Hydatidiform Mole and Choriocarcinoma Support Service**
🖥 www.hmole-chorio.org.uk

### Dealing with psychological effects of early loss of pregnancy

Broach the subject with all women who have suffered a miscarriage or other early loss of pregnancy. Include the woman's partner if possible. Not all women are grieving—adjust your approach accordingly. Legitimize any grief and acknowledge it. Provide information about the condition which caused the loss and reassure where appropriate about the future (if <3 miscarriages, risk of further miscarriage is not significantly ↑, and risk of further ectopic pregnancy is ~1:10).

Discuss worries and concerns of the woman and her partner. Warn of the anniversary phenomenon (sadness at the baby's due date or anniversary of the pregnancy loss) or sadness/jealousy on the birth of another's baby. Inform about self-help organizations, e.g. Miscarriage Association, Ectopic Pregnancy Trust. Provide ongoing support as needed. Different women will want to discuss their feelings at different times after loss. If the woman already has young children, inform the health visitor.

### Further information

**RCOG** 🖥 www.rcog.org.uk
- The management of tubal pregnancy (2004)
- Management of early pregnancy loss (2006)
- Investigation and treatment of couples with recurrent miscarriage (2003)
- Management of gestational trophoblastic neoplasia (2004).

# Ante- and postpartum haemorrhage

## Antepartum haemorrhage

Any bleeding in pregnancy >24wk gestation (or the point of fetal viability) is an antepartum haemorrhage (APH).

### Causes

*Uterine*
- Abruption (📖 p.1099)
- Placenta praevia (below)
- Vasa praevia
- Circumvallate placenta
- Placental sinuses.

*Lower genital tract*
- Cervical
  - Polyp
  - Erosion
  - Carcinoma
  - Cervicitis
- Vaginitis
- Vulval varicosities.

### ⚠ Action
- ALWAYS admit to a specialist obstetric unit. If bleeding is severe admit via an emergency ambulance. Whilst waiting transport, raise legs, give $O_2$ via face mask, gain IV access if possible, take blood for FBC and cross-matching, and start IV infusion.
- NEVER do a vaginal examination—placenta praevia bleeds +++.

**Placenta praevia^G** Occurs when the placenta lies within the lower uterine segment. *Incidence*: 1:4 routine anomaly scans done at 19wk gestation show a low-lying placenta—5% stay low at 32wk; <2% at term.

### Associations
- ↑ with parity
- Age >35y
- Smoking
- Twins
- Pre-term delivery
- Previous Caesarean section
- Endometrial damage (e.g. history of dilatation and curettage, TOP).
- Placental pathology (marginal/vellamentous cord insertions, succenturiate lobes, bipartite placenta).
- Previous placenta praevia (recurrence rate 4–8%).

**Management** If discovered at routine USS at 17–19wk, follow-up USS at 32wk reveals whether the placenta is moving out of the lower segment. When the placenta remains low, management depends on whether the placenta covers the internal os (major placenta praevia) or not (minor placenta praevia). Major placenta praevia always requires delivery by Caesarean section. Normal delivery in a specialist unit may be attempted with minor placenta praevia if the head lies below the lower edge of the placenta.

### Maternal complications
- APH—typically painless bleeding with a peak incidence at 34 wk.
- Malpresentation—35% breech presentation or transverse lie.
- Placental problems—placenta accreta and percreta, especially with a history of previous Caesarean section, abruption.
- Postpartum haemorrhage.

**Fetal complications** IUGR (15%); premature delivery; death.

**Primary postpartum haemorrhage (PPH)** Loss of >500mL blood within 24h of delivery. Affects 1:100 deliveries. May occur in the community after home delivery, delivery in a community obstetric unit, or after rapid discharge from a consultant-led unit.

**Causes** The four Ts
- Tone—uterine atony (90%)
- Tissue—retained products of conception
- Trauma—of the genital tract
- Thrombin—clotting disorders

**Risk factors**
- Age >40y
- Obesity (BMI >35)
- Asian ethnicity
- Anaemia (Hb <9g/dL)
- Pre-eclampsia or gestational hypertension
- Past history of PPH
- Large placental site (e.g. multiple pregnancy, or baby >4kg)
- Low placenta
- Abruption—known or suspected
- Prolonged labour (>12h)
- Pyrexia in labour
- Caesarean section delivery (emergency or elective)
- Operative vaginal delivery and/ or mediolateral episiotomy
- Retained placenta (📖 p.1105).

⚠ **Action**
- Call emergency ambulance for immediate transfer to hospital.
- Gain IV access, take blood for FBC and cross matching and start IV infusion if possible.
- Give ergometrine 0.5mg slowly IV.
- Give high-flow $O_2$ via face mask as soon as possible.
- If the placenta has not been delivered, attempt to deliver it by controlled cord traction.
- Check for trauma and apply pressure to any visible bleeding point/ repair any visible bleeding point. Bimanual pressure on the uterus (rubbing up the fundus) may decrease immediate loss.
- Some community units keep carboprost 250 micrograms (e.g. Hemabate®) for emergency use. Use if available—1mL by deep IM injection—repeat after 15 min. ❶ Contraindicated in women with asthma.

**Secondary PPH** Excessive blood loss PV >24h after delivery. *Peak incidence:* 5–12d after delivery.

**Cause** Postpartum infection—sometimes associated with retained placental tissue or clot.

⚠ **Action**
- If the women is unwell (shocked or toxic) admit to an obstetric unit for further investigation, intravenous antibiotics ± evacuation of retained products of conception.
- If bleeding is slight, manage conservatively. Take a vaginal swab and start oral antibiotics—amoxicillin 500mg tds and metronidazole 400mg tds. Consider referral for USS and/or obstetric review if not settling.

**Further information**

**RCOG** 🖥 www.rcog.org.uk
- Management of postpartum haemorrhage (2009)
- Placenta previa and palcenta previa accreta: diagnosis and management (2005).

# Haemolytic disease and rhesus isoimmunization

15% of women are RhD −ve. Development of anti-D antibodies results from feto-maternal haemorrhage (FMH) in RhD −ve women carrying a RhD +ve fetus. In later pregnancies these antibodies cross the placenta, causing rhesus haemolytic disease of the fetus which becomes successively worse with each pregnancy.

All RhD −ve mothers are tested for D-antibodies at booking, at 28wk, and every 2wk thereafter. Testing is not performed once women are given anti-D prophylaxis. Anti-D titres <4u/ml (<1:16) are unlikely to cause serious disease. If >10u/ml refer for specialist advice.

## Effects on fetus
- Hydrops fetalis (oedematous fetus)
- Intrauterine death

## Effects on neonate
- Jaundice
- Heart failure (oedema, ascites)
- Anaemia
- Yellow vernix
- Hepatosplenomegaly
- CNS signs.

❶ All neonates with haemolytic disease should be managed by specialist paediatricians. Treatment usually involves UV light for jaundice ± exchange transfusion.

**Immunoprophylaxis** Immunoprophylaxis for RhD −ve mothers using anti-D Immunoglobulin (anti-D Ig) is given IM into the deltoid muscle as soon as possible after the sensitizing event—preferably within 72h, although there is evidence of benefit up to 9d. Women already sensitized should not be given anti-D Ig.

**Test for the size of FMH** In the UK blood is taken from the mother (anticoagulated sample) as soon as possible (preferably <2h) after the sensitizing event if >20wk gestation. A Kleihauer acid elution test (which detects fetal haemoglobin (HbF)) identifies women with large FMH who need additional anti-D Ig.

**Other causes** Anti-D antibodies are the most common cause of rhesus disease. Other causes include Rh C, E, c, e, Kell, Kidd, and Duffy. Anti-Du antibodies are relatively common but usually harmless. Follow advice of local transfusion service about follow-up.

❶ Anti-D Ig rarely causes allergic reactions. If the woman is worried about use of blood products, an alternative approach is to check rhesus status of the father—if he is Rh−ve, then the baby is Rh−ve as well, and so anti-D prophylaxis is not required.

## Further information
**NICE** Routine anti-D prophylaxis for women who are rhesus D negative (2008) ▣ www.nice.org.uk

## When should anti-D be administered?

### Following spontaneous miscarriage
- ≥ 20wk—500iu + test the size of FMH.
- 12-19wk gestation—250iu.
- <12wk—only give anti-D if there has been an intervention (e.g. ERPC) to evacuate the uterus.

### Following termination of pregnancy/ectopic pregnancy All non-sensitized RhD –ve women.

### If threatened miscarriage
- All non-sensitized RhD –ve women >12wk gestation.
- If bleeding continues intermittently after 12wk, give anti-D Ig 6-weekly.
- <12wk gestation—only administer if bleeding is heavy, repeated, or there is associated abdominal pain (particularly if close to 12wk).

### Following sensitizing events before delivery
All non-sensitized RhD –ve women after:
- Invasive prenatal diagnosis (amniocentesis, CVS, fetal blood sampling) or other intrauterine procedures.
- APH.
- External cephalic version of the fetus.
- Closed abdominal injury (e.g. RTA).
- Intrauterine death.

<20wk—250iu; >20wk  500iu + Test size of FMH.

### Routine antenatal prophylaxis
- 1–1.5% of RhD –ve women develop anti-D antibodies during pregnancy due to FMH which is usually small and silent—most commonly in the 3rd trimester.
- Routine antenatal prophylaxis ↓ sensitization to <0.2% and should now be routine practice in UK. Give irrespective of whether a woman has had prior anti-D prophylaxis earlier in the pregnancy.
- Administration of 500iu anti-D Ig at 28wk (after blood has been taken for routine antibody screening) and 34wk gestation ↓ incidence of immunization after birth.
- Women who have been given antenatal prophylaxis may still be sensitized by a large FMH so, following any potentially sensitizing event, additional anti-D Ig should be given and a Kleihauer test performed.
- Screening for anti-D antibodies after prophylaxis is uninterpretable.

### Postnatal prophylaxis
- 500–1500iu (500iu in the UK) is given to every non-sensitized RhD –ve woman <72h after delivery of a RhD +ve infant.
- >99% women have FMH of <4mL at delivery—a test to detect FMH >4mL must be done so that additional anti-D Ig can be given as needed
- Risk factors for high FMH include: traumatic delivery, Caesarean section, manual removal of placenta, stillbirth and intrauterine death, abdominal trauma during the 3rd trimester, twin pregnancy (at delivery), unexplained hydrops fetalis.

# A–Z of medical conditions in pregnancy

**Anaemia** Defined as Hb <11g/dL or <10.5g/dL after 28wk. Common in pregnancy (20%). Some ↓ in Hb is physiological because of an ↑ in plasma volume. However, iron requirements ↑ 2–3× and folate requirements ↑ 10–20× during pregnancy. Anaemia is usually due to iron deficiency. Complications include excessive fatigue and poorer fetal outcome. *Risk factors*:

- Starting pregnancy anaemic
- Multiple pregnancy
- Frequent pregnancies
- Poor diet
- Haemoglobinopathy.

*Screening* Haemoglobinopathy and low Hb are routinely screened at booking. Hb is screened again at 28wk.

*Management*
- Routine use of oral iron for all pregnant women is of no proven benefit and may cause harm.
- Women in high-risk groups (e.g. multiple pregnancy) may routinely be given prophylaxis—follow local policies.
- If Hb is <11g/dL at booking or < 10.5g/dL at 28wk, start iron (e.g. ferrous sulphate 200mg tds), and folate (5mg od) if indicated. Repeat Hb in 2wk.

*If there is no response to oral iron* Exclude occult infection (e.g. UTI); check haematinics; consider referral for parenteral iron.

**Antiphospholipid syndrome** Antiphospholipid antibodies (lupus anti-coagulant and/or anticardiolipin antibodies) and a history of ≥1 of:
- arterial thrombosis
- venous thrombosis
- recurrent pregnancy loss (typically second trimester—📖 p.814).

Can be 1° (occurs alone) or 2° to another connective tissue disease—usually SLE. Associated with ↑ risk of thrombosis and ↑ pregnancy loss (<20% pregnancies result in live birth). Treatment is with low-dose aspirin and LMWH usually from 6 to 34wk. Specialist referral is essential.

**Asthma** Affects ~5% of pregnant women.
- Generally improves with pregnancy, especially into third trimester.
- In most cases, treat asthma as usual—most drugs commonly used for treatment of asthma are safe in pregnancy. ❶ Leukotriene receptor antagonists have limited safety data—seek specialist advice.
- Women with very badly controlled asthma are more at risk of early labour and IUGR, and patients on oral steroids may require IV steroids to cover labour.
- Avoid syntometrine for third stage of labour as it contains ergometrine which can cause a severe attack.
- There is a tendency to worsening of asthma after delivery.

**Cardiac disease** Risk of death is highest where pulmonary blood flow cannot be ↑, e.g. Eisenmenger's syndrome (maternal mortality 30–50%), 1° pulmonary hypertension (mortality 40–50%).

**Management** Specialist obstetric care is required for all patients with a pre-existing cardiac condition. Where possible refer pre-conception to a cardiologist for discussion of risks. Antibiotic prophylaxis may be necessary for women with structural cardiac disease for delivery—seek specialist advice.

**Murmurs in pregnancy** Check heart sounds. Murmurs are common. Consider any heart murmurs detected during pregnancy significant and refer for further evaluation—90% will be physiological.

**Depression** A significant cause of maternal death.

**Pre-existing depression** Consider referral for pre-conceptual psychiatric advice. When antidepressants are being used, weigh up the pros and cons of discontinuing treatment during pregnancy.

**Screening for depression** Screen for depression at first presentation, booking, and 4–6wk and 3–4mo postnatally. Ask:
• During the past month, have you often been bothered by feeling down, depressed, or hopeless?
• During the past month, have you often been bothered by having little interest or pleasure in doing things?

If the woman answers 'yes' to either of the initial questions, ask: 'Is this something you feel you need or want help with?'

**Depression in pregnancy** For women with mild/moderate depression consider self-help strategies and talking therapies (e.g. counselling) first. Monitor regularly using depression questionnaires (e.g. PHQ-9 — p.999). Weigh up risks of antidepressant medication against benefits. Involve specialist psychiatric services early.

**Postnatal depression** p.837

| | |
|---|---|
| **Diabetes** p.826 | **Eclampsia** p.1098 |
| **Epilepsy** p.827 | **HIV** p.809 |
| **Hypertension** p.824 | **Infection** p.808 |

**Jaundice** Any cause of jaundice may occur in pregnancy. Investigate as usual and treat according to cause. Common causes are: viral hepatitis; gallstones; Gilbert's or Dubin–Johnson syndrome.

**Jaundice peculiar to pregnancy**
• *Recurrent cholestasis of pregnancy/pruritus gravidarum* p.802
• *Acute fatty degeneration of the liver* Rare. Usually >30wk gestation. The mother develops abdominal pain, jaundice, headache, and vomiting. Admit for specialist care. *Prognosis:* ~15–20% maternal mortality, ~20% fetal mortality.
• *Pre-eclampsia* Jaundice is associated with severe pre-eclampsia ± HELLP syndrome ( p.824).
• *Severe hyperemesis* Jaundice is a complication ( p.801).

**Pre-eclampsia** p.824

**Renal disease** Refer all women for specialist obstetric care. Pre-eclampsia is more common—monitor carefully and refer early.

*Mild renal failure* eGFR 60–89 mL/min and no ↑BP. 96% have successful pregnancies without adverse effect. Low perinatal mortality.

*Moderate and severe renal failure* eGFR <60mL/min and/or ↑ BP. Maternal complications occur in up to 70% and pregnancy-related loss of renal function in about half (10% progress to end-stage renal failure). IUGR in ~40% and pre-term delivery in ~60%.

*Women on dialysis* Conception is uncommon. High rate of miscarriage and intrauterine death. ~40–50% live birth rate. Mothers are prone to volume overload, polyhydramnios, and severe exacerbations of ↑BP ± pre-eclampsia. Women need a 50% ↑ in duration/frequency of dialysis during pregnancy.

*Renal transplant* Risk of first-trimester miscarriage is ↑, but pregnancies that survive are >90% successful. Immunosuppressant drugs must be continued—they are not harmful to the fetus. Pregnancy does not affect long-term survival of the transplanted kidney. Pelvic position of the transplant does not compromise vaginal delivery.

*Rheumatoid arthritis* Symptoms often improve during pregnancy and worsen in the puerperium. Do not use NSAIDs for joint pain >24wk gestation as this can result in closure of the fetal ductus arteriosus. Paracetamol or paracetamol + codeine combinations are safe.

### Disease-modifying drugs
- Sulfasalazine—folic acid supplementation is recommended.
- Azathioprine—associated with IUGR.
- Penicillamine—may weaken fetal collagen.
- Methotrexate is contraindicated.

**Systemic lupus erythematosis (SLE)** Exacerbations are common in pregnancy.
- *Effects on fetus* IUGR; neonatal lupus (from passively acquired maternal antibodies—usually self-limiting skin rash).
- *Effects on mother* Renal complications may worsen and be associated with ↑BP ± pre-eclampsia, oligohydramnios, premature delivery.

*Management* If planning pregnancy refer for review of drugs. Once pregnant refer for specialist obstetric care. Pain control—as for rheumatoid arthritis (above).

### Immunosuppressive drugs
- Azathioprine—may cause IUGR.
- Hydroxychloroquine—risk of deposits in fetal eye/ear.
- Cyclophosphamide and methotrexate are contraindicated.

**Thyroid disease** Refer for specialist obstetric advice.

*Hyperthyroidism* Usually Graves disease. Severity ↓ through pregnancy. May be associated with neonatal goitre, hyper- or hypothyroidism. Continue treatment with carbimazole, aiming to keep plasma $T_4$ at the top of the normal range. Propylthiouracil is preferred postpartum if breast feeding, as less concentrated in breast milk.

*Hypothyroidism* Rare (associated with infertility). If untreated associated with ↑ rate of miscarriage, still birth, and fetal abnormality. $T_4$ needs to be ↑ in pregnancy and normal maintenance dose is ↑ to accommodate this—the fetus is not affected by maternal thyroxine. Check TFTs in each trimester.

**Thromboembolism**[G] Most common direct cause of maternal death in the UK. Pregnancy ↑ risk of thromboembolism 10×—even in very early pregnancy. *Incidence*: ~1:100 pregnancies (20–50% antenatal).

*Major risk factors* Age >35y; obesity—BMI >30kg/m$^2$.

*Other risk factors*

- Smoking
- Parity >4
- Family history of venous thromboembolism
- Previous thromboembolism
- Thrombophilia
- Gross varicose veins
- Sickle cell disease
- Myeloproliferative disorders
- Inflammatory disorders, e.g. inflammatory bowel disease
- Prolonged bed rest/ immobility for any reason

- Other medical disorders, e.g. nephritic syndrome, certain cardiac conditions
- Dehydration—including hyper-emesis and ovarian hyperstimulation
- Severe infection, e.g. pyelonephritis
- Pre-eclampsia
- Prolonged labour
- Caesarean section
- High instrumental delivery
- Any other surgical procedure in pregnancy or puerperium.

⚠ Suspect DVT and/or PE in any woman who is pregnant or in the puerperium who has:
- Leg pain and/or swelling
- Mild unexplained fever
- Chest pain and/or breathlessness.

*Management* If suspected, refer as an emergency for confirmation of diagnosis and initiation of treatment. D-dimer tests are unreliable in pregnancy and should not be used.

If DVT/PE is confirmed, the woman is anticoagulated during the remainder of pregnancy and for ≥6wk postpartum (minimum 3mo total). Avoid warfarin during pregnancy—use low molecular weight heparin (LMWH) instead. Warfarin is safe postpartum and during breastfeeding.

Women should receive a postnatal review with a haematologist before stopping anticoagulation. Advise women to wear graduated compression hosiery for ≥2y after DVT.

*Prevention* Ideally, screen all women with a past history of thromboembolism for thrombophilia prior to conception. Prophylaxis is required if a patient has a thrombophilia or past history of pregnancy or COC-associated thromboembolism. LMWH is used antenatally and for up to 6wk postpartum—refer for expert advice.

**Further information**

**RCOG** 🖳 www.rcog.org.uk
- Thromboprophylaxis during pregnancy, labour and after vaginal delivery (2004)
- Thromboembolic disease in pregnancy and the puerperium (2007)

**NICE** Antenatal and postnatal mental health (2007) 🖳 www.nice.org.uk

# Hypertension in pregnancy

**Chronic hypertension or essential hypertension** Present <20wk into pregnancy. More common in older mothers and may be a FH. May worsen in later pregnancy. Consider changing medication to drugs known to be safe in pregnancy (e.g methyldopa, nifedipine, or $\alpha$-blocker) pre-conceptually or as soon as pregnancy is confirmed. Aim to keep BP <140/90. Pre-eclampsia is ↑ 5×.

**Pregnancy-induced hypertension (PIH)** ↑ BP appearing >20wk into pregnancy and resolving <3mo after delivery. Affects 10% of pregnancies and risk of pre-eclampsia is ↑. Treatment is the same as for chronic hypertension. ↑ risk of developing hypertension later in life.

**Pre-eclampsia$^G$(PET)** Affects 5–7% of primigravida and 2–3% of all pregnancies. Multisystem disease of unknown cause, developing ≥20wk into pregnancy and resolving <10d after the birth. Untreated, may progress to eclampsia (☐ p.1098).

*Risk factors for pre-eclampsia* Evaluate at booking. Refer early (<20 wk) for specialist care if:
- Multiple pregnancy, or pre-eclampsia/eclampsia in previous pregnancy.
- Underlying medical conditions: pre-existing ↑ BP or booking diastolic BP ≥ 90mmHg; pre-existing renal disease or booking proteinuria ≥1+ on >1 occasion; pre-existing DM; antiphospholipid antibodies.
- ≥2 other risk factors: first pregnancy (or first by a new partner); age ≥40y; BMI ≥35 or <18kg/m²; family history of eclampsia/pre-eclampsia (particularly mother/sister); booking diastolic BP ≥80 but <90mmHg.

*Criteria for diagnosis*
- BP>140/90mmHg or >+30/+15mmHg from booking. The earlier in pregnancy the BP rises, the more likely pre-eclampsia will be severe.
- Proteinuria ≥0.3g/24h—urine dipstick is a useful screening tool. If ≥1+ protein then probably significant, but ~25% false +ve rate.

*Interval for routine BP checks* Pre-eclampsia is asymptomatic until its terminal phase, and onset may be rapid. Frequent BP screening is essential. Whenever you check BP, always check urine for protein.
- If no risk factors for pre-eclampsia, routine antenatal care.
- If 1 risk factor for pre-eclampsia but no factor which requires referral in early pregnancy, from 24 to 32wk gestation re-check BP at least every 3wk, and from 32wk gestation, re-check at least every 2wk.
- If >1 risk factor or factor which requires referral in early pregnancy, refer <20 wk and then monitor as directed by the specialist.

*Thresholds for further action* Table 23.5

*Prevention* Low-dose aspirin may benefit high-risk women (i.e. those with past history of pre-eclampsia)—refer for advice.

*Risk of recurrence* in subsequent pregnancy with the same partner—10–15% (usually less severe). Greater risk of ↑ BP later in life.

**Eclampsia** ☐ p.1098        **HELLP syndrome** ☐ p.1098

**Table 23.5** Thresholds for further action

| Findings | | Action |
|---|---|---|
| New hypertension without proteinuria >20wk gestation | Diastolic BP ≥90 and <100mmHg | Refer for specialist assessment* in <48h |
| | Diastolic BP ≥90 and <100mmHg with significant symptoms (below) | Refer for same-day specialist assessment* |
| | Diastolic BP ≥100mmHg | |
| | Systolic BP ≥160mmHg | |
| New hypertension and proteinuria >20wk gestation | Diastolic BP ≥90mmHg and new proteinuria ≥ 1+ on dipstick | Refer for same-day specialist assessment* |
| | Diastolic BP ≥90mmHg and new proteinuria ≥1+ on dipstick and significant symptoms (below) | |
| | Diastolic BP ≥110mmHg and new proteinuria ≥ 1+ on dipstick | Immediate admission |
| | Systolic BP ≥170mmHg and new proteinuria ≥ 1+ on dipstick | |
| New proteinuria without hypertension >20wk gestation | 1+ on dipstick | Repeat pre-eclampsia assessment in <1wk |
| | 2+ on dipstick | Refer for specialist assessment* in <48h |
| | ≥ 1+ on dipstick with significant symptoms (below) | Refer for same-day specialist assessment* |
| Maternal symptoms or fetal signs/ symptoms without new hypertension or proteinuria | Headache and/or visual disturbance with diastolic BP <90mmHg and trace or no proteinuria | Investigate cause of headache. ↓ interval to next pre-eclampsia assessment |
| | Epigastric pain with diastolic BP <90mmHg and trace or no proteinuria | If simple antacids are ineffective, refer for same-day specialist assessment* |
| | ↓ fetal movements or small for gestational age infant with diastolic BP <90mmHg and trace or no proteinuria | Refer for investigation of fetal compromise. ↓ interval to next pre-eclampsia assessment |

⚠ **Significant symptoms**
- Epigastric pain
- Vomiting
- Headache
- Visual disturbance
- ↓ fetal movements
- Small for gestational age infant.

*Most obstetric departments have a day-case 'step-up' assessment unit.
Reproduced with permission from the Pre-eclampsia community guideline, with permission from Action on Pre-eclampsia.

## Further information
**Action on Pre-EClampsia (APEC)** Pre-eclampsia community guideline (2004) 🖳 www.apec.org.uk

## Patient information and support
**Action on Pre-EClampsia (APEC)** ☎ 020 8427 4217 🖳 www.apec.org.uk

# Diabetes and epilepsy in pregnancy

**Pre-existing DM** Affects 2–3:1000 pregnancies. 95% have IDDM.

### Effects on the fetus
- *In utero* Large for dates or IUGR; fetal hyper-insulinaemia; ↑ congenital abnormalities (cardiac, renal, and neural tube defects); hypoxia and intrauterine death (especially >36wk).
- *Postnatally* Hypoglycaemia in first few hours; transient tachypnoea of the newborn or respiratory distress syndrome; neonatal jaundice

### Effects on the mother Problems are more common if poor control.
- *In pregnancy* First trimester miscarriage; premature labour; pre-eclampsia; pyelonephritis; polyhydramnios.
- *In labour* Fetal distress; obstruction (especially shoulder dystocia).

**Management pre-pregnancy** Suggest pre-pregnancy counselling via the diabetic specialist normally involved with care. Pay careful attention to diabetic control (aim BM 4–6mmol/L pre-meals). Advise folate supplementation—5mg od until 13wk. Stop drugs contraindicated in pregnancy, e.g. ACE inhibitors, biguanides, and sulphonylureas. Switch to insulin pre-conception if possible.

**Management during pregnancy** Refer to an obstetrician early. Most women continue to use their pre-pregnancy insulin regime but requirements ↑ 2–3× in pregnancy. USS is routinely used to monitor fetal growth and exclude structural abnormalities. Delivery should always take place in a specialist unit with neonatal care facilities.

**Management postnatally** ↓ insulin to pre-pregnancy levels (if breast-feeding may need less). Oral hypoglycaemics are contraindicated if breast-feeding.

**Gestational diabetes** DM with onset/first recognition in pregnancy. Affects 2% of pregnancies and usually develops in the second trimester. Lower risk of congenital malformation than if pre-existing DM. Intensive management can achieve almost normal rates of macrosomia and neonatal hypoglycaemia, but there is debate whether that is necessary.

**Risk factors** Obesity; family history of type 2 DM; past history of baby>4.5kg; PCOS; unexplained stillbirth/neonatal death.

**Management** Initially diet; if well controlled, then management of pregnancy is otherwise normal. Up to 30% will require insulin. Insulin is stopped immediately postpartum. Check a 6wk postpartum glucose tolerance test. Gestational DM usually recurs in future pregnancies and >30% develop DM in <10y.

**Glycosuria in pregnancy** Routine screening for glycosuria in pregnancy is not recommended. Pregnant women have ↓ renal threshold for glucose and a physiologically ↑ plasma glucose level, so dipstick testing gives a high false +ve rate. However, if glycosuria is detected repeat the urine test—if still +ve arrange for modified GTT.

**Epilepsy in pregnancy** 90% of epileptic women have normal pregnancies and healthy babies.

### Effects on the fetus

*Antenatal* ↑ first trimester miscarriage and ↑ fetal malformation:
- Neural tube defect—↑ risk with sodium valproate or carbamazepine.
- Cleft lip/palate—associated with phenytoin and phenobarbitone.
- Non-specific facial abnormalities—5–30% exposed to anticonvulsants.

*Peri/postnatal* 2x ↑ perinatal mortality; haemorrhagic disease of the newborn is associated with carbamazepine, phenytoin, or phenobarbitone—all mothers on these drugs should have 10mg vitamin K od from 36wk and all babies should have IM vitamin K at birth; withdrawal symptoms—phenobarbitone (jittery, irritable, fits); child has ↑ risk of epilepsy.

### Effects on the mother

*During pregnancy* 10% have ↑ fit frequency. The fetus is at slightly ↑ risk of harm during a generalized tonic–clonic fit but absolute risk of harm is low. There is no evidence that simple partial, complex partial, absence, or myoclonic seizures harm pregnancy in any way, unless the patient falls. Status epilepticus is associated with high infant and maternal mortality.

*During labour/puerperium* 1–2% have fit during labour and a further 1–2% have fit <48h post delivery.

### Management

*Pre-pregnancy* Discuss risks of anti-epileptic medication/epilepsy with all women of child bearing age, whether or not contemplating pregnancy, NICE advises caution in the use of sodium valproate in any woman of child-bearing age because of the risk of harm to the fetus. Advise folate supplementation (prescribe folic acid 5mg od) from the time the pregnancy is being planned until 13wk after conception. Suggest referral to a neurologist for optimization of the anti-epileptic drug regime.

*During pregnancy* Refer for specialist obstetric care—epileptic women are usually managed jointly by an obstetrician and neurologist during pregnancy. Drug doses may need to ↑ during pregnancy if fit frequency rises. Delivery should occur in a specialist centre where any fits can be managed.

*Postnatally* Breastfeeding is not contraindicated with older anticonvulsants, e.g. phenytoin, sodium valproate, carbamazepine (BNF Appendix 5). If drug dose has been ↑ in pregnancy, it may need to ↓ after delivery. All babies should have IM vitamin K due to ↑ risk of haemorrhage. Risk of injury to the child from maternal seizure is low. Discuss child care and minimizing risks to the child from the mother's epilepsy

### Further information

**NICE** 🖥 www.nice.org.uk
- Diabetes in pregnancy (2007)
- The epilepsies: the diagnosis and management of the epilepsies in adults and children in primary and secondary care (2004)

# Intrauterine growth and malpresentation

**Intrauterine growth restriction (IUGR)[G]** Babies may be small because they are premature, small for their gestation, or a combination of the two. Babies small for their gestational age (IUGR—weighing <10th centile for their gestational age) have different problems to those of premature babies.

**Predisposing factors** The major antenatal indicator for IUGR is low maternal weight at booking (<51kg). *Others include*:

- Multiple pregnancy
- Malformation
- Infection
- Maternal smoking
- Maternal DM
- Pre-eclampsia
- Severe maternal anaemia
- Maternal heart or renal disease
- Previous history of small baby.
- Low weekly maternal weight ↑(<0.2kg).

**Antenatal detection** Difficult to detect. About half are not detected until after birth. Most GPs will encounter IUGR when they do a routine antenatal check and find the symphysis–fundal height (SFH) is less than would be expected for the gestation. Other suspicious signs are oligohydramnios and poor fetal movements. Confirm suspicions with USS and then seek specialist obstetric advice. Where the head circumference is relatively spared, suspect placental insufficiency.

## Consequences

- *Labour* More susceptible to hypoxia in labour so require monitoring in a specialist unit where Caesarean section facilities are available and there is paediatric back-up.
- *Postnatal problems* Susceptible to neonatal hypoglycaemia and jaundice. Babies <2kg may have problems with temperature regulation and require incubator facilities.
- *Long-term effects* More prone to cardiovascular disease and NIDDM in later life.

**Oligohydramnios** Liquor volume <500ml. Rare. Associated with:

- Prolonged pregnancy
- PROM (📖 p.830)
- Placental insufficiency
- Fetal abnormality (renal agenesis, urethral aplasia).

Confirm diagnosis with USS, and then refer for specialist obstetric assessment.

**Large for dates** Consider:

- Multiple pregnancy
- Maternal DM
- Fetal abnormality
- Polydramnios
- Molar pregnancy
- Large baby (>90th centile)—may have past history of large babies.

Refer for USS to confirm diagnosis and exclude fetal abnormality or multiple pregnancy. Check maternal fasting blood glucose ± GTT.

**Polyhydramnios** Liquor volume >2L. 1:250 pregnancies. *Causes*:

- *Fetal abnormality* (50%). Hydrops fetalis; anencephaly (no swallowing reflex); spina bifida; oesophageal or duodenal atresia; umbilical hernia; ectopia vesicae.

- *Maternal* (20%). DM; multiple pregnancy.
- *No cause found* (30%).

**Risks** Premature labour; malpresentation; cord prolapse; placental abruption; PPH.

**Management** Refer for USS to confirm diagnosis and exclude fetal abnormality or multiple pregnancy. Check maternal fasting blood glucose ± GTT. Refer for specialist obstetric advice.

**Multiple pregnancy** Detected on early antenatal USS. *Incidence*: twins, 1:105 (1:3 identical); triplets, 1:10 000. *Predisposing factors*:
- Previous twins.
- Family history of non-identical twins.
- Race: most common in African Blacks; least common in Japanese.
- ↑ with maternal age.
- Infertility treatment—induced ovulation (e.g. clomifene); IVF and other assisted reproduction techniques.

**Management** Refer for specialist obstetric care. Monochorionic twins are significantly higher risk than dichorionic twins. *Complications*:
- *In pregnancy* Hyperemesis; anaemia; polyhydramnios; pre-eclampsia (3×); APH; placenta praevia; placental abruption.
- *In labour* Malpresentation; cord prolapse; fetal distress (↑ Caesarean section rate); PPH.
- *Fetus* ↑ perinatal mortality (5×); prematurity; IUGR; malformations (↑ ×2–4); twin–twin transfusion may result in one twin being plethoric (and jaundiced later) and the other anaemic.

**Breech babies**<sup>G</sup> 3–4% of babies at term. Higher incidence <37/wk. Associated with ↑ risk of cerebral palsy as breech presentation is more common in premature infants and those with congenital malformation. *Risk factors*: bicornuate uterus; fibroid; placenta praevia; oligohydramnios.

**Management** Many turn spontaneously, especially if <36wk gestation. If a baby is found to be breech at ≥ 36wk gestation, confirm breech position and position of the placenta on USS and refer for specialist obstetric advice. *Specialist options*: external cephalic version (ECV); vaginal breech delivery; elective Caesarean section.

⚠ 10–15% of breech babies are discovered for the first time late in labour. If delivering at home or in a community unit, arrange transfer to a specialist unit immediately.

**Follow-up** Congenital hip problems are more common in breech babies—refer all breech babies routinely for hip USS even if examination in the first 24h is normal.

## Further information
**RCOG** ⌂ www.rcog.org.uk
- Investigation and management of a small-for-gestational-age fetus (2002)
- Management of breech presentation (2006).

## Information and support for multiple pregnancy
**Twins and multiple births association (TAMBA)** ☎ 0800 138 0509 ⌂ www.tamba.org.uk

# Labour

47% of deliveries are 'normal', i.e. occur without surgical intervention, use of instruments, induction, epidural, or general anaesthetic. Intrapartum care can be provided by GPs as a national enhanced service.

**Braxton–Hicks contractions** Irregular tightenings of the uterus. Start ≥30wk gestation (common after 36wk). May be uncomfortable but not painful.

**Premature rupture of membranes (PROM)** Rupture of membranes before labour starts. Usually presents with a gush of clear fluid (± an audible pop) followed by uncontrolled leakage. If chorioamnionitis is present the woman may have abdominal pain and feel unwell. Difficult to distinguish clinically from profuse vaginal discharge or incontinence of urine. Check temperature, pulse, and BP, and do a routine obstetric examination (including fetal heart).

❶ Do not perform a vaginal examination, as repeated examinations can introduce infection.

## Management
- *Evidence of infection* Admit for specialist obstetric care.
- *<37wk gestation and suspected PROM* Admit to specialist obstetric unit for further assessment.
- *≥37wk gestation* If no signs of spontaneous labour, admit for specialist obstetric assessment within 24h.

**Premature labour** Any labour <37wk gestation. *Prevalence*: 6%—1:4 elective due to maternal/fetal problems. Largest contributor to neonatal morbidity/mortality in industrialized countries.

## Causes of spontaneous premature labour Unknown (40%).
- Cervical incompetence
- Multiple pregnancy
- Uterine abnormality
- DM
- Pyelonephritis or other sexually transmitted or urinary infection
- Polyhydramnios
- APH.

**Presentation** Premature rupture of membranes or contractions. If suspected admit immediately to obstetrics for further assessment.

**Prolonged pregnancy/post-maturity** The due date is based on pregnancy lasting 40wk or 280d. from the date of the LMP, but at 40wk only 58% of babies have delivered. It is normal to deliver between 37wk and 42wk. At 40wk gestation 65% will spontaneously go into labour in the next week, but 15% of women have not gone into labour by 42 wk. Perinatal mortality rate is ↑2× from 42 to 43 wk and 3× >43wk, so induction of labour is indicated if a pregnancy lasts >42wk.

**Initial management** Membrane sweep. If that is ineffective, refer for formal induction of labour (📖 p.832). If referral is declined, ↑ antenatal monitoring to 2× weekly cardiotocography and USS (to measure maximum amniotic pool depth) as markers of fetal well-being.

**Normal labour** Occurs ≥37wk gestation and results in vaginal delivery of a baby in <24h. Often heralded by a 'show' consisting of mucus ± blood and/or spontaneous rupture of membranes ('waters going').
- *First stage of labour* Time from the onset of regular contractions until the cervix is fully dilated.
- *Second stage of labour* Time from complete cervical dilatation until the baby is born. The mother has a desire to push.
- *Third stage of labour* Delivery of the placenta.

**Pain relief for labour** Most women experience pain in labour. Strategies for pain relief include:
- Self-help—keep fit in pregnancy, relaxation techniques, breathing exercises, warm bath.
- TENS—machines are available to hire from most obstetric units and some retail outlets.
- Entonox—takes 30–45 sec to have effect. Advise women to start inhaling it as soon as the contraction starts.
- Injected opioids (e.g. pethidine).
- Epidural.
- Pudendal block—used for instrumental delivery.

Advise women to discuss options with their midwife. Antenatal classes dealing with pain relief significantly ↑ a woman's confidence in managing her labour pains.

**Epidural** Effective method of analgesia available in most hospital units. Initiated once in established labour (cervix >3cm dilated). Regular BP, pulse, and fetal heart monitoring is required. *Particular indications:*
- Occipito-posterior position
- Breech
- Multiple pregnancy
- Pre-eclampsia
- Forceps delivery
- Maternal medical conditions, e.g. cardiac.

### Epidural complications during labour
- Postural hypotension
- Urinary retention
- ↑ need for instrumental delivery because of pelvic floor muscle paralysis.

**Epidural complications post-delivery** Urinary retention, headache (especially if dural puncture).

**Meconium-stained liquor** Passage of fresh meconium (dark green, sticky, and lumpy) during labour may be a sign of fetal distress. Transfer immediately to a consultant unit for further evaluation.

*Management* Paediatrician should be present at delivery. Do not perform oropharyngeal suction if there is no evidence of fetal hypoxia.

**Dystocia** Difficulty in labour. May be due to problems relating to the baby, birth passage, or action of the uterus. Neonatal mortality and maternal morbidity both ↑ with duration of labour. *Possible causes:*
- Pelvic abnormality
- Shoulder dystocia (📖 p.1100)
- Abnormal presentation
- Uterine dysfunction
- Cervical dystocia
- Cephalo-pelvic disproportion.

*Management* If a patient in labour at home or in a community unit fails to progress as expected, admit immediately to a specialist unit for consideration of intervention to speed the labour or Caesarean section. Shoulder dystocia is an obstetric emergency (📖 p.1100).

**Induction of labour^G** Performed when it is felt that the baby is better off out than in (~20% of deliveries). Only undertaken in units with facilities for continuous fetal monitoring and emergency Caesarean section.

*Procedure involves* assessment of the cervix, vaginal prostaglandins, 'sweeping' of the membranes, artificial rupture of the membranes and/or IV oxytocin to maintain contractions.

*Reasons for induction of labour include*
- Post-maturity (most common)—offered from 41–42wk
- Premature rupture of membranes
- Intrauterine death.

**Assisted delivery^G** (Table 23.6) Forceps and ventouse are used in ~11% of deliveries in the UK (range 4–25% between hospitals). Assisted delivery should only be performed with adequate analgesia (usually epidural or pudendal block) and by experienced practitioners.

**Caesarean section^G (LSCS)** (Table 23.7) Rate in England and Wales is 21.5% (range 10–65% between different hospitals). 10% are elective and usually performed at >39wk to minimize risk of respiratory complications, the other 11–12% occur after labour has started. Regional anaesthesia for LSCS is safer for mother and child than general anaesthesia.

*Reasons for emergency LSCS* Failure to progress (25%); presumed fetal compromise (28%); breech (14%).

*Planned LSCS is indicated for*
- Breech (where external cephalic version has failed)
- Multiple pregnancies where the first twin is not cephalic
- Placenta praevia (grade 3–4)
- HIV +ve women and those with 1° HSV in third trimester to ↓ virus transmission.

❶ Maternal request is not, on its own, an indication for LSCS^G but GPs should discuss risks and benefits if a request is made. If the patient still requests a LSCS, refer for a consultant opinion.

**Further information**
**RCOG** Operative vaginal delivery (2006) 🖥 www.rcog.org.uk
**NICE** 🖥 www.nice.org.uk
- Caesarian section guidelines (2004)
- Intrapartum care (2007)
- Induction of labour (2008).

**Table 23.6** Forceps and ventouse

|  | Forceps | Ventouse |
|---|---|---|
| Indication | Delayed 2nd stage of labour | Delayed 2nd stage of labour |
| Procedure | • Wrigley's forceps for 'lift-out' deliveries<br>• Neville–Barnes' forceps for high deliveries<br>• Keilland's forceps if rotation is required | • Vacuum extraction cup is applied to baby's head, suction is applied, and traction aids delivery<br>• Ventouse allows rotation if the baby is malpositioned |
| Early complications | • Maternal trauma (episiotomy always needed)<br>• Fetal facial bruising<br>• Facial nerve paralysis | • 'Chignon' develops on baby's head—resolves in ≤2d<br>• Cephalohaematoma<br>• Retinal haemorrhage<br>• Neonatal jaundice (but no ↑ need for phototherapy) |
| Longer-term complications | ↑ risk of maternal faecal incontinence | |
| Comparison | Ventouse has ↑ failure rate compared with forceps but no ↑ LSCS rate<br>↓ requirement for regional anaesthesia with ventouse deliveries compared with forceps deliveries<br>Forceps result in more maternal trauma than ventouse deliveries | |

**Table 23.7** Comparison of Caesarean section and vaginal birth

|  | Complications |
|---|---|
| ↑ with LSCS | *Mother—this pregnancy*: abdominal pain; bladder or ureteric injury; hysterectomy; maternal death; need for further surgery; need for admission to intensive care/high-dependency unit; thromboembolism; length of hospital stay; need for re-admission<br>*Mother—future pregnancies*: not having more children; antepartum stillbirth, placenta praevia, uterine rupture<br>*Baby*: neonatal respiratory problems |
| No difference | *Mother*: haemorrhage; infection; genital tract injury; faecal incontinence; back pain; dyspareunia; postnatal depression<br>*Baby*: death (except breech); intracranial haemorrhage; brachial plexus injuries; cerebral palsy |
| ↓ with LSCS | *Mother*: perineal pain; urinary incontinence; uterovaginal prolapse |

## Information for women
**NCT** Information on labour and pain relief (including epidurals)
🖥 www.nctpregnancyandbabycare.com

# Maternal postnatal care

Postnatal care from hospital discharge until 14d after delivery, excluding the neonatal check, is provided as an additional service (maternity services) and payment is included in the global sum. 'Opting out' results in a 2.1% ↓ in the global sum.

The *puerperium* is the 6wk period after delivery. Most women in the UK spend ≥6h after delivery in hospital. After discharge home, the midwife continues to visit for 2wk after the birth and then the health visitor takes over. GPs usually see the mother and baby soon after discharge and again for the 6wk postnatal check. Arrange additional reviews as needed.

**The postnatal visit** Discuss problems during pregnancy/delivery and postnatal contraception (Table 23.8). Check:
- *Rhesus status* If the mother is RhD –ve and the baby RhD +ve, ensure anti-D is given <72h after delivery (📖 p.819).
- *Hb on day 5* After delivery (after the postpartum diuresis). If Hb is <10g/dL, continue iron supplements for 3mo.
- *Rubella status* If non-immune, immunize as soon as possible and ensure effective contraception for 3mo afterwards. Reassure that it is safe to breastfeed after immunization.
- *Temperature, pulse, and BP* ↑ BP associated with pre-eclampsia usually resolves <48h after delivery.
- *Fundus* Day 1 = 24wk gestation size (up to umbilicus); day 5 = 16wk gestation size; by day 10, uterus should not be palpable per abdomen. Persistent bulkiness suggests retained products of conception—refer for USS.
- *Pain* Breast, abdominal, perineal, legs.
- *Vaginal loss* Red, then brown, then yellowish over the first week; then serous for 3–6wk. Any fresh red bleeding is abnormal.
- *Moving about* Women should try to become mobile as soon as possible after delivery to ↓ the risk of DVT.
- *Feeding* 📖 p.868.
- *Mental state* Screen for depression at 4–6wk and 3–4mo (📖 p.837).

**Mother's 6wk postnatal check** Discuss any problems in pregnancy or delivery. Discuss any current problems the mother has and specifically enquire about persistent vaginal loss, bladder/bowel control, and any sex-related problems. Discuss any problems with the baby, including worries about hearing/vision. Discuss feeding and contraception.

## Examination/investigation
- BP and weight—if overweight discuss weight control (📖 p.180).
- Abdominal examination—uterus should not be palpable per abdomen.
- Vaginal examination—only if any problems with tears/episiotomy, persistent vaginal bleeding, pain, or to perform overdue cervical smear.
- Screen for depression (📖 p.837).
- Check Hb if anaemic postnatally.
- Check rubella immunization given if not immune antenatally—if not, arrange for vaccination. Check immunity 3mo after vaccination.

**Table 23.8** Postpartum contraception

❶ Contraception is *not* needed until 21d postpartum

| Method | If not breastfeeding* | If breastfeeding† |
|---|---|---|
| COC pill/ combined patch | Start ≥3wk after delivery (patch states >28d) as ↑ risk of thromboembolism. (❶ can be started immediately after miscarriage/termination.)<br>If starting on day 21 (or day 28 for patch) postpartum, immediate protection is provided. If starting after that time, use an additional method for 7d.<br>If PET in pregnancy, start the COC pill *only* when BP and biochemical abnormalities have returned to normal. | Contraindicated <6wk postpartum as it may inhibit lactation and enters breast milk in small quantities.<br>>6wk and <6mo—use only if no other suitable method. |
| POP | Delay until ≥3wk postpartum to avoid ↑risk of heavy bleeding.<br>If started >3wk after delivery, start on first day of period for immediate protection or, if cycle not established, use alternative protection for first 2d. For breastfeeding mothers, ↑ quantity of breast milk. | |
| Injectables/ implants | Preferably delay until ≥6wk postpartum to avoid risk of heavy/ irregular bleeding. If >3 wk (>4wk for implant) postpartum, administer early in period or, if cycle not re established, check pregnancy test before administration and use additional method for 7d. If breastfeeding, delay giving injectable until ≥6wk post partum where possible. | |
| IUCD/IUS | Insert <48h post-delivery (but ↑ risk of expulsion) or delay until >4wk postpartum (Mirena® licence states 6wk)—take care with insertion as the uterus may be soft and perforate easily. Use an additional method for 7d if inserted >4wk postpartum | |
| Cap | Refit any time from 5–6wk postpartum (even after LSCS).<br>❶ May require a different size postpartum. | |
| Condoms | Useful until other methods are established and to prevent transfer of sexually transmitted diseases. | |
| Sterilization | ↑ operative and failure rate at abortion or in postpartum period. Best delayed for a few months. | |

* Ovulation can occur within 10d of abortion and 28d of delivery.

† Advise women <6mo postpartum who are amenorrhoeic and fully breastfeeding that there is only a low chance of pregnancy (~2/1000 women) without contraception. If any supplementary bottle feeding, baby is weaned, or any vaginal bleeding (except occasional spotting), assume that the woman is fertile.

**The baby's 6wk developmental check** 📖 p. 850

**Further information**

**NICE** 🖥 www.nice.org.uk
- Postpartum care (2007)
- Antenatal and postnatal mental health: clinical management and service guidance (2007).

# Common postnatal problems

**Abdominal pain** Cramping 'period like' pains for the first 1–2wk after delivery, especially when breastfeeding. These are due to the uterus contracting down or involuting. Suspect infection if offensive lochia, fever, the uterus stops getting smaller day by day, or is still palpable per abdomen 10d after delivery.

**Breast soreness** The breasts become engorged ('the milk comes in') 3–5d after the birth, and may be quite painful. Support with a well-fitting maternity bra day and night. Express milk if still painful—a warm bath may help. *Other problems:*

**Sore/cracked nipples** Try topical remedies (e.g. Kamillosan®) and/or nipple shields. Consider advice from a breastfeeding advisor—may be a 'positioning problem'.

**Skin infection** Localized soreness, pain around the areola ± nipple, or in the breast after a feed—usually due to candida infection. Treat mother and baby with miconazole oral gel.

❶ Severe knife-like pain in breast during and for up to 1h after feeding suggests deeper infection—treat mother additionally with fluconazole 150mg stat and then 50mg bd for 10d (unlicensed use). Symptoms usually resolve in <3d.

**Blocked duct** Hard tender lump in the breast. Advise the mother to massage that area of the breast while feeding or expressing milk.

**Mastitis** Tender, hot, reddened area of breast ± fever. Treat with flucloxacillin 250mg qds and NSAID (e.g. ibuprofen 400mg tds prn). Continue breastfeeding or express the milk to prevent milk stagnation if too painful for feeding.

**Breast abscess** Admit for incision and drainage.

**Dyspareunia** following perineal trauma. Almost always settles without need for surgery.

**Hair loss** Hair becomes thicker in pregnancy and this hair is all shed at about the same time ~5–6 mo postpartum. Reassure. Hair loss reverts to normal levels within 2–3mo. If severe, persistent, or accompanied by tiredness, consider hypothyroidism (🕮 p.838)—check TFTs.

**Haemorrhoids** Common and painful. *Try:*
• Local ice packs (frozen fingers of rubber gloves are the right shape).
• Topical preparations, e.g. Proctosedyl®.
• Resting lying on one side.
• Keeping stools soft using a stool softener.
• Advising women to wash the haemorrhoids with cool water after opening bowels and gently push them through the anus (if possible).

**Perineal bruising** Can be very painful. Advise regular analgesia, e.g. paracetamol 1g qds ± ibuprofen 400mg tds, ice packs. Ultrasound can help—consider referral to physiotherapy.

**Persistent lochia** Bleeding (lochia) > 6wk postpartum. *Causes:*

- Infection
- Retained products of conception
- Unhealed tears—cervical, vaginal, or perineal
- Resumption of normal cycle
- Side effects of contraception (e.g. POP, depot injection)
- Other cervical or uterine pathology

### Management
- Examine uterus per abdomen and do a bimanual vaginal examination to check involution. Perform a speculum examination and send a vaginal swab for M,C&S.
- If offensive loss or systemic symptoms/signs of infection, treat with antibiotics as for endometritis (□ p.838). Otherwise, arrange USS.
- If not settling and no cause is found, refer to gynaecology.

## Postnatal depression

**Baby blues** Very common—women become tearful and low within the first 10d of delivery. Be supportive. Usually resolves.

**Depression** Common (10–15% mothers), reaching a peak ~12wk after delivery—although symptoms are almost always present at 6wk. Often mothers do not report symptoms. NICE recommends screening all mothers for depression 4–6wk and 3–4mo postnatally by asking:
- During the past month, have you often been bothered by feeling down, depressed or hopeless?
- During the past month, have you often been bothered by having little interest or pleasure in doing things?

If the woman answers 'yes' to either of the initial questions, ask: 'Is this something you feel you need or want help with?'

### Risk factors
- Depression during pregnancy
- A bad birth experience
- Social problems (e.g. poor social support, financial problems)
- Past medical history or family history of depression or postnatal depression
- Alcohol or drug abuse.

### Management
- Talk through the problems. Refer to health visitor for support.<sup>CE</sup>
- Give information, e.g. self-help groups, mother-and-baby groups.
- Consider checking TFTs, especially if presenting with tiredness
- Consider counselling<sup>CE</sup> or referral for cognitive behaviour therapy.
- Consider antidepressant medication. If breastfeeding, tricyclics are relatively safe but most manufacturers advise avoidance (BNF Appendix 5). Sertraline 50mg od is the safest of the SSRIs. In all cases, monitor the baby for unwanted side effects (e.g. drowsiness, respiratory depression). If not breastfeeding, fluoxetine 20mg od is the most effective antidepressant in trials.<sup>CE</sup>
- Monitor progress using depression questionnaires, e.g. Edinburgh Postnatal Depression Scale.

⚠ Refer to the mental health team immediately if any risk of self-harm, suicide, or harm to the baby.

☛ There is evidence that oestrogen (but not progesterone) may help some women with postnatal depression.<sup>C</sup>

***Puerperal psychosis*** Much rarer than postnatal depression (1:500 births). Suspect if severe depression; high suicidal drive; mania; psychotic symptoms. In all cases seek expert help from a psychiatrist. Consider admission—under a Section if necessary. Risk of recurrence is 20%, but 50% will never be mentally ill again.

**Poor abdominal and pelvic muscle tone** Classes for postnatal exercise to re-tone the body are available both on dry land and in the swimming pool at most leisure centres. Pelvic floor exercises can be started <1d after delivery (Box 23.2). Good leaflets explaining these are available from physiotherapists, local maternity units, and the National Childbirth Trust.

**Puerperal pyrexia** Temperature >38°C within 14d of delivery or miscarriage. 90% infections are in the urinary or genital tracts. Ask about:
- Urinary symptoms
- Colour and smell of lochia
- Abdominal pain
- Breast symptoms
- Any other symptoms (e.g. cough, sore throat).

Examine fully, including bimanual vaginal examination, and send MSU and vaginal swabs for M,C&S. *Potential obstetric causes:*

***Superficial perineal infection*** Complicates tear or episiotomy—treat with flucloxacillin 250–500mg qds.

***Endometritis*** Presents with offensive lochia, lower abdominal pain, and a tender uterus. Treat with amoxicillin 250–500mg tds and metronidazole 400mg tds or co-amoxiclav 375mg tds. If not settling in <48h or very unwell admit for IV antibiotics.

***Mastitis*** See breast soreness 📖 p.836

***DVT or PE*** Can present with pyrexia. Refer to exclude if any leg pain/chest pain/breathlessness.

**Superficial thrombophlebitis** Affects 1% women. Presents with a tender (usually varicose) vein. Exclude DVT. Recovery usually occurs within a few days. Meanwhile advise the woman not to stand still and, when sitting, to elevate the leg above waist height. Support the leg, e.g. with an elasticated stocking, and try applying an ice pack to the affected area. NSAIDs (e.g. ibuprofen 400mg prn) may help.

**Tiredness** Very common in the first few months after delivery, but it may be the presenting feature of postnatal depression, anaemia, or hypothyroidism. Check FBC and TFTs.

**Transient autoimmune thyroiditis** Up to 10% women 1–3mo after delivery. Usually presents with fatigue and lethargy.

***Hypothyroidism*** Treat with thyroxine for 6mo then stop for 6wk and repeat TFTs. Follow up with annual TFTs—1:5 go on to develop permanent hypothyroidism.

***Hyperthyroidism*** Refer to an endocrinologist—antithyroid treatment is not normally required but symptom control may be necessary.

## Box 23.2  Pelvic floor exercises—basic techniques

- *Exercise 1* Advise the woman to pull up her pelvic muscles as if stopping herself from passing urine and hold that position for a count of 10.
- *Exercise 2* Advise the woman to pull up her pelvic muscles as in exercise 1, but then relax and contract them rapidly 4 tmes.
- These exercises should be repeated as many times daily as possible long term.

## Further information

**NICE** 🖳 www.nice.org.uk
- Antenatal and postnatal health (2007)
- Postnatal care (2006)

**Clinical Evidence** Howard L *Postnatal Depression* (2006)
🖳 www.clinicalevidence.com

**DTB** The management of postnatal depression (2000) **38**, 33–36
🖳 www.dtb.org.uk

**Cocharane** Lawrie TA *et al.* Oestrogens and progestogens for preventing and treating postnatal depression (2000) 🖳 www.cochrane.co.uk

**Lancet** Gregoire AJP et al. Transdermal oestrogen for treatment of severe postnatal depression (1996) **347**, 930–3.

## General advice and support for postnatal women

**Family Planning Association** ☎ 020 7837 4044 🖳 www.fpa.org.uk

**National Childbirth Trust (NCT)** ☎ 0300 3300 770. Breastfeeding line: 0300 3300 771. Pregnancy and birth line: ☎ 0300 3300 772.
🖳 www.nctpregnancyandbabycare.com

**NHS Direct** 🖳 www.nhsdirect.nhs.uk

**Baby World** 🖳 www.babyworld.co.uk

## Advice and support for women with postnatal depression

**Royal College of Psychiatrists** Information sheet on postnatal depression 🖳 www.rcpsych.ac.uk

**Association for Postnatal Illness** Support and befriending by women who have suffered postnatal depression/puerperal psychosis ☎ 020 7386 0868 🖳 www.apni.org

**Meet-a-Mum Association** Support and information for women with postnatal depression ☎ 0845 120 3746 🖳 www.mama.co.uk

# Stillbirth and neonatal death

Stillbirth is a term applied to those babies born dead after 24wk gestation. Death may occur *in utero* or during labour. Usually present with a lack of fetal movements and on examination no fetal heart can be detected. If suspected, refer as an emergency to the nearest obstetric unit for confirmation of intrauterine death by USS.

**Management** In hospital mothers of babies who have died *in utero* are usually induced. Samples are routinely taken from mother and baby to try to determine cause of death.

**Common causes** Pre-eclampsia; IUGR; renal disease; DM; infection; malformation; post-maturity; abruption; knots in the cord. No cause is found for 1:5 stillbirths.

**After discharge** Make contact with the parents as soon as possible.

*Lactation suppression* Offer cabergoline 1mg as a single dose.

*Registration of stillbirth* A certificate of stillbirth is issued by the obstetrician which must be taken to the Registrar of Deaths within 42d of the stillbirth. Parents are issued with a certificate of burial or cremation and a certificate of registration to keep. The child's name may be entered on the certificate of registration.

*Funeral* Parents have the option of a free hospital funeral. Burial is usually in an unmarked multiple occupancy grave. Parents may pay for a single occupancy grave or cremation. Alternatively parents may pay for a private funeral.

*Benefits* In the UK all maternity benefits are still payable after stillbirth (📖 p.783).

*Follow-up* is routinely arranged by the specialist obstetrician to discuss reasons for the stillbirth and implications for future pregnancies. Primary care follow-up is essential. Stillbirth is a huge burden to come to terms with. Parents do not have the regular contact with medical staff that a baby brings. Ensure regular follow-up by a member of the primary care team. Broach the issues brought up by the baby's death directly. Offer an open door. Give information about support organizations, e.g. SANDS. Advise waiting 6mo–1y before embarking on another pregnancy.

**Neonatal death** Death of an infant <28d old. Rare in the community. In the UK, all deaths of children <18y are subject to review by the local child death review panel (📖 p.925) and should be notified to it immediately. If the death is expected, the GP will be allowed to issue a special death certificate. If unexpected the case will be referred to the police/coroner. Offer lactation suppression with cabergoline 250 micrograms bd for 2d, and follow-up as for stillbirth.

## Patient support and information

**Stillbirth and Neonatal Death Society (SANDS)** ☎ 020 7436 5881
🖥 www.uk-sands.org

❶ In other sections of this book, where management differs from the norm for children, the text is highlighted in a box marked with this symbol.

# Chapter 24

# Child health

# Child health promotion

*Children are one third of our population and all our future.*
US Select Panel for Promotion of Child Health, 1981

Patients ≤15y comprise 20% of the average practice list; school children visit the GP on average 2–3×/y and the under-4s see their GP more often (average 6×/y) and have more home visits than any other age group except the elderly.

**National Service Framework (NSF) for children** Emphasizes child health promotion. It moves from rigid developmental screening to a more flexible assessment of the child within the family context. It includes:

- Immunization—🕮 p.643.
- Childhood screening.
- Health and development reviews—to monitor the child's development, the strengths/weaknesses of the family, and to discuss the parents' hopes and concerns, followed by early intervention as required.
- Health promotion, beginning antenatally and continuing to teenage years, covering the full range of child health issues, e.g. diet, safety, substance abuse (drugs, smoking, and alcohol), teenage sexual health.

Although most child health promotion is still carried out by the health visitor and other members of the primary healthcare team, the need for partnership with parents and involvement of other care providers (e.g. schools and nurseries, social care services) is stressed.

**Childhood screening** The aim of screening is to discover physical developmental or behaviour problems as early as possible so that appropriate management can commence, preventing secondary complications. There has recently been a move away from set times for developmental screening, but the neonatal (🕮 p.846) and 6–8wk check, with emphasis on checking the eyes, heart, and hips as well as developmental milestones (🕮 p.850), are still recommended, as is a comprehensive assessment (usually by the health visitor) by 1y, and again between 2 and 2½y.

Beyond that assessments are carried out according to need. Any consultation can be used to check immunization status, monitor development, and for health promotion. Expected developmental milestones are summarized in Table 24.2 (🕮 p.850). Liaise with the health visitor if:

- Immunizations are not up to date
- You have any worries regarding parenting abilities
- A child does not attend an appointment following referral
- You have concerns about neglect or abuse (but also see 🕮 p.922).

*Neonatal bloodspot screening* 🕮 p.848

**Diploma in Child Health** Designed to give recognition of competence in the care of children to GP vocational trainees, clinical medical officers, and trainees in specialties allied to paediatrics. It is administered by the Royal College of Paediatrics and Child Health (RCPCH). Further details are available at 🖵 www.rcpch.ac.uk

## Health education for new parents

### Reducing the risk of cot death

- Cut smoking in pregnancy.
- Do not let anyone smoke in the same room as your baby.
- Place your baby on his/her back to sleep.
- Do not let your baby get too hot.
- Do not suddenly stop using a dummy before your baby is 6mo old if your baby is used to having one.
- Keep your baby's head uncovered—place your baby with his/her feet to the foot of the cot, to prevent wriggling down under the covers.
- It is safest to sleep your baby in a cot in your bedroom for the first 6mo.
- It is dangerous to share a bed with your baby if either parent:
  - is a smoker, no matter where or when he/she smokes
  - has been drinking alcohol
  - takes medication or drugs that might make him/her drowsy
  - feels very tired.
- It is very dangerous to sleep together with your baby on a sofa, armchair, or settee.
- If your baby is unwell, seek medical advice promptly.

### Protecting your baby from accidents and infections

- Keep small objects out of your baby's reach.
- Stay with your baby when he/she is eating or drinking.
- Make sure your baby's cot and mattress are in good condition and that the mattress fits the cot properly.
- Install at least one smoke alarm.
- Plan a way to escape a fire with your baby.
- Never leave your baby alone in a bath or near water.
- Immunize your baby.
- Make sure your baby cannot reach hot drinks, kettle, or iron flex.
- Only use toys suitable for your baby's age.
- Never shake your baby—ask for help if crying gets too much.
- Use a properly fitted baby car seat that is the right size for your baby.
- Do not use a baby walker.
- Wash your hands before feeding your baby and make sure your baby's bottle and teats are properly sterilized.

## Benefits for parents and children

- *Child benefits* Anyone responsible for the upbringing of a child aged <16y is entitled to child benefit. Claim forms are available from local social security offices or 🖳 www.hmrc.gov.uk
- *Low income benefits* Families with children on low income may be entitled to tax credits and/or income support (📖 p.104).
- *All children <16y (18y if in full-time education) and mothers <1y post-partum* are entitled to free prescriptions and dentistry (📖 p.139). Some families on low incomes are also entitled to free prescriptions.

## Further information

**DH** 🖳 www.dh.gov.uk
- Children's National Service Framework (2004)
- Child health promotion programme (2008).

# The neonatal check

It is essential that a full neonatal check is carried out <72h after delivery. Most neonatal checks are carried out by paediatricians in maternity units before discharge. Neonatal checks can then be provided by GMS GPs as a national enhanced service or by PMS GPs as part of their negotiated services if:

• the baby is discharged <24h after delivery
• the birth occurs at home or in a GP unit, *or*
• there is rapid discharge from the obstetric unit to a peripheral unit.

## Parental concerns

• Discuss any worries the parent(s) might have about the child.
• Review FH, pregnancy, and birth.
• Arrange hepatitis B vaccination if mother is hepatitis B +ve (📖 p.809) or BCG vaccination if in a high-risk group (📖 p.335).

## History

• *Has the baby passed urine?* If no urine in the first 24h suspect renal abnormality and admit for further investigation.
• *Has the baby passed meconium?* If no meconium in the first 24h suspect meconium ileus and admit for further investigation.

**Physical examination** Check the baby systematically (Table 24.1).

**Moro reflex** Elicit if concerned. Support head and shoulders about 15cm from the examination couch. Suddenly allow the baby's head to drop back slightly. The response—extension of the arms followed by adduction towards the chest should be brisk and symmetrical. This reflex disappears by 6mo.

**Discuss neonatal bloodspot screening** 📖 p.848

## Check vitamin K has been given

• Discuss any concerns with the parent(s).
• Deficiency of vitamin K can → *haemorrhagic disease of the newborn* with potentially serious effects including death.
• All parents should be offered IM vitamin K for their baby; if IM vitamin K is declined, they should be offered oral vitamin K. ❶ 1 dose of oral vitamin K does not confer full protection. Formula feeds contain vitamin K supplements but breast-fed babies require further doses— ensure that they get them.
• Babies at high risk of bleeding (premature, low birth weight, unwell babies, and those who have undergone instrumental deliveries) should always have IM vitamin K.

**Health education** 📖 p.845. Discuss:

• Feeding and nutrition
• Sleeping position
• Baby care
• Sibling management
• Crying and sleep problems
• Transport in a car

**Features of common chromosomal abnormalities** 📖 p.859

**Table 24.1** Checklist for the neonatal examination

| | | |
|---|---|---|
| **General appearance** | | |
| Syndrome? Clusters of features, e.g. features of Down's/Turner's syndrome | Weight: small or large for gestation? Pallor, jaundice or cyanosis. ❶ Slight peripheral cyanosis is normal | Skin: birthmarks, meconium staining, purpura, lanugo or evidence of post-maturity |
| **Head and facial features** | | |
| Head circumference Caput succedaneum or cephalhaematoma Fontanelles—number (if 3, ? Down's), size and tension Accessory auricles | Ptosis Subconjunctival haemorrhage, conjunctivitis or sticky eye? Cataract or red reflex? | Sternomastoid swelling Cleft lip Potter's facies Pierre Robin jaw (receding jaw with cleft palate) |
| **Mouth** | | |
| Cleft palate? (📖 p.930) | Profuse saliva* | Epstein's pearls |
| **Arms and hands** | | |
| Proportion of arms/fingers Oedema | Palmar creases Fingers—number, webbing, deformity | Normal movements Erb's or Klumpke's palsy (📖 p.856) |
| **Chest** | | |
| Distortion Breast enlargement | Respiratory rate† Added breath sounds | Air entry/added sounds Recession |
| **Cardiovascular examination** | | |
| Pulses (femoral + brachial) | Heart sounds | Murmurs (📖 p.8/8) |
| **Abdomen** | | |
| Umbilical infection/ discharge or hernia | Anus: patency/position | Masses‡ |
| **Genitalia** | | |
| ♂: penis size and shape, position of urethral orifice, testes (normal, undescended, or maldescended), hernia or hydrocoele ♀: clitoromegaly, vaginal bleeding, posterior vaginal skin tag (common) | | |
| **Back, legs, and feet** | | |
| Sacral pit/spina bifida (📖 p.861) Scoliosis (📖 p.486) | Hips (📖 p.852) Proportion of feet/legs/ body | Club foot (📖 p.505) Toes—number, webbing, deformity |
| **CNS** | | |
| Is the baby behaving normally? | Is the cry normal? | Are all four limbs moving equally and is the Moro reflex symmetrical? |

\* Profuse saliva is associated with oesophageal atresia.
† Respiratory rate <60 breaths/min is normal.
‡ Liver is usually palpable as are the lower poles of the kidneys; the spleen and bladder are never palpable.

# Neonatal bloodspot screening

Neonatal bloodspot screening involves taking a blood sample obtained by pricking a baby's heel. The blood is placed on special filter paper and sent for analysis. The test is usually carried out by the midwife when the baby is 5–8d old and the result is available by 6wk.

⚠ If screening is declined, it is important to flag in the child's notes that the child has not been screened in case the child becomes ill later on.

## What conditions does bloodspot testing detect?

- Throughout the UK babies are screened for phenylketonuria (PKU), congenital hypothyroidism (CHT), and cystic fibrosis (CF)—screening for medium-chain acyl-CoA dehydrogenase deficiency (MCADD) will be extended throughout the UK in 2009.
- Throughout England, babies are screened for sickle cell disease.
- A pilot study of screening boys for Duchenne muscular dystrophy is underway in Wales.

## Phenylketonuria (PKU)

- In the UK 1:10 000 babies has PKU (autosomal recessive trait—higher incidence in Ireland). If there is a FH, prenatal diagnosis is possible.
- Children are unable to break down phenylalanine, an amino acid present in many foods. The baby appears normal at birth but develops severe developmental delay, learning difficulty, and seizures in infancy.
- The bloodspot test detects high levels of blood phenylalanine.
- Treatment is with lifelong dietary restriction of phenylalanine. With treatment, growth and development are normal.

## Congenital hypothyroidism

- In the UK 1:4000 babies is born with congenital hypothyroidism (♀>♂).
- Untreated, children with abnormally low levels of thyroid hormone fail to grow properly and have mild–severe mental disability.
- The bloodspot is used to detect low levels of blood thyroxine.
- Treatment with thyroxine replacement results in normal growth and development. Usually thyroxine replacement is needed lifelong.

## Cystic fibrosis (CF)

- In the UK, 1:2500 babies is born with CF (📖 p.338). Early treatment improves outcome and prolongs both quality and quantity of life.
- Screening detects immunoreactive trypsin (IRT) which is ↑ in children with CF. If IRT is ↑, the blood is DNA tested for the most common gene alterations.
- If a child tests +ve, it is important that parents and siblings receive genetic counselling and are offered genetic testing for the condition. If both parents are carriers of a CF gene, there is a 1:4 chance of any subsequent children they have together being affected.
- Screening will also detect healthy carriers. This has implications not only for the child but also parents and other siblings. Ensure parents have a full explanation of results and understand their meaning.

❶ Not all gene mutations are tested for. Some babies with CF will be missed by newborn screening. Continue to watch for later presentations.

## Sickle cell disease

- In the UK, 1:2400 babies is born with a sickle cell disorder (📖 p.667). Infants with sickle cell disease are at risk of severe overwhelming infections and splenic sequestration crises. Early diagnosis allows prophylaxis with penicillin and vaccines, and parent training to identify children with complications and present early for treatment. This ↓ complications and deaths in young infants.
- Abnormal haemoglobin is screened for using either high-performance liquid chromatography (HPLC), or isoelectric focusing (IEF). If detected, a confirmatory test is performed on the original spot using a different technique from the initial screening test.
- If a child tests positive, it is important that parents and siblings receive genetic counselling and are offered genetic testing for the condition.
- As well as babies with sickle cell disease, this test detects babies with sickle cell trait, other heterozygous states, and other haemoglobin abnormalities (e.g. haemoglobin E, thalassaemia). Even if these have no clinical consequences for the child, the current policy is to inform parents of the results. It is important that parents understand the meaning and significance of results both for the child and for other family members.

## Medium-chain acyl-CoA dehydrogenase deficiency (MCADD)

- In the UK, 1:13 000–20 000 babies is born with MCADD (autosomal recessive trait). Infants are unable to metabolize fats effectively. If they are stressed by fasting or infection, toxic levels of fatty acids build up causing metabolic crises, brain damage, coma, and death.
- The bloodspot test detects high levels of C8 carnitine (a fatty acid of medium length). Rarely, other metabolic disorders are also detected.
- If a child tests +ve, parents and siblings should receive genetic counselling. Treatment prevents long-term consequences, is required lifelong, and involves ensuring that the child does not go without food for >4–6h (longer after adolescence), has a low-fat high-carbohydrate diet, takes L-carnitine supplements, and parents seek medical attention early if the child is unwell.

## Duchenne muscular dystrophy

- In the UK, 1:3500–4500 male infants is born with Duchenne muscular dystrophy (X-linked trait) (📖 p.586).
- The bloodspot test detects increase in CK levels. Babies screening +ve are followed up with repeat CK testing and DNA analysis.
- The screening programme has not been extended beyond Wales as there is no treatable early stage.

## Further information

**UK Newborn Screening Programme Centre**
📖 www.newbornbloodspot.screening.nhs.uk

## Further information for parents

**UK Newborn Screening Programme Centre** Leaflets on screening for parents 📖 www.newbornbloodspot.screening.nhs.uk
**National Society for Phenylketonuria (NSPKU)** ☎ 0208 3264 3010
📖 www.nspku.org

# Summary of developmental milestones

**Table 24.2** Summary of developmental milestones

| Development | 6 week check | 8 months |
|---|---|---|
| *Gross motor* | Controls head when pulled to sitting position (0–3mo)<br>Moro reflex (0–6mo)—should be absent >6mo<br>Holds head in line/slightly higher than body with hips semi-extended during ventral suspension (0–10mo)<br>Lifts head momentarily when lying prone (from birth) | Bears weight on legs (3–7mo)<br>Can be pulled to sit (14wk–6mo)<br>Sits with support (4–6mo)<br>Sits without support (5–8mo)<br>Crawls (6–9mo) |
| *Fine motor/vision* | Stares (from birth)<br>Follows horizontally to 90° (0–6wk) | Reaches out to grasp (palmar grasp) (3–6mo)<br>Transfers and mouths (passes an object from 1 hand to the other and puts it in mouth) (18wk–8mo)<br>Fixes gaze on small objects (5–8mo)<br>Follows fallen toys (4–8mo) |
| *Hearing and speech* | Responds to rattle or bell (from birth)<br>Startle response (from birth) | Vocalizes (4–6mo)<br>Polysyllabic babbling (6–10mo)<br>Laughs (2–5mo)<br>Responds to own name (4–8mo) |
| *Social behaviour/play* | Smiles (0–10wk, mean 5wk)<br>Turns to look at observer's face (from birth) | Puts everything into mouth (4–8mo)<br>Hand and foot regard (4–8mo)<br>Plays peek-a-boo (5½–10mo) |
| ⚠ *Warning signs* | No red reflex<br>No visual fixation or following<br>Failure to respond to sound<br>Asymmetrical neonatal reflexes<br>Excessive head lag<br>Failure to smile | Hand preference<br>Fisting<br>Squint<br>Persistence of primitive reflexes—Moro response, stepping, asymmetrical tonic neck reflex |

**Table 24.2** (*Continued*) Summary of developmental milestones

| 18 months | 3 years | 4 years |
|---|---|---|
| Gets to sitting position (6–11mo) | Climbs and descends stairs | Hops forward on 1 foot for 2m (3–5y) |
| Pulls to standing (6–10mo) | Runs (~15mo) | Stands on 1 foot for 5sec. (2¾–4 ½y) |
| Walks holding on to furniture (7–13mo) | Pedals tricycle (21mo–3y) | Walks heel-to-toe (3½–5¼y); backwards (4–6y) |
| Walks alone (10–15mo) | Jumps in one place (21mo–3y) | Bounces and catches a ball (3¼–5½y) |
| Walks backwards (12–22mo) | Kicks a ball (15–24mo) | |
| Climbs stairs (14–22mo) | Stands on 1 foot for 1sec (22mo–3¼y) | |
| Points with index finger | Picks up 'hundreds and thousands' | Copies a cross (3–4½y) and square (4–5½y) |
| Casts (throws) (9–15mo) | Imitates a vertical line (18–33mo) | Draws a man with 3 parts (with all features) (4½–6y) |
| Delicate pincer grasp (10–18mo) | Copies a circle (2¼–3½y) | Recognizes colours (3–4¾y) |
| Holds 2 bricks and bangs them together (7–13mo) | Threads beads | |
| Scribbles (12–24mo) | Builds a tower of 8 bricks (21mo–3½ y) | |
| Builds a tower of 3–4 bricks (16–24mo) | Matches 2 colours | |
| Turns to sound of name | Uses plurals (30mo–3¼y) | Speaks grammatically (2½–4¼y) |
| Jabbers continually | Uses prepositions (3–4½y) | Counts to 10 |
| Uses 'mama' and 'dada' (11–20mo—half by 15mo) | Joins words into sentences (50% by 23mo; 97% by 3y) | |
| Can say ≥3 words other than 'mama' and 'dada' (10–21mo) | Gives own name | |
| Points to eyes, nose, and mouth (14–23mo) | | |
| Obeys simple instructions (15mo–2½y) | | |
| Holds spoon and gets food to mouth (14mo–2½ y) | Plays alone | Shares toys |
| Explores environment (13–20mo) | Eats with spoon and fork | Brushes teeth |
| Takes off shoes and socks (13–20mo) | Puts on clothes (2¼–3½—with supervision) | Dresses without supervision (3¼–5½y) |
| | Washes and dries hands | Comforts friends in distress (5y) |
| | Separates from mother easily (2–4y) | |
| | Dry in the day (2–4y) | |
| Unable to sit, weight bear, and/or stand without support | Unable to speak in simple sentences | Speech difficult to understand due to poor articulation or because of omission or substitution of consonants (confusion of 's', 'f' and 'th' disappears by 6½y) |
| Persistence of hand regard ± casting. No pincer grip. | Unable to understand speech | |
| Absence of babbling or cooing; inability to understand simple commands | | |

# Screening for hip dysplasia

Congenital dislocation of the hip (CDH) or developmental dysplasia of the hip (DDH) encompasses varying degrees of instability, subluxation, and dysplasia of the hip joint. Affects 3/2000 live births ($\female$:$\male$ $\approx$ 6:1), although 10× that number have unstable hips and even more have 'clicks' detected on routine neonatal screening. Associated with breech presentation at term. Often there is a family history.

## Presentation

- High-risk children (breech babies, family history, foot deformities, sternomastoid tumour) are routinely screened with USS in the neonatal period.
- Otherwise usually detected by clinical examination as part of routine screening. Screening should take place at birth, at the 6wk check, at 6–8mo, and in the second year (15–21mo). Screening tests should be taught *in vivo* by someone experienced in the technique.
- Despite screening some cases slip though the net. They present as toddlers with limp/waddling gait; frequent falls; asymmetric thigh creases, or limited hip abduction noted at later developmental checks.
- Rarely, some go unnoticed until adulthood when they present with premature osteoarthritis.

## Screening a child <3mo

- Screening tests should be performed in a warm room with the baby undressed and lying on a firm surface.
- Flex hips and knees to 90° using one hand for each leg with thumbs on the inner side of the baby's knee and ring and little fingers behind the greater trochanters (Figure 24.1).
- Each hip is tested separately. The examiner's hand on the opposite side from the hip being tested is used to stabilize the pelvis. Hold the thumb over the symphysis pubis and fingers under the sacrum.
- Only test once as repeated testing can damage the hips.

***Ortolani manoeuvre*** Each hip is gently abducted whilst lifting the greater trochanter forward. As a dislocated hip is abducted a clunk or jumping sensation is felt. It is difficult to tell the difference between a click of a normal hip and a clunk of an abnormal one—so refer any clicky or clunky hips for further investigation (usually USS or orthopaedic review).

***Barlow manoeuvre*** This establishes whether the hips are dislocatable. Holding the legs as described above, gently apply pressure along the line of the femur, pushing it backwards out of the acetabulum. The judder of the femoral head slipping in and out of the acetabulum can be felt if the hip is dislocatable.

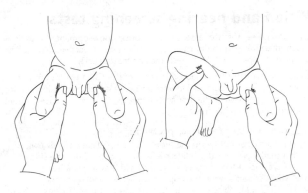

**Fig. 24.1** Screening for congenital dislocation of the hip (Ortolani test)

## Screening a child >3mo

- After 3mo of age, limited abduction is the most common finding in children with CDH. If the infant lies on his/her back with hips flexed at 90°, any hip which cannot abduct >75° should be viewed with suspicion.
- Perform the Ortolani and Barlow tests.
- Other signs:
  - Limb shortening on the affected side—compare knee levels.
  - Asymmetry of the thighs—particularly skin creases.
  - Flattening of the buttock—in a prone position, the affected side may look flatter.

**Management** Refer to an orthopaedic surgeon specializing in paediatric problems. Treatment depends on when the condition is diagnosed:

- *Young babies* Splinting in a pelvic harness to reduce and hold the hip—the hips are held in partial abduction using slings under each thigh attached to a body harness (e.g. von Rosen splint). Usually babies wear a splint for ~3mo.
- *Older babies, toddlers, and adults* Surgery is required.

## Support for parents and children

**Steps** Support for patients with lower limb conditions and their families ☎ 01925 750271 🖳 www.steps-charity.org.uk

# Vision and hearing screening tests

Operational senses are essential for normal development. Conditions which interfere with the normal senses, even if correctable, may lead to permanent impairment if not detected and treated early.

**Vision screening** is carried out as part of the Child Health Promotion Programme. This should include screening by an orthoptist-led service at ~4y. Refer children for further assessment where there is concern about vision, or any parental concern.

### ⚠ *Warning signs for visual problems*
- The child does not fix on the mother's face whilst feeding by 6wk.
- In a child >6wk old, the child's eye wanders about from one side of the eye socket to the other while the child is awake and happy.
- A white spot is seen in the pupil at any age—could be cataract.
- The child holds objects close to his/her face whilst trying to look at them.
- A child >6mo old has a squint in one or both eyes.

### *Tests for squint*
- Sit the child on the parent's lap.
- Stand in front of the child and shine a bright light (e.g. pen torch) at arm's length from the child.
- Fix the child's head in the midline and look for the reflection of the light on the child's corneas.
- The reflection should be symmetrical and near the centre of the pupil (usually slightly towards the nose).
- Turn the child's head to one side keeping the eyes fixed on the light. The reflection should remain symmetrical.
- Repeat, turning the head to the other side.
- If reflections are not symmetrical perform a cover test.

#### *Cover test*
- Sit the child comfortably on the parent's lap.
- Shine a bright light or a place a small bright object at arm's length from the child.
- Cover one eye with a card.
- Watch for any movement of the uncovered eye to fix on the object.
- Then remove the card and watch the covered eye to see if it moves to fix on the object.
- Repeat with the other eye. If either or both eyes move, a squint is present—refer.

**Hearing tests** All newborn babies in the UK are offered hearing tests through the Neonatal Hearing Screening Programme (NHSP).

### ⚠ *Warning signs for hearing problems*
- No startle response to loud noises at 6wk
- The child does not respond to his/her name by 8mo
- Absence of babbling or cooing by 1y
- Inability to understand simple commands by 18mo
- Inability to speak in short sentences by 2½y.

***Neonatal screening*** 2 types of screen are used by the NHSP:
- ***Oto-acoustic emission (OAE) screen*** Involves placing a small soft-tipped earpiece in the outer part of the baby's ear and playing quiet clicking sounds. In a hearing ear, the cochlea produces sounds in response to the clicks that can be recorded and analysed by the computerized screening system. Screening takes a few minutes and can be done at the bedside when the baby is asleep, but it is not always possible to get clear responses, especially if the baby is <24h old.
- ***Automated auditory brainstem response (AABR) screen*** Small sensors are placed on the baby's head and neck and quiet clicking sounds are presented through tiny soft headphones (muffs). A computer analyses the responses to sounds at and around the brainstem.

**When are further hearing tests necessary?** Since introduction of the NHSP there is no longer routine screening of older children for hearing problems, although in some areas school nurses screen children's hearing on school entry. However, some hearing problems, such as glue ear, may arise later. Refer to audiology for further assessment if:
- The newborn hearing test indicates a problem
- The newborn hearing test was missed (refer to audiology for screening at 8mo)
- The child is in a high-risk group for deafness, e.g. cleft lip/palate, Down's syndrome, FH childhood deafness, congenital infection. Refer for screening at 8mo.
- The child becomes at risk of developing deafness, e.g. after bacterial meningitis, skull fracture, or treatment with high doses of gentamicin
- Parental or professional concern about a child's hearing.

**Delayed speech development** may be due to a learning disorder, deafness, or neurological problems. Parents often compare their children's development with others, and this may lead to unnecessary anxiety. The normal range for speech development is wide:
- First words 11–20 mo.
- A 2y-old may use anything from a few words to 2000 words.
- Children start using prepositions at any time from 3 to 4½y.

**Management** If a child's speech is delayed, check other developmental milestones, examine for any neurological deficit, and check his/her hearing. Check your local speech therapy department's referral guidelines, and refer if criteria are met.

### Further information

**NHS** Newborn hearing screening programme
🖳 www.hearing.screening.nhs.uk

### Parent and child information and support

**LOOK** Support for families of blind or visually impaired children
☎ 0121 428 5038 🖳 www.look-uk.org
**National Deaf Children's Society** ☎ 0808 800 8880 🖳 www.ndcs.org.uk

# Birth trauma

## Head trauma

*Caput succedaneum* Swelling, bruising, and oedema of the presenting portion—usually scalp. Unsightly but resolves spontaneously.

*Cephalhaematoma* Uncommon. Haemorrhage beneath the periosteum. Unilateral and usually parietal. Presents as an egg-sized lump on the baby's head. Treatment is not required, but anaemia or hyperbilirubinaemia may follow.

*Depressed skull fracture* Rare. Most result from forceps pressure; rarely, caused by the head resting on a bony prominence *in utero*. May be associated with subdural bleeding, subarachnoid hemorrhage, or contusion/laceration of the brain itself. Seen and felt as a depression in the skull. X-ray confirms diagnosis; may need neurosurgical elevation.

*Intracranial haemorrhage* Rare. Suggested by lack of responsiveness, fits, respiratory distress ± shock. Admit as an emergency.

## Nerve injuries

*Cranial nerve trauma* The facial nerve is injured, most often causing facial asymmetry, especially during crying. Usually resolves spontaneously by 2–3mo of age.

*Brachial plexus injury* Follows stretching caused by shoulder dystocia, breech extraction, or hyperabduction of the neck in cephalic presentations. Often associated with other traumatic injuries, e.g. fractured clavicle or humerus, subluxations of the shoulder or cervical spine.
- *Partial injuries of the brachial plexus* Most recover but site and type of nerve root injury determine prognosis. If persists, refer to paediatric neurology for further investigation.
  - Injuries of the upper brachial plexus (C5–6) affect muscles around the shoulder and elbow—Erb's palsy. *W.H. Erb (1840–1921), German neurologist.*
  - Injuries of the lower plexus (C7–8 and T1) affect primarily muscles of the forearm and hand—Klumpke's palsy. *A.M. Dejerine-Klumpke (1859–1927), French neurologist.*
- *Injuries of the entire brachial plexus* No movement of the arm + sensory loss. Refer immediately for neurological opinion. Prognosis for recovery is poor.

## Fractures

*Mid-clavicular fracture* Most common fracture during birth. Usually occurs due to shoulder dystocia. Most clavicular fractures are greenstick fractures and heal rapidly and uneventfully. A large callus forms at the fracture site in <1wk and remodelling is completed in <1mo. Can be associated with brachial plexus injury and/or pneumothorax.

*Long-bone fractures* The humerus and femur may be fractured during difficult deliveries. Usually long bones heal rapidly without any residual deformity.

**Cerebral palsy** The term cerebral palsy identifies children with non-progressive spasticity, ataxia, or involuntary movements. It affects 0.1–0.2% of children (~1% of premature babies/babies small for dates).

### Causes
- Prematurity
- *In utero* disorders
- Neonatal jaundice
- Birth trauma
- Perinatal asphyxia
- CNS trauma
- Severe systemic disease during early childhood (e.g. meningitis, sepsis).

### Associated disorders
- Fits (25%)
- Squint and other visual problems
- Deafness
- Learning disability, although intelligence is often normal
- Short attention span
- Hyperactivity.

**Classification** 3 main categories, but mixed forms are common.

*Spastic syndromes* (70%). Upper motor neuron involvement.
- Affects motor function and may → hemiplegia, paraplegia, quadriplegia, or diplegia.
- Affected limbs are underdeveloped and have ↑ tone, weakness, and a tendency toward contractures.
- A scissors gait and toe-walking are characteristic.
- In mildly affected children, impairment may occur only during certain activities (e.g. running).
- Dysarthria is common with quadriplegia.

*Athetoid and dyskinetic syndromes* (20%). Basal ganglia involvement.
- Characterized by slow writhing involuntary movements affecting the extremities (athetoid) or proximal parts of the limbs/trunk (dystonic).
- Abrupt jerky distal movements (choreiform) may also occur.
- Movements ↑ with emotional tension and stop during sleep.
- Dysarthria is often severe.

*Ataxic syndromes* (10%). Involvement of the cerebellum. Weakness, inco-ordination, and intention tremor produce unsteadiness, wide-based gait, and difficulty with rapid and fine movements.

**Diagnosis** Diagnosis is rarely made in infancy with certainty, although often abnormalities in tone, reflexes, and posture are noted during routine developmental screening. Refer for paediatric assessment if suspected. Formal diagnosis is usually made by 2y.

**Management** The goal is for children to develop maximal independence within the limits of their handicap. A multidisciplinary coordinated team approach involving physiotherapists, occupational therapists, speech therapists, social workers, teachers, community paediatricians, and the primary health care team in liaison with the child and parents is essential. As with all chronically disabled children, the child and parents need assistance in understanding the disability, setting realistic goals, and relieving their own feelings (📖 p.920).

### Information and support for parents
**SCOPE (Cerebral Palsy)** ☎ 0808 800 3333 🖥 www.scope.org.uk

# Genetic problems

⚠ There are associations between some genetic syndromes and cancer (e.g. Down's syndrome and leukaemia; neurofibromatosis and CNS tumours). Be alert to the potential significance of children with unexplained symptoms in this group[N].

There are 46 chromosomes—22 matching pairs with matching genes (autosomes) and one pair of sex chromosomes which may match (XX—♀) or differ (XY—♂). Genetic abnormalities are the most common cause of developmental delay. There are a huge number of genetic syndromes, but many of them extremely rare. Categorize by the nature of the defect:

## Chromosome number
- *Alteration in number of chromosomes*, e.g. Down's syndrome (extra chromosome number 21).
- *Sex chromosome abnormalities* A sex chromosome is duplicated or deleted, e.g. Turner's syndrome (XO).

## Gross structural changes in chromosomes
- *Translocation* A portion of one chromosome is transposed or translocated onto another. If no genetic information is lost, there is no clinical effect (balanced translocation) although offspring of affected individuals often have problems. 6% of Down's syndrome is due to translocation.
- *Deletion* Loss of a portion of chromosome, e.g. cri-du-chat syndrome (deletion of the short arm of chromosome 5).

## Single-gene abnormalities
*Autosomal dominant inheritance* >1000 diseases are known to be inherited in this way. Individually they are rare and together account for <1% of all disease. Heterozygotes demonstrate the disease. Half the pregnancies of an affected individual will be affected—usually ♂ = ♀. Expression of the gene in a given individual may vary.

*Tuberous sclerosis* Autosomal dominant inheritance but two-thirds arise from new mutations. The abnormality is localized on chromosome 9. Incidence 5–7:100 000. Characterized by hamartomatous lesions in the skin, nervous system, and internal organs. Usual presentation is with:
- Adenoma sebaceum (angiofibromas of the skin—seen as red-brown papules on the face appearing at age 5–10y).
- Epilepsy and developmental delay.

Other features include coarsened skin over the sacrum (shagreen patch), nail fold fibromas, hypopigmented oval patches (ash-leaf spots), and cardiac, renal, lung, and eye abnormalities.

*Sturge–Weber syndrome* Autosomal dominant trait, although most new cases are sporadic mutations. Characterized by unilateral capillary naevus (port wine stain), usually over the forehead and eyelid, epilepsy (90%), developmental delay (50%), hemiparesis and/or homonymous hemianopia (30%), and glaucoma in the affected eye.

*Other examples* Marfan's syndrome (📖 p.291); myotonic dystrophy (📖 p.586); neurofibromatosis (📖 p.588).

**Table 24.3** Structural chromosome problems seen in general practice

| Genetic problem | Features |
|---|---|
| Down's syndrome<br>Trisomy 21 (92%)<br>Translocation (6%)<br>Mosaicism (2%)<br>*Affects 1:600 births* | *Facial abnormalities:* Flat occiput, oval face (mongoloid facies), low-set eyes with prominent epicanthic folds<br>*Other abnormalities:* Single palmar crease, hypotonia, congenital heart disease<br>Developmental delay<br>Life expectancy is ↓ but about half live to 60y |
| Edward's syndrome<br>Trisomy 18<br>*Affects 1:6000 births*<br>♀:♂≈2:1 | *Facial abnormalities:* Low-set malformed ears, receding chin, protruding eyes, cleft lip or palate<br>*Other abnormalities:* Short sternum makes the nipples appear too widely separated; fingers cannot be extended and the index finger overlaps the 3rd digit; umbilical/inguinal hernias; rocker-bottom feet; rigid baby with flexion of limbs<br>Developmental delay<br>Life expectancy ~ 10mo |
| Patau's syndrome<br>Trisomy 13<br>*Affects 1:7500 births* | *Facial abnormalities:* Small head and eyes, cleft lip and palate<br>*Other abnormalities:* Skeletal abnormalities, e.g. flexion contractures of hands ± polydactyly with narrow fingernails; brain malformation; heart malformation; polycystic kidneys<br>50% die in <1mo; usually fatal in the first year |
| Cri-du-chat syndrome<br>Deletion of short arm of chromosome 5<br>*Affects 1:50 000 births* | *Facial abnormalities:* Microcephaly, marked epicanthic folds, moon-shaped face, alert expression<br>*Other abnormalities:* Abnormal cry (cat-like)<br>Developmental delay<br>Usually fatal in the first year |
| Turner's syndrome<br>XO—deletion of one X chromosome<br>Mosaicism may occur (XO, XX)<br>*Affects 1:2500 births* | Female appearance<br>*Facial abnormalities:* Ptosis, nystagmus, webbed neck<br>*Other abnormalities:* Short stature (<130cm); hyperconvex nails; wide carrying angle (cubitus valgus); inverted nipples; broad chest; coarctation of the aorta, left heart defects; lymphoedema of the legs; ovaries rudimentary or absent<br>Lifespan is normal |
| Klinefelter's syndrome<br>XXY or XXYY polysomy<br>*Affects 1:1000 live births* | Male appearance<br>Often undetected until presentation with infertility in adult life<br>*Clinical features:* May present in adolescence with psychopathy, ↓ libido, sparse facial hair, gynaecomastia, small firm testes<br>*Associations:* Hypothyroidism, DM, asthma<br>*Specialist management:* Androgens and plastic surgery may be useful for gynaecomastia |

*Autosomal recessive inheritance* >700 known diseases. Only manifest in the homozygote. Heterozygotes may be asymptomatic or show milder abnormalities. To develop severe disease, the affected gene must be inherited from both parents. The risk of an affected pregnancy is 1:4— usually ♂ = ♀. Affected individuals have unaffected children unless their partner is a heterozygote.

*Glycogen storage diseases* Incidence: ~1:25,000. Lack of ≥1 enzyme involved in glycogen synthesis or breakdown. Characterized by deposition of abnormal amounts or types of glycogen in tissues. Inheritance is autosomal recessive for all forms except type VI, which follows an X-linked inheritance. Symptoms and age of onset vary considerably:
• Predominantly liver involvement (types I, III, IV, VI) → hepatomegaly, hypoglycaemia, metabolic acidosis.
• Predominantly muscle involvement (types V, VII) → weakness, lethargy, poor feeding, heart failure.

Treatment involves frequent small carbohydrate meals; allopurinol (to prevent renal urate stone formation and/or gout) ± limiting anaerobic exercise. A high-protein diet is also helpful for some patients.

*Other examples* PKU (📖 p.848); sickle cell disease (📖 p.667); thalassaemia (📖 p.666); cystic fibrosis (📖 p.338); MCADD (📖 p.849).

*Sex-linked disorders* ~100 are recognized. Most are recessively inherited from the mother and affect only ♂ offspring. A ♂ child of a heterozygote mother has a 1:2 chance of developing the disease. A ♀ child of a heterozygote mother has a 1:2 chance of carrying the disease. A ♀ child can only be fully affected by the disease if the father has the disease and the mother is a carrier, when she has a 1:2 chance of being affected; if not affected, she will be a carrier.

*Fragile X syndrome* Affects 1:1250 ♂ births and 1: 2500 ♀ births. Genetic abnormality carried on the X-chromosome comprising:
• Low IQ (20–70)      • Large jaw          • Short temper
• Large testes         • Facial asymmetry   • Long ears
• High forehead

Half carrier females have a normal IQ, and half have a degree of learning disability. Consider fragile X syndrome in any child with developmental delay of unknown cause. There is some evidence that folic acid supplements ↓ hyperactive and disruptive behaviour in children with fragile X. Antenatal testing is possible for future pregnancies.

*Other examples* Haemophilia (📖 p.668); red-green colour blindness (📖 p.968); Duchenne muscular dystrophy (📖 p.586).

**Polygenic inheritance** Familial trends of disease are often seen but there is no simple inheritance pattern. Usually due to the combination of genes inherited (polygenic inheritance).

*Neural tube defects* Most neural tube defects are detected antenatally by routine antenatal USS. Management is supportive. *Types of defect:*

*Anencepaly* Absent cerebral cortex and skull vault. Incompatible with life—those infants born alive die within hours of birth.

*Cranium defects* Vary in severity from meningocoele (meninges protrude through the defect) to inoperable encephalocoele (brain tissue protrudes through the skull).

*Spina bifida* The vertebral arch is incomplete.
- *Occulta:* covered with skin and fascia. Common and usually asymptomatic although may be associated with mild gait or bladder problems.
- *Cystica:* herniation of the meninges (meningocoele). Uncommon but treatable, usually with minor residual deficit.
- *Whole-cord herniation* (myelomeningocoele) is more common and often results in neurological deficit. It is associated with hydrocephalus, and learning and psychological problems.

⚠ *Folate supplementation* ↓ risk of neural tube defect by 72%. Supplements can be prescribed or are available OTC from chemists and supermarkets. Advise 0.4mg od from when pregnancy is being planned to 13wk unless either parent or an existing child has a neural tube defect, or the mother has coeliac disease, is diabetic or on anti-epileptic medication, when advise 5mg od.

**Other examples** Cleft palate; atopy; ischaemic and congenital heart disease; CDH; club foot; type 1 DM; pyloric stenosis; schizophrenia.

**Management** Depends on the specific problems of each child. A multidisciplinary approach is essential. Support the child and family. Ensure receipt of all available benefits. Tell carers about local facilities, and voluntary and self-help organizations. Review regularly.

## Information and support for families
**Contact a Family** ☎ 0808 808 3555/6 🖳 www.cafamily.org.uk
**Genetics Interests Group** ☎ 020 7704 3141 🖳 www.gig.org.uk
**Unique Rare Chromosome Disorder Support Group** ☎ 01883 330766 🖳 www.rarechromo.org
**Down's Syndrome Association** ☎ 0845 230 0372 🖳 www.downs-syndrome.org.uk
**Turner's Syndrome Support Society** ☎ 0845 230 7520 🖳 www.tss. org.uk
**Tuberous Sclerosis Association** ☎ 0121 445 6970 🖳 www.tuberous-sclerosis.org
**Sturge–Weber Foundation UK** ☎ 01392 464675 🖳 www.sturgeweber.org.uk
**Association for Glycogen Storage Disease (UK)** 🖳 www.agsd.org.uk
**Fragile X Society** ☎ 01371 875 100 🖳 www.fragilex.org.uk
**Association for Spina Bifida and Hydrocephalus (ASBAH)** ☎ 0845 450 7755 🖳 www.asbah.org

# Minor problems of neonates and small babies

Table 24.4 Minor problems of neonates and small babies

| Condition | Features | Management |
|---|---|---|
| Milia | Tiny pearly white papules on the nose ± palate—blocked sebaceous ducts | Disappear spontaneously—reassure |
| Erythema toxicum (neonatal urticaria) | Red blotches with a central, white vesicle<br>Each spot lasts ~24h<br>Spots are sterile; baby is well | If sepsis is suspected, take a swab<br>Otherwise reassure—resolves spontaneously |
| Harlequin colour change | One side of the body flushes red whilst the other stays pale, giving a harlequin effect | A harmless vasomotor effect—reassure |
| Single palmar crease | Common abnormality<br>Associated with several genetic syndromes, e.g. Down's | Usually of no consequence unless associated with other abnormalities. |
| Milaria (heat rash) | Itchy red rash which fades as soon as the baby is cooled (e.g. by undressing) | Reassure—keep the baby cool if the rash appears |
| Peeling skin | Common among babies born after their due date | Apply olive oil, baby oil, or aqueous cream to prevent the skin cracking |
| Petechial or subconjunctival haemorrhage and facial cyanosis | May all occur during delivery | Resolve spontaneously—reassure<br>Ensure the baby has had vitamin K supplements. |
| Swollen breasts | Due to maternal hormones<br>Occur in both sexes and occasionally lactate ('witches' milk') | Breast swelling usually subsides spontaneously<br>May become infected and require antibiotics |
| Sticky eye | Common—usually due to a blocked tear duct<br>Swab to exclude ophthalmia neonatorum | Ophthalmia neonatorum— 📖 p.738<br>Blocked tear duct (📖 p.963) —bathe with boiled water to clear when changing nappies; avoid antibiotics unless overtly infected |
| Sneezing | Neonates clear amniotic fluid from their noses by sneezing | Reassure |
| Red-stained nappy | Common in the first few days of life—usually due to urinary urates but may be due to blood from the cord or vagina (oestrogen withdrawal bleed). | Reassure |

**Table 24.4** (*Continued*) Minor problems of neonates and small babies

| Condition | Features | Management |
|---|---|---|
| Umbilicus | After birth the umbilicus dries, becomes black, and separates at about 1wk old | The umbilical stump can become infected (offensive odour, pus, pre-umbilical flare, malaise), requiring antibiotics<br><br>If a granuloma forms at the site of separation, exclude a patent urachus (refer if present) and treat with silver nitrate cautery |
| Failure to regain birth weight by 2wk of age | Usually due to a feeding problem or minor intercurrent illness | Monitor weight carefully<br><br>Refer to paediatrics if no cause is apparent or if, despite treatment of the underlying cause, the baby is not gaining weight |
| Possetting | Common<br><br>Baby effortlessly brings back 5–10mL of each feed during or soon after the feed | Only of concern if the baby is otherwise unwell or failing to thrive—see gastro-oesophageal reflux<br><br>If thriving, advise parents to feed the child propped up and slow down the speed at which feeds are given |
| Gastro-oesophageal reflux | Similar to possetting but a greater proportion or all of each food is brought back<br><br>Often results in failure to thrive<br><br>More common in babies with cerebral palsy<br><br>Rare complications are oesophageal stricture due to acid reflux or aspiration pneumonia | Advise parents to feed the child propped up<br><br>Thickening agents (e.g. Carobel®) or ready thickened feeds (e.g. SMA Staydown®) may be helpful as may Gaviscon® Infant ± ranitidine<br><br>Babies usually grow out of the condition after a few months and/or when solids are introduced<br><br>Refer to paediatrics if failing to thrive despite simple measures, chestiness, or anaemia |
| Colic | Very common in newborns up to ~3mo<br><br>Repeated bouts of intense unstoppable crying, commonly attributed to abdominal pain (although there is no objective evidence)<br><br>During an attack the baby's body becomes tense and rigid, face goes red, and knees draw up<br><br>Usually occurs in early evening<br><br>Examination is normal | Cause is unknown and symptoms resolve spontaneously with time<br><br>Advise parents to try colic drops or gripe water<br><br>There is no evidence that changing from cow's milk to soya-based formula is helpful<br><br>Refer to paediatrics if diagnosis is in doubt, severe symptoms, other symptoms or signs (e.g. failure to thrive, severe eczema), or fails to resolve by 12wk of age |
| Crying | 📖 p.908 | 📖 p.908 |

# Problems of prematurity

Any baby born at <37wk gestation is considered premature. 5–7% of babies are premature in most developed countries. Prematurity affects all systems of the body, and in general the problems are worse the more premature the baby:

- 32–36 wk gestation—premature. Generally do well—many need only tube feeding and warmth.
- 28–32 wk gestation (1–2% of births)—very preterm. Outlook is variable.
- <28 wk gestation (0.4% of births)—extremely preterm. Some babies as premature as 23–24 wk gestation survive, but there is a high incidence of disability.

**Nutrition** Preterm babies <34 wk suck and swallow poorly, so commonly need nasogastric tube feeding. They are also at particular risk of hypoglycaemia, so need frequent feeds. Breast milk—either the mother's or donated milk—is preferred, sometimes with calorie and mineral supplements. If this is not available, special low birth weight formula is used. Vitamin and iron supplements are routine until >6mo of age.

**Thermoregulation** Poor in preterm infants, as they have a high surface area-to-body weight ratio and little subcutaneous fat. A controlled temperature and adequate insulation with clothes and blankets, where appropriate, is important.

## Respiration

- *Preterm infants >32wk gestation* May have transient tachypnoea at birth because of inability to express fluid from their lungs. Some need oxygen by headbox
- *Preterm infants <32wk gestation* Insufficient surfactant may be produced, causing respiratory distress syndrome and requiring surfactant replacement and mechanical ventilation. Incidence and severity is ↓ by antenatal corticosteroids.
- *Extremely premature babies* May develop chronic lung disease—defined as being ventilator or oxygen dependent at 36wk post-conception—due to *bronchopulmonary dysplasia*. These babies may be sent home on oxygen via nasal cannulae. They are at higher risk from respiratory infections, particularly RSV. Episodes of bradycardia and apnoea are common. Have a low threshold for readmission.

### Prevention of RSV infection

- Take precautions to prevent exposure, e.g. avoiding busy waiting rooms in winter.
- Palivizumab is a monoclonal antibody indicated for the prevention of RSV infection in infants at high risk of infection. Prescribe *only* under specialist supervision. Give the first dose before the start of the RSV season and then give monthly throughout the RSV season.

**Jaundice** The immature liver is less able to process bilirubin, so premature babies are at greater risk of developing neonatal jaundice. They are also more likely to develop kernicterus so have a lower threshold to refer for phototherapy.

**Infection** The immune system is poorly developed, so there is greater risk of infection. Furthermore these babies exhibit few signs, so have a low threshold to refer to paediatrics for a septic screen and antibiotics.

**Anaemia** Low iron stores, ↓ red cell survival, low levels of erythropoietin, and repeated venepuncture lead to anaemia in premature babies. Some very premature babies may need repeated transfusion, and erythropoeitin is often used to ↓ transfusion requirements. Iron supplements are routinely given to most premature babies and should be continued until >6mo old.

**Neurology** Periventricular haemorrhages are common in very preterm babies. Small haemorrhages may have few consequences, but more significant bleeds can lead to cystic leucomalacia, hydrocephalus, and neurodevelopmental problems—in particular cerebral palsy. Hypoxia and severe illness in the neonatal period can also lead to cerebral damage and learning disability.

**Vision** Retinopathy of prematurity—the development of abnormal vascularization at the back of the eye—occurs in very premature babies and is related to duration and concentration of oxygen treatment. This may result in visual impairment—even blindness. Most will have had opthalmological examination whilst in the neonatal unit, but may need follow-up and/or laser treatment once home.

**Hearing** Premature babies are at greater risk of hearing problems and should have neonatal screening and appropriate follow-up.

**Bonding** Separation of mother and premature baby is often necessary. Poor bonding is common—and the problem is added to by fear of losing the baby. In many special care units, periods of 'kangaroo mother care' are used to improve bonding—the baby is nursed skin-to-skin attached to the mother/father's chest. Parents may be (quite understandably) very anxious when their babies first come home after a long period in special care, and may need more support and reassurance than other parents.

**Cot death** Premature babies have ↑ risk of cot death:
- Prevention—📖 p.845
- Management—📖 p.924

### Information and support for parents of premature babies
**Bliss** Support line ☎ 0500 618 140 🖥 www.bliss.org.uk
**Premature Babies** 🖥 www.premature-babies.co.uk

# Neonatal jaundice and pyloric stenosis

**Neonatal jaundice** In the first few days of life, most babies have ↑ serum biliubin levels as the liver takes over the excretion of bilirubin from the placenta. Mild jaundice from age 2-6d is physiological. However, very high levels of unconjugated bilirubin are toxic and can cause encephalopathy (*kernicterus*).

**Which babies with jaundice need referral?** Refer to paediatrics for same day assessment if:

**Jaundice <24h after birth** Any jaundice in the first 24h is assumed to be pathological and needs immediate referral back to hospital to determine cause (usually haemolysis or infection) and for treatment with phototherapy or, in rare severe cases, exchange transfusion.

**Significant jaundice <2wk after birth** This may be difficult to assess, particularly in a dark-skinned baby—check the sclera of the eyes. The opinion of midwives who are dealing with neonates daily can be very valuable. If necessary arrange bilirubin estimation either by asking the community midwife to take a heel-prick sample or by contacting the neonatal on-call doctor. High levels require further investigation and phototherapy. The level at which phototherapy is necessary varies with maturity and age, and may differ slightly between units. Discuss ↑ levels with the neonatal on-call doctor if worried.

**Jaundice persisting >2wk (>3wk in pre-term babies)** Arrange bilirubin estimation. If a split bilirubin test shows >20% conjugated bilirubin *or* >200micromol/L total bilirubin, then refer. Although physiological jaundice may persist for some time, particularly in breast-fed babies, it is important to rule out pathological causes: hypothyroidism (🕮 p.848); haemolysis (🕮 p.664); infection—particularly UTI (🕮 p.876); liver disease—results in high levels of conjugated bilirubin (>20%); galactosaemia.

❶ Early diagnosis is particularly important in congenital biliary atresia so that surgery can be carried out before the liver is irreversibly damaged.

**Jaundice at any time** If the baby is unwell, has persistently pale stools, and/or yellow urine which stains the nappy (baby urine should be almost colourless), refer.

**Persistent physiological or breast milk jaundice** Reassure parents. Repeat bilirubin estimation weekly until it returns to normal and jaundice subsides.

**Galactosaemia** Inborn error of metabolism characterized by ↑ plasma galactose. Clinical manifestations depend on enzyme defect.
- **Galactokinase deficiency** Autosomal recessive inheritance. *Incidence:* 1:40 000. Presents in childhood with cataracts. Treatment involves a galactose-free diet.
- **Classic galactosaemia** Autosomal recessive inheritance. *Incidence:* 1:44 000. The child appears normal at birth but becomes anorexic and jaundiced within a few days or weeks of consuming breast milk or lactose-containing formula. Vomiting, poor growth, hepatomegaly, and septicemia are common and can be rapidly fatal. Treatment

involves eliminating all sources of galactose in the diet. Long-term complications—poor growth, learning difficulty, infertility, speech and neurological abnormalities—are common.

**Neonatal hepatitis** Presents with persistent neonatal jaundice. Always requires specialist investigation and management. Possible causes:

- Congenital infection, e.g. HBV
- Galactosaemia
- Cystic fibrosis
- Glycogen storage diseases.

**Biliary atresia** Incidence: 1:15 000. End stage of a sclerosing process in an initially patent biliary tree. Cause is unclear. Presents with jaundice in neonates. Prognosis has improved with laparotomy and porto-enterostomy which relieves the problem in ~50-70% of babies. Surgery must take place <2mo after birth to stand any chance of success.

**α1-antitrypsin deficiency** May present with jaundice in infancy (📖 p. 433).

**Further information**
**NICE** Neonatal jaundice (scheduled for publication in 2010).
🖥 www.nice.org.uk

**Support for parents**
**Children's Liver Disease Foundation** ☎ 0121 212 3839
🖥 www.childliverdisease.org
**Alpha-1** 🖥 www.alpha-1.org.uk

**Pyloric stenosis** Infantile hypertrophic pyloric stenosis usually develops in the first 3 6wk of life (rare >12wk). Failure of the pyloric sphincter to relax results in hypertrophy of the adjacent pyloric muscle. Typically affects first-born male infants. Pyloric stenosis runs in families and is associated with Turner's syndrome, PKU, and oesophageal atresia.

**Presentation**
- **Projectile vomiting** Milk—no bile. The child is still hungry after vomiting and immediately feeds again. Rarely, there is haematemesis.
- **Failure to thrive**
- **Dehydration and constipation**—'rabbit pellet stools'.
- A **pyloric mass** (feels like an olive) is palpable in the right upper abdomen (95%), especially if the child has just vomited.
- After a test feed, there is **visible peristalsis** of the dilated stomach in the epigastrium.

**Differential diagnosis**
- Posseting/reflux
- Overfeeding
- Gastroenteritis
- Milk allergy
- Infection—especially UTI
- ↑ intracranial pressure
- Uraemia
- Adrenal insufficiency
- Other causes of intestinal obstruction.

**Management** Admit or refer urgently to paediatric surgery. After rehydration and investigation to confirm diagnosis, treatment is surgical with a Ramstedt pyloroplasty. There are usually no long-term consequences.

# Feeding babies

**Breastfeeding** Breastfeeding is the preferred way to feed infants from birth until fully weaned or longer. However, ~1:3 mothers who start breast-feeding have stopped by 6wk. Most wish to continue, but problems with painful breasts/nipples, concern regarding the amount of milk the baby is getting, and lack of support are common reasons for stopping.

Breastfeeding is something that some find natural and others find dif-ficult. Teaching a woman and baby to breastfeed takes time and patience. Be supportive and ask a midwife, health visitor, or the local breastfeeding advisor to help if needed.

### Advantages of breastfeeding

- Encourages a strong bond between mother and baby
- More convenient than bottle feeding—the milk is ready warmed and there is no need for sterilized bottles
- Cheaper than bottle-feeding
- Protects the baby from infection
- ↓ postpartum bleeding
- Helps the mother ↓ weight after pregnancy
- ↓ childhood obesity
- ↓ childhood atopy
- Possible ↓ risk of DM for baby
- Protects the mother against breast and ovarian cancer.

### Common problems with breastfeeding—Table 24.5

**Bottle feeding**

**Cow's milk formula feeds** Prepared from cow's milk altered to simu-late the composition of human milk, with added iron and vitamins. Advise parents to choose a formula suitable for their baby and make up the formula exactly as the manufacturer suggests. Feeding bottles and teats should be well washed and, until >6mo of age, sterilized. Using a cup rather than bottle is advisable from about 6mo. Families on low incomes may be entitled to claim free formula milk for their babies (📖 p.783).

**Follow-on formula** Not essential unless a child is not taking solids and is >6mo old. Baby milks suitable from birth can be used until a switch is made to normal cow's milk.

**Soya protein based formula** Available for children with cow's milk allergy, although this group are frequently also intolerant of soya milk. Soya formula is useful for babies who have transient intolerance after gastro-enteritis, but be careful—it contains large amounts of glucose syrup and can damage the teeth of babies fed on it long term, and it contains phyto-oestrogens which may be harmful particularly to male infants. Soya formula is available on NHS prescription.

**Special artificial formula** Available for children intolerant to soya and cow's milk formulae—prescribe only on consultant recommendation.

**Unmodified cow's milk** Not recommended until the baby is >1y old as unmodified cow's milk is less digestible and contains little iron.

### Further information

**Drugs in Lactation Advisory Service** 🖳 www.ukmicentral.nhs.uk
**UNICEF Baby Friendly Initiative** 🖳 www.babyfriendly.org.uk

**Table 24.5** Common problems with breastfeeding

| Problem | Possible solutions |
|---|---|
| *Painful breasts and/or nipples* | Ensure correct positioning.<br>Treat mastitis or thrush if present. |
| *Feeding difficult despite correct positioning* | Consider tongue tie. If severe, refer for frenulotomy. |
| *It is difficult to know how much milk the baby is taking at each feed* | Encourage demand feeding and tell mothers to exhaust milk supply in one breast before starting the other.<br>Plot weight. If there are concerns about weight gain, consider other causes of failure to thrive—☐ p.870. |
| *Breast milk does not contain all the nutrients the baby needs* | Breast milk has low levels of vitamins K and D, and iron.<br>Ensure babies who have had oral vitamin K at birth receive additional vitamin K supplements.<br>Encourage weaning at 6 mo.<br>Lactating mothers and babies from 6mo can be given vitamin D supplements if needed. Iron drops can be given to babies with low iron reserves (e.g. low birth weight, maternal anaemia). |
| *Only the mother can feed the baby* | Mothers who anticipate that they will be absent from the baby for a period of time can express milk for someone else to feed to the baby in a bottle whilst they are gone. Advise mothers not to attempt this before breastfeeding is well established as the baby might find the two techniques confusing.<br>2 methods are commonly used:<br>• Using a commercially available breast pump, or<br>• By hand into a sterile bowl.<br>Breast milk can be frozen (special bags are available) and defrosted when required. Bottles should be sterilized and the milk warmed in the same way as for bottle feeding. |
| *Disease can be transferred in breast milk* | In general breast milk protects the baby from disease.<br>Some diseases can be transferred in breast milk, e.g. hepatitis B or HIV. Bottle feeding is recommended where uncontaminated water is available. |
| *Drugs taken by the mother may have adverse effects on the baby* | Mothers should take medical advice before taking any drugs (including herbal remedies). For most conditions drugs safe for use whilst breastfeeding are available.<br>Rarely, breastfeeding is contraindicated, e.g. for women taking lithium or on chemotherapy. |

## Sources of support for breastfeeding mothers
**National Childbirth Trust** ☎ 0300 3300 771
🖳 www.nctpregnancyandbabycare.com
**La Leche League** ☎ 0845 120 2918 🖳 www.laleche.org.uk
**Baby Café** 🖳 www.thebabycafe.co.uk
**Association of Breastfeeding Mothers** ☎ 08444 122 949
🖳 www.abm.me.uk
**Breastfeeding Network** ☎ 0300 100 0212
🖳 www.breastfeedingnetwork.org.uk

# Weaning, feeding problems, and failure to thrive

**Weaning** Current guidelines recommend solids should be introduced at 6mo, although they stress individual needs of infants and choices of parents should be considered and supported. Earlier introduction of solids is linked with ↑ rates of infection and ↑ incidence of allergy/intolerance to certain foods, e.g. gluten or eggs.

## Advice for parents on weaning

- Introduce solids to your baby's diet at about 6mo of age.
- Babies are ready when they can sit up, are always hungry even soon after a feed, mouth objects, and are interested in food and chewing.
- Sterilize feeding bowls and cutlery before use until the baby is>6mo old.
- It is not essential to use ready-made baby meals—babies often prefer home-prepared purées and they are cheaper. If making purées, do not add salt or sugar.
- Start with one flavour of finely puréed food, e.g. baby rice or fruit.
- Babies take time to learn how to feed from a spoon and it is usual for most of the food to ooze out of babies' mouths at first and for babies to play with the spoon spilling the contents. Babies often only take 2–3 teaspoonfuls per meal when they start taking solids.
- Gradually offer a wider variety of different foods one by one. Avoid eggs and gluten if your baby is under 6mo old. Do not give your baby raw eggs, shellfish, honey, or nuts.
- Introduce lumpy foods gradually if your baby is >6mo old and once your child has got used to the finely puréed food. Introduce 'finger foods' your baby can feed him/herself, such as pieces of toast, rusks, or biscuits, at the age of 7–9mo.
- Continue giving your baby breast or formula milk. This is your baby's main source of food until he/she is a year old.
- It is usual for your baby's stool to change consistency when weaned.

**Feeding problems** Parents commonly complain that their child is not eating enough or eating the wrong foods. Usually the child continues to grow and develop normally. If so, reassure the parents. Consider referral to the health visitor for advice/support. Advise parents to:
- restrict snacks between meals
- show little emotion when putting food in front of the child at meal times and remove the food after 15–20min without comment about what is or is not eaten.

If the child is not growing or developing normally, look for reasons for failure to thrive (below).

**Failure to thrive** Common problem. Simply means failure to gain weight in infancy as expected. ❶ Breastfed babies need different growth charts. Defined as:
- Weight consistently <3rd centile for age
- Progressive ↓ in weight to <3rd centile or
- ↓ in expected rate of growth based on the child's growth curve.

Usually head circumference is preserved relative to length and length relative to weight.

**Causes** Failure to thrive is the result of insufficient nutrition to allow weight ↑. Causes are many and varied.

*Non-organic causes*
- Lack of food due to neglect, lack of education, poverty, or famine
- Emotional problems, e.g. emotional neglect, unhappy family or other difficulties at home    this is the most common cause.

*Organic causes*
- Chronic infection
- Gastrointestinal disease, e.g. coeliac disease, chronic diarrhoea
- Metabolic disease e.g. DM
- Respiratory disease, e.g. chronic lung disease, cystic fibrosis
- Heart disease
- Physical feeding problems, e.g. cleft palate

**Presentation** Usually detected by the health visitor when performing routine weighing or developmental checks.

### Assessment
- Ask how the child is fed—quantities and times of the day. Check that the parent is making up formula feeds correctly.
- Ask about problems feeding the child—specifically about regurgitation of food and vomiting.
- Ask about other physical problems, e.g. breathlessness, diarrhoea.
- Examine the child carefully from top to toe looking for any physical abnormalities or signs of developmental delay.
- Watch the way the child interacts with you and the parent. Look for evidence of neglect or maltreatment.
- Look to see how large the parents are—two small parents will probably have a small child.

**Management** Treat any reversible causes. Continue to measure weight, length, and head circumference regularly. Try to use the same scales on each occasion. *Refer to paediatrics:*
- If no cause for failure to thrive is found, or if, despite treatment of a reversible cause, the child continues to lose or fails to gain weight—NICE recommends urgent referral.
- If an abnormality requiring specialist paediatric care is found—speed of referral depends on the nature of the abnormality found and degree of failure to thrive.

### Further information
**DH** Infant feeding recommendation ▣ www.dh.gov.uk

### Information and support for parents
**Weaning** Information leaflet available from ▣ www.dh.gov.uk
Lewis S. *Practical Parenting: Weaning and First Foods. Which Foods to Introduce and When* (2003) Hamlyn, London. ISBN: 0600605647
**Parentline** ☎ 0808 800 2222 ▣ www.parentlineplus.org.uk

# Fever and acute illness in the under-5s

Assessing sick children, particularly those too young to tell you what is wrong, can be difficult. Infants <6mo old can be particularly difficult to assess and may deteriorate rapidly over a short period of time. Take parents concerns seriously. Physical signs are often absent or deceptive. One approach is to exclude 'alarm' symptoms and signs that might point to serious illness. In general, the younger the baby, the lower your threshold should be for seeking a paediatrician's opinion.

**Remote assessment** Ask about the features listed in Table 24.6.
- If symptoms/signs suggesting life-threatening disease (e.g. compromised airway, breathing, or circulation, or ↓ level of consciousness), arrange for immediate hospital transfer as an emergency.
- Children with any **Red** features are at high risk of serious illness. If there are no features of an immediately life-threatening illness, arrange for review by a doctor in a face-to-face setting in <2h.
- **Amber** features indicate intermediate risk of serious illness. Arrange for assessment by a doctor in a face-to-face setting the same day.
- Children with all the **Green** features and no **Amber** or **Red** features are at low risk of serious illness and often can be managed with advice.

**Face-to-face assessment** Take a history and perform a *full* physical examination, including temperature, respiratory rate, heart rate, and capillary return. Assess for features of serious disease (Table 24.6). Remember to check under clothing and nappies for rashes. Localizing signs may be absent (e.g. tonsillitis may cause vomiting in small children).

## Further management
- If any **Red** symptoms or signs are present, refer to a paediatrician for immediate or same-day review, depending on clinical state of the child.
- If any **Amber** symptoms or signs are present and a cause is found, treat the cause. If no diagnosis is made, decide on your course of action based on your knowledge of the family and the clinical state of the child. 3 options:
  - Advise the child's parents to call you if there is any deterioration (give advice about symptoms/signs they should watch for) or if the child fails to improve within a defined period of time.
  - Arrange to review the child again within a few hours of initial assessment.
  - Refer for paediatric review.
- If all the **Green** features and no **Amber** or **Red** features are present, give advice about management at home and symptoms/signs that should prompt carers to seek further advice.

**❶** Do not prescribe antibiotics for fever of unknown cause.

**Measuring temperature** For infants <4wk old, measure temperature with an electronic thermometer in the axilla. For children aged ≥4wk use an electronic or chemical dot thermometer in the axilla, or infrared tympanic thermometer in the ear.

**Febrile convulsions** 📖 p.895

**Table 24.6** Traffic light system for assessment of children with fever

| ⚠ Red—high risk | Amber—intermediate risk | Green—low risk |
|---|---|---|
| **Symptoms signs** | | |
| Appears ill | Pallor | Normal colour of skin/lips/tongue |
| Colour—pale, mottled, ashen or blue | ↓ response to social cues | |
| No response to social cues | Wakes only with excessive stimulation | Responds normally to social cues |
| Does not wake or if roused does not stay awake | ↓ activity | Content/smiles |
| Weak, high-pitched, or continuous cry | No smile | Stays awake or awakens quickly |
| Grunting | Nasal flaring | Strong normal cry or not crying |
| Respiratory rate >60 | ↑ respiratory rate (> 50-aged <6mo; > 40 aged > 6mo) | Normal skin turgor |
| Moderate/severe chest indrawing | Oxygen saturation ≤95% in air | Moist mucus membranes |
| ↓ skin turgor | Crackles | None of the amber/red symptoms or signs |
| High temperature aged <6mo (0–3mo >38°C; 3–6mo >39°C) | Dry mucous membranes | |
| Non blanching rash | Poor feeding in infants | |
| Bulging fontanelle | Capillary return ≥3 seconds | |
| Neck stiffness | ↓ urine output | |
| Status epilepticus | Fever for ≥5d. | |
| Focal neurological signs/ seizures | Swelling of a limb/joint | |
| Bile stained vomiting | Non-weight bearing/not using an extremity | |
| | New lump>2cm | |

**Common causes of pyrexia** Childhood infections are the most common cause of fever amongst children in general practice (📖 p.874). Consider UTI if no localizing symptoms/signs. Think of TB and endocarditis, especially in high-risk patients. Do not forget tropical diseases, e.g. malaria in children returning from abroad.

**Other causes of pyrexia** (may present as prolonged fever) include: malignancy (e.g. lymphoma, leukaemia), immunological causes (e.g. Still's disease, Kawasaki's disease), drugs (e.g. antibiotics), and liver or renal disease.

**Acute illness in non-febrile children** Sick children do not have to have a fever. The following are indications for referral for immediate or same-day paediatric review.
• Any symptoms or signs in the **Red** column of Table 24.6.
• Persistent vomiting—more than half of the previous 3 feeds.
• Frank blood in the stools or urine.
• History suggestive of apnoeic episodes.

**Further information**

**NICE** Feverish illness in children: assessment and initial management in children younger than 5 years of age (2007) 🖥 www.nice.org.uk

# Childhood infection

**Table 24.7** A–Z of childhood infection

| Infection | Page | Infection | Page |
|---|---|---|---|
| Chickenpox | 📖 p.650 | Malaria | 📖 p.646 |
| Conjunctivitis | 📖 p.964 | Measles | 📖 p.650 |
| Croup | 📖 p.935 | Mumps | 📖 p.650 |
| Diptheria | 📖 p.655 | Otitis media | 📖 p.944 |
| Epiglottitis | 📖 p.935 | Molluscum contagiosum | 📖 p.632 |
| Erythema infectiosum | 📖 p.650 | Polio | 📖 p.587 |
| Gastroenteritis | 📖 p.418 | Roseola infantum | 📖 p.650 |
| Glandular fever | 📖 p.933 | Rubella | 📖 p.650 |
| Hand, foot, and mouth | 📖 p.650 | Scabies | 📖 p.637 |
| Head lice | 📖 p.636 | Scarlet fever | 📖 p.653 |
| Hepatitis A | 📖 p.430 | Shingles | 📖 p.651 |
| Hepatitis B/C | 📖 p.740 | Sinusitis | 📖 p.940 |
| Herpes | 📖 p.632 | Skin infection | 📖 p.630 |
| HIV | 📖 p.744 | TB | 📖 p.334 |
| Impetigo | 📖 p.630 | Tonsillitis | 📖 p.932 |
| Influenza | 📖 p.330 | UTI in childhood | 📖 p.876 |
| Kawasaki's disease | 📖 p.535 | Warts and verrucas | 📖 p.632 |
| Lyme disease | 📖 p.601 | Whooping cough | 📖 p.336 |

**Viral upper respiratory tract infection (URTI)** Extremely common. Children have >5 URTIs each year. Presents with coryza, runny eyes, and malaise. The child may also have a mild pyrexia and/or a non-specific maculopapular rash.

*Management* Examine to exclude tonsillitis and otitis media. If pyrexia but no other symptoms/signs, check urine to exclude UTI. Most viral URTIs settle within a few days with paracetamol suspension and fluids. Treat complications (e.g. tonsillitis or otitis media) as needed.

**Acute bronchitis** 📖 p.330

**Childhood pneumonia** May be viral, bacterial (pneumococcal, Hib, or staphylococcal) or atypical (e.g. mycoplasma). Presents with fever, malaise, anorexia, cough ± purulent sputum, tachypnoea or other signs of respiratory difficulty, tachycardia, chest pain, and/or abdominal pain. *Examination:* localized crepitations, ↓ breath sounds ± bronchial breathing.

*Management*
- If symptoms are mild, advise paracetamol and fluids and adopt a watch and see approach, or supply with an interval prescription to use if symptoms are not resolving after 4–5d or worsening meanwhile.

- Otherwise, treat with broad-spectrum antibiotic. Commonly used antibiotics are amoxicillin or erythromycin (if penicillin allergic or >5y. as atypical pneumonia is more common). Advise parents to bring the child back for GP review if not improving in 48h or worse in the interim.
- If oxygen saturation <92%, cyanosis, tachypnoea (>70 breaths/min aged 1y; >50 breaths/min aged >1y) or difficulty breathing/grunting, dehydrated (or not feeding or <1y), not responding to antibiotics, or the family are unable to manage—admit for paediatric assessment.

**Prevention** Pneumococcal vaccination is now part of the routine childhood vaccination programme and is given at 2, 4 and 13mo.

**Recurrent chest infection** Consider further investigation and/or referral to look for an underlying cause if a child has a history of ≥2 probable chest infections. Possible underlying causes include:

- Asthma
- Post-infective bronchiectasis
- Oropharyngeal aspiration, e.g. due to reflux
- Congenital heart/lung defects
- Immune disorders, e.g. HIV, hypogammaglobulinaemia, leukaemia
- ✒ Right middle lobe syndrome—narrow diameter of right middle bronchus and acute angle → poor drainage and recurrent chest infections. Often associated with asthma/atopy.
- Sickle cell anaemia
- Foreign body
- TB
- Cystic fibrosis

**Bronchiolitis** Occurs in epidemics—usually in the winter months. Most episodes are due to respiratory syncitial virus (RSV) infection. Usually infects infants <1y old and presents with coryza + fever progressing to irritable cough, rapid breathing ± feeding difficulty.

**Examination** Tachypnoea, tachycardia, widespread crepitations over the lung fields ± high-pitched wheeze.

**Management** Depends on severity of symptoms.
- **Mild**—feeding well, no/mild recession, oxygen saturation >95%. Advise paracetamol suspension as required and fluids. Warn carers about symptoms/signs of worsening illness.
- **More severe**—lethargy, taking <½ usual feeds, dehydrated, intercostal recession ± nasal flaring, grunting, respiratory rate >70, cyanosis, oxygen saturation <95% or apnoeic episodes. Admit as a paediatric emergency for oxygen ± tube feeding. Rarely, ventilation is required.

**High-risk infants** Include premature babies, babies <6wk old, and children with underlying lung disease, congenital heart disease, or immunosuppression. Have a low threshold for admission. Palivizumab, a monoclonal antibody, may be used as prophylaxis. Prescribe *only* under specialist supervision. Give the first dose before the start of the RSV season and then give monthly throughout the RSV season.

**Prognosis** Most recover fully in 10–14d. Up to half wheeze with subsequent viral URTIs.

**Further information**
**British Thoracic Society** Guidelines for the management of community acquired pneumonia in children (2002) 🖳 www.brit-thoracic.org.uk

# Urinary tract infection in childhood[N]

10% of girls and 3.5% of boys have a urinary tract infection (UTI) in childhood—the majority in the first year of life. Amongst neonates, boys have more infections than girls. In all other age groups ♀:♂ ≈ 10:1. 80% of infections are due to *E.coli*.

## Risk factors

- Poor urine flow
- History suggesting/confirmed past UTI
- Recurrent fever of unknown origin
- Antenatally diagnosed renal abnormality
- Family history of vesico-ureteric reflux (VUR) or renal disease
- Constipation
- Dysfunctional voiding
- Enlarged bladder
- Abdominal mass
- Spinal lesion
- Poor growth
- High blood pressure.

**Consequences** 5–15% develop renal scarring <2y after first infection. Infections causing renal scarring are associated with adult pyelonephritis, ↑BP, impaired renal function, and renal failure. Prognosis is worst for children with recurrent infection, VUR, and scarring at first presentation.

**Clinical presentation** Depends on age and site of infection.
- *Infants and toddlers* Usually non-specific with vomiting, irritability, fever, abdominal pain, failure to thrive, and prolonged jaundice.
- *Older children* Dysuria, ↑ frequency, abdominal pain, haematuria, enuresis.
- *Site* Fever >38°C and/or loin pain/tenderness suggests upper UTI/acute pyelonephritis.

## Management

**Presentation with fever** Suspect UTI in any child with fever >38°C with no obvious cause. Use the traffic light system (📖 p.873) to guide management. If any *Red* features, admit/refer for emergency assessment.

**Urine testing** Check sample if signs/symptoms of UTI, unexplained fever, or if a child fails to recover from a fever presumed due to another cause. A clean catch specimen is best. Otherwise collect using a special bag/pad.
- If >3y—dipstick urine. Send a sample for M,C&S if nitrite or leucocyte +ve, strong clinical suspicion of UTI, PMH of UTI, or other risk factors.
- If <3y—dipstick urine if acutely unwell and urgent microscopy is not available. Else (and additionally) send a urine for M,C&S.

## Treatment of children <3y

- With symptoms/signs of UTI—check M,C&S and start antibiotics.
- Well with non-specific symptoms—check M,C&S. Act on result.
- Unwell with non-specific symptoms—check M,C&S. If urgent microscopy is not available, check urine dipstick (Table 24.8).

**Treatment of children >3y** Perform a urine dipstick and act on the results (Table 24.8).

**Antibiotics** Trimethoprim bd for 3d for lower UTI and 7–10d for upper UTI. Review after 24–48h if not improving and send urine for M,C&S if a sample has not already been sent.

**Table 24.8** Management based on urine dipstick testing

| Dipstick result | | Management |
|---|---|---|
| Leucocyte esterase | Nitrite | |
| Positive | Positive | Start antibiotics. If the child is <3y, or is unwell, or has a past history of urinary infection, send a sample for M,C&S |
| Negative | Positive | Start antibiotics; send urine for M,C&S |
| Positive | Negative | Send urine for M,C&S; only start antibiotics if there is strong clinical evidence for UTI or if UTI is proven on laboratory testing |
| Negative | Negative | Do not start treatment for UTI. Look for other possible causes of the child's symptoms. Send urine for M,C&S if: <br>• Clinical features of UTI despite dipstick results <br>• The child appears unwell with no apparent cause <br>• The child is <3y of age <br>• The child has a past history of urine infection. |

**Follow-up** Do not check M,C&S to confirm eradication. Only start pro-phylactic antibiotics (trimethoprim 1–2mg/kg nocte) if >1 UTI. Treat any constipation. Advise to drink plenty of fluids.

**Further investigation**

**Children <6mo responding to antibiotics in <48h** Arrange USS ± micturating cystourethrogram (MCUG) depending on USS findings

**Children of any age with atypical infection** (defined as child very unwell, response to antibiotics took >48h, poor urine flow, abdominal/bladder mass, ↑ Cr, and/or non-*E.coli* infection). Arrange:
• urgent USS
• technetium dimercaptosuccinic acid renal scan (DMSA) scan if <3y of age, *and*
• MCUG if <6mo, or if <3y *and* dilation on USS, poor urine flow, non-*E.coli* infection, or FH of VUR.

**Children of any age with recurrent infection** (defined as ≥2 upper UTI, 1 upper UTI + ≥1 lower UTI or ≥3 lower UTI). Arrange:
• USS (urgent if <6mo old) and DMSA scan, *and*
• MCUG if <6mo.

**Balanitis** 📖 p.472

**Epididymo-orchitis** 📖 p.474

**Horseshoe kidney, ectopic kidney, double ureter** Common malformations of the urinary tract. Usually do not affect kidney function *per se* but predispose to UTI. Recurrent infections may eventually cause renal damage.

**Further information**
**NICE** Urinary tract infection in children (2007) 🖥 www.nice.org.uk

# Congenital heart disease

Common: affects ~ 6:1000 live births. Congenital heart disease is the major cause of heart disease in children.

## Detection

*Antenatal screening* Congenital heart disease may be detected *in utero* by USS. If detected during the routine 10–13wk or 18wk anomaly scan, amniocentesis is routinely offered to screen for Down's syndrome (~ 1:20 have heart disease, especially PDA, ASD, and/or VSD) and other chromosomal abnormalities.

*Clinical examination* Neonatal examination detects ~44% of cardiac malformations found at <1y of age. The rest are detected during routine developmental checks, if a murmur is found incidentally when examining the child for another reason, or when the child becomes symptomatic.

## Presentation

### Murmur on routine examination

- *Ventriculoseptal defect (VSD)* Harsh pansystolic murmur with splitting of the second heart sound
- *Atrioseptal defect (ASD)* Systolic murmur in the pulmonary area with fixed splitting of the second heart sound.
- *Patent ductus arteriosus (PDA)* Loud continuous 'machinery' murmur.
- *Aortic stenosis* Ejection systolic murmur at apex and left sternal edge with soft and delayed second heart sound Slow rising pulse, ↓BP. Rarely, dizziness, faintness, or loss of consciousness on exertion.
- *Pulmonary stenosis* Ejection systolic murmur with ejection click.
- *Coarctation of the aorta* Ejection systolic murmur over the left side and back; absent/delayed femoral pulses and upper limb hypertension.

*Innocent murmurs* Murmurs are a common finding in childhood particularly when examining a febrile child. The majority are not associated with heart disease—so-called 'innocent murmurs'. *Features:*
- Asymptomatic.
- Soft systolic murmur—may vary with position and does not radiate.
- Normal second heart sound.
- No other associated signs of heart disease (normal pulses, no thrill).

Once a murmur has is known to be 'innocent', explain what that means to the parents—otherwise there may be unnecessary ongoing anxiety.

⚠ Unless the child is febrile when the murmur is heard and it disappears once afebrile, refer all children with murmurs for Echo or paediatric evaluation—whether the murmur is detected at routine screening, incidentally when examining the chest for another reason, or when examined because symptomatic.

## Cyanosis

- *<48h old* Likely to be due to transposition of the great arteries or severe pulmonary stenosis.
- *Later presentation* Mostly due to *Tetralogy of Fallot* (Table 24.9).

**Table 24.9** Congenital cardiac abnormalities

| Condition | Features |
|---|---|
| ASD | 📖 p.290 |
| Coarctation of the aorta | 📖 p.290 |
| Tetralogy of Fallot | Large VSD and pulmonary stenosis. |
| | In the newborn period may present with a murmur. |
| | Progressive cyanosis develops over the next weeks/years ± ↓ exercise tolerance ± squatting after exercise. |
| | Treatment is surgical. |
| Hypoplastic left heart | Left ventricle ± mitral valve, aortic valve, and aortic arch are underdeveloped. |
| | Presents within first few days of life with heart failure. |
| | Treatment is surgical. |
| PDA | Ductus arteriosus fails to close after birth. |
| | ♀>♂. Associated with prematurity |
| | Symptoms depend on size of the shunt. Presents with murmur ± failure to thrive ± heart failure. |
| | Treatment is usually surgical closure |
| Transposition of the great arteries | Aorta arises from the right ventricle and pulmonary artery from the left. |
| | Progressive cyanosis develops within a few hours of birth. |
| | Treatment is surgical. |
| Valve disease | 📖 p.288 |
| VSD | 📖 p.290 |

## Heart failure

- Breathlessness particularly when crying/feeding
- Failure to thrive
- Sweating
- Fast respiratory and pulse rates
- Heart enlargement
- Liver enlargement
- Weight ↑ due to fluid retention.

### Causes of heart failure in first week of life include

- Left outflow obstruction
- Severe aortic stenosis
- Coarctation of the aorta
- Hypoplastic left heart.

### Later causes

- Large VSD
- PDA
- Ostium primum ASD.

**Management** In all cases, if new congenital heart disease is suspected, refer for specialist paediatric and/or cardiology opinion. Specialist treatment of valve lesions depends on the gradient measured across the valve. Most other congenital cardiac lesions (except some VSD and ASD) require surgery—staged for complex lesions.

## Information and support

**Children's Heart Federation** ☎ 0808 808 5000
🖥 www.childrens-heart-fed.org.uk

# Diagnosis of asthma in children

Childhood asthma affects ~5% of children in the UK. Peak age of onset is 5y. 40 children/y. in the UK still die from asthma.

**Diagnosis** is clinical—based on recognizing a characteristic pattern of episodic symptoms in the absence of an alternative explanation. Asthma is likely if the child has >1 of the following symptoms:

- Wheeze
- Cough
- Difficulty breathing
- Chest tightness

Particularly if these symptoms:

- are frequent and recurrent
- occur apart from URTIs.
- worse at night/in the early morning
- occur in response to, or are worse after, exercise or other triggers, e.g. pets, cold/damp air, or with emotions/laughter

## Other factors that ↑ the likelihood of asthma include

- Personal history of atopic disorder—probability of asthma in a child with wheeze is ↑ if +ve skin tests, blood eosinophilia ≥4%, and/or ↑ specific IgE to cat, dog, or mite.
- Family history of atopic disorder and/or asthma—the strongest association is with maternal atopy.
- Widespread wheeze heard on auscultation.
- History of improvement in symptoms or lung function in response to asthma therapy.

## Clinical features that ↓ the likelihood of asthma include

- Symptoms with colds only, with no interval symptoms—virus-associated wheeze affects up to 20% of children at some point.
- Isolated cough in the absence of wheeze or difficulty breathing.
- History of moist cough.
- Prominent dizziness, light-headedness, peripheral tingling.
- Repeatedly normal physical examination of chest when symptomatic.
- Normal PEF or spirometry when symptomatic.
- No response to a trial of asthma therapy.
- Clinical features pointing to an alternative diagnosis

**Further action** Based on history and examination, decide how likely the probability of asthma is.

**High probability** Start a trial of treatment (📖 p.882). Review and assess response. Reserve further testing for those with a poor response.

**Intermediate probability** In some children (particularly if <5y) there are not enough features to make a firm diagnosis of asthma, but no features suggesting an alternative diagnosis. There are 3 possible approaches to reaching a diagnosis:

- Watchful waiting with review—if mild, intermittent wheeze, and/or symptoms that occur only with viral URTIs.
- Trial of treatment with review—bronchodilators and/or corticosteroids. Choice depends on frequency and severity of symptoms.
  - If a treatment is beneficial, a diagnosis of asthma is probable. Find the minimum effective dose of therapy. At a later point consider a trial of reduction/withdrawal of therapy.

- If it is unclear if a child has improved, try withdrawing the treatment. If treatment is not beneficial, consider further testing and/or referral.
- Spirometry—possible >5y. ❶ Normal spirometry/PEF testing, if performed when the child is asymptomatic, does not exclude asthma.
  - If evidence of airway obstruction, assess change in FEV$_1$ in response to bronchodilator and/or reponse to treatment. ↑ in FEV$_1$ >12% from baseline and/or beneficial treatment trial supports a diagnosis of asthma. Otherwise consider further testing and/or referral.
  - If no evidence of airways obstruction, consider testing for atopic status, bronchodilator reversibility when symptomatic (using home PEF), and/or bronchial hyper-responsiveness (e.g. exercise challenge in those with symptoms brought on by exercise). Consider specialist referral.

*If low probability of asthma* Consider more detailed investigation and/or specialist referral.

❶ Do a CXR if severe disease or clinical suggestion of another condition.

**Reasons for referral** (*E*=Emergency, *U*=Urgent, *S*=Soon, *R*=Routine)
- Severe exacerbation of asthma or severe URTI—*E*
- Unexpected clinical findings, e.g. focal signs, abnormal voice or cry, dysphagia, inspiratory stridor—*E/U*
- Persistent wet or productive cough—*U/S*
- Failure to thrive—*U/S*
- Diagnosis unclear or in doubt—*U/S/R*
- Failure to respond to conventional treatment (particularly inhaled corticosteroids >400 micrograms/d or frequent use of steroid tablets) *S*
- Excessive vomiting or posseting—*S/R*
- Symptoms present from birth or perinatal lung problem—*S/R*
- Family history of unusual chest disease—*R*
- Nasal polyps—*R*
- Parental anxiety or need for reassurance—*R*.

❶ This is only a rough guide; urgency of referral will depend on the clinical state of the child.

**Differential diagnosis**—Table 24.10, 📖 p.885

**Prognostic factors**
- The earlier the onset of wheeze, the better the prognosis—most children presenting at <2y become asymptomatic by mid-childhood.
- Male gender—risk factor for asthma in prepubertal children, but boys are more likely to 'grow out' of asthma during adolescence.
- Coexistent atopy—risk factor for persistence of wheeze.
- Frequent/severe episodes of wheezing in childhood—associated with recurrent wheeze that persists into adolescence.

**Further information**
**British Thoracic Society/SIGN** British guideline on the management of asthma (2008) 🖥 www.sign.ac.uk

**Information and support for parents and patients**
**Asthma UK** ☎ 0800 121 6244 🖥 www.asthma.org.uk

# Management of asthma in children

**Symptoms/signs of a severe asthma attack in children >2y**
- Unable to complete sentences in one breath or too breathless to talk/feed
- Tachycardia:
  - Pulse >120 bpm if >5y
  - Pulse >130 bpm if 2–5y
- Tachypnoea:
  - respiratory rate >30 breaths/min if >5y
  - respiratory rate >50 breaths/min if 2–5y

**Life threatening signs in children age >2y**
- Central cyanosis
- Silent chest (inaudible wheeze)
- Poor respiratory effort
- Confusion
- Exhaustion
- Hypotension
- Coma

**Symptoms/signs of a singificant asthma attack if <2y**
- Oxygen saturation of <92%
- Marked respiratory distress
- Cyanosis
- Too breathless to feed

*Life-threatening features*
- Episodes of apnoea
- Poor respiratory effort
- Bradycardia

**Management of an acute asthma attack** 📖 p.1091

## Aims of treatment
- To minimize symptoms and impact on lifestyle (e.g. absence from school, limitations on physical ability)
- To minimize the need for reliever medication
- To prevent severe attacks/exacerbations

**Expected PEFR in children** 📖 p.312

**GP services and self-management** 📖 p.318

**Allergen avoidance** 📖 p.319

**Complementary therapy** 📖 p.320

**Drug therapy** Use a stepwise approach (Figure 24.2, and Figure 24.3, 📖 p.884). Start at the step most appropriate to the initial severity of symptoms. The aim is to achieve early control of the condition and then to ↓ treatment by stepping down.

**Exacerbations** Treat exacerbations early. A rescue course of prednisolone 30–40mg od for 1–2wk may be needed at any step and any time.

**Selection of inhaler device** If possible use a metered dose inhaler. Inadequate technique may be mistaken for drug failure. Emphasize that patients must inhale slowly and hold their breath for 10sec after inhalation. Demonstrate inhaler technique before prescribing and check at follow-ups. Spacers or breath-activated devices are useful for children who find activation difficult and essential for children <5y. Dry powder inhalers are an alternative for older children.

**Short-acting β₂ agonists** (📖 p.314), e.g. salbutamol. Work more quickly and/or with fewer side effects than alternatives. Use prn unless

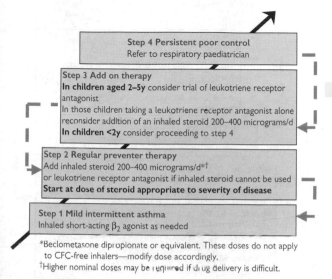

Step 4 Persistent poor control
Refer to respiratory paediatrician

Step 3 Add on therapy
**In children aged 2–5y** consider trial of leukotriene receptor antagonist
In those children taking a leukotriene receptor antagonist alone reconsider addition of an inhaled steroid 200–400 micrograms/d
**In children <2y** consider proceeding to step 4

Step 2 Regular preventer therapy
Add inhaled steroid 200–400 micrograms/d*†
or leukotriene receptor antagonist if inhaled steroid cannot be used
**Start at dose of steroid appropriate to severity of disease**

Step 1 Mild intermittent asthma
Inhaled short-acting β₂ agonist as needed

*Beclometasone dipropionate or equivalent. These doses do not apply
   to CFC-free inhalers—modify dose accordingly.
†Higher nominal doses may be required if drug delivery is difficult.

**Fig. 24.2** Summary of stepwise management in children aged <5y.
Reproduced from the 2008 British guideline on the management of asthma with permission from
the British Thoracic Society and SIGN.

shown to benefit from regular dosing. Using ≥1 canister/mo or >10–12 puffs/d is a marker of poorly controlled asthma.

**Inhaled corticosteroids** (📖 p.314). Most effective preventer for achieving overall treatment goals. May be beneficial even for children with mild asthma. Consider if:
• exacerbations of asthma in the last 2y
• using inhaled β₂ agonists >3×/wk.
• symptomatic ≥3×/wk or ≥1 night/wk.

**Oral steroids** 📖 p.314

**Add-on therapy** Before initiating a new drug, check compliance and inhaler technique, and eliminate trigger factors.
• *Long-acting β₂ agonists* (📖 p.314) Inhaled preparations (e.g.salmeterol) improve lung function/symptoms. Slow-release tablets have similar effect but side effects are greater. Do not use without inhaled steroids. Only continue if of demonstrable benefit.
• *Theophylline* ↑lung function/↓symptoms. Side effects are common.
• *Leukotriene receptor antagonists* (e.g. montelukast) Provide improvement in symptoms and lung function and ↓ exacerbations.

**Stepping down** Review and consider stepping down at intervals ≥3mo. Maintain on the lowest dose of inhaled steroid controlling symptoms. When reducing steroids, cut dose by 25–50% each time.

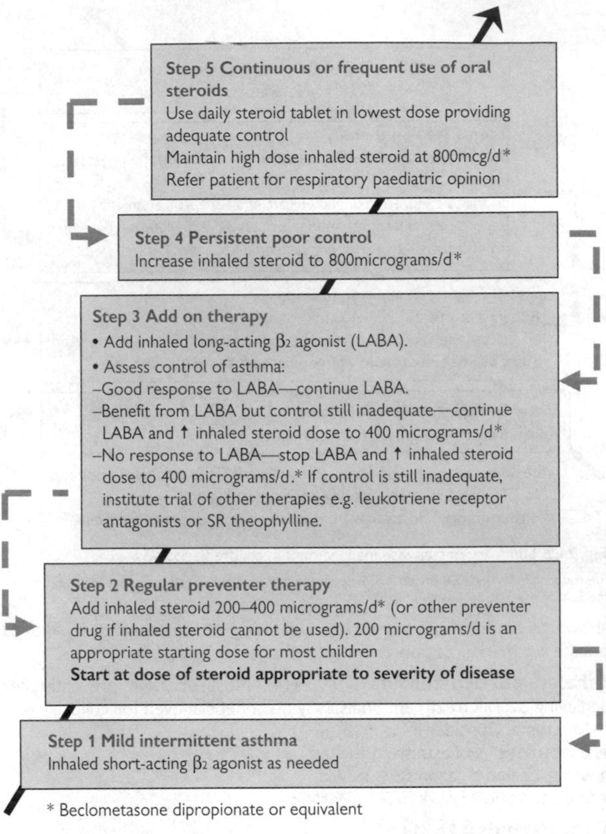

**Step 5 Continuous or frequent use of oral steroids**
Use daily steroid tablet in lowest dose providing adequate control
Maintain high dose inhaled steroid at 800mcg/d*
Refer patient for respiratory paediatric opinion

**Step 4 Persistent poor control**
Increase inhaled steroid to 800micrograms/d*

**Step 3 Add on therapy**
• Add inhaled long-acting β₂ agonist (LABA).
• Assess control of asthma:
–Good response to LABA—continue LABA.
–Benefit from LABA but control still inadequate—continue LABA and ↑ inhaled steroid dose to 400 micrograms/d*
–No response to LABA—stop LABA and ↑ inhaled steroid dose to 400 micrograms/d.* If control is still inadequate, institute trial of other therapies e.g. leukotriene receptor antagonists or SR theophylline.

**Step 2 Regular preventer therapy**
Add inhaled steroid 200–400 micrograms/d* (or other preventer drug if inhaled steroid cannot be used). 200 micrograms/d is an appropriate starting dose for most children
**Start at dose of steroid appropriate to severity of disease**

**Step 1 Mild intermittent asthma**
Inhaled short-acting β₂ agonist as needed

\* Beclometasone dipropionate or equivalent

All doses given refer to beclometasone dipropionate (BDP) administered via metered dose inhaler. For other drugs/formulations, including CFC-free formulations of beclometasone, adjust dose accordingly (see BNF Section 3).

**Fig. 24.3** Summary of stepwise management in children aged 5–12y

Reproduced in modified format from the 2008 British guideline on the management of asthma with permission from the British Thoracic Society and SIGN.

**Table 24.10** Differential diagnosis of wheezing in children

| Clinical clue | Possible diagnosis |
|---|---|
| *Perinatal and family history* | |
| Symptoms present from birth or perinatal lung problem | CF, chronic lung disease, ciliary dyskinesia, developmental anomaly |
| Family history of unusual chest disease | CF, developmental anomaly, neuromuscular disorder |
| Severe upper respiratory tract disease | Defect of host defence |
| *Symptoms and signs* | |
| Persistent wet cough | CF, recurrent aspiration, host defence disorder |
| Excessive vomiting or posseting | Reflux ± aspiration |
| Dysphagia | Swallowing problems ± aspiration |
| Abnormal voice or cry | Laryngeal problem |
| Focal signs in the chest | Developmental disease, post-viral syndrome, bronchiectasis, TB |
| Inspiratory stridor as well as wheeze | Central airways or laryngeal disorder |
| Failure to thrive | CF, host defence defect, gastro-oesophageal reflux |
| *Investigations* | |
| Focal or persistent radiological changes | Developmental disorder, post-infective disorder, recurrent aspiration, inhaled foreign body, bronchiectasis, TB |

Reproduced from the British guideline on the management of asthma (2008) with permission from the British Thoracic Society and SIGN.

## Further information
**British Thoracic Society/SIGN** British guideline on the management of asthma (2008) 🖳 www.sign.ac.uk

## Patient information and support
**Asthma UK** ☎ 0800 121 62 44 🖳 www.asthma.org.uk

# Constipation and malabsorption

**Constipation** Frequent complaint in all age groups of children. Differentiate between normal stools a few days apart (which is normal and needs no treatment) and infrequent hard stools which suggest constipation.

*Infants* Babies show considerable variation in bowel habit according to their diet (and their mothers' diets if breastfed). Babies may change colour alarmingly when opening their bowels and look as if they are straining hard—even to pass a liquid stool. Change from breastfeeding to artificial feeds and/or solids can result in a change in stool colour and consistency, with the stool usually becoming harder and more formed.

*Genuine constipation* may occur as a result of hunger, poor hydration, or use of overstrength feeds. Constipation which causes pain on defecation results in withholding of stool to avoid pain. This is a vicious cycle which can be hard to break.

*Rare causes include* congenital abnormalities, e.g. spinal cord lesions, imperforate anus (after surgical repair), Hirschsprung's disease, hypothyroidism, cerebral palsy.

*Older children* Acute constipation often accompanies acute febrile illness. Once a hard stool causes an anal tear, a cycle of chronic constipation and faecal retention may be started—pain on defecation results in withholding of stool to avoid pain. Symptoms include abdominal pain, anorexia, vomiting, failure to thrive, and a predisposition to UTIs. Eventually the child can no longer cope with the mass of faeces and soft stool leaks out around the hard faecal mass, causing constant faecal soiling.

### Management
- Ensure adequate fluid intake and a high-roughage diet.
- Treatment involves regular senna liquid ± a softener (e.g. lactulose) to dislodge the faecal mass and reinstate a regular bowel pattern. The use of laxatives can make faecal soiling worse initially.
- If not controlled with simple laxatives and diet, refer for paediatric assessment.

### Diarrhoea and vomiting 📖 p.384

**Malabsorption** In all cases refer for investigation and treatment of the cause. Usually presents with:

- Chronic diarrhoea
- Failure to thrive or weight ↓
- Steatorrhoea, *and/or*
- Iron or other nutrient deficiency.

*Causes in children* Common: cow's milk intolerance, coeliac disease. *Rarer*: cystic fibrosis, chronic infection (e.g. giardiasis), inflammatory bowel disease.

### Cow's milk intolerance 2 forms:

*Cow's milk protein intolerance* Affects ~3% of children. Usually occurs in bottle-fed infants <6mo old, but can also affect breastfed babies as cow's milk protein from the mother's diet is secreted in breast milk.

*Presentation* Diarrhoea (occasionally with blood) or, less commonly, constipation, vomiting, and/or failure to thrive.

*Other features* The child often has eczema; there may be a family history of similar symptoms; spilling cow's milk on the baby's skin may cause an urticarial rash; rarely associated with respiratory symptoms such as wheeze or stridor.

*Diagnosis* Often clinical—try withdrawing cow's milk. If this resolves symptoms and they return with reintroduction, cow's milk intolerance is likely. Skin-prick test/RAST have high false +ve and false −ve results.

*Treatment*
- Eliminate cow's milk, usually by replacing cow's milk formula with soya-based formula (e.g. Wysoy®). Take specialist advice if using soya-based formula long term.
- 10% of babies are also intolerant of soya-based formula, and special formulas containing neither are available. Take specialist advice.
- Most children grow out of cow's milk protein intolerance by 12mo.

**Lactose intolerance** Less common in infancy than cow's milk protein intolerance but more common in childhood.

*Presentation in infancy* Severe symptoms of abdominal distention, diarrhoea ± vomiting, and failure to thrive. Stools test +ve for reducing sugars. Treatment is with a lactose-free diet.

*Presentation in later childhood (>2y)* Due to lactase deficiency.
- Common— incidence is very variable depending on place of origin. ~10–15% for people of European origin.
- Symptoms tend to be milder with abdominal pain and/or distention ± diarrhoea and/or vomiting, appearing at any time from 2y of age to adulthood. Symptoms improve when milk products are removed from the diet. Tolerance of milk products is variable—some children tolerate some milk, e.g. milk in other foods (cheese or ice cream)—and others tolerate none.

❶ Soya milk does not contain lactose. Milk from other animals (e.g. goat's milk) does contain lactose. Soya milk contains phyto-oestrogens and has a high glucose content—do not use long term except with specialist advice.

**Cow's milk intolerance following gastroenteritis** Temporary cow's milk intolerance is common after a bout of gastroenteritis in children and can result in continuing diarrhoea (> 2wk). Try excluding cow's milk from the diet (e.g. by switching to soya-based formula or soya milk and avoiding milk products such as yoghurt, cheese, cream, and ice cream). If symptoms improve, wait until all symptoms have gone and then reintroduce cow's milk. If symptoms do not improve, refer for further investigation.

# Gut atresia, hernias, and intussusception

### Oesophageal atresia 📖 p.393

**Duodenal atresia** Usually associated with other abnormalities—particularly Down's syndrome. If not detected on antenatal USS, presents postnatally with bile-stained vomiting. AXR reveals a 'double bubble' with air in stomach and first part of duodenum but none beyond. Requires surgical correction.

**Anorectal atresia (imperforate anus)** 1:4000 live births. Usually the baby fails to pass meconium and no anus is visible. There is often a fistula to the urethra (boys) or vagina (girls). Treatment is surgical. In the period after surgery, anal dilation is vital to prevent stricture and starts 2wk post-op. It requires use of graded dilators by the baby's parents for several months. Faecal incontinence may be a problem but can usually be managed using a combination of dietary manipulation, enemas, and drug treatment.

**Umbilical hernia** Common. Due to a defect in the umbilical ring when the cord separates. More common in people of black ethnic origin and associated with certain syndromes (e.g. trisomy 13, 18). Usually resolves spontaneously. Strangulation is rare. Refer for surgery if an umbilical hernia persists until >2y of age.

### Inguinal hernia
- *Non-acute* History of intermittent groin ± scrotal swelling—the spermatic cord may be thickened on the affected side. Refer to paediatric surgery for repair (herniotomy)
- *Acute* Sudden appearance of an irreducible groin or scrotal swelling—necessitates emergency admission for reduction and repair.

**Diaphragmatic hernia** *Incidence:* 1:2500 live births. A defect in one hemidiaphragm allows the bowel to herniate into the chest cavity → pulmonary hypoplasia *in utero* or lung compression postnatally. Detected antenatally on USS or postnatally when the child develops respiratory distress soon after birth—CXR confirms diagnosis. Corrective surgery is associated with high mortality, but once successfully repaired the child usually has no further difficulties.

### Exomphalos and gastroschisis
- *Exomphalos* Complete return of the gut into the abdominal cavity fails to occur during intrauterine life. At birth there is a swelling at the umbilicus consisting of gut covered by a membrane.
- *Gastroschisis* There is a defect in the abdominal wall through which exposed gut prolapses.

Exomphalos and gastroschisis are usually detected antenatally at routine USS. Delivery then takes place at a specialist centre where surgical repair can be undertaken soon after birth. Once repaired prognosis is good.

**Intussusception** The invagination of one part of the bowel into the lumen of the immediately adjoining bowel. It is the most common cause of intestinal obstruction in young children and usually occurs in previously healthy children. *Incidence:* 2:1000 live births. *Peak age:* 5–18mo. ♂:♀ ≈ 2:1.

### Associations

- Seasonal variation suggests an underlying viral cause—rotavirus and adenovirus have both been implicated
- Intestinal polyps
- Meckel's diverticulum
- Henoch–Schönlein purpura.

### Types

- *Ileo-ileal* Ileum invaginates into adjacent ileum
- *Ileo-colic* Most common type—an ileo-ileal intussusception extends through the ileo-caecal valve
- *Ileo-caecal* The apex of the intussusception is the ileo-caecal valve
- *Colo-colic* Colon invaginates into adjacent colon—may be 2° to bowel tumour.

**Presentation** Very variable. Always have a high index of suspicion.

- Abdominal colic—paroxysms of pain during which the child draws up his/her legs. The child often screams with pain and becomes pale. Episodes are usually 10–15min apart and last 2–3min, but they become more frequent with time.
- Vomiting—early symptom.
- Rectal bleeding—passage of blood ('redcurrant jelly stool') or slime PR is a late sign.
- Sausage-shaped mass in the abdomen—usually in the right upper quadrant, although not always present.

⚠ The child rapidly gets worse if not treated early, becoming toxic and developing an obstructive picture with distended abdomen ± faeculent vomiting.

**Differential diagnosis** Other causes of bowel obstruction, gastroenteritis, constipation, haemolytic uraemic syndrome.

**Management** Admit as an acute surgical emergency. Untreated intussusception is usually fatal. Treatment is with reduction by barium enema or surgery.

# Growth disorders

Take every opportunity to weigh and measure every child. Plot height and weight (and head circumference if <1y) on centile charts. Always correct the age of the child for prematurity at birth.

**Failure to thrive** 📖 p.870　　　　　**Obesity** 📖 p.180

**Calculating expected height** Small parents have small children and tall parents have tall children—always calculate the expected height of the child before deciding the child has short stature or excessive height.

> Expected height = (mother's height + father's height) ÷ 2
> *Then:* add 6cm for a boy or subtract 6cm for a girl.

❶ 3% of 'normal' children fall under the 3rd and 3% above the 97th centile.

**Short stature** Height <3rd centile. Mainly healthy children (80%), but may indicate physical or emotional problems—especially if both parents have heights >3rd centile or serial measurements show that growth has fallen below that expected from the centile chart. *Causes:*
- *Genetic* Achondroplastic dwarfism, familial short stature, Turner's syndrome, familial growth delay (children have delayed pubertal growth spurt but eventually reach normal height).
- *Physical* Low-birth-weight conditions; endocrine causes (e.g. growth hormone deficiency, hypopituitarism, hypothyroidism, DM); chronic illness, e.g. severe asthma, heart disease, chronic infection.
- *Non-organic* Poor nutrition; emotional neglect; eating disorders.

**Assessment**
- Ask how the child eats and about problems with feeding—appetite, food fads, special diets, quantities/times, snacks, etc.
- Ask about other physical problems, e.g. breathlessness, diarrhoea.
- Examine the child carefully from top to toe looking for any physical abnormalities or signs of developmental delay.
- Watch the way the child interacts with you and the parent. Look for evidence of neglect or maltreatment.
- Look to see how large the parents are—two small parents will probably have a small child.

**Management** Treat reversible causes. Continue to measure height and weight regularly. Refer to paediatrics if no cause for short stature, or an abnormality requiring specialist care, is found, or if, despite treatment of a reversible cause, the child fails to grow along his/her growth curve.

**Pituitary dwarfism** ↓ function of the anterior pituitary gland causing short stature or failure to thrive. Skeletal maturation, assessed by bone age, is usually >2y behind chronological age. *Causes:*
- Idiopathic
- Genetic
- Mid-line defect, e.g. cleft palate
- Pituitary tumour, e.g. craniopharyngioma.

**Management** Specialist management is essential. Treatment is with growth hormone ± cortisol, thyroid hormone, and/or gonadal sex steroids.
❶ Growth hormone treatment ↑ risk of slipped femoral epiphysis.

**Excessive height** Most children with height >97th centile come from tall families. Pathological causes of excess height are rare and include pituitary adenoma (gigantism), thyrotoxicosis, precocious puberty, Marfan's syndrome, and homocystinuria. Refer if a child is much taller than predicted height or deviates from his/her growth curve.

**Head growth** At birth, head circumference is 32–37cm (term infant). The anterior fontanelle measures 2.5 × 2.5cm at birth, becoming smaller until it closes any time from 6 to 18mo. Most head growth occurs in infancy. Refer children with head circumference <3rd or >97th centile.

- *Microcephaly* 1:1000 births. Small head out of proportion to the size of the body. Associated with developmental delay. *Causes:* genetic, intrauterine infection (e.g. rubella, CMV), chromosome abnormality, fetal alcohol syndrome, hypoxia.
- *Macrocephaly* Large head circumference. *Causes:*
  - *Hydrocephalus*—suspect if head circumference deviates from the normal curve or if there are signs of ↑ intracranial pressure. Refer.
  - *Megalencephaly*—usually benign and familial. Rarely, associated developmental delay
- *Asymmetrical skull Causes:* postural effects, e.g. children who always sleep on one side; craniosynostosis (premature fusion of skull sutures—if suspected refer for prompt neurosurgical opinion)

## Disorders of puberty

**Delayed puberty** Affects ~2%. No pubertal changes by 13y in girls or 14y in boys, or no progression of puberty over 2y. May be constitutional (>50% boys) or pathological (80% girls). In all cases, refer to a paediatrician for further assessment. *Pathological causes:*

- Failure of the ovaries/testes (1° or hypergonadotrophic hypogonadism)
- Failure of stimulation of normal gonads to produce sex hormones (2° or hypogonadotrophic hypogonadism).

**Precocious puberty** Puberty before the normal age for the population (in the UK: <8y for girls; <9y for boys). Affects 4–5% girls ♀:♂≈5:1. In all cases, refer for further investigation. *Types:*

- *Central or true precocious puberty* (80%)—premature activation of the hypothalamic-pituitary-gonadal axis. No pathological cause is found in 50–60% of males and 90% of females. There may be a family history.
- *Pseudo-precocious puberty* (20%) ↑ level of sex hormones in the absence of excess FSH or LH. There is usually a pathological cause.

## Other problems of puberty

- *Assymetric breast growth in girls* Almost universal. Reassure that usually evens out by the time of full maturation.
- *Gynaecomastia in boys* ~50% during puberty. Small, firm lump under one/both nipples. Reassure. Usually resolves without treatment.
- *Primary amenorrhoea (without delayed puberty)* 📖 p.704
- *Premature pubarche (or adrenarche)* Early appearance of pubic ± axillary hair, and body odour, without other signs of precocious puberty. If no other abnormalities suggesting androgen excess, reassure.

## Information and support for children and parents
**Child Growth Foundation** ☎ 020 8995 0257
🖥 www.childgrowthfoundation.org

# Other childhood endocrine problems

**Diabetes mellitus** 📖 p.352    **Addison's disease** 📖 p.376

**Congenital goitre** Enlarged thyroid gland present at birth ± hypo- or hyperthyroidism. Hypothyroid babies are treated with thyroxine; if there is tracheal compression or hyperthyroidism treatment is surgical.

## Hypothyroidism

**Neonatal (congenital) hypothyroidism** 📖 p.848

**Juvenile (acquired) hypothyroidism** Usually due to autoimmune thyroiditis (Hashimoto's thyroiditis). Often insidious onset with ↑ weight, constipation, dry or coarse hair, and sallow, cool, or mottled coarse skin. In children there may also be growth retardation, delayed skeletal maturation ± delayed puberty. TFTs confirm diagnosis. Refer to paediatrics for specialist management. Treatment is with thyroxine replacement.

## Hyperthyroidism

**Neonatal hyperthyroidism** Rare but potentially life threatening. Occurs in infants of mothers with current or prior Graves' disease due to passage of autoantibodies across the placenta. *Presentation:*

- Feeding problems
- ↑ BP
- Irritability
- Tachycardia
- Exophthalmos
- Goitre
- Frontal bossing
- Microcephaly
- Failure to thrive
- Vomiting
- Diarrhoea.

Refer for specialist management. Affected infants generally recover in <4mo. Long-term consequences include premature fusion of the cranial sutures (craniosynostosis) and developmental delay.

**Juvenile hyperthyroidism** Usually Graves' disease (📖 p.372).

*Features due to hyperthyroidism*
- Weight ↓
- Tremor
- Palpitations (may have AF)
- Hyperactivity
- Diffuse goitre ± thyroid bruit.

*Eye features*
- Double vision
- Eye discomfort ± protrusion exophthalmos and proptosis)
- Lid lag
- Ophthalmoplegia.

TFTs confirm diagnosis. Refer for specialist management. Treatment is with antithyroid medication. Spontaneous resolution in <2y is the norm.

**Congenital adrenal hyperplasia (CAH)** Also known as *adrenogenital syndrome* or *adrenal virilism*. Autosomal recessive trait due to absence or deficiency of any of the enzymes needed for synthesis of cortisol. Each enzyme block causes a characteristic deficiency. 2 patterns:
- Androgens accumulate causing virilization of an affected female fetus.
- Androgen synthesis is impaired causing inadequate virilization of an affected male fetus (much rarer).

*Presentation and management* Ambiguity of the external genitalia. Less severe forms may go unnoticed until puberty. There may be a family history of CAH, ambiguous genitalia, or neonatal death. Rarely, presents with Addisonian crisis. Refer for specialist management. Treatment is usually with glucocorticoid ± mineralocorticoid replacement.

**Male hypogonadism** ↓ function of the testes. 3 types:
- *Primary* Damage to the Leydig cells impairs androgen (testosterone) secretion, e.g. Klinefelter's syndrome, anorchia (absent testes).
- *Secondary (hypogonadotropic)* Disorders of the hypothalamus or pituitary impair gonadotropin secretion which may result in impotency and/or infertility, e.g. panhypopituitarism.
- *Resistance to androgen action* Age of onset dictates presentation:
  - *In utero*—ambiguity of genitalia or female appearance, small penis, incomplete testicular descent.
  - *In childhood*—delayed or impaired puberty, impaired development of male 2° sexual characteristics ± gynaecomastia.
  - *In adulthood*—↓ libido, impotence, loss of muscle power, testicular atrophy, fine wrinkling of the skin around eyes and lips, sparse body hair, osteopoenia, gynaecomastia.

*Management* Refer for specialist investigation. Treatment depends on the nature of the deficiency.

**Androgen insensitivity syndrome (AIS)** X-linked genetic disorder affecting 1:62 000 male births. Abnormalities within androgen receptors result in the individual being genotypically male (46XY) but phenotypically female. External genitalia are female in complete AIS (CAIS), but are often ambiguous in partial AIS (PAIS). The testes fail to descend and are usually found in the groin—rarely within the abdomen. At puberty, breast development occurs and female contours form, but there is little or no pubic or axillary hair. Patients often present with primary amenorrhoea.

*Management* As diagnosis is often made in teenage years, young people with CAIS have usually been treated as female since birth. Specialist support is always required. Testes are usually removed as they have malignant potential, and oestrogens given to complete 2° sexual development.

## Dealing with sexual ambiguity detected at the 6wk check
- Be honest—do not guess the gender of the child.
- Explain that there are rare conditions where girls may be virilized or boys undermasculinized, causing girls to look like boys and vice versa.
- Arrange paediatric assessment as soon as possible for further investigations, gender assignment, and ongoing management.

# Funny turns and febrile convulsions

**Funny turns** Small children are often brought to the GP by their parents because they have had a 'funny turn'. The major questions are: was the episode a fit? If so, what caused it? If not, then is there another serious underlying cause, e.g. heart disease?

**History** A good history from a witness is essential. Ask:
• When and where did the attack happen?
• Were there any precipitating events or warning signs? e.g. viral illness, fever, strong emotions (was the child angry or upset?), head injury
• What happened? Did the child lose consciousness? Jerk his limbs? If so, was the jerking generalized or restricted to one area of the body? What did the child look like during the attack (e.g. colour, floppiness)? Did anything else happen during the attack (e.g. tongue biting)?
• How long did the attack last?
• What happened after the attack? Was the child conscious straight away? Was there disorientation or drowsiness?

*Also check*
• *General history*—is the child well? Does the child have any ongoing medical problems? Past medical history—serious illness, neurological and/or developmental problems, heart problems.
• *Birth history*—problems in pregnancy, birth trauma.
• *Family history*—epilepsy.

**Examination** Full general/neurological examination; developmental milestones. Plot head circumference/weight on centile chart.

**Differential diagnosis** Epileptic attacks—febrile convulsion or child-hood epilepsy (📖 p.896), non-epileptic attacks.

**Non-epileptic attacks** Usually self-limiting and harmless. Frightening for parents/carers, so education about likely duration and cause of attacks and reassurance that the child will come to no harm are important.

*Simple blue breath-holding attacks* Onset usually >6mo of age. Common. Provoked by frustration or upset. *Signs*: +ve Valsalva manoeuvre, cynanosis, stiffening, and coma. No treatment needed—spontaneous recovery. Most children 'grow out' of the attacks by 3y.

*White reflex asystolic (anoxic) attacks* Most common from 6mo to 2y. Usually triggered by minor injury or anxiety. *Signs*: vagal asystole, pallor, rapid coma, stiffening, upward eye movement ± urinary incontinence. No treatment needed—spontaneous recovery.

*Reflex syncope or vasovagal attacks ('faints')* 📖 p.559

*Other causes are rare in children but include*
• Cardiac arrhythmias—refer if recurrent loss of consciousness or collapse on exertion for paediatric cardiology assessment.

| | |
|---|---|
| • Hyperventilation | • Sleep phenomena |
| • Benign monoclonus of infancy | • Hypoglycaemia |
| • Benign paroxysmal vertigo | • Factitious illness. |

**Febrile convulsions** Epileptic seizures provoked by fever in other-wise normal children. *Prevalence:* 3–5% of children aged 6mo–5y (peak age 18mo). There is often a family history. Seizures are usually brief (<5min) and generalized. *Causes (in order of decreasing frequency):* viral infections, otitis media, tonsillitis, UTI, gastroenteritis, LRTI, meningitis, post-immunization.

## Management of the fitting child 📖 p.1066

**Further management** Most children do not require admission. Check temperature, assess respiratory/heart rate, capillary return, and level of consciousness. Examine for a source of infection. If there is no obvious cause and not being admitted, check MSU.

> ⚠ Complex convulsions are more likely to be provoked by a serious condition. Suspect serious pathology if a child has:
> • had a prolonged (>10 min.) or focal febrile convulsion, *or*
> • not recovered within an hour of a febrile convulsion.

*Admit if*
- Complex seizure, the child was drowsy before the seizure, is irritable, systemically unwell or 'toxic', and/or the cause of the fever is unclear.
- Symptoms/signs of meningitis (📖 p.1074), petechial rash, recent or current treatment with antibiotics (may mask symptoms/signs of meningitis), or aged <18mo (meningitis may have non-specific signs).
- The cause of the fever requires hospital management in its own right.
- Early review by a doctor is not possible, inadequate home circumstances, or the carer is anxious or unable to cope.

*For children not being admitted* Reassure parents/carers that febrile convulsions do not harm the child. Antipyretics (e.g. paracetamol) do not prevent convulsions but are useful for symptom control. Advise parents to seek urgent medical help if the child deteriorates in any way, develops a non-blanching rash, fits again, or they are worried. Arrange early review (in <24h). Recommend that immunization schedules are completed.

*Consider out-patient referral if*
- Diagnosis of febrile convulsion is in doubt.
- Febrile convulsions have been frequent, severe and/or complex, and prophylactic treatment (with rectal diazepam or continuous anticonvulsants) might be indicated.
- The child is at ↑ risk of epilepsy, e.g. coexistent neurological or developmental conditions, history of epilepsy in first-degree relative.
- Parents/carers are anxious despite reassurance or request referral.

**Prognosis** Febrile convulsions recur in subsequent febrile illness in ~30% of children. 1% of children having a febrile convulsion go on to develop epilepsy (compared with 0.4% of children who have not had a febrile convulsion).

## Further information

**NICE** The epilepsies: the diagnosis and management of the epilepsies in adults and children in primary and secondary care (2004) 🖥 www.nice.org.uk
**NSF for Coronary Heart Disease** (2005) 🖥 www.dh.gov.uk

# Childhood epilepsy

Childhood epilepsy is a susceptibility to continuing seizures. Prevalence ↑ with age from ~4:1000 children at 7y to ~5:1000 children at 16y. 60% of adult epilepsy starts in childhood.

**Risk factors** Neurological abnormalities or developmental delay; family history; past history of febrile convulsions—1% develop epilepsy.

**Diagnosis** Seizures, faints, and funny turns can be difficult to distinguish and diagnose (📖 p.894). A reliable eye-witness account is key.

⚠ Refer to a specialist paediatrician with training and expertise in epilepsy for diagnosis. All children who have had a first non-febrile seizure should be seen in <2wk.[N].

**Management of the fitting patient** 📖 p.1066

**Long-term management of epilepsy** 📖 p.584

**Epileptic syndromes** In children, epilepsy is considered in terms of the 'epileptic syndrome'. Identifying a syndrome enables predictions about cause, severity, and prognosis. Epileptic syndromes are characterized by a set pattern of seizure type(s) ± other features: physical appearance, age at onset, family history, associated learning disability and/or developmental delay, associated neurological findings, and EEG (should be undertaken in any child with a history of ≥2 epileptic seizures)

❶ It is not possible to identify a syndrome in 30%—and symptoms/signs may take months to evolve until diagnosis can be made in others.

**Benign rolandic epilepsy** Also known as *childhood epilepsy with centrotemporal spikes*. 15–20% of childhood epilepsy. Starts in children aged 2–12y (peak age 7–10y)—usually stops by 13y. Frequently there is a family history. Clonic partial sensorimotor attacks affect the face, tongue, pharynx, hand, and arm. Most common on falling asleep (>½ have seizures only during sleep) or soon after waking. Secondary generalization to tonic–clonic seizures may occur. EEG is characteristic. Use of drug treatment depends on frequency and severity of seizures.

**Juvenile myoclonic epilepsy (JME)** 4–12% of childhood epilepsy. Age of onset 8–24y. (peak age 8–16y.). 50% have FH of epilepsy. Presents with sudden brief bilaterally symmetrical and synchronous involuntary muscle contractions. Upper body > lower body. May cause the patient to throw objects or fall. Consciousness is often maintained. Frequently occurs soon after waking. Triggers may include light (1:2), tiredness, or emotion. Generalized tonic–clonic seizures, often starting with a series of myoclonic jerks, appear <4y after onset of myoclonic seizures in ~90%. Absence seizures also occur in 15–30%. EEG is characteristic.

*Management and prognosis* Usually treated with sodium valproate—fits may not be well controlled with medication. JME does not remit spontaneously. Lifelong medication is needed—relapse rate is ~90% on withdrawal of anti-epileptic medication.

***Lennox–Gastaut syndrome*** Severe early onset form of myoclonic epilepsy (starts age 2–6y) with intractable seizures and a typical EEG. *W.G. Lennox (1884–1960), US neurologist; H.J.P. Gastaut (1915–1995), French neurologist.*

**Absence seizures (petit mal)** 10–12% of childhood epilepsy. Age of onset 4–10y (peak age 5–7y); ♀>♂; ~15% have a family history. The child stops what he/she is doing and may stare into middle-space for a period of seconds (mean 4–20 sec). Can occur 50–100×/d. Deterioration in school performance may be the first sign. Separating absence attacks from day-dreaming can be difficult. EEG is characteristic.

***Management and prognosis*** 80% become seizure free with sodium valproate. ~15% go on to develop JME. ~10% (without other adverse factors) have absence or tonic–clonic seizures in adult life.

**Localization-related epilepsies** Up to 30% of childhood epilepsy. Partial (focal) seizures. May be *symptomatic* (known underlying cause) or *cryptogenic* (symptomatic cause suspected but not found). Clinical features, disabilities, and prognosis depend on cause and location of the brain abnormality.

**Infantile spasms (West's syndrome)** Starts in the first year of life (peak age 4mo). Runs of tonic spasms—usually flexion spasms (*salaam spasms*)—occur every 5–10sec. Characteristic EEG. Associated with loss of vision and social interaction. Treatment is with steroids and anti-epileptics (usually vigabatrin). Poor prognosis: 30–50% have cerebral palsy; 85% have a cognitive disability; 20% death rate.
*W.J. West (1794–1848), British physician.*

### Particular problems to look for in children with epilepsy

- Developmental problems—25% of children with epilepsy have special educational needs, and >20% have moderate/severe learning disability. Specific cognitive disability (e.g. with reading or arithmetic) can occur and may have a serious impact on a child's education if not recognized.
- Social stigmatization (perceived or experienced) is common. Children may have problems making friends and with peers at school because they are not allowed to do everything other children do or have funny turns and are considered 'odd'. This results in psychosocial problems including lack of confidence, poor self-esteem, behavioural problems (e.g. conduct disorder, school refusal), dependence on others, anxiety, and depression.
- Adverse effects of antiepileptic drugs.
- Physical trauma—may occur as a result of having a seizure.

### Further information

**NICE** 🖳 www.nice.org.uk
- The epilepsies: the diagnosis and management of the epilepsies in adults and children in primary and secondary care (2004)
- Newer drugs for epilepsy in children (2004)
- Referral guidelines for suspected cancer (2005).

### Information and support for patients and parents

**Epilepsy Action** ☎ 0808 800 5050 🖳 www.epilepsy.org.uk

# Arthritis in children

Joint and limb pains are common in children. Arthritis is rare.

## Presentation of arthritis in children

**Older children** Usually present with well-localized joint pains ± hot tender swollen joints.

**Babies and young children** May present with immobility of a joint or a limp, but the diagnosis can be extremely difficult.

## Differential diagnosis of joint pains in children

- Juvenile chronic arthritis (JCA)
- Infections, e.g. TB, rubella
- Rheumatic fever
- Henoch–Schönlein purpura
- Traumatic arthritis
- Hypermobility syndrome
- Leukaemia
- Sickle cell disease
- SLE and connective tissue disorders
- Transient synovitis of the hip (irritable hip)
- Septic arthritis
- Perthes' disease
- Slipped femoral epiphysis.

**Septic arthritis** 📖 p.529

**Types of childhood arthritis**—Table 24.11

## Management of children with arthritis

- If suspected, refer urgently to paediatrics for confirmation of diagnosis.
- Once confirmed, ensure that the child is referred to a specialist paediatric rheumatology unit to avoid long-term disability. These units have multidisciplinary facilities for rehabilitation, education, and surgical intervention (if necessary), and support both the family and the child.
- NSAIDs and paracetamol help pain and stiffness, but corticosteroids and immunosuppressants (e.g. methotrexate) are often required for systemic disease.
- Ensure families apply for any benefits that might be available to them
- Tell families about self-help and support groups
- Support families in any applications made to adapt the home or school environment for the child's condition.

## Information and support for parents and children

**Arthritis Research Campaign (ARC)** ☎ 0870 850 5000 🖥 www.arc.org.uk

**Table 24.11** Childhood arthritis

| Type of arthritis | Features |
|---|---|
| **Oligoarthritis or pauciarticular onset arthritis** | |
| *Persistent* | Most common form of JCA (50–60%) but still rare. |
| | Peak age 3y; ♀ >> ♂. |
| | Affects ≤4 joints—especially wrists, knees and ankles. Often asymmetrical. |
| | Associated with uveitis (often with +ve antinuclear antibody) which requires regular screening by slit-lamp examination—rarely, causes blindness. |
| | Generally prognosis is good, with remission in 4–5y. |
| *Extended* | Chronic arthritis with an oligoarticular onset of the disease, which progresses to involve >4 joints. Joints tend to be stiff rather than hot and swollen. |
| **Still's disease\*** | 10% of JCA. |
| | Affects boys and girls equally up to 5y—then girls are more commonly affected. |
| | *Presentation* <br> • Fever—high swinging early-evening temperature <br> • Rash—pink maculopapular rash <br> • Musculoskeletal pain—Arthralgia, arthritis, myalgia <br> • Generalized lymphadenopathy <br> • Hepatosplenomegaly <br> • Pericarditis ± pleurisy (uncommon), |
| | *Investigations* Blood—↑ ESR/CRP; FBC ↑ neutrophils, ↑ platelets. Autoantibodies are –ve. |
| | ⚠ *Differential diagnosis* Malignancy, particularly leukaemia or neuroblastoma; infection. |
| **Polyarticular onset JCA** | Develops with/without preceding systemic illness at any age >1y. |
| | Usually occurs in teenagers producing widespread joint destruction. |
| | Symmetrical arthritis of hands, wrists, PIP joints ± DIP joints. |
| | Rheumatoid factor usually –ve (+ve in 3%—often teenage girls). |
| **Juvenile spondylo-arthropathy** | Affects teenage and younger boys, producing an asymmetrical arthritis of lower limb joints. |
| | Associated with HLA-B27 and acute anterior uveitis. |
| | Represents childhood equivalent of adult ankylosing spondylitis. ~60% of childhood sufferers develop ankylosing spondylitis later in life. |
| **Psoriatic arthritis** | Polyarthritis affecting large and small joints, including fingers and toes. The arthritis can be very erosive. |
| | Psoriasis may be present in the child or first-degree relative (📖 p.622). |

\* G.F. Still (1868–1941), English paediatrician

# Paediatric dermatology

## Birthmarks

### Strawberry naevus (capillary haemangioma)

- Not usually present at birth.
- Occurs anywhere on the skin surface.
- Starts as a small red patch and then grows rapidly over a few months into a bright red vascular lump.
- After initial growth, the naevus stays the same size for 6–12mo, then involutes and disappears by 5–7y.
- No treatment is needed. Parents may need considerable reassurance.
- If interfering with feeding, breathing, or vision, refer for treatment with intralesional steroids or laser.

### Port wine stain (naevus flammeus)

- Present at birth.
- Irregular red/purple macule which often affects one side of the face.
- Permanent—may become darker and lumpy in middle age.
- May be associated with other abnormalities, e.g. intracranial vascular malformation (Sturge–Weber syndrome—📖 p.858).

### Salmon patch (stork mark)

- The most common vascular naevus (~50% neonates).
- Small telangectatic lesion forming a pink macule—most commonly at the nape of the neck or on the upper face.
- Facial lesions resolve spontaneously—those on the neck may persist. No treatment is needed.

### Mongolian blue spot

- Bluish discoloration of the skin, usually over buttocks and lower back in dark-skinned babies.
- Of no clinical significance, but may occasionally be mistaken for bruising and non-accidental injury.
- Usually disappears by 1y.

### Congenital melanocytic naevi ~1.5% of neonates.

- Noted at birth as black or brown raised nodules or plaques.
- May be hairy, irregular, single, or multiple.
- Classified by size: <1.5cm—small; 1.5–20cm—medium; >20cm—large.
- Risk of malignant change to melanoma—the larger the naevus the greater the risk.
- Laser therapy can improve cosmetic appearance.

**Nappy rash** Most common type of nappy eruption. Usually seen in young infants—rare >12mo. An irritant dermatitis due to skin contact with urine or faeces.

### Presentation Glazed erythema in the napkin area, sparing skin folds. Secondary bacterial or fungal infection is common.

### Differential diagnosis

- Seborrhoeic eczema
- Candidiasis
- Napkin psoriasis.

## *Management*
- Advise parents to keep the nappy area dry.
- Give baby as much time as possible with the nappy off.
- Apply aqueous cream as a moisturizer and soap substitute.
- Apply a barrier cream between nappy changes, although this may interfere with the action of some modern nappies.
- Topical treatment with an antifungal combined with hydrocortisone is effective if the nappy rash is not clearing.

### Infantile seborrhoeic eczema
- Starts in the first few weeks of life.
- Affects body folds—axilla, groins, behind ears, neck ± face, and scalp ('*cradle cap*').
- Flexural lesions present as moist shiny well-demarcated scaly erythema
- A yellowish crust is usual on the scalp, neck, and behind the ears.
- Treat flexural lesions with emollients and 1% hydrocortisone ointment, or with clotrimazole and hydrocortisone cream.
- Scalp lesions respond to OTC cradle cap creams, or 2% salicyclic acid in aqueous cream applied od and washed out with baby shampoo.

**Candidiasis** Often complicates nappy rash or infantile seborrhoeic eczema. Erythema, scaling, and pustules involve the flexures. There may be associated satellite lesions. Treatment is with a topical antifungal, e.g. clotrimazole.

**Juvenile plantar dermatosis** Presents with red, dry, fissured, and glazed skin, principally over the forefeet. Sometimes involves the whole sole. Usually starts in primary school years and resolves spontaneously in mid-teens. Due to wearing socks and/or shoes made from synthetic materials. Emollients help but topical steroids are ineffective. Advise cotton socks and leather shoes.

**Accessory nipples** Commonly seen on the milk line in both male and female infants. Usually small and inconspicuous. No treatment is required.

**Acne** 📖 p.620

**Atopic eczema** 📖 p.612

**Head lice** 📖 p.636

**Impetigo** 📖 p.630

**Molluscum contagiosum** 📖 p.632

**Psoriasis** 📖 p.622

**Scabies** 📖 p.637

**Scalded skin syndrome** 📖 p.631

**Urticaria** 📖 p.618

**Warts** 📖 p.632

### Further information
**Electronic Dermatology Atlas** 🖥 www.dermis.net

# Diagnosis of cancer in children[N]

Every year in the UK, 1500 children are diagnosed with cancer and 300 children die as a result of cancer. The most common type of cancer in childhood is acute leukaemia (1:3) followed by brain tumour (1:4). Risk of developing cancer for an individual child is ~1:500 and 75% developing cancer will survive 5y. If a child survives 5y following treatment, there is a 10% chance of death from tumour recurrence or treatment effects.

Diagnosis of childhood malignancy is a particular challenge in primary care. GPs rarely see children with cancer, and the cancers that children get are often unfamiliar to them. Always have a high index of suspicion and, if in doubt, refer for a specialist opinion. Referrals should be made to a paediatrician or specialist in children's cancer.

❶ Some congenital/genetic syndromes may be associated with ↑ risk of childhood cancer (e.g. Down's syndrome—leukaemia; neurofibromatosis and tuberous sclerosis—CNS tumours).

**Abdominal distension** If persistent or progressive, examine the abdomen:
- If a mass is found, refer immediately
- If the child is uncooperative and abdominal examination is not possible, or if examination is difficult, consider referral for urgent abdominal USS.

**Unexplained or persistent back pain** Examine the child and check FBC and blood film. Consider X-ray and/or discussion with a paediatrician. If no cause is found, *refer urgently*.

**Immediate referral/admission** Any child with:
- Hepatosplenomegaly.
- Unexplained petechiae.
- Unexplained urinary retention.
- ↓ conscious level.
- Headache and vomiting that cause early morning waking or occur on waking as these are classic signs of ↑ intracranial pressure ❶ <1% of patients presenting with headache have a brain tumour.
- Children <2y with new-onset seizures (excluding febrile convulsion), bulging fontanelle, extensor attacks, and/or persistent vomiting.
- Mediastinal, hilar, or thoracic mass on CXR.

**Urgent/immediate referral** Any child with:
- New onset seizures.
- Cranial nerve abnormalities.
- Visual disturbances.
- Leg weakness—refer immediately if gait abnormalities or motor or sensory signs.
- Other motor/sensory signs.
- Abdominal mass.
- Skin nodules in a baby that could be metastatic neuroblastoma.
- Proptosis.
- Shortness of breath, particularly if not responding to bronchodilators.
- FBC suggesting malignancy.

**Urgent referral** Refer:
- When a child presents several times (≥3×) with the same problem, but with no clear diagnosis.
- If white papillary reflex (leucocoria).
- If aged ≥2y with persistent headache where you cannot carry out an adequate neurological examination in primary care.
- If aged <2y. with:
  - Abnormal ↑ in head size
  - Arrest/regression of motor development and/or altered behaviour
  - Abnormal eye movements and/or lack of visual following
  - Poor feeding/failure to thrive
  - New squint/change in visual acuity—urgency depends on other factors.
- If unexplained mass at any site that has ≥1 of the following features:
  - Deep to the fascia
  - Non-tender
  - Progressively enlarging
  - Associated with a regional lymph node that is enlarging
  - >2 cm in diameter.
- If lymphadenopathy with ≥1 of the following features (particularly if no evidence of local infection and/or associated with general ill-health, fever or weight loss):
  - Non-tender, firm, or hard lymph nodes
  - Lymph nodes >2 cm in size
  - Lymph nodes progressively enlarging
  - Any axillary nodes (in the absence of local infection or dermatitis)
  - Any supraclavicular nodes.
- If haematuria.
- If persistent localized bone pain/swelling and X-ray showing signs of cancer.
- If unexplained deteriorating school performance or developmental milestones, or unexplained behavioural and/or mood changes.
- If rest pain or unexplained limp—consider X-ray and/or discussion with a paediatrician before, or as well as, referral.
- If family history of retinoblastoma and/or visual problems.

**Investigations** Check FBC and blood film if:
- Pallor and/or fatigue.
- Irritability.
- Unexplained fever.
- Persistent or recurrent URTIs.
- Generalized lymphadenopathy.
- Persistent or unexplained bone pain (additionally consider X-ray).
- Unexplained bruising.

❶ If the blood film or FBC indicates leukaemia, make an ***urgent referral.***

**Consider referral** when there is persistent parental anxiety, even when a benign cause is considered most likely.

**Further information**
**NICE** Referral guidelines for suspected cancer (2005) ⌨ www.nice.org.uk

# Specific childhood cancers

**Acute leukaemia** 📖 p.674     **Brain tumour** 📖 p.566
**Lymphoma** 📖 p.678         **Sarcoma** 📖 p.513

### Gonadal tumours
• Testicular tumours 📖 p.476      • Ovarian tumours 📖 p.720

**Neuroblastoma** Tumour derived from neural crest tissue. 80 cases/y are reported in England and Wales—8% of all paediatric tumours. Neuroblastoma tends to affect children <4y old (50% <2y; 90% <9y). *Sites:* adrenal medulla—50%; abdominal sympathetic ganglia—25%; chest—20%; pelvis—5%; neck—5%.

*Presentation* Variable and often non-specific—depends on site of the tumour and extent of metastases. ~½ present with metastatic disease.
• *General effects* Pallor, fever, anorexia and weight ↓, failure to thrive, diarrhoea, irritability, flushing, ataxia.
• *Local effects of the tumour* Abdominal mass (or thoracic mass on CXR); local spread may cause paraplegia or cauda equina syndrome. Infants <6mo may have rapidly progressive intra-abdominal disease.
• *Effects of metastases* Lymphatic and haematogenous spread, particularly to liver, lungs, and bone, is common. Associated symptoms:
  • Bone pain ± pathological fracture.
  • Breathlessness.
  • Peri-orbital bruising (looks like a black eye), proptosis, or Horner's syndrome.
  • Firm skin nodules (usually babies—'blueberry muffin appearance').

*Investigate with a FBC* if persistent or unexplained bone pain (X-ray is also needed), pallor or fatigue, unexplained irritability, unexplained fever, persistent or recurrent URTI, generalized lymphadenopathy, and/or unexplained bruising.

*If neuroblastoma is suspected* Carry out an abdominal examination (and/or urgent USS), and consider CXR and FBC. If any mass is found, refer urgently.

*Specialist management* Treatment is with surgery, chemotherapy, and/or radiotherapy. Early stage disease has a 95% 5y survival; late stage disease has 20% 5y survival. Children with extra-abdominal tumours and those who are <1y at diagnosis have better prognosis.

**Wilm's nephroblastoma** 70 cases/y in England and Wales. Kidney tumour composed of primitive renal tissue; L>R; bilateral in 10%. Usually affects children <5y old (peak age 2–3y.). ♂>♀. Rarely, associated with Beckwith–Wiedemann syndrome, aniridia, or hemihypertrophy.

### Presentation
• *General effects* Fever, anorexia and weight ↓, anaemia.
• *Local effects of the tumour* Unilateral abdominal mass ± pain ± unexplained haematuria.
• *Effects of metastases* 20% have metastases to liver, lungs, or bone (rare) at presentation. May present with symptoms/signs of metastases.

**Management** If a child presents with abdominal distension, examine the abdomen. *Refer if*: intra-abdominal mass (immediate) or unexplained haematuria (urgent). Treatment is with surgery ± chemotherapy ± radiotherapy depending on histology and stage at diagnosis. Early stage tumours have 80% 5y survival, late stage have 50% 5y survival.

**Retinoblastoma** Rare tumour of the eye. 30 cases/y in England and Wales. Usually affects children <1y old—most are <5y old. May be familial (6%—dominant inheritance) when the tumour is usually bilateral. Usually detected by a white pupillary reflex seen at routine developmental screening. Alternatively, may present with squint or inflammation of the eye. Refer suspected cases to ophthalmology urgently.

*Specialist treatment* Treatment of unilateral tumours is surgical. Bilateral tumours are treated by enucleation or laser ablation of the worst affected eye, and radiotherapy to the other eye. 80% with unilateral tumours and 40% with bilateral tumours survive long term.

**Ongoing care** Once the diagnosis is made, most children embark on an intensive regime of treatment. They are referred to tertiary paediatric oncology units which share care with local hospitals, and have direct access to advice and admission via those units. Outreach nurses provide support in the community (e.g. administration of IV drugs via Hickman lines) with the aim of maintaining as normal a lifestyle as possible.

⚠ Immunosuppression can be a major problem. Any febrile episode in a neutropoenic child requires immediate referral to a specialist unit. Chickenpox can be particularly serious—seek specialist advice from the treating unit if the patient is in contact with any other child with chickenpox.

**The GP's role** Treatment for childhood cancer is increasingly successful with cure rates of >80% for some forms of cancer. The role of the GP is important even if it is peripheral. Keep in touch with the family and up to date with what is going on. Provide support to the child and other family members. Give advice on benefits or local services that might be useful. Ensure prescriptions are supplied promptly.

**Palliative care** Sadly, despite treatment, some children progress to the terminal stages of their cancer. General principles of palliative care apply (📖 pp.1026–1043), but the emotional traumas are often much greater. If possible engage specialist palliative care services early. Try to maintain continuity of care with as few professionals involved as possible. Provide ongoing support to family members after the child has died.

**Further information**
**NICE** Referral guidelines for suspected cancer (2005) 🖥 www.nice.org.uk

**Information and support for patients and their carers**
**Children with Leukaemia** ☎ 020 7404 0808 🖥 www.leukaemia.org.uk
**CLIC and Sargent** ☎ 0800 197 0068 🖥 www.clicsargent.org.uk
**Neuroblastoma Society** ☎ 020 8940 4353 🖥 www.nsoc.co.uk
**Childhood Eye Cancer Trust (CHECT)** ☎ 020 7377 5578
🖥 www.chect.org.uk
**Children's Hospices UK** 🖥 www.childhospice.org.uk

# Behaviour problems

GPs are commonly asked to 'sort out' behaviour problems of children by parents at their wits' end. 2–10% of all children are said to have behaviour problems, depending on how problems are defined and measured.

Differentiation between normal behaviour and behavioural problems can be difficult, especially if you don't know the child or family well. A significant problem is more likely:
- when the behaviour is frequent and chronic
- when >1 problem behaviour occurs, *and*
- if behaviour interferes with social and cognitive functioning.

There is no right or wrong way to deal with these problems, and the approach outlined in Figure 24.4 is just one way to tackle them.

**Managing the problem** For simple problems, parental education, reassurance, and a few specific suggestions tailored to the problem are often sufficient. Follow-up is important to ensure that the problem is resolving. If simple measures are not succeeding within 3–4mo, consider referral to other agencies, e.g. health visitor, school nurse, child psychiatrist, etc. Specific behavioural techniques include:

**Behaviour modification** Behaviour modification is a learning process requiring caregivers to set consistent rules and limits. Parents should try to minimize anger when enforcing rules and ↑ +ve contact with the child.

**Discipline** Ineffective discipline may result in inappropriate behaviour. Scolding or physical punishment may briefly control a child's behaviour if used sparingly, but may ↓ the child's sense of security and self-esteem. Threats to leave or send the child away are damaging. *Options:*
- *+ve reinforcement for appropriate behaviour* This is a powerful tool for controlling a child's behaviour with no adverse effects.
- *Time-out procedure* The child must sit alone in a dull place for a brief period. Time-outs are a learning process for the child and are best used for controlling a single inappropriate behaviour or a few at one time.

**Breaking vicious circle patterns** The child's behaviour (be it normal or abnormal for that developmental stage) evokes a response in the parent or carer which provokes the child to behave in that manner further, thus generating another response from the parent. Try to identify vicious circle patterns and suggest alternative parental responses which make the behaviour futile.

**Sleep problems** 📖 p.910          **Toilet training** 📖 p.912

## Parent information and support

**Green C** *Toddler Taming: A Parents' Guide to the First Four Years* (2000) Vermilion, London. ISBN: 0091875285.
**Green C** *Beyond Toddlerdom: Every Parent's Guide to the 5–10s* (2000) Vermilion, London. ISBN: 0091816246.
**Parentline** ☎ 0808 800 2222 🖥 www.parentlineplus.org.uk

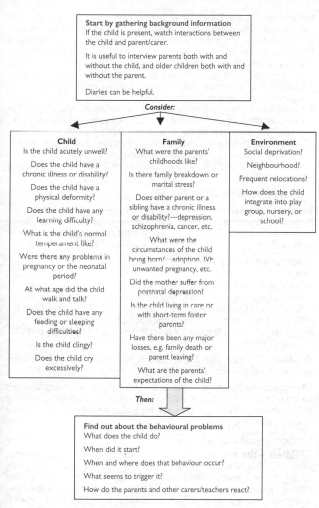

Start by gathering background information
If the child is present, watch interactions between the child and parent/carer.

It is useful to interview parents both with and without the child, and older children both with and without the parent.

Diaries can be helpful.

*Consider:*

**Child**
Is the child acutely unwell?

Does the child have a chronic illness or disability?

Does the child have a physical deformity?

Does the child have any learning difficulty?

What is the child's normal temperament like?

Were there any problems in pregnancy or the neonatal period?

At what age did the child walk and talk?

Does the child have any feeding or sleeping difficulties?

Is the child clingy?

Does the child cry excessively?

**Family**
What were the parents' childhoods like?

Is there family breakdown or marital stress?

Does either parent or a sibling have a chronic illness or disability?—depression, schizophrenia, cancer, etc.

What were the circumstances of the child being born?—adoption, IVF, unwanted pregnancy, etc.

Did the mother suffer from postnatal depression?

Is the child living in care or with short-term foster parents?

Have there been any major losses, e.g. family death or parent leaving?

What are the parents' expectations of the child?

**Environment**
Social deprivation?

Neighbourhood?

Frequent relocations?

How does the child integrate into play group, nursery, or school?

*Then:*

Find out about the behavioural problems
What does the child do?

When did it start?

When and where does that behaviour occur?

What seems to trigger it?

How do the parents and other carers/teachers react?

**Fig. 24.4** Assessment of childhood behaviour problems

## Information and support for children
**Childline** 24h confidential counselling service ☎ 0800 1111
🖥 www.childline.org.uk

**Excessive crying** Babies vary considerably in the amount they cry and the ease with which they are soothed. Likewise, parents vary in their ability to tolerate a crying baby. Babies cry for many reasons—discomfort, hunger, loneliness, separation, boredom, etc. If a baby is crying excessively:

- Take a history from the parent. When does the baby cry? Can he/she be consoled? What do the parents do when the baby cries?
- Examine fully from head to toe to exclude causes of discomfort, e.g. nappy rash, otitis media, eczema, etc.
- Check that the baby is growing along his or her centile line.
- Consider family stress (including postnatal depression—🕮 p.837) as a reason why the parent cannot tolerate the crying.
- Treat any underlying cause found and support the family. Information about behavioural techniques used to manage babies that cry excessively is available from Cry-sis ☎ 08451 228 669 🖳 www.cry-sis.org.uk

**Feeding problems** 🕮 p.870

**Rhythmic behaviour** Head rocking or banging, thumb-sucking, self-stimulation, baby behaviour, and many other variants all occur during normal development. They usually appear if the child is tired, uncertain, or anxious. Reassure parents. Most resolve spontaneously.

**Fears and phobias**
*Fears*
- Fears of the dark, monsters, and spiders are common in 3–4y-olds.
- Fears of injury and death are more common in older children.
- Statements made by the parents in anger or jest may be taken literally by preschool children and can be disturbing.
- Frightening stories, films, or TV programmes may be upsetting and intensify fears.

*Phobias* cause persistent and unrealistic, yet intense, anxiety in reaction to external situations or stimuli.

*Management* Normal developmental-stage-related fears must be differentiated from true phobias. If the phobia is intense and interferes with the child's activity, or if the child does not respond to simple reassurance, refer to child psychiatry.

**School refusal and truancy**
*Children <10y* Younger children may refuse to go to school or recurrently complain of abdominal pain, nausea, or other symptoms that justify staying home. Usually school refusal is a form of separation anxiety, although occasionally it is due to a problem at school, e.g. problems interacting with the teacher or friends, or bullying. Advise parents to consult the school—a star chart with a star from the teacher for each morning the child goes to school without a fuss may help. Relapses can occur if the child is absent or after holidays.

*Older children* School refusal is a more difficult problem. Speak to parents and child together and separately. Try to ascertain if there is a genuine reason why the child avoids school. Liaise with the school. If not succeeding, refer to child psychiatry.

**Conduct disorders** Poor behaviour, e.g. aggression, destructive tendencies, and antisocial behaviour, is a common complaint. Tolerance varies from family to family. Try simple strategies such as rewarding good behaviour and ignoring poor behaviour ± time-out strategies (younger children—📖 p.906). If not succeeding, refer to child psychiatry.

**Childhood depression** 📖 p.919

**Hyperactivity** 📖 p.914

**Tics** Sudden repetitive coordinated movements of no apparent purpose. Commonly involve facial grimacing, head movements, or shoulder movements. Average age of onset ~2y. Tics are present at some point in ~4% of children. Often a family history is present. The majority are precipitated by stress and disappear spontaneously, although some persist into adulthood.

**_Gilles de la Tourette syndrome_** ♂:♀ ≈ 3:1. Characterized by multiple motor tics and irrepressible verbal outbursts—sometimes obscene. There may also be repetitive blinking, nodding, gesturing, echoing of speech, and/or stuttering. Usually begins in childhood. Associated with obsessive–compulsive disorder and ADHD. Probable genetic aetiology.

_Management_ Spontaneous remissions do occur. Haloperidol or clonidine may help those severely affected with tics. Treat any associated obsessive–compulsive disorder (📖 p 994) or ADHD (📖 p 915)
_G. Gilles de la Tourette (1857–1904), French neurologist._

### Parent information and support

**Parentline** ☎ 0808 800 2222 📖 www.parentlineplus.org.uk
**Cry-sis** Support for families with crying and sleepless babies ☎ 08451 228 669
📖 www.cry-sis.org.uk

### Patient information and support

**Childline** 24h confidential counselling service ☎ 0800 1111
📖 www.childline.org.uk

# Sleep problems

Sleeping patterns and habits of children vary considerably and should only be regarded as problems when they are presented as such by the family. First take a careful history. Ask about:

- **Medical problems**, e.g. night cough related to asthma, itching from eczema, obstructive sleep apnoea. Treat appropriately.
- **Physical problems**, e.g. hunger or cold.
- **Night terrors**.
- **Sleep pattern**—usually ≥1 of:
  - difficulty settling
  - waking during the night
  - waking early in the morning
- **Amount of daytime sleep**.

**General advice** In all cases it is helpful to recommend a regular calming bedtime routine (e.g. bath, story, cuddle, bed) and minimal fuss when a child does wake at night, e.g. try to settle back to sleep without taking out of cot, not rewarding waking with games, snacks, etc.

**Resistance to going to bed** The baby/child who cries incessantly when put to bed is a common problem, with a peak age of 1–2y. The child cries when left alone or climbs out of bed and seeks the parents. Causes include:

- Separation anxiety.
- Increasing attempts by the child to control his/her environment.
- Long naps late in the afternoon.
- Rough overstimulating play before bedtime.
- A disturbed parent–child relationship and/or tension in the home.

**Management** Letting the child stay up, staying in the room, and comforting or punishing the child are all ineffective. Options include:

- **Leaving the child to cry** This often works and the crying diminishes after a few nights, but it is very hard for parents to do and can be impossible if they are in shared accommodation.
- **Controlled crying** The child is left to cry for a set length of time (e.g. 2–10min) before the parent returns to settle him/her again with minimum fuss and then leaves. Length of time before returning is gradually ↑. Easier for parents than leaving the child to cry and still effective.
- **Staying with the child until he/she sleeps but gradually withdrawing proximity**, e.g. sit on bed with child, after a few nights sit next to bed, then nearer door, etc. until the child learns to go to sleep alone. This method is gentler than those described above but may take longer.

**Waking during the night** Occurs in half of all children aged 6–12mo and is related to separation anxiety. In older children, episodes often follow a stressful event (e.g. moving home, illness).

**Management** Allowing the child to sleep with the parents, playing, feeding, or punishing the child usually prolong the problem.

- Try the methods used for resistance to going to bed, but advise parents always to check to see that the child is not ill/needing a clean nappy etc. before being left to cry.

- Scheduled waking where a child is woken 15–60min before the time he/she usually wakes and then resettled has also been shown to improve night waking.
- If a child wakes early, another strategy is to make toys or books accessible. The child may then amuse him/herself for a period of time without disturbing his/her parents. Some 2–3y-olds wander around without waking the parents—fitting a stairgate across the child's bedroom door prevents the child coming to any harm doing this.
- Use of sedatives, e.g. promethazine (for children >2y), is often discouraged but can be useful, particularly when parents feel desperate. Only use as a short-term measure.

**Nightmares** Occur during rapid eye movement (REM) sleep. Nightmares can be caused by frightening experiences (e.g. scary stories, television violence), particularly in 3–4y-olds. The child usually becomes fully awake and can vividly recall the details of the nightmare. An occasional nightmare is normal, but persistent or frequent nightmares warrant evaluation by an expert.

**Sleepwalking (somnambulism)** Involves walking clumsily, usually avoiding objects. The child appears confused but not frightened. 15% of children age 5–12y have sleepwalked one or more times. It is most common amongst school-age boys and may be triggered by a stressful event.
- Advise parents/carers not to try to wake the child.
- If the child is in danger, gently steer him/her away from any harm
- If the child sleepwalks frequently, consider taking action to prevent him/her coming to any harm whilst sleepwalking, e.g. stair gate across bedroom door.
- If the sleepwalks occur repeatedly at the same time, waking the child ~15min before the predicted time can break the cycle.

**Night terror** Sudden awakening with inconsolable panic and screaming. Usually occurs in the first 1–3h of sleep. Episodes last seconds → minutes. *Features:*
- Blank or confused stares.
- Incomplete arousal with poor responsiveness to people.
- Amnesia for the episode.

Night terrors are most common in children aged 3–8y and require no treatment apart from simple reassurance. Advise parents not to wake the child as this ↑ the disturbance. If frequent, consider waking the child before episodes occur and keeping the child awake for a few minutes to break the cycle. If the terrors persist beyond 8y, consider a diagnosis of temporal lobe epilepsy.

**Parent information and support**
**Parentline** ☎ 0808 800 2222 ▯ www.parentlineplus.org.uk
**Cry-sis** Support for families with crying and sleepless babies
☎ 08451 228 669 ▯ www.cry-sis.org.uk

# Toilet training

Most children can do without nappies by day from 2–3y and by night from 2–5y. How to approach toilet training will vary from child to child.

## General rules

- *Wait until the child is ready* This usually means that the child can indicate to the parent that he is going to the toilet and has shown an interest in using the potty or toilet. It is helpful to have a potty or child's toilet seat to put on the normal toilet for the child to become familiar with before starting toilet training.
- *Pick a good time* when the child can have a few days at home without nappies in an environment where accidents do not matter. Make sure that the child has plenty of spare clothes available.
- *Keep the potty handy or stay within easy reach of the toilet* When the child says he wishes to go, sit him immediately on the toilet. Reward any result with praise. Do not punish the child for any accidents— advise the parent to ask the child to help clear up any mess and reinforce that it would be better to use the potty/toilet next time.
- *Until the child (and parent) are confident in the child's ability to use the toilet continue using nappies when out and at night* Take the child to the toilet at night before bedtime. When dry nappies are consistently noted in the mornings, try the child without nappies at night—a plastic sheet on the mattress is a good idea. Even when a child has been dry day and night for some time, accidents are common if the child is tired, unwell, or unsettled (whether excited or unhappy).

**❶** If the child does not succeed within a few days, either try training pants or revert to nappies and try again at a later date.

**Nocturnal enuresis** Affects 30% of children aged 4y, 10% at 6y, 3% at 12y, and 1% at 18y. ♂>♀. Tends to run in families.

## Causes

- Enuresis usually represents delay in maturation that resolves with time.
- 1–2% have an underlying physical abnormality—usually UTI. Rare causes (congenital anomalies, sacral nerve disorders, DM, diabetes insipidus, pelvic mass) can be excluded by history, examination, urinalysis for glucose, protein and M,C&S.
- Enuresis is occasionally caused by emotional distress. The child may have been dry and then start wetting the bed at night again. If suspected, ask gently about any problems the child is having and manage those problems before treating the enuresis *per se*.

## Management

- *<6y*—no need for treatment. Most will resolve spontaneously.
- *≥6y*—refer to the school nurse (or paediatric enuresis clinic) who can provide equipment and training to control bedwetting. Techniques used—Table 24.12.

**Table 24.12** Methods of enuresis control

| Method | Features |
|---|---|
| Motivational counselling | The child avoids drinks for 1h (but caffeine for longer) before bed, urinates before going to bed, records wet and dry nights, and changes clothing and bedding when wet. |
| | Rewards (e.g. star chart) are given for dry nights. |
| | The child is reassured throughout that the problem is not his/her fault and just a developmental problem likely to resolve in time. |
| Enuresis alarms | An alarm is triggered when the child starts to pass urine. |
| | In the first few weeks, the child wakes after complete emptying of the bladder; in the next few weeks partial inhibition usually occurs; eventually the child wakes up in response to bladder contractions before he wets the bed. |
| | The alarm should be used for at least 3wk after the last bedwetting episode. |
| | ~70% effective. Relapse occurs in 10–15%. |
| Desmopressin | Synthetic version of antidiuretic hormone. |
| | Taken at night as a tablet |
| | Adverse effects include headache, nausea, nasal congestion, nosebleed, sore throat, cough, flushing, and mild abdominal cramps. |
| | ❶ There is a risk of water overload—advise drinking only one mug of fluid from 1h before desmopressin dose to 8h afterwards. |
| | Effective in the short term (4–6wk), e.g. to cover holidays. |

**Encopresis** Most children are continent of faeces by 2½–3y. Faecal soiling after this age usually occurs during the day.
• If the child has bowel control but passes stool in unacceptable places, the cause is usually emotional. Expert help from child psychiatry is needed—refer.
• If a firm stool is passed occasionally in the toilet but usually in the pants, developmental delay (either mental or social) is likely. Try a firm consistent training programme similar to motivational counselling for enuresis (Table 24.12).
• If soft stool oozes out causing the child to constantly soil himself and smell of faeces, consider overflow incontinence secondary to chronic constipation. Treat underlying constipation. Refer to paediatrics if not settling.

**Information for parents of children with enuresis**
**ERIC** (Enuresis Resource and Information) ☎ 0845 370 8008
🖥 www.eric.org.uk

# Poor progress at school

~20% of school-age children require special educational services at some point in their schooling. ♂: ♀ ≈ 5:1. Consider:

- Does the child have a physical illness affecting his/her schoolwork, e.g asthma, eczema?
- Is the child on any drugs that might affect his/her academic performance (e.g. anticonvulsants)?
- Is the family stable or is there family upset?
- Does another member of the family have a chronic/life-threatening illness?
- Is the child's home environment conducive to doing his/her schoolwork?
- Is this school refusal?
- Is the child happy at school?
- Is there a problem with vision or hearing?
- Is the child of normal intelligence?
- Does the child interact socially with adults and other children?
- Have developmental milestones been met?
- Does the child have specific difficulty with certain aspects of his/her schoolwork, e.g. mathematics, reading, writing?

## Specific learning disorders

### *Speech and language delay* 📖 p.855

***Dyslexia*** Affects 3–5% of the population. ♂ > ♀. There is considerable overlap with other specific learning difficulties such as dyscalculia and dyspraxia. IQ is often normal or high, and the child appears bright and alert. There may be a FH. If suspected, liaise with the child's school via the teacher. Formal testing by an educational psychologist can confirm the diagnosis.

***Dyscalculia*** Rarer than dyslexia but has many of the same features. The core problem is a difficulty in handling numbers and mathematical concepts. Management is the same as for dyslexia.

***Dyspraxia*** Affects 2% of the population in varying degrees—70% are male. IQ is often normal or high. As with dyslexia, children have varying features. Management is as for dyslexia. Common features are:

- Clumsiness
- Poor posture
- Awkward gait
- Reading and writing difficulties
- Difficulty holding a pen or pencil properly
- Poor short-term memory.
- Poor body awareness
- Confusion about which hand to use
- Difficulties throwing/catching balls
- Poor sense of direction
- Difficulty hopping, skipping, and/or riding a bike
- Slow to learn to dress and feed.

### *Severe learning difficulty* 📖 p.916

### *Autistic spectrum disorder* 📖 p.916

***Hyperactivity*** Not easily defined because claims that a child is hyperactive often reflect the tolerance level of the person complaining. More active children with shorter than average attention spans create management problems. Hyperactivity may have an underlying cause (e.g. an emotional disorder, CNS dysfunction, a genetic component) or may be an exaggeration of normal temperament. Often it is stage-related—support until that stage has passed. Simple behaviour management techniques (🕮 p.906) may also help.

## Attention deficit hyperactivity disorder (ADHD)

- Common neurodevelopmental disorder which interferes with normal social functioning, learning, and development.
- Aetiology is probably multifactorial with overstimulation, family environment, and genetic factors all contributing.
- Affects up to 9% of the school age population in the UK; ♂:♀ ≈ 6:1.
- Other emotional, behavioural and learning problems may co-exist.
- Long term ADHD is associated with low academic achievement, substance misuse, unemployment, and antisocial tendencies.

*Presentation* ❶ Many of these behaviours are seen in normal children.
- *Inattention* Poor attention to detail and organization of tasks; appears not to listen; easily distracted; forgetful; lack of concentration on tasks.
- *Impulsivity* Lack of social awareness; shouts out answers to questions; difficulty waiting (unable to take turns or wait in a queue); excessive talking—interrupts others; lack of social awareness.
- *Hyperactivity* Fidgets; inappropriate running, climbing or leaving seat.

Assess how long the problem has been going on, how much it impairs functioning, and whether it occurs in different settings/areas of functioning—a report from school as well as the parents can be useful. ❶ A diagnosis of ADHD should only be made by a specialist.

## *Differential diagnosis*

- Learning disability
- Hearing problems
- Epilepsy
- Autistic disorder
- Thyroid disease
- Drug ingestion
- Psychological problems (depression, emotional trauma, e.g. divorce)

## *Management*

- *Mild/moderate impairment*—watchful waiting to see if problems persist, or refer for parent training/education.
- *Persistent problems/severe impairment*—refer to community paediatrics or child psychiatry for formal diagnosis. Specialist treatment includes behavioural therapy, and drug therapy (e.g. ritalin).
- *In all cases* self-help and local support groups can be helpful.

## Further information

**NICE** Attention deficit hyperactivity disorder (2008) 🖳 www.nice.org.uk

## Information and support for parents and children

**British Dyslexia Association** ☎ 0845 251 9002 🖳 www.bdadyslexia.org.uk
**Dyspraxia Foundation** ☎ 01462 454 986
🖳 www.dyspraxiafoundation.org.uk
**National Attention Deficit Disorder Information and Support Service (ADDISS)** ☎ 020 8952 2800 🖳 www.addiss.co.uk
**Independent Panel for Special Education Advice (IPSEA)**
☎ 0800 018 4016 🖳 www.ipsea.org.uk

# Autism and severe learning difficulty

**Autism** A rare developmental disorder of unknown cause affecting 2:10 000 children, although autistic spectrum disorders are much more common (9:1000). ♂:♀ ≈ 4:1. Autism is a severely disabling condition for both child and family which requires a great deal of support from community services including the GP.

**Diagnosis** Not apparent at birth. Usually detected from 18mo–3y when failure of social interaction and lack of speech becomes apparent. GPs play a vital role in detection and diagnosis.

**Screening** Consider using a screening tool such as the Checklist for Autism in Toddlers (CHAT) for all toddlers with problems with social interaction or speech and language delay at the 18mo check (available from ⌨ www.nas.org.uk).

**Features of autism** Triad of:
• impaired reciprocal social interaction (A symptoms)
• impaired imagination associated with abnormal verbal and non-verbal communication (B symptoms)
• restricted repertoires of activities and interests (C symptoms).

**Management** There is no proven treatment. Behaviour therapy is sometimes tried. Be an advocate for the family if they have any problems. Be approachable and willing to listen. Having a child or living with an adult with autism is very hard. Advise families:
• To set unwavering rules for behaviour.
• To reward and give more attention to good behaviour.
• To contact self-help and support organizations.
• To ensure they receive all benefits payable (e.g. Carer's Allowance, Disability Living Allowance).

**Prognosis** 70% remain severely handicapped—special schooling is often needed; 50% develop useful speech; 20% develop fits in adolescence; 15% lead an independent life.

**Asperger's syndrome (autistic psychopathy)** A variety of autism in which a child, from the age of ~2y, shows obsessive preoccupation with routines and stereotyped behaviour with distress if the environment is altered. Social isolation and linguistic difficulties are absent. Better prognosis than autism. *H. Asperger (1906–1980), Austrian paediatrician.*

**Severe learning difficulty (mental handicap)** Arrested or incomplete development of the mind characterized by subnormality of intelligence. May exist alone or with other disabilities. Often noted by a parent first—take any concerns seriously.

**Causes** Varied—many are rare. Divide into:
• *Congenital*
  • Genetic, e.g. Down's syndrome, Fragile X.
  • Metabolic, e.g. congenital hypothyroidism.
  • Others, e.g. prenatal rubella.
• *Acquired*, e.g. trauma, meningitis, birth injury.

***Management*** Refer to paediatrics/genetics to ensure no treatable cause is missed. *Then:*

* ***Communicate with carers*** Explain referrals, test results and their implications, the local system, and who is responsible for what. Find out about the condition (as far as possible) and tell the carers where to get more information. Ensure carers receive information about benefits and housing/schooling options available.
* ***Refer to other community services***, e.g. paediatrician, district severe learning disability service. Ensure follow-up happens and assist with assessment of special needs for schooling, housing, and employment purposes. Continue prescription of medication started by other team members.
* ***Manage medical problems not related to disability***, e.g. sore throats.
* ***Promote concordance*** with long-term therapy ± education or rehabilitation programmes.
* ***Offer family planning, preconceptual counselling, and/or antenatal diagnosis*** for parents of children with severe learning disability and patients with severe learning disability reaching reproductive age.

### Prognosis

* *IQ 50–70*—80% of people with learning disability. Most lead an independent life and require just special attention to their schooling.
* *IQ 35–49*—special schooling, or extra support within mainstream schooling, and supervision may be needed.
* *IQ <35*—severe learning difficulty. Limited social activity and speech may be impaired. Special schooling and medical services are needed. Support and counselling for families involved is important.

**The chronically disabled child** 📖 p.920

**Information and support for parents and children**
**National Autistic Society of the UK (NAS)** ☎ 0845 070 4004
🖳 www.nas.org.uk
**MENCAP** ☎ 0808 808 1111 🖳 www.mencap.org.uk
**Independent Panel for Special Education Advice (IPSEA)**
☎ 0800 018 4016 🖳 www.ipsea.org.uk

# Adolescence

Changes of adolescence start gradually—from ~10y for girls and ~12y for boys—and are complete by the age of ~17y. Adolescence is characterized by rapid physical development and emotional change. Adjusting to these changes causes problems.

- *Concerns about appearance* Some become very concerned about their appearance. They need reassurance, especially if not growing or maturing as quickly as their friends.
- *Clothes/style* are important to express solidarity with friends and declare independence.
- *Hormonal changes* result in changes in body shape, voice, hair, and skin, body hair growth and menstruation. All can all be hard to adjust to.
- *Acne* may need treatment, especially if scarring.
- *Dieting and consumption of junk food* are common. Rarely, eating disorders develop.

**Consent** 📖 p.52          **Confidentiality** 📖 p.50

**School problems**
- *School refusal* 📖 p.908.
- *Truancy* Usually children who are unhappy at home and frustrated at school. They spend their days with others who feel the same.
- *Poor schoolwork* Emotional problems, e.g. worry about problems at home, often affect schoolwork and make it difficult to concentrate; pressure to do well/pass exams may be counter-productive. Exams are important, but advise parents not to let them dominate life or cause unhappiness.

**Abuse** 📖 p.922.

**Behaviour problems** It is normal for teenagers and their parents to complain about each other's behaviour and to disagree frequently. Parents often feel they have lost control over their child. Adolescents resent parental restrictions on their freedom, but still want parental guidance. Advise parents to lay down sensible ground rules and stick to them. Evidence suggests children are at greater risk of getting into trouble if their parents do not know where they are—advise teenagers to let their parents know where they are going and parents to ask.

**Sexual problems and contraception** 📖 p.768

**Trouble with the law** ♂ > ♀. Most young people do not break the law—when they do, it usually only happens once. Repeated offending may reflect family culture or may result from unhappiness—always ask about emotional feelings when an adolescent is repeatedly getting into trouble.

**Drugs, solvents, and alcohol** Most teenagers never use drugs or inhale solvents, and of those that do, most never get beyond the experimenting stage. Alcohol is the most common drug causing problems for adolescents, but consider the possibility of any form of drug use (📖 p.190) when parents notice sudden serious changes in behaviour.

**Emotional problems** Teenage unhappiness is common (~ ½ 14y-olds feel miserable; ¼ are self-depreciatory; 8% have suicidal thoughts) and does not necessarily indicate depression. However, emotional disorders are often not recognized, even by family and friends. Over-eating, excessive sleepiness, promiscuity, and a persistent over-concern with appearance may be signs of emotional distress. More obviously, phobias and panic attacks appear.

Rarely, changes in behaviour and mood can mark the beginning of more serious psychiatric disorders. Manic depression and schizophrenia, as well as more common disorders such as anxiety, may emerge during adolescent years. Refer for psychiatric assessment if concerned.

*Distinguishing normal adolescent behaviour from mental illness* Teenage behavioural problems may be signs of mental illness if:
• They go on for more than a few weeks.
• They do not vary, e.g. persistently low mood in all circumstances.
• They are severe, e.g. self-harming behaviour, violence.
• There is a significant impact on relationships, school performance, and/or usual activities.

**Childhood depression** Response to childhood stress. Distinguish from depressive symptoms occurring as part of other emotional or conduct disorders. Most common in adolescence ($♀ > ♂$).

*Diagnosis* Difficult, especially among adolescents. Adolescents often do not communicate well with their parents and have little contact with health professionals, resulting in late diagnosis.

*Presenting features*
• Unhappiness and/or tearfulness, apathy, boredom, ↓ ability to enjoy life.
• Antisocial behaviour—$♂>♀$ especially after bereavement.
• ↓ school performance—may admit to poor concentration.
• Separation anxiety reappearing in adolescence.
• Frequent unexplained illness or undue worries about health.
• Self-harm.
• Bipolar depressive disorder is not seen before puberty.

*Management* Unless a mild episode, related to a single precipitating event and no other risk factors for depression, refer for specialist advice. Specialist treatment includes counselling, family therapy, CBT, and drug therapy. ❶ With the exception of fluoxetine, risks of treatment with SSRIs outweigh benefits in children.

**Disorders of puberty** 📖 p.891

**Eating disorders** 📖 p.1012

**Further information**
**NICE** Depression in children and young people (2005) 🖥 www.nice.org.uk

**Information and support for parents and children**
**Parentline** ☎ 0808 800 2222 🖥 www.parentlineplus.org.uk
**Childline** ☎ 0800 1111 🖥 www.childline.org.uk
**Brook Advisory Service** ☎ 0808 802 1234 🖥 www.brook.org.uk
**Sexwise** For under 19s ☎ 0800 28 29 30

# The chronically disabled child

Chronic disability due to a wide variety of causes affects ~10% of children in the UK.

**Effects on the child** Vary from child to child dependent on the nature of the disability, the personality of the child, and the support the child has at home and in the community. Common problems include:

- Physical discomfort—both due to the disability and to painful or embarrassing treatments.
- Alterations in the normal pattern of growth and development and/or physical differences may lead to social isolation and ↓ motivation.
- Frequent hospitalizations and outpatient visits prevent the child integrating into school or ongoing community activities.
- Dependence—the disability may prevent the child reaching his/her own goals and achieving his/her own independence. Many children also realize the additional burden they cause their parents and carers.

**Effects on the family** Vary from family to family depending on financial and/or social support, relationship between parents and other siblings, and many other factors. Stress may cause family break-up, especially when other marital and intra-family problems exist. Common problems:

- Grieving for the loss of the 'ideal child'—conditions that affect the appearance of the child particularly affect attachment between parents and child. The grief might take the form of shock, denial, anger, sadness, depression, guilt, or anxiety, and may occur at any time in the child's development.
- Neglected siblings.
- Inconsistent discipline due to demands placed on the family and sympathy for the child, resulting in behaviour problems.
- Marginalization of one parent—one parent tends to take on the bulk of the caring activities. There is a danger that the other parent will start to feel inadequate and isolated with respect to the care of the child.
- Major expense and time commitment—frequently one parent has to give up work to look after a disabled child, resulting not only in loss of income, but loss of that parent's independence and opportunities for the future.
- Social isolation.
- Confusion over the healthcare, benefits, and social services available.

**Care coordination** Inconsistent policies and funding, inadequate access to facilities (including physical barriers to access), and poor communication and coordination between the healthcare, educational, and community support systems → misery for children with disability and their families. Without coordination of services, care is crisis oriented.

Care coordination requires knowledge about the child's condition, the family, and the community in which they function. In all cases *someone* should be designated responsible for coordinating care—the best person to do that will vary according to circumstances. Regardless of who assists in coordination of services, the family and child must be partners in the process.

**Rehabilitation** The general principles of rehabilitation for adult patients also apply to children—📖 pp.206 and 590.

## Role of the GP

- The GP of any patient with a chronic illness in the community is a team member and may be the key worker who coordinates care.
- The GP provides continuity of care, particularly when the child is under the care of several different secondary care teams, or during the transition from child to adolescent or adult services.
- Maintain an open-door policy and encourage children and carers to seek help for problems early.
- Try to become familiar with a child's disease, even if it is rare. It is impossible to plan care without knowledge of course and prognosis, and an easy way to lose a child's confidence is to appear ignorant of their condition.
- If progress is slower than expected, or stalls, consider other medical problems (e.g. anaemia, infection), behavioural problems, and communication problems (e.g. poor vision/hearing).
- Information alone can improve outcome.

### Information for parents and children

**Benefits information** 🖳 www.direct.gov.uk

**Contact a Family** Support and information for families with disabled children (any disability) ☎ 0808 808 3555 🖳 www.cafamily.org.uk

**Whizz-Kidz** Mobility for non-mobile disabled children ☎ 020 7233 6600 🖳 www.whizz-kidz.org.uk

**Tourism for all** Holidays for families with a disabled child ☎ 0845 124 9971 🖳 www.tourismforall.org.uk

# Safeguarding children

**Refugee children** Many child refugees have traumatic backgrounds. Approach children with sensitivity and consider involving specialist child psychiatric and specialist refugee support services early.

## Circumcision of female children or forced marriage <16y

Both are illegal in the UK. Children may be taken abroad to be circumcised/married. If you suspect that this might be going to happen to any patient, inform social services and/or the police immediately.

**Child abuse** ~3:100 children are abused each year in the UK; there were 4109 reported offences of cruelty or neglect of children in England and Wales in 2002–2003 and every year ~30 000 children's names are added to the Child Protection Register in England alone. Child abuse is defined as depriving children of their human rights—being healthy, staying safe, enjoying and achieving, making a positive contribution, and economic well-being. Classification—Table 24.13.

*Presentation* Always have a high index of suspicion. Suspect abuse if:
- The child discloses it.
- The story is inconsistent with injuries found.
- There is late presentation after an injury or lack of concern about the injury by the parent(s).
- Presentation to an unknown doctor.
- Accompanying adult is not the parent or guardian.
- Sibling has been a victim of abuse.
- Reluctance to allow the child to be examined.
- Characteristic injuries—look for marks consistent with cigarette burns, scalds (especially if symmetrical or doughnut-shaped on buttocks), finger-mark or bite-mark bruises, perineal bruising or anogenital injury, linear marks consistent with whipping, buckle or belt marks.
- Multiple injuries or old injuries coexistent with new.
- Unlikely sites for injuries e.g. mouth, ears, genitalia, eyes.
- Behaviour of the child is suggestive, e.g. withdrawn, 'frozen watchfulness', sexually precocious behaviour, abnormal interaction between child and parents, unwilling to speak about the injury, etc.
- Vaginal discharge, STI, or recurrent UTI in any child <14y.
- Failure to thrive, developmental delay, and/or behavioural problems.

**Table 24.13** Classification of child abuse: >1 type may occur concurrently

| PHYSICAL (7% of children) | EMOTIONAL (6% of children) |
|---|---|
| Hitting, shaking, throwing, burning, suffocating, poisoning, including factitious or induced illness | The child is made to feel worthless, afraid, unloved, or inadequate (e.g. if developmentally inappropriate expectations are imposed) |
| NEGLECT (6% of children) | SEXUAL (4% of children) |
| Failure to meet the child's basic needs, allowing the child to be exposed to danger | Forcing/enticing a child to participate in sexual activities—physical contact or production of pornographic material |

### Risk factors for child abuse

| Parent/carer factors | Child factors |
|---|---|

*Parent/carer factors*
- Mental illness/learning disability
- Substance/alcohol abuse
- Being abused themselves
- Ongoing physical illness
- Unemployment/ poor living conditions.

*Child factors*
- History of sibling abuse
- Learning/behaviour/physical problems
- Unplanned pregnancy/premature birth
- Poor attachment to parents/carers
- Environment high in criticism
- 'Looked after' children.

⚠ **Immediate action** Welfare of the child is *paramount*.—not to report abuse is to collude with the abuser. Do *not* perform a forensic examination unless trained to do so and do *not* ask leading questions.
- Wherever possible, arrange for another health professional to be present during the consultation.
- Take a history from any accompanying adult. If possible also take a history from the child alone
- Examine the child. Ask for an explanation for any injuries noted.
- Keep thorough notes, recording dates and times, history given, injuries noted, and any explanation of those injuries.

**Further action** Depends on the nature of the suspected abuse, suspected abuser (e.g. if someone outside the home is suspected, the child is safe to return home), nature of the injuries, and response of the parents. Follow local guidelines. *Options are*:
- Direct referral to the police—particularly if you feel emergency action may be required to protect the child.
- Hospital admission—protects the child and allows full assessment.
- Contact social services to arrange a Place of Safety Order.
- Liaison with social services child protection team (on-call 24h/d)—follow-up telephone referrals in writing in <24h.

⚠ This guidance appears simple—and is when abuse is overt—but often it is *difficult* to decide if a child is being abused. If you have worries but cannot justify them sufficiently to invoke child protection procedures:
- Check via social services whether the child is on the 'at-risk' register.
- Check notes of siblings and other family members to see if there has been any suggestion of abuse in the family before.
- Discuss your worries with the health visitor and/or other members of the primary health care team or local child protection lead.

If any of these sources ↑ your suspicion, you may be justified in invoking child protection. If you are still unsure, record your worries and reasons for them in the child's notes and alert other involved members of the practice team. Review whenever that child is seen in the practice.

**Responding to child protection enquiries** Under Section 47 of the Children Act (1989), GPs have a legal obligation to share relevant information whether or not they have the consent of the parents.

### Further information

**DH** What to do if you're worried a child is being abused (2006) ▣ www.dh.gov.uk
**NICE** When to suspect child maltreatment (2009) ▣ www.nice.org.uk

# Child death

**Sudden infant death syndrome (cot death)** ~1:1500 babies/y are unexpectedly found dead in the first year of life in the UK. These deaths are most common in winter months and at night (midnight–9a.m.). An identifiable cause for the death can be found for 1:10 deaths—the rest remain unexplained (cot deaths). Theories include cardiac arrhythmia and apnoeic attacks. *Peak age:* 1–4mo. ♂>♀.

### Risk factors for cot death
- Baby sleeping face down
- Smoking (mother and other family members)
- Overheating
- Minor intercurrent illness
- Twin or multiple pregnancy
- Low birth weight
- Social disadvantage
- Young mother
- Large numbers of siblings.

### Reducing the risk of cot death 📖 p.845

### Management

*If you are the first person contacted*
- Check that an ambulance is on its way and go immediately to the scene. Start resuscitation, unless clearly inappropriate. Continue until the baby gets to hospital.
- If it is clear that the baby is dead and can not be resuscitated, inform the parents sympathetically. Contact the police/coroner and the designated paediatrician for unexpected death in childhood. Arrange for the baby to be taken to A&E, not to a mortuary.
- Take a brief history. Record the circumstances of death (e.g. position when found, bedding, vomit) immediately. Listen to the parents. Mention the baby by name and do not be afraid to express your sorrow.
- If the baby is a twin, the surviving twin is at ↑ risk of cot death and should be admitted to hospital for observation.

*If you learn that a baby has died*
- Provide information as requested to the rapid response team, and attend the initial case discussion if possible
- Consider taking part in the scene of death visit to support parents.

### Follow-up
- Review within a few days. There may be some anger directed towards you, as often babies have been seen in general practice within a few days or weeks of the death. Do not be defensive or become angry.
- Discuss suppression of lactation if breastfeeding (📖 p.840).
- Advise parents about likely grief reactions—guilt, anger, ↓ appetite, sleeplessness, hearing the baby cry. Do not forget siblings—they can also be deeply affected. Continue regular review as long as needed and wanted. Be sensitive to anniversaries. Watch for psychiatric illness.
- Ensure parents have received written information about cot death, including details of self-help organizations and helplines. Consider referral for counselling—ideal timing for referral varies.

- Refer for specialist obstetric assessment early in the next pregnancy and make sure parents are put in touch with the Care of Next Infant (CONI) scheme. Discuss the use of apnoea alarms.

**Death of a child in other circumstances** Death of a child is always difficult. Accidents are the most common cause of death, followed by death from childhood cancer. Principles of management used for cot death can be applied.

### Child death review

- All deaths of children <18y (excluding stillbirths) are subject to review by a local child death review panel and should be notified to it.
- Unexpected deaths are investigated by a rapid response team involving police, a senior paediatrician, and other professionals as appropriate.
- This rapid response team notifies and gathers information from other professionals involved with the child, including the GP, carries out an initial case discussion, arranges a visit to the scene of death, and then arranges a post-mortem informed by the investigation.
- Further case discussions take place following the post-mortem. The GP should be invited and sent a report. An appropriate professional is identified to inform the parents of the findings.
- The panel arranges support for the parents throughout this procedure—regard this as additional to GP support.

**Apnoea alarms** Commonly issued to or purchased by parents if they are worried about the risk of cot death. An apnoea alarm cannot be useful unless parents are taught basic life support to a proficient standard. An alarm should not be supplied without this training. There is no evidence that apnoea alarms prevent cot deaths.

**Near-miss cot deaths** Parents may rush a child to A&E or the GP after an episode of pallor ± floppiness. Parents may have attempted mouth-to-mouth resuscitation before the baby starts to respond to them, or may have simply touched the baby or lifted him/her up and received a response. Usually there are no residual symptoms or signs.

*Management* Difficult. Parents may have misinterpreted normal irregularities in sleep, or the child might be unwell and have a physical cause for symptoms, e.g. early stages of a viral infection. Usually parents are very anxious by the time you see the child. Take a careful history and examine the child from top to toe. Treat any cause of symptoms found. Be as reassuring as possible and play down anxieties.

⚠ If the child has any risk factors for cot death, comes from a difficult social background or parents are unable to cope following the episode—admit the child for observation and further assessment.

### Information and parent support
**Foundation for the Study of Infant Deaths (FSID)** ☎ 0808 802 6868
🖳 www.fsid.org.uk
**Child Bereavement Charity** ☎ 01494 446 648
🖳 www.childbereavement.org.uk
**Child Death Helpline** ☎ 0800 282 986 🖳 www.childdeathhelpline.org.uk

# Ear, nose, and throat

# The mouth

## ⚠ Oral surgery referral[N]

*Urgent referral* To exclude malignancy ALL
• Mouth ulcers persisting for >3wk
• Lumps in the mouth persisting >3wk
• Red or white patches in the mouth, including suspected lichen planus, that are painful, swollen or bleeding.

❶ For patients with persistent symptoms/signs related to the oral cavity in whom a definitive diagnosis of a benign lesion cannot be made, refer or follow-up until the symptoms and signs disappear. If the symptoms/signs have not disappeared in ≤6 wk, make an urgent referral.

*Non-urgent referral* Patients with unexplained red and/or white patches of the oral mucosa that are not painful, swollen, or bleeding, including suspected lichen planus.

**Dry mouth** *Causes*: anxiety, drugs, or Sjögren's syndrome. Look for cause and rectify if possible. Prescribe artificial saliva, e.g. glandosane.

**Sore mouth** Treat the cause. *Consider*:
• Oral thrush
• Apthous ulcers
• HSV
• Dry mouth
• Trauma (e.g. burn)
• Side effects of chemo- or radiotherapy
• Anaemia
• Hand, foot, and mouth disease (child)
• Gingivitis

**Mouth ulcers** Treat the cause. *Consider*:
• Apthous ulcers
• Trauma, e.g. sharp tooth, false teeth
• Crohn's disease/UC
• Coeliac disease
• Drugs, e.g. steroids, gold
• Reiter's disease
• Behçet disease
• HSV
• Herpes zoster
• Vincent's angina
• Erythema multiforme
• Self-inflicted, e.g. burns

**Leukoplakia** Thick whitish grey patch usually on the inside of the cheek, tongue, or gum. It is the mouth's reaction to chronic irritation of the mucous membranes. ♂>♀. Common in patients who smoke, patients with ill-fitting dentures, and patients who habitually chew on their cheek. Usually benign but may be an early sign of oral cancer. NICE recommends referral to oral surgery to exclude malignancy in *all* cases.[N]

**Erythroplakia** Reddened area that results when the lining of the mouth thins. The area appears red because the underlying capillaries are more visible. Erythroplakia is a much more ominous predictor of oral cancer than leukoplakia. NICE recommends referral to oral surgery to exclude malignancy in *all* cases.[N]

## Tongue problems
• *Blue tongue* Central cyanosis—📖 p.240.
• *Dry and furred tongue* Suggests dehydration.
• *Geographic tongue* Irregular smoother redder patches which change position over time on the dorsum of the tongue. Caused by loss of papillae. Asymptomatic or causes soreness. Rarely, due to vitamin $B_2$ deficiency.

- *Large tongue* Consider acromegaly, amyloidosis, myxoedema.
- *Smooth tongue* Iron, riboflavin, nicotinic acid, $B_{12}$, or folate deficiency; idiopathic—usually elderly; antibiotic use.
- *Sore tongue* Glossitis of anaemia; Crohn's disease, coeliac disease, carcinoma of the tongue; psychogenic causes.
- *Strawberry tongue* Yellowish-white tongue coating with the dark red papillae of the tongue projecting through. Associated with scarlet fever, although also present in Kawasaki's disease.
- *Ulcer* Assume that any non-healing ulcer is due to carcinoma of the tongue until proven otherwise. Refer for biopsy to oral surgeon. Treatment is with surgery or laser ablation ± radiotherapy.

**Halitosis** Common after sleep. *Short-term halitosis* is associated with acute illness, e.g. tonsillitis, appendicitis (foetor oris), gastroenteritis, diabetic ketoacidosis.

**Chronic halitosis** is usually caused by bacterial putrefaction of food debris and dental plaque, and is related to poor oral hygiene. Associated with gingivitis ± peridontitis. Smoking, alcohol, isosorbide dinitrate, and disulfiram exacerbate the problem.

*Management* Examine the mouth and recommend a dental check. Advise oral hygiene, e.g. regular brushing of teeth/tongue, dental flossing; smoking cessation. Diet advice—avoid garlic, onions, curries. Treat any local infection, e.g. gingivitis. Mouthwashes, e.g. 0.2% aqueous chlorhexidine gluconate, help ↓ dental plaque.

**Aphthous ulcers** Painful white ulcers. Common—affecting ~20%. Usually idiopathic but may be associated with poor health, stress, Crohn's, coeliac, and Behçet disease. Most are short lived. Large ulcers (up to 2cm diameter) can take ~6 wk to heal. Most resolve spontaneously. Topical therapies are effective, e.g. triamcinolone in dental paste qds or hydrocortisone lozenges qds (dissolve in contact with the ulcer). If ulcers are recurrent, check FBC, iron, and folate levels. Refer any ulcer not significantly improving >3wk after presentation to exclude malignancy, or if recurrent ulcers cause distress.

**Oral cancer** Usually squamous cell cancer. >4500 new cases are diagnosed in the UK each year—incidence is increasing. ♂>♀. Major risk factors are smoking and high alcohol consumption. Survival is poor (30–40% 5y survival) mainly because of poor public awareness and late presentation. Usually presents with leukoplakia (white patch), erythroplakia (red patch), or non-healing ulcer (>3wk).

*Management* Refer suspicious lesions to oral surgery for biopsy.

**Lichen planus** 📖 p.624       **Erythema multiforme** 📖 p.600

**Oral thrush** 📖 p.634       **Behçet disease** 📖 p.527

**Herpes simplex virus (HSV) infection (cold sores)** 📖 p.632

**Further information**
NICE Referral guidelines for suspected cancer (2005) 🖥 www.nice.org.uk

**Support and information for patients**
Mouth cancer foundation ☎ 01924 950 950 🖥 www.rdoc.org.uk

# Dental and jaw problems

## Gums
- *Bleeding gums* Consider periodontal disease (most common cause); pregnancy; leukaemia, bleeding disorders; scurvy.
- *Hypertrophied gums* Associated with phenytoin use.
- *Blue line* Along the margin of the teeth—suggests lead poisoning.
- *Gum inflammation* Gingivitis—consider immunodeficiency, vitamin C deficiency, DM, leukaemia, drugs, e.g. phenytoin, nifedipine, ciclosporin.

**Vincent's angina** Pharyngeal infection with ulcerative gingivitis. Management: penicillin V 250mg qds po + metronidazole 400mg tds po.
*J.H. Vincent (1862–1950), French bacteriologist.*

**Peridontal disease** Disease of the peridontal ligament caused by bacterial plaque and exacerbated by smoking and DM. Occurs in the normal population >30y. Leads to gingivitis, dental abscesses, and tooth loss. Encourage patients to register with a dentist[N]—regular dental care helps prevent dental emergencies and peridontal disease. Patients experiencing difficulty finding an NHS dentist should telephone their local primary care organization and ask to be found a dentist.

⚠ Refer urgently to a dentist if unexplained tooth mobility for >3wk.[N]

**Toothache** Pain/excessive sensitivity to temperature may be a problem with exposed dentine or pulp infection—advise to see a dentist.

**Dental abscess** Facial swelling and pain related to bacterial infection. Refer to a dentist. Prescribe analgesia if there will be a delay.

## Complications of tooth extraction
- *Haemorrhage* Apply pressure by placing wet gauze over the tooth socket and get the patient to bite hard for 15min—refer to dentist if not stopping.
- *Painful socket and bad taste in mouth* Infection—refer to a dentist. Give analgesia ± antibiotics (e.g. co-amoxiclav tds) if delay is likely.

**Loss of tooth through trauma** 📖 p.1104

---

 **Cleft lip and palate** *Incidence*: 1:600 live births—half have other abnormalities too (e.g. hypoplastic mandible). Often, though not always, detected at routine antenatal USS. The cleft may be unilateral or bilateral and involve lip and/or palate. Cleft lips are usually repaired in the first few days of life and cleft palates at ~3mo depending on the weight of the baby.

### Problems associated with cleft lip and/or palate
- Feeding difficulties with associated poor weight gain.
- Aspiration pneumonia.
- Hearing problems, particularly glue ear. In some areas children with cleft palate are routinely given grommets at ~18mo. Treat otitis media promptly. Audiology review is important.
- Speech problems—refer for speech therapy.
- Dental problems—universal with cleft palate. Orthodontic treatment is always required.

---

**Temporomandibular joint (TMJ) dysfunction** Common disorder affecting ~70% of the population—only 5% seek treatment. Typically presents in early adulthood. ♂: ♀ ≈ 1:4. Aetiology is complex—malocclusion and trauma play a part, and are exacerbated by psychogenic factors.

***Assessment*** Take a careful history, noting pain—duration, location and nature; precipitating/relieving factors; joint noises; restricted jaw function, e.g. locking, poor bite; and non-specific symptoms, e.g. headache, earache, and tinnitus. Examine the head and neck, including the TMJ and mandibular movement. Do not X-ray as this yields little useful information—CT/MRI may be ordered by specialists.

***Patterns of disease*** There are 3 patterns of disease:
- *Myofacial pain and dysfunction* Due to clenching/teeth grinding. Pain is usually worse in the morning. Stress, anxiety, and depression are key features. Poor sleep is common. May have diffuse muscle tenderness.
- *Internal derangement* The articular disc is in an abnormal position and causes restriction of mandibular movement. Pain is usually continuous and exacerbated by jaw movement.
- *Osteoarthrosis* Degeneration of the joint seen on older patients. Crepitus and sounds from the joint occur on jaw movement.

***Management*** Reassure and explain the benign nature of the disorder. Suggest simple analgesia, e.g. paracetamol ± ibuprofen. Resting the jaw and avoiding stress may help. Refer those with ongoing problems to oral surgery.

***Specialist treatment*** A bite appliance to wear at night helps 70%. Physiotherapy, behavioural therapy, and exercises also help. Drug treatments include NSAIDs, antidepressants, opioids, and muscle relaxants. Surgery is occasionally necessary if medical treatment fails.

**Dislocated jaw** 📖 p.1109          **Fractured mandible** 📖 p.1109

**Information and support**
**British Association of Oral and Maxillofacial Surgeons** Salivary gland disorders; temporomandibular joint disorders 🖥 www.baoms.org.uk
**Cleft Lip and Palate Association (CLAPA)** ☎ 020 7833 4883
🖥 www.clapa.com

# Sore throat

Each GP sees ~120 patients with sore throat every year, mostly children and young adults. 70% of sore throats are viral in origin—the rest are bacterial (mostly Group A β-haemolytic streptococci).

**Clinical picture** Pain on swallowing, fever, headache, tonsillar exudates, nausea and vomiting, and/or abdominal pain (especially in children, due to abdominal lymphadenopathy).

❶ Viral and bacterial infections are indistinguishable clinically but association with coryza, and cough may point to a viral aetiology.

**Differential diagnosis** Glandular fever especially in young adults with persistent sore throat.

**Investigation** Not usually undertaken.
• Throat swabs cannot distinguish commensal organisms (40% carry Group A β-haemolytic streptococci) from clinical infection, are expensive, and do not give instant results, so are rarely used.
• Rapid antigen tests give immediate results but have low sensitivity, limiting usefulness.

**Management** 90% recover in <1 wk without treatment. Complications are rare. Advise analgesia and antipyretics (e.g. paracetamol and/or ibuprofen),↑ fluid intake, and saltwater gargles.

*Use of antibiotics* Antibiotic prescription can probably be avoided in most patients, but educating patients about the reasons for not prescribing is vital to maintaining a good doctor–patient relationship.
• *Benefits* Antibiotics give a modest benefit in symptom relief (16h less symptoms) and may confer slight protection against some complications (e.g. quinsy, otitis media). There is no evidence that antibiotics protect against rheumatic fever or acute glomerulonepritis.
• *Risks* Possibility of side effects with antibiotic use; ↑ in community antibiotic resistance; 'medicalizing' a self-limiting condition—prescribing ↑ faith in antibiotics, encouraging re-attendance with sore throat.

Most patients should be given simple advice and/or a 'delayed prescription' (penicillin V or erythromycin qds) to be collected if no better in 2–3d (70% do not collect the script). Avoid amoxicillin as this causes a rash in those with glandular fever.

*Reasons to give antibiotics immediately[N]*
• Acute sore throat where ≥3 Centor criteria are present: tonsillar exudate, tender anterior cervical lymphadenopathy/lymphadenitis, history of fever, and absence of cough.
• Patient is systemically very unwell.
• Symptoms and signs suggestive of serious illness and/or complications (e.g. peritonsillar abscess, peritonsillar cellulitis).
• High risk of serious complications because of pre-existing comorbidity, e.g. significant heart, lung, renal, liver, or neuromuscular disease, immunosuppression, cystic fibrosis, and young children born prematurely.

**Complications of sore throat** All rare.
- *Quinsy (peritonsillar abscess)* Usually occurs in adults. *Signs*: unilateral peritonsillar swelling, difficulty swallowing (even saliva) and trismus (difficulty opening jaw). Refer for IV antibiotics ± incision and drainage.
- *Retropharyngeal abscess* Occurs in children. *Signs*: inability to swallow, fever. Refer for IV antibiotics ± incision and drainage.
- *Rheumatic fever* 📖 p.284
- *Glomerulonephritis* 📖 p.450

## Indications for referral to ENT
**Urgent referral** Any unexplained sore throat for >1mo.[N]

### Referral for tonsillectomy[G]
- *Recurrent acute tonsillitis* Young children have a lot of throat infections and most will 'grow out' of the problem without the need for surgery. Tonsillectomy is only considered if children miss a lot of school, e.g. >5 attacks/y for 2y causing school absence.
- *Airway obstruction* Very large tonsils causing sleep apnoea.
- *Chronic tonsillitis* >3mo + halitosis.
- *Recurrent quinsy*
- *Unilateral tonsillar enlargement* To exclude malignancy.

⚠ Tonsillectomy carries a small risk of severe haemorrhage. Re-admit any patient with post-operative bleeding for observation.

**Glandular fever (infectious mononucleosis)** Consider in teen-agers or young adults presenting with sore throat lasting >1wk. Caused by Epstein–Barr virus (EBV). Spread by droplet infection and direct contact ('kissing disease') and has a 4–14d incubation period. Presents with sore throat, malaise, fatigue, lymphadenopathy, enlarged spleen, palatal petechiae, and/or rash (10–20%). Send blood for FBC (atypical lymphocytes) and glandular fever antibodies (Monospot or Paul Bunnell).

*Management* Advise rest, fluids, and regular paracetamol; avoid alcohol. Try saltwater or aspirin gargles (only if >16y). Consider a short course of prednisolone for severe symptoms. Treat 2° infection with antibiotics. Counsel re the possibility of prolonged symptoms (up to several months).
⚠ Do not prescribe amoxicillin as it causes a rash.

*Complications* 2° infections; rash with amoxicillin; hepatitis; jaundice; pneumonitis; neurological disturbances (rare).

**Tonsillar tumour** Most often elderly. *Signs*: unilateral tonsillar swelling, dysphagia, sore throat, earache. Refer for excision biopsy.

⚠ Refer any unexplained, sore throat present for >1mo for urgent ENT assessment[N].

## Further information
**NICE** 🖥 www.nice.org.uk
- Respiratory tract infections: antibiotic prescribing (2008)
- Referral guidelines for suspected cancer (2005).

## Information for patients
**Patient UK** Information leaflets on sore throat. UTRI, tonsillitis, tonsils and adenoids, and glandular fever 🖥 www.patient.co.uk

# Hoarseness and stridor

**Hoarseness** Change in quality of the voice affecting pitch, volume, or resonance. Occurs when vocal cord function is affected by a change in the cords, a neurological or muscular problem. *Causes:*

- *Local causes* URTI (most common); laryngitis; trauma—shouting, coughing, vomiting, instrumentation; carcinoma; hypothyroidism; acromegaly.
- *Neurological problems* Laryngeal nerve palsy; motor neuron disease; myaesthenia gravis; multiple sclerosis.
- *Muscular problems* Muscular dystrophy.
- *Functional problems*

**Assessment** Weight ↓, dysphagia, or neck lumps add to suspicions of malignancy. Check TFTs in those with weight gain. Indirect laryngoscopy with a mirror can be difficult and give a poor view. ENT departments have thin fibreoptic scopes for direct visualization in out-patients.

⚠ **Refer urgently for chest X-ray (CXR)^N** if hoarseness persists >3wk, particularly smokers >50y and heavy drinkers.
- *If there is a POSITIVE finding on CXR* refer urgently to a team specializing in the management of lung cancer.
- *If there is a NEGATIVE finding on CXR* refer urgently to a team specializing in the management of head and neck cancer.

**Laryngitis** Hoarseness, malaise ± fever, and/or pain on using voice. Usually viral and self-limiting (1–2wk) but occasionally 2° bacterial infection occurs.

*Management* Advise patients to rest voice, take OTC analgesia (e.g. paracetamol and/or ibuprofen), try steam inhalations. Consider antibiotics if bacterial infection is suspected (e.g. penicillin 250mg qds for 1wk).

**Vocal cord nodules** Can cause hoarseness. Usually precipitated by overuse of the voice—typically in singers. They can be visualized at laryngoscopy. Initial treatment is resting the voice but sometimes nodules have to be removed surgically.

**Functional disorders** Hysterical paralysis of the vocal cord adductors due to psychological stress. Can cause the voice to ↓ to a whisper or be lost completely. More common amongst young women.

*Management* Refer for laryngoscopy to exclude organic cause. Speech therapy and psychological support may help.

**Laryngeal carcinoma** ♂ > ♀. Smoking is the main risk factor. The first sign is usually hoarseness, followed by stridor, dysphagia, and pain.

*Management* Refer urgently to ENT if suspected. Diagnosis is confirmed with laryngoscopy and biopsy. Treatment is with surgery ± radiotherapy. Early tumours confined to the vocal cord have 80–90% 5y survival.

**Post-laryngectomy problems** After laryngectomy patients have a permanent tracheostomy and require practical and psychological support. *Problems include*:

- Excessive secretions.
- Recurrent pneumonia
- Stenosis of the tracheostomy site—refer to ENT/oral surgery if severe.
- Communication difficulties—ensure referred to speech therapy.
- Maintenance of adequate diet—refer to dietician if not maintaining weight and recurrence of tumour has been excluded.

**Stridor** Noise created on inspiration due to narrowing of the larynx or trachea—much more common in children than adults.

⚠ *Signs of severe airways narrowing*

- Distress
- Pallor and cyanosis
- ↑ respiratory rate
- Use of accessory muscles and tracheal tug.

*Causes* Congenital abnormalities of the larynx; epiglottis; croup (laryngotracheobronchitis); inhaled foreign body; trauma; laryngeal paralysis.

---

**Laryngomalacia (congenital laryngeal stridor)**
Common among small babies. Caused by floppy aryatic folds and the small size of the airway. Stridor becomes more noticeable during sleep, excitement, crying, and with concurrent URTIs. Normally resolves without treatment. Parental concern may necessitate referral

**Croup** Common viral infection occurring in epidemics in autumn and spring. Starts with mild fever and runny nose. In younger children (<4y), oedema and secretions in the larynx and trachea result in a barking cough and inspiratory stridor. The cough typically starts at night and is exacerbated by crying and parental anxiety. Some children have recurrent attacks associated with viral URTI.

*Management* Steam helps. There is also evidence that steroids can be helpful—give oral dexamethasone 0.15mg/kg or prednisolone 1–2mg/kg. Admit as a paediatric emergency if there is intercostal recession or cyanosis, or the child's carers are unable to cope.

**Acute epiglottitis in children** Bacterial infection causing a swollen epiglottis. Can potentially obstruct the airway. Much rarer since introduction of routine *Haemophilus influenza* type b (Hib) immunization. Consider if stridor, drooling, fever, and upright 'leaning-forward' posture.

⚠ If suspected do not examine the child's throat as this can precipitate complete obstruction.

*Management* Refer urgently but try to maintain a calm atmosphere to avoid distressing the child. Examination will be undertaken in hospital with full resuscitation facilities on hand. *Treatment:* IV antibiotics.

---

**Adult epiglottitis** Much less common than childhood epiglottitis and less likely to cause complete airway obstruction. Refer for IV antibiotics.

**Inhaled foreign body** Refer to ENT for assessment.

# Neck lumps and salivary gland problems

Neck lumps are common and can be the first sign of serious underlying pathology. Accurate assessment is important to differentiate harmless lumps from those needing further investigation and treatment. Ask about local symptoms in the head/neck and systemic symptoms (e.g. fever, anorexia, weight ↓). Differential diagnosis—Figure 25.1.

⚠ **Refer urgently to ENT[N]**
- Any unexplained lump in the neck of recent onset.
- Any previously undiagnosed lump that has changed over 3–6wk.

**Lymphadenopathy** Most enlarged LNs are reactive LNs—suggested by a short history, soft tender mobile lump, and concurrent infection.

⚠ **Check FBC, blood film, ESR (or CRP/viscosity)**, and consider further investigation, discussion with a specialist and/or referral if:[N]
- Lymphadenopathy present ≥ 6wk.
- LN >2cm in size
- LNs are increasing in size
- Widespread lymphadenopathy
- Associated weight ↓, night sweats and/or splenomegaly.

## Causes of lymphadenopathy
- **Benign infective** Viral infection, e.g. EBV, CMV, adenovirus, HIV; bacterial infection, e.g. streptococcal sore throat, TB; toxoplasmosis, syphilis.
- **Benign non-infective** Sarcoid; connective tissue disease, e.g. RA; skin disease, e.g. eczema, psoriasis; drugs, e.g. phenytoin.
- **Malignant** Lymphoma, CLL, ALL, metastases—head and neck cancer may present with enlarged cervical LNs.

**Branchial cyst** Arises from embryonic remnants of the second branchial cleft in the neck. Most common in young adults. Presents as a smooth swelling in front of the anterior border of the sternomastoid at the junction of its upper and middle thirds—often during a viral URTI. Position is characteristic. *Examination*: fluctuant lump that does not move on swallowing. Treatment is by excision—refer to ENT.

**Thyroglossal cyst** The thyroid gland develops from the lower portion of the thyroglossal duct. If a portion of this duct remains patent it can form a thyroglossal cyst. Usually presents in young adults (peak age 15–30y) with either a painless smooth cystic midline swelling between the isthmus of the thyroid gland and the hyoid cartilage or just above the hyoid cartilage, or, if the cyst is inflamed, a painful tender lump with localized swelling. Examination: the cyst rises as the patient sticks out his/her tongue. Refer to ENT for excision.

## Salivary gland strictures and stones
- **Salivary stones** 80% of calculi are seen in the submandibular duct system. Less frequently they occur in the parotid duct system and rarely in other salivary glands.
- **Strictures** of the salivary gland duct occur as a complication of a pre-existing calculus, due to mucous plugs, or following trauma to the duct wall (e.g. cheek biting).

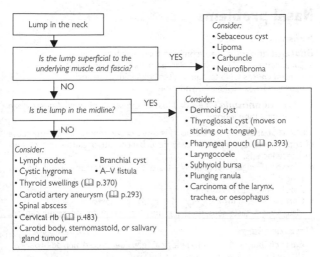

**Fig. 25.1** Differential diagnosis of neck lumps

**Presentation** Pain and swelling on eating due to obstruction of saliva flow. The gland may appear normal or be tender and swollen. Sometimes stones can be visualized at the salivary duct orifice or felt on bimanual palpation. Both stones and strictures predispose to infection in the gland.

**Management** Refer to ENT/oral surgery for confirmation of diagnosis— stones are seen on plain X-rays or sialography. Some stones pass spontaneously, but most require surgical removal—the whole gland may be removed to prevent recurrent problems. Strictures can often be dilated.

**Acute parotiditis** Unilateral parotid swelling and pain caused by bacterial infection. Predisposing factors include DM, immunosuppression/compromise, local fibrosis following radiotherapy, and autoimmune destruction (e.g. Sjögren's syndrome). Precipitating factors include surgery, dehydration, salivary stones/strictures, and poor oral hygiene. Treat with antibiotics (e.g. co-amoxiclav 250/125 tds for 1wk) and rehydration. If not settling, consider abscess formation—refer to ENT/oral surgery for drainage.

**Mumps** 📖 p.650

**Salivary gland tumours** Present with a lump/swelling in a salivary gland—80% in the parotid gland. Treated with surgery ± radiotherapy.

⚠ Refer urgently to ENT/oral surgery if unexplained swelling in the parotid or submandibular gland for > 1mo.[N] Refer sooner if pain, rapid growth, hard fixed mass, weight ↓, or facial nerve palsy.

### Further information
**NICE** Referral guidelines for suspected cancer (2005) 🖥 www.nice.org.uk

# Nasal problems

## Anosmia

**Bilateral anosmia** More common than unilateral. *Causes:*
- *Local causes* URTI, rhinitis, enlarged turbinates, nasal polyps.
- *Central causes* CNS tumours, after head injury, meningitis, hydrocephalus, Kallman's syndrome.

**Unilateral anosmia** One-sided loss of the sense of smell. *Causes:* head injury, frontal lobe lesion

**Taste disturbance** Taste of food is often dependent on smell. Any cause of anosmia can also result in taste disturbance. Other causes of taste disturbance include:
- Glossopharyngeal nerve palsy—taste loss on posterior third of the tongue.
- Facial nerve palsy (🕮 p.545).
- Chronic adrenal insufficiency—↑ sensitivity to taste.
- Malignancy—taste sensations, e.g. metallic taste with pancreatic cancer.

## Nasal discharge
- *Clear discharge* May be physiological (e.g. due to cold air), due to allergy (e.g. hayfever), or viral (e.g. URTI).
- *Clear fluid after trauma* May indicate CSF leak.
- *Green discharge* Indicates active bacterial infection.
- *Yellow discharge* May indicate viral/bacterial infection or allergy.
- *Bloodstained discharge* ⚠ tumour of the nose or post-nasal sinus until proven otherwise—refer urgently to ENT.

❶ The term *rhinorrhoea* is also used to mean nasal discharge. The term *coryza* is usually applied to the watery discharge from nasal mucus membranes that occurs when a patient has a viral infection.

**CSF rhinorrhoea** Clear fluid dripping from the nose after trauma can indicate a fracture of the roof of the ethmoid labyrinth and CSF leak. Fluid tests +ve for glucose. It suggests significant trauma—consider referral for head injury assessment. Spontaneous healing of the CSF leak is the norm, but if it persists refer to neurosurgery for dural closure.

**Nasal obstruction** Common symptom experienced occasionally by many. Usually obstruction is bilateral. ⚠ Assume persistent unilateral blockage is neoplastic until proven otherwise—refer urgently to ENT.

## Causes of nasal obstruction
- *Mucosal swelling* Coryza, rhinitis (🕮 p.940), iatrogenic, nasal polyps.
- *Septal deviation* Trauma, congenital (e.g. 2° to cleft lip).
- *Other* Tumour, enlarged adenoids, foreign body (🕮 p.1104).

**Deviated nasal septum** Common in adults—usually 2° to injury. May be associated with external deformity. Nasal blockage is unilateral. Treat mucosal swelling due to rhinitis first as that may be sufficient to control symptoms. If unsuccessful, refer for surgery (submucous resection).

**Septal haematoma** May occur after injury and causes nasal blockage. Presents as a bilateral soft bulging of the septum. Refer urgently to ENT for evacuation to prevent cartilage destruction.

**Septal perforation** Can cause bleeding, crusting, and discomfort. *Causes:* trauma, nose-picking, cocaine use, post-operative, malignancy. Refer if suspicion of malignancy; otherwise treat symptomatically (e.g. Vaseline or Naseptin for crusting). Surgical closure is often unsuccessful.

**Post-nasal drip** Draining of nasal secretions down the back of the throat. Treat as for chronic sinusitis (📖 p.940). *Symptoms include:*
• Feeling of mucus in the back of the throat.
• Chronic cough—usually worse in the morning and improves in the day.
• Morning sore throat.
• Nasty taste in the mouth/bad breath.

**Causes** URTI, sinusitis, allergic and/or vasomotor rhinitis, nasal polyps, deviated nasal septum.

**Nasal polyps** Most common in ♂ patients aged >40y—associated with asthma, allergic rhinitis, and chronic sinusitis. Consider CF in children <16y. *Symptoms:* nasal blockage; watery discharge; post-nasal drip; change in voice; loss of smell; taste disturbance.

**Signs** Polyps are smooth and pale, usually bilateral, and commonly arise from the middle meatus and middle turbinates. They may completely block the nasal passage. They can be confused with enlarged inferior turbinates but are more mobile and lack sensation.

**Management** Try medical treatment—steroid nasal drops (e.g. Flixonase Nasule® od) until polyps shrink (maximum 1mo) and then steroid nasal spray to ↓ recurrence. Swab and give antibiotics if purulent nasal discharge. Refer for consideration of polypectomy if medical treatment fails. ❶ Polyps often recur after surgery.

⚠ Refer unilateral polyps with an unusual or irregular appearance, especially if ulcerating and/or bleeding, for exclusion of malignancy.

**Nose bleed/epistaxis** 📖 p.1070   **Nasal foreign body** 📖 p.1104
**Snoring and sleep apnoea** 📖 p.346

**Fractured nose** Undisplaced nasal fractures usually heal without intervention. X-ray is unhelpful. Give adequate analgesia. Advise that bruising may be extensive and the nose will feel blocked for 1–2wk.

**Associated injuries** Consider assessment for head injury (📖 p.1108). Always look for associated fractures of the zygoma/maxillary bones ('step' deformity in the orbit, dental malocclusion, difficulty opening the jaw, diplopia). Refer urgently to maxillofacial surgeon if present.

**Assessment for permanent deformity** Can be difficult at the time of the injury because of soft tissue swelling—re-assess 7–10d after injury. Refer promptly any patient with significant deformity, or if the patient is unhappy with the appearance of the nose, to ENT. Reduction should take place <3wk after fracture. Deviation of the nasal septum may not be correctable at the time of manipulation—if symptomatic will need a later submucous resection.

# Sinusitis and rhinitis

**Acute sinusitis** Infection of ≥1 paranasal sinus (maxillary, frontal, ethmoid, or sphenoid). Usually follows URTI—10% are due to tooth infection. Presents with frontal headache/facial pain (may be difficult to distinguish from toothache), typically worse on movement/bending, ± purulent nasal discharge ± fever.

**Management[N]** Most sinusitis resolves spontaneously in 7–10d. *Advise analgesia (paracetamol ± ibuprofen) and fluids for all patients. Steam inhalation may also help.* Treatment options:
- Decongestants—little evidence of effectiveness.
- Steroid nasal sprays (e.g. beclometasone two puffs to each nostril bd).
- Antibiotics (e.g. amoxicillin 250mg tds)—reserve for patients with frontal sinusitis, severe symptoms, symptoms persisting >2½wk., or at high risk of serious complications (e.g. CF or immunosuppression).

**Chronic/recurrent sinusitis** >3mo of symptoms or >3 episodes of sinusitis in any year. Presents with post-nasal drip, frontal headache/facial pain, and/or blocked nose. Associated with nasal polyps (☐ p.939) and vasomotor rhinitis. Treat as for acute sinusitis. Refer to ENT if symptoms are interfering with life—surgery may help.

**Rhinitis** Inflammation of the nasal mucosa. Affects >1:5 people. May be allergic (most children; 1:3 adults) or non-allergic (e.g. *vasomotor*—triggered by physical/chemical agents such as cold air, tobacco, or perfumes; *drug induced*). If allergic cause is suspected, ask about potential allergens—pollen, animals, fungi/moulds, occupational allergens (e.g. flour, latex).

**Symptoms** Nasal discharge, itching, sneezing ± nasal blockage /congestion. Symptoms may be seasonal (only certain times of the year) or perennial (all year); intermittent (<4d/wk or <4wk at a time) or persistent. Make an assessment of severity. Patients have moderate/severe symptoms if ≥1 of troublesome symptoms, abnormal sleep, impairment of daily activities/sport/leisure, or problems at work/school. If symptoms are intrusive and difficult to control, refer for allergy testing.

**Signs** Swollen inferior turbinates; ↓ nasal airway; pale or mauve mucosa; nasal discharge; 'allergic crease' on bridge of nose from persistent rubbing (young sufferers with allergic rhinitis).

**Management of allergic rhinitis** General measures include ↓ in allergen exposure (☐ p.319), nasal douching with saline nose drops ± steam inhalation. Drug treatment—Table 25.2.

**Desensitization** 50–70% success rate. Risk of anaphylaxis is high, so provision is limited to specialist centres. Refer via an allergy clinic.

**Table 25.1** Predominant pollen types at different times of year in the UK

| Jan | Feb | Mar | Apr | May | Jun | Jul | Aug | Sep | Oct | Nov | Dec |
|-----|-----|-----|-----|-----|-----|-----|-----|-----|-----|-----|-----|
| Alder Hazel | | Elm Willow Ash | Silver birch (25%) | Oak | Weed pollen | | | | | | |
| | | | | Grass pollen (60%) | | | | Fungal spores | | | |

**Table 25.2** Drug treatment of allergic rhinitis (BNF 12.2.1, 12.2.2)

| Category | Notes |
|---|---|
| Nasal steroids | Effective if applied properly, and can be used safely long term |
| | Take several days to work—try for >2wk before abandoning. Often started at high dose—when symptoms are controlled, dose is ↓ to the minimum that maintains symptom control |
| | Choose preparations with minimal systemic absorption if using >1mo (e.g. fluticasone, mometasone). If nasal irritation, sore throat, or nose bleeds, switch to a preparation without benzalkonium chloride preservative, e.g. Flixonase Nasule® or Rhinocort® |
| Oral steroids | Only rarely needed. *Consider for:* severe nasal obstruction, short-term rescue medication for uncontrolled symptoms, or control of symptoms for important social/work events (e.g. examinations) |
| | Use 20–30mg prednisolone po for 5–7d in combination with nasal steroids. Injected preparations are not recommended |
| Oral anti-histamines | Choose a non-sedative antihistamine, e.g. loratadine 10mg od. May be used alone or in combination with nasal steroids. Improve associated symptoms (e.g. conjunctivitis) as well as nasal symptoms |
| Topical antihistamines | For example azelastine nasal drops—useful as a rescue therapy |
| | Faster acting than oral antihistamines—onset of action is <15min |
| Leukotriene receptor antagonists | For example montelukast 10mg od |
| | As effective as antihistamines. Useful for patients with concurrent asthma. Combination with antihistamines does not ↑ efficacy |
| Topical/oral decongestants | For example ephedrine nasal drops tds/qds |
| | Effective (drops >> oral preparations) in reducing nasal congestion |
| | Discourage use of nasal drops for >10d as vasoconstriction → mucosal damage → worsening of nasal congestion—a vicious circle termed rhinitis medicamentosa. Not caused by oral preparations |
| Topical anticholinergics | For example ipratropium bromide nasal spray tds—↓ rhinorrhoea but no effect on other nasal symptoms |
| Topical chromones | For example sodium cromoglicate or nedocromil sodium nasal spray—less effective than nasal steroids but may be useful for children or pregnant women wishing to avoid steroids |

**Non-allergic rhinitis** Treat as for allergic rhinitis—treatment is often less successful.

**Hayfever** Rhinitis and/or conjunctivitis and/or wheeze due to an allergic reaction to pollen. Occurs at different times in the year depending on which pollen is involved (Table 25.1).

**Management** When the pollen count is high, keep windows shut (including car windows—consider pollen filter for the car), wear glasses/sunglasses, and avoid grassy spaces. Treat as for allergic rhinitis. Topical chromone eye drops (e.g. nedocromil) may help eye symptoms.

**Further information**
**British Society for Allergy and Clinical Immunology (BSACI)** Guidelines for the management of allergic and non-allergic rhinitis (2008).

# Earache and external ear problems

**Earache** Ear pain is a common presenting symptom. Think of:
- *Local causes*
  - *Outer ear*—otitis externa; furunculosis; impacted wax; pinna pain (perichondritis); malignant disease of the ear.
  - *Middle ear*—otitis media; barotrauma; myringitis; mastoiditis.
- *Referred pain* Trigeminal nerve (dental abscess/caries, impacted molar teeth, TMJ dysfunction); facial nerve (HSV infection, Ramsay Hunt syndrome); vagus nerve (tumours of the piriform fossa, larynx, or post-cricoid area); glossopharyngeal nerve (tonsillitis, quinsy, post-tonsillectomy, tumour of the base of the tongue or tonsil, neuralgia); cervical nerves C2/3 (cervical spondylosis).

⚠ Refer urgently to ENT if unilateral unexplained pain in the head/neck area for >4wk, associated with otalgia (earache) but normal otoscopy.[N]

**Myringitis** Myringitis is inflammation of the tympanic membrane.

*Myringitis bullosa* describes painful vesicles on the tympanic membrane. Associated with mycoplasma or viral URTIs. A similar picture occurs with Ramsay Hunt syndrome (📖 p.546).

**Discharge from the ear** *Otorrhoea* is discharge from the ear. Major causes are: otitis externa, otitis media, and cholesteatoma.

❶ Always exclude a perforated drum in discharging ears—beware of cholesteatoma. If you cannot visualize the drum, review the patient. Clear fluid leaking from an ear after head injury may suggest a CSF leak. Fluid tests +ve for glucose. This implies a head injury with force—refer to A&E for further assessment.

**Otitis externa** Inflammation ± infection of the external ear canal. Common—affects ~10% at some time. Adults > children. Associated with eczema of the ear canal. *Risk factors include:* swimming, humid environment, narrow ear canal, hearing aid use, and mechanical trauma (e.g. cleaning ears out with cotton buds, or after syringing).

*Acute otitis externa* <6wk duration. Presents with ear pain (often severe), discharge (may be offensive), and hearing loss ± lymphadenopathy behind/in front of the ear. If the ear canal is not obscured by debris/discharge, it appears red, swollen, and inflamed. Moving the pinna may be painful. ❶ Acute episodes have a tendency to recur.

⚠ Diabetics and immunosuppressed patients can develop a severe necrotizing form of otitis externa—refer to ENT early.

*Chronic otitis externa* (>3mo duration)—ongoing discharge from the ear ± hearing loss. Causes canal stenosis and permanent hearing ↓.

*Management* Although very common, can be difficult to treat effectively. Take a swab if any discharge.
- Advise analgesia, e.g. paracetamol ± ibuprofen.
- Prescribe ear drops: options are aluminium acetate drops (as effective as antibiotics) and antibiotic and/or steroid drops (e.g. Locorten-Vioform®). ☞ If you cannot see the ear drum to ensure that it is intact, use of potentially ototoxic gentamicin ear drops is controversial.

- There is no evidence that adding oral antibiotics (e.g. flucloxacillin + erythromycin qds) improves outcome[CE]—only use if treatment with drops alone has failed or administration of ear drops may be ineffective, e.g. debris within the canal, very swollen canal, uncooperative child.

❶ Skin of the pinna adjacent to the ear canal is often affected by eczema. Treat with topical corticosteroid cream/ointment—avoid prolonged use.

*If there is no response after 1wk,* consider an alternative eardrop, e.g. Otosporin® (contains neomycin, hydrocortisone, and an antifungal—polymyxin B) ± oral antibiotics. If a swab was taken on the initial visit, prescribe based on the result. Consider gentle syringing to remove infected material. Refer to ENT for aural toilet/advice on further management if there is still no response.

**Furunculosis** Boil in the ear canal. Presents with severe ear pain—may be exacerbated by moving the tragus or opening the jaw. Exclude DM.
- If no surrounding cellulitis, advise OTC analgesia and application of hot compresses—most will settle. If not settling, prescribe topical antibiotics and steroid drops, e.g. Gentisone HC®, 3 drops qds for 1wk.
- If surrounding cellulitis, prescribe flucloxacillin 250–500mg qds for 7d.
- Refer to ENT for incision and drainage if not settling.

**Foreign bodies in the ear** 📖 p.1101

**Ear wax** Normal. Becomes a problem only if causes deafness, pain, or other ear-related symptoms. Wax completely obscuring the lumen is termed 'impacted'. Factors preventing normal extrusion of wax from the ear (e.g. wearing a hearing aid, using cotton buds to clean ears) ↑ the chance of ear wax accumulating.

*Ear syringing* Indicated if impacted wax causes loss of hearing, discomfort, or tinnitus. Avoid syringing if there is deafness in the other ear or a history of perforation of the eardrum (including grommet), previous mastoid operation, or chronic middle ear disease (e.g. chronic suppurative otitis media, cholesteatoma). If ear syringing is contraindicated, refer to ENT for removal under direct vision, e.g. with microsuction.

**Perichondritis of the pinna** Infection of the pinna due to ear piercing or laceration. If not treated quickly can result in destruction of cartilage and 'cauliflower ear'. *Pseudomonas* is a common infecting organism so treat with oral ciprofloxacin 500-750mg bd. If not settling, refer as an emergency to A&E.

**Haematoma of the pinna** 📖 p.1109

---

 **Accessory auricle** *Incidence*: 1.5:100 live births. Small skin lesion consisting of skin ± cartilage in front of the ear. No treatment is necessary but accessory auricles are often removed for cosmetic reasons.

**Bat ears** Common congenital abnormality. A fold of the pinna is absent. The child is noted to have protruding ears. Runs in families. Referral for surgery is indicated if the condition is causing psychosocial problems.

# Otitis media

**Acute suppurative otitis media (OM)** Common acute inflammation of the middle ear. Parental smoking ↑ children's risk of OM—encourage parents to stop smoking. Caused by viral/bacterial infection.

*Presentation* Ear pain—usually unilateral ± fever/systemic upset. Ear discharge may be associated with relief of pain if there is a spontaneous perforation of the eardrum. *Examination*: red bulging drum. If perforation has occurred, the external canal may be filled with pus, obscuring the drum. ❶ If you can't see the drum, review the patient after treatment.

## Management[N]

- In 80%, symptoms resolve in ≤ 4d without treatment. Advise fluids and paracetamol and/or ibuprofen for analgesia and fever control. Symptoms resolve 24h earlier with antibiotics, but antibiotics carry the risk of side effects and use ↑ community antibiotic resistance. Consider using a 'delayed' approach—prescribing if symptoms are no better in 4d.
- Consider prescribing immediately (e.g. amoxicillin tds) for children with bilateral OM or acute OM with otorrhoea
- Prescribe immediately if very systemically unwell or at high risk of serious complications because of pre-existing comorbidity (e.g. significant heart, lung, renal, liver, or neuromuscular disease; immunosuppression; CF; young children born prematurely).
- If recurrent attacks (>4 episodes in 6mo) or acute perforation does not heal in <1mo, refer to ENT.

**Chronic suppurative otitis media** Persistent drainage (>1mo) from the ear associated with tympanic membrane perforation and conductive hearing loss. Not usually painful.
- *Central perforation* 'Safe disease'. Treat as for otitis externa (📖 p.942). Refer to ENT if there is persistent discharge, deafness, vertigo, or earache. Surgery to close the drum may help.
- *Attic or marginal perforation* 'Unsafe disease'. May indicate *cholesteatoma*. Refer to ENT for further assessment.

**Serous/secretory otitis media (glue ear)** Non-infected fluid accumulates in the middle ear due to dysfunction/obstruction of the Eustachian tube, e.g. 2° to throat or ear infection, or tonsillar hyperplasia. Most common cause of hearing loss in childhood. More common in children with Down's syndrome or cleft lip/palate. *Symptoms*: deafness ± earache, difficulties with speech/language, ± behavioural problems. *Signs*: dull concave drum with visible peripheral vessels ± fluid level and/or air bubbles behind the drum.

> **Management in children** Untreated, 75% have no symptoms in <3mo, 5% have bilateral hearing loss persisting >12mo. Glue ear resolves as the child grows older—treatment is aimed at ↓ impact of symptoms until natural resolution. If not resolving, refer to community audiology/ENT depending on local policy. Specialist treatment options include watchful waiting or grommet insertion.

**Grommets** Air-conducting tubes inserted through the eardrum to drain the middle ear. Most are extruded spontaneously <9mo after insertion. May need reinsertion if deafness recurs. Patients can swim/bathe but should avoid diving. If discharge from the ear, treat with antibiotic/steroid ear drops ± aural toilet (see otitis externa, 🕮 p.942).

**Management in adults** Uncommon in adults—usually follows URTI and spontaneously resolves in <6wk. If not resolving or no history of preceding URTI, refer to ENT to exclude post-nasal space tumour.

**Mastoiditis** Rare complication of acute OM—infection spreads to the mastoid. *Symptoms*: persistent throbbing earache; creamy profuse ear discharge; increasing conductive deafness; fever and general malaise. *Signs*: tenderness ± swelling over the mastoid; ear may stick out; drum is red/bulging or perforated. If the eardrum is normal, it is not mastoiditis. Refer to ENT as an emergency. Treatment is with IV antibiotics.

**Cholesteatoma** Skin or stratified squamous epithelium growing in the middle ear. Thought to result from formation of a *retraction pocket* in the pars flaccida of the eardrum. Local expansion as the drum desquamates can damage adjacent structures (e.g. facial nerve, semicircular canals—resulting in vertigo). If infected there is an offensive discharge from the ear. *Signs*: perforation of the pars flaccida of the drum with pearly white discharge within it and conductive deafness. Refer to ENT. Treatment is with suction to clear out the cholesteatoma and/or surgery. Following surgery, the ear should be dry and trouble free—if not, refer back to ENT. Lifelong follow-up is required as cholesteatoma recurs.

**Tympanosclerosis** Thickening and calcification of the tympanic membrane as a result of scarring from recurrent ear infections or after grommet insertion. Usually asymptomatic. No action is needed.

**Barotrauma** Caused by changes in atmospheric pressure (e.g. air travel, diving) in those with poor Eustachian tube function. Presents with a sensation of pressure/pain in one/both ears, hearing loss ± vertigo. There is fluid behind the drum (or perforated drum), haemorrhagic areas in the drum ± conductive hearing ↓. Usually resolves spontaneously in 2–3wk. If perforation has not healed in <1mo refer to ENT.

**Prevention** Valsalva manoeuvre, yawning, or sucking boiled sweets during flight, particularly during take-off/landing, encourages the Eustachian tube to open to allow pressure to equalize. Decongestants may help, e.g. pseudoephedrine 120mg 30min prior to flight. Patients with otitis media should not fly.

### Further information

**NICE** Respiratory tract infections: antibiotic prescribing (2008)
🖳 www.nice.org.uk
**SIGN** Diagnosis and management of childhood acute otitis media in primary care (2003) 🖳 www.sign.ac.uk
**Clinical Evidence** Williamson I. Otitis media with effusion (2004)
🖳 www.clinicalevidence.com

# Deafness

**Congenital deafness** Usually detected on neonatal screening (📖 p.855). *Causes:*
- Genetic (50%)
- Intrauterine infection, e.g. rubella
- Drugs given in pregnancy, e.g. streptomycin
- Birth asphyxia
- Meningitis
- Severe neonatal jaundice.

**Childhood deafness** Temporary deafness due to middle ear infections is common, but permanent deafness is rare (1–2:1000). ↓ hearing is often noticed by parents or teachers—take concerns seriously and refer for assessment. Deafness causes long-term speech, language ± behavioural problems, and early intervention makes a difference.

*Management* History, examination, assess development (including speech and language), consider referral for audiology or to ENT. *Causes:*
- *If no earache*—bilateral glue ear (📖 p.944); impacted wax; hereditary cause; sequel of meningitis, head injury, or birth complications.
- *If earache*—acute otitis media (📖 p.944); impacted wax.

**Adult deafness** Common and debilitating, leading to isolation and depression. Presentation tends to be late. *Causes:* Table 25.3.

*Presentation* Usually hearing loss develops insidiously with increasing problems understanding others when there is background noise. Tinnitus may be the presenting problem.

*Useful screening questions*
- Do other people mumble a lot?
- Do you find yourself frequently saying 'pardon'?
- Does the family say the TV is too loud?
- Do you miss hearing the door bell or phone?
- Do you occasionally get the wrong end of the stick in a conversation?

*Management* Examine the drum; exclude wax; consider post-nasal space tumour. If no self-limiting cause is found, refer for a hearing test to quantify hearing loss and assess suitability for hearing aid.

⚠ *Refer to ENT if*
- Conductive deafness of unknown cause.
- Sudden deafness if no wax visible.
- Asymmetrical deafness—refer urgently to ENT[N] to exclude rare dangerous diagnoses, e.g. acoustic neuroma, cholesteatoma.

**Benefits for deaf people** 📖 p.224

**Presbyacusis** Very common. Causes bilateral symmetrical sensorineural deafness in the over-50s. Deafness is gradual in onset. High frequencies are more severely affected, so speech discrimination, particularly of high-pitched voices, is lost first. Examination is normal. Refer for an audiogram to confirm diagnosis and then for a hearing aid if appropriate.

**Otosclerosis** Bilateral conductive deafness due to adherence of the stapes footplate to the bone around the oval window. May be FH (50%). If deteriorates in pregnancy, avoid prescribing combined contraceptives. Refer to ENT for assessment to replace the stapes with an implant.

**Table 25.3** Causes of adult deafness

| Conductive deafness | Sensorineural deafness |
| --- | --- |
| Impacted wax (🕮 p.943) | Presbyacusis |
| Debris/foreign body in the ear canal | Infections (measles, meningitis) |
| Perforation of the eardrum | Ménière's disease (🕮 p.949) |
| Middle ear effusion (glue ear) | Drugs, e.g. aminoglycosides, furosemide |
| Otosclerosis | Acoustic neuroma |
| | Noise-induced deafness |

**Noise-induced deafness** Caused by exposure to noise >85dB. May occur in work or non-work settings\ (e.g. firearm sports). Immediate indications are ringing in the ears/muffling of hearing after exposure. Refer to audiology. Avoid further excessive noise exposure. Hearing aids may help. If employment related may be eligible for compensation (🕮 p.118; war veterans—🕮 p.225). Employees should be protected from noise and provided with ear protection if working in noisy environments.

**Acoustic neuroma** Slow-growing neurofibroma arising from the acoustic nerve. *Symptoms*: unilateral sensorineural deafness, tinnitus ± facial palsy. *Management*: refer to ENT. Treatment is surgical.

⚠ Refer urgently to ENT to exclude acoustic neuroma if unilateral or asymmetrical sensorineural deafness.[N]

**Hearing aids** can help anyone with reduced hearing, but they never restore perfect hearing. Aids may be:
• *Body worn, behind-the-ear, or in-the-ear.*
• *Analogue or digital* Most traditional aids are analogue aids and amplify all sounds including background noise. Digital aids can be programmed to filter out background noise and customized to the individual's pattern of hearing loss, whistle less, and can have different settings for different sound environments, e.g. TV, crowded rooms.
• *Bone conduction aids* for those with conductive hearing loss or if unable to wear conventional aids because of surgery/malformation.
• *CROS/BiCROS aids* for those with unilateral complete deafness. CROS hearing aids pick up sound from the side with no hearing and feed it to the better ear. BiCROS aids amplify sound from both sides and feed it into the ear that has some hearing.

**Cochlear implants** benefit patients of any age with profound bilateral sensorineural hearing loss. Two components—one external (worn behind the ear) and the other internal (surgically implanted). Intense speech therapy is needed for several years to interpret signals from the implant.

**Information and support for deaf patients and their carers**
**National Deaf Children's Society** ☎ 0808 800 8880 🖥 www.ndcs.org.uk
**Royal National Institute for the Deaf** ☎ 0808 808 0123 Text phone 0808 808 9000 🖥 www.rnid.org.uk
**British Deaf Association** Helpline ☎ 01772 259 725 Text phone 05603 115295 🖥 www.bda.org.uk
**Hearing Concern LINK** ☎ 01323 638230 🖥 www.hearingconcernlink.org

# Tinnitus and vertigo

## Dizziness and giddiness 📖 p.559

**Tinnitus** Ringing or buzzing heard in the ears or head. Occasional tinnitus is common (15% of population), but 2% are severely affected. Patients with tinnitus which interferes with daily life and sleep are prone to depression. *Cause:* often unknown. May accompany hearing loss, or be due to noise exposure, head injury, Ménière's disease, anaemia, ↑BP, or drugs (loop diuretics, tricyclics, aminoglycosides, aspirin, NSAIDs).

**Management** Reassure patients that there is no sinister cause. Refer to audiology for a hearing aid if there is deafness. Drugs are not helpful, but look for and treat associated depression. Psychological support is important—consider referral to a hearing therapist and/or support group (e.g. Tinnitus Association). Masking with background music/radio or an aid that produces white noise (available via ENT) can help. Surgical sectioning of the cochlear nerve is a last resort → deafness.

### Indications for referral to ENT
- Objective tinnitus—noise can be heard by an observer. Rare and may be due to vascular malformations or TMJ problems
- Unilateral tinnitus—especially if associated with deafness. Refer to exclude acoustic neuroma.

**Vertigo** An illusion that the surroundings are spinning. Ask about duration and frequency, associated nausea, deafness and tinnitus, and recent viral symptoms. *Causes:*
- Episodic vertigo lasting a few seconds or minutes—commonly due to benign positional vertigo.
- Episodic vertigo lasting minutes to hours—consider Ménière's disease.
- Prolonged vertigo (>24h)—peripheral lesion, e.g. viral labyrinthitis or trauma, or central lesion (usually associated with other signs), e.g. multiple sclerosis, stroke, tumour.

### Examination
- Look for neurological signs, especially cerebellar signs, cranial nerve lesions and Romberg's sign.
- Assess BP, nystagmus, eardrums, and hearing.
- Hallpike manoeuvre:
  - Move the patient quickly from a sitting position to a supine position with the head turned to one side and extended over the end of the bed—look for nystagmus and ask about vertigo.
  - Repeat with the head turned to the other side.

**Nystagmus** Involuntary oscillatory eye movements—can be congenital or due to labyrinthine or visual system problems. Refer all cases, unless associated with self-limiting labyrinthitis, for assessment.

⚠ Sudden attacks of vertigo can be dangerous. Consider risks of swimming, dangerous machinery, and ladders. Advise patients to stop driving and inform the DVLA—if Group 1 licence can resume once symptoms are controlled; Group 2 licences are restored if symptom free >1y.

**Benign positional vertigo** Sudden onset of vertigo lasting only a few seconds or minutes. Occurs with sudden changes in posture. Common after head injury or viral illness. Possibly caused by otoliths in the labyrinth. Diagnosis is based on history and a +ve Hallpike test. Normal tympanic membrane.

*Management* Usually self-limiting (few weeks), though may continue intermittently for years. Reassure. Labyrinthine sedatives are not helpful. Teach the patient to minimize symptoms by sitting and lying in stages. Habituation may occur by maintaining the trigger position until vertigo settles. If not settling, perform or refer to ENT for Epley's manoeuvre[C] (rapid repositioning of head to move otoliths out of the labyrinth) and/or refer to physiotherapy for exercises.

**Viral labyrinthitis** Usually follows a viral URTI.
- *Symptoms and signs* Sudden onset of vertigo, prostration, nausea and vomiting; no associated loss of hearing; normal tympanic membrane.
- *Treatment* Labyrinthine sedatives, e.g. cyclizine or prochlorperazine.
- *Natural history* Usually resolves in 2–3wk. If persists >6 wk, refer.

**Ménière's syndrome** Overdiagnosed in patients with recurrent vertigo and deafness. It is a complex of symptoms including clustering of attacks of vertigo and nausea, tinnitus, a sense of fullness in the ear, and sensorineural deafness which may be progressive. *Aetiology*: idiopathic dilation of endolymphatic spaces.

*Management*
- Refer all suspected cases to ENT or neurology to confirm diagnosis.
- Provide information and advise about support organizations.
- Treat acute attacks with labyrinthine sedatives, e.g. cyclizine or prochlorperazine. Consider buccal/rectal routes of administration if vomiting. Do not use long term.
- Encourage patients to mobilize after an acute attack.
- Betahistine taken regularly may help in some patients, as may thiazide diuretics, a low-salt diet, vestibular rehabilitation, tinnitus maskers, and/or hearing aids.
- There is some indication that stress may precipitate attacks.
- Look out for and treat concurrent anxiety and depression.
- Labyrinthectomy is a last resort and can help vertigo, but results in deafness on that side.

*P. Ménière (1799–1862), French ENT surgeon.*

---

 **Vertebro-basilar insufficiency** Common in older patients. History of dizziness on extension and rotation of the neck. Normal tympanic membranes. May have associated cervical spondylosis and neck pain. Provide lifestyle advice. ☞ Some advocate use of a cervical collar.

---

**Information and support for patients**
**Royal National Institute for the Deaf (RNID)** ☎ 0808 808 0123
🖥 www.rnid.org.uk
**British Tinnitus Association** ☎ 0800 018 0527 🖥 www.tinnitus.org.uk
**Ménières Society** ☎ 0845 120 2975 🖥 www.menieres.co.uk

# Ophthalmology

'The eye is the window of the mind'
*Richard II*, William Shakespeare (1564–1616)

❶ Community-based optometrists are a valuable resource available to GPs to help differentiate eye conditions and refine referral pathways. Getting an optometrist's opinion can also assist in setting the appropriate priority level for referral or prevent unnecessary referrals.

# Assessment of the eye

**History** Ask about pain, redness, watering, a change in appearance of the eye, altered vision, and if the problem is unilateral or bilateral. Distinguish between blurred and double vision. Enquire about trauma, previous similar episodes, systemic illness, and eye disease in the family.

## Examination

- The eyelids should be symmetrical. Check the skin around the lids, the position of the eyelashes, and any inflammation, crusting, or swelling of the lid or lid margin.
- Then examine the eye surface—it should be bright and shiny. Use a fluorescein stain if any indication of corneal damage.
- Note any redness—if most marked around the lid lining and periphery of the eye, conjunctivitis is likely, whereas a duskier redness around the margin of the cornea (ciliary congestion) suggests disease of the cornea, iris, or deeper parts of the eye (uvea).

**Examining the ocular media** Takes practice. Darken the room and ensure that you have good batteries in the ophthalmoscope. Check the red reflex (opacities within the eye appear as a shadow). Then focus onto the retina—use a systematic approach to avoid missing anything, i.e. start at the optic disc (look for shape, colour, and size of the cup) and then follow each of the four main vessels to the periphery. End by examining the macula: ask the patient to look directly at the light. Dilating the pupils with a short-acting mydriatic (e.g. 0.5–1% tropicamide) makes examination much easier—warn patients that they may have temporarily blurred vision and should not drive home.

**Visual acuity** Test and record the central (macular) vision of each eye separately (with glasses on if worn) for both near and distance. Cover the non-test eye carefully. On a full-size Snellen chart, line 6 can be read by the normal eye at 6m (Figure 26.3—📖 p.955). Near vision can be checked using a newspaper or a near-vision test card (Figure 26.2—📖 p.954). If patients have forgotten their glasses, use a 'pin-hole'.

**Visual fields** Test peripheral vision by sitting in front of the patient and comparing their visual field with your own (one eye at a time)—the most basic test is to check that the patient can see hand movement in each of the four quadrants. Refer for formal tests. Visual field defects—📖 p.969.

**Eye movements** If the patient complains of double vision, move an object to the nine positions of gaze (Figure 26.1) to check when the double vision occurs.

**Pupils** Should be round, central, and of equal size. They should respond equally to light and accommodation. *Pupil abnormalities*:

- **Fixed dilated pupil** Causes: trauma (e.g. blow to the iris), mydriatics, acute glaucoma, 3rd nerve palsy, coning.
- **Afferent pupillary defect** Pupils are the same size but there is an absent constriction response to light in the affected eye; constriction occurs if light is shone into the other eye (consensual response). *Causes*: optic neuritis, retinal disease.

- **Argyll Robertson pupil** Occurs in patients with DM or neurosyphilis. Bilateral small irregular pupils with no light response. *D. Argyll Robertson (1837–1909), Scottish ophthalmologist.*
- **Holmes–Adie pupil** Accommodation is partially paralysed, causing blurring of near vision, slight pupil dilation, and a very slow pupil response to light and accommodation (minutes). Occurs unilaterally in young adults. It is not associated with serious neurological disease. *G.M. Holmes (1876–1965), Irish neurologist; W.J. Adie (1886–1935), British neurologist.*
- **Horner's syndrome** 📖 p.308.

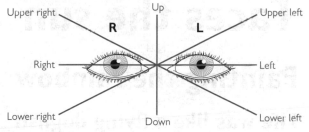

**Fig. 26.1** The 9 positions of gaze (straight ahead is one position)

**Table 26.1** Eye referrals

| | |
|---|---|
| Emergency referral (direct to A&E or emergency eye clinic) | Sudden loss of vision |
| | Acute glaucoma |
| | Perforating injury, intraocular foreign body |
| | Chemical burns |
| | Retinal detachment |
| | Corneal ulcer |
| | Sudden onset of diplopia or squint + pain |
| | Temporal arteritis with visual symptoms—📖 p.532 |
| Same day (<24h) | Hyphema or vitreous haemorrhage |
| | Orbital fracture |
| | Sudden onset of ocular inflammation, e.g. iritis or ophthalmic herpes zoster |
| | Corneal foreign bodies or abrasions |
| Urgent (<2wk) | Central visual loss |
| | Sinister 'floaters' |
| | Flashing lights without a field defect |
| | Chronic glaucoma with pressure >35mmHg |
| Routine referral | Gradual loss of vision |
| | Chronic glaucoma (unless pressure >35mmHg) |
| | Chronic red eye conditions |
| | Painless diplopia or squint |
| | Chalazion/stye/cyst |
| | Ptosis |
| | Headaches and migraine* |

\* Urgent if sinister cause suspected (📖 p.560)

N.48

# She waved

N.36

# Faces the sun

N.24

# Painting the rainbow

N.18

## Life was like a flying dogfish

N.14

### Quietly a storm drove purple ducks across the road. The chimney top

N.12

### Glowed in the dusk and my sister let her biscuit fall through ashes. September was

N.10

**In drizzling mood when hedgehogs threw pinecones in the dark. Squirrels played classical music.**

N.8

**We won a feather duster by encouraging Jessica to bake an enormous apple pie and pirouette between the tables.**

N.6

**Queuing had never appealed to the young porcupines but swimming held great drama for the blue and pink ostrich.**

N.5

Delight was exceeding the pleasures of everyday ambulation and breaking the pattern of a melancholy existence to see the trees.

**Fig. 26.2** Near-vision reading card—reading types are read at 30cm with reading glasses if used

Reproduced from Collier *et al.* *Oxford Handbook of Clinical Specialties* 6e (2003), with permission from Oxford University Press.

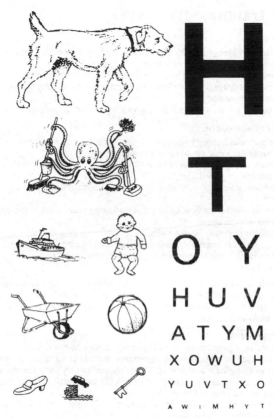

❶ These Snellen charts are for illustration purposes only. Lines on a full-sized chart are read from a distance of 6m with distance glasses if worn. Read from the top of the chart to the bottom. *Interpretation:*

| Able to read | 6 | Normal vision | 6/6 |
|---|---|---|---|
| *down to the* | 9 | Can see at 6m what a normal person can see at 9m | 6/9 |
| *line labelled:* | 12 | Can see at 6m what a normal person can see at 12m | 6/12 |
| | 18 | Can see at 6m what a normal person can see at 18m | 6/18 |
| | 36 | Can see at 6m what a normal person can see at 36m | 6/36 |
| | 60 | Can see at 6m what a normal person can see at 60m | 6/60 |
| *Counts fingers* | | Counts fingers held at 0.5m distance | CF |
| *Hand movement* | | Perceives hand moving at 0.25m distance | HM |
| *Perceives light* | | Can see a torch light when shone into the eye | PL |
| *No perceived light* | | Blind | No PL |

**Fig. 26.3** Snellen charts

Reproduced from Collier *et al. Oxford Handbook of Clinical Specialities* 6e (2003), with permission from Oxford University Press.

# Eye trauma

### In all cases

- Measure and record acuity and examine both eyes carefully—you may be asked to write a legal report on your findings.
- If the patient is unable to open the injured eye, try to instill local anaesthetic drops and then examine. If unable to do so, refer to eye casualty for assessment
- Encourage accident prevention, e.g. wearing protective goggles.

### Corneal abrasions

- Take a careful history to exclude high-speed particles, (e.g. from strimmer etc.) that could cause penetrating injury.
- Abrasions may cause severe pain—if so, apply a few drops of local anaesthetic (e.g. oxybuprocaine 0.4%) before examining.
- Use fluorescein stain with blue light illumination to detect abrasion (Plate 7).
- If the abrasion is vertical, ensure that no foreign body is left in the eye by everting the upper lid.
- Abrasions normally heal in <48h.
- Prescribe chloramphenicol eye drops qds until healing is complete.
- Eye padding is not needed except to protect the eye after a local anaesthetic.

**Superficial foreign bodies** Cause discomfort, a 'foreign body sensation', and watering. They can be difficult to see, so examine very carefully (Plate 8), including everting the eyelids. The foreign body sensation may come from an abrasion.

### Management

- If metal or a penetrating injury is suspected, refer to eye casualty.
- Superficial foreign bodies can be removed with a corner of clean card after instilling local anaesthetic. If that fails, you can try using the tip of a sterile green needle (bent if necessary), but be careful. Refer to eye casualty if you are not confident.
- After removal, treat with topical antibiotics, e.g. chloramphenicol every 2h for 3d then qds for 5d.
- If left >12h, a rust ring may form around a metal foreign body—refer to eye casualty for removal.

**Arc eye** Due to corneal epithelial damage as a result of exposure to UV light. Seen in welders, sunbed users, skiers, mountaineers, and sailors who don't use adequate eye protection. Symptoms include severe eye pain, watering, and blepharospasm a few hours after exposure.

**Management** Pad the eye and give analgesics and cyclopentolate 1% eye drops bd (causes pupil dilation). Recovery should occur within 24h—if not refer. Advise patients on suitable protective wear for future exposure.

**Blunt injury** Caused by fists, squash balls, etc. The result may be anything from a 'black eye' to globe rupture. Globe rupture is usually obvious with a wound and severely ↓ vision. More minor injuries include subconjunctival haemorrhage (🕮 p.965) or corneal abrasion.

### Refer urgently if

- Visual acuity is affected
- Double vision
- Lacerated conjunctiva
- **Hyphaema** blood in the anterior chamber
- Unable to see posterior limit of a subconjunctival haemorrhage—may indicate orbital fracture
- Persistent pupil dilation—usually recovers spontaneously but may indicate a torn iris
- Any signs of retinal damage (oedema, choroidal rupture), or
- If you cannot assess the eye, e.g. if lid swelling or pain prevents examination.

**'Blow-out' fracture of the orbit** Uncommon fracture due to blunt trauma to the eye (e.g. squash ball injury).

**Signs** Enophthalmos (often masked by swelling), infra-orbital nerve loss, and inability to look upwards due to trapping of inferior rectus muscle.

**Action** Refer for X-ray and assessment of eye trauma via A&E.

**Penetrating wounds** Refer urgently to eye casualty if penetrating injury is a possibility, i.e. history of flying object or working with hammers, drills, lathes, or chisels where a metal fragment may fly off. X-ray/CT scan can confirm diagnosis and help locate the foreign body.

### Symptoms/signs

- Wound may be tiny.
- Vision may initially be normal or may be very poor, depending on the size of the foreign body.
- Eye is painful and waters.
- Photophobia, hyphaema, and/or pupil distortion.

⚠ **Do not remove large foreign bodies (dart or knife)**—support the object with padding whilst transferring the patient supine to eye casualty or A&E. Cover the other eye to prevent damage from conjugate movement.

**Chemical burns** can cause great damage, particularly alkali injuries. Use topical anaesthetic (e.g. oxybuprocaine 0.4%) before examining. Hold the lids open, brush out any powder, and irrigate with large amounts (1–2L) of clean saline or water immediately. Do not try to neutralize the acid or alkali. Refer urgently to eye casualty.

# Eye pain, papilloedema, and orbital disease

**Eye pain** *Consider:*
- *Painful conditions* Corneal abrasion, foreign body, keratitis, iritis, scleritis, acute glaucoma, ophthalmic shingles, arc eye.
- *Eye discomfort* Conjunctivitis, entropion, trichiasis, dry eye, episcleritis, optic neuritis.
- *Referred pain* Tension type headache, migraine, refractive error, trigeminal neuralgia, ophthalmic shingles, giant cell arteritis, ocular muscle imbalance, ↑ ICP.
- *Photophobia* Painful vision in normal light. One of the three principle features of meningism. Associated with meningitis. Discomfort in the light can also be due to eye disease, e.g. conjunctivitis and migraine.

**Papilloedema** (Plate 9). *Causes:*
- Intracranial space-occupying lesion
- Encephalitis
- SAH
- Benign intracranial hypertension
- Malignant hypertension
- Optic neuritis
- Disc infiltration, e.g. leukaemia
- Ischaemic optic neuropathy
- Retinal venous obstruction
- Metabolic causes, e.g. hypocalcaemia

⚠ Always refer any patient with papilloedema for immediate specialist medical opinion.

**Swelling around the eyes** Oedema around the eyes gives the face a bloated appearance. Swollen eyelids may partially close the eyes. In severe cases the whole face becomes oedematous. It is associated with nephrotic syndrome, allergic reactions (e.g. pollen, dust or insect bites), angio-oedema, and periorbital cellulitis.

**Exophthalmos** The eyes protrude from the orbit and thus have a staring appearance. Stand at the same level as the patient and look at the patient's eyes. There should be no white of the sclera visible below the iris. If the eye is pushed forward, as in exophthalmos, white sclera is seen below the iris and the patient can look upwards without moving his/her eyebrows (distinguishes from lid retraction).
- *Bilateral* Caused by Graves' disease (📖 p.372)
- *Unilateral* Caused by Graves' disease, orbital disease (e.g. tumours; cellulitis); vascular disease (e.g. cavernous sinus thrombosis, carotid-cavernous fistula); sinus disease (e.g. tumour)

 **Microphthalmos** 1:1000 live births. Small eyes. Associated with Down's syndrome and other genetic abnormalities.

## Orbital inflammation

*Preseptal cellulitis* Infections of the upper lid may cause significant swelling and redness around the eye. Typically affects children following mild trauma. The eye is unaffected—infection is localized to skin and superficial tissues. Treat as localized cellulitis with oral antibiotics (e.g. flucloxacillin). Monitor carefully as can progress to orbital cellulitis.

**Orbital cellulitis** Typically due to spread of infection from the paranasal sinuses. Usually presents with pain, double/blurred vision, and general malaise. *Signs*: fever, eyelid swelling, proptosis, and inability to move the eye. Severe cases can lead to septicaemia, meningitis, and cavernous sinus thromboses. If suspected, refer immediately to ophthalmology for IV antibiotics/surgical drainage.

**Thyroid eye disease** 📖 p.373

**Orbital tumours** The eye is in a confined space within the orbit. Any ↑ in mass, pushes the eye forwards. *Symptoms/signs*:
• Unilateral proptosis is a tumour until proven otherwise.
• Orbital pain—especially in rapidly growing malignant tumours.
• Lid swelling/distortion.
• Limitation of eye movements ± diplopia.
• ↓ visual acuity—involvement of optic nerve, retina, or vascular supply.

⚠ If suspected—refer for urgent ophthalmology opinion.

**Tumours may be**
• *Primary*—benign or malignant. Any orbital structure may be involved, e.g. lacrimal gland (carcinoma or adenoma); retina (retinoblastoma in children, melanoma), optic nerve (neurofibroma, astrocytoma, meningioma); lymphoid tissue (lymphoma); connective tissue (rhabdomyosarcoma— rapid growing causing proptosis, ocular inflammation, and poor vision due to optic nerve involvement)
• *Due to spread from adjacent structures*, e.g. post-nasal space tumour.
• *Due to blood-borne metastases*, e.g. breast, leukaemia, neuroblastoma, Ewing's sarcoma.

**Information for patients and carers**
**Eye Care Trust** Information on anophthalmia and microphthalmia
🖳 www.eyecaretrust.org.uk
**Micro- and Anophthalmic Children's Society (MACS)** ☎ 0800 169 8088
🖳 www.macs.org.uk

# Lid disease

**Ingrowing lashes (trichiasis)** Causes an irritable foreign body feeling in the eye ± recurrent infection. In severe cases, the ingrowing lashes may damage the cornea. Refer to ophthalmology.

**Loss of eyelashes (madarosis)** Usually due to blepharitis (📖 p.962) in which case the condition is bilateral and associated with other symptoms/signs of blepharitis. Other causes include plucking/rubbing (may be unilateral or bilateral), alopecia areata, and discoid lupus (scarring madarosis). Sometimes no cause is found. Treat the cause.

**Depigmentation of the eyelashes (poliosis)** Vitiligo can affect the eyelids. There is usually a family history. Associated with other autoimmune disease, e.g. thyroid disease.

**Entropion** In-turning of the eyelids due to degenerative changes or secondary to scarring. Most commonly affects the lower lid. ↑ with age (rare <40y). The eyelashes rub on the cornea and irritate the eye. Taping the lower lid to the cheek can give temporary relief. If left untreated, can cause corneal vascularization, ulceration, and infection. Refer for rapid surgical correction.

**Ectropion** Turning out of the lower eyelid. Causes eye irritation and watering. Most common in the elderly or those with facial nerve palsy (📖 p.545). Refer for consideration of surgery.

**Ptosis** From the Greek meaning 'to fall', ptosis describes drooping of the upper eyelid. When the normal eye is looking straight forward, the margin of the upper lid is situated ~2mm above the pupil. Ask the patient to look downwards as far as possible and then upwards as far as possible. The lid margin should move >8mm. The lid margin moves <4mm in patients with severe ptosis. To determine the cause, look at the pupil.
• *Dilated pupil*—oculomotor nerve palsy. Refer urgently to neurology
• *Constricted pupil*—Horner's syndrome, tabes dorsalis
• *Normal pupil*—old age, congenital, myasthenia gravis, muscular dystrophy, myopathy, botulism. Treat the cause where possible.

>  **Congenital ptosis** Unilateral/bilateral weakness of the levator muscle. Children may compensate by tilting their heads upwards to see better. About half have associated superior rectus muscle weakness. Refer for surgical correction if obstructing vision as may cause amblyopia.

## Neurological causes of ptosis
• *Oculomotor (3rd nerve palsy)*—Often ptosis is complete and the pupil dilated. Refer urgently to neurology to exclude tumour.[N]
• *Horner's syndrome*—📖 p.308
• *Tabes dorsalis*—2° to syphilis.

## Muscular and mechanical causes of ptsosis
• *Senile*—most common cause of ptosis. Due to age-related changes in the levator muscle. Refer if causing problems.
• *Myaesthenia gravis*—📖 p.556

- *Muscular dystrophy,* e.g. myotonic or oculopharyngeal dystrophy.
- *Myopathy,* e.g. Graves disease.
- *Mechanical* Swelling of the eyelid due to allergy, mass effect of tumour.

## Causes of localized eyelid swelling

- Stye
- Chalazion
- Sebaceous cyst
- Papilloma
- Xanthelasma
- Marginal cyst of Zeis/Moll
- Dermoid cyst—usually upper inner or outer angles of the orbit
- BCC (rodent ulcer)—usually at the lid margin
- Lacrimal gland and lacrimal sac disorders (📖 p.962).

**Stye** Common eyelid infection—2 forms.

*External stye (hordeolum externum)* Most common form of stye. Infection of a lash follicle or associated gland of Moll (sweat gland) or Zeis (sebum gland) usually by *Staphylococcus aureus*. Confined to the skin and always points outwards. Treat with hot compresses and topical antibiotics (e.g. chloramphenicol ointment).

*Marginal cyst of Zeis or Moll* Non-infected swellings of the glands of Zeis/ Moll. No treatment needed unless troublesome, when refer.

*Internal stye (hordeolum internum)* Abscess of a meibomiam gland. Often causes less swelling than external stye. May point inwards onto the conjunctiva (seen as red patch with yellow centre before it bursts) or outwards through the skin. Treat in the same way as external stye with hot compresses and topical antibiotics.

*Chalazion/meibomiam cyst* Following an internal stye, the meibomiam gland may become blocked, forming a cyst. Cysts may resolve spontaneously but often become infected (treat with topical antibiotics) and/or chronic. If recurrent infection or chronic cyst, refer to ophthalmology for incision and curettage. ❶ Refer early if <7y as large cysts can affect refraction and generate amblyopia.

**Squamous cell papilloma** Benign skin tumour, which may form a horn-like lesion. Refer for excision/curettage.

**Blepharitis** 📖 p.962

**Xanthelasma** 📖 p.241

**Basal cell carcinoma (rodent ulcer, BCC)** 📖 p.629

## Further information

**NICE** Referral guidelines for suspected cancer (2005) 🖥 www.nice.org.uk

## Information for patients

**Eye Care Trust** Patient information on eyelid and tear gland disorders 🖥 www.eyecaretrust.org.uk

**Good Hope NHS Hospital Trust** Patient information on stye and chalazion 🖥 www.goodhope.org.uk/departments/eyedept

# Blepharitis and tear duct problems

**Blepharitis** Chronic low-grade inflammation of meibomian glands and lid margins. Presents with long history of irritable burning dry red eyes. Eyelids have red margins ± scales on the eyelashes—on elevation of the upper lid, look for inflamed meibomian glands. Associated with dry eyes, internal stye (🕮 p.961), and ingrowing eyelashes.

**Differential diagnosis** Lid papilloma and warts can become inflamed and mimic blepharitis.

**Management** Prolonged treatment is often needed.
- Removal of scales and crusts from the lid margins.
- Treat dry eye symptoms with preservative-free tear supplements, e.g. Liquifilm®.
- Exacerbations—treat with fusidate eye drops rubbed into the lid margins. Steroid ointment may occasionally be useful (only use on specialist advice and for ≤ 2wk). Systemic tetracycline may be necessary in severe cases.

### Blepharitis: eye care instructions

1 Apply a warm, moist hand towel to the closed lids for 10–20 minutes in the morning and at bedtime.
2 Following the warm compress at bedtime, mix a solution of half baby shampoo and half warm water in the cap from a bottle of the baby shampoo. Put the solution on a wet wash cloth or cotton wool bud, and gently scrub from side to side on the upper eyelids and lashes for 15–20 seconds.
3 Pull the lower lid down and away from the eyeball and gently scrub side to side along the edge of the lower eyelid and lashes for 15–20 seconds. Avoid scrubbing the eyeball.
4 Rinse the cloth and clean any remaining shampoo from the lids with clear warm water.
5 When instructed, place a 1cm strip of fucithalmic ointment under the lower lids at bedtime and rub the excess onto the lid edges.
6 If there is a problem with dandruff of the scalp and eyebrows, shampooing frequently with a shampoo containing selenium sulphide or pyrithione zinc (such as Head & Shoulders™) will be helpful.
7 Continue this treatment for 2–3 months or until the problem is controlled. After an initial treatment period, it will probably be necessary to continue to use warm compresses and lid scrubs from time to time to keep the lid scales under control.

Alternatives to baby shampoo include bicarbonate of soda solution or sterile impregnated Lid-Care® wipes.

**Dry eye syndrome (keratoconjunctivitis sicca)** Tear secretion ↓ with age. Dry eyes cause eye irritation and redness which is often worse in centrally heated buildings. The eye feels gritty, vision is occasionally blurred, and there is reflex watering of the eye in severe cases.

**Causes** ↓ tear production (e.g. age, Sjögren's syndrome), ↑ evaporation of tears (e.g. exposure keratitis), or mucin deficiency in the tears.

## Management
- Treat with artificial tears, e.g. Viscotears®, hypromellose, Liquifilm®. If one preparation does not work, try another. Always use preservative-free drops—hypersensitivity can be a problem with prolonged use.
- If simple medication fails, try combined short- and long-acting drops, e.g. Celluvisc® tds and Liquifilm® tds.
- Refer to ophthalmology if continuing symptoms despite treatment.

❶ Long-acting drops (e.g. Celluvisc®, Viscotears®) blur vision for a time. Short-acting drops (e.g. Liquifilm®) only give relief for ~30min and may need very frequent application.

**Watering eyes (epiphoria)** Due to overproduction of tears or outflow obstruction. Caused by emotion, corneal irritation (e.g. blepharitis, corneal abrasion, foreign body, conjunctivitis, entropion), iritis, acute glaucoma, ectropion, blocked tear duct.

**Acute dacryocystitis** Acute infection of the tear sac—can spread to surrounding tissues. Treat immediately with antibiotics, e.g. flucloxacilin. Abscess can form—if it does surgical drainage is required, so refer.

**Chronic dacryocystitis** Seen in the middle-aged and elderly. Presents with a watery eye which discharges mucus regularly. The eye does not look inflamed. Refer for syringing of the lacrimal system or surgery.

---

**Infantile dacryocystitis (blocked tear duct)** Delay in canalization/obstruction of the lacrimal duct causing persistent watering or sticky eyes in 20% of babies. Vision is normal and there is no conjunctival inflammation. If the lower lid conjunctiva is reddened, swab to exclude chlamydia (🕮 p. 738).

**Management** Advise parents to bathe the lids with cooled boiled water. Avoid antibiotic eye drops unless there is clear infection. Spontaneous resolution is the norm. 4% fail to clear by 1y—refer to a paediatric ophthalmologist. Treatment is by probing the duct to clear it.

---

## Information for patients
**Eye Care Trust** Patient information on blepharitis, eyelid and tear gland disorders 🖥 www.eyecaretrust.org.uk
**Good Hope NHS Hospital Trust** Patient information on blepharitis, dry eyes, watery eyes and blocked lacrimal duct in children
🖥 www.goodhope.org.uk/departments/eyedept

# The red eye and conjunctivitis

⚠ **'Red flag' signs of a potentially dangerous red eye**
- ↓ visual acuity.
- Pain deep in the eye—not surface irritation as with conjunctivitis.
- Absent or sluggish pupil response.
- Corneal damage on fluorescein staining.
- History of trauma.

Refer the patient to be seen by a specialist the same day

**Differential diagnosis** Think systematically about the structures within the eye to come to a differential diagnosis (Table 26.2).

**Conjunctivitis** Inflammation of the conjunctiva is the most common eye problem seen in general practice (Plate 10)—1:8 children have an episode of acute infective conjunctivitis every year. Presents with red sore eye; eye discharge (clear, mucoid or muco-purulent); sticking of the eyelids especially on waking; no change in visual acuity. Examination may reveal enlarged papillae under the upper eyelid and/or pre-auricular lymph node enlargement.

**Bacterial or viral conjunctivitis** Clinically difficult to distinguish—doctors get it right only ~50% of the time. Both present with acute red eye, usually starting in one eye and often spreading to involve both, together with watery/purulent discharge. The eyes are often crusted ± stuck together on waking. Visual acuity is not impaired. Both may occur in association with viral URTI.

*Management*
- Recent evidence shows that in ~85% of cases, acute infective conjunctivitis clears in <7d with or without treatment.
- Advise patients to bathe the affected eye(s) with boiled cooled water morning and night.
- If symptoms are not improving in >5d, take a swab for M,C&S (± chlamydia) and treat empirically with chloramphenicol qds or sodium fusidate bd for 5d. ❶ Chloramphenicol is available OTC.
- If still not clearing, act on swab results or consider alternative diagnosis, e.g. allergy, dry eyes.

⚠ Advise patients to seek medical advice if: ↓ visual acuity, eye becomes painful rather than sore/gritty, or symptoms are not improving in 5d.

**Allergic conjunctivitis** Bilateral symptoms appear seasonally (e.g. hay fever) or on contact with an allergen (e.g. animal fur). Presents with red watery itchy eyes ± photophobia ± family/personal history of atopy. *Signs*: follicles in the lower tarsal conjunctiva and 'cobblestones' under the upper lid.

**Management** Treat with topical or systemic antihistamines (e.g. sodium cromoglicate eye drops). Avoid topical steroids because of long-term complications (cataract, glaucoma, fungal infection). Consider cold compress and wash-out with cold water during acute exacerbations. Refer if symptoms are persistent despite treatment, or if vision is affected.

**Table 26.2** Differential diagnosis of red eye

| Structure | Condition |
|---|---|
| *Inflammation of the orbit* | Thyroid eye disease/exomphalos—📖 p.373 |
| | Orbital cellulitis—📖 p.959 |
| | Tumour—📖 p.959 |
| *Lid disease* | Stye—📖 p.961 |
| | Chalazion—📖 p.961 |
| | Blepharitis—📖 p.962 |
| | Allergic eye disease |
| *Scleral inflammation* | Scleritis/episcleritis—📖 p.967 |
| | Post-operative inflammation |
| *Conjunctival disease* | Viral infection |
| | Bacterial infection |
| | Chlamydial infection |
| | Allergy |
| | Subconjunctival haemorrhage |
| *Corneal disease* | Foreign body/trauma—📖 p.956 |
| | Corneal abrasion—📖 p.956 |
| | Dry eye syndrome—📖 p.962 |
| | Ophthalmic shingles—📖 p.967 |
| | Corneal ulceration—📖 p.966 |
| | Arc eye—📖 p.956 |
| *Uveal/iris inflammation* | Anterior uveitis—📖 p.967 |
| | Posterior uveitis/toxoplasma |
| *Other causes of red eye* | Acute glaucoma—📖 p.975 |
| | Post operative endophthalmitis—📖 p.977 |

***Ophthlamia neonatorum*** 📖 p.738

***Herpes simplex keratoconjunctivitis*** 📖 p.966

**Subconjunctival haemorrhage** Spontaneous painless localized haemorrhage under the conjunctiva (Plate 11). Common in the elderly. Looks alarming but is generally painless (may cause some aching of the eye). Clears spontaneously in 1–2wk but may recur. *Associations:* ↑BP, clotting disorders, leukaemia, ↑ venous pressure. Check BP. If severe/recurrent, check FBC and clotting screen.

❶ Consider referral if follows trauma, especially if the posterior edge of the haemorrhage cannot be seen (it may be associated with orbital haematoma, penetrating injury, or orbital fracture).

**Pterygium/pinguecula** 📖 p.966

**Information for patients**
**Eye Care Trust** 🖥 www.eyecaretrust.org.uk

# Corneal, scleral, and uveal disease

**Corneal abrasions** 📖 p.956        **Arc eye** 📖 p.956

**Superficial foreign bodies** 📖 p.956        **Corneal arcus** 📖 p.241

**Pinguecula/pterygium** Common. Found particularly in people who work outdoors in hot dusty climates. Creamy coloured raised triangular plaque on the conjunctiva on either side of the cornea—nasal side > temporal side. If it grows over the edge of the cornea termed pterygium else termed pinguecula (Plate 12). No need to treat unless encroaching over the pupil and causing visual loss → refer for surgical excision—recurrence is possible. ❶ Differential diagnosis is carcinoma *in situ*—if any atypical features, refer for excision biopsy.

**Corneal vascularization** Growth of blood vessels onto the cornea. Occurs in patients with severe lid disease, rosacea, or due to excessive contact lens wear. If a contact lens wearer, advise to remove contact lenses for at least 2mo. Refer to ophthalmology for specialist management to prevent long term damage.

### Keratitis, keratoconjunctivitis, and corneal ulceration

- Keratitis is inflammation of the cornea.
- Keratoconjunctivitis is inflammation of the conjunctiva and cornea.

*Presentation* Presents with a very painful eye, blurred vision, photophobia, and profuse watering. On examination there is ↓ visual acuity, circumcorneal injection (blood vessel dilatation concentrated around the limbus), conjunctivitis (particularly the quadrant most associated with the injury/infection) ± a creamy white disc-shaped lesion on the central or inferior cornea. The pupil may be small due to reflex miosis. Corneal ulcers stain green with fluorescein—use a bright light with a blue filter to see them.

*Causes* Bacterial—2° to trauma, foreign body, dry eyes, entropion, blepharitis; viral—herpes simplex, herpes zoster, or adenovirus; fungal; protozoal—history of foreign travel/contact lens wear; non-infective, e.g. 2° to autoimmune disease or trauma.

*Management* Treatment depends on cause. Delay in treatment may result in loss of sight so refer for same-day ophthalmology assessment.

**Herpes simplex infection and dendritic ulcer** HSV keratitis is common and can be recurrent in the same eye with the virus lying dormant within the trigeminal nerve between attacks. Presents with acute keratitis or keratoconjunctivitis. Occasionally may present as an irritable eye with little discomfort. Examination and fluorescein staining reveals a characteristic corneal ulcer with a delicate branching pattern (dendritic ulcer). Refer for urgent (same-day) ophthalmology opinion. Treatment is with 3% aciclovir ointment 5×/d continued for 3d after healing.

⚠ There is a danger of massive amoebic ulceration and blindness if steroid eye drops are administered to patients with dendritic ulcer.

**Ophthalmic shingles** Zoster in the ophthalmic branch of the oculo-motor (3rd) nerve. Pain, tingling, or numbness around the eye precedes a blistering rash and inflammation. In 50% the eye is affected with conjunc-tivitis, scleritis, episcleritis, keratitis, iritis, visual loss, and/or oculomotor nerve palsy. Nose tip involvement makes eye involvement likely (nerve supply is the same as the globe). Prescribe oral aciclovir (800mg 5×/d) and refer immediately. The cornea may become anaesthetic/scarred and require grafting.

**Episcleritis** The episclera is the thin layer of vascular tissue overlying the sclera. Episcleritis is unilateral in 2:3 cases. It presents with diffuse inflammation of the eye with minimal tenderness and no discharge. Try treatment with an NSAID (e.g. ibuprofen 400mg tds or ketorolac 0.5% eye drops qds). If NSAID is ineffective, refer to ophthalmology for considera-tion of treatment with steroids.

**Scleritis** Inflammation of the sclera. Can be unilateral or bilateral. ♀ > ♂. *Peak age*: 40–60y. Affects the anterior or posterior segment and may be diffuse, nodular, or necrotizing. Presents with painful red eye. Vision may be blurred due to corneal, iris, or posterior segment involvement, and visual acuity ↓. The eye is tender to touch, and may have a deep purple hue. Look for scleral nodules. There may be accompanying uveitis and keratitis.

*Associations* In ~50% associated with systemic illness, e.g. herpes zoster, rheumatoid arthritis, systemic lupus erythematosis, polyarteritis nodosum, Wegener's granulomatosis, trauma, infection, or surgery.

*Management* Refer urgently to ophthalmology. Treated with steroids. Complications include cataract, glaucoma, and retinal detachment.

**Iritis (anterior uveitis)** Most common in young/middle-aged adults. Acute onset of pain, photophobia, blurred vision, and ↓visual acuity, watering, circumcorneal redness, small or irregular pupil ± keratitic precipitates on the posterior surface of the cornea ± *hypopyon* (anterior chamber pus, causing a white 'fluid-level' line). Pain ↑ as eyes converge and pupils constrict. May be secondary to corneal graft rejection or eye infections, e.g. toxoplasmosis, herpes virus keratitis. In 30% associated with seronegative arthropathies, e g ankylosing spondylitis.

*Management* Refer urgently to ophthalmology. Complications include posterior synechiae (irregular pupil shape), glaucoma, and cataract. Relapses are common.

### Information for patients
**Eye Care Trust** ⌨ www.eyecaretrust.org.uk
**Good Hope NHS Hospital Trust**
⌨ www.goodhope.org.uk/departments/eyedept
**Uveitis Information Group** ☎ 01806 577310 ⌨ www.uveitis.net

# Visual field loss and blindness

**Visual field loss** Not all patients who have a visual field loss are aware of it. ❶ If you suspect visual field loss, refer to a community optometrist or ophthalmology for formal field testing. *Causes*: Figure 26.4.

**Blindness** is defined as inability to perform any work for which eyesight is essential (not the total absence of sight). In practice this means <3/60 vision (may be >3/60 if patient has severe visual field defect, e.g. glaucoma). 157 000 people are registered blind in England.

**Partial sightedness** does not have a standard definition but usually implies vision in the range 3/60–6/60. 155 000 people are registered partially sighted in England.

### Major causes of blindness in the UK
- *Elderly* Macular degeneration; glaucoma.
- *Younger patients* Diabetic retinopathy; uveitis; inherited retinal disease; retinovascular disease.

❶ Worldwide, chlamydial infection causing trachoma is a common cause.

**Registration of blindness and partial sight** Voluntary in England. Refer patients with low vision for assessment. Application is made by a consultant ophthalmologist to social services.

**Support** Many patients benefit from links with national support organizations who provide information, and active local organizations who support the blind and partially sighted with drivers and guides.

**Driving** 📖 p.133

## Colour blindness
**Congenital colour blindness** Inherited as a sex-linked characteristic. ♂:♀ ≈ 20:1. The Ishihara test consists of series of cards with a number in coloured dots against a contrasting background of more coloured dots. Coloured dots are paired to detect different patterns of colour blindness. Lack of red–green discrimination is most common. Colour blindness prohibits certain types of employment (e.g. airline pilot).

**Impaired colour recognition** Occurs later in life. Red is the most common colour affected. May be an early sign of an optic nerve disorder. Patients complain of colour looking 'washed out' (desaturated) in one eye compared with the other—refer.

## Information and support for patients and carers
**Royal National Institute for the Blind** Information and talking book service ☎ 0303 123 9999 🖥 www.rnib.org.uk
**Partially Sighted Society** ☎ 0844 477 4966 🖥 www.partsight.org.uk
**LOOK** For families of blind/visually impaired children ☎ 0121 428 5038 🖥 www.look-uk.org
**National Blind Children's Society** ☎ 01278 764 764 🖥 www.nbcs.org.uk

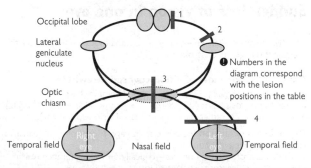

| Defect (lesion position) | Description and causes |
|---|---|
| Bilateral homonymous hemianopia (1) | Normal eyes; normal papillary responses; no conscious vision (cortical blindness) *Cause:* bilateral damage to the visual cortex—usually CVA. |
| Homonymous hemianopia (1) | Half the visual field is affected symmetrically in both eyes. Macular fibres may be preserved (macular sparing) if the posterior cerebral artery is functional. *Cause:* strokes involving the middle cerebral artery. |
| Quadrantinopia (2) | Loss of a homonymous (symmetrical) quadrant of vision indicates temporal lobe disease with superior defect and parietal lobe disease with inferior loss. *Causes:* vascular events, tumours, trauma. |
| Bitemporal hemianopia (3) | The temporal side of the visual field is affected in both eyes. If one nerve is completely affected, a junctional scotoma results. *Causes:* compressive chiasmal lesions, e.g. pituitary tumour, craniopharyngioma, or meningioma. |
| Altitudinal defect (4) | Field defect respecting the horizontal. *Cause:* optic nerve disease, e.g. optic neuropathy, optic neuritis. |
| Enlarged blind spot (4) | Blind spot is enlarged if the optic disc is enlarged. *Causes:* papilloedema, disc inflammation, infiltration with lymphoma. |
| Central scotoma (4) | Loss of central vision with normal visual field around it. May be unilateral or bilateral.<br>• *Bilateral causes:* toxic (e.g. tobacco), $B_{12}$ deficiency, MS, age-related macular degeneration, inherited.<br>• *Unilateral causes:* glioma of optic nerve, vascular lesion. |
| Tunnel vision | Loss of peripheral vision in all directions. *Causes:* glaucoma, retinitis pigmentosa, retinal detachment, functional visual loss (visual fields having no anatomical correspondence). |
| Loss of vision from one eye | Due to lesions of the retina or optic nerve anterior to the optic chiasm. *Causes:* retinal detachment, retinal vein occlusion, optic neuropathy, infiltration of the nerve, demyelination, compression of the nerve. |

**Fig. 26.4** Visual field loss, position of lesion, and causes

# Sudden loss of vision in one eye

⚠ Always refer as an emergency to ophthalmology—unless you are certain it is migraine or stroke

### Causes of sudden loss of vision covered elsewhere

- Acute glaucoma (📖 p.975)
- Stroke/amaurosis fugax (📖 p.570)
- Wet AMD (rapid rather than sudden loss of vision—📖 p.972).
- Migraine (📖 p.562)
- Temporal arteritis (📖 p.532)

**Retinal vein occlusion** Incidence ↑ with age. More common than arterial occlusion. *Presents with*:

- Sudden loss of vision in one eye—typically on waking (branch retinal vein occlusion causes partial visual loss).
- Fundus like 'a stormy sunset'—scattered haemorrhages, engorged veins, disc swelling ± cotton wool spots.
- ± painful eye due to neovascular glaucoma ± afferent pupil defect.

#### *Causes*

- Glaucoma
- Arteriosclerosis
- ↑BP
- Polycythaemia
- Hypercholesterolaemia
- ↑ homocysteine.

**Management** Refer as an emergency to ophthalmology. Laser treatment may prevent neovascular glaucoma ('90-day glaucoma' due to iris neovascularization) and vitreous haemorrhage due to retinal neovascularization. Macular oedema may be helped by intraocular steroids.

**Retinal artery occlusion** Usually due to thromboembolism. Sudden visual loss in one eye (counting fingers or light perception) and afferent pupil defect. The retina appears white ± cherry red spot at the macular. A retinal embolus may be visible. Exclude temporal arteritis (📖 p.532).

⚠ *If the patient presents <1h after onset* Applying then releasing firm eyeball pressure can sometimes dislodge an embolus into one of the smaller branches and thus preserve some vision.

**Management** Refer as an emergency to ophthalmology. There is no reliable treatment.[C] Usual outcome is optic atrophy and blindness. Treat any risk factors for atherosclerosis or embolism, i.e. ↑BP, hyperlipidaemia, smoking, DM, carotid/cardiac disease.

**Vitreous haemorrhage** Presents with sudden ↓ in vision, loss of red reflex, and difficulty visualizing the retina. *Risk factors*: DM with new vessel formation, bleeding disorders, retinal tear/detachment, central retinal vein occlusion, trauma, head injury, tumour. Refer urgently to ophthalmology. Treatment is with vitrectomy and repair of retinal damage with laser therapy or cryotherapy.

**Retinal detachment** Affects 1:5000 people each year. *Presents with*:
- Painless loss of vision—'like a curtain' coming across the vision.
- Rate of detachment can vary. Upper retinal detachments tend to occur more quickly, causing loss of lower part of vision.

- 50% have premonitory symptoms—flashing lights or spots before eyes due to abnormal retinal stimulation prior to the detachment.
- If the macular is detached, central vision is lost and does not completely recover even after retinal reattachment.
- Examination reveals visual field loss (± central visual loss), afferent pupil defect, and a grey retina which may balloon forwards.

### Causes
- Idiopathic
- After cataract surgery
- Retinopathy of prematurity
- Trauma
- Myopia
- Inherited eye disease
- DM

**Management** Refer urgently to ophthalmology for treatment to secure the retina.

**Floaters** Small dark spots in the visual field usually caused by opacities in the vitreous. Floaters continue to move when the eye comes to rest. *Risk factors*: myopia, cataract operation, trauma. Usually harmless and may settle with time.

⚠ Sudden showers of floaters in one eye ± flashing lights can indicate retinal detachment which may be difficult to see on examination. Floaters associated with eye pain/inflammation may indicate posterior uveitis.

### General rules for referral
- If long-standing floaters/flashes, no need for referral.
- If symptoms are of recent onset (<6wk) and no other symptoms, refer urgently to ophthalmology out-patients.
- If symptoms are of recent onset (<6wk) and associated with any visual field loss, ↓ acuity, or pain/inflammation of the eye, refer as an ophthalmology emergency.

**Optic neuritis** Disc swelling due to inflammation or demyelination. Presents with rapid visual loss (hours–days) and ↓ colour vision (red desaturation), discomfort on eye movements, temporary worsening of symptoms when hot, and optic disc swelling. Refer urgently to ophthalmology for confirmation of diagnosis. Steroids may help in severe cases. Visual loss usually stabilizes after week 2 and recovers over 6wk.

**Causes** Multiple sclerosis (1:4 patients with MS present with optic neuritis—📖 p.576); DM; viral infections, e.g. influenza, measles, chickenpox; familial, e.g. Leber's disease.

**Anterior ischaemic optic neuropathy (ANION)** Occurs when the short ciliary arteries are damaged. Two forms:
- *Arteritic* Due to arterial inflammation (e.g. temporal arteritis, SLE).
- *Non-arteritic* Results from arterial emboli.

**Presentation** Central vision drops suddenly and irreversibly. Examination reveals a complete or altitudinal visual field defect. The disc appears swollen and pale ± haemorrhages. May be accompanied by symptoms of the underlying condition (e.g. temporal arteritis—📖 p.532).

**Management** Refer as an ophthalmology emergency. Treatment depends on cause.

# Gradual loss of vision

## Causes of gradual loss of vision covered elsewhere
- Chronic glaucoma (📖 p.974)
- Cataract (📖 p.976)
- Diabetic retinopathy (📖 p.365).

**Age-related macular degeneration (AMD)** Most common cause of blindness in the UK—2% of people >65y old are blind in one or both eyes due to AMD. Always a bilateral disease but one eye is usually more severely affected than the other. *Risk factors:* ↑ age, +ve family history, smoking, ↑ BP.

***Presentation*** Difficult to detect in primary care. Signs are often minimal.
*Symptoms*
- In all cases, there is deterioration/distortion of central vision—affects reading/face recognition first—worst with changes in lighting.
- A dark patch that rapidly fades may be noticed on waking—can be interpreted as 'seeing a shadowy figure' and be very frightening.
- With severe visual loss pateints may see visual hallucinations—usually of faces or stars. These can also be very frightening.

***Classification***
***Dry (geographic) AMD*** All patients start with this form of AMD. Caused by atrophy of the neuroretina. The cells of the macula break down resulting in drusen formation (yellowish lipid deposits). As number/size of drusen ↑, central vision ↓.

***Wet AMD*** Accounts for 50% of blindness due to AMD. In some patients with dry AMD, drusen lift the retinal pigment epithelium away from its blood supply. New blood vessels grow from the choroid and may bleed forming scars → irreversible loss of central vision.

***Management*** If progressive loss of vision, refer to ophthalmology for confirmation of diagnosis—urgently if recent onset or rapid ↓ in vision. For those with dry AMD or scarring due to wet AMD, there is no effective treatment. Treatment of other coexisting conditions (e.g. cataract and glaucoma) can help. Provision of visual aids, registration of blindness, and social support are important.

***Ranibizumab*** is a monoclonal antibody to the vascular growth factor that stimulates new vessel growth. It is approved as an effective treatment by NICE for the treatment of patients with active wet AMD and visual symptoms. It is only administered in secondary care settings. Injections are given into the eye 1×/mo for 3mo with further injections thereafter if visual acuity ↓.

**Central serous retinopathy (CSR)** Typically occurs in hypermetropic middle-aged patients. Vision is blurred and distorted, particularly for reading. The cause is a serous leakage of fluid from abnormal choroidal vessels. The condition is generally self-limiting, but can be bilateral and chronic. Refer to ophthalmology

**Macular hole** Typically ♀ in mid-60s. Presents with gradual visual loss/distortion and colour loss. If it occurs in the non-dominant eye, the patient may be relatively asymptomatic. Refer to ophthalmology. Vision takes 4–12mo to recover following treatment.

**Macular dystrophies** Several inherited retinal diseases (e.g. Best's disease; Stargardt's macular dystrophy; Bull's eye maculopathy) present with progressive loss of central vision either in early adulthood or aged 40–60y. Ask if there is a history of visual loss in a family.

**Retinitis pigmentosa** Familial disorder resulting in retinal degeneration. Usually first noticed in adolescence and progresses to blindness. Two forms exist—the autosomal dominant form is more common and milder than the autosomal recessive form. Refer to ophthalmology for confirmation of diagnosis.
- *Symptoms* Night blindness, loss of visual field, difficulty in light adaptation, gradual loss of central vision.
- *Signs* Black pigment flecks in the retina, optic atrophy, attenuated blood vessels.

**Epiretinal membrane** Presents with distortion and blurred central vision, particularly for near vision. Associated with previous peripheral vascular disease, retinal detachment/break, branch retinal vein occlusion, uveitis, trauma, or tumour. Refer to ophthalmology for vitrectomy and membrane peel.

**Optic atrophy** *Signs*: gradual visual loss, pale optic disc. *Causes*: glaucoma, MS, ischaemia (e.g. retinal artery occlusion), retinal damage (choroiditis, retinitis pigmentosa), toxic (tobacco ambylopia, methanol, arsenic, quinine) Refer for confirmation of diagnosis to ophthalmology or neurology.

**Compressive lesions of the optic pathway,** e.g. meningioma, glioma, abscess, arteriovenous malformation can cause visual field defects—type depends on the site of the lesion (📖 p.969).

### Uveal and retinal tumours

*Melanoma* Most common tumour affecting the eye. Usually detected during routine examination by an optometrist. Other presentations include gradual central visual loss and/or retinal detachment. Can affect the iris, ciliary body or choroids. Refer for urgent ophthalmology opinion.

*Secondaries* Metastasis to the eye can occur from tumours of the breast, lung, or kidney. Appear as pale elevations of the choroid. Symptoms are variable but include visual loss and retinal detachment. Refer urgently for confirmation of diagnosis.

*Retinoblastoma* 📖 p.905

### Futher information
**NICE** Macular degeneration (age-related)—ranibizumab and pegaptanib (2008) 🖥 www.nice.org.uk

### Information and support for patients
**Macular Disease Society** ☎ 0845 241 2041 🖥 www.maculardisease.org
**British Retinitis Pigmentosa Society** ☎ 0845 123 2354
🖥 www.brps.org.uk

# Glaucoma

**Chronic simple glaucoma (open-angle) (COAG)** Common. Affects ~2% of all >40y-olds. Accounts for ~1:4 ophthalmology out-patient appointments and 10% of new blindness registrations.

### Risk factors
- ↑ intraocular pressure (IOP) >21mmHg—the major risk factor—but 30% of newly diagnosed glaucoma patients have 'normal' pressure.
- Family history (↑ risk ×10)
- Abnormal BP (↑ in elderly)
- ↑ age
- Myopia
- Black race
- ↑ plasma viscosity.

**Presentation** May be detected during routine optometrist examination or through routine screening for diabetics or patients with family history. Otherwise patients present late, as glaucoma is asymptomatic and visual acuity is preserved until visual fields are severely impaired. *Signs*: optic nerve damage (glaucomatous disc cupping), visual field loss (sausage-shaped blind spots) and ↑ intraocular pressure

### Variants
- *Ocular hypertension* ↑ IOP with little field loss
- *Normal tension glaucoma* Field loss and disc cupping but normal IOP.

**Management** Advise all patients >40y to have regular optometry check-ups. Those with a family history of glaucoma should have biannual checks of their intraocular pressures (*tonometry*), and annual visual field checks, at an optician from age 40y. Refer patients with ↑ pressures or in whom you notice (or are doubtful about) disc cupping to ophthalmology for assessment. Patients with ↑ IOP must be followed up lifelong. Aim is to ↓ IOP to slow disease progression (even with 'normal' pressures).

### Medical treatment
- Topical prostaglandin (e.g. latanoprost od in the evening)—↑ outflow of aqueous.
- Topical β-blockers (e.g. timolol bd)—↓ aqueous secretion. Caution in patients with asthma or heart failure. *Side effects*: allergy and dry eyes.
- Topical carbonic anhydrase inhibitors (e.g. dorzolamide tds, or bd if in combination with a β-blocker)—↓ aqueous secretion. *Side effects*: blurred vision, tiredness, dyspepsia.
- Topical α-agonists (e.g. brimonidine bd)—↓ aqueous secretion and ↑ outflow. *Side effects*: local reactions, headache, dry mouth, tiredness.

**Surgery** Trabeculoplasty is considered when the 'target' IOP is not met with medical treatment (especially in patients <50y). *Side effects:* failure, worsening cataract.

**Acute closed-angle glaucoma (AACG)** Uncommon. Affects 0.1% of patients >40y—typically elderly long-sighted women with early cataract. Closed-angle glaucoma may present in one of 3 ways:

• *Latent* Usually picked up when screening the opposite eye after an episode of acute or subacute glaucoma. The patient is asymptomatic and IOP normal, but the anterior chamber is shallow with a narrow angle.

• *Subacute* Episodic haloes around bright lights, impaired vision ± frontal headache/eye pain. Attacks are precipitated by the pupil dilating, e.g. at night or when entering a darkened room, and relieved by sleep or entering a brighter environment. Examination between attacks is normal, but during an attack the pupil is semi-dilated and the cornea slightly clouded. Patients with subacute glaucoma are at risk of an acute attack.

• *Acute* Blockage of aqueous drainage from the anterior chamber causes a sudden ↑ in IOP from 15–20 to 60–70mmHg. There may be a history of previous subacute attacks. The patient complains of eye pain with acute loss of vision in one eye ± abdominal pain/nausea/vomiting.

**Examination** Vision ↓; cornea looks hazy (due to oedema); pupil is fixed and dilated (often slightly oval in shape with long axis vertical); circumcorneal redness; eyeball feels hard (due to ↑ pressure); poor fundal view ± cataract

**Management** Refer acute or subacute glaucoma as an emergency to ophthalmology. Specialist treatment is with meiosis to open drainage channels (e.g. pilocarpine 4% drops) and acetazolamide ± apraclonidine and/or latanoprost drops to ↓ aqueous production. Surgery or laser treatment (peripheral iridotomy) to allow free aqueous circulation is undertaken once IOP has been ↓. Patient may need prophylactic surgery on the contralateral eye to prevent AACG in that eye too. AACG may damage the trabecular meshwork and patients are at risk of developing chronic glaucoma following an attack. Regular check-ups are necessary.

**Neovascular glaucoma** May occur in patients with diabetic retinopathy, central or branch retinal vein obstruction, or ocular ischaemia. Blood vessels grow across the iris and the iridiocorneal angle, preventing fluid drainage. Pressures can be very high (40–70mm Hg) and the patient may suffer pain from corneal oedema. Treatment is surgical and, in severe cases, if the eye is blind, it is removed.

 **Congenital glaucoma** 1:10 000 live births. ♂ > ♀. Usually bilateral. Presents with irritation of the eye (watering, rubbing), photophobia, large eyes with large fixed pupils ± cloudy cornea. Refer urgently for paediatric ophthalmic opinion. Surgery is needed to prevent blindness.

**Further information**
**NICE** Diagnosis and management of chronic open angle glaucoma and ocular hypertension (2009) ▣ www.nice.org.uk

**Information and support for patients**
**International Glaucoma Association** ☎ 01233 648170 ▣ www.iga.org.uk

# Cataract

Lens opacity is found in 75% >65y-olds. Most do not need treatment.

### Risk factors for cataract

- Old age
- DM
- +ve family history
- Prolonged steroid treatment
- ↑BP
- Excessive alcohol

- Smoking
- Prenatal rubella/toxoplasma (congenital cataract)
- Hypocalcaemia
- Eye trauma
- Radiation exposure.

### Presentation

*In adults*

- Blurred vision and gradual loss of vision.
- Dazzles and halos around objects—especially in sunlight.
- Frequent spectacle changes due to changing refractive index.

❶ Unilateral cataract may not be noticed by the patient, but loss of binocular vision affects judgment of distance.

 *In children* Cataracts present with squint, white pupil, nystagmus, amblyopia, or loss of binocular vision. May be hereditary or associated with Down's syndrome, galactosaemia, or congenital rubella.

*Signs* A shadow in the red reflex/ absent red reflex; difficulty visualizing the fundus.

### Types of cataract

- Congenital cataract—localized and usually polar.
- Nuclear cataracts—central; most common in old age.
- Cortical lens opacities.
- Subcapsular cataracts—usually linked to old age or steroid use.
- Dot cataracts—common in DM.
- Traumatic cataract.
- Mature cataract.

### Management

*Adult cataract* Check fasting blood glucose to exclude DM. Advise patients to have their visual acuity checked regularly. Refer to ophthalmology if ↓ sight (or any other symptom) interferes with social functioning, driving, or independence.

*Surgical treatment* Removal of the natural lens ± posterior chamber lens implantation. Usually done as a day-case procedure under LA. Healing takes 2–6wk depending on the technique used. 75–95% without other ocular pathology have 6/12 vision or better 3mo post-op. Patients require testing for new spectacles 6wk post-op to allow refractive changes to settle.

*Complications of cataract surgery*
- Intraocular infection (endophthalmitis)—rare (0.1%). Presents with pain and blurred vision ± red eye ± tenderness. Refer back to the operating surgeon urgently—antibiotics injected within 2–3h can preserve vision. Delayed referral (>12h) will lead to blindness.
- Posterior capsule rupture.
- Broken or protruding sutures—cause sensation of a foreign body on the cornea or pain. May need to be removed.
- Vitreous haemorrhage.
- Glaucoma.
- Posterior capsule opacification—5–30% <5y post-op. Symptoms are similar to the original cataract—treatment is with laser therapy to create a hole in the capsule.

 ***Childhood cataract*** Refer immediately to ophthalmology.

**Information for patients**
**Eye Care Trust** 🖥 www.eyecaretrust.org.uk
**Royal College of Ophthalmologists** 🖥 www.rcophth.ac.uk
**Good Hope NHS Hospital Trust**
🖥 www.goodhope.org.uk/departments/eyedept

# Refractive errors and squint

**Glasses check** Look through the patient's glasses.
- If image is magnified (prescription '+'), the patient is long sighted
- If image is reduced (prescription '–'), the patient is short sighted.

**Amblyopia (lazy eye)** Poor vision in the absence of ocular or visual pathway disorder. Squint, ptosis, cataract, unequal refractive errors, or astigmatism can cause the image from one eye to be disregarded. This neglect leads to amblyopia. If this persists after 7–8y of age, it becomes irreversible. Referral of children for treatment of these problems is vital. Treatment is with glasses ± patching, and squint surgery if necessary.

## Refraction errors

*Hypermetropia (long sight)* Most common refractive error. Common in infants and lessens with age. Distant objects focus behind the retina so continuous ciliary muscle contraction (to make the lens more convex) is needed to achieve a focused image. This can lead to convergent squint. Other symptoms include eye tiredness and headache. Convex lenses are used for correction.

*Myopia (short sight)* Close objects can be focused on the retina but distant objects focus in front of the retina. There is often a +ve family history. Concave lenses are used to correct the defect. Contact lenses may be necessary in high myopia (>8.00 diopters). Myopia is unusual <6y old. It tends to worsen until the late teens. Regular (6 monthly) eye checks are needed to ensure correct lenses are prescribed. In adults increasing myopia can indicate developing cataracts. High myopia (8–20 diopters) predisposes to retinal detachment—recommend these patients have an annual eye examination (more frequent if floaters).

*Astigmatism* The degree of curvature across the cornea or lens differs in the vertical and horizontal planes. Thus objects are distorted longitudinally or vertically. Lenses can be used to correct this defect.

*Presbyopia* Age-related loss of accommodation. The lens becomes larger and stiffer (less easy to deform) between 45 and 65y. Focusing on close objects (accommodation) is more difficult, and glasses may become necessary for near work (e.g. reading).

**Refractive procedures** are increasingly being undertaken as an alternative to spectacles. *LASIK (laser assisted in-situ keratomileusis)* is a combination of surgery and laser therapy. It can be used for higher degrees of refractive error and astigmatism. Complications are rare.

**Squint** Common abnormality of coordinated eye movement. May be congenital or acquired. 3% of children have a congenital squint. During examination note the light reflexes from different parts of the cornea—they should be symmetrical. If not, there is a squint.

*Childhood screening for squint* 📖 p.854

*Pseudosquint*
- *Wide epicanthic folds* give the appearance of a squint—corneal reflections are symmetrical.

- *Intermittent deviation of the eyes in neonates* Common. Check red reflex is present. Normally settles by 3mo—squint after this time is significant. Refer.

**Non-paralytic squint** Usually congenital. There is a full range of eye movement in both eyes and no double vision. Squint is due to an imbalance in the muscles of the eye. May be convergent (esotropia) or divergent (exotropia). Esotropia (Plate 13) is the most common form in childhood and is often associated with long-sightedness.

**Predisposing factors** Family history of squint, high refractive errors, neurological disease (e.g. cerebral palsy), cataract, Down's syndrome, Turner's syndrome, retinoblastoma, optic atrophy, craniofacial anomalies, retinal disease.

**Management** Refer all non-paralytic squints as soon as recognized for ophthalmology assessment. Without treatment children with squint risk developing ambylopia, failure of binocular vision, and long-term visual problems. Visual maturity occurs at 7–8y. Eye-patching, correction of refractive errors (spectacles), and realignment surgery can improve sight up to this age.

**Paralytic squint** Caused by damage to the extraocular muscles or the nerve supplying them. Usually acquired and caused by cranial nerve palsy. Results in diplopia—maximal when looking in the direction requiring the action of the paralysed muscle. The image from the eye which is not moving correctly is peripheral to the image from the normal eye. Refer for urgent neurology/ophthalmology opinion.[N] Once sinister causes have been excluded, management involves treatment of the underlying condition ± patching and/or prism spectacles ± surgery.

**Gaze palsies** Inability to perform coordinated movements of the two eyes together in the same direction. In all cases, refer to neurology—treatment depends on cause (Table 26.3).
- Horizontal gaze palsy—loss of conjugate eye movements to one side.
- Vertical gaze palsy—loss of conjugate eye movements upwards.

**Table 26.3** Ocular nerve palsies

| Nerve | Effect of paralysis | Causes of nerve palsy |
|---|---|---|
| 3rd Oculo-motor nerve | Ptosis and ophthalmoplegia—eye looks down and out. Surgical causes are also associated with pain, proptosis, and pupil dilation. | *Surgical:* Berry aneurysm (posterior communicating artery), cavernous sinus lesions. *Medical:* microvascular disease, e.g. DM |
| 4th Trochlear nerve | Superior obique muscle is paralysed. Causes diplopia and torticollis. The eye cannot look down and inwards. | Trauma (30%), DM (30%), idiopathic |
| 6th Abducens nerve | Lateral rectus paralysed. Causes diplopia. The eye is turned in and cannot move laterally from the midline. | Tumour, trauma to the base of the skull, vascular. |

# Contact lenses and drugs for the eye

**Contact lenses** 20% are worn because they are more suitable for the eye condition than spectacles; 80% for cosmetic/convenience reasons. Some are worn just to change eye colour. Contact lenses are used in high myopia or hypermetropia, presbyopia, and after cataract removal because thick spectacle lenses cause visual field distortion. They are also useful when the cornea has been damaged, e.g. after ulceration or trauma and in keratoconus (a rare corneal degenerative disease).

**Types of lens** Hard, gas-permeable (larger hard lenses are designed to allow air to reach the cornea), and soft lenses are available. Some soft lenses are 'daily disposable' or 'monthly disposable'. Hard and gas-permeable lenses can correct for minor astigmatism; normal soft lenses cannot as the lens is too flexible. A high astigmatism requires spectacles or a special (toric) soft lens (delicate and needs careful cleaning). Patients with poor tear secretion do not tolerate contact lenses well.

**Care of lenses** Careful cleaning of the lenses and contact lens container is vital—particular solutions are used for each type of lens and these should not be interchanged. Contact lenses can be stained by fluorescein or rifampicin—ask before prescribing.

## Complications
- Eye infection.
- Corneal abrasion or vascularization (painful watery eye after lens removal).
- Sensitization to cleaning agents (redness, stinging, swollen eyelids).
- Giant papillary conjunctivitis.
- Losing the lens within the eye.
- Keratitis.
- Acanthamoeba infection.

**Drugs and the eye** Many eye complaints can be treated with topical medication.
- Ointments last longer in the eye than drops but can cause blurring of vision—they are particularly useful at night.
- Antibiotics should generally be given as drops, enabling clearance through the naso-lacrimal system. In severe infections drops should be used every 2h, reducing to qds after 48h.
- Antibiotic preparations (e.g. chloramphenicol, fusidic acid) can potentially become contaminated with bacteria so should be changed regularly.

**Mydriatics** (e.g. tropicamide, cyclopentolate) dilate the pupil and cause cycloplegia → blurred vision. They are used to dilate the pupil for examination and to prevent adhesions to the lens in iritis. They can precipitate acute closed-angle glaucoma in susceptible patients.

**Miotics** (e.g. pilocarpine) constrict the pupil and ↑ aqueous drainage. They are used in glaucoma. They can cause systemic side effects, e.g. sweating, ↑ BP, pulmonary oedema.

***Local anaesthetic drops*** (e.g. oxybuprocaine, proxymetacaine ) can help examination of painful eyes and foreign body removal. Protect the eye with an eyepad until the anaesthetic has worn off to prevent corneal damage (corneal reflex is suppressed).

***Steroid eye drops*** Used in scleritis, episcleritis, iritis. Prescribe only after slit-lamp examination and on the advice of an ophthalmologist. They can cause severe eye damage if used when a dendritic ulcer is present. Long-term use may cause glaucoma and thinning of the cornea/sclera, and may facilitate fungal infection.

***ß-blocking drops*** (e.g. timolol, betaxolol) are used in glaucoma. Beware of systemic side effects—bronchospasm, bradycardia.

**$\alpha_2$-receptor agonists** (e.g. brimonidine) are used in glaucoma. May cause dry mouth, headache, fatigue

***Prostaglandin analogues*** (e.g. latanoprost, bimatoprost) used in glaucoma. May cause lash growth and ocular inflammation.

# Mental health

# Mental health assessment

When assessing a patient with mental health problems in primary care, the objectives are to:

- Establish a constructive relationship with the patient to enable patient and doctor to communicate effectively and serve as the basis for any subsequent therapeutic relationship.
- Assess the patient's emotions and attitudes.
- Determine if the patient has a mental disorder and, if so, which.
- Find out (where possible) what caused the mental disorder.
- Establish how it might be treated.

## Psychiatric history

*Informants* Often worries about a patient with a psychiatric disorder are flagged up to a GP by a concerned relative or friend. Talk to the informant (although be careful to maintain confidentiality of the patient), establish the concerns and circumstances, and review old notes before seeing the patient.

*The consultation* Use open questions at the start, becoming directive when necessary—clarify, reflect, facilitate, listen. Be open and ready to ask about suicide, sex, drugs, etc. Ask about:

- *Occupation*—unemployed? Happy in job?
- *Home situation*—housing, relationships, social support, debt ,etc.
- *Presenting complaint*—chronological account, past history of similar symptoms. Ask directly about thoughts of suicide and self-harm.
- *Family history*—psychiatric illness, recent loss or serious illness of a family member, bereavement, depression, suicide or attempted suicide, psychosis, alcoholism, drug use.
- *Personal history*—abuse (as a child, domestic violence), substance misuse, serious illness (including past psychiatric history and major physical illness), recent significant events (e.g. childbirth, house move).
- *Attitudes and beliefs*—How does the patient see him/herself? What does he/she think is wrong? How does he/she think other people view the situation? What does the patient want you to do about it?

## Mental state examination *Check:*

- Appearance and behaviour—signs of self-neglect or malnutrition, attitude, movements, social interaction.
- Speech—spontaneity, rate, amount, continuity (flight of ideas, loosening of associations).
- Mood—depressed or over-elated. Consider screening for depression, e.g. screening questions for patients with chronic disease (📖 p.998), screening questions for pregnant or postnatal women (📖 p.998), PHQ-9 (📖 p.999).
- Thinking—form, content, flow, possession.
- Perception—illusions, hallucinations, pseudohallucinations.
- Cognition—cognitive screen, e.g. 6 CIT (📖 p.1009).
- Insight—patient's understanding of his/her illness, its effects, and need for treatment.

## Action
- Summarize the history back to the patient and give an opportunity for him/her to fill in any gaps.
- Draw up a problem list and management plan with the patient.
- Set a review date.

---

### High-risk groups for psychiatric illness

#### Women
- More vulnerable to depression and eating disorders
- During pregnancy and in the postpartum period
- When looking after children <5y old, especially lone parents who also go out to work.
- When subjected to domestic violence
- During the menopause.

#### Men
- More at risk of suicide.

#### People with long-term physical health problems, e.g.
- Diabetes
- Heart disease
- Chronic disabling lung disease
- Cancers
- Disabling neurological disorders: stroke, PD, MS, MND.

#### Substance abusers
- Drug abuse
- Alcoholism.

#### People suffering adverse life events
- Bereavement
- Divorce
- Unemployment
- Financial problems.

**Minority ethnic groups** More likely to suffer mental health problems due to social and economic deprivation, isolation from their usual culture, racism, and past exposure to war or torture (>50% of refugees have mental disorders).

**Carers** All carers are at high risk of depression (~40% of carers of stroke victims are depressed). This starts early after the onset of care-giving. It is good practice to:
- Identify all carers and mark their records
- Check carers' mental and physical health annually
- Inform carers that they are entitled to a needs assessment
- Ask patients if you can share information with their carers
- Inform carers about support groups and carer centres.

**Residents of care homes and nursing homes** 50% have depression.

---

# Mental health symptoms and signs

**Acute confusion** 📖 p.1008                    **Anxiety** 📖 p.990

**Depression** 📖 p.998

**Abnormal beliefs** Decide whether a belief is normal in the context of the patient. If not, decide if the belief is a:
- *Delusion*, i.e. a belief that does not seem to have a rational basis and which is not amenable to argument, or
- *Over-valued idea*, i.e. a belief that is odd but understandable given the patient's background.

**Compulsions** Forced behaviours repeated despite inappropriateness, unreasonableness, and associated discomfort, in response to an obsession. Can be disabling, e.g. repeated handwashing hundreds of times a day. Obsessive–compulsive disorder—📖 p.994.

**Perceptions (abnormal)** *Consider*:
- *Illusion* Misinterpretation of visual or other information e.g. a person seeing a shadow of a tree moving in the breeze might interpret it as a person moving. Can happen if ↓ level of consciousness, or occasionally if visual impairment—particularly AMD.
- *Hallucination*
- *Pseudo-hallucination* Vivid perception which is recognized as not being real, e.g. delirium tremens
- *Depersonalization* Feeling of being unreal—like an actor playing yourself. Associated with a wide range of mental illness, e.g. depression, schizophrenia.
- *Derealization* Feeling of everything around you being unreal—as if in a dream. Often linked to depersonalization.

**Hallucinations** Sensory experiences in the absence of stimuli. May be visual, auditory, gustatory, olfactory, or tactile.
- *Visual, tactile, and auditory hallucinations* suggest mental illness:
  - Visual and tactile hallucinations suggest organic disorder, e.g. dementia, acute confusional state, metabolic encephalopathy, drug abuse.
  - Auditory hallucinations suggest psychosis.
- Hallucinations experienced when the patient is falling asleep (*hypnagogic hallucination*) or waking up (*hypnapompic hallucination*) are features of narcolepsy.
- *Olfactory and gustatory hallucinations* often occur together. May be suggestive of psychosis, but also occur with temporal lobe epilepsy and olfactory bulb tumours.

**Thought disorders** Consider disorders of:

### Content
- *Ideas of reference* The patient feels that he/she is noticed by everyone around him/stands out from the crowd; media content, e.g. television or radio, refers to him/herself, or that others are talking or thinking about him/her. Becomes a delusion of reference when insight is lost. Associated with schizophrenia, depressive states, and acute and chronic cognitive impairment.
- *Delusions*.

## Flow

- *Flight of ideas* Leaps from idea to idea. There is always some association between ideas but it may seem odd, e.g. rhymes. Associated with manic illness.
- *Perseveration* Persistence of a verbal or other behaviour beyond what is apparently intended, expected, or needed. Associated with dementia and brain damage, e.g. cerebral palsy, CVA.
- *Loosening of association* Series of thoughts appear only distantly (or loosely) related to one another or completely unrelated. Associated with schizophrenia.
- *Thought block* Abrupt and complete interruption in the stream of thought leaving a blank mind. Associated with schizophrenia.

## Form

- *Preoccupation* The patient thinks about a topic frequently but can terminate the thoughts voluntarily. Common symptom, e.g. in anxiety states. Ask about preoccupation with suicide in depressed patients.
- *Obsession* Thought or image repeated despite its inappropriateness or intrusiveness and associated discomfort. The thought and efforts to stop it can be disabling.

## Possession

- *Thought insertion* Thoughts do not belong to the patient but have been planted there by someone else. One of the first-rank symptoms of schizophrenia.
- *Thought withdrawal* Opposite of thought insertion. The patient perceives that a thought is missing and has been removed by someone else. A first-rank symptom of schizophrenia.
- *Thought broadcasting* The patient believes that his/her thoughts can be heard by other people, either directly or via the newspapers, radio, etc. Associated with schizophrenia.

**Delusions** Beliefs held unshakably despite available counter-evidence and which are unexpected in view of circumstances and background. The belief is usually (but not always) false.

- *Primary delusions* Belief arrives in the head fully formed. e.g. thought insertion; strongly suggestive of schizophrenia.
- *Secondary delusions* Belief arises on the basis of experience, e.g. someone who has lost their job several times through no fault of their own may believe they are unemployable.

**Paranoid delusions** Delusions (usually primary) which concern the relationship between the patient and other people. Associated with schizophrenia, depressive states, and acute and chronic cognitive impairment.

- *Delusions of persecution* Most common type of paranoid delusion. Belief that a person or organization is intentionally harassing or inflicting harm upon the patient. Associated with schizophrenia, depressive states, and acute and chronic cognitive impairment
- *Delusions of grandeur* Beliefs of possessing exaggerated power, importance, knowledge, or ability. Associated with manic depression.

# Counselling and cognitive behavioural therapy

**Counselling** 1:3 problems brought to the GP have a psychosocial component. To cater for these patients, most PCOs (81%) have some provision for practice-based counselling and 50% of practices have counselling services. Counselling services may also be available via community psychiatric or clinical psychology services.

*What is counselling?* There are no universally agreed definitions of the term 'counselling' or 'counsellor', and the distinction between counselling and psychotherapy is often unclear. Usually the key element in counselling is reflective listening to encourage patients to think about and try to resolve their own difficulties. It does not involve giving advice. Most counsellors use brief (time-limited) therapy offering patients a mean of 7 sessions, each usually lasting ~50min.

*Who is a counsellor?* There is no formal registration requirement in the UK for counsellors or psychotherapists. The GMC advises that GPs should only refer to practitioners who are members of a recognized disciplinary body and thus subject to ethical and disciplinary codes (Table 27.1).

*Does counselling work?* Many patients regard antidepressants as harmful or addictive, and are increasingly reluctant to take them. They see counselling as an attractive alternative—a view supported by most GPs. Evidence shows that counselling subjectively improves the condition for which the patient has been referred, and non-directive counselling is more effective than GP care in reducing anxiety and depression in the short term but not the long term. However, counselling does not ↓ drug costs, and practices with counsellors make more referrals to 2° care psychiatric services[5]. More research into cost-effectiveness is needed.

*Who should be referred?* Counsellors see a wide range of patients (Table 27.2). About two-thirds of patients referred for counselling have significant levels of anxiety or depression.

**Problem solving therapy** Another short-term therapy (typically 5–6× 45min sessions)—it involves drawing up a list of problems, and generating and agreeing solutions, broken down into steps, for patients to work on as homework between sessions. Shown to be as effective as antidepressants for moderate depression.[R]

## Cognitive behavioural therapy (CBT)

- *Behavioural therapies* aim to change behaviour. Usually the therapist uses a system of graded exposure (systematic desensitization) combined with teaching a method of anxiety reduction.
- *Cognitive therapy* focuses on people's thoughts and the reasoning behind their assumptions on the basis that incorrect assumptions → abnormal reactions which then reinforce these assumptions further (a vicious cycle).

**Table 27.1** UK recognized professional bodies for counsellors and psychotherapists

**Counsellors**
- British Association for Counselling and Psychotherapy (BACP)
- UK Register of Counsellors
- Association of Counsellors and Psychotherapists in Primary Care

**Psychologists**
- British Psychological Society (chartered and counselling psychologists)

**Psychotherapists**
- UK Council for Psychotherapy
- British Confederation of Psychotherapists

**Table 27.2** Conditions suitable for referral to a counsellor

| Conditions suitable for referral | Conditions unsuitable for referral |
|---|---|
| Anxiety | Psychotic illness |
| Depression—especially minor depression (📖 p.998) | Phobias |
| | Obsessive–compulsive disorder |
| Relationship problems | Eating disorder |
| Bereavement | Personality disorder |
| After traumatic events | |
| Substance abuse | |

**What is CBT used for?** CBT is of proven effectiveness in the treatment of mild depression, anxiety disorders, phobias, panic disorder, and eating disorders, and for the treatment of delusions and hallucinations in psychotic illness.

**How can patients be referred for CBT?** CBT is usually provided by highly trained psychotherapists accessed via psychiatry services. Guided self-help programmes based on CBT are also effective for mild depression and can be delivered:
- Using books, e.g. Gilbert P *Overcoming depression* (2000) Constable & Robin, London. ISBN: 1841191256
- *Beating the Blues* (🖥 www.beatingtheblues.co.uk)
- Via the Internet, e.g. *Living Life to the Full* (🖥 www.livinglifetothefull.org) or *The Mood Gym* (🖥 www.moodgym.anu.edu.au)

**Further information**
**NICE** Depression (2004, amended 2007) 🖥 www.nice.org.uk
**Bower P, Rowland N, Hardy R.** The clinical effectiveness of counselling in primary care *Psychol Med* (2003) **33**, 203–15.

# Anxiety

Anxiety is only considered abnormal when it occurs in the absence of a stressful event, impairs physical, occupational, or social functioning, and/or is excessively severe or prolonged. Differentiating between anxiety disorders—Figure 27.1.

**Generalized anxiety disorder (GAD)** Long-term condition, fluctuating in severity and nature, often beginning in adolescence. Lifetime prevalence ~5%. Features include the following.

### Psychological symptoms
- Fearful anticipation
- Irritability
- Sensitivity to noise
- Restlessness
- Poor concentration
- Worrying thoughts
- Insomnia
- Nightmares
- Depression
- Obsessions
- Depersonalization.

### Physical symptoms
- Dry mouth
- Tremor
- Dizziness
- Headache
- Epigastric discomfort
- Difficulty swallowing
- Frequent or loose motions
- Chest discomfort/constriction
- Difficulty breathing/hyperventilation
- Palpitations/awareness of missed beats
- Frequency or urgency of micturition
- Erectile dysfunction
- Menstrual problems
- Parasthesiae
- Tinnitus
- Excessive wind.

### Associations
- Anxiety often accompanies depression (📖 p.998) and may be a feature of early schizophrenia.
- Other conditions which can cause anxiety and/or mimic symptoms of anxiety include drug/alcohol withdrawal, caffeine abuse, thyrotoxicosis, hypoglycaemia, temporal lobe epilepsy, phaeochromocytoma.

**Management** Check TFTs. Use a stepped treatment approach.[N]
- **Step 1** Recognize and diagnose. Consider using an anxiety scale (e.g. Hamilton Anxiety Scale) to record baseline morbidity.
- **Step 2** Primary care management—general measures (avoid caffeine; identify potential causes of anxiety); problem solving; benzodiadepines (diazepam 2–5mg tds prn or equivalent) short term—avoid using >2–4wk because of risk of dependence. Discuss longer-term options:
  - Referral for CBT.
  - Drug treatment—SSRIs are the drugs of choice.
  - Self-help—other forms of CBT (e.g. book-based or computer-based), exercise, self-help groups.
- **Step 3** Review. If not improving, offer another type of treatment or venlafaxine MR 75mg/d—ensure BP monitoring.
- **Step 4** Refer to specialist mental health services if significant symptoms despite treatment with two different interventions.

**Phobias** As GAD but limited to certain situations. 2 main features:
- **Avoidance** of the circumstances that provoke anxiety.
- **Anticipatory anxiety** if there is a prospect of meeting that situation

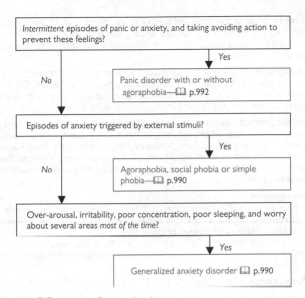

**Fig. 27.1** Differentiation of anxiety disorders

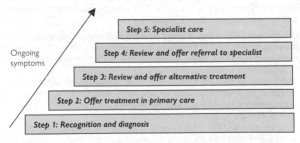

**Fig. 27.2** Stepwise approach to anxiety management

Figures 27.1 and 27.2 are reproduced with permission in modified format from NICE CG22 *Anxiety: management of anxiety (panic disorder, with or without agoraphobia, and generalized anxiety disorder) in adults in primary secondary and community care* (2004) London: NICE. Available from 🖳 www.nice.org.uk

**Simple phobia** Inappropriate anxiety in the presence of ≥1 object/situation, e.g. flying, enclosed spaces, spiders. Common in early life. Most adult phobias are a continuation of childhood phobias. *Lifetime prevalence:* 4% ♂; 13% ♀.

**Management** Treatment is only needed if symptoms are frequent, intrusive, or prevent necessary activities. Exposure therapy is effective. Obtain directly (via trained psychotherapist), by referral to psychiatry, or through the private sector (e.g. British Airways 'Fear of Flying' course).

**Social phobia** Intense and persistent fear of being scrutinized or negatively evaluated by others, resulting in fear and avoidance of social situations (e.g. meeting people in authority, using a telephone, speaking in front of a group). Must be significantly disabling, not simple shyness. May be generalized (person fears most social situations) or specific (related to certain activities only).

**Management**
- *Drug therapy* SSRIs. Continue ≥12mo, or long term if symptoms remain unresolved, there is a comorbid condition (e.g. depression, GAD, panic attacks), a history of relapse, or early onset.
- *Psychological therapies* CBT (cognitive restructuring) ± exposure. Obtain directly or via local psychiatric services depending on local arrangements.

**Agoraphobia** Usually onset is aged 20–40y with an initial panic attack.

**Symptoms** Panic attacks, fear of fainting and/or loss of control are experienced in crowds, away from home, or in situations from which escape is difficult. Avoidance results in patients remaining within their home where they know symptoms will not occur. Other symptoms include depression, depersonalization, and obsessional thoughts.

**Management** Difficult to manage in general practice. Diagnosis is often delayed as patients will not come to the surgery and ongoing management complicated by refusal to be referred to psychiatric services. Prognosis is best when there is good marital/social support. *Options:*
- *Behavioural therapy* e.g. exposure, training in coping with panic attacks. Available by direct referral or via psychiatric services according to local arrangements. Home visits may be required, but should be resisted as part of therapy.
- *Drug treatment* SSRIs (citalopram and paroxetine are licensed), MAOIs, and TCAs (imipramine and clomipramine are commonly used). Relapse rate is high. Benzodiazepines can be used if frequent panic attacks, particularly if initiating other treatment, but beware of dependence.

**Panic disorder** Panic attacks are very common, but panic disorder is uncommon: lifetime prevalence—1% of ♂, 3% of ♀.

**Definitions**
- *Panic attack* ≥4 symptoms in one attack.
- *Panic disorder* Chronic disorder; diagnosis depends on >4 attacks in 4wk or one attack followed by a persistent fear of having another.

**Symptoms** Intense feeling of apprehension or impending disaster. Anxiety builds up quickly and unexpectedly without a recognizable trigger, and patients often present with any combination of:

- Shortness of breath/ smothering sensations
- Choking
- Palpitations and ↑ heart rate
- Chest discomfort or pain
- Sweating
- Dizziness, unsteady feelings, or faintness.
- Nausea or abdominal pain
- Depersonalization/derealization
- Numbness or tingling sensations
- Flushes or chills
- Trembling or shaking
- Fear of dying
- Fear of doing something crazy or uncontrolled.

**Examination** Obvious distress; sweating; tachycardia; hyper-ventilation. ↑BP is common and usually settles when the episode is over. Otherwise examination is normal.

**Associations** Depression (56% are depressed); GAD; agoraphobia; substance abuse; suicide (↑ risk).

**Differential diagnosis** Alcohol withdrawal; other psychiatric disorders (e.g. psychosis); hyperthyroidism; temporal lobe epilepsy; cardiac arrythmia; labyrinthitis; hypoglycaemia; hyperparathyroidism; phaeochromocytoma (very rare).

**Management of acute panic attack** 📖 p.1116

**Management of panic disorder** Use a stepped treatment approach (Figure 27.2, 📖 p.991). Primary care treatment options include:

- **Psychological treatment** CBT (📖 p.988) is effective—availability may be limited in the community.
- **Drug treatment** SSRIs are usually used first line—paroxetine and citalopram are licenced in UK. Warn patients about possible transient ↑ in anxiety on starting treatment. Minimize initial side effects by starting at a low dose and ↑ slowly. Review <2wk after starting treatment and at 4, 6, and 12wk. If an SSRI is not suitable or ineffective, offer a TCA, e.g. imipramine or clomipramine 10–25mg nocte (unlicensed), or another form of treatment. If effective, continue treatment for 6mo, reviewing every 8–12wk. Minimize discontinuation symptoms by tapering dose over an extended time period.
- **Self-help options** Self-help groups; bibliotherapy, i.e. book- or computer-based forms of CBT; exercise.

❶ Do not use benzodiazepines for treatment of patients with panic disorder—they are associated with a less good long-term outcome.

### Further reading
**NICE** Management of anxiety (panic disorder, with or without agoraphobia, and generalised anxiety disorder) in adults in primary, secondary and community care (2004, amended 2007) 🖳 www.nice.org.uk

### Patient information and support
**Triumph over Phobia (TOP) UK** ☎ 0845 600 9601 🖳 www.topuk.org
**Anxiety Care** ☎ 020 8478 3400 🖳 www.anxietycare.org.uk
**No More Panic** 🖳 www.nomorepanic.co.uk

# Other anxiety-type disorders

**Stress** 📖 p.996    **Post-traumatic stress disorder** 📖 p.996

**Mixed anxiety and depression** Combinations of anxiety and depression are common—particularly amongst women. Prevalence ~10%. When anxiety and depression occur together, symptoms are more severe, there is ↑ functional impairment, illness is more chronic/persistent, and there is poorer response to treatment given. Treat as for anxiety and/or depression depending on the predominating features. Refer for psychiatric assessment if management strategies are not working.

**Somatization or hysteria** Physical symptoms in response to emotional distress. Characterized by an excessive preoccupation with bodily sensations combined with a fear of physical illness. Common feature of depression, anxiety, schizophrenia, and substance use.

*Somatization disorder* Chronic condition. History of numerous unsubstantiated physical complaints. Starts at <30y and often persists many years. ♀: ♂ ≈ 10:1; lifetime prevalence 0.1–0.2% although mild symptoms are much more common.

*Clinical features*
- >2y history of multiple symptoms with no physical explanation.
- Persistent refusal to be reassured that there is no explanation for the symptoms.
- Impaired social/family functioning due to these symptoms and/or associated behaviour.

*Management*
- Reattribution involves acknowledging/taking symptoms seriously, offering any necessary examination and investigations, asking about psychosocial problems, and explaining the link between symptoms and stress.
- Treat comorbid psychiatric problems (e.g. depression, anxiety, panic).
- Beware of risks of drug interaction—self-medication with multiple OTC (or even prescription) drugs is common.
- Beware of side effects of medication—these patients do not tolerate prescribed drugs well and have a heightened awareness of side effects.
- Refer to psychiatry if risk of suicide, marked functional impairment, impulsive or antisocial behaviour.

**Obsessive–compulsive disorder (OCD)** Recurrent obsessive thoughts and compulsive acts. Lifetime prevalence ≈2% although minor obsessional symptoms are much more common. ♂:♀ ≈2:3. Tends to present in young adults. Patients may have symptoms for years before seeking help as they know that their thoughts/actions are irrational and are embarrassed to tell anyone. Relatives may highlight the problem.

*Features*
- *Obsessional thinking*—recurrent persistent thoughts, impulses and images causing anxiety or distress.
- *Compulsive behaviour*—repetitive behaviours, rituals or mental acts done to prevent or ↓ anxiety.
- *Other features*—indecisiveness and inability to take action, anxiety, depression, and depersonalization.

### Screening questions[N]
- Do you wash or clean a lot?
- Do you check things a lot?
- Is there any thought that keeps bothering you that you would like to get rid of but can't?
- Do your daily activities take a long time to finish?
- Are you concerned about orderliness or symmetry?
- Do these problems trouble you?

**Management** Consider treatment with an SSRI (e.g. fluoxetine 20–40mg od), self help CBT—including exposure-response prevention (ERP), and/or refer for individual or group CBT. Involve the family/carers in ERP where appropriate. Inform patients and carers about self-help organizations. If these strategies are unsuccessful in controlling symptoms, refer for specialist care.

**Prognosis** Two-thirds improve within 1y of presentation. Symptoms worsen with stress. 15% have a deteriorating course.

---

**Heartsink patients** Characterized by:
- Frequent presentation—the top 1% of attenders at GP surgeries generate 6% of GP workload.
- Highly complex and often multiple problems—some real, others not.
- Exasperation generated between patient and doctor.

**❶** It is a two-way process. Some GPs report more heartsink patients than others. The problem relates to the GP's perception of patients as well as the patients themselves.

**GP risk factors** Perception of high workload, low job satisfaction, lack of training in counselling or communication, and lack of postgraduate skills.

### Management strategy
- Do a detailed review of notes ± chart of life.
- Agree patient contacts, e.g. limit to one partner, agree frequency of appointments, etc.
- Agree an agenda within consultations, e.g. problem list—only one problem per visit.
- Employ reattribution techniques as for somatization disorder.
- Avoid unnecessary investigation and referral.
- Be aware of your own reaction to the patient.
- Acknowledge that even heartsink patients can be genuinely ill.
- Consider psychiatric diagnoses—especially chronic anxiety, depression, somatization disorder. Screening questionnaires can be useful.
- Consider referral for cognitive behavioural therapy.

---

### Further information
**NICE** Obsessive compulsive disorder: core interventions in the treatment of obsessive compulsive disorder and body dysmorphic disorder (2005) 🖥 www.nice.org.uk

### Patient information and support
**OCD Action** ☎ 0845 390 6232 🖥 www.ocdaction.org.uk

# Chronic stress

We all suffer from stress, and most of the time the pressures of everyday life are a motivating force. A problem only arises when those pressures exceed the individual's ability to cope with them.

**Causes of stress** Virtually anything we do can cause stress. The most common causes of stress-related morbidity in the UK are:
- Work problems
- Financial problems
- Exam stress
- Family problems
- Legal problems

**The stress epidemic** 105 million working days are lost each year in the UK due to stress (11% of all sickness absence). The Health and Safety Executive estimate that ~0.5 million people in the UK are experiencing work-related stress at a level they believe is making them ill, up to 5 million people feel 'very' or 'extremely' stressed by their work, and work-related stress costs society >£4 billion every year.

**Presentation** Most patients do not consult their GP with stress unless they feel that it is affecting their health. Common symptoms include:
- Mood swings
- Anxiety
- Depression
- Low self-esteem
- Poor concentration and/or memory
- Fatigue and/or lethargy
- Poor or ↑ appetite
- ↑ smoking, alcohol and/or caffeine consumption
- Sleep disturbance
- Headaches
- Loss of libido
- Menstrual abnormalities
- Dry mouth
- Other unexplained aches/pains, e.g. muscular pains, chest pains
- Worsening of pre-existing conditions, e.g. irritable bowel syndrome, eczema, asthma, psoriasis, migraine.

**The GP's role** is to identify stress as a cause of presenting symptoms, educate patients about stress and the links between symptoms and stress, identify sources of stress, provide support and self-management strategies, treat medical problems arising out of stress (e.g. depression), and provide certification if stress is so great that unable to work

**Post-traumatic stress disorder (PTSD)** May occur in 25–30% of those who have experienced/witnessed traumatic events, e.g. major accident, fire, assault, military combat. It can affect people of all ages.

*Symptoms* Most develop symptoms immediately after the event but it is common for sufferers not to present until months/years afterwards. In ~15% onset of symptoms is delayed. 65% experience chronic symptoms.
- *Intrusive recollections*—thoughts, nightmares, flashbacks.
- *Avoidant behaviour* of people, places, situations, or circumstances resembling/associated with the event; refusal to talk/think about the event; excessive rumination about questions about the event (e.g. Why me? How could it have been prevented?)
- *↑ arousal* ↑ anxiety/irritability, insomnia, ↓ concentration, ↑ vigilance.
- *Numbing of emotions* Inability to experience feelings; feelings of detachment; giving up previous activities; amnesia for parts of the event.

*Associations* Depression, anxiety; drug/alcohol abuse and dependence.

***Management*** Treat any other associated psychiatric illness.
- *Watchful waiting* If mild symptoms present <4 wk. Be supportive and listen. Arrange follow up in <1mo.
- *Trauma-focused psychological treatment* CBT and/or eye movement desensitization and reprocessing (EMDR). Refer via CMHT if severe symptoms <4wk, or ongoing intrusive symptoms >4 wk after trauma.
- *Drug treatment*, e.g. paroxetine, mirtazapine. Not first-line treatment. Reserve for those refusing psychological therapy, or with continuing symptoms despite therapy.

❶ Debriefing after traumatic events is unhelpful.

**The stressed GP** 📖 p.8

**10 tips for chronic stress relief**
- Ensure you get enough sleep and rest. Avoid using sleeping tablets to achieve this—see insomnia 📖 p.196.
- Look after yourself and your own health, e.g. don't skip meals, sit down to eat, take time out to spend time with family and friends, make time for hobbies and relaxation, do not ignore health worries.
- Avoid using nicotine, alcohol, or caffeine as a means of stress relief.
- Work off stress with physical exercise — ↓ levels of adrenaline released and ↑ release of natural endorphins which → a sense of well-being and enhances sleep.
- Try relaxation techniques.
- Avoid interpersonal conflicts: try to agree more and be more tolerant.
- Learn to accept what you can't change.
- Learn to say 'No'.
- Manage your time better—prioritize and delegate; create time buffers to deal with unexpected overruns and emergencies.
- Try to sort out the cause of the stress, e.g. talk to line manager at work, arrange marriage or debt counselling, arrange more child care.

**Time management made easy** This technique aims to transform an overwhelming volume of work into a series of manageable tasks.
- Make a list of all the things you need to do.
- List them in order of genuine importance.
- Note whether you really need to do the task, what you need to do personally, and what can be delegated to others.
- Note a time scale in which each task needs to be done, e.g. immediately, within a day, a week, a month, etc.

**Further information**
**Health and Safety Executive (HSE)** 🖥 www.hse.gov.uk/stress
**NICE** Post-traumatic stress disorder (PTSD): the management of PTSD in adults and children in primary, secondary and community care (2005) 🖥 www.nice.org.uk

**Patient advice and support**
**Stress Management Society** ☎ 0844 3578629 🖥 www.stress.org.uk
**International Stress Management Association (UK)** 🖥 www.isma.org.uk

# Depression

2.3 million people suffer from depression in UK at any time; 1:5 seeking help in primary care have psychological problems; 1:10 suffer from depression. ♂:♀ ≈ 1:2.

**Recognition** ~30-50% cases are not detected, although most of those are mild cases which are more likely to resolve spontaneously. Diagnosis of mental illness is stigmatizing. Polls show 60% think people with depression would feel too embarrassed to consult their GP. This can lead to 'collusion' between patient and doctor during consultation to avoid diagnosis of mental health problems, doing little to tackle the problem.

### Screening questions for depression[N]

- During the last month, have you often been bothered by feeling down depressed or hopeless?
- During the last month, have you often been bothered by having little interest or pleasure in doing things?

If +ve response to either question, investigate further, e.g with PHQ-9

**Causes and comorbidity** Associated with:

- *Psychiatric disorders*, e.g. anxiety disorders, alcohol abuse, substance abuse, eating disorders.
- *Physical disorders*, e.g. PD, MS, dementia, endocrine disease (thyroid disorders, Addison's disease), hypercalcaemia, RA, SLE, cancer, AIDS and other chronic infections, cardio- and cerebrovascular disease, learning disability.
- *Drugs causing symptoms of depression* β-blockers, anticonvulsants, $Ca^{2+}$ channel blockers, corticosteroids (although prednisolone is sometimes used, especially in terminal care, for the artificial 'high' it can give), oral contraceptives, antipsychotic drugs, drugs used for PD (e.g. levodopa).

### History

- Onset including precipitating events.
- Nature of symptoms, severity, and affect on life.
- Past history of similar symptoms/past psychiatric history.
- Current life events—stressors at home and at work.
- Family history.
- Coexisting medical conditions.
- Current medication—prescribed and non-prescribed.

❶ Sleep disturbance and fatigue have high predictive value for depression and should prompt enquiry about other symptoms.

*Assessing severity of depression* Most easily done using a patient self-complete measure, such as the Patient Health Questionnaire (PHQ-9). Each of the nine items in the PHQ is scored from 0 (not at all) to 3 (nearly every day). PHQ-9 scores:

- 5–9—mild depression
- 10–14—moderate depression
- 15–19—moderately severe depression
- ≥20—severe depression.

## Patient Health Questionnaire (PHQ-9)

| Name: | | | Date: | | |
|---|---|---|---|---|---|
| **Over the last 2 weeks, how often have you been bothered by any of the following problems? (use ✓ to indicate your answer)** | | **Not at all** | **Several days** | **More than half the days** | **Nearly every day** |
| 1. | Little interest or pleasure in doing things | 0 | 1 | 2 | 3 |
| 2. | Feeling down, depressed, or hopeless | 0 | 1 | 2 | 3 |
| 3. | Trouble falling or staying asleep, or sleeping too much | 0 | 1 | 2 | 3 |
| 4. | Feeling tired or having little energy | 0 | 1 | 2 | 3 |
| 5. | Poor appetite or overeating | 0 | 1 | 2 | 3 |
| 6. | Feeling bad about yourself— or that you are a failure or have let yourself or your family down | 0 | 1 | 2 | 3 |
| 7. | Trouble concentrating on things, such as reading the newspaper or watching television | 0 | 1 | 2 | 3 |
| 8. | Moving or speaking so slowly that other people could have noticed. Or the opposite— being so fidgety or restless that you have been moving around a lot more than usual | 0 | 1 | 2 | 3 |
| 9. | Thoughts that you would be better off dead, or of hurting yourself in some way | 0 | 1 | 2 | 3 |
| | **Add columns:** | ☐ | ☐ | ☐ | ☐ |
| | | | | **Total:** | |
| 10. | If you ticked off *any* problems, how *difficult* have these problems made it for you to do your work, take care of things at home, or get along with other people? | Not difficult at all | | | |
| | | Somewhat difficult | | | |
| | | Very difficult | | | |
| | | Extremely difficult | | | |

The Patient Health Questionnaire (PHQ-9) was developed by Spitzer RL, Williams BW, Kroenke K, and colleagues, with an educational grant from Pfizer Inc. Copyright© 2005 Pfizer Inc. All rights reserved. Reproduced with permission.

*Assessment of suicidal intent* ❶ Always ask patients directly about suicidal ideas and intent—📖 p.1114.

> *Risk factors for suicide*
> - ♂>♀
> - Age 40-60 y
> - Living alone
> - Divorced > widowed > single > married
> - Unemployment
> - Chronic physical illness
> - Past psychiatric history
> - Recent admission to psychiatric hospital
> - History of suicide attempt/self harm
> - Alcohol/drug misuse

*Cultural considerations* Some cultures have no terms for depression and may present with physical symptoms (somatization) or use less familiar 'cultural-specific' terms to describe depressive symptoms, e.g. 'sorrow in my heart'.

## Definitions

*Major depression* 2 key features:
- Depressed mood *and/or*
- ↓ interest or pleasure, which must be disabling to the patient.

Major depression can be diagnosed if:
- ≥5 of the 9 depressive symptom criteria on the PHQ-9 have been present >$^1/_2$ the days in the past 2 wk., *or*
- ≥5 symptoms from the following list are present most of the time for ≥2wk, at least 1 of which must be a key feature:
  - Low mood
  - Loss of interest or pleasure
  - Fatigue or loss of energy
  - Change in appetite or weight
  - Insomnia or hypersomnia
  - Poor concentration or difficulty making decisions
  - Low self-esteem, sense of worthlessness or guilt
  - Psychomotor agitation or retardation
  - Feelings of hopelessness and recurrent thoughts of death or suicide

*Mild to moderate depression* Some of the above symptoms (but not enough to make diagnosis of major depression) associated with some functional impairment.

*Dysthymia* A chronic form of minor depression. Depressed mood for *most* of the day, for more days than not, for ≥2y *and* the presence of ≥2 of the above symptoms.

## Examination
- *General appearance* Self-neglect, smell of alcohol, weight ↓
- *Assessment of mood* Looks depressed and/or tired; speech monotone or monosyllabic; avoids eye contact; tearful, anxious, or jumpy/fidgety; feeling of distance; poor concentration, etc.
- *Psychotic symptoms* Hallucinations, delusions etc. (📖 p.1004).

**Suicide and deliberate self-harm** 📖 p.1114.

**Management of depression** Depends on severity (Fig. 27.3a,
📖 p.1003).
- *Major depression and dysthymia*—antidepressants or high intensity
  psychological treatments e.g. CBT.
- *Acute milder depression*—education about depression, e.g. information
  leaflets; support, self-help, and/or guided self-help based on CBT;
  simple problem-solving strategies; *or* watchful waiting (review in <2wk).
- *Persistent milder depression*—consider antidepressants if symptoms for
  a long period (e.g. >2y.)
- *Milder depression with history of major depression*—consider
  antidepressants or watchful waiting. Always review in <2wk and
  monitor regularly for development of major depression.

**Referral to specialist psychiatry or crisis team**
(*U*=Urgent; *S*=Soon; *R*=Routine)
- High suicide risk—*U*
- Psychotic major depression—*U*
- History of biopolar disorder—*R/S*
- Atypical symptoms—*R/S*
- Failure or partial response following ≥2 attempts to treat—*R*
- Recurrent depression—*R*

---

**Management of other specific types of depression**

***Seasonal affective disorder (SAD)*** 'Winter blues'—recurrent disorder involving 'seasonal' episodes of depression, usually in the winter
months. Affects ≈2% adults. ♀:♂ ≈ 2:1. Peak incidence third decade.

***Symptoms*** Depression + ↑ sleep, ↑ food intake (with carbohydrate craving)
and weight gain. 30% experience elatory mood swings in summer.

***Management*** SSRIs (particularly sertraline); phototherapy (30–90min/d
in early morning—effects should be seen within 3wk). Light boxes can
be borrowed from psychiatry departments, hired, or bought (contact
SAD Association for more information 🖥 www.sada.org.uk).

***Recurrent brief depression (RBD)*** Recurrent depressive episodes
of short duration (2–7d) which meet criteria for major depression. High
prevalence in primary care. Episodes occur as often as monthly. ~50%
also have seasonal variation. At present there is no effective treatment—
antidepressants are ineffective.

---

**Further Reading**
**NICE** Depression (2009) 🖥 www.nice.org.uk

**Patient information and support**
**Depression Alliance** ☎ 0845 123 2320 🖥 www.depressionalliance.org
**Samaritans** 24h emotional support via telephone ☎ 08457 909 090
🖥 www.samaritans.org

# Treatment for depression

**Antidepressant drug therapy** (BNF 4.3)

***When should antidepressants be started?*** Don't prescribe at the first visit as symptoms may improve significantly over the following weeks. Watchful waiting is a useful first-line strategy (*'Don't just do something, sit there!'*).

***What should I tell the patient?*** Giving patients information ↑ compliance. When starting antidepressant drugs explain the reasons for prescribing; timescale of action—unlikely to have any effect for 2wk, effects build up to maximum effect at 4–6wk; and likely side effects including possible exacerbation of anxiety in the first 2wk of treatment.

***Which drugs are available?*** The major groups are:
- ***Selective serotonin re-uptake inhibitors (SSRIs)***, e.g.fluoxetine 20mg od—usually first choice as less likely to be discontinued due to side effects. Warn of possible anxiety and agitation and advise patients to stop if significant. GI side effects including dyspepsia are common.
- ***Serotonin and noradrenaline re-uptake inhibitors (SNRIs)***, e.g. venlafaxine 75mg MR od, duloxetine 60mg od. Avoid if uncontrolled hypertension. Venlafaxine is also contraindicated if high risk of arrhythmia.
- ***Tricyclic antidepressants (TCAs)***, e.g. lofepramine 70mg od/bd/tds— titrate dose up from low dose until patient feels the drug is helping or until side effects intrude.[S] Common side effects include drowsiness, dry mouth, blurred vision, constipation, urinary retention, and sweating.
- ***Monoamine oxidase inhibitors (MAOIs)***, e.g. phenelzine 15mg tds. MAOIs should not be started until at least 1–2wk after a tricyclic has been stopped (3wk in the case of clomipramine or imipramine). Other antidepressants should not be started for 2wk after treatment with MAOIs has been stopped (3wk if starting clomipramine or imipramine).

***Follow-up*** Review the patient every 1–2wk until stable, assessing response, compliance, side effects, and suicidal risk. Continue treatment for >6mo. after remission as this greatly ↓ risk of relapse. Patients with ≥2 past episodes of major depression should be advised to continue for 2y. Reassure patients that antidepressant medication is not addictive.

***Discontinuation reactions*** Occur once a drug has been used ≥8wk. ↓ risk by tapering dose over ≥4wk. Warn about possible reactions:
- Withdrawal of SSRIs—headache, nausea, paraesthesia, dizziness, and anxiety.
- Withdrawal of other antidepressants (especially MAOIs)—nausea, vomiting, anorexia, headache, 'chills', insomnia, paraesthesiae, anxiety/ panic, and restlessness.

**St John's wort** May be effective in mild depression but formulations vary widely in potency. Interacts with many drugs including antidepressants (especially SSRIs), warfarin, oral contraceptives, and theophylline.

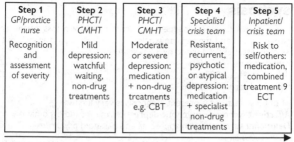

*PHCT* = Primary healthcare team
*ECT* = electro-convulsive therapy
*CMHT* = Community mental health team

**Fig. 27.3a** Stepped care for depression

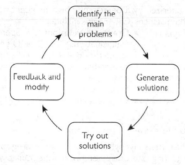

**Fig. 27.3b** Simple problem solving strategy to use in the surgery

### Other treatments

***Exercise*** Beneficial in mild/moderate depression.

### *Counselling* ☐ p.988

***Specific psychological therapies*** Simple problem-solving strategies (Figure 27.3b) can be used in the surgery. Other psychological therapies such as CBT (☐ p.988), behaviour therapy, interpersonal psychotherapy, and problem-solving therapy (☐ p.988) can be used as first-line therapies in mild/moderate depression. Some of these are freely accessible to patients via the internet, e.g. *The Mood Gym* (🖥 www.moodgym.anu.edu.au). Excessive waiting lists may be a limiting factor where referral to psychological services is required.

### Further reading

**NICE** Depression (2009) 🖥 www.nice.org.uk

### Patient information and support

**Depression Alliance** ☎ 0845 123 2320 🖥 www.depressionalliance.org
**Samaritans** 24h emotional support via telephone ☎ 0845 7909 090
🖥 www.samaritans.org

# Psychosis

The archetypal layman's 'madness'. Characterized by a loss of the link between reason and the outside world. Psychosis is not a diagnosis but a class of illnesses characterized by 3 key features:

- hallucinations—📖 p.986
- delusions—📖 p.987 *and*
- thought disorder 📖 p.986.

If ≥1 of these features is present, diagnosis is very limited:

- *Affective psychoses*—psychotic depression, mania, and hypomania
- *Delusional psychosis*—schizophrenia and paranoid psychoses (📖 p.1006) *or*
- *Organic psychoses*—the dementias (📖 p.1010) and acute confusional states (📖 p.1008).

**Mania and hypomania** Most of us experience ups and downs in our mood according to the circumstances we find ourselves in.

*Mania* is characterized by a persistently high or euphoric mood out of keeping with circumstances. Other signs include:

- ↑ pressure of speech
- ↑ energy and activity
- ↑ appetite
- ↑ sexual desire
- ↑ pain threshold
- ↓desire or need for sleep
- ↓ insight
- Grandiose delusions
- Hallucinations
- Labile mood—elation to irritability and hostility when thwarted
- Over-assertiveness
- Spending sprees
- Disinhibition
- Self-important ideas
- Poor concentration—easily distracted.

*Hypomania* is a less severe form of mania.

**Differential diagnosis** Hypoglycaemia; alcohol or drug abuse; prescribed drug side effects (e.g. steroids); temporal lobe epilepsy; frontal lobe dysfunction (e.g. due to tumour or stroke); thyrotoxicosis.

---

### Acute management

- Treatment in hospital is usually required for the first episode or acute relapses.
- If unwilling to accept voluntary admission, use compulsory admission under the Mental Health Act (📖 p.1118).
- Sedation whilst awaiting admission may be required—use chlorpromazine 50–100mg po or 50mg IM (↓ dose for elderly patients and avoid if the patient is epileptic, or has been drinking or taking barbiturates).

---

**Chronic management** Requires long-term follow-up.

- *Regular reviews* Case registers help ensure that regular reviews take place. Check a written care plan has been drawn up by the psychiatric service. Assess symptoms, compliance with medication, efficacy of treatment, medication side effects, risks of suicide.
- *Educate* the patient and relatives/friends about early signs of relapse and action in case of relapse.

- *Reinforce compliance with treatment*
- *Ensure adequate social support* Self-help groups, day centres, benefits.
- *Monitor drugs for toxic side effects*
- *Advise patients to inform the DVLA* Driving should cease during the acute illness (all vehicles) and until stable with insight for 3 years (LGV/PCV drivers)—📖 p.133.

**Drug treatment** (BNF 4.2.3)
- Lithium is the drug of choice. Initiate only under consultant supervision.
- Check levels weekly until the dose is constant for 4wk, then monthly for 6mo, then every 3mo thereafter as long as the dose remains constant.
- If levels are slowly rising suspect nephrotoxicity.
- Check plasma creatinine, eGFR, and TFTs every 6mo.
- Avoid changing proprietary brands as bioavailability varies.
- *Toxic effects*: blurred vision, diahorrea and vomiting ↓ $K^+$, drowsiness, ataxia, coarse tremor, dysarthria, hyperextension, fits, psychosis, coma, and shock.
- *Alternative drugs*: sodium valproate; carbamazepine.

**Bipolar disorder or manic depression** Consists of episodes when the patient has mania (bipolar I) or hypomania (bipolar II) against a background of depression. Lifetime prevalence ~1%. ♂:♀ ≈ 1:1. Peak incidence is in late teens and early 20s—90% develop the disorder before 30y.

**Management** as for mania.

**Schizophrenia** 📖 p.1006

**Further information**
**NICE** Bipolar disorder (2006) 🖥 www. mdf.org.uk

**Patient information and support**
**Manic Depression Fellowship** ☎ 0808 802 1983 🖥 www.mdf.org.uk
**Royal College of Psychiatrists** Patient information sheets
🖥 www.rcpsych.ac.uk

# Schizophrenia

A frightening and disabling condition in which the sufferer is unable to distinguish his/her internal world from the outside world. Lifetime prevalence ~1%. Peak age of onset: ♂ 15–25y; ♀ 25–35y.

**First-rank symptoms** Reliable markers in ~70% of patients. ≥ 1 symptom is suggestive of schizophrenia.

- Auditory hallucinations in the form of a commentary
- Hearing thoughts spoken aloud
- Hearing voices referring to the patient, made in the 3rd person
- Somatic hallucinations
- Thought broadcasting

- Thought withdrawal, insertion, and interruption
- Delusional perception
- Feelings or actions experienced as made or influenced by external agents (passivity feelings)

**Acute schizophrenia** Typically presents in a young people with +ve symptoms (delusions, hallucinations, and/or thought disorder). The patient lacks insight, so initial approach may come from a relative or friend.

**Assessment** See the patient:
- Try to elicit any history of drug abuse—amphetamines can give a picture identical to schizophrenia.
- Ask about physical and psychological symptoms, in particular thoughts and perceptions.
- Assess the patient's behaviour and appearance. Look for evidence of self-care, loss of affect, poverty of thought, and social withdrawal.
- Ask friends, neighbours, or relatives present to tell you about of the patient's behaviour.

**Differential diagnosis** Illicit drugs, temporal lobe epilepsy, acute confusional state, dementia, affective disorders, personality disorder.

**Management** (BNF 4.2.1)
- Seek expert psychiatric help. Is the patient is a risk to self/others?
  - Patients who are a risk need acute admission either voluntarily or under the Mental Health Act (🕮 p.1118).
  - Patients who are no immediate risk may be assessed urgently by the community psychiatric services as an outpatient.
- Start antipsychotic treatment, if necessary before psychiatric assessment—delay in treatment ↑ patient risks and → poorer prognosis.
- Oral atypical antipsychotic drugs (e.g. amisulpride, olanzapine, risperidone) are first-line treatment for newly diagnosed schizophrenia.
- Stick to a single drug and start at the lower end of the dose range, e.g. risperidone 1mg bd on day 1 and ↑ to 2mg bd on day 2. Don't use loading doses.
- Advise patients to inform the DVLA—driving should cease during the acute illness (all vehicles) and until stable with insight for 3y (LGV/PCV drivers) (🕮 p.133).

**Follow-up** Liaise with the community psychiatric services and reinforce the management plan agreed. Following acute episodes there is ↓ risk of relapse if antipsychotic medication continues for 6–24mo. Provide contacts for patient and relative support groups.

**Chronic schizophrenia** Characterized by thought disorder and –ve symptoms (poverty of thought, apathy, inactivity, lack of volition, social withdrawal and loss of affect). Aim to treat the disease, prevent relapse and improve quality of life.

## Long-term health problems

- ↑ death from suicide (1:10 schizophrenics), accidents, cardiovascular disease, and respiratory disease.
- ↑ obesity due to side effects of antipsychotic drugs, poor diet, sedentary lifestyle, and lack of exercise.
- Substance abuse—¾ smoke; ↑ prevalence of alcohol and drug abuse.
- Rarely patients drink excessive amounts of water → hyponatraemia.

**Regular reviews** Case registers ensure regular reviews take place.
- *Check that there is a written care plan* from the psychiatric service.
- *Check mental health*—assess symptoms, compliance with medication, efficacy of treatment, medication side effects, risks of suicide.
- *Check physical health*—watch for weight ↑, DM, and hyperprolactinaemia, especially on atypical antipsychotics. Check BP and lipids. ECG if palpitations—look for QT prolongation on atypical antipsychotics.
- *Promote lifestyle changes*—↑ exercise; ↓ smoking; improve diet; encourage sensible drinking and avoidance of illicit drugs, e.g. cannabis and amphetamines which exacerbate symptoms and ↑ risk of relapse.
- *Review social support*—assistance may be needed with: finances, housing, employment, structured daily activity, transport, social network. Those who can help include social services, community mental health team, housing officer, disablement resettlement officer.

**Referral to psychiatry** *U*=Urgent; *S*=Soon; *R*=Routine
- ↑ in risk to self or others—*U*.
- Poor response to treatment—*U/S/R*.
- Problems with adherence: consider depot administration—*S/R*.
- Suspected comorbid substance misuse—*R*.
- Patient new to your practice—*R*.
- Patient is on conventional antipsychotics (e.g. sulpiride, thioridazine) and suffering significant side effects or persistent symptoms. Refer for consideration of change of medication to atypical antipsychotic—*R*.
- For family interventions to ↓ 'expressed emotion' (smothering, or hostility and criticism about the patient by the family)—effective in ↓ relapse—*R*.
- For CBT—persistent symptoms despite antipsychotics, to ↑ insight—*R*.

## Further information

**NICE** Schizophrenia (2009) 🖥 www.nice.org.uk

## Patient information and support

**National Association for Mental Health (MIND)** 0845 766 0163
🖥 www.mind.org.uk
**Rethink (National Schizophrenia Fellowship)** ☎ 0845 456 0455
🖥 www.rethink.org

# Acute confusional states (delirium)

Common condition seen in general practice—particularly amongst elderly patients. May occur *de novo* or be superimposed upon chronic confusion of dementia (📖 p.1010) causing sudden worsening of cognition.

## Presentation
- Global cognitive deficit with onset over hours/days.
- Fluctuating conscious level—typically worse at night/late afternoon.
- Impaired memory—on recovery amnesia of the events is usual.
- Disorientation in time and place.
- Odd behaviour—may be underactive, drowsy, and/or withdrawn *or* hyperactive and agitated.
- Disordered thinking—often slow and muddled ± delusions (e.g. accuse relatives of taking things).
- Disturbed perceptions—hallucinations (particularly visual) are common.
- Mood swings.

***Examination*** Can be difficult. If possible do a thorough general physical examination to exclude treatable causes.

## Possible causes
- *Infection* Particularly UTI, pneumonia. Rarely encephalitis, meningitis.
- *Drugs* Opiates, sedatives, L-dopa, anticonvulsants, recreational drugs.
- *Metabolic* Hypoglycaemia, uraemia, liver failure, hypercalcaemia, other electrolyte imbalance (rarer).
- *Alcohol or drug withdrawal.*
- *Hypoxia,* e.g. severe pneumonia, exacerbation of COPD, cardiac failure.
- *Cardiovascular* MI, stroke, TIA.
- *Intracranial lesion* Space-occupying lesion, ↑ ICP, head injury (especially subdural haematoma).
- *Thyroid disease.*
- *Carcinomatosis.*
- *Epilepsy* Temporal lobe epilepsy, post-ictal state.
- *Nutritional deficiency* $B_{12}$, thiamine or nicotinic acid deficiency.

## Differential diagnosis
- Deafness—may appear confused.
- Dementia—longer history and lack of fluctuations in conscious level. In practice may be difficult to distinguish especially if you come across a patient who is alone and can give no history
- Primary mental illness, e.g. schizophrenia (📖 p.1006), anxiety state (📖 p.990)

**Management** is aimed at treating all remediable causes.
## Admit if
- The patient lives alone
- The patient will be left unsupervised for any duration of time
- Carers (or residential home) are unprepared/unable to continue looking after the patient, *and/or*
- History and examination have indicated a cause requiring acute hospital treatment—admit as an emergency.

### Possible investigations to consider in the community
- Cognitive function test e.g. 6CIT (Table 27.3).
- Urine—dipstick for glucose, ketones, blood, protein, nitrates and white cells, send for M,C&S.
- Check BM to exclude hypoglycaemia.
- Blood—FBC, ESR, U&E, eGFR, LFTs, TFTs.
- ECG.
- CXR.

### Management at home
- Acute confusion is frightening for carers—reassure and support them.
- Treat the cause, e.g. antibiotics for UTI or chest infection
- Try to avoid sedation as this can make confusion worse. Where unavoidable use haloperidol 1–2mg prn or lorazepam 0.5–1mg prn.
- Involve district nursing services, e.g. to provide incontinence aids, cot sides, moral support.
- If the cause does not become clear despite investigation or the patient fails to improve with treatment, admit for further investigation and assessment.

**Table 27.3** The 6 Cognitive Impairment Test (6CIT)—Kingshill Version 2000

| | Question | Response | Score |
|---|---|---|---|
| 1. | What year is it? | Correct: 0; Incorrect: 4 | |
| 2. | What month is it? | Correct: 0; Incorrect: 3 | |
| **Remember the following address:** | | e.g. John Brown, 42 West Street, Bedford | |
| 3. | What time is it (to the nearest hour)? | Correct: 0; Incorrect: 3 | |
| 4. | Count backwards from 20 to 1 | Correct: 0; 1 error: 2; >1 error: 4 | |
| 5. | Months of the year backwards | Correct: 0; 1 error: 2; >1 error: 4 | |
| 6. | Repeat the memory phrase | Correct: 0; 1 error: 2; 2 errors: 4; 3 errors: 6; 4 errors: 8; all incorrect: 10 | |
| | Total | | |

**Instructions on scoring** Ring the appropriate score results for each question; add up the scores to produce a result out of 28.

**Score**
- 0–7 — Not significant
- 8–9 — Probably significant—refer, possible dementia
- 10–28 — Significant—refer, likely dementia

# Dementia

Generalized impairment of intellect, memory, and personality, with no impairment of consciousness. Prevalence ↑ with age (rare <60y; 5% >65y; 20% >80y). Common causes: Alzheimer's disease (60%); vascular (multi-infarct) dementia; dementia with Lewy bodies.

## Presentation

*History* Patients may be aware of 'being a bit forgetful' but usually relatives complain about their behaviour. Early symptoms are loss of short-term memory and inability to perform normally simple tasks. Alternatively, patients present later with failure to cope at home or self-neglect. To diagnose dementia there must be a clear history of progressive impairment of memory and cognition ± personality change. Always assess level of support in the home, housing, and ability to cope (both patient and carers).

*Examination* Check general appearance—look for evidence of self-neglect, malnutrition, abuse; screen for cognitive deficit, e.g. with 6CIT (Table 27.3, 📖 p.1009).

**Investigation** Aimed at detecting treatable causes: check FBC, U&E, eGFR, LFTs, $Ca^{2+}$, TFTs, glucose, $B_{12}$, folate. Consider MSU, CXR, ECG.

## Differential diagnosis

- Acute confusion—📖 p.1008
- Depression—📖 p.998
- Communication difficulties—deafness, dysphasia, or language difficulties.

## Prevention[N]

- Do not use statins, HRT, vitamin E, or aspirin for 1° prevention.
- 2° prevention: review and treat vascular and other risk factors.
- Offer referral to genetic counselling to those thought to have a genetic cause for their dementia, and refer unaffected relatives.

## Management

- *Refer* All patients should be referred to a psychogeriatrician/memory assessment clinic for formal diagnosis, exclusion of treatable causes, ongoing specialist support and assessment, and care planning. Refer to a social worker and/or CPN for community support.
- *Apply principles of rehabilitation* (📖 p.206, 📖 p.590)
- *Support carers* (📖 p.222). Advise re benefits (📖 p.224), self-help groups, respite care. Warn that dementia is progressive and prepare carers for a time when the patient does not recognize them.
- *Discuss whilst sufferer still has capacity,* along with carers, the use of advanced statements, lasting power of attorney (📖 p.124), advanced decisions to refuse treatment, and preferred place of care plans.
- *Treat concurrent problems* (e.g. UTI, chest infection, anaemia, depression)—they make dementia worse. Consider possible side effects of medication.
- *Management of memory loss* Notebook to record 'tasks must do'; medication dispensers.

- *Management of agitation*
  - Maintain a constant environment if possible.
  - Arrange for door catches to prevent wandering.
  - Take up loose carpets to prevent falls.
  - Consider fire and electrical safety.
  - Avoid sedatives wherever possible as they may worsen confusion—if needed use very low dose, review regularly, and consider newer atypical drugs, e.g. risperidone.

**Alzheimer's disease** Most common form of dementia. Each GP has ~16 patients with Alzheimer's disease at any time. *Cause:* unknown—defective genes found on chromosomes 14,19, and 21.

**Risk factors** FH, Down's syndrome (onset at ~30y.), late onset depression, hypothyroidism, history of head injury.

**Presentation** Presents with steady ↓ in memory and cognition. *Onset:* any age—normally >40y. ♀:♂ ≈ 0.7.

**Management** Specific treatment with anticholinesterase inhibitors (e.g. donepezil, galantamine, rivastigmine) is now available. There is some evidence that these drugs ↓ rate of decline. They are *only* prescribed for patients presenting with moderate dementia[N] and only under specialist supervision—refer.

**Prognosis** Mean survival ~7y from outset.

*A. Alzheimer (1864–1915). German neuropathologist/psychiatrist.*

**Lewy body dementia** Fluctuating but persistent cognitive impairment, parkinsonism, and hallucinations. No specific treatment. Avoid antipsychotics as they can be fatal. Use benzodiazepines if tranquillization is necessary. *F.H. Lewy (1885–1950), German neurologist.*

**Pick dementia** Dementia characterized by personality change associated with frontal lobe signs such as gross tactlessness. Lack of restraint may lead to stealing, practical jokes, and unusual sexual adventures. Treatment is supportive. *A. Pick (1851–1924), Czech neurologist/psychiatrist.*

**Vascular (multi-infarct) dementia** Multiple lacunar infarcts or larger strokes cause generalized intellectual impairment. Tends to occur in a stepwise progression with each subsequent infarct. The final picture is one of dementia, pseudobulbar palsy, and shuffling gait with small steps. Treatment is as for secondary prevention of TIA/stroke (☐ p.572).

## Further information
**NICE** Dementia (2006) 🖳 www.nice.org.uk

## Patient information and support
**Alzheimer's Society** ☎ 0845 300 0336 🖳 www.alzheimers.org.uk
**Benefits enquiry line** ☎ 0800 882 200
**Carers UK** ☎ 0808 808 7777 🖳 www.carersuk.org

# Eating disorders

### Identification of and screening for eating disorders

Target groups for screening include:
- Young women with low BMI compared with age norms.
- Patients consulting with weight concerns who are not overweight.
- Women with menstrual disturbances or amenorrhoea.
- Patients with GI symptoms.
- Patients with symptoms/signs of starvation—sensitivity to cold, delayed gastric emptying, constipation, ↓ BP, bradycardia, hypothermia.
- Patients with physical signs of repeated vomiting—pitted teeth ± dental caries, general weakness, cardiac arrythmias, renal damage, ↑ risk of UTI, epileptic fits, ↓$K^+$.
- Children with poor growth.
- Young people with type 1 DM and poor treatment adherence.

### *Screen target populations with simple screening questions*
- Do you worry excessively about your weight?
- Do you think you have an eating problem?

⚠ Patients who are pregnant or have DM are particularly at risk of complications if they have comorbid eating disorders. Refer early for specialist support and ensure that everyone involved in care is aware of the eating disorder.

**Anorexia nervosa** Prevalence 0.02–0.04%. ♀>>♂. Usually begins in adolescence. Peak prevalence at 16–17y. *Features:*
- Refusal to maintain body weight >85% of that expected (BMI <17.5kg/m²).
- Intense fear of gaining weight, although underweight.
- Disturbed experience of body weight or shape or undue influence of shape on self-image.
- Amenorrhoea in women for ≥3 mo and ↓ sexual interest.

Patients tend to have a set daily calorific intake, e.g. 600–1000 calories, and may employ strategies, e.g. bingeing and vomiting, purging, or excessive exercise, to try to lose weight. Depression and social withdrawal are common, as are symptoms 2° to starvation.

### *Management[N]*
- Give ongoing support and information.
- Check electrolytes.
- Refer to a specialist eating disorders clinic (if available) or psychiatry. Treatment involves family therapy for adolescents, psychotherapy, and possible admission for re-feeding.

*Follow-up* Patients with enduring anorexia nervosa not under 2° care follow-up should be offered an annual physical and mental health check.

⚠ Many patients with anorexia nervosa have compromised cardiac function. Avoid prescribing drugs which adversely affect cardiac function (e.g. antipsychotics, TCAs, macrolide antibiotics, some antihistamines). If prescribing is essential then follow up with ECG monitoring.

**Bulimia nervosa** Prevalence 1–2%. Mainly ♀ aged 16–40y. Features:
- Recurrent episodes of binge eating, far beyond normally accepted amounts of food.
- Inappropriate compensatory behaviour to prevent weight ↑, e.g. vomiting; use of laxatives, diuretics, and/or appetite suppressants. Bulimics can be subdivided into those who purge and those who just use fasting and exercise to control their weight.
- Self-image unduly influenced by body shape (see anorexia).
- Normal menses and normal weight. If low BMI classified as anorexia.

### Management
- Give ongoing support and information.
- Check electrolytes.
- First-line treatment:
  - Evidence-based self-help programme, e.g. Overcoming Bulimia— available from 🖳 www.overcomingbulimiaonline.com
  - Antidepressant medication—fluoxetine 60mg od is the drug of choice.
- If unsuccessful, refer to a specialist eating disorders clinic (if available) or psychiatry. CBT may help.

### Advice for patients purging
- *Vomiting* Advise patients to avoid brushing their teeth after vomiting, rinse with a non-acid mouthwash after vomiting, and ↓ acid oral environment (e.g. by limiting acid foods).
- *Laxatives* Where laxative abuse is present, advise patients to gradually ↓ laxative intake. Laxative abuse does not significantly ↓ calorie absorption.

**Binge eating disorder** A pattern of consumption of large amounts of food, even when a patient is not hungry. Common. Usually associated with obsessive feelings about food and body image, feelings of guilt/disgust about the amounts consumed, and/or a feeling of lack of control.

### Management
- Give ongoing support and information.
- Provide an evidence-based self-help programme as a first step and/or antidepressant medication (SSRIs are the drug group of choice).
- If unsuccessful refer for specialist help. CBT might be helpful.
- In all cases, provide concurrent advice and support to tackle any comorbid obesity.

### Further information
**NICE** Core interventions in the treatment and management of anorexia nervosa, bulimia nervosa and related eating disorders (2004) 🖳 www.nice.org

### Patient support and information
**Beating Eating Disorders (BEAT)** ☎ 0845 634 1414 (adults) 0845 634 7650 (youths) 🖳 www.b-eat.co.uk

# Other psychological conditions

**Personality (behavioural) disorder** Patients may prefer the term 'personality difficulties'. Personality changes through life, and personality disorder should not be diagnosed aged <18 y. *Features*:

- Pervasive and maladaptive patterns of behaviour, thinking, and control of emotions.
- These patterns of behaviour, thinking and control of emotions must be enduring and not limited to episodes of mental illness.
- There must be significant distress/disturbance in social function.

*Types of personality disorder* 3 main types:

- Schizoid—paranoid ideas, difficulty mixing.
- Histrionic—impulsive, unstable, 'borderline'.
- Dependent—anxious, obsessive.

*Management*

- Be clear about professional boundaries and avoid conflict.
- Involve family or friends in the care plan if appropriate.
- Consider referral to psychiatry:
  - For diagnostic clarification
  - If there is a risk of harm to self or others
  - For treatment of co-morbid mental illness
  - For specialist treatment of personality disorder.
- SSRIs can help impulsive behaviour.
- Low-dose atypical antipsychotics may help paranoid ideas.
- Mood stabilizers may help emotional instability.

⚠ Risk of overdose is ↑ amongst patients with personality disorder

**Factitious disorder (Munchausen syndrome)** Intentional production or feigning of physical or psychological symptoms to assume the sick role (± hospital admission). Can be difficult to detect. Differs from *malingering* as there is no external reward (e.g. financial). Associated with personality disorder.

*Common presentations*

- *Physical* Dermatitis artefacta; pyrexia of unknown origin (PUO); bruising disorders; brittle DM; diarrhoea of unknown cause; neurological symptoms, e.g. pseudo-paralysis or pseudo-fits (neurologica diabolica); abdominal pain (laparotomophilia migrans); chest pain (cardiopathia fantastica).
- *Psychological* Feigned psychosis, fictitious bereavement, fictitious overdose.

*Management* Exclude any other basis for presenting pathology. Explain findings to the patient, exploring possible causes. Assess psychological and social difficulties. Consider referral to psychiatry.
*Baron H.K.F.F. von Munchausen (1720–1797), German traveller/soldier.*

**Munchausen syndrome by proxy** Caregiver—typically a mother with child—seeks repeated medical investigations and needless treatment for the person he/she is caring for. The child or person being cared for may actually be harmed by the carer to achieve these aims. Commonly reported symptoms include neurological symptoms, bleeding, rashes.

*Management* Often difficult to detect and even harder to prove. A form of abuse that must be taken seriously and handled with care (印 p.922). Involve all relevant agencies early (e.g. social services, paediatrics).

**Malingering** Intentional production or feigning of physical or psychological symptoms to assume the sick role for a known external purpose. Malingering is not considered mental illness or psychopathology, although it can occur in the context of other mental illnesses. Forms:
- *Pure malingering*—the individual falsifies all symptoms.
- *Partial malingering*—the individual has symptoms but exaggerates the impact they have upon daily functioning.
- *Simulation*—the individual acts out the symptoms of a specific disability.
- *False imputation*—the individual has valid symptoms but is dishonest as to the source of the problems, e.g. attributing neck pain to a RTA to obtain compensation.

### Differential diagnosis
- True medical or psychiatric illness yet to be diagnosed.
- Factitious disorder/Munchausen syndrome.
- Somatization disorder.

### Common motivating factors
- Avoidance of going to jail or release from jail.
- Avoidance of work.
- Avoidance of family responsibility.
- Desire to obtain narcotics.
- Desire to be awarded money in litigation.
- Need for attention.

*Management* Difficult. As doctors we tend to believe our patients.
- Exclude causes for the presenting symptoms through careful history/ examination.
- Avoid prescribing drugs for symptoms and unnecessary referrals as these might perpetuate symptoms.
- Avoid certifying the patient as unfit to work or perform activities—if the patient is unhappy about this, suggest a second opinion.
- Tactfully explain your findings and conclusions to the patient and explore the reasons for the behaviour.
- Provide support to find more appropriate ways to solve problems.

### Patient/relative information and support
**Borderline Personality Disorder (BPD) Central** ▣ www.bpdcentral.com
**Self injury and Related Issues (SIARI)** ▣ www.siari.co.uk

# Cancer and palliative care

# Principles of cancer care

If cancer is suspected as a result of signs or symptoms locally at the original site or at distant sites, an accurate and comprehensive assessment of both the patient and the disease must be undertaken before a treatment decision is reached. Treatment can be:

- *Radical* Curative intent—surgery and/or drug/radiotherapy.
- *Adjuvant* Given after surgery when micrometastatic disease is suspected—decision to proceed is based on the likelihood of relapse.
- *Palliative* When cure is not possible (&book; p.1026).

## Assessment of the tumour

- *Histological nature of the tumour* Tissue of origin, cancer type (e.g. adenocarcinoma, squamous cell cancer), degree of differentiation, and tumour grade. High-grade poorly differentiated tumours tend to have a poorer outcome than low-grade well-differentiated tumours.
- *Biological behaviour of the tumour* Tumour markers produced by cancers may be a useful adjunct to histological classification and staging and can be used to influence and monitor efficacy of treatment (Table 28.1). ❶ Tumour markers can be ↑ in non-malignant conditions.
- *Anatomical extent of the tumour* Usually determined through a combination of clinical, radiological, biochemical, and surgical assessment. Routine blood tests including liver function tests and bone profiles may also indicate the presence of metastases.

**Cancer staging** Staging allows the plan of treatment to be made.

***TMN classification*** Widely used classification of tumours. Exact criteria for staging depend on the primary organ site:

- *T*—Primary tumour. Graded $T_1$–$T_4$ with increasing size of primary.
- *N*—Regional lymph nodes. Advancing nodal disease is graded $N_0$–$N_3$.
- *M*—Presence ($M_1$) or absence ($M_0$) of metastases.

### Stage grouping

- *Stage 1* Clinical examination reveals a tumour confined to the primary organ. The lesion tends to be operable and completely resectable.
- *Stage 2* Clinical examination shows evidence of local spread into surrounding tissue and first draining LNs. The lesion is operable and resectable but there is a higher risk of further spread of disease
- *Stage 3* Clinical examination reveals an extensive primary tumour with fixation to deeper structures and local invasion. The lesion may not be operable and may require a combination of treatment modalities.
- *Stage 4* Evidence of distant metastases beyond the site of origin. The primary site may be surgically inoperable.

## Other factors

- *Patient's performance status* The Eastern Co-operative Oncology Group (ECOG) Performance Status Scale is widely used (Table 28.2). Patients with ECOG score >2 are usually deemed unsuitable for most chemotherapy interventions
- *Mortality, morbidity, and efficacy of the therapeutic procedure*
- *Patient preference*

**Table 28.1** Tumour markers and associated conditions

| Tumour marker | Associated conditions | |
| --- | --- | --- |
| | **Malignant conditions** | **Non-malignant conditions** |
| CEA | GI tract cancers (particularly colorectal cancer) | Cirrhosis<br>Pancreatitis<br>Smoking |
| CA 19-9 | Colorectal cancer<br>Pancreatic cancer | Cholestasis |
| CA 125 | Ovarian cancer<br>Breast cancer<br>Hepatocellular cancer | Cirrhosis<br>Pregnancy<br>Peritonitis |
| α FP | Hepatocellular cancer<br>Germ cell cancers<br>(not pure seminoma) | Cirrhosis<br>Pregnancy<br>Hepatitis<br>Open neural tube defects |
| hCG | Germ cell cancers<br>Choriocarcinoma and<br>hydatidiform mole | Pregnancy |
| PSA | Prostate cancer | Benign prostatic hypertrophy<br>Prostatitis<br>Prostate instrumentation (including rectal examination)<br>Acute urinary retention<br>Physical exercise<br>Old age |

**Table 28.2** ECOG Performance Status Scale

| Classification | Description |
| --- | --- |
| ECOG 0 | Fully active; able to carry on all activities without restriction |
| ECOG 1 | Restricted in physically strenuous activity but ambulatory and able to carry out work of a light or sedentary nature |
| ECOG 2 | Ambulatory and capable of all self-care; confined to bed or chair 50% of waking hours |
| ECOG 3 | Capable of only limited self-care; confined to bed or chair 50% or more of waking hours |
| ECOG 4 | Completely disabled; cannot carry on any self-care; totally confined to bed or chair |

As published in Oken MM, Creech RH, Tormey DC *et al.* Toxicity and response criteria of the Eastern cooperative oncology group. *Am J Clin Oncol* (1982) **5**: 649–55, with permission from the Eastern Cooperative Oncology Group, Robert Comis MD, Group Chair.

**The GP's role** Treatment of cancer is increasingly successful but also increasingly complex. It is largely a specialist activity, but the role of the GP is important at this time, even if peripheral.
- Keep in touch with the family and up to date with treatment—provide support (e.g. advice on benefits/local services), preventive care (e.g. flu vaccination for patients and/or carers), and general medical care.
- Liaise with the secondary care teams involved, and provide continuity if care is passed from one specialist team to another.
- If the patient does not survive, provide ongoing support to the family.

# Surgery for cancer

Surgery has 3 main roles in cancer management.

**Diagnosis and staging** Advances in imaging and laparoscopic techniques have dramatically reduced the number of patients requiring open surgery to confirm a cancer diagnosis. However, surgical staging remains important in the following.

- Breast cancer—'sentinel' axillary node biopsy is needed to accurately predict the state of nodal disease.
- Ovarian cancer—tumour deposits on the peritoneal surface are poorly visualized with conventional imaging. Direct visualization is required using laparotomy or laparoscopy.
- Certain abdominal malignancies—laparoscopic assessment of the extent and spread of tumour is performed prior to major resection.

## Curative surgery

**Non-metastatic disease** Surgery with curative intent is dependent on complete resection of the tumour with a margin of normal tissue. Local control of tumours with a propensity to spread to lymph nodes may be improved with resection of the draining group of nodes, e.g. vulval tumours. However, even if the tumour was completely resected, surgery can still fail to cure either as a result of:

- Development of metastatic disease as a result of the presence of micro-metastatic deposits unidentifiable at the time of surgery.
- Development of local relapse as a result of inadequate margins. Surgical margins can be limited by patient-related factors (e.g. only a partial lobectomy may be possible in patients with lung cancer because of poor underlying respiratory function) or by tumour-related margins (e.g. invasion of the tumour into vital structure such as the aorta).

**Metastatic disease** Surgery may be curative in a limited number of tumours with metastases. However, this is much less common, requires careful patient selection, and is best performed by a specialist team. Circumstances in which curative surgery may be offered include:

- Isolated brain metastases from breast cancer with a long disease-free interval.
- Liver metastases from colorectal cancer.
- Pulmonary metastases from osteosarcoma or soft tissue sarcoma.

**Palliative surgery** Surgery can be effective in achieving good symptom control in the palliative setting, but decision to proceed must be carefully considered, particularly as patients may have limited life expectancy, poor performance status, and rapid tumour progression. Ideally, such decisions should be multidisciplinary and involve surgeons specialized in oncology and experienced in palliative management (Table 28.3).

**Table 28.3** Situations in which palliative surgery should be considered

| Situation | Comments |
|---|---|
| Cancers causing obstructive symptoms e.g. bowel, ovary, ureter, bronchus | Surgery to relieve the obstruction may be warranted even if the underlying disease is incurable with locally advanced disease or distant metastases. |
| | *Bowel obstruction*—this occurs most commonly in patients with colonic or ovarian cancer. |
| | *Oesophageal or bronchial obstruction*—laser therapy of an intra-luminal mass may restore the lumen. |
| | *Obstructive hydronephrosis*—nephrostomy or ureteric catheters may relieve the obstruction. |
| | *Placement of a stent*—may help to relieve the symptoms of dysphagia, dyspnoea, jaundice, and large bowel obstruction. |
| Fistulae | Fistulae, often arising as a result of pelvic tumours or as a side effect of radiotherapy, can be associated with distressing malodours and excessive discharge. |
| | Surgery may provide excellent palliation but may not be useful in those with multiple sites of fistulae or rapidly advancing intra-abdominal disease where life expectancy is limited. |
| Jaundice | Radiological and/or endoscopic stent placement can relieve obstructive jaundice secondary to extrinsic pressure from lymph nodes on the biliary system or intrinsic pressure from cholangiocarcinoma or pancreatic carcinoma. |
| | *Complications:* Infection or blockage necessitate replacement. |
| | *Surgical relief* by choledochoenterostomy avoids the problems associated with stents and may be indicated in a small minority with excellent performance status and slowly growing disease. |
| Spinal cord compression and brain tumours | Urgent referral for neurological assessment for decompressive surgery is indicated for confirmed spinal disease or operable brain tumours. |
| GI bleeding | A wide range of endoscopic techniques have been developed to stop bleeding from benign and malignant causes, including sclerotherapy with adrenaline, laser coagulation, and radiological embolization. |
| | These techniques may avoid the need for major surgery in patients who have a limited life expectancy. |
| Bone metastases | Prophylactic fixation of a long bone may reduce either pain and/or the risk of pathological fracture in patients with: |
| | • Lesions in weight-bearing bones |
| | • Destruction of > 50% of the cortex |
| | • Pain on weight-bearing |
| | • Lytic lesions |
| | In all cases fixation should be followed by radiotherapy to control growth and promote healing. |
| Pain | If the expected morbidity of the procedure is low, surgical debulking of large slowly growing tumours can reduce pain. |
| | Neurosurgical approaches such as cordotomy are only rarely considered. |

# Chemotherapy

Chemotherapy is the use of chemical agents in the cure or palliation of malignant disease.

**Drug groups** Include:
- Antibiotics, e.g. bleomycin
- Alkylating agents, e.g busulfan
- Antimetabolites, e.g. methotrexate, 5-fluorouracil
- Alkaloids, e.g. vincristine
- Platinum derivatives—DNA intercalating agents, e.g. cisplatin
- Enzymes, e.g. asparaginase
- Hormones, e.g. sex hormones, corticosteroids
- Biological agents, e.g. interferon, monoclonal antibodies (e.g. rituximab)
- Others, e.g. hydroxycarbamide, retinoids.

These agents work in a variety of ways to inhibit tumour growth and/or cause tumour cell damage. Normal cells may be damaged at the same time as tumour cells, resulting in the high levels of toxicity experienced by patients.

**Choice of agent** depends on known activity of the agent, cost, and patient factors. It is a specialist decision.

**Types of tumour** Response to chemotherapy depends on type and grade of tumour being treated. Broadly tumours can be divided into:
- *Those likely to respond*—leukaemia, lymphoma (Hodgkins and intermediate/high grade non-Hodgkin's), testicular tumours, small-cell lung cancer, embryonal tumours, choriocarcinoma, ovarian cancer, sarcoma, breast cancer, prostate cancer.
- *Those that may respond*—low-grade non-Hodgkin's lymphoma, GI cancer, brain/CNS tumours, melanoma, bladder cancer, uterine cancer.
- *Those unlikely to respond*—non-small-cell lung cancer, renal cancer, pancreatic cancer, head and neck cancer, cervical cancer, liver cancer

**Combination chemotherapy** Often different chemotherapeutic agents are combined to increase their chances of effect. Agents acting in different ways may potentiate each other's actions, and using combinations reduces the risk of resistance (if one agent does not have any effect, another may). Choosing agents with different side-effect profiles reduces cumulative toxic effects.

**Intermittent chemotherapy** Particularly useful for cytotoxic drugs. Intermittent treatment exploits the difference in recovery rates between normal and malignant tissues. Gaps between cycles of treatment allow normal tissue (particularly the immune system) to recover, but the malignant tissue does not recover to such a large extent (Figure 28.1). The population of malignant cells diminishes relative to the normal cells with each cycle.

**Adjuvant chemotherapy** Given to prevent relapse after primary treatment of a non-metastatic tumour for which relapse rate is known to be high. An example is adjuvant chemotherapy for breast cancer.

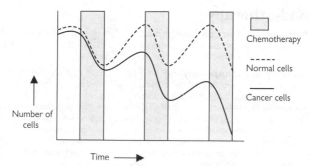

**Fig. 28.1** Action of cytotoxic chemotherapy on normal and cancer cell populations

**Neutropoenic sepsis** Neutropoenic sepsis is defined as fever >38.0°C for ≥2h when the neutrophil count is <1.0 × 10⁹/L. *Causes:*
- Chemotherapy (most common cause).
- Radiotherapy—if large volumes of bone marrow are irradiated, e.g. pelvic radiotherapy.
- Malignant infiltration of the bone marrow, e.g. prostate/breast cancer.

**Risks of neutropoenia** Bacterial and fungal infection. Risk of infection ↑ sharply as neutrophil counts fall below 1.0 × 10⁹/L, with greatest risk at counts <0.1 × 10⁹/L. Neutropoenia for >5d is a further risk factor.

**Presentation and primary care management** Symptoms/signs may be minimal—have a high index of suspicion. Neutropoenic septic patients can deteriorate rapidly and become hypotensive or moribund within hours. Early referral for investigation and specialist management is critical.
- If a high-risk patient complains of chills, fever, rigors, sore throat, or generalized aches, check an urgent FBC.
- Mouth ulcers and ↑ fatigue can be signs of neutropoenia.

⚠ Development of fever in a patient with neutropoenia is a medical emergency caused by infection until proven otherwise.

**Information for patients about side effects of chemotherapy**
Chemocare 🖥 www.chemocare.com
Cancer Research UK ☎ 0808 800 4040 🖥 www.cancerhelp.org.uk
Macmillan Cancer Support ☎ 0808 808 0000 🖥 www.macmillan.org.uk

# Radiotherapy

**Mechanism of action** Ionizing radiation damages cells. Radiotherapy aims to deliver a dose of irradiation to an area which allows normal tissues, but not the cancer, to recover from the damage.

**Delivery of radiotherapy** may be used alone or with chemotherapy. Once the maximum dose of radiotherapy has been received by any area, that area cannot usually be irradiated again.

- *External beam*—external source of ionizing radiation (e.g. gamma rays) is aimed at a target point in the body. Patients may be immobilized, e.g. with special boards/moulds, to ensure delivery of treatment to the correct place. Can be single dose (e.g. for palliative reasons) or fractionated into several doses spread over weeks. Fractionation ↑ effect.
- *Brachytherapy* Delivery of radiation by placing a radioactive source within or close to the malignancy, e.g. caesium-137 in the uterus.

**Table 28.4** Managing post-radiotherapy skin reactions

| RTOG score* | Description | Skin appearance | Treatment |
|---|---|---|---|
| 0 | Normal | Normal | Aqueous cream bd to delay onset of reaction |
| 1 | Faint erythema | Skin slightly pink or red | Aqueous cream tds or prn |
| 2A | Tender or bright erythema (dry desquamation) | Skin red, dry, and scaly— some itch and tingling | Frequent aqueous cream (qds or prn) Diprobase® cream or soft white paraffin (avoid excess build-up) Hydrocortisone cream may be used sparingly on itchy areas. Review after 7d—discontinue if the skin breaks |
| 2B | Patchy moist desquamation, oedema | Skin inflamed with patches of epidermis broken down and moist | Apply hydrogel dressings to moist areas with appropriate 2° dressing; e.g Surgipad® or foam dressing Apply aqueous cream to other parts of the field |
| 3 | Confluent moist desquamation | Epidermis blisters and sloughs; underlying dermis exposed and sore; oozing of serous fluid | Apply hydrogel or foam dressing suitable for the amount of exudate Review frequently Swab and treat with oral antibiotics (e.g. flucloxacillin 500mg qds) if any signs of infection |
| Post radio-therapy | Reaction may continue for several weeks post treatment. Continue with use of aqueous creams until skin returns to normal. If RTOG 2B/3 apply principles of moist wound healing as above or (if patient is not allergic to silicone) a silicone dressing. If infection is suspected apply silver impregnated dressings or silver sulfadiazine cream. | | |

* RTOG stands for radiotherapy and oncology group.

## Treatment may be

- *Curative*, e.g. childhood tumours, lymphoma, seminoma, head and neck tumours, bladder cancer, squamous/basal cell skin cancer.
- *Adjuvant* pre-operatively to ↓ size/extent of otherwise inoperable tumours, or post-operatively to treat microscopic foci remaining after tumour removal (e.g. in treatment of breast cancer).
- *Palliative* for control of distressing symptoms. Only symptomatic sites of disease are targeted, e.g. bone metastases, haemorrhage, obstruction of a viscus, neurological complications, fungating tumours.

**Table 28.5** Non-skin side effects of radiotherapy

| Side effect | Description/action |
|---|---|
| Sore mouth/ throat | Associated with radiotherapy to the head/neck. |
| | *Advice*: visit the dentist prior to treatment; avoid smoking, alcohol, and spicy foods; rest voice when radiotherapy reaction becomes established. |
| | *Consider treatment with*: normal saline/bicarbonate mouthwashes, antiseptic mouth washes (e.g. chlorhexidine, though alcohol may sting), soluble aspirin (can be gargled) or paracetamol, benzydamine, topical local anaesthetics (e.g. xylocaine gel), topical steroids (e.g. triamcinolone in dental paste, hydrocortisone pellets), coating agents (e.g. sucralfate). |
| | If insufficient fluid/food intake, consider nutritional support via NG tube and/or referral for gastrostomy (if weight loss > 10%). |
| Dysphagia | May result from thoracic radiotherapy. Avoid smoking, spirits, and spicy food. Consider treatment with antacid, sucralfate, soluble paracetamol or aspirin, NSAID po/PR. |
| Nausea and vomiting | Radiotherapy to the abdomen often causes nausea as a result of serotonin release. Consider prophylactic antiemetic therapy with a serotonin inhibitor, e.g. ondansetron. |
| Diarrhoea | Frequently accompanies abdominal/pelvic radiotherapy. |
| | *Management*: dietary modification (e.g. ↓ dietary fibre) may help. Supply with loperamide—1mg initial dose then 2mg every 2h until symptoms settle (4mg every 4h at night). Proctitis may accompany rectal/prostatic irradiation. Treat with rectal steroids. |
| Pneumonitis | Acute pneumonitis can develop 1–3mo after treatment and is associated with a fever, dry cough, and breathlessness. Differential diagnosis: pneumonia |
| | *Investigation*: CXR—shows lung infiltration confined within the treatment volume.. |
| | *Management*: steroids—start with 40mg od prednisolone and reduce over a period of weeks as improvement occurs. |
| | ❶ Pulmonary fibrosis may occur >12mo after treatment. |
| Cerebral oedema | Can occur after cranial irradiation, especially if no surgery to the tumour. Steroid dose is ↓ after completion of radiotherapy. Consider ↑ dose again. |
| Somnolence syndrome | Occurs within a few weeks of brain irradiation. Presents with nausea/vomiting, anorexia, dysarthria, ataxia, profound lethargy. Treatment is supportive. Recovery may occur spontaneously. |

# Palliative care in general practice

> *Any man's death diminishes me because I am involved in mankind.*
> Devotions, Meditation 17, John Donne (1572–1631)

Palliative care starts when the emphasis changes from curing the patient and prolonging life to relieving symptoms and maintaining well-being or 'quality of life'. GPs have 1–2 patients with terminal disease at any time and get more personally involved with them than with any others.

The problems arising are a complex mix of physical, psychological, social, cultural, and spiritual factors involving both patients and carers. To respond adequately, good lines of communication and close multidisciplinary teamwork are needed. Local palliative care teams are invaluable sources of advice and support, and frequently produce booklets with advice on aspects of palliative care for GPs.

Symptom control must be tailored to the needs of the individual. A few basic rules apply:
- Carefully diagnose the cause of the symptom.
- Explain the symptom to the patient.
- Discuss treatment options.
- Set realistic goals.
- Anticipate likely problems.
- Review regularly.

**The Gold Standards Framework** aims to improve quality and of palliative care provided by the primary care team by developing practice-based organization of care of dying patients. The framework focuses on: optimizing continuity of care, teamwork, advanced planning (including out-of-hours), symptom control, and patient, carer, and staff support. Evaluation data show that the framework ↑ the proportion of patients dying in their preferred place and improves quality of care as perceived by the practitioners involved.

⚠ Death is the natural end to life—not a failure of medicine.

## Further information

**Gold Standards Framework** 🖳 www.goldstandardsframework.nhs.uk
**NICE** Improving supportive and palliative care for adults with cancer (2004) 🖳 www.nice.org.uk
**Hospice Information** 🖳 www.helpthehospices.org.uk
**Doyle D, Woodruff R** *The IAHPC Manual of Palliative Care* (2004, 2nd edn) IAHPC Press, Houston, Texas. ISBN: 0975852515
🖳 www.hospicecare.com/manual/IAHPCmanual.htm

## Patient advice and support

**Macmillan Cancer Support** ☎ 0808 808 0000 🖳 www.macmillan.org.uk

**Syringe drivers** Although drugs can usually be administered by mouth to control the symptoms of terminal illness, occasionally that is not possible. Portable syringe drivers give a continuous subcutaneous infusion and can provide good control of symptoms with little discomfort or inconvenience to the patient. *Indications*:
- The patient is unable to take medicines by mouth because of nausea and vomiting, dysphagia, severe weakness, or coma.
- There is bowel obstruction and further surgery is inappropriate.
- The patient does not want to take regular medication by mouth.

### Drugs that can be used in syringe drivers

**Mixing drugs in syringe drivers** Provided that there is evidence of compatibility, drugs can be mixed in syringe drivers. Diamorphine can be mixed with:
- Cyclizine
- Hyoscine hydrobromide
- Hyoscine butylbromide
- Midazolam
- Dexamethasone
- Levomepromazine
- Haloperidol
- Metoclopramide.

### Common problems with syringe drivers
- *If the syringe driver runs too slowly* Check that it is switched on; check the battery; check the cannula is not blocked.
- *If the syringe driver runs too quickly* Check the rate setting.
- *Injection site reaction* If there is pain or inflammation, change the injection site.

**Table 28.6** Drugs that can be used in syringe drivers

| Indication | Drugs |
|---|---|
| Nausea and vomiting | Haloperidol 2.5–10mg/24h |
| | Levomepromazine 5–200mg/24h (causes sedation in 50%) |
| | Cyclizine 150mg/24h (may precipitate if mixed with other drugs) |
| | Metoclopramide 30–100mg/24h |
| | Octreotide 300–600 micrograms/24h (consultant supervision) |
| | Hyoscine butylbromide 20–60mg/24h |
| Respiratory secretions | Hyoscine hydrobromide 0.6–2.4mg/24h |
| | Glycopyrronium 0.6–1.2mg/24h |
| Restlessness and confusion | Haloperidol 5–15mg/24h |
| | Levomepromazine 50–200mg/24h |
| | Midazolam 20–100mg/24h (and fitting) |
| Pain control | Diamorphine: ⅓–½ dose oral morphine/24h |
| | Morphine: ½–⅔ dose of oral morphine/24h |
| | Oxycodone: half dose oral oxycodone/24h |

❶ Subcutaneous infusion solution should be monitored regularly both to check for precipitation (and discoloration) and to ensure the infusion is running at the correct rate.

⚠ Incorrect use of syringe drivers is a common cause of drug errors.

# Pain and general debility

**Pain control** Pain control is the cornerstone of palliative care. Cancer pain is multifactorial—be aware of physical and psychological factors.

*Principles of pain control* 📖 p.214

*Pain-relieving drugs* 📖 p.216

*Management of specific types of pain* Table 28.7

**Weakness, fatigue, and drowsiness** Almost a universal symptom.

*Reversible causes*
- Drugs—opioids, benzodiazepines, steroids (proximal muscle weakness), diuretics (dehydration and biochemical abnormalities), antihypertensives (postural hypotension).
- Emotional problems—depression, anxiety, fear, apathy.
- Biochemical abnormalities—hypercalcaemia, DM, electrolyte disturbance, uraemia, liver disease, thyroid dysfunction.
- Anaemia
- Infection
- Poor nutrition
- Prolonged bed rest
- Raised intracranial pressure (drowsiness only).

**Management** Treat reversible causes. Provide advice on modification of lifestyle. If drowsiness and fatigue persist, consider a trial of dexamethasone 4–6mg/d or antidepressant. Although steroids make muscle wasting worse, they may improve general fatigue and mobility. Provide psychological support to patients and carers. Consider referral to physiotherapist, review of aids and appliances, review of home layout (possibly with referral to OT), and/or review of home care arrangements.

**Hypercalcaemia** Occurs with 10% of tumours, particularly myeloma (>30%) and breast cancer (40%).

*Presentation and differential diagnosis* 📖 p.374

⚠ Always suspect hypercalcaemia if someone is iller than expected for no obvious reason. Untreated hypercalcaemia can be fatal.

**Management** Depending on the general state of the patient, make a decision whether or not to treat the hypercalcaemia. If a decision is made *not* to treat, provide symptom control and do not check the serum calcium again. If you decide to treat:
- *Asymptomatic patient with corrected calcium <3 mmol/L* Monitor
- *Symptomatic and/or corrected calcium > 3mmol/L* Arrange treatment with IV fluids and bisphosphonates via oncologist/palliative care team immediately. Check serum calcium 7–10d post-treatment. 20% do not respond and there is no benefit from re-treating them. Effect of bisphosphonate lasts 20–30d. Consider maintenance with oral bisphosphonates started 1wk after the initial IV treatment or regular IV bisphosphonate. Many who are initially responsive to bisphosphonates become unresponsive with time.

**Table 28.7** Management of specific types of pain

| Type of pain | Management |
|---|---|
| Bone pain | • Try NSAIDs and/or strong opioids.<br>• Consider referral for palliative radiotherapy, strontium treatment (prostate cancer) or IV bisphosphonates (↓ pain in myeloma, breast and prostate cancer).<br>• Refer to orthopaedics if any lytic metastases at risk of fracture, for consideration of pinning. |
| Abdominal pain | • *Constipation* is the most common cause—☐ p.1033<br>• *Colic*: try loperamide 2–4mg qds or hyoscine hydrobromide 300 micrograms tds s/ling. Hyoscine butylbromide 20–60mg/24h can also be given via syringe driver.<br>• *Liver capsule pain*—dexamethasone 4–8mg/d. Titrate dose to the minimum that controls pain. Alternatively try NSAID + PPI cover<br>• *Gastric distention*—may be helped by an antacid ± an anti-foaming agent (e.g. Asilone). Alternatively a prokinetic may help, e.g. metoclopramide or domperidone 10mg tds before meals.<br>• *Upper GI tumour*—often neuropathic element of pain. Coeliac plexus block may help—refer to the palliative care team.<br>• *Consider drug causes*—NSAIDs are a common iatrogenic cause.<br>• *Acute/subacute obstruction*—☐ p.1031. |
| Neuropathic pain | • Often burning/shooting and may not respond to simple analgesia.<br>• Titrate to the maximum tolerated dose of opioid.<br>• If inadequate add a nerve pain killer, e.g. amitriptyline 10–25mg nocte increasing as needed every 2wk to 75–150mg. Alternatives include carbamazepine, gabapentin, pregabalin, phenytoin, sodium valproate, and clonazepam.<br>• If pain is due to nerve compression as a result of tumour, dexamethasone 4–8mg od may help.<br>• Other options: TENS, acupuncture, nerve block. |
| Rectal pain | • Topical drugs, e.g. rectal steroids.<br>• Tricyclic antidepressants, e.g. amitriptyline 10–100mg nocte.<br>• Anal spasms: glyceryl trinitrate ointment 0.1–0.2% bd.<br>• Referral for local radiotherapy. |
| Muscle pain | • Paracetamol and/or NSAIDs.<br>• Muscle relaxants, e.g. diazepam 5–10mg od, baclofen 5–10mg tds, dantrolene 25mg od increasing at weekly intervals to 75mg tds.<br>• Physiotherapy, aromatherapy, relaxation, heat pads. |
| Bladder pain/ spasm | • Treat reversible causes. ↑ fluids. Toilet regularly.<br>• Try oxybutinin 5mg tds, tolterodine 2mg bd, propiverine 15mg od/bd/tds, or trospium 20mg bd.<br>• Amitriptyline 10–75mg nocte is often effective.<br>• If catheterized, try instilling 20mL intravesical bupivacaine 0.25% for 15 min tds or oxybutinin 5mL in 30mL od/bd/tds.<br>• NSAIDs can also be useful.<br>• Steroids, e.g. dexamethasone 4–8mg od may ↓ tumour related bladder inflammation.<br>• In the terminal situation hyoscine butylbromide 60–120mg/24h or glycopyrronium 0.4–0.8mg/24h sc can be helpful. |
| Pain of short duration | e.g. dressing changes—try a short-acting opioid, e.g. fentanyl citrate 200 micrograms lozenge sucked for 15min prior to procedure or breakthrough dose of oral morphine 20min prior to procedure. |

# Anorexia, nausea and vomiting

**Anorexia** Treat nausea, mouth problems, pain, and other symptoms. ↓ psychological distress and treat depression. Advise small appetizing meals frequently in comfortable surroundings.

### Drugs that may be helpful
- Alcohol pre-meals.
- Metoclopramide or domperidone 10mg tds pre-meals to prevent feeling of satiety caused by gastric stasis.
- Dexamethasone 2–4mg od or prednisolone 15–30mg od.

### General principles of management of nausea and vomiting
- *Assess* Try to identify likely cause (Table 28.8).
- *Review medication* Could medication be the cause? Which antiemetics have been used before and how effective were they?
- *Try non-drug measures*
- *Choose an antiemetic* If cause can be identified, choose an appropriate antiemetic (Table 28.8). Use the antiemetic ladder (Figure 28.2). Administer antiemetics regularly rather than prn and choose an appropriate route of administration.
- *Review frequently* Is the antiemetic effective? Has the underlying cause of the nausea/vomiting resolved? Avoid changing antiemetic before it has been given an adequate trial at maximum dose.

❶ If there is >1 cause for nausea/vomiting you may need >1 drug.

### Route of administration
- For prophylaxis of nausea and vomiting—use po medication
- For established nausea or vomiting—consider a parenteral route e.g. syringe driver (📖 p.1027)—persistent nausea may ↓ gastric emptying and drug absorption. Once symptoms are controlled consider reverting to a po route.

**Non-drug measures** Do not forget non-drug measures to ↓ nausea.
- Avoidance of food smells and unpleasant odours.
- Relaxation/diversion/anxiety management.
- Acupressure/acupuncture.

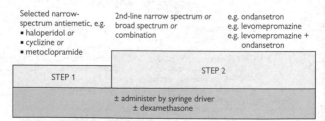

**Fig. 28.2** The antiemetic ladder

**Table 28.8** Causes of vomiting and choice of antiemetic

| Mechanism of vomiting | Antiemetic |
| --- | --- |
| Drug/toxin–induced or metabolic e.g. hypercalcaemia | Haloperidol 1.5–5mg nocte<br>Levomepromazine 6.25mg nocte<br>If persistent nausea due to opioids, consider changing opioid |
| Chemotherapy/radiotherapy | Granisetron 1mg bd or ondansetron 8mg bd po or 16mg od pr—chemotherapy- or radiotherapy-induced vomiting<br>Haloperidol 1.5–5mg nocte—radiotherapy-induced vomiting<br>Dexamethasone 4–8mg daily po/sc—often given as part of a chemotherapy regime<br>Metoclopramide 20mg qds |
| ↑ intracranial pressure | Dexamethasone 4–16mg/d<br>Cyclizine 50mg bd/tds (or 150mg/d via syringe driver) |
| Anxiety, fear, or pain | Benzodiazepines, e.g. diazepam 2–10mg/d or midazolam SC<br>Cyclizine 50mg bd/tds<br>Levomepromazine 6–25mg/d |
| Motion/position | Cyclizine 50mg tds po/sc/IM<br>Hyoscine po (300 micrograms tds) or transdermal (1mg/72h)<br>Prochlorperazine po (5mg qds) or buccal (3–6mg bd) |
| Gastric stasis* | Domperidone 10mg tds or metoclopramide 10mg tds (particularly if multifactorial with gastric stasis and a central component) |
| Gastric irritation | Stop the irritant if possible, e.g. stop NSAIDs<br>Proton pump inhibitors, e.g. lansoprazole 30mg od or omeprazole 20mg od<br>Antacids<br>Misoprostol 200 micrograms bd—if caused by NSAIDS |
| Constipation | Laxatives/suppositories/enemas |
| Intestinal obstruction | Refer for surgery if appropriate<br>Cyclizine, haloperidol, or levomepromazine<br>Dexamethasone 4–8 mg/d—antiemetic and ↓ obstruction.<br>If vomiting cannot be controlled consider referral for venting gastrostomy or antisecretory agents (e.g. octreotide) |
| Cough induced | 📖 p.1036 |
| Unknown cause | Cyclizine 50mg tds or 150mg/d via syringe driver<br>Levomepromazine 6–25mg/d<br>Dexamethasone 4–8mg daily po/sc<br>Metoclopramide 10mg tds/qds po |

*Vomits of undigested food without nausea soon after eating.

❶ Drugs with antimuscarinic effects (e.g.cyclizine) antagonize prokinetic drugs (e.g. metoclopramide)—if possible, do not use concurrently.

## Other GI problems

**Mouth problems** Review medication making the mouth sore or dry. Refer to the DN for advice on mouth care (e.g. use a toothbrush to keep the tongue clean). Treat oral thrush—fluconazole 50mg od for 7d and soak dentures in Milton fluid for ≥ 12h to prevent reinfection. Consider mouthwashes, e.g. saline, Oraldene®, chlorhexidine gluconate, benzydamine (for pain). Try ¼–½ ascorbic acid 1g effervescent tablet/d— place on tongue and allow to dissolve.

### Specific measures
- Painful mouth—benzydamine mouthwash ± lidocaine 10% spray.
- Ulcers or painful areas—triamcinolone in dental paste, or hydrocortisone pellets qds after eating and nocte
- Oral cancer pain—topical NSAIDs, e.g. piroxicam melt
- Chemotherapy-induced ulcers—sucralfate suspension
- Dry mouth—review medication that might be causing dry mouth, e.g. antidepressants, opioids. Try salivary stimulants, e.g. iced water, pineapple chunks, chewing gum, boiled sweets, or mints. Consider saliva substitutes, e.g. Glandosane spray®
- Radiotherapy-induced dryness—pilocarpine
- Excessive salivation—amitriptyline 10–100mg nocte, hyoscine or glycopyrronium via syringe driver.

**Dysphagia** May be due to physical obstruction (by tumour bulk) or functional obstruction (neurological deficit).
- Treat the cause if possible, e.g. celestin tube for oesophageal tumour
- If the patient is hungry and wishes to be fed, consider referral for a percutaneous endoscopic gastrostomy (PEG)
- If the patient does not wish to have a PEG ask whether he/she would like subcutaneous fluids and treat symptomatically with mouth care, anxiolytics, analgesia, and sedation.

**Hiccup** A distressing symptom. Treatment is often unsatisfactory.
- *General measures* Rebreathing with a paper bag; pharyngeal stimulation by drinking cold water or taking a teaspoonful of granulated sugar.
- *Peripheral hiccups* Irritation of the phrenic nerve or diaphragm—try metoclopramide (10mg tds), antacids containing simeticone, dexamethasone (4–12mg/d) or ranitidine (150mg bd).
- *Central hiccups* Due to medullary stimulation, e.g. ↑ICP, uraemia—try chlorpromazine (10–25mg tds/qds), dexamethasone (4–12mg/d), nifedipine (10mg tds), or baclofen (5mg bd).

**Ascites** Free fluid in the peritoneal cavity. Common with ovarian cancer (50% patients). Presents with abdominal distention. *Signs*: shifting dullness to percussion ± fluid thrill. Depending on clinical state, consider referring for radio- or chemotherapy if appropriate.

### Symptom control
- Give analgesia for discomfort.
- Refer for paracentesis and/or peritoneo-venous shunt.
- Try diuretics—furosemide 20–40mg od and/or spironolactone 100–400mg od. May take a week to produce maximal effect. ❶ Monitor albumin level—if low, diuretics make ascites worse.

- Dexamethasone 2–4mg daily may help. Discontinue if not effective.
- 'Squashed stomach syndrome'—try prokinetics, e.g. domperidone or metoclopramide 10mg tds.

**Constipation** Passage of hard stools less frequently than the patient's own normal pattern. It is a very common symptom. Occult presentations are common in the very elderly and frail and include:

- Confusion
- Urinary retention
- Abdominal pain
- Overflow diarrhoea
- Loss of appetite
- Nausea/vomiting.

⚠ Constipation can herald spinal cord compression (📖 p.486). If suspected do a full neurological examination.

**Management** Pre-empt constipation by putting everyone at risk (e.g. patients on opioids) on regular aperients. Treat reversible causes, e.g. give analgesia if pain on defecation, alter diet, ↑ fluid intake.
- Treat with regular stool softener (e.g. lactulose) ± regular bowel stimulant (e.g. senna) or a combination drug (e.g. co-danthrusate). Titrate dose against reponse.
- If that is ineffective, consider adding rectal measures. If soft stools and lax rectum, try bisacodyl suppositories (❶ must come into direct contact with rectum). If hard stools, try glycerol suppositories—insert into the faeces and allow to dissolve.
- If still not cleared, refer to the district nurse for lubricant ± stimulant enema (usually acts in ~20 min). Once cleared, leave on a regular aperient with instructions to ↑ aperients if constipation recurs.

**Gut fistulae** Connections from the gut to other organs—commonly skin, bladder or vagina. Bowel fistulae are characterized by air passing through the fistula channel. If well enough for surgery, refer to a surgeon. If not fit for surgery, consider referring to palliative care for octreotide.

**Diarrhoea** Clarify what the patient/carer means by diarrhoea. Less common than constipation but can be distressing for the patient and difficult for the carer, especially if incontinence results.

**Management**
- ↑ fluid intake—small amounts of clear fluids frequently.
- Screen for infection (including pseudomembranous colitis if diarrhoea after a course of antibiotics) and treat if necessary.
- Ensure no overflow diarrhoea 2° to constipation, no excessive/erratic laxative use, and no other medication is causing diarrhoea.
- Consider giving aspirin (300–600mg tds)—↓ intestinal electrolyte and water secretion caused by prostaglandins. May particularly help with radiotherapy-induced diarrhoea.
- Consider ondansetron 4mg tds for radiotherapy-induced diarrhoea.
- Consider giving pancreatic enzyme supplements, e.g. Creon® 25000 tds prior to meals if fat malabsorption (e.g. 2° to pancreatic carcinoma).
- Otherwise treat symptomatically with codeine phosphate 30–60mg qds or loperamide 2mg tds/qds.
- Refer to palliative care if unable to control symptoms.

# Skin, neurological, and orthopaedic problems

**Bed sores** Due to pressure necrosis of the skin. Immobile patients are at high risk, especially if frail ± incontinent. Likely sites of pressure damage—shoulder blades, elbows, spine, buttocks, knees, ankles, and heels. Bed sores heal slowly in terminally ill patients and are a source of discomfort and stress for both patients and carers (who often feel guilty that a pressure sore is a mark of poor care).

- If at risk refer to the DN for palliative care nursing team for advice on prevention of bed sores—protective mattresses and cushions, incontinence advice, advice on positioning and movement.
- Warn carers to make contact with the DN or palliative care nursing team if a red patch does not improve 24h after relieving the pressure on the area.
- Treat any sores that develop aggressively and admit if not resolving.

**Wound care** Large wounds can have a major impact on quality of life. Patients with advanced disease have major risk factors for development and poor healing of wounds—immobility, poor nutrition, skin infiltration ± breakdown due to malignancy. Skin infiltration causing ulceration or fungating wounds can be particularly distressing.

***Management*** The primary aim is comfort. Healing is a secondary aim and may be impossible. Always involve the DN and/or specialist palliative care nursing team early. Many hospitals also have wound care specialist nurses who are invaluable sources of advice.

***Specific management problems*** Table 28.9

**Raised intracranial pressure** Occurs with 1° or 2° brain tumours. Characterized by

- Headache—worse on lying
- Vomiting
- Confusion
- Diplopia
- Convulsions
- Papilloedema.

***Management***
- Unless a terminal event, refer urgently to neurosurgery for assessment. Options include insertion of a shunt or cranial radiotherapy.
- If no further active treatment is appropriate, start symptomatic treatment—raise the head of the bed, start dexamethasone 16mg/d (stop if no response in 1wk), analgesia.

**Spinal cord compression** 📖 p.486

**Bone fractures** Common in advanced cancer due to osteoporosis, trauma as a result of falls, or metastases. Have a high index of suspicion if a new bony pain develops. Treat with analgesia. Unless in a very terminal state, confirm the fracture on X-ray and refer to orthopaedics or radiotherapy urgently for consideration of fixation (long bones, wrist, neck of femur) and/or radiotherapy (rib fractures, vertebral fractures).

⚠ In the elderly, fracture of a long bone can present as acute confusion.

**Table 28.9** Common wound management problems

| Problem | Management |
| --- | --- |
| Pain | Exclude infection; ensure the dressing is comfortable; limit frequency of dressing changes |
| | Ensure adequate background analgesia; consider additional analgesia for dressing changes and/or topical opioids on the dressing |
| Excessive exudate | Use high-absorbency dressings with further packing on top ± plastic pads to protect clothing |
| | Change the top layer of the dressing as often as needed but avoid frequent changes of the dressing placed directly on the wound |
| | Protect the surrounding skin with a barrier cream/spray |
| Necrotic tissue | Use desloughing agents |
| | Referral for surgical debridement may be necessary |
| Bleeding | Prevent bleeding during dressing changes by:<br>• Avoiding frequent dressing changes<br>• Using non-adherent dressings or dressings which liquefy and can be washed off (e.g. Sorbsan®) *and*<br>• Irrigating the wound with saline to remove dressings.<br>If there is surface bleeding, put pressure on the wound; if pressure is not working try:<br>• Kaltostat®<br>• Adrenaline mg/mL or (1:1000) on a gauze pad, *or*<br>• Sucralfate liquid — place on a non-adherent dressing and apply firmly to the bleeding area.<br>Consider referral for radiotherapy or palliative surgery (e.g. cautery) |
| Odour | Treat with systemic and/or topical metronidazole |
| | Charcoal dressings can be helpful |
| | Seal the wound, e.g. with additional layer of clingfilm dressing |
| | Try disguising the smell with deodorisers (e.g. Nilodor®) used sparingly on top of the dressing—short-term measure. Long term the deodorant smell often becomes associated with the smell of the wound for the patient |
| Infection | Usually chronic and localized |
| | Irrigate the wound with warm saline or under running water in the shower/bath |
| | If the surrounding skin is inflamed, swab the wound and send for M,C&S. Then start oral antibiotics, e.g. flucloxacillin 250–500mg qds or erythromycin 250–500mg qds. Alter antibiotics depending on sensitivities of the organisms grown |

# Respiratory problems

**Cough** Troublesome symptom. Prolonged bouts of coughing are exhausting and frightening, especially if associated with beathlessness and/or haemoptysis.

**Haemoptysis** 📖 p.305

**Breathlessness** Affects 70% of terminally ill patients. It is usually multifactorial. Breathlessness always has a psychological element—being short of breath is frightening. Causes—Figure 28.3.

## Management of cough and breathlessness

### General non-drug measures

- Reassure. Explain reasons for breathlessness/cough and adaptations to lifestyle which might help, e.g. sitting up straight.
- Breathing exercises can help—refer to physiotherapy.
- Exclude treatable causes (Box 28.1 and Figure 28.3).
- Steam inhalations or nebulized saline can help with tenacious secretions.
- Try a stream of air over the face if the patient is breathless, e.g. fan, open window

### General drug measures

- Try simple linctus 5–10mL prn for cough.
- Oral or subcutaneous opioids ↓ subjective sensation of breathlessness—start with 2.5mg morphine sulphate solution every 4h and titrate upwards. Opioids may also help with cough—try pholcodine 10mL tds or morphine sulphate solution as for breathlessness. If already on opioids, ↑ dose by 25%. Titrate dose until symptoms are controlled or side effects.
- Try benzodiazepines—2–5mg diazepam od/bd for background control of breathlessness + lorazepam 1–2mg s/ling prn in between. Diazepam acts as a central cough suppressant—try 2–10mg tds for cough.
- Oxygen has a variable effect and is worth a try
- Hyoscine hydrobromide 400–600 micrograms every 4-8h (or 0.6–2.4mg/24h via syringe driver) and/or ipratropium inhalers/nebulized ipratropium ↓ secretions.

### Specific measures

- **Chest infection** Treat with nebulized saline to make secretions less viscous ± antibiotics (if not considered a terminal event).
- **Post-nasal drip** Steam inhalations, steroid nasal spray or drops ± antibiotics.
- **Laryngeal irritation** Try inhaled steroids, e.g. beclometasone 100 micrograms/actuation 2 puffs bd
- **Bronchospasm** Try bronchodilators ± inhaled or oral steroids.
  ❶ Salbutamol may help cough even in the absence of wheeze.
- **Gastric reflux** Try antacids containing simeticone
- **Lung cancer** Try inhaled sodium cromoglicate 10mg qds; local anaesthesia using nebulized bupivacaine or lidocaine can be helpful—refer for specialist advice (avoid eating/drinking for 1h afterwards to avoid aspiration). Palliative radiotherapy or chemotherapy can also relieve cough in patients with lung cancer—refer.

**Stridor** Coarse wheezing sound which results from obstruction of a major airway, e.g. larynx.

### Management

- Corticosteroids (e.g. dexamethasone 16mg/d) can give relief.
- Consider referral for radiotherapy or endoscopic insertion of a stent if appropriate.
- If a terminal event, sedate with high doses of midazolam (10–40mg repeated prn).

**Fig. 28.3** Causes of breathlessness

Reproduced from Lynch J and Simon C, *Respiratory Problems* (2007) with permission from Oxford University Press

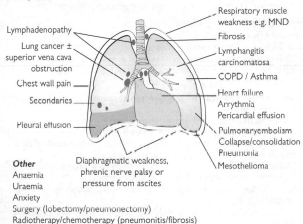

Lymphadenopathy

Lung cancer ± superior vena cava obstruction

Chest wall pain

Secondaries

Pleural effusion

Respiratory muscle weakness e.g. MND

Fibrosis

Lymphangitis carcinomatosa

COPD / Asthma

Heart failure
Arrythmia
Pericardial effusion

Pulmonaryembolism
Collapse/consolidation
Pneumonia
Mesothelioma

Diaphragmatic weakness, phrenic nerve palsy or pressure from ascites

**Other**
Anaemia
Uraemia
Anxiety
Surgery (lobectomy/pneumonectomy)
Radiotherapy/chemotherapy (pneumonitis/fibrosis)

---

### Box 28.1 Reversible causes of cough

- Infection
- Bronchospasm
- Gastro-oesophageal reflux
- Aspiration
- Drug-induced, e.g. ACE inhibitors
- Treatment-related, e.g. total body irradiation.
- Malignant bronchial obstruction/ lung metastases
- Heart failure
- Secretions
- Pharyngeal candidiasis

# Haematological and vascular problems

**Bleeding/haemorrhage** In all patients likely to bleed (e.g. in end-stage leukaemia) pre-warn carers and give them a strategy.

*Severe life-threatening bleed* Decide whether the cause of the bleed is treatable or a terminal event. This is best done in advance, but bleeding cannot always be predicted.
- *Severe bleed—active treatment* 🕮 p.1070
- *Severe bleed—no active treatment*
  - Stay with the patient.
  - Give sedative medication, e.g. midazolam 20–40mg sc/IV or diazepam 10–20mg PR and diamorphine 5–10mg sc/IV.
  - Support carers as big bleeds are extremely distressing.

### *Non-life-threatening bleed*
*First aid measures*
- In all cases: reassure; monitor frequently.
- Surface bleeding—pressure on wound; if pressure is not working try Kaltostat® or adrenaline (1mg/mL or 1:1000) on a gauze pad.
- Nose bleeds—nasal packing or cautery.

*Follow-up treatment* Follow-up is directed at cause if appropriate.
- Anticoagulants—check INR.
- Treat infection that might exacerbate a bleed.
- Consider ↓ bleeding tendency with tranexamic acid 500mg qds.
- Upper GI bleeding—stop NSAIDs, start PPI at double standard dose, and consider referral for gastroscopy.
- Lower GI bleeding—consider rectal steroids to ↓ inflammation or rectal tranexamic acid ± referral for colonoscopy.
- Radiotherapy—consider referral if haemoptysis, cutaneous bleeding, or haematuria.
- Referral for chemotherapy or palliative surgery (e.g. cautery) are also options

**Anaemia** Do not check for anaemia if no intention to transfuse.
- *If Hb <10g/dL and symptomatic* Treat any reversible cause (e.g. iron deficiency, GI bleeding 2° to NSAIDs). Consider transfusion.
- *If transfused* Record whether any benefit is derived (as if not, further transfusions are futile) and the duration of benefit (if <3wk—repeat transfusions are impractical). Monitor for return of symptoms; repeat FBC and arrange repeat transfusion as needed.

**Superior vena cava (SVC) obstruction** Due to infiltration of the vessel wall, clot within the superior vena cava, or extrinsic pressure. 75% are due to 1° lung cancer (3% of patients with lung cancer have SVC obstruction). Lymphoma is the other major cause.

### *Presentation*
- Shortness of breath/stridor.
- Headache worse on stooping ± visual disturbances ± dizziness and collapse.

- Swelling of the face, particularly around the eyes, neck, hands, and arms, and/or injected cornea.
- Examination: look for non-pulsatile distention of neck veins and dilated collateral veins (seen as small dilated veins over the anterior chest wall below the clavicles) in which blood courses downwards.

### Management

- Treat breathlessness (opioids—5mg morphine sulphate solution every 4h ± benzodiazepine depending on the level of anxiety).
- Start corticosteroid (dexamethasone 16mg/d.).
- Refer urgently for oncology opinion. Palliative radiotherapy has a response rate of 70%. Stenting ± thrombolysis is also an option.

**Lymphoedema** Due to obstruction of lymphatic drainage resulting in oedema with high protein content. Affects ≥1 limbs ± adjacent trunk. If left untreated, lymphoedema becomes increasingly resistant to treatment due to chronic inflammation and subcutaneous fibrosis. Cellulitis causes rapid ↑ in swelling. *Causes:*

- Axillary, groin or intrapelvic tumour
- Extensive axillary or groin surgery
- Post operative infection/radiotherapy.

### Presentation

- Swollen limb ± pitting
- Impaired limb mobility and function
- Discomfort/pain related to tissue swelling and/or shoulder strain
- Neuralgic pain, especially when axillary nodes are involved
- Psychological distress.

### Management Table 28.10

**Table 28.10** Management of lymphoedema

| | |
|---|---|
| *Avoid injury to limb* | In at-risk patients (e.g. patients who have had breast cancer with axillary clearance) or those with lymphoedema, injury to the limb may precipitate or worsen lymphoedema. Do not take blood from the limb or use it for IV access or vaccination |
| *Skin hygiene* | Skin care with moisturizers, e.g. aqueous cream, Emulsiderm. |
| | Topical treatment of fungal infection |
| | Systemic treatment of bacterial infection |
| *External support* | Intensive—with compression bandages |
| | Maintenance—with lymphoedema sleeve (contact breast care specialist nurse for more information on obtaining sleeves) |
| *Exercise* | Gentle daily exercise of affected limb, gradually increasing range of movement |
| | ❶ Must wear a sleeve/bandages when doing exercises |
| *Massage* | Very gentle fingertip massage in the line of drainage of lymphatics |
| *Diuretics* | If the condition has developed or deteriorated since prescription of corticosteroid or NSAID or if there venous component, consider trial of diuretics |
| | Otherwise diuretics are of no benefit |

# Psychiatric problems

**Anxiety** All patients with terminal disease are anxious at times for a variety of reasons, including fear of uncontrolled symptoms and of being left alone to die. When anxiety starts interfering with quality of life, intervention is justified.

## Management
*Non-drug measures*—often all that is needed:
- Acknowledgement of the patient's anxiety.
- Full explanation of questions + written information as needed.
- Support—self-help groups, day care, patients' groups, specialist home nurses (e.g. Macmillan Nurses).
- Relaxation training and training in breathing control.
- Physical therapies, e.g. aromatherapy, art therapy, exercise.

### Drug measures
- *Acute anxiety* Try lorazepam 1–2mg SL prn or diazepam 2–10mg prn
- *Chronic anxiety* Try an antidepressant, e.g. sertraline 50mg od. Alternatives include regular diazepam, e.g. 5–10 mg od/bd, haloperidol 1–3mg bd/tds, or β-blockers, e.g. propranolol 40mg od/tds—watch for postural hypotension.

If anxiety is not responding to simple measures, seek specialist help from either the psychiatric or palliative care team.

**Depression** A terminal diagnosis commonly makes patients sad. 10–20% of terminally ill patients develop clinical depression but, in practice, it is often difficult to decide whether a patient is depressed or just appropriately sad about his/her diagnosis and its implications. Many symptoms of terminal disease (e.g. poor appetite) are also symptoms of depression, so depression screening questionnaires are often unhelpful. If in doubt, a trial of antidepressants can help.

*Assessment of suicide risk* Ask about suicidal ideas and plans in a sensitive but probing way. It is a common misconception that asking about suicide can plant the idea into a patient's head and make suicide more likely. Evidence is to the contrary.

## Management
*Non-drug measures*
- Support, e.g. day and/or respite care; carers' group; specialist nurse support (e.g. Macmillan Nurse, CPN); ↑ help in the home.
- Relaxation often ↑ the patient's feeling of control over the situation.
- Explanation of worries/problems/concerns about the future.
- Physical activity—exercise; writing.

### Drug measures
- Consider starting an antidepressant—📖 p.1002
- All antidepressants take ~2wk to work.
- If immediate effect is required, consider using flupentixol 1mg od (beware as can cause psychomotor agitation).

If not responding or suicidal refer for psychiatric opinion.

**Terminal anguish and spiritual distress** Characterized by overwhelming distress. Often related to unresolved conflict, guilt, fears, or loss of control.

### Anxiety can be increased if
- Patients are unaware of the diagnosis, but feel people are lying to them.
- They are experiencing breathlessness, haemorrhage, or constant nausea or diarrhoea.
- Weak religious conviction—convinced believers and convinced non-believers have less anxiety.
- There are young dependent children or other dependent relatives.
- Patients have unfinished business to attend to, such as legal affairs.

**Action** Listening can itself be therapeutic. Talk to the patient, if possible, about dying and try to break down fears into component parts. Address fears that can be dealt with. As a last resort, and after discussion with the patient (where possible) and/or relatives, consider sedation.

**Confusion** 📖 p.1008

**Insomnia** 📖 p.196

# The last 48 hours

It is notoriously difficult to predict when death will occur. Symptoms and signs of approaching death include:
- Day-by-day deterioration
- Gaunt appearance
- Difficulty swallowing medicines
- ↓ intake of food and fluids
- Profound weakness—needs assistance with all care, may be bedbound.
- Drowsy or ↓ cognition—often unable to cooperate with carers.

## Goals of treatment in the last 48 hours
- Ensure patients are comfortable—physically, emotionally, and spiritually
- Make the end of life peaceful and dignified. What is dignified for one patient may not be for another—ask.
- Support patients and carers so that the experience of death for those left behind is as positive as possible.

**Patient's wishes** Dying is a unique and special event for each individual. Helping to explore a patient's wishes about death and dying should not be a discussion left to the last 24h.

**Advance directives/living wills/lasting power of attorney** 📖 p.124

**Out of hours providers** Alert out of hours providers if a patient is dying at home. This will ensure appropriate response to calls, and avoid unnecessary and unwanted admissions. Consider a 'just-in-case' box to leave at the patient's home containing drugs that might be needed should the patient deteriorate outside normal working hours.

**Different cultures** Different religious and cultural groups have different approaches to the dying process. Be sensitive to cultural and religious beliefs. If in doubt, ask a family member.

**Assessment of patient needs** Ask which problems are causing the patient/carers most concern, and address those concerns where possible. Patients often under-report symptoms.

**Physical examination** Keep examination to a minimum to avoid unnecessary interference. Check sites of discomfort/pain suggested by history or non-verbal cues: mouth, bladder, and bowel.

**Psychological assessment** Find out what the patient wants to know. Gently assessing how the patient feels about their disease and situation can shed light on their needs and distress.

**Investigations** Any investigation at the end of life should have a clear and justifiable purpose (e.g. excluding a reversible condition where treatment would make the patient more comfortable). The need for investigations in the terminal stage of illness is minimal.

**Review of medication** Comfort is the priority. Stop all unnecessary medication.

**Symptom control** Dying patients tolerate symptoms very poorly because of their weakness. Nursing care is the mainstay of treatment. However, GPs have a role:
- Ensure that new problems do not develop, e.g. use of appropriate mattresses and measures to prevent bed sores.

- Treat specific symptoms, e.g. dry mouth.
- Think ahead—discuss treatment options that might be available later, e.g. use of a syringe driver, buccal, PR or transcutaneous preparations to deliver medication when/if the oral route is no longer possible, use of strong analgesia which may also have a sedative effect.
- Ensure that a clear management plan is agreed between the medical and nursing team and the patient/family members. Anticipate probable needs of the patient so that immediate response can be made when the time comes: define clearly what should be done in the event of a symptom arising/worsening; ensure drugs or equipment that may be needed are in the home; inform the out-of-hours service.

**Excessive respiratory secretion (death rattle)** Noisy moist breathing. Can be distressing for relatives. Reassure that the patient is not suffering or choking. Try repositioning and/or tipping the bed head down (if possible) to ↓ noise. Treat prophylactically—it is easier to prevent than remove accumulated secretions. *Suitable drugs*:

- Glycopyrronium—non-sedative. Give 200 micrograms sc stat and review after 1h. If effective, give 200 micrograms sc every 4h or 0.6–1.2mg/24h via syringe driver.
- Hyoscine hydrobromide—sedative in high doses, give 400 micrograms sc stat and review response after 30min. If effective, give 400–600 micrograms every 4–8h or 0.6–2.4mg/24h via syringe driver. If patient is conscious and respiratory secretions are not too distressing, it may be more appropriate to use a transdermal patch (Scopaderm® 1.5mg over 3d) or sublingual tablets (Kwells®). Dry mouth is a side effect.

**Terminal breathlessness** Distressing symptom for patients/carers. Support carers in attendance and explain management:

- Diamorphine or morphine: dose depends on whether the patient is being converted from oral morphine (or an alternative opioid), to diamorphine. If no previous opioid, start diamorphine 5mg/24h sc. If previously on oral morphine, divide the total 24h dose by 3 to obtain the 24h s/cut dose. ↑ dose slowly as needed.
- Midazolam 5–10mg/24h sc.
- If sticky secretions—try nebulised saline + physiotherapy.

**Terminal restlessness** *Causes*:

- *Pain/discomfort* Urinary retention, constipation, pain which the patient cannot tell you about, excess secretions in throat.
- *Opioid toxicity* Causes myoclonic jerking. The dose of morphine may need to be ↓ if a patient becomes uraemic.
- *Biochemical causes* ↑ $Ca^{2+}$, uraemia. ❶ if it has been decided not to treat abnormalities, do not check for them.
- *Psychological/spiritual distress*.

**Management** Treat reversible causes, e.g. catheterization for retention, hyoscine to dry up secretions. If still restless, treat with a sedative. This does not shorten life but makes the patient/relatives more comfortable. *Suitable drugs*: haloperidol 1–3mg tds po; chlorpromazine 25–50mg tds po; diazepam 2–10mg tds po, midazolam (10–100mg/24h via syringe driver or 5mg stat) or levomepromazine (50–150mg/24h via syringe driver or 6.25mg stat).

**Terminal anguish and spiritual distress** 📖 p.1041

# Chapter 29

# Emergencies in general practice

# Emergency patient encounters

**Emergency calls** Nearly all requests for emergency care are made by telephone. General rules:

- *Train surgery staff* to handle distressed callers, recognize serious problems, and act appropriately when such calls are received.
- *Where possible use a single number for patients to access help.* If using an answering machine ensure that the message is easily heard and contains clear instructions. Worried patients find it difficult to cope with complicated telephone referral systems or messages.
- *Appear helpful* rather than defensive from the outset. Keep calm and friendly, even in the event of provocation. Worried callers often appear abrupt or demanding.
- *Record* the time of the call, date, patient's name, address, and a contact telephone number, brief details of the problem, and action taken (even if calls are being recorded).
- *Collect only information you need to decide what action is necessary* If the patient needs to be seen, collect enough information to decide where and how quickly the patient should be seen, and whether extra equipment or help is needed.
- *If giving advice* make it simple and in language the patient can understand. Repeat to make sure that it has been understood. Consider asking the patient/carer to repeat what you have told them. Always tell callers to ring back if symptoms change or they have further worries.
- *If a visit is indicated* ensure that the address is right and ask for directions if you are not sure where to go. Try to give a rough arrival time.
- *In some cases* (e.g. major trauma, large GI bleeds, MI, stroke, burns, overdoses) call for an emergency ambulance at once.
- *If a call seems inappropriate* consider the reason for it, e.g. depression might provoke recurrent calls for minor ailments.

⚠ If in doubt—see the patient.

## Emergency home visits

- Try to stick to the problem you have been called about.
- Take a concise history and examine as appropriate.
- Make a decision on management and explain it to the patient and any carers in clear and concise terms that they can understand. Repeat advice several times ± write it down.
- Record history, examination, management suggested, and advice given for the patient's notes.
- Always invite the patient and carers to ring you again should symptoms change, the situation deteriorate, or further worries appear.
- For inappropriate calls, take time to educate the patient and/or carers about self-management and use of emergency GP visiting services.
- Always consider hidden reasons for seemingly unnecessary visits.

## Being prepared

- Ensure that you have a reliable car with a full tank of fuel.
- Have a good street map of the area ± Ordinance Survey map ± an electronic in-car navigation system.

- Carry a large strong torch in the car.
- Carry a mobile telephone.
- Check that your drug box is fully stocked and all items are in date.
- Check that all equipment carried is operational and carry spare batteries.
- Carry a list of emergency telephone numbers.
- Know which chemists have extended opening hours and/or carry the chemist's rota.

### Safety and security
- In all cases ensure that someone else knows where you are going, when to expect you back, and what to do if you don't return on time.
- If you are going to a call that you are worried about, either take someone with you to sit in the car or call the police to meet you there before going in.
- If you reach a call and find you are uncomfortable, make sure you can get out. Note the layout of the property and make sure that you have a clear route to the door.
- Set up your mobile phone to call the police or your base at a single touch of a button. Consider carrying an attack alarm.
- If possible, have separate bags for drugs and consultation equipment.
- Leave the drug box locked out of sight in the boot of the car when doing a visit.

**Referral letters** Good communication is essential when referring patients to other doctors and agencies, especially in emergency situations. Ensure that all referral letters include:
- Address of the referrer (including telephone number if possible).
- Name and address of registered GP if not the referrer.
- Date of referral.
- Name, address, and date of birth of the patient (and any other identifiers available, e.g. hospital or NHS number).
- Name of the person to whom the patient is being referred (or department if not a named individual).
- Presenting condition—history, examination, investigations already performed with results, treatments already tried with outcomes.
- Relevant past medical history and family history.
- Current medication and any intolerances/allergies known.
- Reason for referral (what you want the recipient of the letter to do), e.g. to investigate symptoms, to reassure parents.
- Any other relevant information, e.g. social circumstances.
- Signature (and name in legible format) of referrer.

**❶** Consider using carbonized paper to keep copies of emergency referral letters.

**The doctor's bag** 📖 p.98

# Managing a resuscitation attempt outside hospital

⚠ Ventricular fibrillation complicating acute MI is the most common cause of cardiac arrest that members of the primary health care team will encounter. Success is greatest when the event is witnessed and attempted defibrillation is performed with the minimum of delay.

**Resuscitation equipment** (Table 29.1)
- Resuscitation equipment is used relatively infrequently. Staff must know where to find equipment at the time it is needed and should be trained to use the equipment to a level appropriate to the individual's expected role.
- Each practice should have a named individual with responsibility for checking the state of readiness of all resuscitation drugs and equipment, on a regular basis, ideally once a week. In common with drugs, disposable items like adhesive electrodes have a finite shelf-life and will require replacement from time to time if unused.

**Training** Training and practice are necessary to acquire skill in resuscitation techniques. Resuscitation skills decline rapidly and updates and retraining using manikins are necessary every 6–12mo to maintain adequate skill levels. Levels of resuscitation skill needed by different members of the primary health care team differ according to the individual's role:
- All those in direct contact with patients should be trained in basic life support and related resuscitation skills such as the recovery position.
- Doctors, nurses, and other paramedical workers such as physiotherapists should also be able to use an automatic external defibrillator (AED) effectively. Other personnel (e.g. receptionists) may also be trained to use an AED.

⚠ It is unacceptable for patients who sustain a cardiopulmonary arrest to await the arrival of the ambulance service before basic resuscitation is performed and a defibrillator is available.

**Performance management** Accurate records of all resuscitation attempts and electronic data stored by most AEDs during a resuscitation attempt should be kept for audit, training and medico-legal reasons. The responsibility for this rests with the most senior member of the practice team involved. Process and outcome of all resuscitation attempts should be audited—at both practice and PCO level—to allow deficiencies to be addressed, and examples of good practice to be shared.

## Ethical issues
- It is essential to identify individuals for whom cardiopulmonary arrest is a terminal event and where resuscitation is inappropriate.
- Overall responsibility for a 'Do not attempt to resuscitate' (DNAR) decision rests with the doctor in charge of the patient's care.
- Seek opinions of other members of the medical and nursing team, the patient and any relatives in reaching a DNAR decision.

- Record that the patient should not be resuscitated in the notes, the reasons for that decision, and what the relatives have been told.
- Ensure that all members of the team involved with the patient's care are aware of the decision and have it recorded in their notes.
- Review the decision not to attempt resuscitation regularly in the light of the patient's condition.

## Further information

**Resuscitation Council (UK)** (2001) Cardiopulmonary resuscitation guidance for clinical practice and training in primary care ⌨ www.resus.org.uk
**BMA, RCN and Resuscitation Council (UK)** (2001) Decisions relating to cardiopulmonary resuscitation ⌨ www.resus.org.uk

**Table 29.1** Resuscitation equipment needed

| Equipment | Notes |
|---|---|
| Defibrillator with electrodes and razor | An automated external defibrillator should be available wherever and whenever sick patients are seen. |
| | Regular maintenance is needed even if the machine is not used. |
| | After the machine is used, manufacturer's instructions should be followed to return it to a state of readiness with minimum delay. |
| Pocket mask with 1-way valve | All personnel should be trained to use one |
| Oropharyngeal airway | Suitable for use by those appropriately trained. Keep a range of sizes available. |
| Oxygen and mask with reservoir bag | Should be available wherever possible. |
| | Oxygen cylinders need regular maintenance—follow national safety standards |
| Suction | Simple mechanical portable hand-held suction devices are recommended. |
| Drugs | Adrenaline (epinephrine) 1mg IV |
| | Atropine 3mg IV (give once only) for bradycardia, asystole, and pulseless electrical activity |
| | Amiodarone 300mg IV for VF resistant to defibrillation |
| | Naloxone for suspected cases of respiratory arrest due to opioid overdose |
| | ⚠ There is no evidence for the use of alkalizing agents, buffers, or calcium salts before hospitalization |
| | Drugs should be given by the IV route, preferably through a catheter placed in a large vein, e.g. in the antecubital fossa, and flushed in with a bolus of IV fluid. |
| | Many drugs can be given via the bronchial route if a tracheal tube is in place; the dose for adrenaline (epinephrine) and atropine is double the IV dose. |
| Other | Saline flush, gloves, syringes and needles, IV cannulae, IV fluids, sharps box, scissors, tape |

# Adult basic life support

**Basic paediatric life support** 📖 p.1056

**Adult basic adult life support (ABLS)** (Figure 29.1) is a holding operation—sustaining life until help arrives. ABLS should be started as soon as the arrest is detected—outcome is less good the longer the delay.

**1. Danger** Ensure safety of rescuer and patient.

**2. Response** Check the patient for any response.
- Is he **A**lert? Yes/No
- Does he respond to **V**ocal stimuli? Yes/No
- Does he respond to a **P**ainful stimulus (pinching the lower part of the nasal septum)? Yes/No
- Is the patient **U**nconscious? Yes/No.

*If he responds by answering or moving* Do not move the patient unless in danger. Get help. Reassess regularly.

*If he does not respond* Shout for help; turn the patient on to his back.

**3. Airway** Open the airway—place one hand on the patient's forehead and tilt his head back. With fingertips under the point of the patient's chin, lift the chin to open the airway.

⚠ Try to avoid head tilt if trauma to the neck is suspected.

**4. Breathing** With airway open, look, listen and feel for breathing for no more than 10sec—look for chest movement, listen at the victim's mouth for breath sounds, feel for air on your cheek.

*If breathing normally* Turn the patient into the recovery position (📖 p.1067), get help, and check for continued breathing.

*If not breathing* or only making occasional gasps/weak attempts at breathing: get help, and then start chest compressions.

❶ In the first few minutes after cardiac arrest, a victim may be barely breathing, or taking infrequent noisy gasps. Do not confuse this with normal breathing. If you have any doubt whether breathing is normal, act as if it is *not* normal.

**5. Circulation** Start chest compressions if not breathing:
- Kneel by the side of the victim and place the heel of one hand in the centre of the victim's chest. Place the heel of the other hand on top of the first hand. Interlock the fingers of your hands and ensure that pressure is not applied over the victim's ribs. Do not apply any pressure over the upper abdomen or the bottom end of the bony sternum
- Position yourself vertically above the victim's chest and, with arms straight, press down on the sternum 4–5cm
- After each compression, release all the pressure on the chest without losing contact between your hands and the sternum. Compression and release should take an equal amount of time
- Repeat at a rate of ~100×/min.

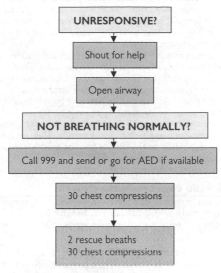

**Fig. 29.1** Adult basic life support (ABLS) algorithm

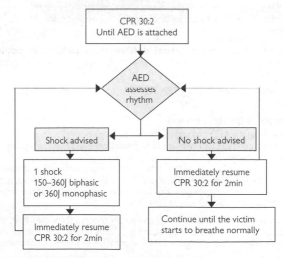

**Fig. 29.2** Automated external defibrillator (AED) algorithm

Figures 29.1 and 29.2 are reproduced from the *Resuscitation Guidelines* (2005) with permission from the Resuscitation Council UK ⊞ www.resus.org.uk

6. **Combine chest compression with rescue breaths**
   - After 30 compressions open the airway using head tilt and chin lift.
   - Pinch the soft part of the victim's nose closed, using the index finger and thumb of your hand on his forehead. Allow the victim's mouth to open, but maintain chin lift.
   - Give a rescue breath—take a normal breath and place your lips around the victim's mouth (mouth-to-nose technique is an alternative) making sure that you have a good seal. Blow steadily into his mouth for ~1sec whilst watching for the chest to rise.
   - Maintaining head tilt and chin lift, take your mouth away from the victim and watch for the chest to fall as air comes out.
   - Take another normal breath and blow into the victim's mouth again to give a total of two effective rescue breaths. Then return your hands without delay to the correct position on the sternum and give a further 30 chest compressions.
   - Continue chest compressions and rescue breaths in a ratio of 30:2.

*If rescue breaths do not make the chest rise*
- Check the victim's mouth and remove any visible obstruction.
- Recheck that there is adequate head tilt and chin lift.
- Don't attempt >2 breaths each time before returning to chest compressions.

**❶ Chest-compression-only CPR** If you are unable or unwilling to give rescue breaths, give continuous chest compressions only at a rate of 100/min.

⚠ Only stop to recheck the victim if the patient makes a movement or takes a spontaneous breath; otherwise resuscitation should not be interrupted

**Use of automated external defibrillators (AEDs) in adults**
(Figure 29.2) Program AEDs to deliver a single shock followed by a pause of 2min for the immediate resumption of CPR.

*If a patient arrests* Start CPR according to the guidelines for basic life support.

*As soon as the AED arrives*
- Switch on the AED and attach the electrode pads. If >1 rescuer is present, continue CPR whilst this is done. (Some AEDs automatically switch on when the AED lid is opened).
  - Place one AED pad to the right of the sternum, below the clavicle.
  - Place the other pad in the mid-axillary line with its long axis vertical.
- Follow the voice/visual prompts. Ensure that nobody touches the victim whilst the AED is analysing the rhythm.

*If a shock is indicated* Ensure that nobody touches the victim. Push the shock button as directed (fully automatic AEDs deliver the shock automatically). Immediately resume CPR and continue to follow the prompts.

*If no shock is indicated* Immediately resume CPR and continue to follow the prompts.

**Use of AEDs in children** 📖 p.1058

**When to go for assistance** It is vital for rescuers to get assistance as quickly as possible. If you are the only rescuer, go for assistance before starting CPR.

### When >1 rescuer is available
- One should start resuscitation while another goes for assistance
- Another should take over CPR every 2min to prevent fatigue. Ensure minimum of delay during change-over of rescuers.

**Duration of resuscitation** Continue resuscitation until:
- Qualified help arrives and takes over
- The victim starts breathing normally *and/or*
- You become exhausted.

**Pad position for external defibrillators** Place 1 pad to the right of the sternum below the clavicle. Place the other pad vertically in the midaxillary line approximately level with the V6 ECG electrode position or female breast (although clear of any breast tissue).

## Further information

**Resuscitation Council (UK)** Resuscitation guidelines (2005)
www.resus.org.uk

# Adult advanced life support

Advanced life support has 3 basic stages (Figure 29.3):
• Revive the patient using basic life support (📖 p.1050). Basic life support should be started if there is any delay in obtaining a defibrillator, but must not delay shock delivery.
• Restore spontaneous cardiac output using an automated external defibrillator (📖 p.1052) or a manual defibrillator.
• Review possible causes for cardiac arrest and take further action as needed.

**Precordial thump** Appropriate *only* if the arrest is witnessed and and a defibrillator is not to hand—may dislodge a pulmonary embolus or 'jerk' the heart back into sinus rhythm. Use the ulnar edge of a tightly clenched fist and deliver a sharp impact to the lower half of the sternum from a height of ~20cm then immediately retract the fist.

## VF/VT arrest
• Attempt defibrillation (1 shock 150–200J biphasic or 360J monophasic).
• Immediately resume chest compressions (30:2) without reassessing rhythm or feeling for the pulse. Continue CPR for 2min and then pause briefly to check the monitor.
• If VT/VF persists give a second shock (150–360J biphasic or 360J monophasic). Continue CPR for 2min and then pause briefly to check the monitor.
• If VF/VT persists give adrenaline (epinephrine) 1mg IV (or intraosseously if IV access cannot be attained) followed immediately by a third shock (150–360J biphasic or 360J monophasic). Resume CPR immediately, continue for 2 min, and then pause briefly to check the monitor.
• If VF/VT persists give amiodarone 300mg IV (lidocaine 1mg/kg is an alternative if amiodarone is not available) followed immediately by a fourth shock (150–360J biphasic or 360J monophasic). Resume CPR immediately and continue for 2min.
• Give adrenaline (epinephrine) 1mg IV immediately before alternate shocks (i.e. approximately every 3–5min).
• Give a further shock after each 2min period of CPR and after confirming that VF/VT persists.

## Non-VT/VF arrest
• Start CPR 30:2. Without stopping CPR, check that the leads are attached correctly.
• Give adrenaline (epinephrine) 1mg IV as soon as IV access is achieved.
• If asystole or pulseless electrical activity with rate <60bpm, give atropine 3mg IV (once only).
• Continue CPR 30:2 until the airway is secured; then continue chest compression without pausing during ventilation.
• Recheck the rhythm after 2min and proceed accordingly.
• Give adrenaline (epinephrine) 1mg IV every 3–5min (alternate loops).

**Fine VF** Fine VF that is difficult to distinguish from asystole is very unlikely to be shocked successfully into a perfusing rhythm. Continuing good quality CPR may improve the amplitude and frequency of the VF and improve the chance of successful defibrillation to a perfusing rhythm.

**Organized electrical activity** If organized electrical activity is seen during the brief pause in compressions, check for a pulse.
• If a pulse is present, start post-resuscitation care (📖 p.1067).
• If no pulse, continue CPR and follow the non-shockable algorithm.

### Further information
**Resuscitation Council (UK)** (2005) Resuscitation guidelines.
🖥 www.resus.org.uk

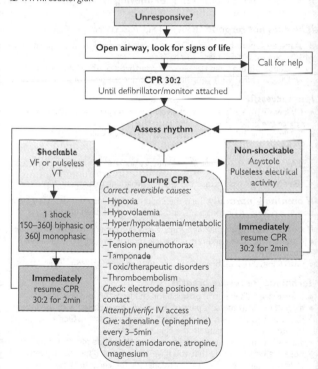

**Fig. 29.3** Adult advanced life support algorithm

Reproduced from the *Resuscitation Guidelines* (2005), with permission from the Resuscitation Council UK 🖥 www.resus.org.uk

# Paediatric basic life support

Basic paediatric life support (Figure 29.4) is a holding operation until help arrives.

**1. Danger** Ensure safety of rescuer and patient.

**2. Response** Check the child for any response.
- Is he **A**lert?
- Does he respond to **V**ocal stimuli?
- Does he respond to **P**ainful stimuli (pinch lower part of nasal septum)?
- Is he **U**nconscious?

*If he responds by answering or moving* Do not move the child unless in danger. Get help. Reassess regularly.

*If he does not respond* Shout for help. Assess airway (below)

**3. Airway** Open the airway. Do not move the child from the position in which you found him unless you have to.
- Gently tilt the head back—with your hand on the child's forehead.
- Lift the chin—with your fingertips under the point of the child's chin.

*If unsuccessful*
- Try jaw thrust—place the first two fingers of each hand behind each side of the child's jaw bone and push the jaw forward.
- Try lifting the chin or jaw thrust after carefully turning the child onto his back.

⚠ Avoid head tilt as much as possible if trauma to the neck is suspected

**4. Breathing** Look, listen, and feel for breathing (maximum 10sec).

*If breathing normally* Turn the child carefully into the recovery position (📖 p.1067) if unconscious, and check for continued breathing

*If not breathing* or making agonal gasps (infrequent irregular breaths):
- Carefully turn the child onto his back and remove any obvious airway obstruction.
- Give 5 initial rescue breaths—note any gag or cough response.

### Technique for rescue breaths
- Ensure head tilt (neutral position for children<1y) and chin lift.
- If age ≥1y, pinch the soft part of the child's nose closed with the index finger and thumb of the hand which is on his forehead. Open the child's mouth a little, but maintain the chin upwards.
- Take a breath and place your lips around the child's mouth (mouth and nose if <1y*), ensuring that you have a good seal. Blow steadily into the child's airway over ~1–1.5sec watching for the chest to rise.
- Maintaining head tilt and chin lift, take your mouth away, and watch for the chest to fall as air comes out.
- Take another breath and repeat this sequence five times.

❶ If you have difficulty achieving an effective breath, consider airway obstruction—📖 p.1082.

*If the nose and mouth cannot both be covered place your lips around the mouth alone as for an older child, or nose alone (close the child's lips to prevent air escape).

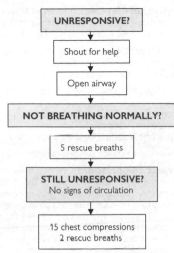

**Fig. 29.4** Paediatric basic life support (PBLS) algorithm

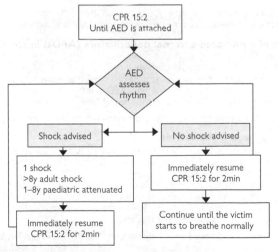

**Fig. 29.5** Automated external defibrillator (AED) algorithm

Figures 29.4 and 29.5 are reproduced from the *Resuscitation Guidelines* (2005), with permission from the Resuscitation Council UK 🖳 www.resus.org.uk

**5. Circulation (signs of life)** Check (maximum 10sec) for:
- Any movement, coughing or normal breathing (not agonal gasps).
- Pulse—child ≥ 1y carotid pulse; child <1y brachial pulse.

*If circulation is present* Continue rescue breathing until the child starts breathing effectively on his own. Turn the child into the recovery position (📖 p.1067) if unconscious, and reassess frequently.

*If circulation is absent* or slow pulse (<60bpm) with poor perfusion, or you are not sure:
- Give 15 chest compressions. Then give 2 rescue breaths followed by 15 further chest compressions.
- Continue the cycle of 2 breaths followed by 15 chest compressions.

❶ Lone rescuers may use a ratio of 30 compressions to 2 rescue breaths.

*Technique for chest compressions* Compress the sternum one finger's breadth above the xiphisternum by ~¹/₃ of the depth of the chest. Release the pressure; then repeat at a rate of ~100 compressions/min.
- Children <1y with a lone rescuer—use the tips of 2 fingers.
- Children <1y with ≥2 rescuers—place both thumbs flat on the lower third of the sternum with tips pointing towards the child's head and encircle the lower part of the child's ribcage with the tips of the fingers supporting the infant's back. Press down with both thumbs.
- Children >1y—place the heel of 1 hand over the lower third of the sternum. Lift the fingers. Position yourself vertically above the chest with arm straight, and push downwards. For larger children use both hands with fingers interlocked to achieve satisfactory compressions.

⚠ Stop to recheck for signs of a circulation only if the child moves or takes a spontaneous breath—otherwise continue uninterrupted.

**Use of automated external defibrillators (AEDs) in children** (Figure 29.5)
- Children >8y—use the standard adult AED.
- Children aged 1–8y—paediatric pads or a paediatric mode should be used if available—if not, use the adult AED as it is.
- Children <1y—AED use is currently not advised.

*If a patient arrests* Start CPR according to the guidelines for PBLS

*As soon as the AED arrives*
- Switch on the AED and attach the electrode pads. If >1 rescuer is present, continue CPR whilst this is done. (Some AEDs automatically switch on when the AED lid is opened).
  - Place one AED pad to the right of the sternum below the clavicle.
  - Place the other pad in the mid-axillary line with its long axis vertical.
- Follow the voice/visual prompts. Ensure that nobody touches the victim whilst the AED is analysing the rhythm.

*If a shock is indicated* Ensure that nobody touches the victim. Push the shock button as directed (fully automatic AEDs deliver the shock automatically). Immediately resume CPR and continue to follow the prompts.

*If no shock is indicated* Immediately resume CPR and continue to follow the prompts.

**When to go for assistance** It is vital for rescuers to get assistance as quickly as possible when a child collapses.

*When >1 rescuer is available* One should start resuscitation while another rescuer goes for assistance.

*Lone rescuer* Perform resuscitation for 1 minute before going for assistance (and consider taking a young child/infant with you to minimize interruption in CPR). The only exception to this is a *witnessed sudden collapse*—in this case cardiac arrest is likely to be due to arrhythmia and the child may need defibrillation so seek help immediately.

**Duration of resuscitation** Continue resuscitation until:
• child shows signs of life (spontaneous respiration, pulse, movement)
• further qualified help arrives
• you become exhausted.

### Cervical spine injury
• If spinal cord injury is suspected (e.g. if the victim has sustained a fall, been struck on the head or neck, or has been rescued after diving into shallow water), take particular care during handling and resuscitation to maintain alignment of the head, neck, and chest in the neutral position.
• A spinal board and/or cervical collar should be used if available.

**Resuscitation of the newborn** p.1062

**Further information**
**Resuscitation Council (UK)** Resuscitation guidelines (2005)
www.resus.org.uk

# Paediatric advanced life support

Cardiac arrest in children is rare. Unless there is underlying heart disease, it is usually a consequence of respiratory arrest which results in asystole or pulseless electrical activity and has poor prognosis. Therefore good airway management and providing high-flow oxygen for very sick children is important in preventing cardiac arrest.

**Basic paediatric life support** Follow the algorithm in Figure 29.6.

**Unable to ventilate?** Consider foreign body in the airway and initiate airway obstruction sequence (📖 p.1082).

### Checking the pulse
- *Child*—feel for the carotid pulse in the neck
- *Infant*—feel for the brachial pulse on the inner aspect of the upper arm.

**Once the airway is protected** If the airway is protected by tracheal intubation, continue chest compression without pausing for ventilation. Provide ventilation at a rate of 10/min and compression at 100/min. When circulation is restored, ventilate the child at a rate of 12–20 breaths/min.

### Adrenaline (epinephrine) dose
- IV or intraosseous (IO) access—10 micrograms/kg adrenaline (0.1mL/kg of 1:10 000 solution)
- If circulatory access is not present and cannot be quickly obtained, but the child has a tracheal tube in place, consider giving adrenaline 100 micrograms/kg via the tracheal tube (1mL/kg of 1:10 000 or 0.1 mL/kg of 1:1 000 solution). This is the least satisfactory route of administration.

⚠ Do not give 1:1000 adrenaline IV or IO.

**VF/pulseless VT** Less common in paediatric life support.
- Defibrillation:
  - Give one shock of 4J/kg *or*
  - If using an AED for a child of 1–8y deliver a paediatric attenuated adult shock energy.
  - If using an AED for a child >8y use the adult shock energy.
- For VF/pulseless VT persisting after the third shock, try amiodarone 5mg/kg diluted in 5% dextrose.

**Bradycardia** When bradycardia is unresponsive to improved ventilation and circulatory support, try atropine 20 micrograms/kg (maximum dose 600 micrograms; minimum dose 100 micrograms).

**Magnesium** Magnesium treatment is indicated in children with documented hypomagnesemia or with polymorphic VT (torsade de pointes), regardless of cause. Give IV magnesium sulphate over several minutes at a dose of 25–50mg/kg (to a maximum of 2g).

**Intravenous fluids** In situations where the cardiac arrest has resulted from circulatory failure, a standard (20mL/kg) bolus of crystalloid fluid should be given if there is no response to the initial dose of adrenaline.

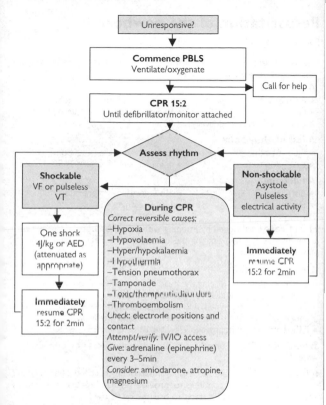

**Fig. 29.6** Paediatric advanced life support (PALS) algorithm

Reproduced from the *Resuscitation Guidelines* (2005), with permission from the Resuscitation Council UK ▯ www.resus.org.uk

---

### Estimating the weight of a child for drug/fluid doses
- May not be necessary—use a recent weight from the parent-held child record if available.
- Otherwise for children >1y, weight (in kg) ≈ 2 × (age + 4).

# Resuscitation of the newborn

Follow the algorithm in Figure 29.7.

**Rapid assessment of the infant at birth** Start the clock. Assess colour, tone, breathing, heart rate.

### A healthy baby
- Born blue
- Good tone
- Cries seconds after delivery
- Good heart rate (120–150bpm)
- Rapidly becomes pink during first 90sec.

### A less healthy baby
- Blue at birth
- Less good tone
- ± slow heart rate (<100bpm)
- ± inadequate breathing by 90–120sec.

### An ill baby
- Born pale
- Floppy
- Slow/very slow heart rate(<100bpm)
- Not breathing.

**Heart rate** Best judged by listening with a stethoscope—in many cases it can also be felt by palpating the umbilical cord. Feeling for peripheral pulses is not helpful.

### Airway
- Open the airway by placing the head in a neutral position, where the neck is neither extended nor flexed.
- If the occiput is prominent and the neck tends to flex, place a support under the shoulders—but do not over-extend the neck.
- If the baby is very floppy, apply jaw thrust or chin lift as needed.

**Breathing** Inflation breaths are breaths with pressures of ~30cm of water for 2–3sec.

*If heart rate ↑* You have successfully inflated the chest. If the baby doesn't start breathing alone, continue to provide regular breaths at a rate of ~30–40 breaths/min until it starts to breathe on its own.

*If heart rate does not ↑* Either you have not inflated the chest or the baby needs more help. By far the most likely is that you have failed to inflate the chest (the chest does not move). *Consider:*
- Is the baby's head in the neutral position?
- Do you need jaw thrust?
- Do you need a longer inflation time?
- Do you need a second person's help with the airway?
- Is there an obstruction in the oropharynx, e.g. meconium (laryngo-scope and suction)?
- What about an oropharyngeal (Guedel) airway?

**Chest compressions** Only commence after inflation of the lungs.
- Grip the chest in both hands in such a way that the thumbs of both hands can press on the sternum at a point just below an imaginary line joining the nipples and with the fingers over the spine at the back.
- Compress the chest quickly—↓ the AP diameter of the chest by ~$1/3$ with each compression. The ratio of compressions to inflations is 3:1.

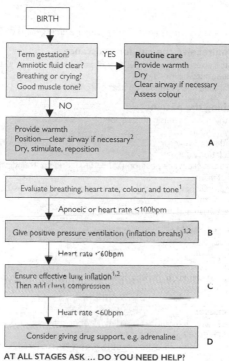

**Fig. 29.7** Newborn life support algorithm

Reproduced from the *Resuscitation Council* (2005), with permission from the Resuscitation Council
🖳 www.resus.org.uk

**Drug support** For a few babies inflation of the lungs and effective chest compression are not sufficient to produce effective circulation. IV or intraosseous drugs may be helpful. *Doses:*

• Adrenaline (epinephrine)—10 micrograms/kg (0.1mL/kg of 1:10 000 solution). increasing to 30 micrograms/kg (0.3mL/kg of 1:10 000 solution) if ineffective.
• Sodium bicarbonate—1–2mmol/kg (2–4mL 4.2% bicarbonate solution).
• Glucose—250mg/kg (2.5 mL/kg of 10% dextrose).

For emergency volume replacement (e.g. history of a bleed)—use 10mL/kg 0.9% saline given over 10–20sec. Repeat if needed.

**Further information**
**Resuscitation Council (UK)** Resuscitation guidelines (2005)
🖳 www.resus.org.uk

# Coma

Patients in coma/pre-coma nearly always require emergency admission.

## When you receive the call for assistance

- Advise the attendant (unless history of possible spinal injury) to turn the patient onto his/her side
- Call an ambulance to meet you at the scene.

## On reaching the patient

- Assess the need for basic life support:
  - Airway patent?
  - Breathing satisfactory?
  - Circulation adequate?
- Turn into the recovery position (📖 p.1067) if no contraindications, e.g. spinal injury.
- Call for ambulance support if you have not already done so.
- Ensure that the patient is warm.
- Try to establish a diagnosis (see assessment).

## As soon as possible

- Insert an airway
- Give oxygen
- Establish IV access
- Transfer to hospital unless the condition has resolved, e.g. hypoglycaemia, fit

## Possible causes

- *Drugs* Sedatives or hypnotics, opioids, alcohol, solvents, carbon monoxide poisoning.
- *Vascular* Stroke, low cardiac output (e.g. post MI, ruptured AAA).
- *CNS* Fit or post-ictal state, hydrocephalus (e.g. blocked shunt), cerebral oedema (e.g. meningitis, SAH, head injury), concussion, extradural or subdural haematoma.
- *Metabolic* Hypo- or hyperglycaemia, hypothermia, hypopituitarism.
- *Infection* Meningitis or septicaemia, pneumonia.

## Assessment and management See Figure 29.9

**Table 29.2** The Glasgow Coma Scale

| Eye opening | Spontaneous | 4 | To pain | 2 |
|---|---|---|---|---|
| | To voice | 3 | None | 1 |
| Best verbal response | Oriented | 5 | Incomprehensible | 2 |
| | Confused | 4 | None | 1 |
| | Inappropriate words | 3 | | |
| Best motor response | Obeys command | 6 | Flexion | 3 |
| | Localizes pain | 5 | Extension | 2 |
| | Withdraw | 4 | None | 1 |

Total score = eye opening + best verbal + best motor response scores.

Reprinted from Teasdale and Jennett, Assessment of coma and impaired consciousness: a practical scale, *Lancet* (1974) **304**, 81–84, copyright with permission from Elsevier.

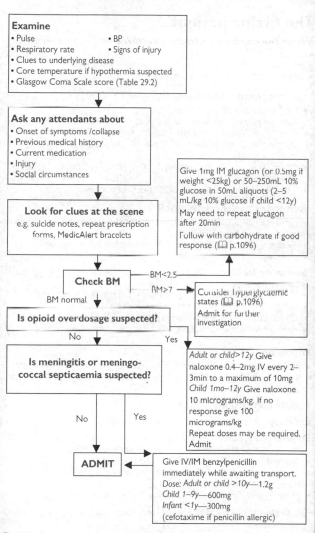

**Examine**
- Pulse
- BP
- Respiratory rate
- Signs of injury
- Clues to underlying disease
- Core temperature if hypothermia suspected
- Glasgow Coma Scale score (Table 29.2)

**Ask any attendants about**
- Onset of symptoms /collapse
- Previous medical history
- Current medication
- Injury
- Social circumstances

**Look for clues at the scene**
e.g. suicide notes, repeat prescription forms, MedicAlert bracelets

**Check BM**

BM normal

**Is opioid overdosage suspected?**

No

Yes

**Is meningitis or meningo-coccal septicaemia suspected?**

No          Yes

**ADMIT**

BM<2.5 → Give 1mg IM glucagon (or 0.5mg if weight <25kg) or 50–250mL 10% glucose in 50mL aliquots (2–5 mL/kg 10% glucose if child <12y)
May need to repeat glucagon after 20min
Follow with carbohydrate if good response (📖 p.1096)

BM>7 → Consider hyperglycaemic states (📖 p.1096)
Admit for further investigation

*Adult or child>12y* Give naloxone 0.4–2mg IV every 2–3min to a maximum of 10mg
*Child 1mo–12y* Give naloxone 10 micrograms/kg. If no response give 100 micrograms/kg
Repeat doses may be required.
Admit

Give IV/IM benzylpenicillin immediately while awaiting transport.
Dose: *Adult or child >10y*—1.2g
*Child 1–9y*—600mg
*Infant <1y*—300mg
(cefotaxime if penicillin allergic)

**Fig. 29.8** Assessment and management of the unconscious patient

# The fitting patient

**When the call for assistance is received** Instruct the attendant:
- to stay with the fitting patient
- to move anything from the vicinity that might cause injury
- to turn the patient onto his/her side.

## ⚠ Management of a major fit
- Ensure that the airway is clear.
- Turn the patient into the recovery position (Figure 29.9).
- Prevent onlookers from restraining the fitting patient.
- Do not give drugs for the first 10min—the fit is likely to stop spontaneously.
- After 10min treat with diazepam 5–10mg IV or PR (5mg if 2–3y or elderly; 2.5mg if <2y).
- If the fit is not controlled, treat as status epilepticus.

## Admit any patient with a fit if
- there is suspicion that the fit is secondary to other illness, e.g. meningitis, subdural haematoma
- recovery after the fit is incomplete (other than feeling sleepy)
- status epilepticus.

**Status epilepticus** If >1 seizure without the patient regaining consciousness *or* fitting continues >20min:
- Give diazepam 5–10mg IV or PR (5mg if 2–3y or elderly; 2.5mg if <2y).
- Repeat every 15min until fits are controlled.
- Check BM to exclude low blood sugar.
- Arrange immediate admission even if fits are controlled.

## Follow up
- Refer any adult who has a first fit to neurology for urgent assessment.
- Refer any child who has a first fit not related to fever to paediatrics for urgent assessment.

**Febrile convulsions** 📖 p.895

**Epilepsy** Children—📖 p.896; Adults—📖 p.582

**Delirium tremens (DTs)** Major alcohol withdrawal symptoms; usually occur 2–3d after an alcoholic has stopped drinking. *Features:*
- *General* Fever, tachycardia, ↑BP, ↑ respiratory rate.
- *Psychiatric* Vivid visual and tactile hallucinations, acute confusional state, apprehension.
- *Neurological* Tremor, fits, fluctuating level of consciousness.

⚠ *Action* DTs have 15% mortality and always warrant emergency hospital admission.

## Further information
**NICE** 🖥 www.nice.org.uk
- The epilepsies: the diagnosis and management of the epilepsies in adults and children in primary and secondary care (2004)
- Referral guidelines for suspected cancer (2005)

**Fig. 29.9** The recovery position. When a patient is unconscious but has circulation and is breathing, it is important to:
- Maintain a good airway.
- Ensure that the tongue does not cause obstruction.
- Minimize the risk of inhalation of gastric contents.

For this reason the victim should be placed in the recovery position. This allows the tongue to fall forward, keeping the airway clear.

***Putting a patient into the
recovery position***
- Remove the patient's glasses.
- Kneel beside the patient and make sure that that both legs are straight (A)
- Place the arm nearest to you out at right angles to the body, elbow bent with the hand palm uppermost (A)
- Bring the far arm across the chest, and hold the back of the hand against the patient's cheek nearest to you (B)
- With your other hand, grasp the far leg just above the knee and pull it up, keeping the foot on the ground (B)
- Keeping the patient's hand pressed against his cheek, pull on the leg to roll the patient towards you onto his side (C)
- Adjust the upper leg so that both the hip and knee are bent at right angles (D)
- Tilt the head back to make sure that the airway remains open (D)
- Adjust the hand under the cheek, if necessary, to keep the head tilted
- Check breathing regularly.

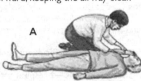
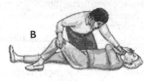
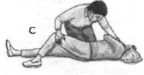
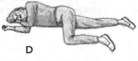

⚠ Monitor the peripheral circulation of the lower arm. If the patient has to be kept in the recovery position for >30min, turn the patient onto the opposite side.

**The unconscious child** The child should be in as near a true lateral position as possible with his/her mouth dependent to allow free drainage of fluid. The position should be stable. In an infant this may require the support of a small pillow or rolled-up blanket placed behind his/her back to maintain the position

**Cervical spine injury** If spinal cord injury is suspected (e.g. the victim has sustained a fall, has been struck on the head or neck, or has been rescued after diving into shallow water), take particular care during handling and resuscitation to maintain alignment of the head, neck, and chest in the neutral position. A spinal board and/or cervical collar should be used if available.

# Anaphylaxis

Severe systemic allergic reaction that is life-threatening. Common causes:
- *Foods* Nuts, milk, fruit, fish and shellfish, eggs, pulses (beans, peas).
- *Drugs* Antibiotics, aspirin and other NSAIDs, opioids.
- *Insect stings* Wasp or bee
- *Latex*

**Features** Often history of anaphylaxis/severe allergic reaction. Anaphylaxis is likely when *all* of the following criteria are met.
- *Sudden onset/rapid progression* of symptoms over minutes.
- *Life-threatening:*
  - **A**irway problems—difficulty breathing/swallowing, feeling that throat is closing, hoarseness, stridor, and/or
  - **B**reathing problems—↑ respiratory rate, wheeze, shortness of breath, oxygen saturation <92%, cyanosis (late sign), confusion due to anoxia, respiratory arrest, and/or
  - **C**irculation problems—shock (pallor, clammy, tachycardia—bradycardia is a late feature), ↓ BP, faintness/dizziness, collapse, agitation/confusion, loss of consciousness. May cause myocardial ischaemia and ECG changes even if normal coronary arteries.
- *Skin and/or mucosal changes* Flushing, erythema, urticaria, and/or angioedema, rhinitis and/or conjunctivitis—subtle/absent in 1:5. ❶ Skin or mucosal changes alone are *not* a sign of an anaphylactic reaction, although they may develop into one.

**Other symptoms** Abdominal symptoms, e.g. abdominal pain, vomiting or incontinence; anxiety ± sense of impending doom.

### Differential diagnosis
- *Life threatening* Severe asthma, septic shock.
- *Non-life threatening* Simple faint, hyperventilation/panic attack, breath-holding attacks in small children, lone urticaria/angio-oedema.

**Action** If suspected when the initial call for help comes in, call an emergency ambulance immediately—then visit. Ask if the patient has had a similar event before. If so, ask if he/she has an Epipen or similar. If yes, advise to use it immediately. Patients with airway/breathing problems may prefer to sit up; if low blood pressure, lie flat (on left side if pregnant) with legs elevated; if unconscious and breathing place in recovery position (📖 p.1067). On attendance, follow the algorithm in Figure 29.10.

**Follow up** Warn patients or parents of the possibility of recurrence. Advise sufferers to wear a device (e.g. MedicAlert bracelet) that will inform bystanders or medical staff should a future attack occur. Refer all patients after their first anaphylactic attack to a specialist allergy clinic. Consider supplying sufferers (or parents) with an EpiPen® or similar which can be used to administer IM adrenaline (epinephrine) immediately should symptoms recur. If you supply an EpiPen®, teach anyone likely to need to use it how to operate the device. IM epinephrine is very safe.

### Further information
**Resuscitation Council UK** Emergency medical treatment of anaphylactic reactions for first medical responders (2008) 🖥 www.resus.org.uk

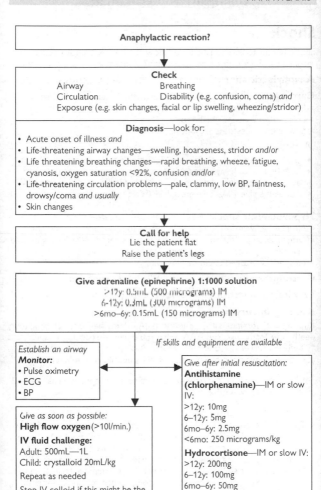

**Anaphylactic reaction?**

**Check**

Airway            Breathing

Circulation       Disability (e.g. confusion, coma) *and*

Exposure (e.g. skin changes, facial or lip swelling, wheezing/stridor)

**Diagnosis**—look for:
- Acute onset of illness *and*
- Life-threatening airway changes—swelling, hoarseness, stridor *and/or*
- Life threatening breathing changes—rapid breathing, wheeze, fatigue, cyanosis, oxygen saturation <92%, confusion *and/or*
- Life-threatening circulation problems—pale, clammy, low BP, faintness, drowsy/coma *and usually*
- Skin changes

**Call for help**
Lie the patient flat
Raise the patient's legs

**Give adrenaline (epinephrine) 1:1000 solution**
>12y: 0.5mL (500 micrograms) IM
6–12y: 0.3mL (300 micrograms) IM
>6mo–6y: 0.15mL (150 micrograms) IM

*Establish an airway*
**Monitor:**
- Pulse oximetry
- ECG
- BP

*Give as soon as possible:*
**High flow oxygen** (>10l/min.)

**IV fluid challenge:**
Adult: 500mL—1L
Child: crystalloid 20mL/kg

Repeat as needed

Stop IV colloid if this might be the cause of anaphylaxis

*If skills and equipment are available*

*Give after initial resuscitation:*
**Antihistamine (chlorphenamine)**—IM or slow IV:
>12y: 10mg
6–12y: 5mg
6mo–6y: 2.5mg
<6mo: 250 micrograms/kg

**Hydrocortisone**—IM or slow IV:
>12y: 200mg
6–12y: 100mg
6mo–6y: 50mg
<6mo: 25mg

**Fig. 29.10** Emergency treatment of anaphylaxis

## Information and support for patients

**Allergy UK** ☎ 01322 619898 🖳 www.allergyuk.org
**Anaphylaxis Campaign** ☎ 01252 542029 🖳 www.anaphylaxis.org.uk
**MedicAlert Foundation** Supply MedicAlert bracelets. ☎ 0800 581 420
🖳 www.medicalert.org.uk

# Shock

Shock is due to inadequate blood flow to the peripheral circulation. It results in ↓ BP (± tachycardia), peripheral cyanosis, and ↓ urinary output.

**Anaphylactic shock** 📖 p.1068          **Septic shock** 📖 p.1074

**Cardiogenic shock**, e.g. due to MI, arrhythmia, tamponade. *Signs:*
• Hypotension—systolic BP <80–90mmHg.
• Pulse rate may be normal, ↑, or ↓.
• Severe breathlessness ± cyanosis.

### Action

• Sit the patient up if possible. Call for ambulance assistance.
• Gain IV access. Treat underlying cause, e.g. atropine for bradycardia; diamorphine, furosemide, and GTN spray (if tolerated) for acute LVF
• If available give 100% oxygen, unless COPD when 24%.

**Hypovolaemic shock** Usually due to haemorrhage. Signs:
• *Initially* Tachycardia (pulse >100bpm), pallor, sweating ± restlessness.
• *Later* Decompensation—sudden fall in pulse rate and BP. Young people may decompensate very rapidly—if tachycardic treat as a medical emergency—speed could be life-saving.

**Gastrointestinal bleeding** 📖 p.1072          **Lacerations** 📖 p.1103

**Very heavy menstrual bleeding** 📖 p.707

### Bleeding aneurysm

**Ruptured abdominal aortic aneurysm (AAA)** In the community setting, death rate from ruptured AAA ~90% (80% before reaching hospital and 10% during surgery). Consider ruptured AAA in any patient with ↓BP and atypical abdominal symptoms (especially if pulsatile abdominal mass).

⚠ In a patient with a known AAA, abdominal pain represents a ruptured AAA unless proven otherwise.

### Dissecting thoracic aneurysm

• Typically presents with sudden tearing chest pain radiating to the back.
• Consider if ↓BP and chest pain (especially if pain radiates to the back).
• As dissection progresses, branches of the aorta are sequentially occluded, causing hemiplegia (carotid artery), unequal pulses and BP in the two arms (subclavian artery), paraplegia (spinal arteries), acute renal failure (renal arteries), aortic incompetence (proximal extension), and MI (cardiac arteries).

### Action

• Lie the patient down flat and raise legs above waist height.
• Call for ambulance assistance. Gain IV access and (if possible) take blood for FBC and cross-matching—try to insert 2 large-bore cannulae.
• If available, start IV fluids. Give rapidly over 10–15 min.
• If available give 100% oxygen, unless COPD when give 24%.

**Nose bleed/epistaxis** Usually due to ruptured blood vessels on the nasal septum. *Causes:*
• *Young* Nose-picking, coryza, allergic rhinitis, blood dyscrasias.

- *Elderly* Degenerative arterial disease, ↑ BP, nose-picking, coryza, allergic rhinitis, medication (warfarin or aspirin), blood dyscrasias, telangiectasia, tumour. Often no cause is found.

*Action* Figure 29.11. Recurrent minor nosebleeds—refer to ENT.

**Terminally ill patients** Bleeding can be a terminal event in patients with cancer. Where possible, make a decision in advance about whether to treat severe bleeding and prepare carers.
- *If a decision is made to treat*—treat as for hypovolaemic shock and admit to hospital as an emergency. ❶ If bleeding from a lung tumour, protect the airway and lie the patient on the side of the tumour.
- *If a decision is made not to treat*—stay with the patient and give sedative medication (e.g. midazolam 20–40mg sc or IV, or diazepam 10–20mg PR ± analgesia). Support the carers.

**Other rarer causes of shock** Admit as medical emergencies.
- *Neurogenic*—due to cerebral trauma or haemorrhage e.g. head injury, subarachnoid haemorrhage
- *Poisoning*                                    • *Liver failure*

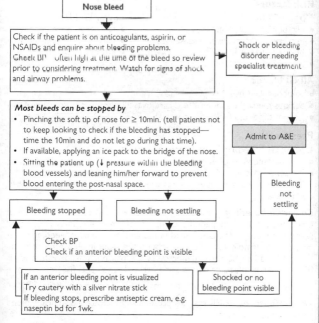

**Fig. 29.11** Acute management of nosebleed in the community

# Gastrointestinal bleeding

Take all GI bleeds seriously. GI bleeding is fatal in ~1:10 elderly patients admitted to hospital.

## Causes of GI bleeding

### Upper GI bleed
- Peptic ulcer
- Gastritis
- Mallory–Weiss tear
- Oesophagitis
- Oesophageal or gastric cancer
- Oesophageal varices
- Drugs—steroids, anticoagulants, NSAIDs
- Angiodysplasia
- Haemangioma
- Bleeding disorders
- Swallowed blood from nosebleed.

### Lower GI bleed
- Diverticulitis
- Colitis: infectious/inflammatory
- Large bowel tumour or polyp
- Haemorrhoids
- Anal fissure
- Angiodysplasia (arteriovenous malformations are common)
- Haemangioma
- Bleeding disorders
- Blood from upper GI bleed.

## Risk factors

### Upper GI bleed
- History of alcohol abuse
- History of chronic liver disease
- History of NSAID use
- History of oral steroid use.

### Lower GI bleed
- Change in bowel habit
- History of diverticulitis
- History of UC.

### All GI bleeds
- Anticoagulant use
- Serious medical conditions (e.g. cardiovascular/respiratory/renal disease)
- Recent tiredness (? due to anaemia).

## Presentation

**Upper GI bleeding** Typical presentation:
- Haematemesis—vomiting of blood.
- Melaena—passage of offensive black tarry stool consisting of digested blood PR. Always indicates a significant bleed. ❶ Iron tablets may cause black stools.

**Lower GI bleeding** Passage of fresh blood PR Brisk bleeding is a medical emergency, but often patients complain of small amounts of bleeding related to passage of stool. Mixed blood and stool implies bleeding proximal to the sigmoid colon; blood around the stool implies a more distal bleed; blood on the toilet paper or in the pan not mixed with stool is often from anal bleeding due to haemorrhoids or an anal fissure.

❶ Very heavy upper GI bleeds can present with fresh red bleeding PR.

**Other features** which may be present and indicate a significant bleed (may precede bleeding):
- Faintness or dizziness, especially on standing.
- Patient feels cold or clammy.
- Collapse ± cardiac arrest.

### Examination
- Colour—pallor, peripheral cyanosis.
- BP, pulse, and JVP—tachycardia, ↓ BP/JVP and/or postural drop.
- Depending on clinical state, perform abdominal ± rectal examination.
- If history is suggestive of haemorrhoids/anal fissure, check anus.
- Examine any vomitus/stool.

### Action
- When a call for help is received, arrange immediate emergency transfer of the patient to hospital if a significant acute GI bleed is suspected.
- Attend the patient if diagnosis from history is unclear or (if possible) once the ambulance has been called to assist.
- Regard as an emergency until proved otherwise.

**On arrival** Briefly assess the severity of the bleed from history and examination. If a significant GI bleed is suspected:
- Lie the patient flat and lift legs higher than body (e.g. feet on a pillow).
- Insert a large-bore IV cannula—the opportunity may be lost by the time the ambulance crew arrive. If possible take a sample for FBC and X-match on insertion.
- If available, give oxygen.
- If available, start IV fluids.
- Transfer as rapidly as possible to hospital.

❶ Except for patients with haemorrhoids/anal fissure, all patients presenting with GI bleeding, even if the bleeding does not cause any circulatory compromise, require further investigation to establish the cause. Refer urgently to a lower GI team if:
- ≥60y with rectal bleeding persisting ≥ 6wk without anal symptoms, even without change in bowel habit
- ≥40y with a combination of rectal bleeding persisting ≥6wk combined with a change in bowel habit towards looser stools/↑ stool frequency.

**Coffee-grounds vomit** Vomiting of altered blood—looks like coffee granules. Implies upper GI bleeding—although less severe than fresh red blood. History and examination is as for acute GI bleed. Always admit to hospital for further assessment.

**Management in terminally ill patients** If a terminally ill patient has a severe life-threatening bleed, make a decision as to whether the cause of the bleed is treatable or a terminal event. This is best done in advance, but bleeding can't always be predicted.

*If active treatment is indicated*—treat as for acute GI bleeding (above).

*If no active treatment is indicated*
- Stay with the patient
- Give sedative medication, e.g. midazolam 20–40mg sc/IV or diazepam 10–20mg PR ± analgesia.
- Support carers as big bleeds are extremely distressing.

❶ Unless a patient is very near to death, admit all non-life-threatening GI bleeds. Palliative treatment options include laser treatment and arterial embolization—both can be performed on frail patients.

# Meningitis and encephalitis[ND]

Meningitis and encephalitis present in similar fashion. Usually rapid onset (<48h). Typical symptoms may be preceded by a prodrome of fever, vomiting, malaise, poor feeding, and lethargy which is often indistinguishable from a viral infection. Particularly significant early signs include:
- Severe leg pain—so bad that the child cannot stand/walk.
- Cold hands or feet when the child is running a fever.
- Pale skin ± blueness around the lips.

## Typical symptoms/signs
### Meningism
- Headache
- Photophobia
- Stiff neck—cannot put chin on chest
- Kernig's sign +ve—with hips fully flexed resists passive knee extension.

### ↑ intracranial pressure
- Irritability
- Vomiting
- Drowsiness/↓ consciousness
- ↓ pulse rate
- Fits
- ↑ BP
- Abnormal tone/posturing
- Bulging fontanelle (baby).

### Septicaemia/septic shock
- Fever
- Tachypnoea
- Arthritis
- Peripheral shutdown—cool peripheries, mottled
- Hypotension
  skin, cyanosis
- Tachycardia
- ± rash—petechiae suggest meningococcus.

⚠ Small children, or immunocompromised patients may not present with typical signs. Go on gut feeling.

### ⚠ Action
- Call an emergency ambulance and get the patient to hospital as soon as possible.
- If shocked, lie the patient flat and raise legs above waist height.
- If symptoms/signs of meningitis or meningococcal septicaemia, give IV/IM benzylpenicillin immediately while awaiting transport. *Dose:*
  - Child ≥10y: 1.2g
  - Child 1–9y: 600mg
  - Infant <1y: 300mg
- Cefotaxime is an alternative for patients allergic to penicillin (child >12y, 1g; child <12y, 50mg/kg).
- If possible gain IV access whilst awaiting the ambulance and take blood for cultures. Consider starting IV fluids/plasma expander. Give 10mL/kg rapidly over 10–15 min.
- If available give 100% oxygen.

## Contact tracing/prophylaxis for meningococcal meningitis

- Undertaken by the local public health department.
- For a single case only very close contacts ('kissing contacts'), e.g. immediate family members, require prophylactic antibiotics.
- Prophylaxis—rifampicin 600mg bd for 2d (child 10mg/kg bd for 2d unless <1y when dose is 5mg/kg bd for 2d) or ciprofloxacin 500mg as a single dose (unlicensed and not suitable for children).
- Rifampicin colours urine red.

**❶** Meningitis and acute encephalitis are notifiable diseases.

## Meningitis vaccination

- Group C strains are responsible for 40% of meningococcal disease.
- Group B strains are responsible for most of the rest.
- Group A strains—common in other parts of the world; rare in the UK.

***Meningococcal A&C vaccine*** No protection against group B strain. Immunize individuals travelling abroad to high-risk areas with the Meningococcal A&C vaccine, even if they have received Meningitis C conjugate vaccine beforehand.

## *Meningitis C conjugate vaccine*

- For infants doses are given at 2, 3, and 4mo as part of the routine childhood vaccination programme
- For infants >4mo, two doses are required and >1y of age only one dose is necessary to confer lasting immunity.
- Vaccine may be given to HIV +ve patients.
- A gap of 6mo is recommended between a dose of the Meningococcal A&C vaccine, usually given for travel purposes, and Meningitis C conjugate vaccine.
- Do not use Meningitis C conjugate vaccine for travel purposes as the greatest risk is from group A infection.

## Telephone helplines for families

**Meningitis Research Foundation** ☎ 080 8800 3344
🖳 www.meningitis.org.uk
**Meningitis Trust** ☎ 0800 028 1828 🖳 www.meningitis-trust.org

# Chest pain and palpitations

**Chest pain** Common symptom.

⚠ Always think—could this be an MI, PE, dissecting aneurysm, or peri-cariditis?

### On receiving the call for assistance Ask:
- Nature and location of the pain.
- Duration of the pain.
- Other associated symptoms—sweating, nausea, shortness of breath, palpitations.
- Past medical history (particularly heart disease, high cholesterol).
- Family history (particularly heart disease).
- Smoker?

### Action
- Consider differential diagnosis (Table 29.3).
- If MI is suspected call for ambulance assistance before (or instead of) visiting.
- Otherwise visit (or arrange surgery appointment), assess, and treat according to cause.

### Further assessment

*History* Ask about:
- Site and nature of pain. Any history of trauma?
- Duration.
- Associated symptoms (e.g. breathlessness, nausea).
- Provoking and relieving factors.
- PMH, FH (e.g. heart disease), drug history, smoking history.

### Examination
- Check BP in both arms
- General appearance—distress, sweating, pallor
- JVP and carotid pulse
- Respiratory rate
- Apex beat
- Heart sounds
- Lung fields
- Local tenderness
- Pain on movement of chest
- Skin rashes
- Swelling or tenderness of legs (?DVT).

*Investigations* ECG and CXR may be helpful.

**Palpitations** The uncomfortable awareness of heart beat. Can be physi-ological (e.g. after exercise, at times of stress) or signify arrhythmia. Can cause a feeling of faintness or even collapse (e.g. Stokes–Adams attack, due to AV block). Ask the patient to tap out the rhythm.
- *Bradycardia* 📖 p.280
- *Occasional missed beat* suggests ventricular ectopics (📖 p.276).
- *Tachycardia* 📖 p.276

**Table 29.3** Causes of acute chest pain

| Diagnosis | Features |
|---|---|
| MI (📖 p.1078) | Band-like chest pain around the chest or central chest pressure/dull ache ± radiation to shoulders, arms (L>R), neck, and/or jaw |
| | Often associated with nausea, sweating, and/or shortness of breath |
| Unstable angina (📖 p.1078) | As for MI |
| Pericarditis (📖 p.285) | Sharp constant sternal pain relieved by sitting forwards |
| | May radiate to left shoulder ± arm or into the abdomen |
| | Worse lying on the left side and on inspiration, swallowing, and coughing |
| Dissecting thoracic aneurysm (📖 p.1070) | Typically presents with sudden tearing chest pain radiating to the back |
| | Consider in any patient with chest pain (especially if radiates through to the back) and ↓BP |
| PE (📖 p.1086) | Acute dyspnoea, sharp chest pain (worse on inspiration), haemoptysis, and/or syncope; tachycardic and mild pyrexia |
| Pleurisy | Sharp localized chest pain, worse on inspiration |
| | May be associated with symptoms and signs of a chest infection |
| Pneumothorax (📖 p.1087) | Sudden onset of pleuritic chest pain or ↑ breathlessness ± pallor and tachycardia |
| Oesophageal spasm, oesophagitis | Central chest pain. May be associated with acid reflux (although not always) |
| | May be described as burning, but often indistinguishable from cardiac pain |
| | May respond to antacids |
| Musculoskeletal pain | Localized pain—worse on movement |
| | May be a history of injury |
| Shingles | Intense, often sharp, unilateral pain |
| | Responds poorly to analgesia |
| | May be present several days before rash appears |
| Costochondritis | Inflammation of the costochondral junctions—tenderness over the costochondral junction and pain in the affected area on springing the chest wall |
| Bornholm's disease | Unilateral chest and/or abdominal pain, rhinitis. Coxsackie virus infection |
| | Treat with simple analgesia |
| Idiopathic chest pain | No cause apparent |
| | Common |
| | Affects young people > elderly people, ♀ > ♂ |

⚠ If a patient is acutely unwell with chest pain and the cause is not clear, err on the side of caution and admit for further assessment

# Myocardial infarct and unstable angina

⚠ Diagnosis of myocardial infarct (MI) is sometimes not obvious. Always have a high index of suspicion.

**Typical presentation** Sustained central chest pain not relieved by sublingual GTN.

### Other features that may be present
- Collapse ± cardiac arrest.
- Breathlessness.
- Anxiety/fear of dying.
- Nausea ± vomiting.
- Sweating.
- Pain in one or both arms, jaw, back, or upper abdomen.

❶ May occasionally be silent, especially in patients with DM.

**Examination** Pulse, BP, JVP, heart sounds, chest (? pulmonary oedema)

### Investigation
**ECG** ST elevation (Figure 29.12) *or* R waves and ST depression in leads V1–V3 (posterior infarction) *or* new LBBB.

### Action
**When the call for assistance is made** If MI is suspected, arrange immediate transfer to hospital—for thrombolysis to be effective, it must be given as soon as possible after the onset of pain. Seeing the patient before arranging transfer introduces unnecessary delays.

If possible attend the patient once the ambulance has been called to assist—there is a lot a GP can do that an ambulance crew cannot. If the patient is seen:
- Give aspirin 300mg po (unless contraindicated).
- Insert IV cannula.
- Give IV analgesia (e.g. morphine 2.5–5mg). Repeat in 15min as necessary.
- Give IV antiemetic (metoclopramide 10mg).
- Give sublingual GTN to act as a coronary artery vasodilator (if systolic BP >90 and pulse <100bpm).
- If available, give oxygen.
- If bradycardia, give atropine 300 micrograms IV and further doses of 300 micrograms if needed to a maximum of 1.2mg.

**Thrombolysis in general practice** May be appropriate in places where transfer to hospital takes >30min. Special training and equipment are necessary.

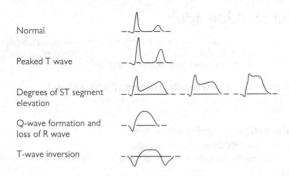

Normal

Peaked T wave

Degrees of ST segment
elevation

Q-wave formation and
loss of R wave

T-wave inversion

**Fig. 29.12** Sequence of ECG changes after MI

Reproduced from Morris A, Brady WJ, *British Medical Journal*, ABC of clinical electrocardiography:
acute myocardial infarction —part 1 (2002) with permission from the BMJ publishing group.

## Late calls

• If the patient is seen <24h after an acute episode—admit for specialist
  assessment.
• If the patient is seen >24h after an acute episode but still has residual
  pain or other symptoms—admit.
• If the patient is seen >24h after an acute episode and is well, start
  regular aspirin, supply with GTN spray, and warn to call for assistance
  (by calling ambulance and/or emergency GP) if chest pain lasts >20min
  despite GTN spray. Refer to cardiology for follow-up.

**Unstable angina** Pain on minimal or no exertion, pain at rest (may
occur at night), or angina which is rapidly worsening in intensity, frequency,
or duration. 15% suffer MI in <1mo.

**Management** It is often difficult to tell the difference between acute MI
and unstable angina in general practice. Treat as for acute MI and admit if
attacks are severe, occur at rest, or last >20min even with GTN spray.

# The choking adult

△ If blockage of the airway is only partial, the victim will usually be able to dislodge the foreign body by coughing. If obstruction is complete, urgent intervention is required to prevent asphyxia.

## Is foreign body airways obstruction (FBAO) likely?
• Sudden onset of respiratory distress whilst eating?
• Is the victim clutching his/her neck?

## Is the patient coughing effectively?
### Signs of an effective cough include
• In response to the question 'Are you choking?', the victim answers and says 'Yes'.
• Fully responsive—able to speak, cough, and breathe.
▶▶ Encourage the victim to cough and monitor.

### Signs of an ineffective cough include
• In response to the question 'Are you choking?', the victim either responds by nodding or is unable to respond.
• Breathing sounds wheezy.
• Unable to breathe.
• Attempts at coughing are silent.
• Unconscious.
▶▶ Call for assistance (e.g. dial 999) and assess conscious level

## If victim IS conscious but has absent/ineffective coughing
• Give up to 5 back blows as needed.
• If back blows don't relieve the obstruction, give up to 5 abdominal thrusts as needed.

### Following back blows, or abdominal thrusts Reassess:
• *If the object has not been expelled and the victim is still conscious* Continue the sequence of back blows and abdominal thrusts.
• *If the object is expelled successfully* Assess clinical condition (including abdominal examination if abdominal thrusts are used). If there is any suspicion that part of the object is still in the respiratory tract or there are any intra-abdominal injuries as a result of abdominal thrusts, refer to A&E for assessment.

## If the victim becomes UNCONSCIOUS
• Support the victim carefully to the ground
• Immediately call an ambulance
• Begin CPR (📖 p.1050) with 30 chest compressions at a rate of 100/min—even if carotid pulse is present

**Foreign body in the throat** Occurs after eating—fish bone or food bolus are most common. Can cause severe discomfort, distress, and inability to swallow saliva.

**Management** Refer immediately to A&E or ENT for investigation (lateral neck X-ray ± laryngoscopy). Most fish bones have passed and the discomfort comes from mucosal trauma. Food boluses often pass spontaneously (especially if the patient is given a smooth muscle relaxant), but occasionally need removal under GA.

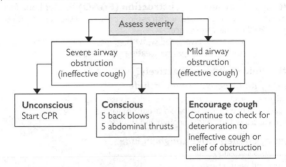

**Fig. 29.13** Algorithm for the management of choking in adults

Reproduced from the *Resuscitation Guidelines* (2005) with permission from the Resuscitation Council UK. ⌨ www.resus.org.uk

### Back blows for adults
* Stand to the side and slightly behind the victim.
* Support the chest with one hand and lean the victim well forwards so that when the obstructing object is dislodged it comes out of the mouth.
* Give up to 5 sharp blows between the shoulder blades with the heel of the other hand.

### Abdominal thrusts for adults
* Stand behind the victim and put both arms around the upper part of the abdomen.
* Lean the victim forwards.
* Clench your fist and place it between the umbilicus and the bottom of the sternum.
* Grasp this hand with your other hand and pull sharply inwards and upwards. Repeat up to 5 times as needed.

### Further information
**Resuscitation Council (UK)** Resuscitation Guidelines (2005)
⌨ www.resus.org.uk

# The choking child

⚠ If the child is breathing spontaneously, encourage his/her own efforts to clear the obstruction. ONLY intervene if ineffective.

**Is foreign body airways obstruction (FBAO) likely?** Look for:
• Sudden onset of respiratory distress in a previously well child—often witnessed by the child's carer.
• Respiratory distress associated with coughing, gagging, or stridor.
• Recent history of playing with or eating small objects.

## Is the child coughing effectively?
### Signs of an effective cough include
• Fully responsive—crying or verbal response to questions.
• Loud cough and able to take a breath before coughing.
▶▶ Encourage the child to cough and monitor.

### Signs of an ineffective cough include
• Unable to vocalize.
• Quiet or silent cough.
• Unable to breathe ± cyanosis.
• Decreasing level of consciousness.
▶▶ Call for assistance (e.g. dial 999) and assess conscious level.

**If the child IS conscious but has absent/ineffective coughing**
Give up to 5 back blows as needed. If back blows don't relieve the obstruction, give up to 5 chest thrusts (infants <1y) or up to 5 abdominal thrusts (children ≥ 1y) as needed. Then reassess.
• *If the object has NOT been expelled and the victim is still conscious* Continue the sequence of back blows and chest (for infant) or abdominal (for children) thrusts. ❶ Don't leave the child.
• *If the object is expelled successfully* Assess clinical condition (including abdominal examination if abdominal thrusts used). If there is any suspicion that part of the object is still in the respiratory tract or there are any intra-abdominal injuries as a result of abdominal thrusts, refer to A&E.

**If the child is UNCONSCIOUS ❶** Don't leave the child
• Place on a firm flat surface—call out/send for help if not arrived.
• Open the mouth and look for any obvious object. If one is seen, make an attempt to remove it with a single finger sweep.
• Open the airway and attempt 5 rescue breaths. Assess effectiveness of each breath—if a breath doesn't make the chest rise, reposition the head before making the next attempt.
• If there is no response to the rescue breaths, proceed immediately to chest compression—regardless of whether the breaths were successful. Follow the PBLS sequence (📖 p.1056) for 1min before summoning help if not already there.

**If it appears that the obstruction has been relieved** Open and check the airway. Deliver rescue breaths if the child is not breathing. If the child regains consciousness and is breathing effectively, place him/her in a safe side-lying (recovery) position and monitor breathing and conscious level whilst awaiting the arrival of the emergency services.

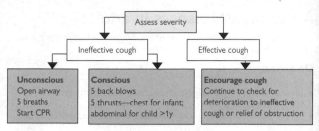

**Fig. 29.14** Algorithm for management of paediatric foreign body airway obstruction (PFBAO)

Reproduced from *Resuscitation Guidelines* (2005) with permission of the Resuscitation Council (UK) 🖳 www.resus.org.uk

### Back blows for small children/infants
- Place the child in a head-downwards, prone position (e.g. across your lap). Support the head if needed by holding the jaw.
- Deliver a smart blow with the heel of one hand to the middle of the back between the shoulder blades. Repeat up to 5 times as needed.

### Back blows for older children
- Support the child in a forward-leaning position.
- Deliver a smart blow with the heel of one hand to the middle of the back between the shoulder blades from behind. Repeat up to 5 times as needed.

### Chest thrusts for infants <1y
- Turn the child into a supine position with head down (e.g. by holding the child's occiput and laying the child along your arm, supported on your thigh).
- Deliver 5 sharp chest thrusts (like chest compressions but slower rate (~20/min)) to a point one finger's breadth above the xiphisternum.

### Abdominal thrusts for children ≥1y
- Stand behind the child (kneel if small child). Place your arms under the child's arms and encircle his/her torso.
- Clench your fist and place it between the umbilicus and xiphisternum.
- Grasp your clenched hand with your other hand and pull sharply inwards and upwards. Repeat up to 5 times as needed.

❶ Ensure that pressure is not applied to the xiphoid process or the lower rib cage as this may cause abdominal trauma.

### Further information
**Resuscitation Council (UK)** Resuscitation guidelines (2005)
🖳 www.resus.org.uk

# Acute breathlessness in adults

Attend as soon as possible after receiving the call for help. If there is likely to be any delay, call for emergency ambulance assistance.

## On arrival

- Be calm and reassuring.
- Breathlessness is frightening and panic only adds to the sensation of being breathless.
- Direct history and examination to finding the cause as quickly as possible.
- Treat according to the cause.
- If no cause can be found, don't delay—admit to hospital as an acute medical emergency.

**Causes** Table 29.4

**Acute left ventricular failure (acute LVF)** Severe acute breathlessness due to pulmonary oedema. Urgent action is needed to save life.

### Presenting features

- Sudden acute breathlessness
- Fatigue
- Cough ± haemoptysis (usually pink and frothy)
- Tends to occur at night
- Some relief gained from sitting/standing.

### Signs

- Dyspnoea
- Tachycardia—gallop rhythm may be present
- Coarse wet-sounding crackles at both bases
- Ankle/sacral oedema if right heart failure also present.
- ± hypotension.

### Action

- If severe call for ambulance support.
- Sit the patient up.
- Be reassuring—it is very frightening to be very short of breath.
- Give 100% oxygen if available and no history of COPD (24% if history of COPD).
- Give IV furosemide 40–80mg slowly (or bumetanide 1–2mg).
- Give IV morphine or diamorphine 2.5–5mg over 5min.
- Give metoclopramide 10mg IV (can be mixed with diamorphine).
- Give GTN spray 2 puffs sublingually.

**Admission** Depends on severity and cause of attack, response to treatment and social support. Always admit if:

- Alone at home.
- Inadequate social support.
- Suspected cause of acute LVF warrants admission (e.g. acute MI).
- Very breathless and no improvement over 30min with treatment at home.
- Hypotension or arrhythmia.

**Table 29.4** Causes of acute breathlessness

| Diagnosis | Features |
|---|---|
| Asthma<br>p.1088 | Breathlessness and wheeze. Usually in association with a past history of asthma though can present de novo<br><br>Signs of a severe attack include: inability to speak in sentences, tachycardia, pulsus paradoxus,↑ respiratory rate, use of accessory muscles of respiration, drowsiness, or exhaustion |
| Anaphylaxis<br>p.1068 | One or both of:<br>• Respiratory difficulty e.g. wheeze, stridor<br>• Hypotension<br>*Other features may include:* erythema, angio-oedema, generalized pruritus or itching of the palate and/or external auditory meatus, rhinitis, nausea ± vomiting, palpitations, urticaria, conjunctivitis, sense of impending doom |
| Acute left ventricular failure | *Symptoms* — Sudden acute breathlessness / Fatigue / Cough ± haemoptysis / Tends to occur at night / Some relief from sitting/standing<br><br>*Signs* — Dyspnoea / Tachycardia ± gallop rhythm / Coarse crackles at both bases / Ankle/sacral oedema if right heart failure also present / ± hypotension |
| Arrhythmia<br>p.276 | Usually palpitations (though not always) associated with chest pain, collapse, or funny turns, sweating, breathlessness, and/or hyperventilation. May be a PMH/FH of similar symptoms or thyroid disease |
| PE<br>p.1086 | Acute dyspnoea, sharp chest pain (worse on inspiration), haemoptysis, and/or syncope; tachycardic and mild pyrexia |
| Acute exacerbation of COPD<br>p.326 | Worsening of previously stable COPD. Presents with ≥1 of<br><br>↑ dyspnoea / ↓ exercise tolerance / ↑ fatigue / ↑ fluid retention / ↑ wheeze / Chest tightness<br>↑ cough / ↑ sputum purulence / ↑ sputum volume / Upper airways symptoms, e.g. cold, sore throat / New onset cyanosis / Acute confusion |
| Pneumonia<br>p.332 | Breathlessness, cough, fever, sputum, ± sharp localized chest pain, worse on inspiration |
| Pneumothorax<br>p.1087 | Sudden onset of pleuritic chest pain or ↑ breathlessness ± pallor and tachycardia |
| Choking<br>p.1080 | Think of aspirated foreign bodies in any history of sudden onset of stridor or symptoms of respiratory distress |
| SVC obstruction<br>p.1038 | Acute breathlessness, headache worse on stooping, swelling of the face and/or neck with fixed elevation of JVP—admit for assessment |
| Air hunger due to shock<br>p.1070 | Inadequate blood flow to the peripheral circulation—usually associated with ↓ BP (± tachycardia) and peripheral cyanosis |
| Hyperventilation<br>p.1116 | Breathlessness associated with fear, terror and a sense of impending doom |

# Pulmonary embolism and pneumothorax

**Pulmonary embolism** Venous thrombi, usually from a deep vein thrombosis in the leg, pass into the pulmonary circulation and block blood flow to the lungs. Without treatment 20% with proximal deep vein thrombosis develop pulmonary embolus (PE). Fatal in ~1:10 cases, causing ~20 000 deaths/y in UK hospitals.

### Risk factors
- Immobility—long flight or bus journey, post-op, plaster cast
- Smoking
- COC pill
- Pregnancy or puerperium
- Malignancy
- Past history or family history of DVT, PE, or clotting tendency.

### Presentation

**Symptoms** Acute dyspnoea, pleuritic chest pain, haemoptysis, syncope. Large clots can rapidly be fatal.

### Signs
- Hypotension
- Tachycardia
- Cyanosis
- Tachypnoea
- Pleural rub
- ↑JVP.

Look for a source of emboli—though often DVT is not clinically obvious.

⚠ Have a high level of suspicion. Patients may have minimal symptoms/ signs apart from some pleuritis pain and dyspnoea. PE in the community can be linked with surgical procedures done 2–3wk previously.

### Differential diagnosis
- Pneumonia and pleurisy.
- MI/unstable angina.
- Other causes of acute breathlessness—acute LVF, asthma, exacerbation of COPD, pneumothorax, shock (e.g. due to anaphylaxis), arrythmia, hyperventilation.
- Other causes of acute chest pain—aortic dissection, rib fracture, musculoskeletal chest pain, pericarditis, oesophageal spasm, shingles.

**Immediate action** If suspected, give oxygen as soon as possible and admit as an acute medical emergency.

**Further management** In all cases of proven PE, anticoagulation is started in hospital or by a hospital-at-home service before discharge to general practice. Warfarin should be continued for 6mo. Aim to keep the INR ≈ 2.5 (range 2–3).

**Spontaneous pneumothorax** *Risk factors:*
- Previous pneumothorax
- Smoking
- Ascent in an aeroplane
- Diving.

### Cause
- *In patients <40y* Usually due to rupture of a pleural bleb. Typical patient is tall, thin, and male ($\male$:$\female$ $\approx$ 6:1).
- *Patients >40y* Usually due to COPD (70–80%).
- *Rarer causes* Asthma, pneumonia, TB, lung cancer, pulmonary fibrosis.

**Presentation** Sudden onset of pleuritic chest pain or ↑ breathlessness ± pallor and tachycardia. Look for resonant percussion note, ↓ or absent breath sounds—signs may be absent if the pneumothorax is small.

### Management
- Refer for CXR.
- If pneumothorax is confirmed, seek specialist advice about further management.
- Small pneumothoraces usually resolve spontaneously (50% collapse takes ~40d to resorb). Monitor until completely resolved.
- Larger pneumothoraces may require admission for aspiration or a chest drain.
- Smoking cessation ↓ risk of recurrence.

**Traumatic pneumothorax** Trauma may not initially be obvious—ask about injections around the chest area, e.g. acupuncture (to neck and shoulders as well as chest); aspiration of breast lump, etc. Presentation and management is as for spontaneous pneumothorax.

**Tension pneumothorax** Complication of traumatic pneumothorax; rare after spontaneous pneumothorax. A valvular mechanism develops—air is sucked into the pleural space during inspiration but cannot be expelled during expiration. The pressure within the pleural space ↑, the lung deflates further, the mediastinum shifts to the opposite side of the chest, and venous return ↓. Can rapidly be fatal.

### Clinical features
- Agitated and distressed patient often with a history of chest trauma
- Tachycardia
- Sweating
- Signs of a large pneumothorax—↓ breath sounds and ↓ chest movement on the affected side
- Mediastinal shift—trachea deviated away from the side of the pneumothorax.

**Action** If tension pneumothorax is suspected:
- Sit the patient upright if possible.
- Insert a large bore cannula through the second intercostal space of the chest wall in the mid-clavicular line on the side of the pneumothorax to relieve the pressure in the pleural space.
- Transfer as an emergency to hospital.

# Acute asthma in adults

Many deaths from asthma are preventable. Delay can be fatal. Factors leading to poor outcome include:
- Doctors failing to assess severity by objective measurement.
- Patients or relatives failing to appreciate severity.
- Under-use of corticosteroids.

⚠ Regard each emergency asthma consultation as acute severe asthma until proven otherwise

## Risk factors for developing fatal or near-fatal asthma
### A combination of severe asthma recognized by ≥1 of
- Previous near fatal asthma
- Previous admission for asthma—especially if within 1y
- Requiring ≥3 classes of asthma medication
- Heavy use of $\beta_2$ agonist
- Repeated attendances at A&E for asthma care, especially if within 1y
- Brittle asthma

### and adverse behavioural or psychosocial features recognized by ≥1 of
- Non-compliance with treatment or monitoring
- Failure to attend appointments
- Self-discharge from hospital
- Psychosis, depression, other psychiatric illness, or deliberate self-harm
- Current or recent major tranquillizer use
- Denial
- Alcohol or drug misuse
- Obesity
- Learning difficulties
- Employment/income problems
- Social isolation
- Childhood abuse
- Severe marital/legal/domestic stress

## Assess and record
- Peak expiratory flow rate (PEFR)
- Symptoms and response to self-treatment
- Heart and respiratory rates
- Oxygen saturation by pulse oximetry (if available).

⚠ Patients with severe or life-threatening attacks may not be distressed and may not have all the characteristic abnormalities of severe asthma. The presence of any should alert the doctor.

## Levels of severity of acute asthma exacerbations
### Moderate asthma exacerbation
- Increasing symptoms
- PEFR >50–75% predicted
- No features of acute severe asthma.

### Acute severe asthma Any one of:
- PEFR 33–50% best or predicted
- Respiratory rate ≥25 breaths/min
- Heart rate ≥110/min
- Inability to complete sentences in one breath.

***Life-threatening asthma*** Any one of the following with severe asthma:

- PEFR <33% best/predicted
- O2 saturation <92%
- Silent chest
- Cyanosis
- Feeble respiratory effort
- Bradycardia
- Dysrhythmia
- Hypotension
- Exhaustion
- Confusion
- Coma.

***Near-fatal asthma*** Respiratory acidosis and/or requiring mechanical ventilation with ↑ inflation pressures.

### Brittle asthma

- ***Type 1*** Wide PEFR variability (>40% diurnal variation for >50% of the time for a period of >150d) despite intense therapy.
- ***Type 2*** Sudden severe attacks on a background of apparently well-controlled asthma.

**Management** Figure 29.15, 🕮 p.1090

### Admit to hospital if

- Life-threatening features.
- Features of acute severe asthma present after initial treatment.
- Previous near fatal asthma.

### Lower threshold for admission if

- Afternoon or evening attack.
- Recent nocturnal symptoms or hospital admission.
- Previous severe attacks.
- Patient unable to assess own condition.
- Concern over social circumstances.

### If admitting the patient to hospital

- Stay with the patient until the ambulance arrives.
- Send written assessment and referral details to the hospital.
- Give high dose β₂ bronchodilator via an oxygen-driven nebulizer in the ambulance.

### Follow-up after treatment or discharge from hospital

- GP review within 48h
- Monitor symptoms and PEFR
- Check inhaler technique
- Written asthma action plan
- Modify treatment according to guidelines for chronic persistent asthma
- Address potentially preventable contributors to admission.

### Further information

**BTS/SIGN** British guideline on the management of asthma (2008)
🖥 www.sign.ac.uk

| Moderate asthma | Acute severe asthma | Life-threatening asthma |
|---|---|---|
| INITIAL ASSESSMENT | | |
| PEFR>50% best or predicted | PEFR 33–50% best or predicted | PEFR<33% best or predicted |
| FURTHER ASSESSMENT | | |
| Speech normal<br>Respiration <25 breaths/min<br>Pulse <110bpm | Can't complete sentences<br>Respiration ≥25 breaths/min<br>Pulse ≥110bpm | Oxygen saturation <92%<br>Silent chest, cyanosis, or feeble respiratory effort<br>Bradycardia, dysrhythmia, or hypotension<br>Exhaustion, confusion, or coma |
| MANAGEMENT | | |
| Treat at home or in the surgery *and* ASSESS RESPONSE TO TREATMENT | Consider admission | Arrange immediate admission |
| TREATMENT | | |
| *High dose* $\beta_2$ *bronchodilator*<br>Ideally via oxygen-driven nebulizer (salbutamol 5mg or terbutaline 10mg)<br>Alternatively use inhaler via spacer (1 puff 4–10× repeated at intervals of 10–20min)<br>*If PEFR >50–75% predicted/best* Give prednisolone 40–50mg<br>Continue or step up usual treatment<br>*If good response to first nebulized treatment* (symptoms improved, respiration and pulse settling, and PEFR>50%) continue or step up usual treatment and continue prednisolone | Oxygen 40–60% if available<br>*High dose* $\beta_2$ *bronchodilator*<br>Ideally via oxygen-driven nebulizer (salbutamol 5mg or terbutaline 10mg)<br>Alternatively use inhaler via spacer (1 puff 4–10× repeated at 10–20min intervals)<br>*Prednisolone 40–50mg or IV hydrocortisone 100mg*<br>*If no response in acute severe asthma:* ADMIT | Oxygen 40–60% if available<br>*Prednisolone 40–50mg or IV hydrocortisone 100mg immediately*<br>*High dose* $\beta_2$ *bronchodilator and ipratropium*<br>Ideally via oxygen-driven nebulizer (salbutamol 5mg or terbutaline 10mg, and ipratropium 0.5mg)<br>Alternatively use inhaler via spacer (1 puff 4–10× repeated at 10–20min intervals)<br>*ADMIT immediately* |

**Fig. 29.15** Management of acute severe asthma in adults

Reproduced from the *British guideline on the management of asthma* (2008) with permission from the British Thoracic Society and SIGN

# Acute asthma in children

## Assess and record
- Pulse rate—increasing heart rate generally reflects ↑ severity.
- Respiratory rate and breathlessness.
- Use of accessory muscles—best noted by palpation of neck muscles.
- Amount of wheezing.
- Degree of agitation and conscious level.

## Levels of severity
*Child >5y* Figure 29.16, 🕮 p.1092
*Child 2–5y* Figure 29.17, 🕮 p.1093
*Child <2y* Assessment of children <2y can be difficult.
- *Moderate asthma*
  - $O_2$ saturation ≥92%
  - Audible wheezing
  - Using accessory muscles
  - Still feeding
- *Severe asthma*
  - $O_2$ saturation <92%
  - Cyanosis
  - Marked respiratory distress
  - Too breathless to feed
- *Life threatening asthma*
  - Apnoea
  - Bradycardia
  - Poor respiratory effort

⚠ If a patient has signs and symptoms across categories, always treat according to the most severe features.

## Management
*Child >5y* Figure 29.16, 🕮 p.1092
*Child 2–5y* Figure 29.17, 🕮 p.1093
*Child <2y* Intermittent wheezing attacks are usually in response to viral infection and response to bronchodilators is inconsistent.
- *If mild/moderate wheeze*
  - A trial of bronchodilators can be considered if symptoms are of concern—use a metered dose inhaler and spacer with a face mask.
  - If no response consider alternative diagnosis (aspiration pneumonitis, pneumonia, bronchiolitis, tracheomalacia, CF, congenital anomaly) and/or admit.
- *If severe wheezing* Admit to hospital
- *If any life-threatening features* Admit immediately as a blue-light emergency.

## Follow-up after treatment or discharge from hospital
- GP review within 1 week.
- Monitor symptoms, PEFR, and check inhaler technique.
- Written asthma action plan.
- Modify treatment according to guidelines for chronic persistent asthma.
- Address potentially preventable contributors to admission.

| ASSESS ASTHMA SEVERITY | | |
|---|---|---|
| **Moderate exacerbation** | **Severe exacerbation** | **Life-threatening asthma** |
| Oxygen saturation ≥92% | Oxygen saturation <92% | Oxygen saturation <92% |
| PEFR≥50% best or predicted | PEFR<50% best or predicted | PEFR<33% best or predicted |
| Able to talk | Too breathless to talk | Silent chest |
| Heart rate ≤120bpm | Heart rate >120bpm | Poor respiratory effort |
| Respiratory rate ≤30 breaths/min | Respiratory rate >30 breaths/min | Agitation |
| | Use of accessory neck muscles | Altered consciousness |
| | | Cyanosis |
| β₂ agonist 4–6 puffs via spacer | Oxygen via face mask | Oxygen via face mask |
| Consider soluble prednisolone 30–40mg | β₂ agonist 4–6 puffs via spacer ± face mask, repeated as needed after 10–20min, or nebulized salbutamol 2.5–5mg (or terbutaline 5–10mg) | Nebulize: −salbutamol 5mg or terbutaline 10mg + −ipratropium 0.25mg |
| | Soluble prednisolone 30–40mg | Soluble prednisolone 30–40mg or IV hydrocortisone 100mg |
| **Increase β₂ agonist dose by 2 puffs every 2min up to 10 puffs according to response** | **Assess response to treatment 15min after β₂ agonist** | |
| IF POOR RESPONSE ARRANGE ADMISSION | IF POOR RESPONSE REPEAT β₂ AGONIST AND ARRANGE ADMISSION | REPEAT β₂ AGONIST VIA OXYGEN-DRIVEN NEBULIZER WHILST ARRANGING IMMEDIATE HOSPITAL ADMISSION |

| GOOD RESPONSE | POOR RESPONSE |
|---|---|
| Continue β₂ agonist via spacer or nebulizer as needed (max. every 4h) | Stay with the patient until ambulance arrives |
| **If symptoms are not controlled repeat β₂ agonist and refer to hospital** | Send written assessment and referral details |
| Continue prednisolone for up to 3d | Repeat β₂ agonist via oxygen-driven nebulizer in the ambulance |
| Arrange follow-up clinic visit | |

⚠ *Lower threshold for admission if*
• Attack in late afternoon or at night.
• Recent hospital admission or previous severe attack.
• Concern over social circumstances or ability to cope at home.

**Fig. 29.16** Management of acute asthma in children aged >5y

Reproduced from the *British guideline on the management of asthma* (2008) with permission from the British Thoracic Society and SIGN

| ASSESS ASTHMA SEVERITY | | |
|---|---|---|
| **Moderate exacerbation** | **Severe exacerbation** | **Life-threatening asthma** |
| Oxygen saturation ≥92% | Oxygen saturation <92% | Oxygen saturation <92% |
| Able to talk | Too breathless to talk | Silent chest |
| Heart rate ≤130bpm | Heart rate >130/min | Poor respiratory effort |
| Respiratory rate ≤50 breaths/min | Respiratory rate >50 breaths/min | Agitation |
| | Use of accessory neck muscles | Altered consciousness |
| | | Cyanosis |
| β₂ agonist 4–6 puffs via spacer | Oxygen via face mask | Oxygen via face mask |
| Consider soluble prednisolone 20mg | β₂ agonist 4–6 puffs via spacer ± face mask, repeated as needed after 10–20min, or nebulized salbutamol 2.5mg (or terbutaline 5mg) | Nebulize: <br>–salbutamol 2.5mg or terbutaline 5mg <br>+ <br>–ipratropium 0.25mg |
| | Soluble prednisolone 20mg | Soluble prednisolone 20mg or IV hydrocortisone 50mg |
| Increase β₂ agonist dose by 2 puffs every 2min up to 10 puffs according to response | Assess response to treatment 15min. after β₂ agonist | |
| IF POOR RESPONSE ARRANGE ADMISSION | IF POOR RESPONSE REPEAT β₂ AGONIST AND ARRANGE ADMISSION | REPEAT β₂ AGONIST VIA OXYGEN-DRIVEN NEBULIZER WHILST ARRANGING IMMEDIATE HOSPITAL ADMISSION |

| GOOD RESPONSE | POOR RESPONSE |
|---|---|
| Continue β₂ agonist via nebulizer or spacer as needed (max every 4h) | Stay with the patient until the ambulance arrives |
| **If symptoms are not controlled repeat β₂ agonist and refer to hospital** | Send written assessment and referral details |
| Continue prednisolone for up to 3d | Repeat β₂ agonist via oxygen-driven nebulizer in the ambulance |
| Arrange follow-up clinic visit | |

⚠ **Lower threshold for admission if**
• Attack in late afternoon or at night.
• Recent hospital admission or previous severe attack.
• Concern over social circumstances or ability to cope at home.

**Fig. 29.17** Management of acute asthma in children aged 2–5y

Reproduced from the *British guideline on the management of asthma* (2008) with permission from SIGN/British Thoracic Society and SIGN.

## Further information

**BTS/SIGN** British guideline on the management of asthma (2008)
🖥 www.sign.ac.uk

# Acute abdominal pain

❶ Signs may be masked in elderly patients or those on corticosteroids. Small children with abdominal pain are difficult to assess.

**History** Consider:
- Site of pain (Figure 29.18).
- Onset: How long? How did it start? Change over time?
- Character of pain: Type of pain—burning, shooting, stabbing, dull, etc.
- Radiation.
- Associated symptoms, e.g. nausea, vomiting, diarrhoea.
- Timing/pattern, e.g constant, colicky, relationship to food.
- Exacerbating and relieving factors including previous treatments tried and results.
- Severity.

## Examination
- Temperature
- Pulse
- BP
- Jaundice
- Anaemia
- Site of pain (Figure 29.18)
- Guarding/rebound tenderness
- Rectal/vaginal examination as necessary

**Management** Treat the cause (Table 29.5)—if unsure admit as a surgical emergency to hospital.

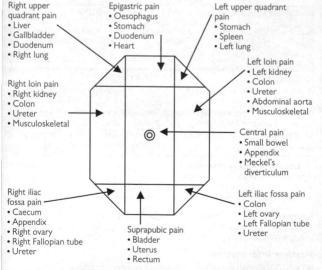

Right upper quadrant pain
- Liver
- Gallbladder
- Duodenum
- Right lung

Epigastric pain
- Oesophagus
- Stomach
- Duodenum
- Heart

Left upper quadrant pain
- Stomach
- Spleen
- Left lung

Right loin pain
- Right kidney
- Colon
- Ureter
- Musculoskeletal

Left loin pain
- Left kidney
- Colon
- Ureter
- Abdominal aorta
- Musculoskeletal

Central pain
- Small bowel
- Appendix
- Meckel's diverticulum

Right iliac fossa pain
- Caecum
- Appendix
- Right ovary
- Right Fallopian tube
- Ureter

Suprapubic pain
- Bladder
- Uterus
- Rectum

Left iliac fossa pain
- Colon
- Left ovary
- Left Fallopian tube
- Ureter

**Fig. 29.18** Site of abdominal pain gives important clues about the organ involved

**Table 29.5** Differential diagnosis of acute abdominal pain

| Renal and gynaecological causes | | | |
|---|---|---|---|
| Renal colic | 📖 p.452 | Dysmenorrhoea | 📖 p.712 |
| UTI/pyelonephritis | 📖 p.456 | Endometriosis | 📖 p.714 |
| Hydronephrosis | 📖 p.462 | Pelvic inflammatory disease | 📖 p.736 |
| Henoch–Schönlein purpura | 📖 p.534 | Ovarian torsion/bleed/rupture | |
| Ectopic pregnancy | 📖 p.813 | Gynaecological malignancy | |
| **GI causes** | | | |
| Irritable bowel syndrome | 📖 p.426 | Perforated bowel | |
| Constipation | 📖 p.386 | Appendicitis | 📖 p.402 |
| Diverticular disease | 📖 p.408 | Meckel's diverticulum | 📖 p.403 |
| Gallbladder disease | 📖 p.436 | Pancreatitis | 📖 p.438 |
| Liver disease | | Bowel obstruction | 📖 p.408 |
| Inflammatory bowel disease | 📖 p.422 | Intussusception | 📖 p.889 |
| Gastroenteritis | 📖 p.418 | Strangulated hernia | 📖 p.400 |
| Gastritis | 📖 p.395 | Volvulus | 📖 p.408 |
| Peptic ulcer | 📖 p.396 | GI malignancy | |
| **Other causes** | | | |
| Spinal arthritis | 📖 p.484 | Mesenteric adenitis | 📖 p.402 |
| Muscular pain | | MI | 📖 p.1078 |
| CCF | 📖 p.268 | Pneumonia | 📖 p.332 |
| Sickle cell crisis | 📖 p.667 | Subphrenic abscess | 📖 p.402 |
| Ruptured spleen | | DM ketoacidosis | 📖 p.1096 |
| Torsion of the testis | 📖 p.474 | Porphyria | 📖 p.609 |
| Leaking/ruptured AAA | 📖 p.1070 | Addison's disease | 📖 p.376 |
| Shingles/post-herpetic neuralgia | 📖 p.651 | Lead poisoning | |

**Acute abdominal pain in pregnancy** 📖 p.1098

**Ruptured spleen** May occur immediately following trauma or present days/weeks later. Diseased spleens (e.g. glandular fever, malaria, leukaemia) rupture more easily.

### Presentation
- History of abdominal trauma.
- Blood loss: tachycardia, ↓ BP ± postural drop, pallor.
- Peritoneal irritation: guarding, abdominal rigidity, shoulder-tip pain.
- Paralytic ileus: abdominal distention, lack of bowel sounds.

⚠ **Action** If suspected, admit as a blue-light surgical emergency.

# Endocrine emergencies

**Hypoglycaemia** Known diabetic on oral/insulin therapy. Short history. May present with coma, fits or odd/violent behaviour, tachycardia ± ↑ BP. There may or may not have been warning signs/symptoms—sweating, hunger, tremor. ❶ Younger children may present atypically with behavioural changes or headache.

**Investigation** Blood sugar (on blood testing strip) <2.5mmol/L.

### ⚠ Action

- If conscious give simple carbohydrate, e.g. 3 glucose tablets, 100mL of sugar-containing soft drink, e.g. Lucozade®, GlucoGel®
- If unable to take oral carbohydrate, give IM glucagon 1mg IM (chidren <25kg, 0.5mg)—takes ≤5min to act (may have poor effect if the patient is starved or drunk) *or* IV glucose (adult: 50–250mL 10% solution in 50mL aliquots; child: 2–5mL/kg 10% solution).
- Once the patient has regained consciousness, supplement with simple carbohydrate as for the conscious patient and as symptoms improve give complex carbohydrate, e.g. biscuits.
- Repeat glucose testing in <15min. Then monitor frequent blood sugars hourly over the next 4h, and every 4h for the following 24h.
- Maintain a high glucose intake for several hours if the patient has a severe episode of hypoglycaemia due to a sulphonylurea.
- Review reasons for the hypoglycaemia.

**Hyperglycaemic ketoacidotic coma** Usually occurs in patients with type 1 DM, but may rarely occur in patients with type 2 DM. May be the way in which DM presents (i.e. can occur in young patients not known to be diabetic). Presents with a 2–3d history of deterioration often precipitated by infection. Typically the patient is dehydrated with Kussmaul breathing (deep sighing breaths), ketotic (fruity) smelling breath, shock (↓ BP and postural drop, tachycardia) ± coma. ⚠ Can present with vomiting and abdominal pain mimicking acute abdomen—always check for ketotic breath and Kussmaul breathing.

**Investigation** BM is usually >20mmol/L and urine (if available) tests +ve for ketones.

⚠ **Action** Arrange to admit to hospital as an emergency. If shocked/ coma, lie flat, elevate feet, and resuscitate.
- Airway—check airway is clear.
- Breathing—give 100% $O_2$ if available.
- Circulation—gain IV access if possible and give 1L (child: 10mL/kg) 0.9% saline rapidly. Repeat up to 3× as needed.

**Hyperglycaemic hyperosmolar non-ketotic coma** Only occurs in patients with type 2 DM. Presents with <1wk history of deterioration, ↓ level of consciousness, dehydration ++, ↓ BP with postural drop. Often precipitated by other illness, e.g. infection, MI. May be a presenting feature of type 2 DM. Blood sugar (on blood testing strip) >35mmol/L.

⚠ **Action** Admit to hospital immediately.

## Myxoedema coma
### Presentation

- >65y old
- History of thyroid surgery/radioactive iodine
- May be precipitated by MI, stroke, infection, or trauma
- Looks hypothyroid
- Hypothermia
- Hyporeflexia
- Heart failure
- Cyanosis
- Bradycardia
- Coma
- Seizures.

**Investigation** Finger-prick blood glucose may be ↓.

### ⚠ Action
- Keep warm
- Treat heart failure with diuretics ± opioids and nitrates (📖 p.1084)
- Admit to hospital as an emergency.

## Hyperthyroid crisis (thyrotoxic storm)
### Risk factors

- Recent thyroid surgery/radioactive iodine
- Infection
- Trauma
- MI

### Presentation

- Fever
- Agitation and/or confusion
- Coma
- Tachycardia/AF
- Diarrhoea and vomiting
- Acute abdomen
- May have goitre ± thyroid bruit.

### ⚠ Action Admit to hospital as an emergency.

**Hypoadrenal (Addisonian) crisis** May occur in patients on long-term steroids (treatment or replacement) if the steroids are stopped suddenly or not ↑ during intercurrent illness, or may be a presenting feature of congenital adrenal hyperplasia or Addison's disease. Presents with vomiting, hypotension, and shock.

**Management** Give IM or IV hydrocortisone:
- Adults and children >12y: 100mg.
- Children 1mo–12y: 2–4mg/kg.

Admit to hospital for further management.

### Prevention of Addisonian crises
- Warn all patients taking long-term steroids not to stop their steroids abruptly and to tell any doctor treating them about their condition.
- Advise patients to carry a steroid card or Addison's disease self-help group emergency card, and to wear a MedicAlert bracelet or similar in case of emergency.
- Double dose of steroid prior to dental treatment or if intercurrent illness (e.g. URTI).
- If vomiting, replace oral steroid with IM hydrocortisone.

# Obstetric emergencies

### Resuscitation of the newborn 📖 p.1062

**Eclampsia** Occurs when a pregnant woman has a fit as a result of pre-eclampsia. Usually BP is very high and, if the baby is not yet born, it becomes distressed. There is a serious risk of stroke in the mother. Women with pre-eclampsia have a 2% chance of eclamptic seizure. 44% occur after the baby is born—usually <24h after delivery. Give IV or PR diazepam and admit as an acute blue-light emergency.

**HELLP syndrome** Occurs in pregnancy or <48h after delivery. Associated with severe pre-eclampsia.
- **H**aemolysis
- **E**levated **L**iver enzymes
- **L**ow **P**latelets

*Signs* Hypertension (80%); right upper quadrant pain (90%); nausea and vomiting (50%); oedema.

*Management* Admit as for pre-eclampsia (📖 p.824).

**Obstetric shock** *Causes:*
- Haemorrhage—APH (📖 p.816); placental abruption (remember, bleeding may be internal and not seen per vaginum); PPH (📖 p.817)
- Ruptured uterus
- Inverted uterus
- Pulmonary embolus
- Anaphylaxis (usually drugs)
- Amniotic fluid embolism
- Broad ligament haematoma
- Septicaemia.

#### ⚠ Action
- Call for help
- Arrange immediate admission to the nearest specialist obstetric unit (or A&E, if necessary)
- Gain IV access and start IV fluids, give O₂ via face mask (if available)
- Treat the cause if apparent

**Fetal distress** Signifies hypoxia. *Signs:*
- Passage of meconium during labour.
- Fetal tachycardia (>160bpm at term).
- Fetal bradycardia (<100bpm—seek urgent obstetric assistance).

#### ⚠ Action
- Give the mother O₂ via a face mask and turn her onto her side.
- Transfer immediately to a specialist obstetric unit for further assessment ± delivery.

**Acute abdominal pain in pregnancy** Non-obstetric causes of abdominal pain may be forgotten or signs may be less well localized than in the non-pregnant patient (📖 p.1094).

**Appendicitis** 1:1000 pregnancies. Mortality is higher in pregnancy and perforation more common (15–20%). Fetal mortality is 5–10% for simple appendicitis but rises to 30% when there is perforation. Because of the pregnancy, the appendix is displaced and pain is often felt in the para-umbilical region or subcostally. Admit immediately if suspected.

**Cholecystitis** 1–6:10 000 pregnancies. Pregnancy encourages gallstone formation. Symptoms include RUQ pain, nausea, and vomiting. Diagnosis can be confirmed on USS. Treatment is the same as outside pregnancy aiming for interval cholecystectomy after birth.

**Fibroids** Torsion or red degeneration. Fibroids ↑ in size in pregnancy. They may twist if pedunculated. Red degeneration occurs usually after 20wk and may occur until the puerperium. It presents as abdominal pain ± localized tenderness ± vomiting and low-grade fever. Confirm diagnosis with USS. Treatment is with rest and analgesia. Pain resolves within 1wk.

**Ovarian tumours/torsion** 1:1000 pregnancies. Both torsion and rupture of a cyst may cause abdominal pain, as may bleeding into a cyst. USS can confirm the presence of a cyst. Management depends on the nature of the cyst and the severity of the pain. Admit for assessment.

### If <20wk gestation, also consider
- *Miscarriage* 📖 p.813
- *Ectopic pregnancy* 📖 p.813

### If >20wk gestation, also consider
- *Labour* 📖 p.830
- *Pubic symphysis dehiscence* 📖 p.498
- *Abruptio placentae*
- *Uterine rupture*
- *Haematoma of the rectus abdominis* Rarely, bleeding into the rectus sheath and haematoma formation occurs spontaneously or after coughing in late pregnancy. May cause swelling and abdominal tenderness. USS can be helpful. If unsure of diagnosis, admit to exclude acute surgical or obstetric cause of pain.

**Uterine rupture** Rare in the UK (1:1500 deliveries). Associated with maternal mortality of 5% and fetal mortality of 30%. 70% are due to dehiscence of Caesarean section scars. Rupture occurs most commonly during labour, but occasionally may occur in the third trimester or after an otherwise normal delivery.

**Presentation** Pain is variable but usually severe bursting constant lower abdominal pain ± heavy vaginal bleeding. Generally associated with profound shock in the mother and fetal distress. If in labour, the presenting part may disappear from the pelvis ± contractions stop.

⚠ **Action** Admit as an acute emergency to a specialist obstetric unit.

**Abruptio placentae** 1:80–200 pregnancies. Part of the placenta becomes detached from the uterus. Consequences depend on the degree of separation and the amount of blood loss. *Presentation:*
- Typically constant pain—may be felt in the back if posterior placenta.
- Woody, hard, and tender uterus.
- Shock ± PV bleeding.
- Fetal heart absent or signs of fetal distress— fetal tachycardia or bradycardia.

⚠ **Action** If suspected, admit as an acute emergency to the nearest specialist obstetric unit.

**Shoulder dystocia** Affects <1% deliveries but is a life-threatening emergency. Occurs when the anterior shoulder impacts upon the symphysis pubis after the head has delivered and prevents the rest of the baby following. Most cases of shoulder dystocia are unanticipated. *Clues:*
- Prolonged first or second stage of labour.
- 'Head bobbing'—the head consistently descends and then returns to its original position during a contraction or pushing in the second stage.

If shoulder dystocia occurs in the community there is not usually time to transfer a woman to a specialist unit.

⚠ **Action** Call for help. Consider episiotomy. Then try any of the following procedures (no particular order).
- Roll the mother onto her hands and knees and try delivering posterior shoulder first.
- Flex and abduct the mother's legs up to her abdomen (upside down squatting position)—try delivery again.
- Deliver the posterior arm—put a hand in the vagina in front of the baby; ensure the posterior elbow is flexed in front of the body and pull to deliver the forearm. The anterior shoulder usually follows.
- External pressure—ask an assistant to apply suprapubic pressure with the heel of the hand. A rocking movement can help.
- Adduction of the most accessible (preferably anterior) shoulder. Simultaneously put pressure on the posterior clavicle to turn the baby. If unsuccessful continue rotation through 180° and try again.

**Cord prolapse** 1:200–300 births. The cord passes through the os in front of the presenting part of the baby. If the presenting part squashes the cord, umbilical blood flow is restricted, causing fetal hypoxia and distress (fetal mortality 10-17%). *Risk factors:*
- Malpresentation—breech/transverse/oblique
- Cephalo-pelvic disproportion
- Multiple pregnancy
- Preterm rupture of membranes
- Polyhydramnios
- Pelvic tumours.

⚠ **Action**
- Minimize handling of the cord to prevent spasm.
- Try to keep the cord within the vagina.
- Call for help.

Aim to prevent the presenting part from occluding the cord. Try:
- Displacing the presenting part upwards with the examining hand.
- Get patient into knee–elbow position—head down.
- If possible, drop the head end of the bed.
- Fill the bladder with 500–750 mL normal saline via a catheter and clamp the catheter.

Admit as an emergency to the nearest specialist obstetric unit—usually treated with emergency Caesarean section.

**Retained placenta** The third stage of labour is complete in <10min in 97% of labours. If the placenta has not been delivered in <30min (to allow for cervical spasm), it will probably not deliver spontaneously.

### ⚠ Action
- Avoid excessive cord traction.
- Check that the placenta is not in the vagina—remove if it is.
- Check the uterus.

*If the uterus is well contracted* Cervical spasm is probably trapping an otherwise separated placenta—wait for the cervix to relax to enable removal of the placenta.

*If the uterus is bulky* The placenta may have failed to separate. Try:
- Rubbing up a contraction.
- Putting the baby to the breast (stimulates uterine contraction).
- Giving a further dose of Syntometrine®.
- If the placenta will still not deliver, admit as emergency for manual removal.

**Uterine inversion** Rare.

⚠ **Action** Do not remove the placenta if attached until the uterus is replaced. If noted early, try to replace the uterus. Otherwise admit as an emergency. The mother may become profoundly shocked, so set up an IV infusion before transfer, if possible, and give $O_2$ via a face mask.

**Broad ligament haematoma** Presents in a recently delivered woman as obstretric shock without excessive PV bleeding. Examination reveals pain and tenderness on the affected side. The uterus is deviated from that side.

⚠ **Action** Admit to the nearest specialist obstetric unit as an acute emergency.

**Amniotic fluid embolism** Very rare. Mortality ~80%. Presents with shock, cyanosis, and dyspnoea. May occur at the height of a contraction.

### ⚠ If suspected
- Call for help
- Resuscitate—Airway; Breathing; Circulation
- Transfer to the nearest A&E or obstetric unit as an emergency.

# Accidents and injuries

**Road accidents** Doctors are not legally obliged to attend an accident that they happen to pass, but most feel morally obliged to do so.

## Immediate action

- Assess the scene.
- Ensure that police and ambulance have been called.
- Take steps to ensure your own safety and that of others, e.g. park your vehicle defensively, turn on hazard lights, use warning triangles.
- Ensure all vehicle ignitions are turned off.
- Triage casualties into priority groups—decide who to attend first.
- Forbid smoking.

## Immediate treatment

- Check the need for basic resuscitation:
  - **A**irway patent?
  - **B**reathing adequate?
  - **C**irculation intact?
- Resuscitate as necessary (□ p.1051 or inside back cover).
- Control any haemorrhage with elevation and pressure.
- DO NOT attempt to move anyone who potentially could have a back or neck injury until skilled personnel and equipment are available.
- Do not give anything by mouth.
- Use coats and rugs to keep victims warm.
- If available give analgesia (e.g. opioids, but not if significant head injury or risk of intraperitoneal injury; entonox—from ambulance).
- If shocked set up IV fluids if available.
- Take directions from the paramedics—they are almost certainly more experienced than you in these situations.

## Medico-legal issues

- Ensure that your medico-legal insurance covers emergency treatments.
- Keep full records of events, action taken, drugs administered, origin of drugs, batch numbers, and expiry dates.
- A GP can charge a fee to the victims for any assistance given.

**Road safety** Road accidents are responsible for 30–40% of all fatal accidents. *Prevention:*

- Wear seatbelts and appropriate protective clothing (e.g. helmet if riding a pedal or motor cycle).
- Avoid alcohol/other drugs that hamper performance when driving.
- Supervise children close to roads; teach them the Green Cross Code.
- Keep speed down
- Keep vehicles well maintained
- When cycling, use cycle tracks if available
- Do not drive if tired or ill
- Ensure that children are properly strapped in.

**Burns and scalds** □ p.1110    **Drowning** □ p.1122

**Head & facial injury** □ p.1108  **Fractures** □ p.1106

**Whiplash** □ p.483    **Poisoning and overdose** □ p.1112

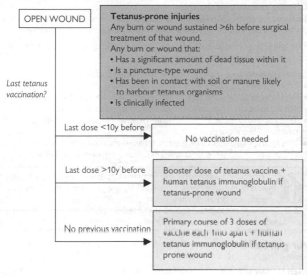

Fig. 29.19 Who should have tetanus vaccination?

**Muscle injuries and sprains** 📖 p.510

**Subungual haematoma** 📖 p.195

**Haematoma of the pinna** 📖 p.1109

**Wounds** Most patients with significant lacerations present directly to A&E. If a patient presents to general practice, perform immediate care (elevate bleeding limb and apply pressure to arrest bleeding). Advise nil by mouth and transfer to A&E.

### Minor lacerations
- Ensure that there is no foreign body in the wound. If in doubt refer for X-ray/surgical exploration (especially important if injury with glass).
- Wash wound and clean away debris and any necrotic material.
- Check that there is no damage to underlying nerves, tendons, bone, or blood supply before dressing or closing a wound.
- Aim to oppose the skin edges without tension to allow healing.
- Do not attempt to close a wound if you are not confident that you can achieve an adequate result.
- Always refer cuts through the lip margin to A&E; consider referral to A&E for any facial wounds and wounds in children.
- Check tetanus status (Figure 29.19).
- In assault cases take particular care to document all injuries carefully, e.g. with photographs, drawings, and measurements of wounds.
- Consider non-accidental injury in children (📖 p.922).

*Closing the wound* Options:

*Skin closure strips (Steri-Strips™)* Use for small cuts in non-hairy skin not under tension. Can be used in addition to sutures for larger wounds.

*Skin 'glue' (e.g. Histoacryl®)* Quick (takes 30sec to set) and can be used on hairy skin such as the scalp.

*Suturing* Undertake training before attempting suturing.
• Infiltrate wound edges with 1% lidocaine (max. 2mg/kg).
• Addition of adrenaline (epinephrine) can help haemostasis but must not be used on digits or extremities as necrosis can occur.
• Take care to oppose edges accurately—start interrupted sutures in the middle of the wound.
• Use appropriate suture (e.g. adult face 5-0 monofilament nylon—remove after 5d; limbs or trunk 3-0 nylon—remove after 1–2wk).

> **Pretibial lacerations** The shin has poor blood supply especially in the elderly. Flap wounds are common; they may heal poorly ± break down to form ulcers. *Management:* wash wound; carefully realign the flap and secure with Steri-Strips™ without tension and bandage; advise elevation of the leg; review regularly to check healing.

**Air gun pellets** Common. Refer for X-ray. Can be difficult to remove—leave in place if not in a harmful position. If in a joint, refer for removal.

**Fish hooks** Infiltrate with lidocaine. Push the hook forwards through the skin until the barb is exposed. Cut the barb off and then ease the hook back through the skin the same way it entered.

**Knocked-out teeth** Ask the patient to suck tooth clean, reinsert or store in milk or saliva, and send to a dentist.

**Coin and other foreign body ingestion** Most coins will pass through the gut without any problems. If asymptomatic, they can be left to take their course (advise checking stools to ensure passed). If symptomatic, refer for X-ray and consideration for endoscopic removal. If there is any indication of aspiration, refer urgently.

**Foreign bodies in the ear** Most common in children. Try to remove under direct vision with forceps, but avoid pushing objects deeper into the canal and causing damage. Don't poke around with forceps in an uncooperative child. Removal under GA may be needed. Insects can be drowned in oil and syringed out.

**Foreign bodies in the nose** Common in young children. Any child with smelly discharge from one nostril has a foreign body in the nose until proven otherwise—refer for exploration under GA. Do not try to remove a foreign body yourself unless the object is very superficial and the child is cooperative. You might push the object further in and cause trauma.

**Removal of ticks** Use a commercially available tick remover when possible. If a tick remover is not available, grip the tick as close as possible to the skin with a pair of tweezers and firmly pull the tick out of the skin.

**Animal bites** ~200 000 people are bitten by dogs each year in the UK. Animal bites are contaminated and wound infection is common. Clean carefully with soap and water. Check tetanus status. Do not suture unless cosmetically essential and there is minimal tissue damage—refer if in doubt. Give prophylaxis against infection (e.g. with co-amoxiclav or erythromycin).

**Human bites** are especially prone to infection. Also consider risk of hepatitis B and HIV. If HIV prophylaxis is indicated, it needs to be started immediately—refer urgently to A&E for local policy implementation.

**Snake bites** The adder is the only poisonous snake in the UK. Bites are only rarely lethal. Attempt to identify the snake species and refer the patient urgently to hospital. Do not apply a tourniquet or try cutting or sucking the wound.

**Insect stings** Response depends on the insect involved and the individual's response to the stings. Ranges from blisters through papules to urticarial wheals—secondary infection is common.

**Anaphylaxis** Follow algorithm in Figure 29.10 (📖 p.1069) and admit to hospital as a blue-light emergency.

**Immediately after the sting** Remove any sting present in the wound. Often no further treatment is needed.
- *If severe local reaction occurs* Apply an ice pack; give oral antihistamine (e.g. chlorpheniramine 4mg stat), continue antihistamine every 4–6 h as needed.
- *If 2° bacterial infection occurs* Treat with oral or topical antibiotics.

**Remove sources of insects**, e.g. remove fleas from carpets with household flea spray (multiple bites on ankles and lower legs).

**Weaver fish sting** Common on sandy beaches. The fish lurks under the sand and so is usually trodden on—presents with severe pain in the foot. Immerse the affected area in uncomfortably hot (but not scalding) water. Give analgesia. Pain resolves after 2–3d.

**Jellyfish sting**
- Remove the patient from the sea as soon as possible.
- Scrape or wash off adherent tentacles.
- Alcoholic solutions including suntan lotions should **not** be applied because they may cause further discharge of stinging hairs.
- Ice packs ↓ pain and a slurry of baking soda (sodium bicarbonate), but not vinegar, may be useful for treating stings from UK species.

**Home safety** Every year >4000 people die due to accidents in the home and nearly 3 million seek treatment in A&E departments. Most accidents inside the home occur in the living/dining room followed by the kitchen. Accidents inside the home include fires, choking/suffocation, drowning, falls, poisoning, injury by hot substances, and electrical injuries.

**Prevention** Spot the dangers; take safety advice (e.g. from HV if young children in the house); fit smoke alarms and safety devices (e.g. stairgates for toddlers); ensure adequate supervision of children or elderly confused people; maintain equipment correctly.

# Fractures

- *Symptoms* Pain at the affected site—worse on movement, ↓ function.
- *Signs* Swelling, bruising, deformity, local tenderness, impaired function, crepitus, abnormal mobility.

⚠ **Action**
- Immobilize the affected part and give analgesia.
- If available and the patient is shocked, start an IV infusion.
- Refer to A&E for assessment, X-ray, and treatment.

**Ottawa Rules for ankle or foot injury** Foot and ankle injuries are common. It can be difficult to distinguish between a sprain and a fracture. The Ottawa Rules ↓ need for X-ray by a quarter.

*Ankle injury* Refer for an ankle X-ray if there is pain in the malleolar area *and*
- Bone tenderness at the posterior tip of the lateral malleolus, or
- Bone tenderness at the posterior tip of the medial malleolus, or
- Unable to weight bear at the time of the injury and when seen.

*Foot injury* Refer for a foot X-ray if there is pain in the midfoot *and*
- Bone tenderness at the fifth metatarsal base, or
- Bone tenderness at the navicular, or
- Inability to weight-bear at the time of injury and when seen.

*Otherwise diagnose a sprain* Treat sprains with rest, ice, compression, elevation, and analgesia (paracetamol ± NSAIDs). If severe (or the patient is an athlete), refer to physiotherapy.

**Fractures** Table 29.7

>  Always consider assessment and treatment for osteoporosis in all men and women >50y who have had a Colles' fracture, hip fracture and/or vertebral collapse.

**Head and facial injury** 📖 p.1108

**Fracture complications** Often occur after the patient has been discharged from hospital and may present as a primary care emergency. Patients should not have persistent pain—beware of compartment syndrome. Refer back to the fracture clinic or A&E if:
- Persistent pain
- Limb swelling that is not settling
- Offensive odour or discharge
- Cast edges are abrading the skin or the cast has deteriorated in structural strength, e.g. because of getting wet.

**Compartment syndrome** Crush injury, fracture, prolonged immobility, or tight splints, dressings, or casts can result in ↑ pressure within muscle compartments and eventually vascular occlusion. Presents with swelling, severe pain (↑ on passive stretch of muscles), distal numbness, redness, mottling, blisters. ❶ Pulses may be present distally. Loosen any restricting bandage/cast. Refer as an emergency to orthopaedics—fasciotomy may be needed to relieve the pressure.

**Table 29.6** Common fractures seen in primary care

| Fracture | Features and management |
|---|---|
| Clavicle | Common injury (5% all fractures). Usually results from a fall onto an outstretched arm. 80% fractures are in the middle third, 15% in the lateral third, and 5% in the medial third. |
| | Refer to A&E for confirmation of diagnosis and fracture clinic follow-up. Treatment is with sling support and analgesia. Most heal well. |
| | *Complications*: pneumothorax, malunion, and nerve/vessel damage. |
| Colles' | Most commonly due to a fall onto an outstretched hand in an elderly lady. Pain and swelling of the wrist ('dinner-fork' deformity). |
| | Refer any suspected fracture for X-ray and reduction. |
| | *Complications* include rupture of the extensor pollicis longus tendon, carpal tunnel syndrome, and reflex sympathetic dystrophy. |
| Scaphoid | Caused by falling onto an outstretched hand. Pain, swelling, and tenderness in the anatomical snuff box. |
| | Symptoms may be mild and fracture is easily missed—refer suspected cases for scaphoid view X-rays. If X-ray is inconclusive and pain continues, repeat 2wk later—bone scan or MRI can help if still –ve. |
| | Non-union and avascular necrosis of the proximal fragment is a potential complication, which can lead to long-term problems of arthritis and pain. |
| Fingers | Common injuries. Often associated with sport. Refer all suspected fractures for X-ray ± reduction. |
| Hip | Common amongst the elderly and carries high morbidity and mortality (~25%). ♀ > ♂. Usually occurs through the neck of the femur. |
| | *Risk factors*: maternal hip fracture, osteoporosis, unsteadiness, sedative medication, poor eye sight, polypharmacy. |
| | There may be a history of a fall but not always. Suspect in any patient who is elderly or has risk factors for osteoporosis who is 'off legs'. Occasionally patients can still weight-bear with difficulty. |
| | *Signs*: external rotation, shortening and adduction of leg |
| | Refer urgently to A&E for X-ray. |
| Ankle | History is of a fall over an obstacle or trip down a step. The ankle rapidly becomes swollen and tender—often bilaterally. |
| | Decide whether an X-ray is needed. If so, refer to A&E. |
| Metatarsals | The most common fracture is the base of the fifth metatarsal in an 'ankle twisting' injury. March or stress fractures occur in people who do a lot of walking or running and affect the neck/shaft of the second metatarsal. |
| | Decide whether an X-ray is needed. If so, refer to A&E. Undisplaced fractures are usually treated with analgesia and support. |
| Toes | Caused by stubbing the toe or dropping a heavy object on it. |
| | *Undisplaced suspected fractures*: do not X-ray unless diagnosis is in doubt. Support the injured toe by 'buddy strapping' it to the adjacent toe. Give analgesia. |
| | *Fracture displacement and/or dislocation*: refer for X-ray and reduction. |

# Head and facial injury

## Severe head injury

- Perform basic life support (📖 p.1050).
- Protect the cervical spine (below and 📖 p.1067).
- Transfer to A&E by ambulance.

## Less severe head injuries

*History* If possible take the history from a witness as well as the patient. Ask about circumstances of injury, loss of consciousness (LOC), seizures, current symptoms, and behaviour.

*Examination* Check scalp and head for injury; neurological examination (including fundi); other injuries—accompanying neck injuries are common.

### ⚠ *Refer to A&E if*[N]

- Glasgow Coma Scale <15 at any time since injury (📖 p.1064).
- Loss of consciousness.
- Focal neurological deficit since injury—problems speaking, understanding, reading, writing; ↓ sensation; loss of balance; weakness; visual changes; abnormal reflexes; problems walking; irritability or altered behaviour, especially in young children.
- Any suspicion of skull fracture; penetrating head injury; blood or CSF in the nose, ear, or wound; serious scalp laceration or haematoma.
- Amnesia for events before or after injury.
- Persistent headache.
- Vomiting.
- Seizure.
- Any previous cranial neurosurgical interventions.
- High-energy head injury (e.g. pedestrian hit by motor vehicle, fall >1m or >5 stairs).
- History of bleeding or clotting disorder or on anticoagulant therapy
- Difficulty in assessing the patient (e.g. very young, elderly, intoxicated, or epileptic) or concern about diagnosis.
- Suspicion of non-accidental injury.
- Inadequate supervision at home.

❶ If Glasgow Coma Scale is <15, neck pain/tenderness, focal neurological deficit, paraesthesia in the extremities, or any other clinical suspicion of cervical spine injury, immobilize the neck and refer to A&E.

### *If examination is normal*

- Warn the patient (+ carer) that they may suffer from mild headaches, tiredness, dizziness, tinnitus, poor concentration, and poor memory for the next few days.
- Advise rest and paracetamol (but not codeine-based analgesics) for the headache.
- Young children can be difficult to assess—sleepiness is common and is not a worrying sign as long as the child is rousable.
- Give written head injury information regarding warning signs to trigger reconsultation—drowsiness, severe headache, persistent vomiting, visual disturbance and/or unusual behaviour.

**Injury to the face** Mostly due to RTAs and violent incidents. Carefully document injuries as your notes may be required for legal procedings. Look for other injuries, e.g. airway problems, head injury, neck injury. Palpate the face for signs of a fracture, if present refer to maxillofacial surgeons for assessment. Check tetanus status. Post-traumatic stress disorder (📖 p.996) is common after facial injury.

## Specific injuries

- *Facial lacerations* Best sutured by an experienced surgeon. Refer to A&E.
- *Fractured mandible* A blow to the jaw can cause unilateral or bilateral fractures. Presents with pain (worse on moving jaw), bruising ± bleeding inside the mouth ± discontinuity of the teeth (displaced fracture) ± numbness of the lower lip (if the inferior dental nerve has been damaged). Refer for X-ray.
- *Dislocated jaw* Presents with pain and the mouth is stuck open— refer for X-ray and reduction.
- *Fractured zygoma/malar complex* A blow on the cheek may fracture the zygomatic arch in isolation or more usually cause a 'tripod' fracture. Signs: bony tenderness, flattening of the malar process (best seen from above—may be masked by swelling), epistaxis, subconjunctival haemorrhage extending posteriorly and infra-orbital numbness, ± jaw locked. Refer for X-ray. Advise not to blow nose.
- *Middle third facial fractures (Le Fort)* Usually bilateral. Signs: epistaxis, CSF rhinorrhea, crepitus on palpation, swelling, open bite, and risk of airway compromise. Refer for X-ray.
- *Haematoma of the pinna* Usually after trauma (e.g. rugby). Must be evacuated urgently (aspirated via large-bore needle or surgically) to prevent necrosis of the cartilage and 'cauliflower' ear—refer.
- *Nasal fracture and other nasal injuries* 📖 p.939
- *'Blow-out' fracture of orbit* 📖 p.957
- *Whiplash* 📖 p.483
- *Avulsed tooth* 📖 p.1104
- *Dog bite* 📖 p.1105

**Post-concussion syndrome** Seen following even quite minor head injury. Due to neuronal damage. Features include all or some of:

- Headache
- Dizziness
- Poor concentration
- Fatigue
- Depression
- Memory problems.

Treatment is supportive and symptoms usually resolve with time (although can take months or even years).

## Further information

**NICE** Triage, assessment investigation and early management of head injury in infants, children and adults (2007) 🖥 www.nice.org.uk

# Scalds and burns

### Assess

- Cause, size, and thickness of the burn.
- Use the 'rule of nines' to estimate the extent of the burn (Box 29.1).
- Partial-thickness burns are red, painful, and blistered; full-thickness burns are painless and white or grey.
- Always consider non-accidental injury in children (🕮 p.922).

### ⚠ Action

- Remove clothing from the affected area and place under cold running water for >10min or until pain is relieved.
- Do not burst blisters.
- Prescribe/give analgesia.
- Refer all but the smallest (<5%) partial-thickness burns for assessment in A&E.
- Refer all electrical burns for assessment in A&E.
- Refer all chemical burns for assessment in A&E unless burn area is minimal and pain free.
- Consider referral to A&E for smoke inhalation.

### *If managing the burn in the community*

- Check tetanus immunity and give immunization ± prophylaxis as necessary—🕮 p.1103
- Apply silver sulfadiazine cream or paraffin-impregnated gauze and non-adherent dressings. Review for healing and infection every 1–2d.
- Cover burns on hands in silver sulfadiazine and place in a plastic bag—elevate the hand in a sling and encourage finger movement.
- Refer if burns are not healed in 10–12d.

## Prevention of scalds and burns

- Prevention through public education is important.
- Children often sustain burns by pulling on the flex of boiling kettles or irons, pulling on saucepan handles, or climbing onto hot cookers.
- Refer any children who have sustained accidental burns to the health visitor for follow-up.

## Smoke inhalation

- Refer all patients who have potentially inhaled smoke for assessment—a seemingly well patient can deteriorate later.
- Smoke can cause thermal injury, carbon monoxide poisoning, and cyanide poisoning.
- Airway problems occur due to thermal and chemical damage to the airways causing oedema—suspect if singed nasal hairs, a sore throat, or a hoarse voice.
- Carbon monoxide poisoning may result in the classic cherry-red mucosa—but this may be absent.
- Cyanide poisoning is commonly due to smouldering plastics and causes dizziness, headaches, and seizures.

**Box 29.1 Rule of Nines** Ignore areas of erythema only.

| | |
|---|---|
| Palm | 1% |
| Arm (all over) | 9% |
| Leg (all over) | 18% (14% children) |
| Front | 18% |
| Back | 18% |
| Head (all over) | 9% (14% children) |
| Genitals | 1% |

The Rule of Nines is inaccurate for children <10y. For children and for small burns, estimate the extent of the burn by comparison with the area of the patient's hand. The area of the fingers and palm ≈1% of total body surface area burn.

**Sunburn** Susceptibility depends on skin type.
- Tingling is followed 2–12h later by erythema. Redness is maximum at 24h and fades over 2–3d. Desquamation and pigmentation follow.
- Severe sunburn may cause blistering, pain, and systemic upset. Treatment is symptomatic with calamine lotion prn (some advocate application of vinegar) and paracetamol for pain
- Rarely, dressings are required for blisters or, in severe cases, hospital admission for fluid management.
- Predisposes to skin cancer and photo-ageing.

**The sun safety code** Take care not to burn in the sun.
- Cover up with loose cool clothing, a hat, and sunglasses
- If swimming outdoors or on the beach, dress in a UV-protective sunsuit. When out of the water, add a T-shirt, sunglasses, and sun hat.
- Seek shade during the hottest part of the day.
- Apply sunscreen (≥SPF 25) on sun-exposed parts of the body.

## Burns in special situations
### Chemical burns
- Usually caused by strong acids or alkalis.
- Wear gloves to remove contaminated clothing.
- Irrigate with cold running water for ≥ 20min.
- Do not attempt to neutralize the chemical—this can exacerbate injury by producing heat.
- Refer all burns to A&E unless the burn area is minimal and pain free.

### Electric shock
- Causes thermal tissue injury and direct injury due to the electric current passing through the tissue.
- Skin burns may be seen at the entry and exit sites of the current.
- Muscle damage can be severe with minimal skin injury.
- Cardiac damage may occur and rhabdomyolysis can → renal failure.
- Refer all patients for specialist management.

# Poisoning or overdose

## On receiving the call for assistance
- Try to establish what has happened—substances involved, ongoing dangers, state of the patient.
- Advise the caller to stay with the patient until you arrive.
- If the patient is unconscious, arrange for an ambulance to meet you at the scene.
- Arrange for the patient to be removed from any source of danger, e.g. contaminated clothing or inhaled gases. DO NOT put yourself or anyone else in danger attempting to do this. If necessary call the fire brigade, who have protective clothing and equipment, to help remove a patient from a dangerous environment.

## Assessment of the unconscious patient
### Assess the need for basic life support
- **A**irway patent?
- **B**reathing satisfactory?
- **C**irculation adequate?

Resuscitation (📖 p.1050) takes priority over everything else.

### Additionally
- If breathing is depressed and opioid overdose is a possibility give naloxone 0.4–2mg IV every 2–3min to a maximum of 10mg (child: 10 micrograms/kg and then, if no response, 100 micrograms/kg).
- Check BM—if low give 50–250mL 10% glucose IV in 50mL aliquots.

### General examination
- BP
- Pulse
- Temperature
- Level of coma (📖 p.1064)

- Pupil responses
- Evidence of IV drug abuse
- Obvious injury.

❶ The coma may not be due to poisoning/overdose.

### *If unconscious, turn into the recovery position* 📖 p.1067. Check no contraindications first, e.g. spinal injury.

### Note down any information about the exposure
- *Product name* As much detail as possible—if unidentified tablets, see if any are left and send them to the hospital in their own container (if there is one) with the patient.
- *Time of the incident*
- *Duration of exposure/amount ingested*
- *Route of exposure*—swallowed, inhaled, injected, etc.
- *Whether intentional or accidental*
- *Take a general history from any attendant*—medical history, current medication, substance abuse, alcohol, social circumstances.

## Assessment of the conscious patient
- Note down any information about the exposure as for the unconscious patient.

- Record symptoms that the patient is experiencing as a result of exposure.
- Examination—pulse, BP, temperature (if necessary), level of consciousness or confusion, evidence of IV drug abuse, any injuries.
- If non-accidental exposure, assess suicidal intent (📖 p.1115).
- Take a general history from the patient and/or any attendant—medical history, current medication, substance abuse, alcohol, social circumstances.

### Consider admission if

- The patient's clinical condition warrants it (unconsciousness, respiratory depression, etc.).
- The exposure warrants admission for treatment or observation:
  - *Symptomatic poisoning* Admit to hospital.
  - *Agents with delayed action* Aspirin, iron, paracetamol, tricyclic antidepressants, co-phenotrope, paraquat, and modified-release preparations. Admit to hospital even if the patient seems well.
  - *Other agents* Consult poisons information.
- You judge that there is serious suicidal intent (📖 p.1115) or the patient has another psychiatric condition which warrants acute admission.
- There is a lack of social support.

---

 **Overdose and poisoning in children** Peak incidence of accidental poisoning is at 2y old—mainly household substances, prescribed or OTC drugs, or plants. Teenagers may take deliberate overdoses, especially of OTC medication (e.g. paracetamol).

⚠ Poisoning can be a form of non-accidental injury (📖 p.922).

---

**Deliberate self-harm (DSH)** Deliberate non-fatal act committed in the knowledge that it was potentially harmful and, in the case of drug overdose, that the amount taken was excessive. 90% DSH is due to self-poisoning and it accounts for 20% of admissions to general medical wards—the most frequent reason for admission for young ♀ patients. Paracetamol or aspirin are the most common drugs used. Self-harm is often aimed at changing a situation (e.g. to get a boyfriend back), communication of distress ('cry for help'), or a sign of emotional distress, or it may be a failed genuine suicide attempt.

### Management 📖 p. 1114

❶ People who have self-harmed should be treated with the same care, respect, and privacy as any other patient.

### Poisons information
**UK National Poisons Information Service** ☎ 0844 892 1111 (Ireland: ☎ 01 809 2566)
**TOXBASE Poisons database** 🖥 www.toxbase.org

# Suicide and attempted suicide

Calls to patients who have deliberately self-harmed themselves, are threatening suicide, or whose relatives are worried about suicide risk are common primary care emergencies.

• *Assessment*—Figure 29.21.     • *Management*—Figure 29.20.

**Compulsory admission** 📖 p.1118

**Suicide prevention** The UK suicide rate is 1:6000. Suicide risk can be ↓ by early recognition, assessment, and treatment of those likely to attempt suicide (many visit their GP just weeks before suicide), planning follow-up care for those discharged from psychiatric hospital, and ↓ availability and lethality of suicide methods (e.g. avoiding TCAs and monitoring antidepressant repeat prescriptions carefully).

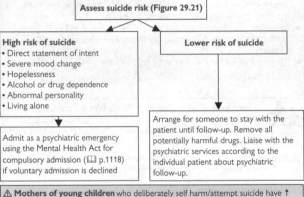

Assess suicide risk (Figure 29.21)

**High risk of suicide**
• Direct statement of intent
• Severe mood change
• Hopelessness
• Alcohol or drug dependence
• Abnormal personality
• Living alone

**Lower risk of suicide**

Admit as a psychiatric emergency using the Mental Health Act for compulsory admission (📖 p.1118) if voluntary admission is declined

Arrange for someone to stay with the patient until follow-up. Remove all potentially harmful drugs. Liaise with the psychiatric services according to the individual patient about psychiatric follow-up.

⚠ **Mothers of young children** who deliberately self harm/attempt suicide have ↑ risk of child abuse. Assess risks, offer support, arrange for health visitor or social services to visit.

**Fig. 29.20** Management of patients who have deliberately self-harmed or have threatened or attempted suicide

## Further information

**NICE** Self-harm: the short-term physical and psychological management and secondary prevention of self-harm in primary and secondary care (2004) 🖥 www.nice.org.uk
**DH** National Suicide Prevention Strategy for England (2002) 🖥 www.dh.gov.u

## Information and support for patients and relatives

**Self Injury and Related Issues (SIARI)** 🖥 www.siari.co.uk
**Samaritans** 24h emotional support via telephone ☎ 08457 90 9090 🖥 www.samaritans.org
**Survivors of Bereavement by Suicide** ☎ 0844 561 6855 🖥 www.uk-sobs.org.uk

**If any self-harm** Assess the situation and admit to A&E as needed

**Ask about suicidal ideas and plans** in a sensitive but probing way. It is a common misconception that asking about suicide can plant the idea into a patient's head and make suicide more likely. Evidence is to the contrary.

**Ask about present circumstances**
What problems are making the patient feel this way?
Does he/she still feel like this?
Would the act of suicide be aimed to hurt someone in particular?
What kind of support does the patient have from friends, relatives, and formal services e.g. CPN?

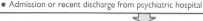

**Assess suicidal risk** Ask patient and any relatives/friends present. *Risk factors:*
- ♂>♀
- ↑ with age
- Social isolation
- History of deliberate self harm (100x ↑ risk)
- Depression
- Alcohol or substance abuse
- Personality disorder
- Schizophrenia
- Serious medical illness (e.g. cancer)
- Divorced ˃ widowed ˃ never married ˃ married
- Certain professions: vets, pharmacists, farmers, doctors
- Admission or recent discharge from psychiatric hospital

**Assess psychiatric state** Features associated with ↑ suicide risk are:
- Depression
- Agitation
- Presence of suicidal ideation
- Hopelessness—good predictor of subsequent and immediate risk
- Early schizophrenia with retained insight, especially young patients who see their ambitions restricted
- Presence of delusions of control, poverty, and/or guilt

**Useful questions for assessing suicidal ideas and plans**
- Do you feel you have a future?
- Do you feel that life's not worth living?
- Do you ever feel completely hopeless?
- Do you ever feel you'd be better off dead and away from it all?
- Have you ever made any plans to end your life (if drug overdose—have you handled the tablets)?
- Have you ever made an attempt to take your own life? If so, was there a final act, e.g suicide note?
- What prevents you doing it?
- Have you made any arrangements for your affairs after your death?

**Fig. 29.21** Assessment of patients who have deliberately self-harmed or have threatened or attempted suicide

# Disturbed behaviour

## ⚠ Look after your own safety

- If the patient is known to be violent, get back up from the police before entering the situation.
- Tell someone you are going in and when to expect an 'exit' call. Advise them to call for help if that call is not made.
- Do not put yourself in a vulnerable situation—sit where there is a clear, unimpeded exit route.
- Do not make the patient feel trapped.
- Do not try to restrain the patient.

## Acute hyperventilation/panic attack

*Features* Fear, terror and feeling of impending doom accompanied by some or all of the following:

- Palpitations
- Shortness of breath
- Choking sensation
- Dizziness
- Paraesthesiae
- Chest pain/discomfort
- Sweating
- Carpopedal spasm.

## *Differential diagnosis*

- Dysrhythmia
- Asthma
- Anaphylaxis
- Thyrotoxicosis
- Temporal lobe epilepsy
- Hypoglycaemia
- Phaeochromocytoma (very rare).

### ⚠ Action

*Talking down* Explain the nature of the symptoms to the patient:

- Racing of the heart is due to adrenaline produced by the panic
- Paraesthesiae/feelings of dizziness are to overbreathing due to panic
- Count breaths in and out gently slowing breathing rate.

*Rebreathing techniques*

- Place a paper bag over the patient's mouth and ask him to breath in and out through the mouth.
- A connected but not switched on $O_2$ mask or nebuliser mask is an alternative in the surgery.
- This raises the partial pressure of $CO_2$ in the blood and symptoms due to low $CO_2$ (e.g. tetany, paraesthesiae, dizziness) resolve. This demonstrates the link between hyperventilation and the symptoms too.

*Propranolol* 10–20mg stat may be helpful—DO NOT USE for asthmatics or patients with heart failure or on verapamil.

*Recurrent panic attacks* 📖 p.992

**Violent or agitated behaviour** When a patient becomes very agitated or violent or starts to behave oddly, the GP is usually called - by the patient, relatives or friends or police attending the disturbance.

### *Causes of disturbed behaviour*

- *Physical illness causing acute confusional state* Infection (e.g. UTI, chest infection); hypoglycaemia; hypoxia; head injury; epilepsy—📖 p.582.

- **Drugs** Alcohol (or alcohol withdrawal); prescribed drugs (e.g. steroid psychosis); illicit drugs (e.g. amphetamines).
- **Psychiatric illness** Schizophrenia; mania; anxiety/depression; dementia; personality disorder (e.g. attention-seeking; uncontrolled anger).

### Assessment

- Before seeing the patient gather as much information as possible from notes, relatives—even neighbours.
- Ask the patient and family for any history of drugs or alcohol excess.
- Listen to the patient and talk calmly—choose your words carefully.
- Try to look for organic causes—this can be difficult in the heat of the moment—physical examination except from a distance may be impossible. Don't put yourself at risk.
- Suspect an organic cause where there are visual hallucinations.
- Discuss and explain your suggested management with the patient and any attendants.
- If the patient is an immediate danger to himself or others, admission is warranted.
- If the cause of the behaviour is unclear, admission for investigation is needed.
- Instigate management of treatable causes identified e.g. admit if MI suspected; treat UTI.
- Consider sedation to cover the period before admission or to alleviate symptoms if admission is inappropriate.

**Acute management** After assessing the problem, decide if hospitalization is required and whether this can be done on a voluntary or involuntary basis.

### Suitable drugs to use for sedation

- **Oral** diazepam 5–10mg PO or lorazepam 1mg PO/sublingually; chlorpromazine 50–100mg PO.
- **Intramuscular** chlorpromazine 50mg; haloperidol 1–3mg.

❶ *Avoid sedating* patients with COPD, epilepsy or if the patient has been taking illicit drugs, barbiturates or alcohol.

### Compulsory admission under the Mental Health Act 📖 p.1118

⚠ **Acute dystonia** can occur soon after giving phenothiazines or butyophenones. *Signs:*

- Torticollis
- Tongue protrusion
- Grimacing
- Opisthotonus.

Dystonia can be relieved with IM procyclidine 5–10mg (repeated prn after 20min to a maximum dose of 20mg).

# Compulsory admission and treatment of patients with mental illness

Most people requiring inpatient care for mental disorder agree to hospital admission and become 'informal' patients. A minority (~5%) require compulsory admission and detention under the Mental Health Act 2007* and are termed 'sectioned', in reference to the section of the Mental Health Act under which they are detained (Figure 29.22).

## Procedure for 'sectioning' a patient

### Applications can be made for
- Admission for assessment under Section 2 (📖 p.1121).
- Admission for treatment under Section 3 (📖 p.1121).
- Emergency admission under Section 4 (📖 p.1121).
- Guardianship under Section 7 (📖 p.1121).

### Applications can be made by
- An approved mental health professional (AMHP).
- The nearest relative of the person concerned. The nearest relative is defined in the Act as the first surviving person out of:
  - Spouse (or cohabitee for >6mo)
  - Oldest child (if >18y)
  - Parent
  - Oldest sibling (if >18y)
  - Grandparent
  - Grandchild (>18y)
  - Uncle or aunt (>18y)
  - Nephew or niece (>18y)
  - Non-relative living with the patient for ≥5y.

The applicant (AMHP or nearest relative) must have seen the patient <2wk (<24h in the case of Section 4) before the date of the application.

❶ Wherever possible, the AMHP should be chosen rather than the nearest relative to avoid affecting family relationships.

### Applications must be based on
- Two medical recommendations (except Section 4 which only needs one). Doctors, or other approved clinicians may examine the patient together or separately, but there must be <6d between examinations. Recommendations must be signed on or before the date of application.
- Where two medical recommendations are required, the clinicians should not be from the same hospital or practice *and* one of the clinicians must be 'approved' under the Mental Health Act.
- If practicable, one clinician must have prior knowledge of the patient (ideally a GP—but GPs are not obliged to attend outside the practice area). If neither clinician has prior knowledge of the patient, the applicant must state on the application why this was so.
- Medical recommendation(s) and application must concur on at least one form of mental disorder.

*Applies in England and Wales only. In Northern Ireland similar provisions apply under the Mental Health (Northern Ireland) Order 1986. Scotland—see 📖 p.1120.

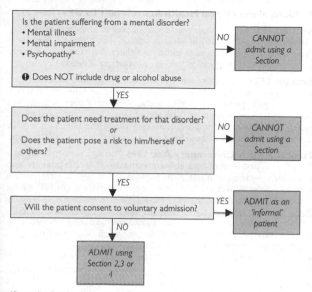

*Personality disorder characterized by inability to make loving relationships, antisocial behaviour, and lack of guilt

**Fig. 29.22** Deciding whether a Section is needed

In practice 'sectioning' means calling in the duty social worker (or other social services approved mental health professional) and duty psychiatrist. It can be a time-consuming and frustrating business. Always try to obtain voluntary admission—it is better for you and the patient.

Keep a supply of forms you might need for sectioning—Forms 3, 7, and 10 (GP recommendation for Sections 2, 4, and 3 respectively) and Form 5 (Application for Section 4 for a 'nearest relative').

Deputizing doctors should always try to contact the patient's own GP.

❶ The Mental Health Act only allows for compulsory assessment and treatment of a patient's mental health problems—the patient may refuse consent for investigation and/or treatment of other health problems whilst 'sectioned'.

**Sections of the Mental Health Act relevant to GPs** (Table 29.7)

**Section 115** allows an approved social worker to enter and inspect any premises (except hospital) in which a person with a mental disorder is living if he/she has reasonable cause to believe that that person is not under proper care. Application through a magistrate is needed.

**Section 135** gives right of entry of a police officer who believes that a person with a mental disorder is being ill-treated or suffering from self-neglect to enter premises and remove that person to a place of safety. The police officer who attends must be accompanied by an approved mental health professional and approved clinician unless the person is already 'sectioned' and absent without leave. Requires application to a magistrate.

**Mental Health Community Act 1995** This Act aims to 'provide a system of supervision of care in the community of certain patients who have been detained in hospital'. In England and Wales, the responsible medical officer applies for 'after-care under supervision' (ACUS) to the responsible health authority every 6mo for the first year and then annually. Application can only be made in respect of a patient (≥16y old) currently liable to be detained in hospital because of a mental disorder where:
- there could be serious risk of harm to the patient or others if the patient were not to receive further care services *and*
- supervision would help to ensure receipt of further care services.

If patients refuse treatment, they cannot be treated against their will but can be conveyed to a day centre or hospital.

**Scotland** The Mental Health Act (Care and Treatment)(Scotland) 2003 provides for compulsory admission under Part 5 for 72h. The application is made by a fully registered medical practitioner in consultation with a mental health officer, unless this is impracticable. In hospital Part 6 (lasting 28d) can be applied and then, if necessary, Part 7 (Compulsory Treatment Order) for 6mo.

*Further information* 🖥 www.scotland.gov.uk

**Further information**
**DH** Mental Health Act 2007—Overview 🖥 www.dh.gov.uk

**Table 29.7** Sections of the Mental Health Act relevant to primary care

| Section | Notes | Application |
|---------|-------|-------------|
| **Section 2**<br>Admission for assessment | Most commonly used section in the community.<br>Admission for 28d for assessment.<br>Not renewable after that time.<br>Patients may appeal within 2wk of detention via the Mental Health Tribunal | Application must be made by the nearest relative or an AMHP on the recommendation of two doctors—one approved and one who has prior knowledge of the patient.<br>If application is made by the AMHP, the nearest relative should be informed before application or as soon as possible afterwards.<br>Application is valid for 14d. |
| **Section 3**<br>Admission for treatment | Admission for treatment for ≤6mo<br>The exact mental disorder must be stated.<br>Detention is renewable for a further 6mo and annually thereafter. | Application must be made by the nearest relative or an AMHP on the recommendation of two doctors—one approved, and one who has prior knowledge of the patient.<br>Application is valid for 14d. |
| **Section 4**<br>Emergency admission for assessment | Used in situations where admission is urgent and compliance with Section 2 would cause undesirable delay<br>Admission to hospital for 72h only.<br>Not renewable.<br>Usually converted to a Section 2 on arrival at hospital. | Application must be made by the nearest relative or an AMHP<br>If application is made by the AMHP, the nearest relative should be informed before application or as soon as possible afterwards.<br>Medical recommendation is from either an approved clinician (not necessarily a doctor) or a doctor with prior knowledge of the patient.<br>Application is only valid for 24h. |
| **Section 7**<br>Guardianship | A Guardian has power to:<br>• Require a person to live at a particular place<br>• Require a person to go to specific places at specific times for medical treatment, work, education, or training<br>• Require a doctor, AMHP, or other specified person be given access to the person under Guardianship.<br>❶ Guardians can insist that a person sees a doctor but cannot force treatment. | Application must be made by the nearest relative or an AMHP on the recommendation of 2 clinicians—one approved and one who has prior knowledge of the patient.<br>Application is valid for 14d. |

# Miscellaneous emergencies

### Acute limb ischaemia
#### Causes
- Acute thrombotic occlusion of pre-existing stenotic segment (60%)
- Embolus (30%)
- Trauma, e.g. compartment syndrome or traumatic vessel damage.

#### Presentation
- **P**ain
- **P**allor
- **P**araesthesia
- **P**ulselessness
- **P**aralysis
- **P**erishing cold

#### Action
Admit acutely under the care of a vascular surgeon. Treatment can be surgical (e.g. embolectomy) or medical (e.g. thrombolysis).

**Drowning** Most common in drunk adults and children poorly supervised around water. Children can drown in a few centimetres of water.

#### Action
- Call for help.
- Start basic life support (**A**irway, **B**reathing, **C**irculation)—📖 p.1050 (adults), 📖 p.1156 (children).

⚠ Attempted resuscitation of a seemingly dead child is worthwhile as cooling ↓ metabolic rate and recovery can occur after prolonged immersion.

**Prevention** Drowning is the third most common cause of accidental death among the under 16s. More than half of those who drown can swim. 44% of drownings occur in rivers or streams, 3% in garden ponds, 2% in swimming pools, and 5% in home baths. Alcohol is a contributory factor in 14% of cases. The best way to ↓ drowning is prevention: spot the dangers; take safety advice; do not go near water alone; learn how to help others.

**Hypothermia** Defined as a core temperature <35°C. *Causes:*
- Not feeling the cold, e.g. neuropathy, confusion, dementia.
- Inadequate heat in the home, e.g. poor housing, poverty, and fear of high fuel bill.
- Immobility.
- Hypothyroidism.
- DM.
- Alcohol.
- ↑ heat loss e.g. psoriasis, erythroderma.
- Inadequate protection from the cold, e.g. unsuitable clothing whilst doing outdoor sports.
- Drugs: antipsychotics, antidepressants, barbiturates, tranquillizers —may lower the level of consciousness and ↓ ability to shiver.
- Falls: if unable to rise from the floor may remain still and cold until discovered.
- Unconsciousness, e.g. overdose, stroke.

**Presentation** Skin pale and cold to touch; puffy face; listlessness, drowsiness and/or confusion.

**When severe** ↓ breathing—slow and shallow; ↓ pulse volume—faint and irregular; stiff muscles; loss of consciousness.

### Investigation

• Rectal temperature on low-reading thermometer <35°C.
• ECG—J wave on the end of the QRS complex.

### Action

• Remove from the cold environment.
• Wrap in blankets—including head.
• *Do not* use direct heat (e.g. hot-water bottles) as this can cause rapid fluid shifts and potentially fatal pulmonary oedema.
• Transfer to hospital.
• Consider the cause of the incident and liaise with the hospital, primary healthcare team, and social services to prevent recurrence in the future.

**Heat stroke and heat exhaustion** Exercising in excessive heat leads to dehydration, salt depletion, and metabolite accumulation. *Signs:* headache, nausea, confusion, incoordination, cramps, weakness, dizziness, malaise. *Treatment:* rest, fluid and salt replacement. Admit for IV fluids and supportive measures in severe cases.

### Sunburn 📖 p.1111

**Acute altitude sickness** Altitude sickness is a potentially fatal complication of rapidly climbing to altitudes >8000 ft. Two main forms: pulmonary oedema and cerebral oedema. Presents with fatigue, headache, dizziness, nausea/loss of appetite, breathlessness, palpitations, and/or insomnia. Treatment is with oxygen therapy and descent to a lower altitude. Prevent by gradual ascent. Use of prophylactic acetazolamide is controversial.

**Wound dehiscence** Breakdown of a surgical wound—usually abdominal. May be partial or complete.

• *Partial breakdown*—skin remains intact but muscle layers break down → incisional hernia. Typically the patient feels something 'give' ± sudden ↑ in pain and pink fluid discharge. Refer for urgent reassessment by the operating surgeon.
• *Complete dehiscence*—wound breaks down entirely. The patient becomes shocked and distressed. Lie flat; give strong opiate analgesia; cover the wound with a sterile pack soaked in saline; admit as a 'blue-light' emergency.

### Risk factors

• Malnutrition
• Obesity
• ↑ intra-abdominal pressure, e.g. from coughing
• Wound infection
• Haematoma formation
• Ascites draining through a wound.

# Index

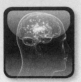